ANATOMY & PHYSIOLOGY

FOR HEALTH PROFESSIONS

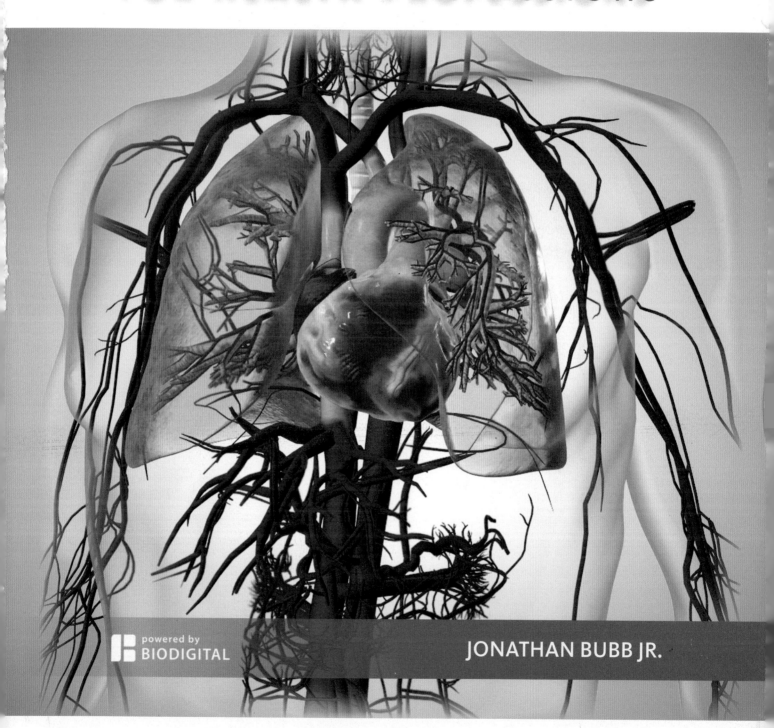

powered by
BIODIGITAL

JONATHAN BUBB JR.

ANATOMY & PHYSIOLOGY

FOR HEALTH PROFESSIONS

powered by
BIODIGITAL

JONATHAN BUBB JR.

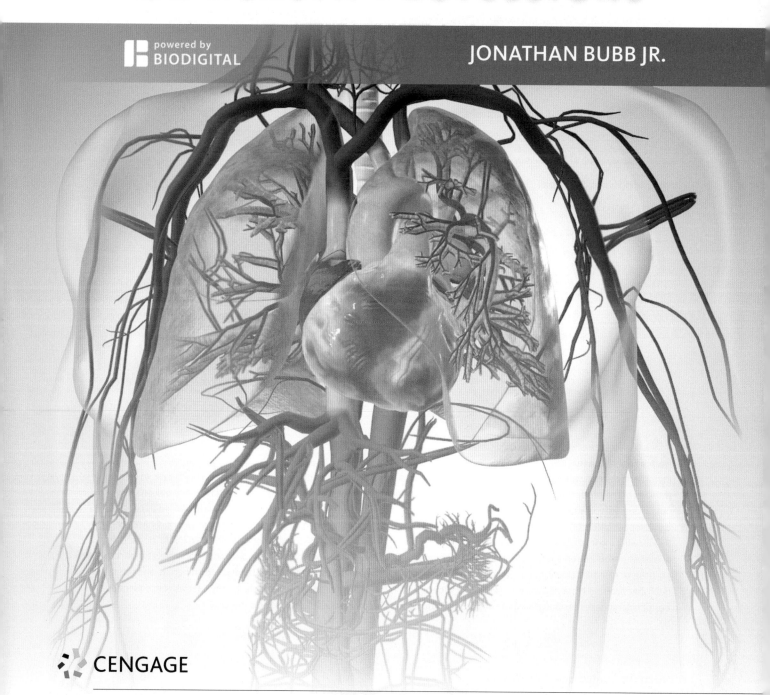

CENGAGE

Australia • Brazil • Canada • Mexico • Singapore • United Kingdom • United States

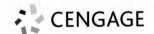

Anatomy & Physiology for Health Professions
Jonathan Bubb Jr

SVP, Higher Education & Skills Product: Erin Joyner

Senior Product Director: Matthew Seeley

Senior Product Team Manager: Laura Stewart

Product Assistant: Anne Van Vorst

Director, Learning Design: Rebecca von Gillern

Senior Manager, Learning Design: Leigh Hefferon

Senior Learning Designer: Deb Myette-Flis

Marketing Director: Sean Chamberland

Marketing Manager: Courtney Cozzy

Director, Content Creation: Juliet Steiner

Senior Content Creation Manager: Patty Stephan

Senior Content Manager: Kenneth McGrath

Digital Delivery Lead: Allison Marion

Production Service: SPi Global

Designer: Felicia Bennett

Cover and interior design: Felicia Bennett

Cover image credit: BioDigital

For product information and technology assistance, contact us at
Cengage Customer & Sales Support, 1-800-354-9706 or
support.cengage.com.

For permission to use material from this text or product, submit all requests online at **www.cengage.com/permissions.**

Library of Congress Control Number: 2020924034

ISBN: 978-0-3576-4917-6
SSO ISBN: 978-1-3374-0379-5

Cengage
200 Pier 4 Boulevard
Boston, MA 02210
USA

Cengage is a leading provider of customized learning solutions with employees residing in nearly 40 different countries and sales in more than 125 countries around the world. Find your local representative at **www.cengage.com.**

To learn more about Cengage platforms and services, register or access your online learning solution, or purchase materials for your course, visit **www.cengage.com.**

Notice to the Reader

Publisher does not warrant or guarantee any of the products described herein or perform any independent analysis in connection with any of the product information contained herein. Publisher does not assume, and expressly disclaims, any obligation to obtain and include information other than that provided to it by the manufacturer. The reader is expressly warned to consider and adopt all safety precautions that might be indicated by the activities described herein and to avoid all potential hazards. By following the instructions contained herein, the reader willingly assumes all risks in connection with such instructions. The publisher makes no representations or warranties of any kind, including but not limited to, the warranties of fitness for particular purpose or merchantability, nor are any such representations implied with respect to the material set forth herein, and the publisher takes no responsibility with respect to such material. The publisher shall not be liable for any special, consequential, or exemplary damages resulting, in whole or part, from the readers' use of, or reliance upon, this material.

Printed in the United States of America
Print Number: 01   Print Year: 2021

Contributors

JENNIFER COLLINS
Masters in Instructional Design, University of Wisconsin Stout
Writer, instructional designer
Raleigh, NC
Chapters 4, 13, 17, 18

SCOTT E. DOBRIN
Assistant Professor of Biology
Collegium of Natural Sciences
Eckerd College
St. Petersburg, Florida
Chapter 6

JULIE A. DOLL, MASTER OF SCIENCE
Anatomy Instructor
Midwestern University
Chicago, Illinois
Chapters 3, 11

BRUCE S. FORCIEA, D.C.
Anatomy and Physiology Instructor,
Moraine Park Technical College, Unitek College
Milwaukee, WI
Chapters 5, 9, 10

COLIN KING, MS, PA-C
Physician Assistant
Department of Cardiac Surgery
Thomas Jefferson University Hospital
Philadelphia, PA
Chapters 7, 8

DR. SHAUN N. MARTINS, BS, DC
Human Anatomy Adjunct Professor
Los Positas Community College
Livermore, California
Chapters 1, 2, 14

ANGELA SPARKMAN, MS BIOLOGY, A MASTER OF EDUCATION, AND MT(ASCP) CERTIFICATION
Associate Professor, Life Sciences
Ivy Tech Community College
New Albany, Indiana
Chapter 12

Contents

Chapter 1

Tissues of the Human Body

Chapter Introduction

KEY TERMS

connective tissue One of the four primary tissue types, forms and functions vary and include support, storage, and protection.

epithelial tissue The center of the artery, called the tunica interna endothelium.

muscle tissue One of four primary tissue types, contracts and creates a force resulting in movement.

nervous tissue Tissue that consists of neurons and supporting neuroglial cells and makes up the central and peripheral nervous system.

All of the tissues in the human body work together seamlessly to ensure all of the body systems function properly. There are four main types of tissues in the body that perform different functions:

- **Epithelial tissue** (supports body and organ function): The center of the artery, called the tunica interna endothelium (Figure 1-1), is an example of epithelial tissue.
- **Connective tissue** (covers organs and body structures): The outer layer of arteries, the tunic adventitia (Figure 1-1), is a tough outer covering of connective tissue.
- **Muscle tissue** (moves organs and body structures): This, combined with elastic tissue, makes up the middle layer of the artery, the tunica media (Figure 1-1) This enables the artery to rebound quickly when constricting and relaxing.
- **Nervous tissue** (controls organs and body structures): This type of tissue allows the nervous system to relay information about the tissues being cold or responding to anxiety and triggers the arteries to constrict.

Each of these specialized tissues is comprised of cells that work together. Understanding what makes up each type of tissue and each tissue's functions will help you better understand the organs and systems of the human body.

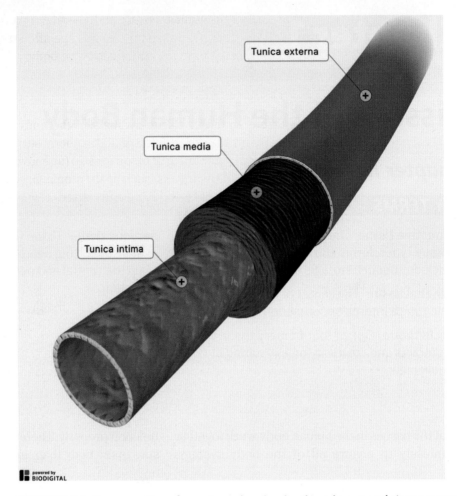

FIGURE 1-1 Cross section of an artery showing its three layers and tissue types. The inner layer shown in yellow (the tunica interna) is made of endothelium. The middle layer (called the tunica media) is elastic tissue and smooth muscle. The outer layer (the tunica externa) is collagenous connective tissue.

UNIT OBJECTIVE 1.1

Classify epithelial tissue according to cell shape, arrangement, and function.

KEY TERM

epithelium One of four primary tissue types, lines and covers all free body surfaces, both inside and out; functions are protection, absorption, filtration, and secretion.

UNIT INTRODUCTION

As noted previously, one type of tissue found in the body is epithelial tissue. This is the tissue found at the center of the constricting and relaxing artery you explored, which is shown in yellow in Figure 1-1. As noted previously, this tissue, called the tunica interna endothelium, is a type of epithelial tissue, or **epithelium**. This specialized tissue has specific structural characteristics and performs special functions throughout the body.

EPITHELIAL TISSUE

You'll find epithelial tissue throughout the body (Figure 1-2), as it lines and covers the inside and outside of all free body surfaces. This includes the outer layer of skin, inner lining of blood vessels (as shown in Figure 1-1), and the inner lining of all hollow organs, such as the stomach, small intestine, and bladder. It also forms most of the body's glands, arteries, veins, and capillaries.

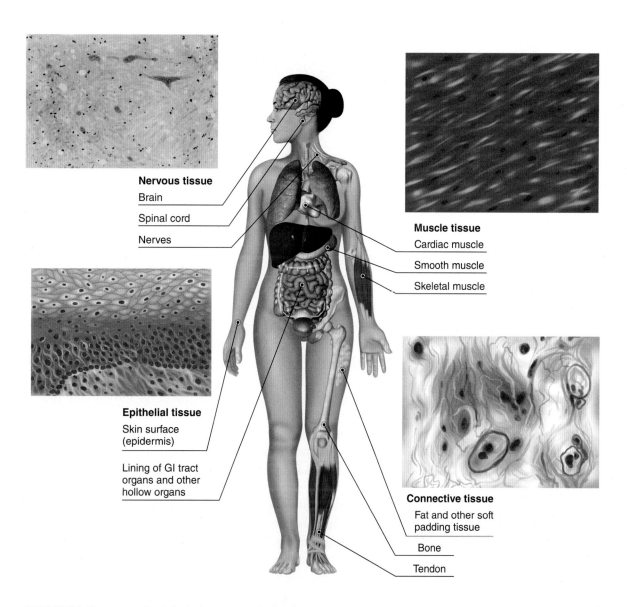

Nervous tissue
Brain
Spinal cord
Nerves

Muscle tissue
Cardiac muscle
Smooth muscle
Skeletal muscle

Epithelial tissue
Skin surface (epidermis)
Lining of GI tract organs and other hollow organs

Connective tissue
Fat and other soft padding tissue
Bone
Tendon

FIGURE 1-2 Areas of epithelial tissue in the body.

LEARNING OBJECTIVE 1.1.1 **Describe the structural characteristics of epithelial tissue.**

KEY TERMS

apical surface Side of epithelial tissue that is exposed to the cavity of an internal organ or exterior of the body.

basement membrane Material secreted by both the epithelial cells above it and the connective tissue cells below it; forms the basal surface and anchors epithelium in place.

cell membrane junctions Hold cells tightly together to prevent loss of chemicals and water and cells from being pulled apart and allow chemicals and water to pass between cells; three common types are tight junctions, desmosomes, and gap junctions.

desmosomes Junctions that are scattered throughout the cell membrane and act as anchors to prevent cells from being pulled apart due to mechanical stress.

gap junctions Hollow, water-filled cylinders that allow things like nutrients and ions to pass between neighboring cells; most commonly found in cardiac cells and embryonic cells.

tight junctions Junctions that encircle cells, fusing them together into leakproof sheets; prevent substances from leaking into spaces between cells and, in the small intestine, prevent digestive enzymes from getting into the bloodstream.

Special Characteristics of Epithelial Tissue

Epithelium generally contains the following unique characteristics:

- Epithelial tissues are avascular. This means they have no blood supply of their own. They depend on capillaries in underlying tissue to supply them with nutrients and oxygen and get rid of waste products, through a process called diffusion. Note that the capillary in Figure 1-3 is located in the dermal layer below the epithelium.

- With the exception of glandular epithelium, specialized cell membrane junctions bind epithelial cells tightly together at many points. Figure 1-3 shows tight junctions, desmosomes, and gap junctions. All of these junctions, except gap junctions, seal close any spaces between cells. Closing the space between cells prevents such things as leakage of enzymes in the digestive tract and water loss through the skin. This also forms a barrier in the skin to keep things out, and this prevents cells from being pulled apart. Tight junctions encircle cells, fusing them together into leakproof sheets. Desmosomes are scattered throughout the cell membrane, acting as anchors to prevent cells from being pulled apart by mechanical stress. Gap Junctions are water-filled, hollow cylinders that join neighboring cells and allow things, such as nutrients and ions, to pass from one cell to another. These are most common in the heart and embryonic cells.

- Membranes and skin always have one unattached or free side called the apical surface. It is the exposed surface of the skin or

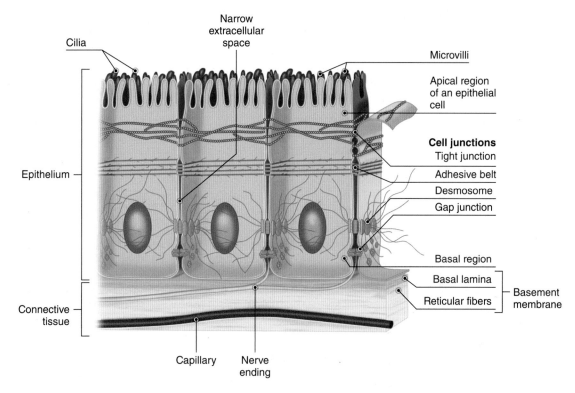

FIGURE 1-3 Special characteristics of epithelial tissue with cell junctions.

cavity of an internal organ. Some apical surfaces are smooth and some have modifications such as cilia or microvilli. In Figure 1-3 you can see the apical surface of the cavity and the microvilli on the surface. Microvilli greatly increase surface area for more efficient and faster absorption.

- Epithelium is anchored in place by a **basement membrane**. The basement membrane is a substance secreted by the basal epithelial cells and the underlying connective tissue cells that make up the dermis, to hold the epithelium in place. This side is called the basal surface or region and can be seen in Figure 1-3.
- With sufficient nutrients, epithelial cells regenerate quickly. They retain the ability to undergo mitosis and replace damaged cells. In epithelial tissues like the skin and digestive tract, new epithelial cells are constantly replacing cells that die.

LEARNING OBJECTIVE 1.1.2 Identify the functions of epithelial tissue.

Functions of Epithelial Tissue

Epithelial tissue has four main functions. Each function reflects the tissue's role as a boundary or interface tissue that primarily supports functions of the body and of other tissues. These functions are protection, absorption, filtration, and secretion. Here are a few examples of each function.

1. Protection: The epithelial layer of skin acts as a barrier and keeps bacteria and chemicals from entering the body. Note that Figure 1-4 illustrates the many layers of epithelium and the second layer of skin, the dermis. While relatively thin, the outermost layers of epithelium are tough and water resistant.

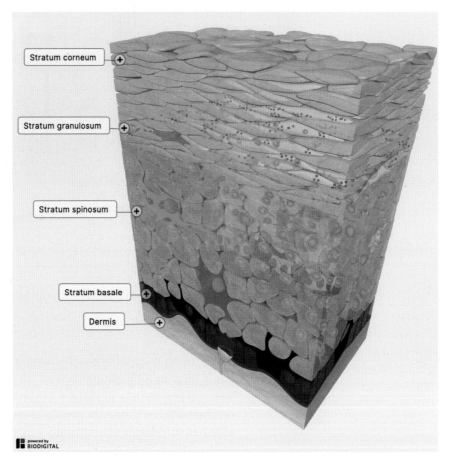

Stratum corneum

Stratum granulosum

Stratum spinosum

Stratum basale

Dermis

powered by
BIODIGITAL

FIGURE 1-4 Cross section of the skin showing layers of epithelium (except for the stratum lucidum) and the dermis.

2. Absorption: The digestive system is lined with epithelium that is specialized for absorption. Study Figure 1-5, which shows tissue from the small intestine. Note the finger-like projections on the innermost layer of the small intestine. These projections are a result of folds in this layer of tissue. These folds greatly increase the surface area of this tissue (by millions of times!). More surface area enables faster, more efficient absorption of nutrients in the small intestine.

3. Filtration: The kidneys contain epithelium whose role is absorption *and* filtration. As you can see in Figure 1-6, a coronal cross section of a kidney, the structure of the kidney forces fluid to be filtered through several sections. For more information on kidney function, see Chapter 15.

4. Secretion: Secretion is a specialty of glandular epithelium. Glandular epithelium produces substances, such as hormones, sweat, mucus, and enzymes. An example of this process is the thyroid gland releasing its hormones.

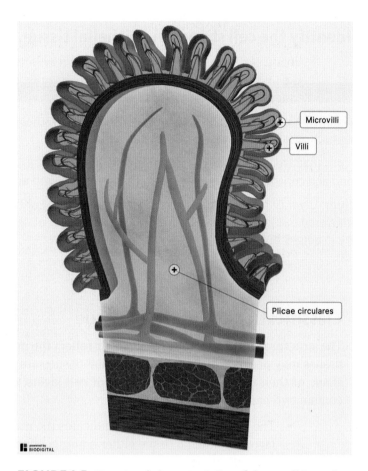

FIGURE 1-5 Structural characteristics of the small intestine that increase its surface area.

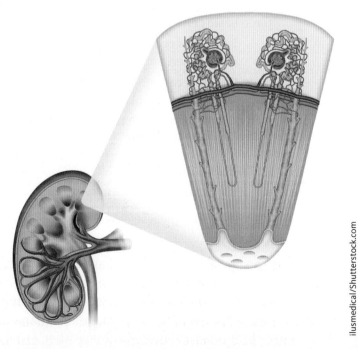

FIGURE 1-6 Coronal cross section of the kidney, with an enlargement of one section to illustrate a nephron.

KEY TERMS

columnar cells Epithelial cells that are taller than they are wide with elongated, oval-shaped nuclei.

cuboidal cells Epithelial cells that are cube-shaped with nuclei that are round and central in the cell.

pseudostratified epithelium Layer of epithelium that appears to be multilayered but is only one cell layer thick; cells vary in height but all touch the basement membrane.

simple epithelium Epithelium that is one cell layer thick.

squamous cells Epithelial cells that are flat and hexagonal shaped with disc-shaped nuclei.

stratified epithelium Epithelium that consists of more than one layer of cells.

Classification of Epithelial Tissue

The structure and organization of the cells reflect the many functions epithelial tissues may perform in the body. Epithelial tissues are classified based on the shape of their cells and by the number of cell layers they form. Their names contain two parts:

- The first part of their name indicates the number of cell layers. Epithelial tissue either consists of one layer (**simple epithelium**), more than one layer of the same cell shape (**stratified epithelium**), or multiple layers containing cells of different shapes (**pseudostratified epithelium**).
- The second part of their name indicates the cell shape. There are three basic cell shapes. All three can be seen in Figure 1-7.
  - **Squamous cells** are flat and hexagonal shaped with disc-shaped nuclei.
  - **Cuboidal cells** are cube shaped and about as wide as they are tall with spherical nuclei.
  - **Columnar cells** are taller than they are wide with elongated, oval-shaped nuclei.

Simple epithelial tissue consists of one layer of cells, where all of the cells are the same shape. Tissues classified as stratified epithelium are a little trickier to name because the cell shape changes in between the layers of cells. However, the shape of the cells in the apical layer is always used to name stratified epithelia.

CLINICAL TIP Determine the apical surface as well as the number of cell layers to identify the cell type and name the epithelial tissue. If the nucleus is visible in the apical cells, you can also use its shape to help you determine if the epithelial tissue is made of squamous, cuboidal, columnar, or pseudostratified cells. Remember, stratified epithelium is named by the cell type on the apical surface only.

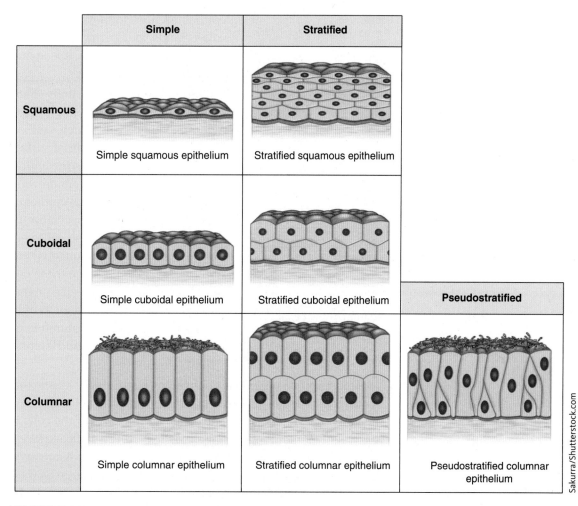

FIGURE 1-7 This table shows the characteristics of squamous, cuboidal, and columnar epithelium, along with how they appear when arranged simply, stratified, and in a pseudostratified manner.

LEARNING OBJECTIVE 1.1.4 Describe the simple, stratified, pseudostratified, and ciliated epithelium.

SIMPLE EPITHELIA

There are four types of simple epithelia. As you read about the different types of epithelium, refer to the images shown for each one.

1. Simple squamous epithelium (Figure 1-8). Tissue composed of simple squamous epithelium that is one cell layer thick. The cells are shaped like flat tiles with disc-shaped nuclei. It is specialized for diffusion and filtration in the capillary walls, lungs, and kidneys as well as secretion in serous membranes.

2. Simple cuboidal epithelium (Figure 1-9). Tissue composed of simple cuboidal epithelium that is one cell layer thick. This tissue's cube-shaped cells have a round nucleus in the center of the cell. Simple cuboidal

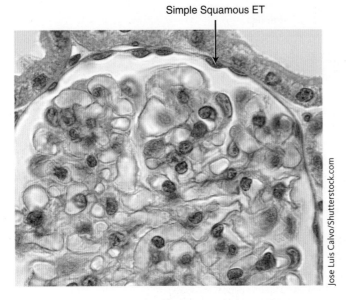

Simple Squamous ET

Jose Luis Calvo/Shutterstock.com

FIGURE 1-8 Simple squamous epithelium of the renal cortex. The arrow is pointing to the simple squamous cell layer.

epithelium lines kidney tubules, the ducts of small glands, and forms the secretory cells of many glands in the body. It is specialized for secretion and absorption.

3. Simple columnar epithelium (Figure 1-10). Tissue composed of a single layer of tall, column-shaped cells. Each cell's elongated nucleus sits toward the basal surface. Simple columnar epithelium lines the entire digestive tract and parts of the female reproductive tract. Like simple cuboidal epithelium, simple columnar epithelium is specialized for secretion (in the stomach these cells secrete acid, digestive enzymes, and mucous) and absorption (in the small intestine these cells absorb nutrients). Some contain cilia on their surface and aid in the active movement of molecules. For example, ciliated columnar epithelium lines the uterine tubes and helps move the ovum to the uterus.

4. Pseudostratified columnar epithelium (Figure 1-11). Tissue that appears to be composed of multiple layers because the cells appear to vary in height; however, it is only one cell layer thick. All of the cells rest on the basement membrane, but not all of the cells reach the surface of the epi-thelium. The cells that do reach the surface vary in diameter, with some being large on the apical surface and others being large on the basement membrane side. The nuclei also lie at different levels, which gives the false impression that the tissue is stratified. Pseudostratified columnar epithelium is specialized for absorption and secretion. This tissue type is found in the male reproductive tract and the ducts of some large glands. A ciliated variety is found in the upper respiratory tract.

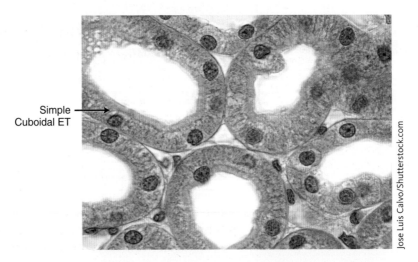

Simple Cuboidal ET

Jose Luis Calvo/Shutterstock.com

FIGURE 1-9 Simple cuboidal epithelium of the proximal convoluted tubule of the kidney. The arrow is pointing to one of the cuboidal cells.

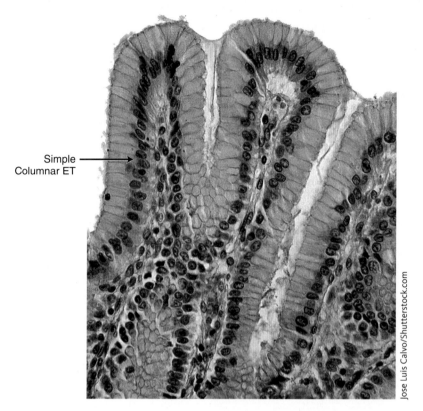

Simple
Columnar ET →

Jose Luis Calvo/Shutterstock.com

FIGURE 1-10 Simple columnar epithelium found in the lining of the
stomach. The arrow is pointing to a columnar cell.

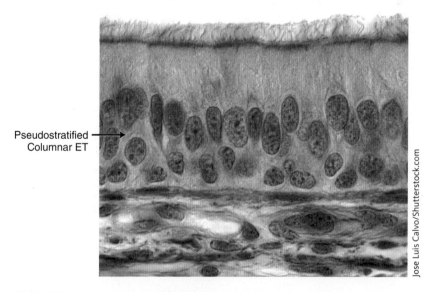

Pseudostratified →
Columnar ET

Jose Luis Calvo/Shutterstock.com

FIGURE 1-11 Pseudostratified columnar epithelium. Notice how the
position of cell nuclei make it look like there are two cell
layers, while there is actually only one layer.

Identify the locations of each epithelial tissue type in the body.

STRATIFIED EPITHELIA

Stratified epithelium consists of two or more layers of cells. The cells at the basement membrane are constantly dividing and being pushed upward to form the apical layer of cells. These multilayered tissues are specialized for protection. Remember that the number of cell layers as well as the cell shape at the apical surface is used to name these tissue types. There are four types of stratified epithelium.

Stratified Squamous ET

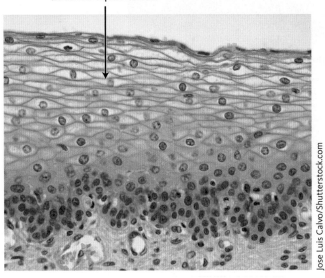

Jose Luis Calvo/Shutterstock.com

FIGURE 1-12 Non-keratinized stratified squamous epithelium. The arrow is pointing to the layers of squamous epithelium.

1. Stratified squamous epithelium (Figure 1-12). The most common type of stratified epithelium in the body. It is specialized to withstand large amounts of friction and is found in the mouth, esophagus, vagina, and surface of the skin. The cells on the apical surface are squamous, while the cells below are cuboidal or columnar. The stratified squamous epithelium that makes up the surface of the skin is keratinized (they have become filled with keratin, which causes the cell to die). This makes the cells tough and waterproof. In other areas of the body, this tissue type is nonkeratinized.

2. Stratified cuboidal epithelium (Figure 1-13) and stratified columnar epithelium (Figure 1-14). Rare types of tissues in the body. Stratified cuboidal epithelium is found in the ducts of sweat glands, mammary glands, and salivary glands. Stratified columnar epithelium is found in parts of the pharynx, anus, and uterus; part of the male urethra; and the ductus deferens. Both epithelial types are specialized for secretion and absorption.

3. Transitional epithelium (Figure 1-15). Tissue found in the hollow urinary organs. It lines the ureters, bladder, and part of the urethra. As organs like the bladder stretch, the cells of transitional epithelium change shape. When the organ relaxes, the tissue is no longer stretched and it takes on a scalloped appearance. Transitional epithelium functions not only to stretch, but also to form an impermeable barrier that keeps urine from leaking through the wall of the bladder.

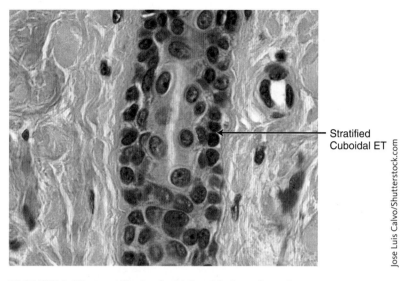

Stratified
Cuboidal ET

Jose Luis Calvo/Shutterstock.com

FIGURE 1-13 Stratified cuboidal epithelium found in an eccrine sweat gland. The arrow is pointing to the bottom layer of the stratified cuboidal epithelium.

Stratified Columnar ET

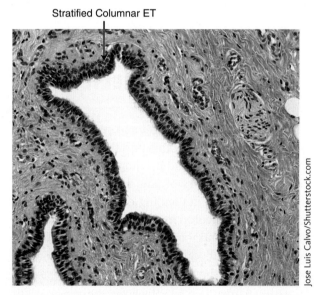

Jose Luis Calvo/Shutterstock.com

FIGURE 1-14 Stratified columnar epithelium. This type of epithelium is very rare, but is the dense collection of cells seen surrounding the white opening at the center of the image.

Transitional ET

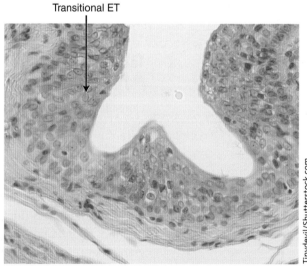

Tinydevil/Shutterstock.com

FIGURE 1-15 Transitional epithelium. The arrow is pointing to the mass of cells that are currently in a relaxed state. When the tissue starts to stretch this layer will become much thinner.

LEARNING OBJECTIVE **1.1.6** Identify the locations of glandular epithelium, endothelium, and mesothelium.

LEARNING OBJECTIVE **1.1.7** Describe the function of glandular epithelium, endothelium, and mesothelium.

KEY TERMS

endocrine gland Ductless gland that secretes a hormone into the bloodstream.

endothelium Simple squamous epithelium found lining blood vessels, lymphatic vessels, and the heart.

exocrine glands Gland that secretes a substance onto the surface of the body using a duct.

glandular epithelium Tissue type that makes up endocrine and exocrine glands.

hormones Chemical substances, secreted by endocrine glands, that target another tissue in the body.

ischemic Decrease in blood supply.

mesothelium Single layer of epithelial cells that forms part of serous membranes in the body.

sebaceous glands Exocrine gland located in the skin that produces sebum, or oil; usually associated with hair follicles.

serous membranes To Come.

vasoconstriction Narrowing of blood vessels.

GLANDULAR EPITHELIUM, ENDOTHELIUM, AND MESOTHELIUM

Consider the role of the thyroid and the glands that target and stimulate thyroid tissue, which results in the release of thyroid hormones into the bloodstream.

Like many other glands in the body, the thyroid is comprised of **glandular epithelium**. Glandular epithelium forms secretory organs called glands, which are classified as either exocrine or endocrine depending on how they secrete their product. As an embryo forms, glands develop from the folding of the glandular epithelium. A duct forms when the gland maintains an opening with epithelium. Glands with secretory ducts are called **exocrine glands**. All exocrine glands secrete their products onto surfaces through ducts. This may mean that the substance is being secreted within a lumen, like in the gastrointestinal tract, or onto the surface of the skin. The internal surface of the gastrointestinal tract and the outer surface of the skin are both considered a surface of the body. Exocrine glands are common in the body. A few examples include the following:

- Sweat glands
- Sebaceous glands
- Mucous secreting glands (Goblet cells)
- Salivary glands
- The liver
- The pancreas
- Mammary glands

If the gland does not have a duct it is classified as an **endocrine gland**. Endocrine glands secrete **hormones** directly into the fluid that surrounds the cells. The hormones are then able to enter nearby capillaries and travel through the bloodstream to their target organs.

The glandular epithelium of the hypothalamus creates hormones that target the pituitary gland, which, in turn, targets and stimulates the thyroid gland. For example, consider hyperthyroidism; in response to the hormones released from the glandular epithelium of the pituitary gland, the thyroid glandular epithelium releases too much thyroid hormone.

Recall that Raynaud's phenomenon is caused by abnormal **vasoconstriction**. The arteries, comprised of a variety of tissues, respond to cold and stress by constricting. This most often occurs in the fingers (Figure 1-16), but can also include the toes, nose, and ears. As blood flow is decreased, the tissues become **ischemic** due to low oxygen levels. The affected areas first turn white, then grayish blue, and will feel cold and numb. As the attack subsides and blood flows back into the area, the color returns to normal. A tingling, painful, throbbing sensation and possibly swelling may occur as blood returns. The inner lining of epithelial tissue that covers the lumen of arteries is called **endothelium** (Figure 1-1). It forms a

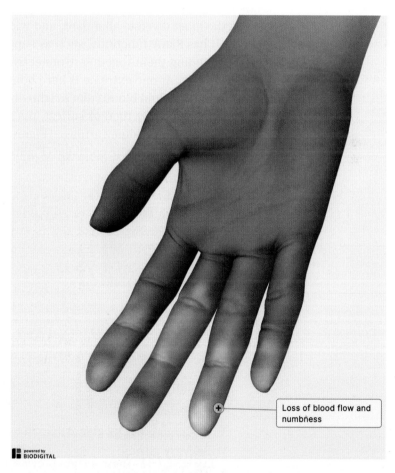

Loss of blood flow and numbness

powered by
BIODIGITAL

FIGURE 1-16 A patient's hand who is experiencing Raynaud's disease and the characteristic loss of blood flow to the fingers and resulting numbness.

slick surface that decreases friction as blood and fluid move through the vessel lumen. For more information on the function of the endothelium, see Chapter 9.

Another important type of epithelial tissue is the **mesothelium**. It is comprised of simple squamous epithelium and makes up one of the layers of **serous membranes**. Serous membranes line cavities of the body that do not open to the exterior, such as the pericardium around the heart, the pleural membranes around each lung, and the peritoneal cavity. A small amount of serous fluid is secreted between the layers of serous membranes, which lubricates them so they become slippery. This decreases friction and helps protect the internal organs as they rub against each other. The serous membranes also help anchor organs in place.

UNIT OBJECTIVE 1.2

Compare the major types of connective tissue.

UNIT INTRODUCTION

Another tissue type found in the human body is connective tissue. Connective tissue is the most diverse, abundant, and widespread type of tissue present in the body. It has many functions, such as supporting and protecting body parts as well as binding them together. Connective tissue ranges widely, from very rigid to very soft. At one extreme is hard bone, and at the other extreme is soft adipose tissue and fluid blood (that's right—blood is considered a fluid connective tissue!). From most rigid to softest, the major connective tissue types are bone (Figure 1-17A), hyaline cartilage (Figure 1-17B), dense regular connective tissue (Figure 1-17C), elastic cartilage (Figure 1-17D), and blood.

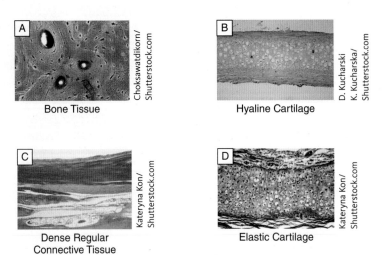

Bone Tissue

Choksawatdikorn/Shutterstock.com

Hyaline Cartilage

D. Kucharski K. Kucharska/Shutterstock.com

Dense Regular Connective Tissue

Kateryna Kon/Shutterstock.com

Elastic Cartilage

Kateryna Kon/Shutterstock.com

FIGURE 1-17 These images provide a microscopic look at bone (A), hyaline cartilage (B), dense regular connective tissue (C), and elastic cartilage. (D).

LEARNING OBJECTIVE 1.2.1 Describe the basic structure of connective tissue.

KEY TERMS

adipocytes Specialized cells found in adipose connective tissue that store fat.

collagen An abundant structural protein found throughout the body.

elastic Type of cartilage found in the epiglottis and external ear that contains many elastic fibers in its extracellular matrix.

extracellular matrix Ground substance and protein fibers found in connective tissue that make up the extracellular matrix.

ground substance Nonliving material secreted by connective tissue cells; along with the protein fibers in connective tissue, it makes up the extracellular matrix.

osteocytes Specialized bone cells that maintain bone tissue.

reticular Netlike structure containing fibers, fibroblasts, and white blood cells that forms an internal framework for the spleen, thymus, lymph nodes, and bone marrow.

CHARACTERISTICS OF CONNECTIVE TISSUE

There are several distinguishing characteristics of connective tissue:

- Cells. Each type of connective tissue contains specific types of cells. For example, adipose tissue has **adipocytes**, and bone tissue has **osteocytes**. Most connective tissue cells are scattered throughout the tissue. This is different from epithelial tissue, where the cells are very close with little to no space between them.

- Protein fibers. Three types of protein fibers are found in connective tissue: **collagen** fibers (strong and resistant to stretch), **elastic** fibers (flexible and able to stretch and recoil), and **reticular** fibers (form an internal framework of soft organs like the spleen). The type and amount of each fiber found in connective tissue indicate to what extent that tissue is used for strength and support.

- **Extracellular matrix** and **ground substance**. Everything outside of the cells, including protein fibers, makes up the extracellular matrix (Figure 1-18). The extracellular matrix also contains a material called the ground substance. Ground substance is a nonliving material secreted by connective tissue cells. It primarily consists of water, proteins, and carbohydrates. It may be viscous (found in blood), semisolid (found in cartilage), or solid (found in bone).

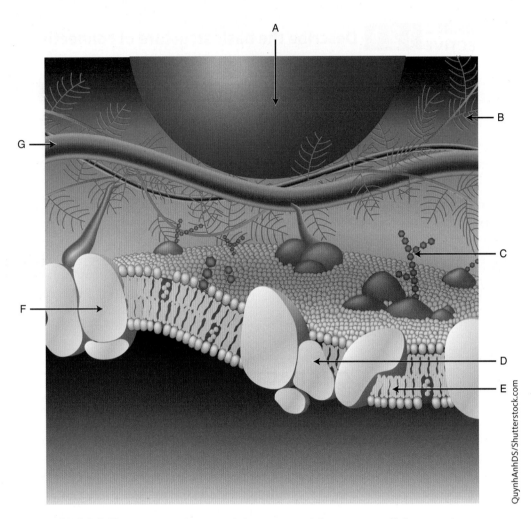

QuynhAnhDS/Shutterstock.com

FIGURE 1-18 Diagram of extracellular matrix. A) large extracellular protein,
B) chondroitin sulfate proteoglycan, C) carbohydrate cell marker
molecule, D) Peripheral protein, E) Phospholipid forming cell
membrane, F) Transmembrane protein, G) Blood vessel.

LEARNING OBJECTIVE 1.2.2 **Identify the locations of loose connective tissue.**

KEY TERMS

adipose Loose connective tissue commonly known as fat.

areolar Loose connective tissue with predominantly fibroblast cells, collagen, and elastic fibers; has a large amount of ground substance around the cells.

loose connective tissue Contains fewer cells and fibers than dense connective tissue; types are areolar, adipose, and reticular.

reticular Netlike structure containing fibers, fibroblasts, and white blood cells that forms an internal framework for the spleen, thymus, lymph nodes, and bone marrow.

LOCATIONS OF LOOSE CONNECTIVE TISSUE

Loose connective tissue is the most common type of connective tissue found in humans. It generally has more cells and fewer fibers than other connective tissue types. Loose connective tissue is soft tissue found in almost all areas of the body. It surrounds nerves and blood vessels, attaches epithelial tissue to underlying tissues, and holds organs in place. There are three main types of loose connective tissue: areolar, reticular, and adipose.

LEARNING OBJECTIVE 1.2.3 Describe the structure of areolar loose connective tissue.

KEY TERMS

lamina propria Thin layer of loose connective tissue that lies beneath the epithelium.

macrophages Type of white blood cell found in areolar connective tissue; functions as part of the body's immune system and engulfs and breaks down cells and cellular debris.

mast cells Type of cell found in areolar connective tissue; contains structures rich in histamine and heparin, which have important functions in immune response and blood thinning, respectively.

AREOLAR CONNECTIVE TISSUE STRUCTURE

Areolar connective tissue is the soft packing material of the body. It helps hold internal organs together, cushions and protects the organs it surrounds, and keeps organs in their proper positions. It has a fluid matrix containing all types of fibers with a lot of space around cells. The fluid matrix also provides water and salts for surrounding tissues (Figure 1-19), and the majority of body cells use the fluid matrix to obtain their nutrients and get rid of their waste products. Areolar connective tissue contains many cell types that serve a variety of functions. These cells include fibroblasts, plasma cells, macrophages, and mast cells.

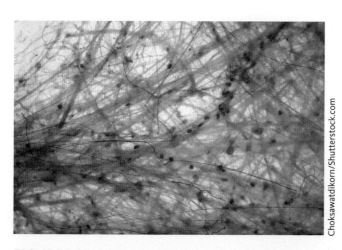

Choksawatdikorn/Shutterstock.com

FIGURE 1-19 Areolar connective tissue. Notice how it appears to be going in many directions and is scattered unevenly.

- Macrophages. A type of white blood cell. They have the ability to surround and absorb foreign debris in the body. These cells play an important part in the body's immune system response.

- Mast cells. These cells contain heparin and histamine. Heparin plays a role in thinning blood in the body, and histamine is an important part of immune responses, such as allergic and anaphylactic reactions.

A layer of areolar loose connective tissue called the lamina propria under-lies all mucous membranes. It is found in the epidermis and in the subcutaneous layer with adipose cells.

LEARNING OBJECTIVE 1.2.4 Describe the structure of reticular loose connective tissue.

KEY TERM

reticular cells Cells found in a netlike structure containing fibers, fibroblasts, and white blood cells that forms an internal framework for the spleen, thymus, lymph nodes, and bone marrow.

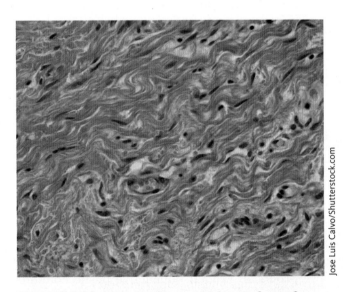

FIGURE 1-20 Reticular fibers, which are a form of dense irregular connective tissue. These fibers are tightly packed but not uniform in their direction.

Jose Luis Calvo/Shutterstock.com

RETICULAR CONNECTIVE TISSUE STRUCTURE

Recall that there are three fiber types present in the body. Of those three fibers, reticular fibers are the least common in the body; however, it is the primary fiber that makes up reticular connective tissue. In fact, reticular connective tissue is made up of a network of reticular fibers and reticular cells. These networks form a netlike structure that makes up the internal structure of lymphatic tissue and provides a framework that provides support to structures such as the lymph nodes, spleen, bone marrow, and liver (see black fibers in Figure 1-20). Reticular connective tissue is soft and requires additional support to maintain its shape.

LEARNING OBJECTIVE 1.2.5 Describe the structure of adipose loose connective tissue.

KEY TERM

adipose cells Specialized cells that store fat and make up adipose connective tissue.

ADIPOSE CONNECTIVE TISSUE

Adipose connective tissue is basically an areolar tissue where specialized **adipose cells** are the primary cell type. This loose connective tissue is commonly called fat, as adipose cells specialize in fat accumulation and storage. This large accumulation of fat within the cell displaces the cell's nucleus, pushing it out to the side in the cell cytoplasm (Figure 1-21). Adipose is deposited around the kidneys and eyeballs for protection; beneath the skin for insulation and protection; and areas of the body for potential energy.

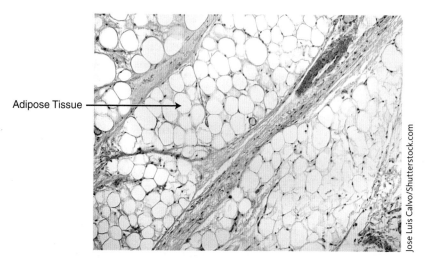

Adipose Tissue →

Jose Luis Calvo/Shutterstock.com

FIGURE 1-21 White adipose cells full of fat molecules. The entire cell is almostly entirely composed of fat.

There are two types of adipose connective tissue: yellow adipose tissue and brown adipose tissue.

- White adipose tissue is the most abundant adipose tissue in the body. It is present at birth and remains in the body throughout adulthood. It first appears as white in color; however, it slowly becomes yellow over time as pigments, such as carotene (vitamin A), are ingested and stored there. The main functions of yellow adipose tissue include storing energy, protecting internal structures, and insulating the body to help maintain homeostasis.
- Brown adipose tissue is found primarily in infants. It is a specialized tissue that can generate heat. As such, it plays a significant role in helping maintain normal body temperature in infants.

LEARNING OBJECTIVE 1.2.6 **Identify the locations of dense connective tissue.**

DENSE CONNECTIVE TISSUE

Dense connective tissue forms strong, ropelike structures, such as ligaments and tendons, throughout the body. It also makes up the dermis of the skin, where it forms parallel bundles rather than ropelike structures, as is found in the ligaments and tendons (see Figure 1-17C). There are two types of dense connective tissue: dense regular connective tissue and dense irregular connective tissue.

LEARNING OBJECTIVE 1.2.7 Describe the structure of dense regular connective tissue.

Structure of Dense Regular Connective Tissue

Dense regular connective tissue is composed primarily of collagen fibers with rows of fibroblast cells. Fibroblasts make the proteins that the collagen fibers are composed of. The collagen fibers are arranged parallel to each other (Figure 1-22), which gives the tissues (ligaments and tendons) much strength and flexibility.

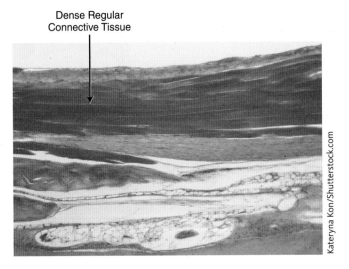

Dense Regular Connective Tissue

FIGURE 1-22 Dense regular connective tissue.

Kateryna Kon/Shutterstock.com

LEARNING OBJECTIVE 1.2.8 Describe the structure of dense irregular connective tissue.

Structure of Dense Irregular Connective Tissue

Dense irregular connective tissue is composed primarily of collagen fibers and fibroblasts, but unlike dense regular connective tissue, the collagen fibers run in all different directions and are clumped together. Dense irregular connective tissue makes up the dermis of the skin and provides tensile strength in all directions.

LEARNING OBJECTIVE 1.2.9 Identify the types of cartilage.

LEARNING OBJECTIVE 1.2.10 Identify the locations of hyaline, elastic, and fibrocartilage.

LEARNING OBJECTIVE 1.2.11 Describe the structure of hyaline, elastic, and fibrocartilage.

KEY TERMS

chondrocytes Mature cells found in cartilage.

elastic Type of cartilage found in the epiglottis and external ear that contains many elastic fibers in its extracellular matrix.

epiphyseal plate During bone development, hyaline cartilage is replaced by bone at the epiphyseal plate.

fibrocartilage Type of durable cartilage with many fibers and very little extracellular matrix found in the intervertebral discs, the menisci of the knee, and the pubic symphysis; acts as a shock absorber and resists compression.

hyaline Most common type of cartilage but also the weakest; flexible and resilient; found in the fetal skeleton, nose, trachea, larynx, costal cartilage, and articular ends of long bones.

lacunae Small spaces within the extracellular matrix of bone and cartilage where osteocytes and chondrocytes are found.

CARTILAGE

Cartilage provides flexible support that is firm yet not as rigid as bone. It is found in several locations in the body and is comprised of specialized cells known as **chondrocytes**. As extracellular matrix is secreted, the chondrocytes become trapped in cavities called **lacunae**. The extracellular matrix of cartilage is softer and more flexible than bone. There are three types of cartilage: **hyaline**, **elastic**, and **fibrocartilage**.

- Hyaline cartilage. The most common type of cartilage, hyaline cartilage provides flexible but firm support in the body. It is found in the trachea, bronchi, where the ribs attach to the sternum (costal cartilage), and at the ends of bones at joints (Figure 1-23). It also makes up a majority of the fetal skeleton. By the time a baby is born, most of its hyaline cartilage has been replaced by bone, with the exception of the **epiphyseal plates**, or growth plates. Hyaline cartilage has a gel-like matrix composed primarily of collagen fibers. It has a glassy, blue-white appearance under a microscope and the collagen fibers are difficult to see.

- Elastic cartilage. Much like hyaline cartilage, elastic

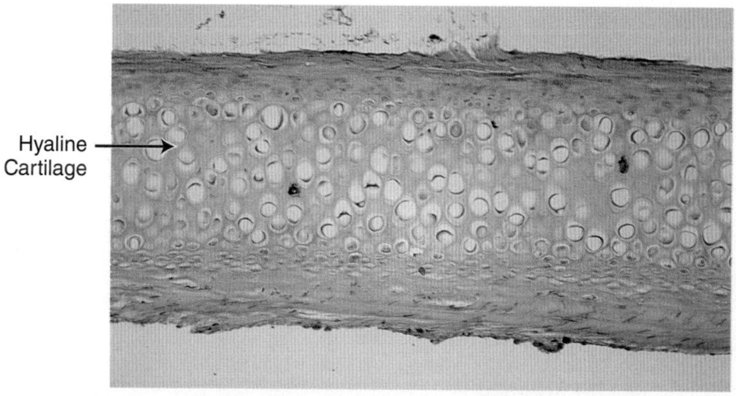

Hyaline Cartilage

D. Kucharski K. Kucharska/Shutterstock.com

FIGURE 1-23 Hyaline cartilage. The arrow is pointing to the hyaline cartilage cells located along the horizontal axis of the image.

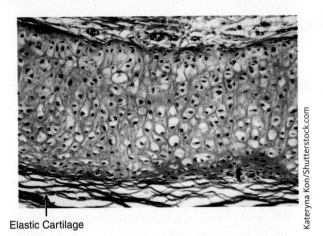

Elastic Cartilage

Kateryna Kon/Shutterstock.com

FIGURE 1-24 Elastic tissue of the outer ear. The arrow is pointing to the elastic tissue that is directly beneath a layer of hyaline cartilage.

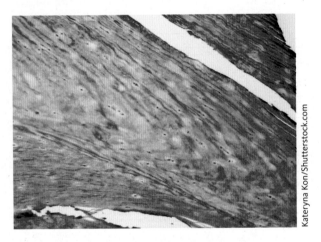

Kateryna Kon/Shutterstock.com

FIGURE 1-25 Fibrocartilage. Notice how the connective tissue appears to have fibers running the length of the image.

cartilage provides firm but flexible support throughout the body. It is found in the epiglottis, larynx, and external ear (Figure 1-24). Elastic cartilage contains numerous elastic fibers (also easily seen under a microscope) in its extracellular matrix, forming a web-like appearance around the chondrocytes (see Figure 1-24). It is resilient and very flexible. Although it is similar to hyaline cartilage, it contains more elastic fibers. It is not as common in the body as hyaline cartilage, and it looks very different when viewing the tissue under a microscope. The network of elastic fibers stain dark and are easily seen under a microscope. It does not appear smooth or stain blue as hyaline cartilage does.

- Fibrocartilage. Strong, flexible, and found in between bones where more strength is needed in the joint, fibrocartilage is also found in the intervertebral discs (circular structures found between the vertebrae), pubic symphysis (a pad of cartilage between the anterior pelvic bones where they meet), and the menisci (c-shaped pads) of the knee joints (Figure 1-25). The dense, interwoven collagen fibers of fibrocartilage are easily seen under a microscope. It is also very strong and resilient.

LEARNING OBJECTIVE **1.2.12** **Identify the connective tissue properties of blood.**

KEY TERMS

blood plasma Watery ground substance containing dissolved proteins, of the fluid connective tissue called blood.

erythrocytes Red blood cells found in blood that contain hemoglobin and carry oxygen throughout the body.

leukocytes White blood cell; circulates throughout the body and plays an important part in the body's immune response and reaction to foreign bodies and disease.

thrombocytes Commonly called platelets, found in the blood and play a role in blood clotting and wound healing.

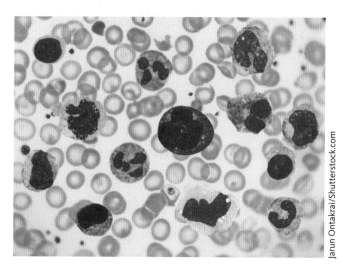

Jarun Ontakrai/Shutterstock.com

FIGURE 1-26 Human blood smear. The smaller round cells with a somewhat clear center are red blood cells (RBCs), while the large cells with differently shaped nuclei are the white blood cells.

CONNECTIVE TISSUE PROPERTIES OF BLOOD

As previously mentioned, blood is considered a fluid connective tissue. It contains cells, such as **erythrocytes** (red blood cells) and **leukocytes** (white blood cells); cell fragments called **thrombocytes** (platelets); and a nonliving, fluid extracellular matrix called **blood plasma** (see Figure 1-26). Recall that one of the structures that define connective tissue is the presence of fibers. Since it is a connective tissue, many soluble fibers can be found within blood. These fibers must remain dissolved in order for blood to move easily throughout the body. The soluble fibers only become visible when they are needed during specialized functions, such as during the blood-clotting process. Plasma, the fluid extracellular matrix of blood, transports nutrients, waste products, and hormones throughout the body.

LEARNING OBJECTIVE | **1.2.13** | **Identify the connective tissue features of bone.**

KEY TERM

osteocytes Specialized bone cells that maintain bone tissue.

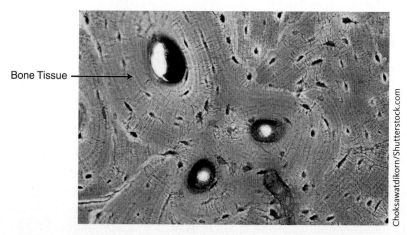

Bone Tissue →

Choksawatdikorn/Shutterstock.com

FIGURE 1-27 Compact bone tissue. The arrow is pointing to the layers of an osteon.

CONNECTIVE TISSUE FEATURES OF BONE

Bone is the hardest connective tissue. It is composed of specialized cells called **osteocytes** that sit in cavities called lacunae in the extracellular matrix. The lacunae are surrounded by many layers of hard extracellular matrix. This matrix contains many collagen fibers and mineral salts, which include calcium carbonate and calcium phosphate (Figure 1-27). Bones have many functions in the body, including enabling body movement, supporting the body, protecting the body's organs (the skull protects the brain, the ribcage protects the heart and lungs), and producing red blood cells. Bone and the many functions of bone are discussed in further detail in Chapter 3 of this course.

LEARNING OBJECTIVE **1.2.14** Explain the general functions of connective tissue.

FUNCTIONS OF CONNECTIVE TISSUE

Although there are many categories of connective tissue, there are three main types of connective tissue found in the adult. The functions of these types of connective tissue tend to overlap with one another:

- Connective tissue (both loose and dense) has a variety of functions, as touched on previously in this chapter. These functions include storage of energy, providing support to internal structures, binding structures together, and providing insulation to the body.
- Supportive connective tissue (cartilage and bone) stores energy and provides support throughout the body.
- Fluid connective tissue (blood) has storage and transportation functions.

Given the diversity and abundance of connective tissues in the body, they perform a wide variety of functions, including:

- Support: Connective tissue sheets form capsules that surround and protect organs like the kidneys and spleen. For example, bone offers support and a framework for skeletal muscle, and cartilage supports body structures such as the nose, ears, trachea, and bronchi.
- Storage: Bone stores calcium and phosphorus. Fat is the major energy reserve in the body.
- Transport: Blood transports waste products, nutrients, oxygen, hormones, and blood cells between areas of the body.
- Binding: Dense irregular connective tissue binds skin to underlying muscle and bone. Tendons bind muscles to bone, and ligaments bind bone to bone.
- Protection: Many bones structurally protect the organs that underlie them. For example, the skull protects the brain, and the ribcage protects the heart and lungs. As mentioned previously, connective tissue sheets form capsules that surround and protect organs like the kidneys and spleen. Many connective tissues also contain white blood cells, which offer immune protection.

UNIT OBJECTIVE 1.3

Compare the structure and functions of the three types of muscle tissue.

muscle tissue One of four primary tissue types, contracts and creates a force resulting in movement.

UNIT INTRODUCTION

Muscle tissue is another tissue type found in the human body. It is specialized to contract. When muscle tissue contracts, it results in movement of the body and its structures. There are three types of muscle tissue that serve different functions throughout the body. These are referred to as smooth muscle tissue, skeletal muscle tissue, and cardiac muscle tissue.

LEARNING OBJECTIVE 1.3.1 **Identify the structure of smooth muscle.**

peristalsis Process of smooth muscle contraction along the GI tract that forces material to move further along the tract.

smooth muscle tissue Involuntary, nonstriated type of muscle tissue with tapered cells that contain a single nucleus; found in the hollow organs of the body.

STRUCTURE OF SMOOTH MUSCLE

Smooth muscle tissue is found in the walls of hollow organs like the stomach, intestines, bladder, uterus, airways, and blood vessels (Figure 1-28). Smooth muscle has many important roles in the body, including playing a vital role in supporting normal respiration, maintenance of blood pressure, and digestion of food. Smooth muscle has the following characteristics:

- It is controlled involuntarily, meaning that you cannot consciously control the movement of smooth muscle.
- Smooth muscle cells are tapered at the ends and contain one nucleus per cell (see Figure 1-28).
- There are no visible striations when looking at smooth muscle tissue under a microscope (see Figure 1-28). This is how it gets its name.

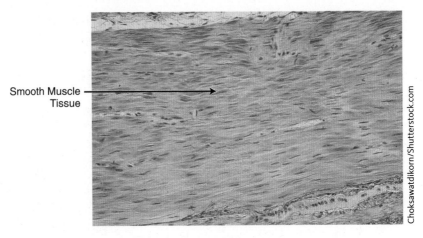

Smooth Muscle Tissue

Choksawatdikorn/Shutterstock.com

FIGURE 1-28 A sample of smooth muscle. Notice how it differs from skeletal muscle and cardiac muscle.

- The contraction of smooth muscle is slower and sustained for longer periods of time than the contraction of skeletal and cardiac muscle. One example of this is called peristalsis. Peristalsis is a wavelike contraction of smooth muscle. When it occurs in the digestive tract, this typical smooth muscle contraction keeps food moving.

LEARNING OBJECTIVE 1.3.2   Identify the structure of skeletal muscle.

KEY TERMS

muscle fibers Long, cylindrical cells that make up skeletal muscle tissue.

skeletal muscle tissue Voluntary, striated, multinucleated type of muscle tissue; its contraction causes movement of the skeleton.

striations Ridges or visible lines.

STRUCTURE OF SKELETAL MUSCLE

Skeletal muscle tissue is packaged together by sheets of connective tissue into organs called skeletal muscles (Figure 1-29). Skeletal muscles attach via tendons at joints in the skeleton. When contracted, they cause movement by pulling on bones and skin. Contraction and relaxation of skeletal muscle also produces heat as a by-product. This is why we shiver when we are cold—to help increase our body temperature. Long chains of skeletal muscle cells are called muscle fibers and have the following characteristics:

- You can control it voluntarily.
- The muscle cells are elongated, cylindrical, and multinucleated.

- The muscle cells have visible **striations** (or parallel lines/ridges) under a microscope (see Figure 1-29).

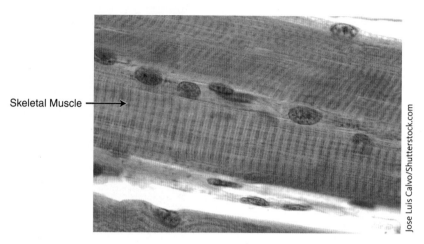

Skeletal Muscle —→

Jose Luis Calvo/Shutterstock.com

FIGURE 1-29 Skeletal muscle fibers. Notice how the muscle fibers are striated, have multiple nuclei, and the nuclei are found along the edge of the cell and not in the middle.

LEARNING OBJECTIVE 1.3.3 Identify the structure of cardiac muscle.

KEY TERMS

cardiac muscle tissue Involuntary, striated, branched type of muscle tissue found in the heart; the cells have a single nucleus and are tightly adhered to each other by intercalated discs.

intercalated discs Specialized cell junctions found in cardiac muscle.

myocardium Thick middle layer of the heart wall consisting of cardiac muscle.

STRUCTURE OF CARDIAC MUSCLE

Cardiac muscle tissue is only found in the heart wall (and forms the myocardium). It has the following characteristics (Figure 1-30):

- It is controlled involuntarily, which means that you cannot consciously control the beating of the heart.
- Cardiac muscle cells are short, branched, and have a single nucleus per cell.
- Cardiac muscle cells fit tightly together and contain intercalated discs, which are gap junctions that hold the cells tightly together. Intercalated discs are vital for the transmission of electrical signals that keep the heart beating in a normal rhythm. They prevent the loss of electrical signal as it travels from cardiac cell to cardiac cell. They also help maintain the strength of the electrical signal as it passes through the myocardium of the heart.
- The muscle cells have visible striations under a microscope.

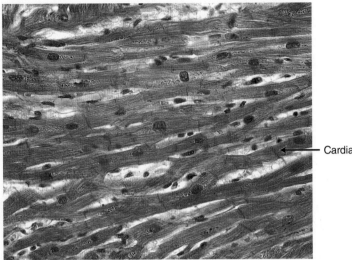

Jose Luis Calvo/Shutterstock.com

Cardiac Muscle

FIGURE 1-30 Cardiac muscle cells. The cardiac muscle cells are striated, branched, and contain intercalated discs between the individual cells. The arrow is pointing to one of the intercalated discs.

LEARNING
OBJECTIVE **1.3.4** Explain the functions of smooth, skeletal, and cardiac muscle.

FUNCTIONS OF SMOOTH, SKELETAL, AND CARDIAC MUSCLE

Each muscle tissue plays a special role in the body system based on how it functions:

- Smooth muscle contracts involuntarily and is responsible for many functions, such as:
    - Moving materials through internal organs (like food through the digestive system)
    - Regulating the size of organs (like contraction of the bladder to expel urine)
    - Forcing fluid through tubes (like blood through blood vessels, which helps regulate blood pressure)
    - Controlling the amount of light that enters the eye (expanding and constricting pupils).
- Cardiac muscle is only found in the heart and it moves involuntarily. It relaxes and contracts the heart in a regular rhythm in response to electrical signals. These highly coordinated contractions pump blood throughout our bodies.
- Skeletal muscle is a voluntary type of muscle tissue that controls body movement. However, there may be some cases in which skeletal muscle may also be classified as being involuntarily controlled. It may be involuntarily controlled by our nervous

system during a reflex or during certain processes, such as the contraction of the diaphragm for breathing. Contracting skeletal muscles move the skeleton and our body and produces heat that keeps us warm.

UNIT OBJECTIVE 1.4

Describe the organization of nervous tissue and how this relates to the tissue's function.

KEY TERMS

action potentials Rapid change in voltage generated by muscle and nervous tissue.

nervous tissue Tissue that consists of neurons and supporting neuroglial cells and makes up the central and peripheral nervous system.

neuroglia Supporting cells found in nervous tissue.

neurons Cells found in nervous tissue that detect stimuli, process information, and transmit electrical impulses from one area of the body to another.

UNIT INTRODUCTION

Nervous tissue makes up the nervous system and is the last type of tissue we discuss in this chapter. It is found in the brain, spinal cord, and nerves and is discussed in detail in Chapter 6 of this course. Nervous tissue is composed of nerve cells, or neurons, and many supporting cells called neuroglia. Neurons are the conducting tissue of the nervous system, and they transmit electric signals throughout the body. The electric signals are called action potentials. Neuroglial cells are specialized cells that are the major support cells of the brain and spinal cord.

LEARNING OBJECTIVE 1.4.1 Identify dendrites, soma, axon, myelin sheath, nodes of Ranvier, and axon bulbs of a neuron.

KEY TERMS

axon Single, long extension of the cell membrane of a neuron; carries outgoing signals to other cells.

axon bulbs End of the axon where neurotransmitters are released.

dendrites Specialized regions of the neuron that have neurotransmitter receptors and serve as the input zone.

myelin sheath Insulating layer around parts of an axon that greatly increases the speed of an action potential.

nodes of Ranvier Small spaces in between areas of myelination on an axon; nerve impulse jumps from node to node.

soma Cell body of a neuron containing the nucleus and other cell organelles.

STRUCTURE OF A NEURON

A neuron is composed of the following parts (Figure 1-31):

- **Soma.** Another name for the cell body where the nucleus and other organelles are located.
- **Dendrites.** Extensions of the cell membrane surrounding the soma. They are numerous and short compared to the axon.
- **Axon.** A single, long extension of the cell membrane that communicates with other neurons and target tissues.
- **Myelin sheath.** A lipid layer that is added to the outside of axons to increase the speed of the electric signal.
- **Nodes of Ranvier.** The spaces between the myelin sheath along the length of the axon.
- **Axon bulbs.** Extensions at the end of the axon where branching occurs. These enable the neuron to communicate with numerous other neurons and target tissues. Neurotransmitters are released here.

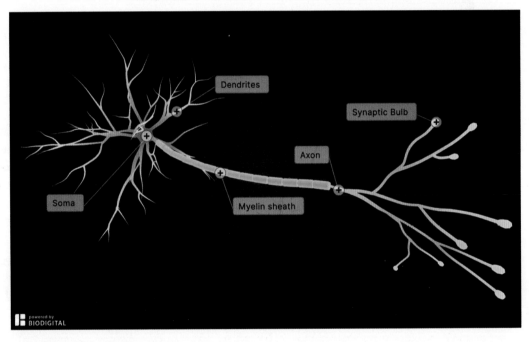

FIGURE 1-31 Image of a neuron showing the soma, dendrites, axon, myelin sheath, and synaptic bulbs.

The largest portion of a neuron is comprised of a cell body (also called a soma), dendrites, and an axon (Figure 1-31). The cell body contains the nucleus and other organelles (Figure 1-31).

LEARNING OBJECTIVE 1.4.2 Explain the function of dendrites in a nerve cell.

LEARNING OBJECTIVE 1.4.3 Explain the function of the soma in a nerve cell.

FUNCTIONS OF THE SOMA AND DENDRITES

Dendrites receive incoming action potentials from other neurons and pass them on to the soma (cell body) (Figure 1-31). Dendrites are short projections of the cell membrane and contain cytoplasm. The action potential the dendrite receives can only travel toward the soma of the neuron. Each cell body has many short dendrites, which allows one neuron to communicate with several other neurons simultaneously.

The soma, or cell body, of the neuron contains cytoplasm, the neuron's organelles, and the neuron's nucleus. It is the site of most cell functions that keep the neurons alive and functioning normally. These functions include providing energy for the neuron and breaking down the neuron's waste. In some cases, the soma is also able to directly receive action potentials from other neurons (Figure 1-31). When this occurs, incoming action potentials can communicate directly with the soma and do not have to pass through a dendrite.

LEARNING OBJECTIVE 1.4.4 Explain the function of axons in a nerve cell.

KEY TERMS

oligodendrocytes Specialized neuroglial cells that myelinate the axons of neurons in the brain and spinal cord.

Schwann cells Specialized neuroglial cells that myelinate neurons outside of the brain and spinal cord.

axon bulbs End of the axon where neurotransmitters are released.

FUNCTION OF THE AXON

An axon is a single extension of the cell membrane and contains cytoplasm and organelles. Each neuron has a single axon. The axon conducts action potentials away from the soma to the dendrite or soma of the next neuron. Axons are longer than dendrites (in some cases extending 6 feet!). At the end of the axon, where branching often occurs, there are many small extensions called axon bulbs (see Figure 1-31). It is within these bulbs that neurotransmitters are released. These neurotransmitters send the action potential on to another neuron. The branching at the end of the axon enables one neuron to signal many other neurons simultaneously.

Many axons in the body are surrounded by a myelin sheath. The myelin sheath is an insulating layer that is made out of a fatty substance. It protects and insulates the axon as well as increases the speed of the action potential by thousands of times. Small gaps in the myelin sheath along the neuron's axon are called nodes of Ranvier. These nodes, combined with areas of the myelin sheath, encourage the action potential to travel faster along the axon. This is because the action potential can jump between sections of the myelinated axon from node of Ranvier to node of Ranvier. This jumping prevents the action potential from having to travel down the entire length of the axon (Figure 1-31).

Neuroglial cells produce myelin. In the brain and spinal cord, specialized neuroglial cells called **oligodendrocytes** myelinate the axons. In these axons, oligodendrocytes myelinate neurons and there are no nodes of Ranvier. This is because the distance that the action potential must travel is very short, so the action potential reaches the target quickly, without the need for nodes of Ranvier. Outside of the brain and spinal cord, specialized neuroglial cells called **Schwann cells** myelinate axons. Because the axon may be several feet long, there is a need for action potentials to be able to travel very quickly. In these neurons, the Schwann cells myelinate nerves and nodes of Ranvier are present.

LEARNING OBJECTIVE 1.4.5 **Explain the general functions of nervous tissue.**

KEY TERMS

cerebrospinal fluid Fluid produced in the lateral ventricles of the brain that surrounds the brain and spinal cord to protect and remove waste products.

conduct Ability of nerves to transmit impulses.

stimulated Ability to respond to a stimulus and change it into an impulse.

FUNCTIONS OF NERVOUS TISSUE

The characteristic functions of nervous tissue are its ability to be **stimulated** (receive impulses) and its ability to **conduct** (pass impulses on). The main purpose of the neuron is to receive messages and pass them along to the next appropriate neuron or target tissue of the body. When the cell body or dendrite of a neuron receives an action potential, its cell membrane becomes stimulated and this triggers the neuron to conduct an action potential down its axon. Recall that nervous tissue is composed of both neurons and neuroglial cells. Neuroglial cells make up the majority of brain and spinal cord tissue. Neuroglial cells have many important functions, such as:

- Myelinating of axons
- Forming a barrier between the blood and the neurons
- Producing **cerebrospinal fluid**
- Removing foreign substances in the tissue.

Chapter 2

The Integumentary System

Chapter Introduction

The integument, or skin, is the body's largest organ. It is the first line of defense against pathogens, chemicals, and pollutants. It plays a crucial role in protection from ultraviolet radiation and production of vitamin D. It undergoes much abuse yet remains pliable and tough. Changes in skin color, texture, or growth may reflect systemic infections or disease.

UNIT OBJECTIVE 2.1

Identify the layers of the integument.

UNIT INTRODUCTION

In order to fulfill its role in the body, integument is composed of different structures and layers. Each layer is composed of different tissues and contains structures, such as nails, hair, and glands that support the many functions of integument.

LEARNING OBJECTIVE 2.1.1 Identify the epidermis, dermis, and hypodermis.

LEARNING OBJECTIVE 2.1.2 Describe the structure of the epidermis, dermis, and hypodermis.

KEY TERMS

dermis Deepest layer of skin that is composed of irregular connective tissue.

epidermis Superficial layer of skin that covers the dermis; composed of stratified squamous epithelium.

hypodermis Layer of loose areolar connective tissue below the layer of dermis, mainly adipose tissue, that connects skin to muscle and bone.

integumentary Skin and its accessory organs.

subcutaneous tissue Same tissue as the hypodermis.

THE INTEGUMENTARY SYSTEM

The **integumentary** system, also called the integument, consists of the skin and its accessory structures (nails, hair, and sweat and oil glands). It acts as a barrier between the body and the external environment (Figure 2-1). It has many functions, which include the following:

1. *Protection*: The skin protects against microorganism invasion, water loss, abrasion and other mechanical damage, and ultraviolet light.
2. *Temperature regulation*: Sweat glands located in the skin, along with the amount of blood flow to capillaries in the skin, help regulate body temperature.
3. *Vitamin D production*: Several proteins are manufactured in the skin and when exposed to ultraviolet light, a molecule is made that can become vitamin D.
4. *Sensation*: Many sensory receptors are located in the skin that detect touch, pressure, pain, heat, and cold.
5. *Excretion*: Sweat glands excrete small amounts of waste products in sweat. These secretions are acidic and help prevent bacterial growth on the skin.

Skin is a vital organ that helps prevent the loss of heat, water, and molecules from the body. It also acts as a barrier that prevents water, other chemicals, and microorganisms from entering the body. Structurally the skin is tough, yet pliable, and is composed of two kinds of tissue layers (Figure 2-1).

- The outermost layer is the **epidermis**. It is made of epithelial tissue.
- The epidermis rests on the **dermis**, which is made of irregular connective tissue.

The skin rests on the **hypodermis**, a **subcutaneous tissue** that is a loose connective tissue. It is primarily composed of adipose. Although the hypodermis is not considered a layer of the skin, it does help to anchor, insulate, and protect the two skin layers above it.

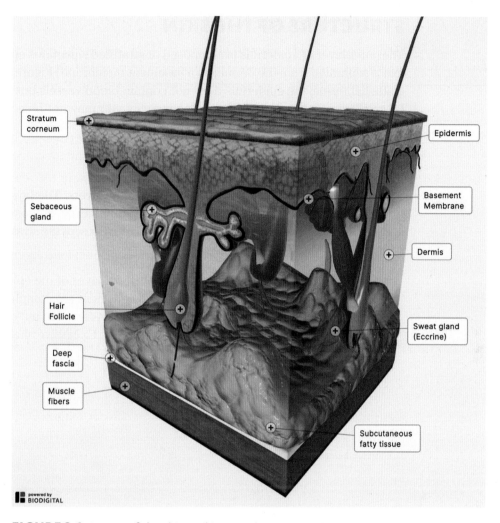

FIGURE 2-1 Layers of the skin and its accessory structures.

LEARNING OBJECTIVE 2.1.3 Identify the layers of the epidermis and dermis.

KEY TERMS

dermal papillae Projections of the dermis that push upward into the epidermis; increase surface area and allow for more diffusion of nutrients and oxygen into the epidermal cells.

sebaceous glands Exocrine gland located in the skin that produces sebum, or oil; usually associated with hair follicles.

stratum basale Also called the stratum germanitivum; deepest layer of the epidermis.

stratum corneum The outer dead layer of the skin.

stratum granulosum Layer in the epidermis filled with keratin granules.

stratum lucidum Translucent layer of epidermis between the stratum granulosum and stratum corneum; only present in thick skin.

stratum spinosum Layer of epidermis above the stratum basale.

STRUCTURE OF THE SKIN

The outer layer of epidermis is composed of stratified squamous epithelial cells and is separated from the dermis by a basement membrane (Figure 2-2). Like all epithelial tissue, the epidermis does not contain blood vessels but is nourished by capillaries in the dermis. This explains why you may not bleed even if you get a superficial scratch.

Layers of the Epidermis

The epidermis is composed of up to five strata, or layers. The layers, from the innermost to the outermost layers, are the stratum basale, spinosum, granulosum, lucidum, and corneum (Figure 2-2 for all layers except the stratum lucidum, which is only found in thick skin).

- **Stratum corneum.** The most superficial layer of the epidermis, it is the thickest layer, and the dead cells here are completely filled with keratin. The cells in this layer are referred to as "cornfield" or "horny" cells and slough off continually. Excessive shedding of this layer is called dandruff.

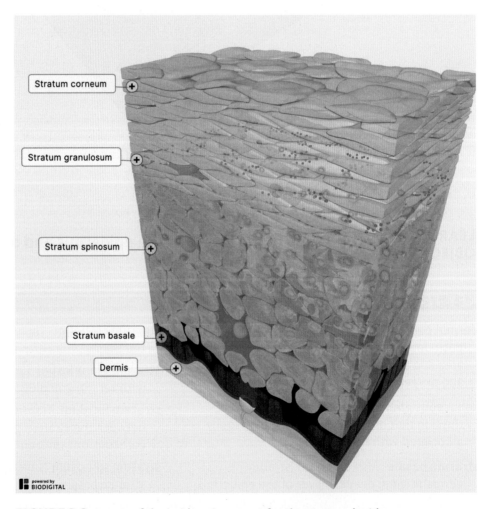

FIGURE 2-2 Layers of the epidermis, except for the stratum lucidum.

- **Stratum lucidum.** As the dead cells leave the stratum granulosum, they form the transparent stratum lucidum. This layer is only present in hairless, thick skin, which is found on the palms of the hands and soles of the feet.
- **Stratum granulosum.** The next layer up is the stratum granulosum. In this layer, the cell organelles, including the nucleus, degenerate, which causes the cells to die.
- **Stratum spinosum.** As the new epidermal cells move up, they become part of the stratum spinosum. A limited amount of cell division occurs here.
- **Stratum basale.** The deepest cell layer, it is also called the stratum germinativum. The stratum basale sits on the basement membrane and is the most nourished layer of the epidermis because it is closest to the blood vessels in the dermis. Some of the stem cells here are constantly dividing to become epidermal cells while others maintain the population of stem cells.

Layers of the Dermis

The second layer of the skin is called the dermis. The connective tissue that comprises the dermis contains nerve endings, smooth muscles, hair follicles, lymphatic vessels, sebaceous (oil) glands, sweat glands, and blood vessels (Figure 2-1). The dermis is divided into two regions called the papillary layer and the reticular layer.

- The upper papillary layer gets its name from the dermal papillae, which are upward projections toward the epidermis. These unique projections form fingerprints and increase friction, which enhances the gripping ability of the hands and feet.
- The second layer, the reticular layer, is the main layer of the dermis. It is composed primarily of collagen and elastic fibers, which make it resistant to stretching in many directions. The blood vessels in the dermis help regulate body temperature. When body temperature is too high, the capillaries here become engorged with blood and the skin turns red and hot. This allows body heat to escape from the skin.

UNIT OBJECTIVE 2.2

Identify the roles and functions of keratin and melanin in the integument.

UNIT INTRODUCTION

The proteins keratin and melanin play an important role in the integumentary system. Epithelial cells called keratinocytes produce keratin. Its function is to make the outermost layer of the skin a protective barrier for the body. It makes the cells tough and waterproof. Melanin is a protein pigment produced by melanocytes that determines skin, eye, and hair color. It protects us from the sun's ultraviolet light by absorbing it.

LEARNING OBJECTIVE 2.2.1 Explain the roles and function of melanin.

LEARNING OBJECTIVE 2.2.2 Identify the cells that secrete melanin.

KEY TERMS

melanin Pigments ranging from yellow to black that are found in the retina, skin, and hair.

melanocytes Cells found in the stratum basale that produces melanin.

melasma Dark spots that form on the face during pregnancy due to hormonal fluctuations.

MELANIN

Melanocytes, found in the stratum basale, produce a group of pigments called melanin. Melanin ranges in color from yellow to brown to black. Melanin is responsible for skin, eye, and hair color and protects us from the sun's ultraviolet light. Certain areas of the body contain more melanin, such as the nipples and areolae of the breasts, the axillae, and genitalia. Other structures, such as freckles and moles, also contain more melanin. Other parts of the body contain less melanin, such as the lips, palms of the hands, and soles of the feet. Melanin production is controlled by the following:

- Genetics: Many different genes determine the amount and type of melanin an individual produces.
- Exposure to light: Ultraviolet light from the sun stimulates the production of melanin. This results in what we call a "tan."
- Hormones: An increase in hormones can stimulate the production of more melanin. This is common during pregnancy when surges in hormones may produce dark spots on the face known as melasma.

All races have about the same number of melanocytes. The variations we see in skin color are determined by the color and amount of melanin that the melanocytes produce.

LEARNING OBJECTIVE 2.2.3 Explain the roles and function of keratin.

LEARNING OBJECTIVE 2.2.4 Identify the cells that secrete keratin.

KERATIN

The deepest layer of the epidermis, the stratum basale (Figure 2-2), has stem cells that continually produce new epithelial cells. As new cells form, they push old cells to the surface where they are sloughed off. As the cells move toward the surface, they fill with keratin. The cells that produce this keratin are called keratinocytes (Figure 2-2). This process is called keratinization.

The shape and chemical composition of keratinocytes continually change. During keratinization, these cells die and produce an outer layer of hard, dead cells that form the protective barrier of the epidermis. Keratin is the protein substance that makes the epidermis tough and waterproof.

UNIT OBJECTIVE 2.3

Identify the accessory structures of the integument.

UNIT INTRODUCTION

The Integumentary system contains the body's largest organ, our skin. Our skin contains many accessory structures that serve a variety of purposes. These accessory structures include nerve endings, blood vessels, sweat glands, sebaceous glands, hair follicles, and nails. All of these structures work together to make up the integumentary system.

LEARNING OBJECTIVE 2.3.1 Identify hair follicles in the skin.

HAIR FOLLICLES IN THE SKIN

Hair is an epithelial structure that forms from stratum basale epithelial cells that make up the hair follicle (Figure 2-1). Just like skin, hair forms as new cells develop and push older cells to the surface. Older cells become keratinized and die. Thus, the majority of the hair shaft is dead keratinocytes (Figure 2-1).

Describe factors affecting hair growth.

FACTORS AFFECTING HAIR GROWTH

Hair is found everywhere on the body except the lips, nipples, palms of the hands, and soles of the feet. Humans do not have the ability to form new hair follicles as they grow—they are born with the number of hair follicles that they will have for their entire lives. The main factors affecting hair growth are the following:

- Hormones: After puberty, male hormones stimulate increased hair growth on the face and body. Women produce a smaller amount of these hormones and generally have less hair growth on the face and body.
- Genetics: Some people are genetically predisposed to growing more or less hair.
- Age: As humans age, hair gets thinner and hair growth rates get slower. The amount of hair an individual has and the rate at which hair grows may vary widely from person to person.

LEARNING OBJECTIVE 2.3.3 **Identify factors affecting hair color and texture.**

FACTORS AFFECTING HAIR COLOR AND TEXTURE

Hair color is determined by varying amounts of different types of melanin. Melanin pigment may be yellow, brown, black, or rust colored. These pigments combine to form all of the varieties of human hair color. A lack of melanin production results in white hair, as seen in individuals with albinism. Gray or white hair also results when pigment production stops due to the death of melanocytes. This occurs naturally as we age.

Hair also comes in different shapes and lengths. Humans have short hair in the eyebrows and longer hair on their heads. When the hair shaft shape is round, the hair is straight and usually coarse. When the hair shaft shape is oval, hair is wavy and smooth. When the hair shaft shape is flat, the hair is curly.

LEARNING OBJECTIVE 2.3.4 **Describe the structure of hair follicles and nails.**

KEY TERMS

cuticle Edge of the skinfold covering the proximal nail.

external epithelial root sheath External layer of the epithelial root sheath.

free edge Distal end of the nail that appears white.

hair bulb Swelling at the base where the hair originates in the dermis.

internal epithelial root sheath Internal layer of the epithelial root sheath; surrounds the hair but does not extend the length of the hair follicle.

lunula Whitish area at the proximal end of the nail.

nail bed Layer of living epidermis below the nail body.

nail body Part of the nail we see.

root Found at the proximal end of the nail.

STRUCTURE OF HAIR FOLLICLES AND NAILS

Hair follicles contain an inner and an external epithelial root sheath (Figure 2-1).

- The **inner epithelial root sheath** is made of epithelial tissue and forms the hair.
- The **external epithelial root sheath** is composed of dermal connective tissue and supplies the **hair bulb** with a nearby blood supply for nutrients.

Hair follicles have a small muscle (arrector pili) that anchors it to the nearby dermal tissue (Figure 2-1). The arrector pili are stimulated by cold temperatures and emotions, such as fear. When these small muscles contract, the hair is elevated and pulled straight. This may also cause raised bumps, known commonly as "goose bumps," to appear on the surface of the skin.

The nails are modified, highly keratinized epidermis. Each nail has a **free edge**, a **nail body**, and a **root** (Figure 2-3). The edge of the skinfold covering the proximal end of the nail is called the eponychium (or **cuticle**). The stratum basale of the epidermis extends under the nail body and makes up the **nail bed** (Figure 2-3). The cells of the nail bed form new nail cells. The **lunula** is a semilunar, white area found at the proximal end of the nail. It is formed as a result of air mixed with keratin in the cells of the nail bed. The nails appear pink due to the dense concentration of blood vessels in the underlying dermis.

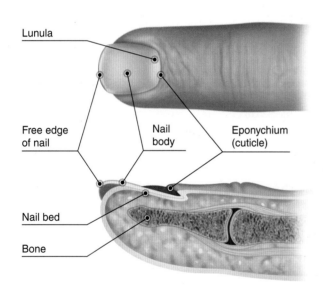

FIGURE 2-3 Anatomy of a nail.

Lunula

Free edge of nail

Nail body

Eponychium (cuticle)

Nail bed

Bone

CLINICAL TIP Nails can reflect how well oxygenated a patient is. When a person's oxygen levels are adequate, nails will appear pink in color. When a person's oxygen levels are low, their nail beds may appear blue.

UNIT OBJECTIVE 2.4

Describe the glands of the integument.

UNIT INTRODUCTION

In addition to the many accessory structures previously discussed, the integumentary system also contains glands that help moisten the body, protect the body, and aid in thermoregulation. These glands are sudoriferous glands and sebaceous glands. Sudoriferous glands are also known as sweat glands and function as protection and thermoregulation. Sebaceous glands are also called oil glands and function to moisten and protect the skin.

LEARNING OBJECTIVE 2.4.1 Identify sudoriferous glands.

LEARNING OBJECTIVE 2.4.2 Explain the role of sudoriferous glands.

KEY TERMS

apocrine Type of sweat gland found only in the axillary and genital areas that does not function until puberty; also secretes proteins and fatty acids.

eccrine Type of sweat gland that is more common than apocrine sweat glands and found everywhere on the body; the sweat that they secrete plays an important role in preventing bacterial growth and thermoregulation.

sudoriferous glands Also called sweat glands; eccrine and apocrine are the two types.

thermoregulation Regulation of body temperature.

STRUCTURE AND FUNCTION OF SUDORIFEROUS GLANDS

Sudoriferous glands, more commonly known as sweat glands (Figure 2-1), are distributed throughout the skin. There are two types of sweat glands in the human body:

- Eccrine sweat glands: Common and found everywhere on the body, the sweat that they secrete plays an important role in thermoregulation. Sweat from eccrine sweat glands is a secretion containing water, salts, traces of metabolic wastes (urea, ammonia, uric acid), and lactic acid. It is acidic (pH from 4 to 6), which helps protect the skin from pathogens.

- Apocrine sweat glands: Found in the axillary and genital areas of the body, they are larger sweat glands that have ducts that empty into hair follicles (Figure 2-1). Secretions from apocrine sweat glands include all the substances found in the sweat secreted by eccrine glands, but they also contain proteins and fatty acids. Apocrine glands do not function until puberty and play a minimal role in thermoregulation. Hormones, stress, and sexual arousal.

CLINICAL TIP	To help you remember the different locations of eccrine and apocrine sweat glands, think of it this way: eccrine = everywhere and apocrine = axillary. The first letter for each sweat gland matches where it is found in the body.

LEARNING OBJECTIVE 2.4.3 Identify sebaceous glands.

LEARNING OBJECTIVE 2.4.4 Explain the role of sebaceous glands.

KEY TERMS

sebaceous glands Exocrine gland located in the skin that produces sebum, or oil; usually associated with hair follicles.

sebum Oily substance secreted by sebaceous glands that helps keep the skin soft and moist and prevents the hair from becoming too brittle.

STRUCTURE AND FUNCTION OF SEBACEOUS GLANDS

Sebaceous glands, also called oil glands, are found everywhere in the skin except on the palms of the hands and soles of the feet. They secrete an oily substance called sebum that usually empties into a hair follicle (Figure 2-1). Sebum has several functions:

- Helps keep the skin soft and moist and prevents hair from becoming too brittle.
- Contains chemicals that kill bacteria that helps protect the skin. Bacteria are always present on the skin, but sebum and sweat both prevent the overgrowth of these bacteria.

Sebaceous glands become more active during puberty when some hormone levels are higher than normal. This increase in hormones results in an increase in sebum production. In some individuals, the hair follicles where the sebum exits on to the skin can become blocked and infected. This results in the skin condition known as acne. Acne is discussed in greater detail later in this chapter.

LEARNING OBJECTIVE 2.4.5 Identify ceruminous glands.

LEARNING OBJECTIVE 2.4.6 Explain the role of ceruminous glands.

KEY TERMS

cerumen Also called ear wax, secreted by ceruminous glands in the external ear canal and helps protect the skin there.

ceruminous glands Found in the skin that lines the external ear canal; modified apocrine sweat glands that produce a substance called cerumen, also known as earwax.

STRUCTURE AND FUNCTION OF CERUMINOUS GLANDS

Ceruminous glands are found in the skin that lines the external ear canal. These are modified apocrine sweat glands that produce a substance called cerumen, also known as earwax. Cerumen contains numerous chemicals that kill bacteria and that help protect the external ear canal from pathogens and physical damage.

LEARNING OBJECTIVE 2.4.7 Identify mammary glands.

LEARNING OBJECTIVE 2.4.8 Explain the role of mammary glands.

KEY TERM

Mammary glands Enlarged, modified sweat glands found in the breasts of females.

STRUCTURE AND FUNCTION OF MAMMARY GLANDS

Mammary glands are enlarged, modified sweat glands found in the breasts of females (Figure 2-4). These glands are surrounded by connective tissue and fat, which comprise the rest of the breasts. In females, the mammary glandular tissue develops during puberty in response to high levels of estrogen. During pregnancy and childbirth, additional hormones trigger the production and release of milk. Males also have mammary glandular tissue; however, the tissue never fully develops and therefore cannot function as it does in the female.

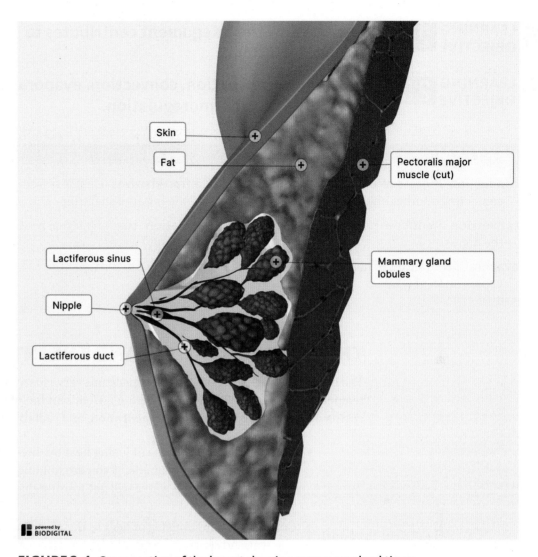

FIGURE 2-4 Cross section of the breast showing mammary gland tissue.

UNIT OBJECTIVE 2.5

Identify the role of the integument in maintaining homeostasis and associated pathologies.

UNIT INTRODUCTION

The integumentary system's main function is to act as a protective barrier for your body. It helps maintain homeostasis by preventing pathogens and other foreign chemicals from entering your body. It also helps maintain normal body temperature. There are many pathologies associated with altered function of the integumentary system. Having a detailed understanding of how the integument contributes to thermoregulation will help you better understand how to care for patients with integument-altering conditions.

LEARNING OBJECTIVE 2.5.1 Describe how the integument contributes to thermoregulation.

LEARNING OBJECTIVE 2.5.2 Explain how conduction, convection, evaporation, and radiation affect thermoregulation.

KEY TERMS

conduction Process of losing heat by directly contacting another object.

convection Transfer of heat to the air surrounding the body.

evaporation Transfer of heat through the vaporization of water.

infrared waves Heat loss from radiating heat in the infrared spectrum.

radiation Loss of internal heat by infrared (or energy) waves.

THERMOREGULATION AND THE INTEGUMENT

The body must regulate core body temperature very closely. Normal core body temperature is 36.5−37.5°C (97.7−99.5°F). Heat can be lost through the processes of conduction, convection, evaporation, and radiation.

- Conduction. The process of losing heat by directly contacting another object. For example, if you are holding a glass of ice water, eventually the water will get warmer due to the heat from your hands.
- Convection. The transfer of heat to the air surrounding the body. The warmed air rises and cooler air moves in to take its place. This also occurs in water.
- Evaporation. The transfer of heat through the vaporization of water. Eccrine sweat glands play an important role in this process. They have nerve endings that trigger them to secrete sweat onto the surface of the skin when the external temperature or body temperature is too high. This sweat evaporates off the skin surface, taking heat with it.
- Radiation. The loss of internal heat by infrared (or energy) waves. When the body temperature is too high, blood vessels in the skin dilate. This flushes capillaries with warm blood. The capillaries are close to the surface of the skin, so this causes heat loss via radiation. The heat radiates from the surface of the skin.

When exercising, most excess heat is lost by evaporation; otherwise, the body gets rid of most excess heat through the process of radiation.

LEARNING OBJECTIVE 2.5.3 Identify the role of the integument in protection.

HOW THE INTEGUMENT PROTECTS YOU

The integumentary system's main function is to act as a protective barrier for the body. The skin is our largest organ and is your immune system's first line of defense. It is tough, yet flexible, and is mostly impenetrable. The integumentary system helps your body:

- Retain fluids and prevent dehydration
- Eliminate waste products (think back to our discussion of what is contained in sweat)
- Regulate body temperature to maintain homeostasis
- Protect body from pathogens, like bacteria, viruses, and fungi

LEARNING OBJECTIVE 2.5.4 Give examples of molecules that can and cannot pass through the skin.

KEY TERMS

lipid soluble Dissolves in lipids.   **water soluble** Dissolves in water.

MOLECULES THAT DO AND DO NOT PASS THROUGH SKIN

Although the skin is relatively impenetrable, there are some molecules that can pass through it. For example, absorption through the skin is one route that some medications can use to enter the body. Whether a molecule will be absorbed through the skin depends on several factors:

- Concentration of the molecule: The higher concentration there is of a molecule, the more likely it will be absorbed into the skin.
- Duration of contact: The longer the skin comes in contact with a molecule, the more likely it is to be absorbed.
- Molecule size: If the molecule is small enough, it will fit between the skin cells and gain entry.
- Solubility: Another factor is whether the substance is water soluble (dissolves in water) or lipid soluble (dissolves in lipids). Recall that cell membranes are composed of lipids and that water and lipids repel each other. If the substance dissolves in water, and if that water comes in contact with the lipid bilayer of a cell membrane, then that substance will be repelled. However, if the substance dissolves in lipids and it comes in contact with the lipid bilayer of a cell membrane, it will pass through to the inside of the cell.

UNIT OBJECTIVE 2.6

Describe pathologies affecting keratin and melanin.

UNIT INTRODUCTION

As previously mentioned, keratin and melanin serve very important roles in maintaining homeostasis. If they are not functioning normally in the integumentary system, several pathologies may result. Understanding the relationship between normal and altered keratin and melanin functioning will help you better understand and care for patients with related pathologies.

LEARNING OBJECTIVE 2.6.1 Identify common pathologies affecting keratin and melanin.

LEARNING OBJECTIVE 2.6.2 Explain common pathologies affecting keratin and melanin.

KEY TERMS

asymptomatic Showing no signs or symptoms.

autoimmune disease Disease caused by your immune system mistakenly attacking your own body.

hives Also called urticaria, red, round, itchy welts on the skin usually in response to an allergic reaction.

impetigo Highly contagious bacterial skin infection that forms blisters and yellow, crusty sores.

psoriasis Skin disease characterized by shiny, silver or red patches.

urticaria Also called hives, red, round, itchy welts on the skin usually in response to an allergic reaction.

vitiligo Skin condition in which a loss of pigment occurs in areas of skin or hair that result in white patches.

COMMON PATHOLOGIES AFFECTING KERATIN AND MELANIN

The skin is the first thing a health care provider sees when meeting a patient. It should always be part of a patient's initial examination. There are several common skin pathologies that you'll likely encounter when you begin your career in the health care field, including impetigo, urticaria (commonly called hives), psoriasis, vitiligo, and albinism.

- Impetigo. A highly contagious bacterial infection of the skin characterized by a red rash with fluid-filled blisters that erupt easily and form a yellow crust (Figure 2-5). It is common in children and is usually found on the face, arms, and legs.

- Urticaria (hives). Raised, itchy welts on the skin (Figure 2-6). They are common after exposure to an allergen; however, if they are chronic (lasting more than 6 weeks), they may also be a sign of an endocrine condition, infection, or cancer.

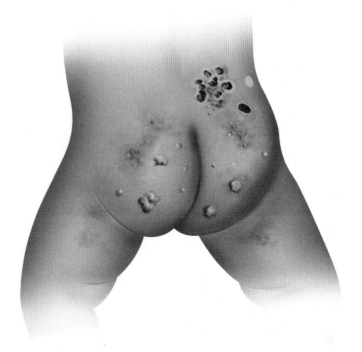

FIGURE 2-5 Impetigo's characteristic red rash and yellowish crust that forms after blisters burst.

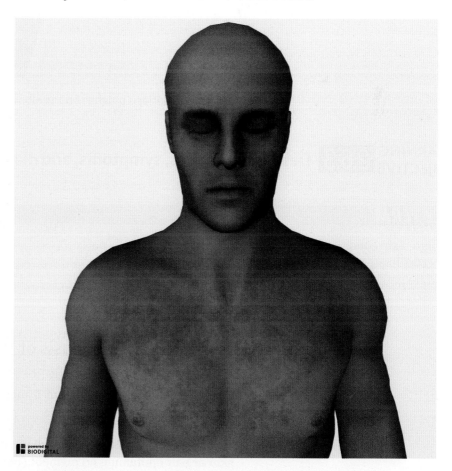

FIGURE 2-6 Digital rendering of urticaria (hives) on the chest.

- Psoriasis. A chronic skin disorder characterized by scaly, silver or red, sharply defined patches (Figure 2-7). Psoriasis is considered an **autoimmune disease**. It is commonly located on the scalp, elbows, knees, and back. It may be itchy or **asymptomatic**.

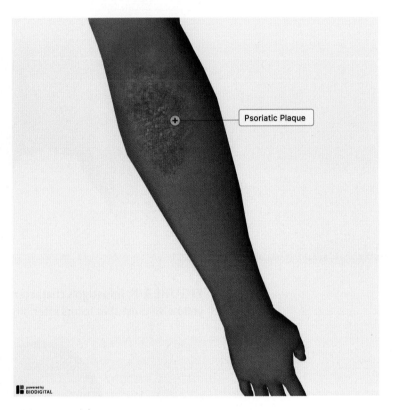

Psoriatic Plaque

FIGURE 2-7 Psoriasis patches on the elbows.

LEARNING OBJECTIVE **2.6.3** Describe the signs, symptoms, and diagnosis of vitiligo.

KEY TERM

vitiligo Skin condition in which a loss of pigment occurs in areas of skin or hair that results in white patches.

Signs, Symptoms, and Diagnosis of Vitiligo

Vitiligo is a skin condition caused by a lack of melanin production or the death of melanocytes. It can start at any age, but it most commonly appears before the age of 20.

- Signs and symptoms: Vitiligo is characterized by white patches of skin or hair containing no pigment (Figure 2-8). It is commonly found on the face, hands, arms, and feet, but it may appear anywhere on the body. It is not contagious or harmful, and the rate at which it may spread is unpredictable. It affects all races equally, but it is more noticeable in individuals with darker skin.

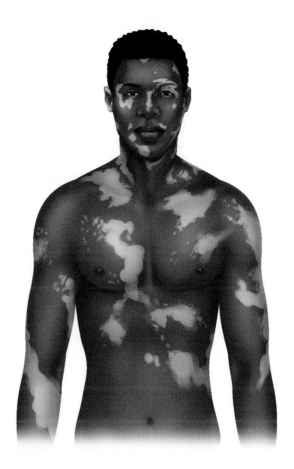

FIGURE 2-8 Vitiligo in an individual with dark skin.

- Diagnosis: Diagnosis of vitiligo may involve a variety of tests. Diagnosis typically begins with a thorough physical examination of the patient and exploration of the patient's medical history and the medical history of the patient's family. This is done to determine whether the patient has a history of skin trauma where the vitiligo has occurred or a history of autoimmune disease in the patient and his or her family. The health care provider will also explore if any members of the patient's family have vitiligo. The patient may also undergo examination and blood tests to rule out other conditions, such as dermatitis or psoriasis. Diagnosis may also include taking a small biopsy of the affected area.

LEARNING OBJECTIVE 2.6.4 Describe the signs, symptoms, and diagnosis of albinism.

Signs, Symptoms, and Diagnosis of Albinism

Albinism is a group of genetic disorders in which a person has little to no production of melanin.

- Signs and symptoms: The most recognizable form of albinism results in white hair and very pale skin (Figure 2-9). Skin and hair color may range from white to brown. Some people may develop moles (with or without pigmentation) and freckles when exposed to sunlight. People with albinism are at an increased risk of getting skin cancer. In addition to influencing color of skin, hair, and eyes, melanin also plays a role in the formation of the optic nerve. This means that people with this disorder often have vision problems as well. Eye color ranges from very light blue to brown. Interestingly, melanin production may change over one's lifetime and begin or increase during childhood.

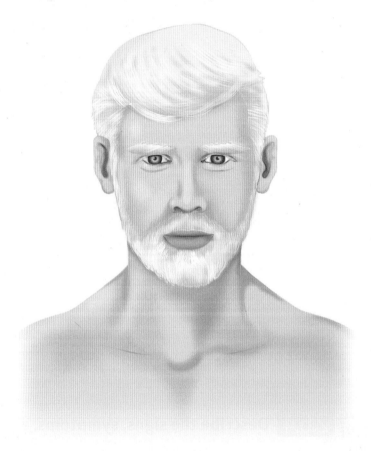

FIGURE 2-9 An individual with albinism.

- Diagnosis: Diagnosis is based on the patient's medical history and a physical examination that includes checking pigmentation of the skin and hair. Diagnosis may also include an eye examination with an eye specialist (ophthalmologist) to rule out other eye conditions that may be causing visual disturbances. Comparison of a child's pigmentation to other family members is also an important part of the diagnostic process.

LEARNING OBJECTIVE 2.6.5 Describe the signs, symptoms, and diagnosis of epidermolysis bullosa.

KEY TERM

epidermolysis bullosa Rare genetic disorder that causes the skin to become loose and very thin, forming large red areas that blister and peel away.

Epidermolysis Bullosa

Epidermolysis bullosa is a group of rare inherited diseases that cause extremely fragile skin that blisters easily (Figure 2-10). Blisters may form in response to rubbing, scratching, or heat. They may form inside the mouth and other internal areas, like the stomach. Most forms of epidermolysis bullosa are inherited and begin to present in infancy or early childhood.

- Signs and symptoms: Patients with this condition may have the following signs and symptoms:
    - Fragile skin that blisters easily
    - Thick nails or nails that do not form
    - Itchy, painful skin
    - Skin that appears thin
    - Blistering and scarring of the scalp
    - Hair loss
    - Blisters inside the mouth and throat
    - Difficulty swallowing
    - Thickened skin on the palms and soles of the feet
    - Dental problems

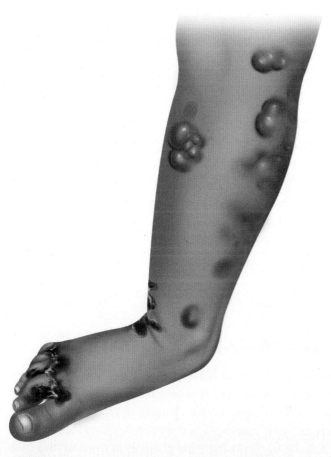

FIGURE 2-10 Epidermolysis bullosa on the leg of an infant.

- Diagnosis: Diagnosing the condition involves a variety of laboratory tests and may depend on when the disorder begins to present. In pregnant patients who have a family history of the condition, prenatal genetic testing and counseling may be performed. Infants, children, and adults who are suspected of having the condition may also undergo genetic testing, which involves taking a small blood sample. A skin biopsy may also be taken to determine the layers of skin that are impacted by the condition.

UNIT OBJECTIVE 2.7

Describe pathologies related to the integumentary system's accessory structures.

UNIT INTRODUCTION

The many accessory structures of the integumentary system play an important role in maintaining homeostasis. If they are not functioning properly, signs and symptoms of pathologies may be observed not only on the skin, but also in an individual's hair and nails.

LEARNING OBJECTIVE 2.7.1 Identify pathologies of the hair and nails.

KEY TERMS

alopecia Partial or complete loss of hair from parts of the body that would normally have hair; male and female pattern baldness is an example.

Beau's lines Horizontal grooves across the nails caused by a temporary disruption in nail growth from things such as illness, malnutrition, or chemotherapy.

dandruff Small pieces or flakes of dead skin on the scalp or in the hair.

folliculitis Inflammation of the hair follicles from something like a bacterial infection.

seborrheic dermatitis Common skin condition that forms round, red, scaly patches and dandruff in areas where there are many sebaceous glands like the face, scalp, nose, and back.

spoon nails Nail disease resulting in spoon-shaped nails that look scooped out; usually caused by iron-deficiency anemia.

yellow nail syndrome Rare medical syndrome caused by the underdevelopment of lymphatic vessels, respiratory disease, and possibly titanium exposure; nails stop growing and appear yellowish-green.

PATHOLOGIES OF THE HAIR AND NAILS

When recording a routine patient medical history, it is important to note any changes they may have experienced in their hair and nails, as these structures may easily show symptoms of underlying disease. During physical examination, the hair and nails are easily accessible and commonly show observable changes in the patient's overall health status. Knowing what changes in the hair and nails indicate about the body's functions will help you better assist the health care team.

Pathologies of the Hair and Scalp

Pathologies of the hair and scalp include hair shedding, alopecia, dandruff, seborrheic dermatitis, and folliculitis.

- Hair shedding. The loss of large amounts of hair. It is usually temporary and may occur due to sudden weight loss, iron deficiency, fever, or stress.
- Alopecia. The partial or complete absence of hair from areas of the body where it normally grows. It is most commonly the result of male and female pattern baldness, but it can also be due to an autoimmune disease. Alopecia areata is an autoimmune disease where the person's immune system attacks and destroys hair follicles. It is most common in individuals with Down syndrome, diabetes, thyroid disease, or vitiligo.
- Dandruff. A scalp condition resulting in flakes of skin in the hair. It often causes the scalp to be itchy. It is not related to hygiene. Individuals with skin conditions such as psoriasis, eczema, or seborrheic dermatitis are more likely to have dandruff.
- Seborrheic dermatitis. A skin condition that causes red skin, scaly patches of dead skin, and dandruff (Figure 2-11). It is commonly found on the scalp, sides of the nose, ears, eyebrows, eyelids, and chest. In babies it is called cradle cap.

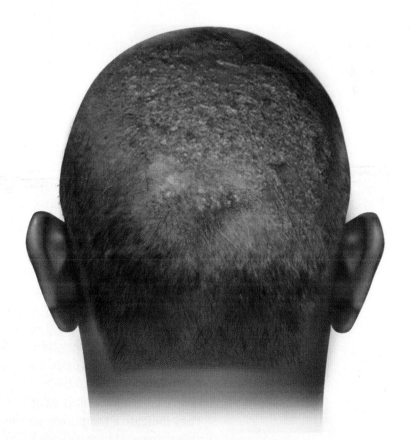

FIGURE 2-11 Seborrheic dermatitis of the scalp.

- Folliculitis. The inflammation of hair follicles that is usually the result of a bacterial or fungal infection. It may first appear as red bumps or whitehead pimples near the hair follicle (Figure 2-12). The infection can spread and turn into itchy, crusty sores. While it's not life-threatening, it can cause permanent hair loss and scarring.

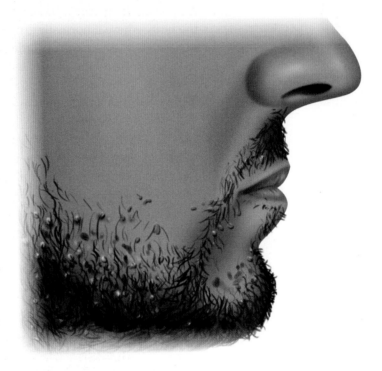

FIGURE 2-12 Folliculitis.

Pathologies of the Nails

Pathologies of the nails include yellow nail syndrome, spoon nails, and Beau's lines. Changes in the appearance, shape, or structure of the nails are clinically significant and may indicate underlying pathologies.

- Yellow nail syndrome: Occurs when nail growth slows or stops. The thickened nails appear yellow or green and may be an outward sign of respiratory disease or caused by hand swelling.
- Spoon nails: Appear as if they have been scooped out. In this condition, nails are very thin. This malformation is frequently an outward sign of iron deficiency, certain liver conditions, heart disease, or hypothyroidism.
- Beau's lines: Horizontal indentations that run across the nail. They indicate a temporary interference with nail growth. They may be caused by injury to the nail, severe illness, or zinc deficiency.

LEARNING OBJECTIVE 2.7.2 Describe the signs, symptoms, and diagnosis of congenital hypertrichosis.

congenital hypertrichosis Rare genetic disease resulting in hair growth that covers the entire body.

Congenital Hypertrichosis

Congenital hypertrichosis is a genetic disorder that results in excessive hair growth in patches or all over the body.

- Signs and symptoms: Patients with this condition have excessive hair growth at birth and may also have the following:
    - Excessive early childhood growth
    - Learning disabilities or attention-deficit disorder
    - Long, narrow face with a high forehead
    - Red cheeks
    - Pointed chin
- Diagnosis: Diagnosis is based on excessive hair growth at birth and genetic testing. The growth may regress during adolescence or increase throughout a patient's lifetime, depending on the form of congenital hypertrichosis a patient has.

LEARNING OBJECTIVE 2.7.3 Describe the signs, symptoms, and diagnosis of onychomycosis.

athlete's foot Fungal infection affecting the skin around the toes and toenails.

onychomycosis Fungal infection of the nail resulting in nail discoloration, thickening, and crumbling.

Onychomycosis

Onychomycosis is nail fungus (Figure 2-13). It may occur under the nails of the hands or feet. It is commonly called **athlete's foot** when it infects the skin around the toenails. It begins as a yellow or white spot under the nail and quickly spreads deeper. It is contagious and may infect several nails. Onychomycosis may lead to other serious infections if a patient has a suppressed immune system

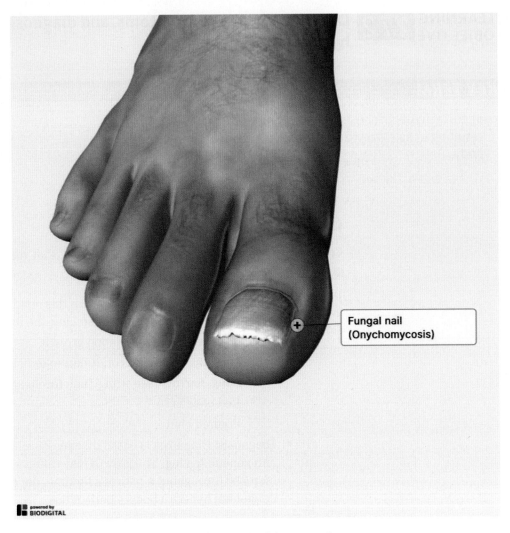

Fungal nail
(Onychomycosis)

powered by
BIODIGITAL

FIGURE 2-13 Onychomycosis (nail fungus) of the toe nails.

due to other medical conditions or in patients on certain medications. It may also be more severe in patients who have conditions that cause decreased blood flow to the feet, such as diabetes.

- Signs and symptoms:
    - ° Discoloration of the nail
    - ° Thickened nails that may crumble at the edge
    - ° Brittle, dry, crumbly nails
    - ° Distortion of nail shape
    - ° Slightly foul smell of infected area
- Diagnosis: Diagnosis involves a physical examination and possibly testing nail clippings or scrapings from under the infected nail in a laboratory. Yeast and bacteria can also infect nails, and psoriasis can mimic nail fungus.

LEARNING OBJECTIVE **2.7.4** **Describe the signs, symptoms, and diagnosis of pachyonychia congenita.**

KEY TERMS

follicular keratosis Skin condition caused by excessive production of keratin that results in blocked hair follicle openings and tiny, rough bumps on the skin.

pachyonychia congenita Rare genetic disorder that causes skin and nails to become thick and abnormally shaped.

Pachyonychia Congenita

Pachyonychia congenita is a rare genetic disorder that affects keratin production throughout the body. Depending on which genes are affected, the symptoms may vary from person to person. In some forms of the disease, a person has fingernails and toenails that become abnormally thick and abnormally shaped. However, when different keratin genes are affected, the person may experience patches on the tongue and inside the cheek.

- Signs and symptoms: As mentioned previously, exact signs and symptoms of the disease will vary based on the person's exact genetic mutation. Most often, patients experience abnormally thick and abnormally shaped nails. This condition may also result in the following:
    - Thick, white patches on the tongue and inside of the cheeks
    - Painful blisters and callouses on the soles of the feet or palms of the hands
    - Follicular keratosis around hair follicles
    - Cysts in the axillary region, groin, scalp, or back
    - Excessive sweating of palms of the hands and soles of the feet
    - Baby being born with teeth
    - Effects in the larynx, causing hoarseness or breathing difficulties
- Diagnosis: As with most conditions, physical examination is an important part of diagnosis. The health care provider will look for the signs and symptoms mentioned above and rule out other causes and conditions that may lead to similar symptoms. Taking a thorough patient and family medical history is important to determine if other members of the patient's family have the condition. Since this condition is caused by genetic mutations, diagnosis also involves genetic testing. Genetic testing may not

only confirm the presence of the condition, but also identify the exact genes affected. This can assist in management of the condition.

UNIT OBJECTIVE 2.8

Describe pathologies related to glands of the integumentary system.

UNIT INTRODUCTION

Recall that the integumentary system includes sweat glands and sebaceous glands. If these glands are not functioning properly, homeostasis is interrupted and an individual may suffer from one of the pathologies listed in Common Pathologies of the Integumentary Glands.

LEARNING OBJECTIVE 2.8.1 Identify common pathologies affecting glands of the integument.

KEY TERMS

bromhidrosis Condition of offensive body odor, usually associated with the breakdown of sweat from apocrine sweat gland secretion.

sebaceous hyperplasia Disorder characterized by enlarged sebaceous glands that appear as bumps on the face.

COMMON PATHOLOGIES OF THE INTEGUMENTARY GLANDS

The glands of the integument include sebaceous glands and sweat glands. Common disorders of the sebaceous glands include acne and **sebaceous hyperplasia**. The most common disorder of the sweat glands is **bromhidrosis**.

- Acne (Figure 2-14). A common chronic disorder that most commonly occurs in adolescence and young adulthood. It is discussed in more detail in Acne Vulgaris.
- Sebaceous hyperplasia. A common condition resulting in enlarged sebaceous glands on the forehead or cheeks. It occurs in middle-aged and older adults. It appears as small bumps under the skin and is benign.
- Bromhidrosis. The most common type of pathology associated with the sweat glands, this condition causes the breakdown of apocrine sweat by bacteria. It is a condition that causes abnormal body odor, which comes from the by-products of the bacteria.

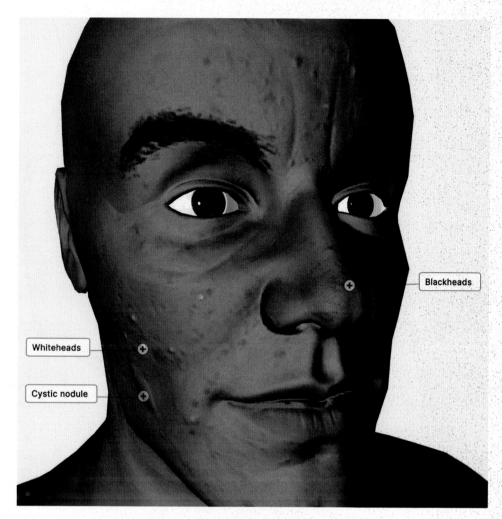

FIGURE 2-14 Digital depiction of the different stages of acne.

LEARNING OBJECTIVE 2.8.2 **Describe the signs, symptoms, and diagnosis of acne vulgaris.**

Acne Vulgaris

Acne vulgaris is a common condition that affects the hair follicles and sebaceous glands on the face, neck, chest, and back. It is caused by overproduction of oil that mixes with dead skin cells. The combination of dead cells and oil clogs skin pores and causes pores to become infected by bacteria. This results in inflammation and redness of the skin and the formation of pustules (Figure 2-15), blackheads (Figure 2-16), and whiteheads (Figure 2-17). Acne can scar the skin if not treated. It is most common during hormonal changes, such as during puberty, and in individuals with a genetic predisposition for the condition.

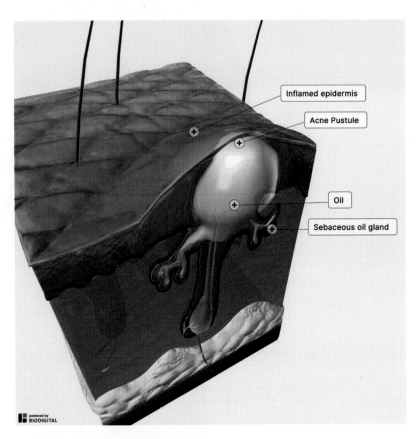

FIGURE 2-15 Acne pustule.

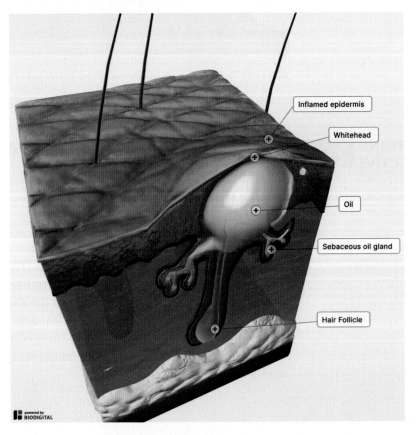

FIGURE 2-16 Acne whitehead.

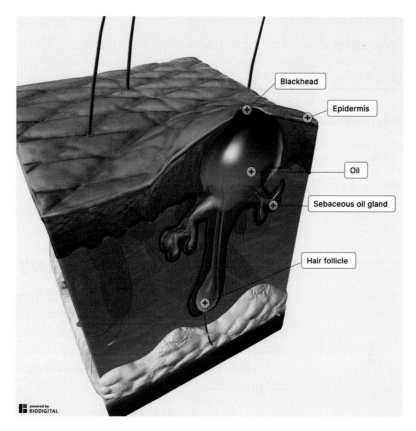

FIGURE 2-17 Acne blackhead.

UNIT OBJECTIVE 2.9

Describe the two major types of skin wounds and the steps of the healing process.

UNIT INTRODUCTION

Skin wounds and burns are common injuries that you will encounter when you begin your health care career. Understanding the different types of lacerations and burns will better enable you to assist in caring for patients with these conditions.

| **LEARNING OBJECTIVE** **2.9.1** | Describe the types of skin lacerations and burns. |

| **LEARNING OBJECTIVE** **2.9.2** | Contrast first degree, second degree, and third-degree burns. |

KEY TERMS

abrasions Scrapes caused by rubbing the skin against another surface that are on the surface of the skin and do not bleed.

avulsions Occurs when the skin is torn away and the tissues below are exposed, causing extensive bleeding.

first-degree burns Superficial burns that only affect the epidermis. Skin may look red, swollen and be sensitive.

lacerations Cut that is a deep tear in the skin; bleeding is common.

punctures Wound caused by a small, pointed object that results in a hole in the skin; do not always bleed.

skin grafting Surgical procedure that involves removing skin from one area of the body and attaching it to another injured area; common procedure for burned areas.

second-degree burns Burns that affect the epidermis and dermis. Skin is red, painful, and blistered.

third-degree burns Burns that affect the epidermis, dermis and underlying tissues such as fat and muscle. Area appears blistered and black. Skin regeneration is not possible and skin grafts are needed.

SKIN WOUNDS AND BURNS

Skin wounds and burns may occur at different severities and in response to exposure to different events and substances. Knowing what caused the skin injury is of vital importance during the assessment process and during formation of the treatment plan.

Open skin wounds fall into four categories: abrasion, avulsion, laceration, and puncture.

- Abrasions are scrapes caused by rubbing the skin against another surface. They are only on the surface of the skin (the epidermis) and do not typically bleed.

- Avulsions occur when the skin is torn away and the tissues below are exposed. These wounds often have extensive bleeding.

- Lacerations are cuts. They are deep tears in the skin usually from a sharp object. Bleeding is common with these wounds.

- Punctures are wounds caused by a small, pointed object that results in a hole in the skin. These do not always bleed.

Burns of the skin may be caused by excess sun exposure, exposure to high temperatures, or exposure to many other substances. Common household products, like bleach and chlorine used in pool maintenance, can result in chemical burns. When caring for patients with different types of burns, it is important to understand details not only about the skin, but the entire integumentary system to be sure you help provide comprehensive care.

There are three common types of burns: first degree, second degree, and third degree (Figure 2-18ABC).

- First-degree burns are superficial burns and only affect the epidermis (Figure 2-18A). When this type of burn occurs, the skin appears red, swollen, and may be itchy and sensitive. Sunburns without blisters are an example of a common first-degree burn (Figure 2-19). First-degree burns typically heal in 2–3 days.

- Second-degree burns are partial-thickness burns and affect the epidermis and the dermis (Figure 2-18B). In this type of burn, the skin is red, painful, and blistered. Healing occurs slower than first degree burns.

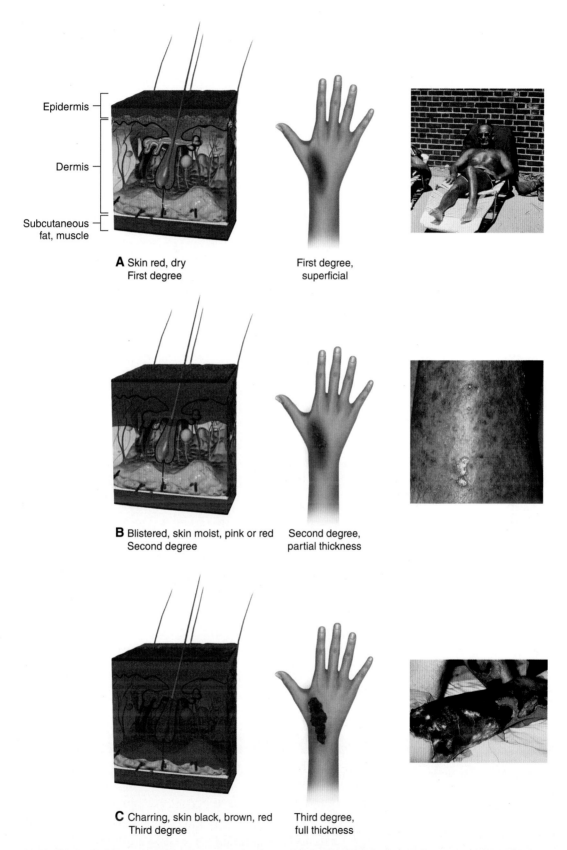

Epidermis

Dermis

Subcutaneous
fat, muscle

A Skin red, dry
First degree

First degree,
superficial

B Blistered, skin moist, pink or red
Second degree

Second degree,
partial thickness

C Charring, skin black, brown, red
Third degree

Third degree,
full thickness

FIGURE 2-18ABC Explanations of each type of burn. Each degree of burn is shown through artistic renderings identifying the layers of skin affected and photograph of that type of burn.

- **Third-degree burns** are full-thickness burns and affect the epidermis, dermis, and underlying tissue, such as muscle and fat (Figure 2-18C). The area is blistered and appears black. Nerve endings in the tissue are destroyed, so patients initially do not experience pain when this type of burn occurs. Regeneration of skin tissue is not possible and **skin grafting** must be done.

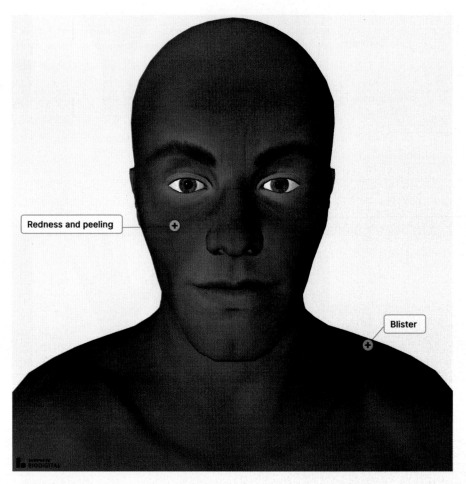

Redness and peeling

Blister

FIGURE 2-19 Sunburn.

LEARNING OBJECTIVE 2.9.3 **Explain the "Rule of Nines."**

KEY TERMS

electrolytes Minerals, typically salts, that carry a charge and are responsible for many essential processes in the body.

Rule of Nines Standardized method used to quickly assess the extent of burns on the surface area of the body; applied to second- and third-degree burns and divides the body into 11 areas, each accounting for 9% of the total body surface area, with one additional area around the genitals, accounting for 1%.

DETERMINING THE EXTENT OF BURNS

Burns result in tissue damage and cell death. They are an immediate threat to life because they cause dehydration and expose the patient to potential infection. Without the skin barrier, a patient's body will have difficulty maintaining homeostasis. This may include loss of body fluids, loss of **electrolytes**, and increased ability of pathogens to easily enter the body.

Therefore, it is important to quickly assess how extensive a patient's burns are. The "**Rule of Nines**" is a standardized method used to quickly assess the extent of burns on the surface area of the body (Figure 2-20). This rule is only used with patients who have second- and third-degree burns. It divides the body into 11 areas. Each area accounts for 9% of the total body surface area. One additional area around the genitals accounts for 1%. Knowing the percent of total body surface burned allows health care professionals to recommend appropriate interventions and treatment.

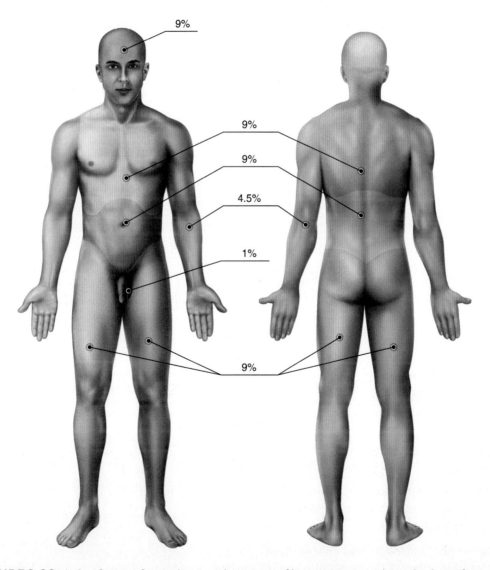

FIGURE 2-20 Rule of Nines for evaluating the extent of burns. Diagram shows body surface area percentages, in multiples of nine.

LEARNING OBJECTIVE 2.9.4 Describe the four steps involved in wound healing.

FOUR STEPS OF WOUND HEALING

When the skin is injured, the body sets a cascade of chemical reactions into motion to begin wound healing. The cascade is divided into four overlapping steps: hemostasis, defensive/inflammatory, proliferative, and maturation.

- Step 1: **Hemostasis**. In this step, the body stops bleeding by activating the blood-clotting system almost immediately after the injury.
- Step 2: Defensive/**inflammatory**. This step is a protective mechanism. White blood cells arrive at the site of injury to destroy any pathogens and get rid of dead cells. Swelling, redness, heat, and pain are the hallmarks of inflammation and are associated with this step. This step peaks 24–48 hours after the injury occurs. It does not usually last longer than 3 days.
- Step 3: **Proliferative**. During this step, the injured area is quickly filled with and covered with new cells. This often lasts from 4 to 24 days after initial injury.
- Step 4: **Maturation**. In this step, the collagen fibers that were quickly added in step 3 reorganize to slowly gain strength and flexibility in the new skin. This phase often lasts from 21 days to 2 years after initial injury.

LEARNING OBJECTIVE 2.9.5 Contrast keloid, hypertrophic, and contracture scarring.

KELOID, HYPERTROPHIC, AND CONTRACTURE SCARRING

There are several different types of scars that can occur after injuring the skin (Figure 2-21).

- **Keloid** scars (Figure 2-21) result from an overly aggressive healing process. They grow larger than the wound and are usually smooth on top and pink or purple in color. They are irregularly shaped and may continue to enlarge over time. They are more common in people who have darker skin.
- **Hypertrophic scarring** scars are raised, red scars similar to keloids but they do not grow beyond the boundary of the wound.
- **Contracture** scars (Figure 2-22) are common in patients with burns. They tighten the skin and may impair the patient's ability to move. They may also extend deeper than the skin and affect muscles and nerves.

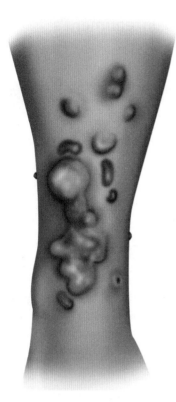

FIGURE 2-21 Keloidal scarring of the leg and ankle.

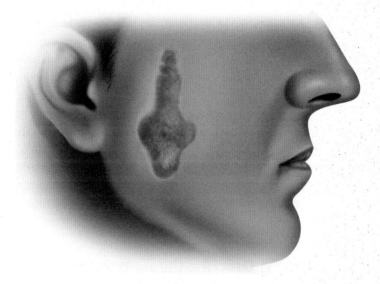

FIGURE 2-22 Contracture scar on the face.

UNIT OBJECTIVE 2.10

Describe the pathologies relating to the role of the integumentary system in maintaining homeostasis.

UNIT INTRODUCTION

As previously mentioned, the integument plays a vital role in helping maintain homeostasis in the human body. It does this by playing a part in thermoregulation and protecting underlying structures and organs. When the integument is compromised, the body may have difficulty maintaining homeostasis.

LEARNING OBJECTIVE 2.10.1 Identify common disorders that alter the integument's ability to maintain homeostasis.

KEY TERMS

anhidrosis Disorder of the sweat gland that inhibits normal sweating.

homeostasis A dynamic equilibrium that keeps the internal state of the body balanced.

hyperhidrosis Condition in which patient experiences excessive sweating.

COMMON INTEGUMENT DISORDERS

The body must be able to maintain an internal temperature, within the range of $36-37.5°$, regardless of changes in the environment. The brain closely regulates and monitors this range. Maintaining a steady internal temperature is known as homeostasis. As discussed throughout this chapter, the integument plays a large role in maintaining homeostasis. In some cases, structures of the integument may become compromised. For example, anhidrosis refers to the inability to sweat. Patients with this condition have sweat glands that have failed. Since we know that sweat glands play a role in cooling the body (as discussed previously), patients with this condition have difficulty maintaining homeostasis because they have a hard time staying cool.

Hyperhidrosis can also disrupt thermoregulation. Hyperhidrosis is the opposite of anhidrosis. Patients with this condition have overactive sweat glands and, thus, sweat excessively. Not only does this disrupt the integument's ability to use sweat appropriately, but may also damage integument by making skin more prone to infection and inflammation due to being moist for long periods of time. It may even cause skin to crack or be damaged.

LEARNING OBJECTIVE 2.10.2 Describe the signs, symptoms, and diagnosis of hypothermia and hyperthermia and their effects on homeostasis.

LEARNING OBJECTIVE 2.10.3 Compare and contrast the ways in which the body alters normal homeostatic mechanisms to compensate for common integumentary system pathologies.

KEY TERMS

heat illness Category of hyperthermia; signs and symptoms include normal to elevated core temperature; fatigue; nausea; vomiting; increased heart rate; signs of dehydration; mental status intact; and responsiveness to a cool environment, electrolytes, and fluids.

heat stroke Category of hyperthermia; patient usually has an elevated core temperature greater than 40.5°C; hot, dry skin; increased heart rate; weakness; vomiting, nausea, headache; the blood's ability to coagulate may be impaired; and skeletal muscle may be injured, leading to renal failure.

hyperthermia Having a core temperature greater than 38.5°C.

hypothermia Having a core temperature below 36°C.

Hypothermia

Hypothermia is defined as a core body temperature of 35°C or less. It is usually caused by prolonged exposure to cold temperatures, which can increase heat loss by as much as 25 times faster than normal. It can also result from use of certain medications, thyroid conditions, diabetes, severe trauma, or drugs and alcohol. The signs and symptoms of hypothermia are:

- Shivering
- Slurred speech
- Confusion and memory loss
- Slow, shallow breathing
- Drowsiness
- Slow, weak pulse
- Loss of coordination

In severe hypothermia, the person may be unconscious without obvious signs of a pulse or breathing.

Diagnosis includes physical examination and recognizing the symptoms listed above. Emergency departments have a specialized thermometer that can precisely detect core body temperature to help with identification and treatment of this condition.

Hyperthermia

Hyperthermia is defined as having a core temperature greater than 38.5°C. It is more common during the summer months when temperatures are high, but may be caused by more serious medical conditions that need to be ruled out immediately. It can be categorized as heat illness or heat stroke.

The signs and symptoms of heat illness include:

- Normal to elevated core temperature
- Fatigue
- Nausea, vomiting, and diarrhea
- Increased heart rate
- Signs of dehydration
- Mental status intact
- Responsive to cool environment, electrolytes, and fluids

Signs and symptoms of heat stroke include:

- Elevated core temperature usually greater than 40.5°C
- Hot, dry skin

- Increased heart rate
- Increased blood pressure
- Weakness, vomiting, nausea, and headache
- Blood's ability to coagulate may be impaired
- Skeletal muscle may be injured, leading to renal failure

Diagnosis includes a physical exam recognizing the signs and symptoms listed above as well as rapid cooling techniques such as using ice packs, a cooling blanket, and an ice bath.

Both hypothermia and hyperthermia are life-threatening conditions that require immediate treatment.

UNIT OBJECTIVE 2.11

Distinguish among the major types of skin cancer and disorders.

UNIT INTRODUCTION

There are two common conditions that affect the skin. One of the most commonly known skin conditions is skin cancer, which is one of the most prevalent types of cancer. Specifically, there are three common types:

- Basal cell carcinoma
- Squamous cell carcinoma
- Melanoma

Another common condition affecting the skin is staphylococcus scalded skin syndrome. This bacterial infection may be very painful and cause serious damage to the skin.

LEARNING OBJECTIVE **2.11.1** Identify common disorders affecting the skin.

LEARNING OBJECTIVE **2.11.2** Describe the three common types of skin cancer.

LEARNING OBJECTIVE **2.11.3** Contrast the three common types of skin cancer.

KEY TERMS

basal cell carcinoma Most common type of skin cancer; appears as flattened, round spots that are shiny and pale; rarely spreads.

melanoma Type of skin cancer that develops from melanocytes; appears as a freckle or mole that changes in color, size, or shape and grows quickly;

may also look like a blood blister; commonly spread and if left untreated may be fatal.

squamous cell carcinoma Type of skin cancer that appears as scaly, red, painful areas that bleed and do not heal and that grow slowly and rarely spread.

COMMON TYPES OF SKIN CANCER

There are three common types of skin cancer: basal cell carcinoma, squamous cell carcinoma, and melanoma. Become familiar with your skin so that any changes can be recognized right away.

- **Basal cell carcinoma** (Figure 2-23) is the most common type of skin cancer. This slow-growing cancer usually develops in areas of the skin exposed to the sun. It usually appears as a flattened, round spot that is shiny and pale. It may be scaly, bleed, and fail to heal. It rarely spreads to other parts of the body but must be removed.

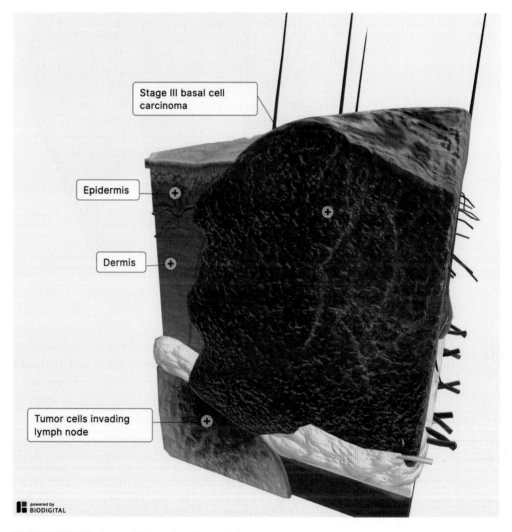

FIGURE 2-23 Stage III basal cell carcinoma.

- **Squamous cell carcinoma** (Figure 2-24) is slightly less common and usually develops on areas of the skin exposed to the sun. They appear as scaly, red, painful areas that bleed and do not heal. They grow slowly and are more likely to grow into deeper layers of the skin and spread to other parts of the body.

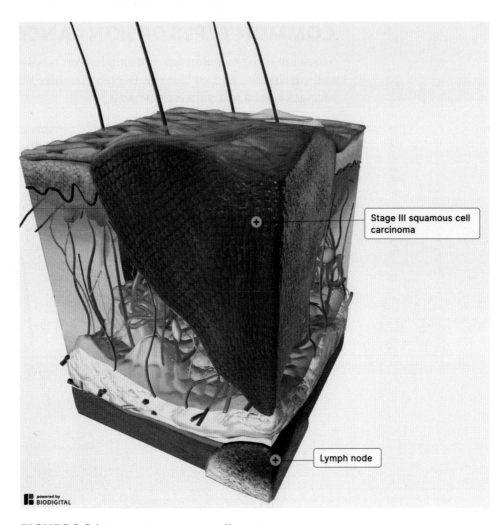

FIGURE 2-24 Stage III squamous cell carcinoma.

- Melanoma cancers (Figure 2-25) develop from melanocytes and are much less common than basal cell and squamous cell carcinomas. They grow quickly and are much more likely to spread to other parts of the body. They may appear as a mole or freckle that changes in color, size, or shape; as a lump with little or no pigment; or look like a blood blister.

Use the ABCDE signs of melanomas to detect any changes in existing moles or new moles and freckles when they appear (Figures 2-26 to 2-29). ABCDE stands for asymmetry, border, color, diameter, and evolution:

- Asymmetry (Figure 2-26): A lesion that is not a mirror image of itself when divided in half.
- Border (Figure 2-27): A mole with an irregular border.
- Color (Figure 2-28): A mole that contains different colors.
- Diameter (Figure 2-29): A change in the diameter or size of a mole.
- Evolution: Monitoring whether a mole grows or changes in size, shape, or color over time.

If left untreated, melanomas may be fatal.

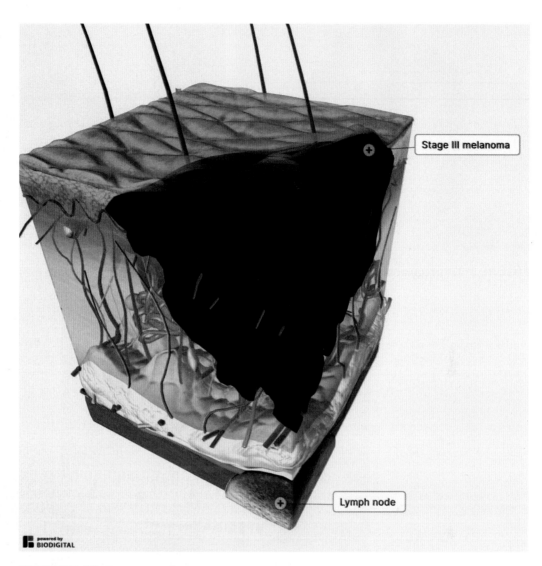

FIGURE 2-25 Stage III melanoma.

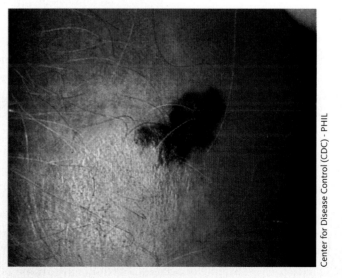

FIGURE 2-26 Asymmetrical appearance of a cancerous mole.

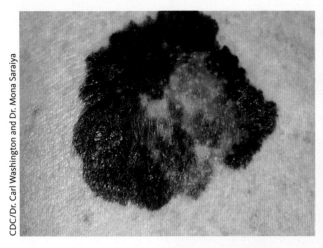

CDC/Dr. Carl Washington and Dr. Mona Saraiya

FIGURE 2-27 Irregular border of a cancerous mole.

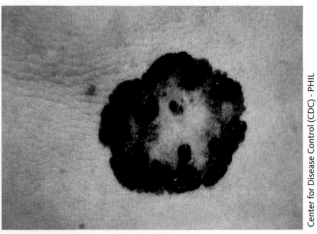

Center for Disease Control (CDC) - PHIL

FIGURE 2-28 A cancerous mole exhibits multiple colors.

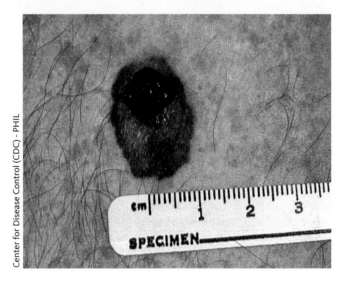

Center for Disease Control (CDC) - PHIL

FIGURE 2-29 Change in the diameter or size of a cancerous mole.

LEARNING OBJECTIVE 2.11.4 Describe the signs, symptoms, and diagnosis of staphylococcus scalded skin syndrome.

KEY TERM

staphylococcus scalded skin syndrome is a serious bacterial skin infection that is usually caused by *Staphylococcal aureas bacteria.*

STAPHYLOCOCCUS SCALDED SKIN SYNDROME

Staphylococcus scalded skin syndrome is a serious bacterial skin infection that is usually caused by *Staphylococcal aureas* bacteria. The bacteria release toxins that cause the skin to blister and peel over large parts of the body. The skin appears to be scalded or burned, hence its name. It can happen at any age but children under 5 years of age are at the highest risk.

The signs and symptoms include:

- Irritability
- Fatigue
- Fever
- Red skin
- Fluid-filled blisters that break easily
- Moist skin that is painful where blisters have broken
- Large areas where the top layer of skin has peeled away

The diagnosis requires a physical examination and recognizing the symptoms listed above along with a skin biopsy. Cultures may be done of the blood, urine, nose, throat, and skin to check for bacteria and other pathogens.

Chapter 3

The Skeletal System

Chapter Introduction

Bone fractures and breaks are among the most common injuries treated by the health care team. They are especially common in certain populations, such as older adults (those who are 65 years of age or older) who are prone to falls and injuries from falls. To better understand your role in caring for patients, it is important for you to understand the structure of bones and the skeletal system of the human body.

UNIT OBJECTIVE 3.1

Describe the structure and classification of bones.

UNIT INTRODUCTION

There are many different types of bones throughout the human body. All bones are comprised of the same types of bone tissue but the tissue from which they arise is different. In general, bones are classified by their shape, function, and structure.

LEARNING OBJECTIVE 3.1.1 Identify compact bone and cancellous bone.

KEY TERMS

cancellous bone Also called spongy or trabecular bone, found at the ends of long bones, in parts of the pelvis, ribs, skull, and spinal column.

compact bone Also called cortical bone, most rigid bone type in the body.

woven bone Temporary bone that forms after a bone breaks.

TYPES OF BONE TISSUE

All bones in the body are comprised of a rigid outer region (composed of compact bone) and a brittle inner region (composed of cancellous bone tissue). The two main types and one temporary type of bone tissue in the human skeletal system are:

- Compact bone. The strongest bone in the body, it is also referred to as cortical bone; its main functions are to support, protect, and enable body movement (Figure 3-1).

- **Cancellous bone.** Also called spongy or trabecular bone (Figure 3-1AB), it has a spongy appearance and is found at the ends of long bones and in parts of the pelvis, ribs, skull, and spinal column. It is more fragile than compact bone and creates a support for bone marrow, which produces red and white blood cells.

- **Woven bone.** When a bone breaks, temporary woven bone forms to help repair the fracture. This type of bone and its role in fracture repair are discussed in further detail later in the chapter.

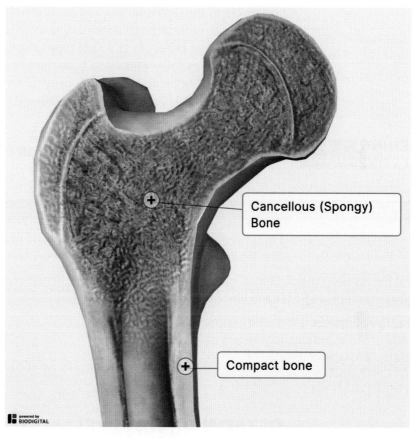

Cancellous (Spongy) Bone

Compact bone

FIGURE 3-1 Digital illustration of the femur, a long bone in the body. The main purpose of this bone is to support the body's weight; thus, the outer section of the bone is comprised of compact bone.

LEARNING OBJECTIVE 3.1.2 **Describe the structure of compact bone.**

KEY TERMS

lamellar bone Mature bone.

matrix Intracellular substance that makes bones dense and builds up bone during mineralization.

osteoblasts Immature bone cells found around the perimeter of bone tissue that help build new

bone tissue and contribute to the density of bones.

periosteum Fibrous outer layer of bone.

COMPACT BONE

As mentioned previously, compact bone is the strongest type of bone in the body. It is considered to be mature bone, or lamellar bone. Its strength comes primarily from its structural elements.

Periosteum

The periosteum refers to the fibrous outer layer of the bone. Its main functions are to provide the neurovasculature and nutrients to bone tissue and also play a role in the development and healing of bone, including supplying blood and nerves to cortical bone surrounding the medullar cavity. It is comprised of several different types of cells. One type of cell, osteoblasts, contributes to the density of bones (also known as bone mass). These cells release the organic components of bone matrix, which provide a network of fibers necessary for mineralization. This process will be discussed later.

LEARNING OBJECTIVE 3.1.3 Describe the structure of an osteon or Haversian system.

KEY TERMS

canaliculi Small ducts found in between lacunae that help route nutrients to cells in lacunae and lamellae.

central (haversian) canal Central canal of bone that contains nerve fibers and blood vessels.

lacunae Small spaces within the extracellular matrix of bone and cartilage where osteocytes and chondrocytes are found.

lamellae Layers of compact bone tissue that resemble the layers of a tree trunk.

osteon Circular areas where bone tissues come together.

OSTEON OR HAVERSIAN SYSTEM

Bone matrix comes together in a circular arrangement and forms what is known as an osteon (Figure 3-2). At the center of these circular layers is a middle canal called the central (haversian) canal (Figure 3-2AB). The central canal contains many items crucial to bone development and bone structure, which include nerve fibers and the blood vessels that supply the bone with nutrients. Much like the layers of a tree trunk, these layers of compact bone tissue then form around the haversian canal in a circle. These layers are called lamellae. Each lamella contains spaces (lacunae) where bone cells live (Figure 3-2AB). In between these lacunae are canaliculi, which are small ducts that help route nutrients to the cells in the lacunae and lamellae. Canaliculi contain small cytoplasmic projections from osteocytes, which allow for communication between cells in separate lacunae (Figure 3-2AB).

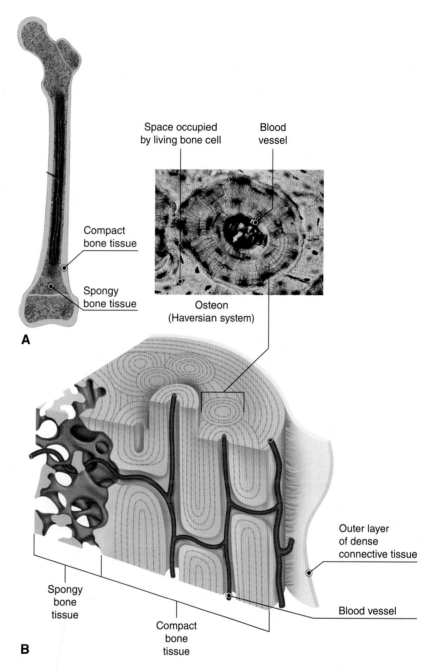

FIGURE 3-2AB Structure of compact and spongy bone. Make special note of the central (haversian) canal, osteon, and lamellae.

LEARNING OBJECTIVE 3.1.4 Describe the structure of cancellous bone.

KEY TERM

trabeculae Tissue that provides structural support to spongy bone.

CANCELLOUS BONE

Like compact bone, cancellous bone is also considered to be lamellar (i.e., layered). It too is comprised of matrix layers; however, unlike the columns of osteons in compact bone tissue, the bony trabeculae of cancellous bone are made up of a single osteon. This makes cancellous bones less dense, lighter, and more fragile than compact bones. It is found in the medullary cavity of bones and is lined with endosteum, a thin membrane that is very similar to periosteum in compact bone. (Figure 3-3).

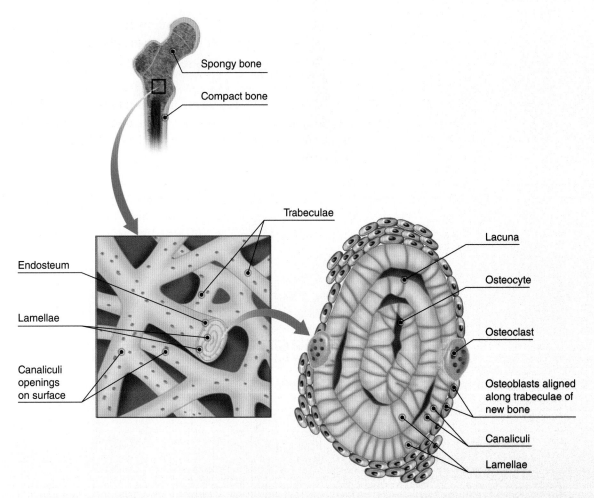

FIGURE 3-3 Magnified cross section of spongy bone trabeculae. On the far right is a cross section of a single trabecula and its parts.

LEARNING OBJECTIVE **3.1.5**   **Identify red bone marrow and yellow bone marrow.**

LEARNING OBJECTIVE **3.1.6**   **Describe the two types of bone marrow.**

KEY TERMS

bone marrow Substance found in medullary cavity that primarily produces new blood cells.

hematopoiesis Process of creating new blood cells.

medullary cavity Hollow inner cavity of bones.

red bone marrow Bone marrow reddish in appearance that produces platelets, red blood cells, and white blood cells.

yellow bone marrow Bone marrow yellow in color that contains a high number of fat cells and contributes to formation of bones and cartilage.

BONE MARROW

Bone marrow (Figure 3-4) is found in the hollow inner cavity of bones (known as the **medullary cavity**). Its main function is to produce new blood cells, but it also plays a role in the immune response of the body.

There are two types of bone marrow:

- **Red bone marrow.** Bone marrow found mostly in the bones of the skull, pelvis, spine, ribs, sternum, and long bones of the legs and arms. Red bone marrow, which has a reddish appearance, primarily produces platelets, red blood cells, and white blood cells through a process called **hematopoiesis**.
- **Yellow bone marrow.** Bone marrow that is yellowish in color found mostly in long bones. It contains a high number of fat cells and contributes to the formation of bones and cartilage in the body.

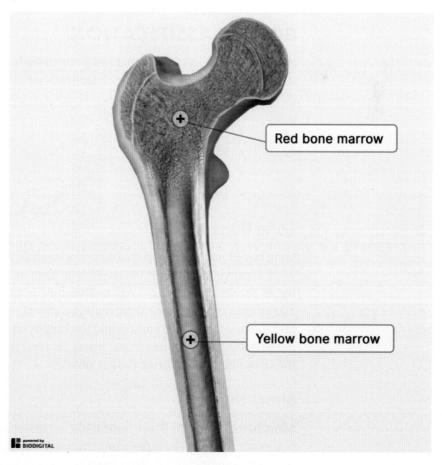

FIGURE 3-4 Cross section of a femur with the locations of red and yellow bone marrow.

LEARNING OBJECTIVE 3.1.7 Identify the five classifications of bones based on their shapes.

LEARNING OBJECTIVE 3.1.8 Describe the five classifications of bones based on their shapes.

LEARNING OBJECTIVE 3.1.9 Give examples of bones that fall into each of the five structural classifications.

KEY TERMS

diaphysis Shaft in the middle of a long bone.

epiphysis Flared ends of a long bone.

flat bones Relatively thin bones that are responsible for protecting inner organs.

irregular bones Complex bones of varying shapes that do not fit into other bone classifications.

long bones Hard, dense bones responsible for bearing most of the body's weight, providing support to the skeletal system, and enabling the body's mobility.

patella Small sesamoid bone commonly called the kneecap.

sesamoid bones Bones that form within tendons.

short bones Bones, found in the wrists and ankles, that are roughly as wide as they are long.

BONE CLASSIFICATION

In the human skeletal system, bones are classified according to their shape and structure. There are five major classifications of bone:

- Long bones
- Short bones
- Flat bones
- Sesamoid bones
- Irregular bones

Long Bones

Long bones are hard, dense bones responsible for bearing most of the body's weight, providing support to the skeletal system, and enabling the body's mobility. As shown in Figures 3-5 AB and 3-6, long bones have a distinctive shape that allows them to carry out their main functions—a large **diaphysis** (shaft in the middle) and two flared ends called the **epiphysis**. Some examples of long bones in the body are the bones in the lower limbs (femur, tibia, fibula) and bones in the upper limbs (humerus, radius, ulna).

Short Bones

Short bones (Figure 3-6) are bones that are about as wide as they are long. These bones are found in the wrists and ankles. Their main purpose is to provide support and stability with limited motion.

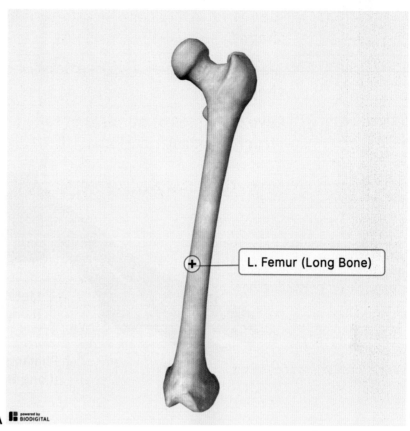

A

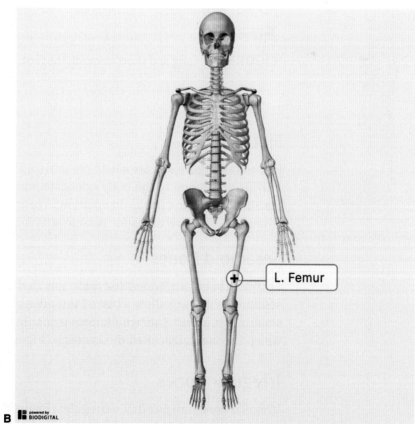

B

FIGURE 3-5AB Isolated view of the femur (A), which is a long bone, as well as the femur's location in the female human skeleton (B).

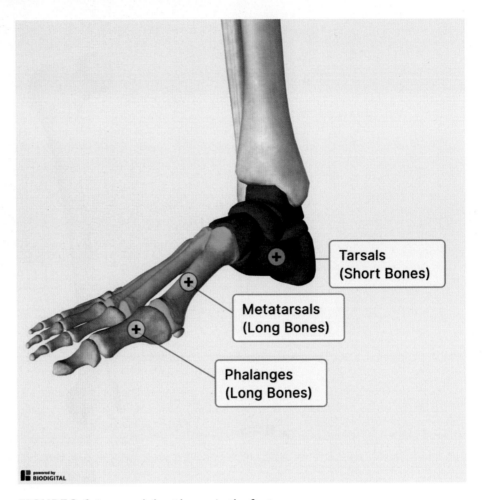

FIGURE 3-6 Long and short bones in the foot.

Flat Bones

Flat bones (Figure 3-7) are relatively thin (or flat). This shape allows the bone to provide protection to the body's delicate inner organs. Flat bones are found in the skull, chest, and pelvis. In addition to protection, flat bones, like other types of bones, also allow areas for muscle attachment.

Sesamoid Bones

Sesamoid bones are bones that are embedded in tendons. The main purpose of a sesamoid bone is to allow a place for tendons to connect. As such, their shape is small and rounded. One well-known example of a sesamoid bone is the patella, which is commonly called the kneecap (Figure 3-8).

Irregular Bones

Irregular bones are just that—irregular (Figure 3-9AB). Their shape is often complex and does not fit into any of the other bone classifications. Some examples of irregular bones include the bones of the spine (also called vertebrae) and the coccyx.

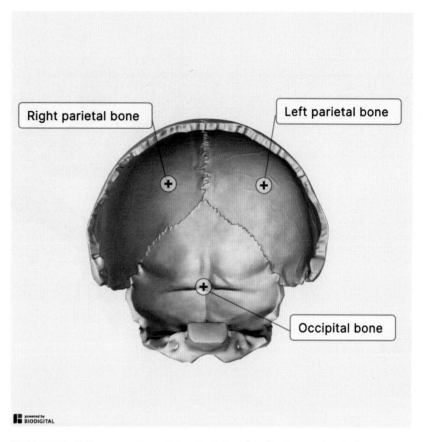

FIGURE 3-7 Cross section of the skull showing flat bones that help protect the brain.

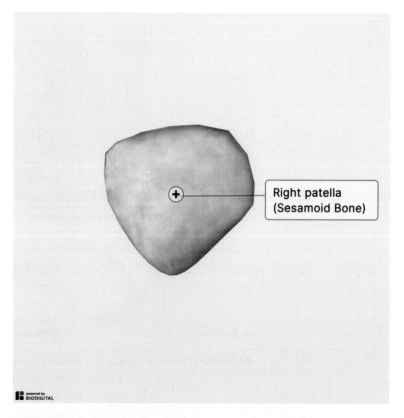

FIGURE 3-8 The patella, which is commonly called the kneecap.

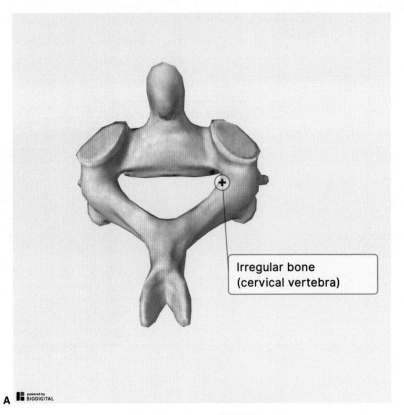

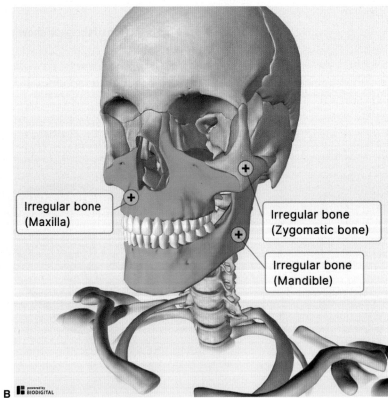

FIGURE 3-9AB Irregular bones have many different shapes and
sizes and are found throughout the body.
(A) Irregular bone in the spine (a cervical vertebra).
(B) Irregular bones in the jaw.

LEARNING OBJECTIVE 3.1.10 Identify the following parts of a bone: diaphysis, metaphysis, epiphysis, epiphyseal plate, articular cartilage, periosteum, endosteum, and medullary cavity.

KEY TERMS

articular cartilage Hyaline cartilage covering bone ends at movable joints.

epiphyseal plate During bone development, hyaline cartilage is replaced by bone at the epiphyseal plate.

metaphysis Narrow portion of a long bone between the epiphysis and diaphysis.

REGIONS OF THE LONG BONE

Some bones, such as flat bones and irregular bones, are too small or uniquely shaped to share many characteristics with one another. However, long bones share some of their basic structures. These structures are as follows (Figure 3-10):

- Diaphysis. The diaphysis, or shaft, of the femur is meant to support high levels of stress and body weight.

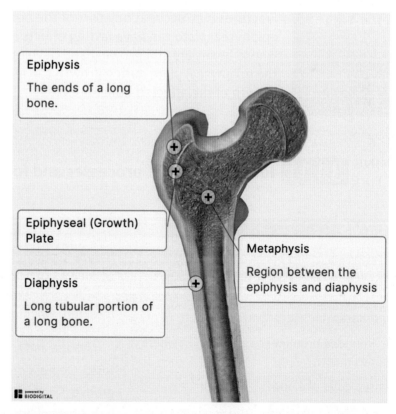

Epiphysis

The ends of a long bone.

Epiphyseal (Growth) Plate

Diaphysis

Long tubular portion of a long bone.

Metaphysis

Region between the epiphysis and diaphysis

powered by BIODIGITAL

FIGURE 3-10 Femur with the regions of the long bone labeled.

- **Metaphysis.** Narrow portion of a long bone between the epiphysis and diaphysis.
- Epiphysis: Each epiphysis helps to distribute the weight supported by the diaphysis.
- **Epiphyseal plate.** Sometimes called the growth plate, part of the long bone that enables the bone to grow longer. It is comprised of cartilage and is located between the epiphysis and the metaphysis of long bones.
- Medullary cavity. Hollow center of the long bone where bone marrow is located.
- **Articular cartilage.** Layer of tissue that provides cushion between bones. In healthy bones, it lines each epiphysis of the femur. In bones with certain diseases, such as arthritis, this cartilage may become damaged and worn down.
- Periosteum. Membrane that covers all portions of the outer surface of the bone except for the articular surfaces of bones making up a joint. It is a connective tissue layer that transmits blood and nerve supply to underlying compact bone.
- Endosteum. Membrane that lines the inner surface of bones in the medullary cavity.

CLINICAL TIP	Fractures may occur at any part of the bone. However, fractures in the epiphyseal plate can have lasting effects in adolescents and children whose bones are still growing and developing. Fractures and breaks in the epiphyseal plate during growth can lead to stunted or abnormal growth of the affected bone.

LEARNING OBJECTIVE 3.1.11 Identify types of processes and fossae on bones.

KEY TERMS

articular process Helps bones connect to one another and is associated with movable joints.

bony landmarks Individual parts of bones.

condyle Rounded prominence at the point where two bones meet.

crest Raised edge of a bone.

eminences Bumps in bones.

epicondyle Area of the bone between the condyle and the shaft of the bone.

fissure Openings for nerves, blood vessels, and tendons to pass through. Usually elongated and larger than foramina.

foramen Openings for nerves, blood vessels, and tendons to pass through. Usually round or ovoid in shape and smaller than fissures.

fossa Depression in a bone.

groove Deep depression in the bone.

line Ridge of bone that is less prominent than a crest.

notch Small indentation in bone.

process Projection from a bone.

sinus Space (cavity) within a bone.

spinous process Sharp edge or point in a bone.

transverse process Lateral prominence of bone.

tubercle Small rounded eminences in bones.

tuberosity Small rounded eminences in bones. Significantly larger than tubercles.

BONY LANDMARKS

Another way that you can describe and refer to bones is to identify individual parts of the bones. These parts are often referred to as bony landmarks. There are two main categories of bony landmarks: processes and fossae.

Processes

A process is defined as a projection from a bone. There are several different types of processes found in the body, which can be seen in Figure 3-11AB.

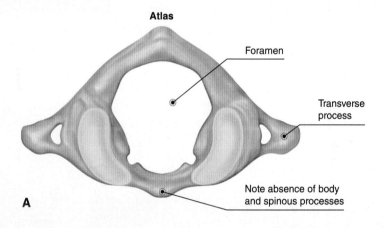

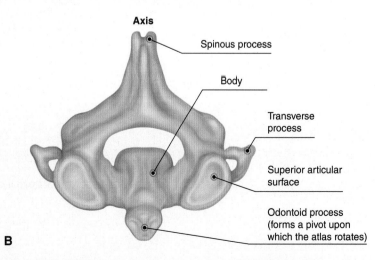

FIGURE 3-11AB Atlas (C-1) and axis (C-2), which are the two bones in the spinal column that allow rotation of the neck. They have numerous processes and fossae to visualize.

- **Articular process.** Articulation refers to the point where two bones meet and is sometimes called a joint; help bones connect to one another and are associated with movable joints (Figure 3-11).
- **Crest.** Raised edge of a bone (Figure 3-12).
- **Tubercle** and **tuberosity.** Small rounded **eminences**, or small bumps (Figure 3-13).
- **Line.** Ridge of bone that is less prominent than a crest.
- **Transverse process.** Lateral prominence of bone (Figure 3-11).
- **Spinous process.** Sharp edge or point (Figure 3-11).
- **Condyle/epicondyle.** Rounded prominence at the point where two bones meet (Figure 3-13).

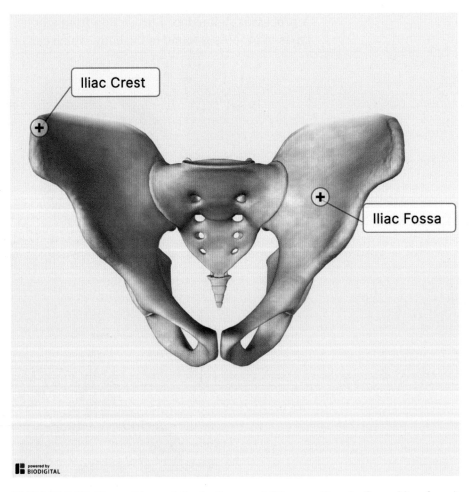

Iliac Crest

Iliac Fossa

FIGURE 3-12 The pelvis contains both a crest (iliac crest) and a fossa (iliac fossa).

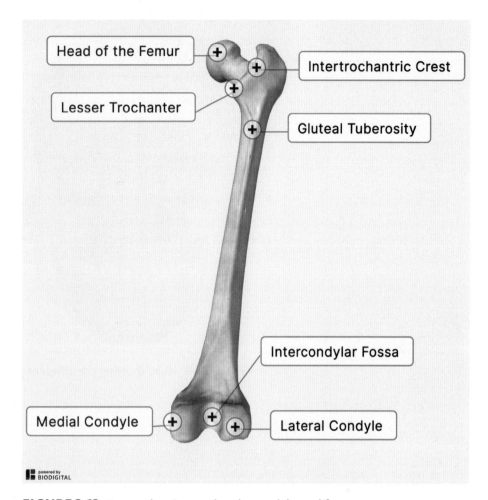

Head of the Femur

Intertrochantric Crest

Lesser Trochanter

Gluteal Tuberosity

Intercondylar Fossa

Medial Condyle

Lateral Condyle

powered by
BIODIGITAL

FIGURE 3-13 Femur showing a tubercle, condyle, and fossa.

Fossae

The other main type of bony landmark is a fossa. A **fossa** is a depression in a bone. There are several distinct types of fossae in the human skeleton. Explore the figures to learn more about each fossa.

- Articular fossa (Figure 3-13).
- **Fissure** and **foramen** (Figure 3-11). Openings that allow structures to pass through them. For example, there is a large opening (foramen) at the center of each vertebra that allows the nerves of the spinal cord to pass through the spinal column.
- **Sinus**. Space (cavity) within a bone, like the paranasal sinuses (Figure 3-14).
- **Notch**. Small indentation (Figure 3-15).
- **Groove**. Deep depression in the bone (Figure 3-16).

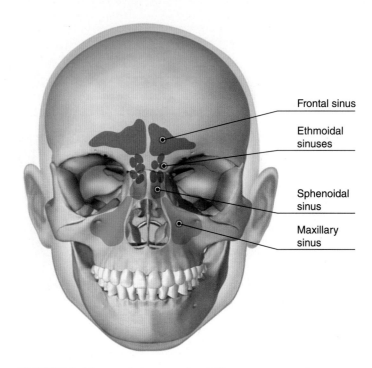

FIGURE 3-14 Head showing the different paranasal sinuses.

Frontal sinus

Ethmoidal sinuses

Sphenoidal sinus

Maxillary sinus

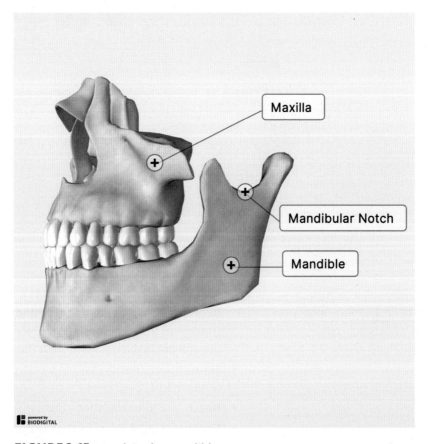

Maxilla

Mandibular Notch

Mandible

FIGURE 3-15 Notch in the mandible.

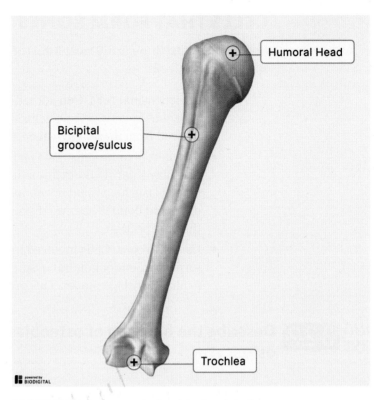

FIGURE 3-16 Groove (sulcus) in the right humerus.

UNIT OBJECTIVE 3.2

Describe the process of osteogenesis.

UNIT INTRODUCTION

Bones are formed through several different processes. These bone-forming processes occur during different life stages and rely on several different types of specialized cells. These specialized cells are activated when certain hormones are released. Once activated, specialized bone cells use vitamins and minerals to grow and maintain the bones of the body.

LEARNING OBJECTIVE **3.2.1** Identify the cells involved in bone formation.

KEY TERMS

cartilage cells Cells involved in endochondral ossification.

mesenchymal cells Type of stem cell that is not yet specialized from which all connective tissue is derived.

osteoclasts Cells that help break down old bone tissue; phagocytic bone cells that are formed from white blood cells.

osteogenesis Process through which bones are formed.

CELLS THAT FORM BONES

Bones are formed through different forms of **osteogenesis**. This process involves special types of cells:

- **Mesenchymal cells.** Considered bone precursor cells, type of stem cells that are not yet specialized cells. All connective tissues are derived from mesenchymal cells.
- Specialized bone cells. Two main types of specialized bone cells that play a part in bone formation: osteoblasts and **osteoclasts**. Osteoblasts help build new bone tissue, and osteoclasts help break down old bone tissue. We discuss these cells in greater detail in the next section.
- **Cartilage cells.** Cells involved in a particular kind of bone formation, endochondral ossification, in which bone forms from a hyaline cartilage model. This process is discussed later in this unit.

LEARNING OBJECTIVE 3.2.2 Describe the function of osteoblasts, osteoclasts, and osteocytes.

KEY TERMS

osteoblasts Immature bone cells found around the perimeter of bone tissue that help build new bone tissue and contribute to the density of bones.

osteocytes Specialized bone cells that maintain bone tissue.

osteoid Organic component of bone matrix comprised of protein mixture, matrix vesicles, and collagen that helps to grow new bone.

phagocytic Cell possessing the ability to absorb or "eat" another cell.

MAJOR CELLS FOUND IN BONE TISSUE

Bone tissue contains three types of cells:

- Osteoblasts. Immature bone cells found around the perimeter of bone tissue. They are considered part of periosteum. When osteoblasts are active, they are cube shaped. When they are dormant, they appear flat. Osteoblasts form from stem cells called osteoprogenitor cells and are responsible for secreting the soft, organic component of bone matrix known as the **osteoid**. Osteoid primarily consists of a protein mixture, matrix vesicles, and collagen. These substances help create new bone.
- Osteocyte. Mature bone cells. As we discussed in the previous unit, osteocytes are found within the matrix of bone tissue. More specifically, osteocytes are found in lacunae between the concentric lamellae of osteons (Figure 3-3). Osteocytes are oval

shaped with cytoplasmic projections (in canaliculi of osteons). These cells help maintain bone tissue. They sense stresses on bone and stimulate activity of other bone cells.

- Osteoclasts. **Phagocytic** bone cells. Phagocytic means that the cell can absorb or "eat" other cells, cellular debris, and pathogens. Osteoclasts are derived from white blood cells and are found around the perimeter of bone. They are large, round cells with multiple nuclei (Figure 3-3). Their primary function is to break down bone tissue, which is an important part of remodeling bones. In some conditions, such as osteoporosis, osteoclasts become too active, which cause bones to break down too much and leads to weak bones.

LEARNING OBJECTIVE 3.2.3 Describe the process of intramembranous ossification.

LEARNING OBJECTIVE 3.2.4 Identify bones that are made through intramembranous ossification.

KEY TERMS

intramembranous ossification Process through which flat bones, short bones, and irregular bones are formed.

mesenchyme Viscous tissue consisting of mesenchymal cells and watery matrix.

osteoprogenitor cells Cells that are considered precursors to fully formed bone cells.

viscous Watery or sticky.

INTRAMEMBRANOUS OSSIFICATION

As previously mentioned, there are different forms of osteogenesis that create new bone tissue. One form is called **intramembranous ossification**. In intramembranous ossification, bone tissue arises directly from **mesenchyme**. Mesenchyme is a **viscous** (thick or sticky) tissue that consists of mesenchymal cells and watery matrix. There are several main steps in this process (Figure 3-17ABCD):

1. The mesenchyme condenses to form clusters of connective tissue that will form bone.
2. Blood vessels bring **osteoprogenitor cells**, the precursor cells of bone tissue, to the condensed mesenchyme.
3. Osteoprogenitor cells become osteoblasts.
4. Osteoblasts then secrete bone matrix components and form woven bone tissue.
5. Woven bone is then remodeled into mature, lamellar bone.

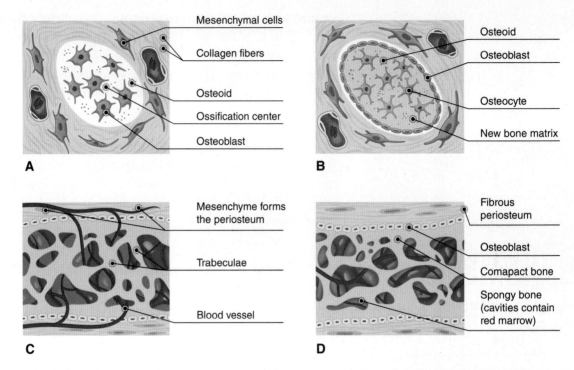

A

Mesenchymal cells
Collagen fibers
Osteoid
Ossification center
Osteoblast

B

Osteoid
Osteoblast
Osteocyte
New bone matrix

C

Mesenchyme forms
the periosteum
Trabeculae
Blood vessel

D

Fibrous
periosteum
Osteoblast
Comapact bone
Spongy bone
(cavities contain
red marrow)

FIGURE 3-17ABCD Intramembranous ossification.

Bones Made from Intramembranous Ossification

Intramembranous ossification is responsible for forming many of the bones in the body. Some examples include a variety of:

- Flat bones
  - Ilium of pelvis
  - Scapula
  - Sternum
  - Skull bones, such as the frontal bone
- Short bones
  - Carpals
  - Tarsals
- Irregular bones
  - Vertebrae
  - Bones of the face, such as the zygomatic bone

LEARNING OBJECTIVE **3.2.5** Describe the process of endochondral ossification.

LEARNING OBJECTIVE **3.2.6** Identify bones that are made through endochondral ossification.

ENDOCHONDRAL OSSIFICATION

A second form of osteogenesis is called endochondral ossification. In this process, bone arises from a cartilage model. The cartilage model is comprised of hyaline cartilage tissue. There are several main steps in this process (Figure 3-18):

1. Mesenchyme condenses and forms a cartilage model of long bones of the fetal skeleton.

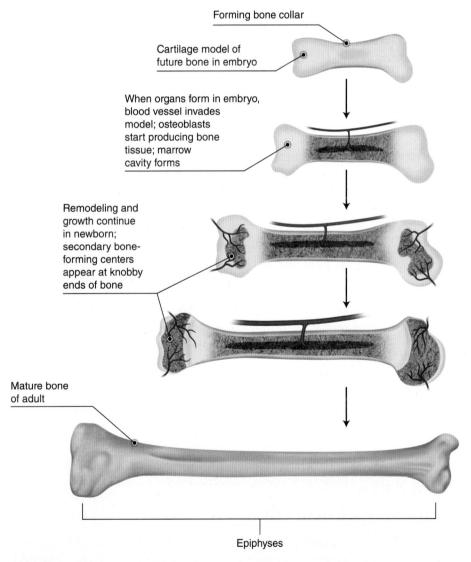

FIGURE 3-18 During endochondral ossification, a secondary ossification center remains in the metaphysis/epiphyseal plate. This lets the bone continue to grow until a person reaches adult height.

2. Blood vessels then invade the cartilage model and bring osteoprogenitor cells. This is the establishment of the primary ossification center.
3. Osteoprogenitor cells differentiate into osteoblasts that secrete bone matrix components.
4. The bone matrix calcifies, and the cartilage cells die.
5. A secondary ossification center remains at the metaphysis/epiphyseal plate of the long bone. This is the growth plate where long bones continue to grow in length until the skeleton has reached its adult length.

Bones Made from Endochondral Ossification

As previously mentioned, endochondral ossification forms the long bones of the body, which include the following:

- Femur, tibia, fibula
- Humerus, radius, ulna

LEARNING OBJECTIVE 3.2.7 Identify the hormones that contribute to bone growth.

LEARNING OBJECTIVE 3.2.8 Describe the function of the hormones that contribute to bone growth.

KEY TERMS

inhibiting Act of stopping something.

mineralization Process of making bones more rigid.

HORMONES AFFECTING BONE GROWTH

Hormones play an important part in both stimulating bone growth and in telling bones when they should stop growing. Vitamin D, calcitonin, and growth hormone are the hormones that are primarily responsible for bone growth. Parathyroid hormone is responsible for stopping, or inhibiting, bone growth.

Vitamin D

Vitamin D is derived from cholesterol in the skin in response to sun exposure. Once synthesized, vitamin D stimulates mineralization, or stiffening, of bone tissue by encouraging the intestines to absorb calcium. Individuals who are deficient in vitamin D may have weak and/or irregularly shaped bones due to inadequate bone mineralization.

Calcitonin

Calcitonin is a hormone that is secreted from the thyroid gland. When the body contains excess calcium in the blood, it releases calcitonin. Calcitonin, in turn, stimulates osteoblasts, which are bone-forming cells. Calcitonin is discussed in greater detail later in this chapter.

Growth Hormone

Growth hormone is derived from the anterior pituitary gland in the brain. It has a variety of functions in the body depending on its interactions with other hormones and molecules. In bones, growth hormone interacts with IGF-I to promote bone growth and turnover. Before puberty, growth hormone promotes lengthening of bones at the epiphyseal plates. Excess growth hormone circulating in adults can cause a condition called acromegaly, which is discussed later in this chapter.

When calcium is present in high levels in the body, calcitonin returns its concentration to homeostatic levels by encouraging bones to absorb calcium. It does so by stimulating the activity of osteoblasts, which are bone cells that are responsible for building up new bone tissue and for storing calcium.

Parathyroid Hormone

Parathyroid hormone is secreted by the parathyroid glands.

Parathyroid hormone stimulates bones to stop absorbing calcium, which increases the concentration of calcium available in blood. To increase levels of calcium in the blood, parathyroid hormone stimulates activity of osteoclasts, which are bone cells that break down bone tissue and release stored calcium.

UNIT OBJECTIVE 3.3

Describe the major bones and bony landmarks of the human skeleton.

UNIT INTRODUCTION

In addition to being classified by the process through which they are formed, bones can also be classified and divided based on their function, their shape, and any bony landmarks they have. In this unit, we discuss the two main divisions of the skeletal system as well as identify common bony landmarks of bones throughout the body.

LEARNING OBJECTIVE 3.3.1 Identify the major divisions of the skeletal system.

LEARNING OBJECTIVE 3.3.2 Identify the axial and appendicular skeleton.

KEY TERMS

appendicular skeleton Division of bones in the human skeleton where muscles can attach and move the body.

axial skeleton Division of bones in the human skeletal system that functions as an anchor or base for the body and provides protection to vital organs.

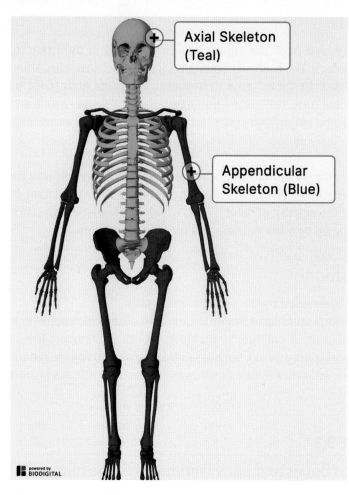

Axial Skeleton
(Teal)

Appendicular
Skeleton (Blue)

FIGURE 3-19 Adult male skeleton showing the axial skeleton (light blue) and the appendicular skeleton (dark blue).

ADULT SKELETAL SYSTEM

It is important to note that the adult human skeletal system is divided into two major divisions: the axial skeleton and the appendicular skeleton (Figure 3-19).

Axial Skeleton

The axial skeleton functions as an anchor or base for the body. It also protects the body's vital organs. Bones that are a part of this skeletal division include the following:

- Vertebral column
- Skull
- Rib cage

Appendicular Skeleton

The appendicular skeleton provides areas where muscle can attach and move the body. Bones that are considered part of the appendicular skeleton include the following:

- Long bones of the upper and lower limbs
- Bones of the hands and feet
- Pelvic and pectoral girdle

LEARNING OBJECTIVE **3.3.3** **Identify the bones of the cranium.**

KEY TERMS

cranium Flat bones that surround the brain and make up the head.

neurocranium Upper and back part of the skull.

viscerocranium All bones not included in the neurocranium.

CRANIUM

The bones found in the cranium are divided into two main classifications (Figure 3-20): the neurocranium and the viscerocranium. The neurocranium is the upper and back part of the skull, while the viscerocranium refers to all bones not included in the neurocranium.

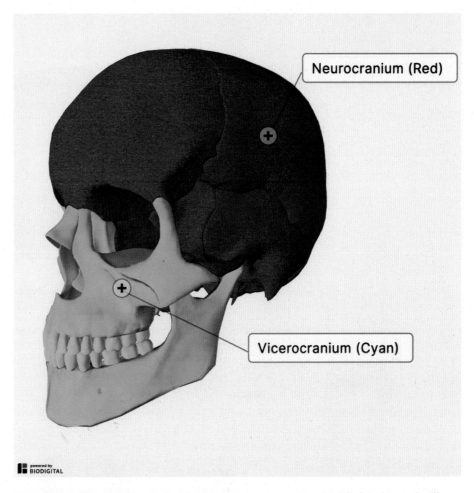

FIGURE 3-20 Human skull showing the neurocranium highlighted in red. All other bones represent the viscerocranium.

CLINICAL TIP	An easy way to distinguish between the neurocranium and viscerocranium is to imagine you are wearing a standard bicycle helmet. Any bones covered by the helmet comprise the neurocranium. Bones that are not covered by the helmet comprise the viscerocranium.

The main bones of the neurocranium are labeled in Figure 3-21AB. They include the following:

- Frontal bone
- Occipital bone
- Parietal bones
- Temporal bones
- Sphenoid bone
- Ethmoid bone

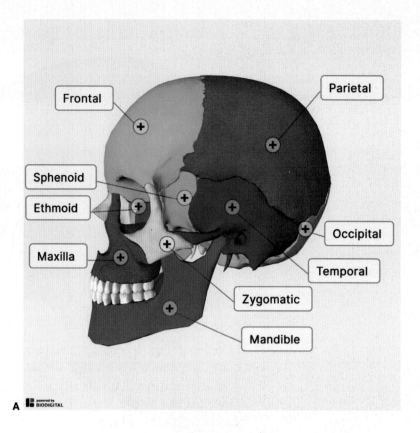

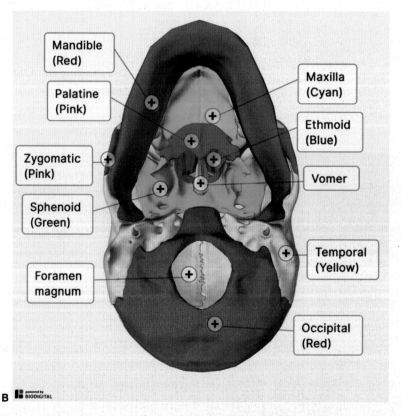

FIGURE 3-21AB (A) Main bones of the cranium. (B) Inferior view of the skull showing the foramen magnum (highlighted in light blue).

LEARNING OBJECTIVE 3.3.4 Describe the structure and important landmarks of the cranial bones.

KEY TERMS

coronal suture Immovable, fibrous joint between the frontal bone and the right and left parietal bones.

external acoustic meatus Opening in temporal bone that allows for the ear canal.

foramen magnum Bony landmark that is a large hole that transmits the spinal cord.

foramina of brain case Opening inside the skull that allows arteries, veins, and cranial nerves to pass through.

sagittal suture Immovable, fibrous joint between the right and left parietal bones.

sutures Immovable joints between skull bones.

LANDMARKS OF CRANIAL BONES

As you can see in Figure 3-22AB, cranial bones vary in shape. The bones that surround the brain (such as the frontal bone) are mostly smooth, flat bones. There are a few bones that are irregularly shaped, including the temporal, ethmoid, and sphenoid bones. In addition to having unique shapes, these irregularly shaped bones feature many foramina that allow arteries, veins, and nerves to pass through the skull.

There are several important landmarks that you should be sure to note about these bones:

- **Foramen magnum** (found at the base of the occipital bone) (Figure 3-21B). Large hole that provides space for the spinal cord to pass through.
- **Foramina of brain case** (Figure 3-22B). Openings inside the skull that allow arteries, veins, and cranial nerves to pass through.
- **Sutures** (Figure 3-22A). Immovable joints between skull bones. Two main sutures to remember:
   - **Coronal suture** (Figure 3-22A). Joins frontal bone with parietal bones.
   - **Sagittal suture** (Figure 3-22A). Joins left and right parietal bones.
- **External acoustic meatus** (found in the temporal bone) (Figure 3-22B). Allows for the opening of the ear canal.

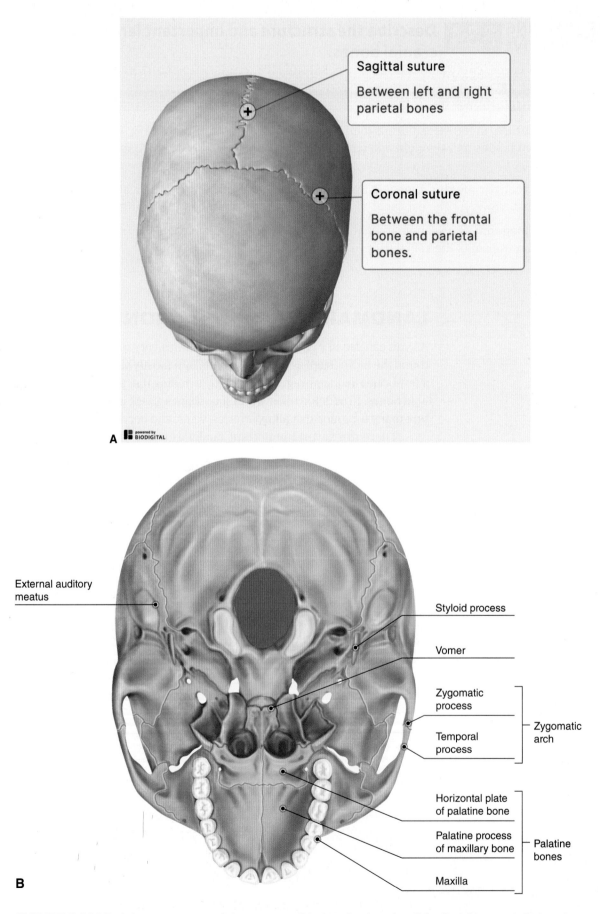

FIGURE 3-22AB (A) Main sutures of the cranium. (B) Main landmarks of the facial bones, inferior view.

LEARNING OBJECTIVE 3.3.5 Identify the facial bones.

LEARNING OBJECTIVE 3.3.6 Describe the structure and important landmarks of the facial bones.

FACIAL BONES

As previously mentioned, the bones of the face comprise the viscerocranium. These bones include the following:

- Zygomatic bone (Figure 3-23)
- Mandible (Figure 3-23)
- Maxilla (Figure 3-23)
- Lacrimal bone (Figure 3-23)
- Nasal bones (Figure 3-23)
- Palatine bones (Figure 3-22B)
- Vomer (Figure 3-22B)
- Inferior nasal concha (Figure 3-24)

It is worth noting that all facial bones are irregular bones. As such, they vary in their size and shape. In general, facial bones feature some foramina and many processes. There are some important landmarks to keep in mind when studying the bones of the face:

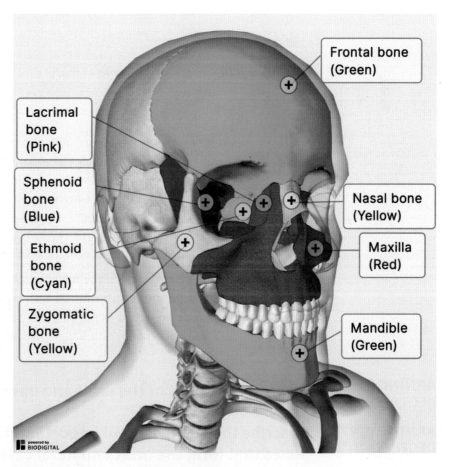

FIGURE 3-23 Main facial bones of the viscerocranium.

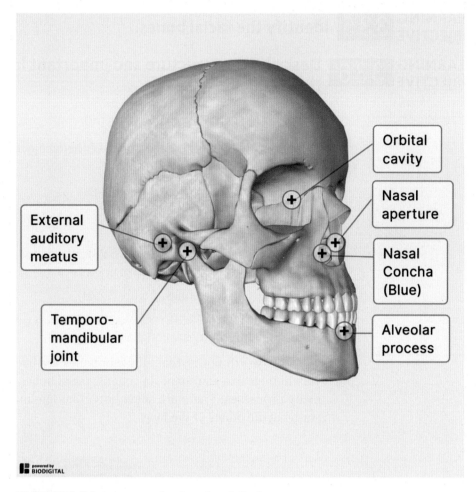

FIGURE 3-24 Important landmarks of the face.

- Alveolar processes (Figure 3-24). Located on the mandible and maxilla, provide attachment sites for teeth.
- Zygomatic arch (Figure 3-22B). Found on the temporal bone and zygomatic bone, what creates our "cheekbones."
- Nasal aperture (Figure 3-24). Opening into the nasal cavity.
- Orbital cavity (Figure 3-24). Holds each of our eyes, which are referred to as orbits.
- Nasal cavity: Inside of the nose; space through which air passes between your external nose and the pharynx.
- Temporomandibular joint (Figure 3-24). Joint between the mandible and temporal bone; sometimes referred to informally as the jaw.

LEARNING OBJECTIVE 3.3.7 Identify the bones of the orbit and nasal cavity.

LEARNING OBJECTIVE 3.3.8 Describe the structure and important landmarks of the bones that form the orbit and nasal cavity.

BONY ORBIT AND NASAL CAVITY

The bony orbit (the part of the skull surrounding the orbit) is comprised of the following bones (Figure 3-25):

- Frontal bone
- Zygomatic bone
- Maxilla
- Sphenoid bone
- Ethmoid bone
- Palatine bone
- Lacrimal bone

Many of these bones contain specialized landmarks that help enable the function of the organs and tissues these bones protect.

- Orbital plates. Flat surfaces on the bones of the bony orbit that create a cone-shaped cavity almost completely surrounding the orbits.

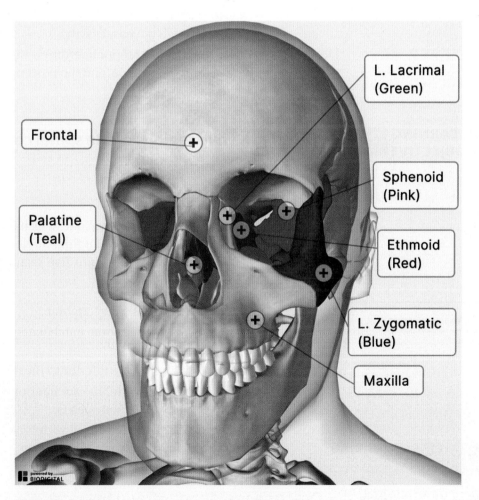

FIGURE 3-25 Important landmarks of the bony orbit and nasal cavity.

- Superior and inferior orbital fissures. Large foramina that transmit nerves and blood vessels to the eye and surrounding tissues.
- Lacrimal groove. Depression located on the medial side of the bony orbit. It opens to the lacrimal sac, which drains tears toward the nasal cavity.

The nasal cavity is comprised of several bones as well. These bones are as follows:

- Ethmoid bone
- Inferior nasal concha
- Maxilla
- Palatine bone
- Vomer

Several important landmarks on bones of the nasal cavity enable appropriate functioning of tissues and organs in this area of the body:

- Nasal septum. Separates the left and right nasal cavities.
- Nasal conchae (superior, middle, and inferior). Rotate air as it passes through the nasal cavity.
- Nasal apertures. Anterior aperture is the opening to the nasal cavity from the outside, and the posterior aperture opens to the pharynx.

LEARNING OBJECTIVE 3.3.9 **Identify the five regions of the spinal column.**

SPINAL COLUMN

The occipital condyles of the occipital bone, which form the main joint between the skull and cervical spine, allow the first cervical vertebra to attach to the skull. The spinal column is divided into five regions, listed from superior to inferior (Figure 3-26):

- Cervical. Superior seven vertebrae.
- Thoracic. Twelve vertebrae immediately inferior to the cervical vertebrae.
- Lumbar. Five vertebrae inferior to the thoracic vertebrae.
- Sacral. Five fused vertebrae are inferior to the lumbar vertebrae that form part of the bony pelvis.
- Coccygeal. Three to five fused vertebrae found inferior to the sacral vertebrae that form the tailbone.

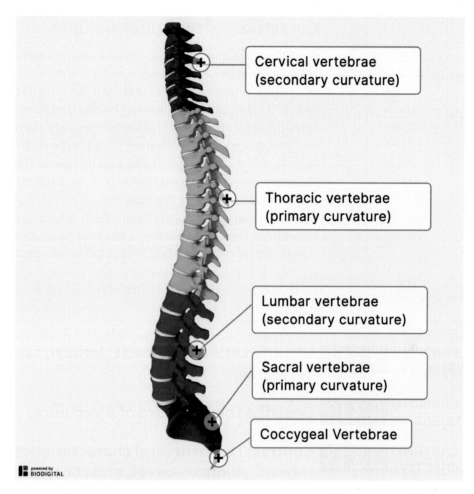

FIGURE 3-26 Regions of the spinal column and the primary and secondary curvatures of the spine. From superior to inferior, the image shows the cervical region and curvature (dark blue), the thoracic region and curvature (light blue), the lumbar region and curvature (pink), the sacral region and curvature (dark blue), and the coccygeal region (light blue).

LEARNING OBJECTIVE **3.3.10** **Identify the primary and secondary curvatures of the spinal column.**

KEY TERMS

curvatures Curves in the spinal column.

kyphotic curvature Primary curvature of the spine.

lordotic curvature Secondary curvature of the spine.

primary curvatures Curvature of the thoracic and sacral vertebrae that forms during fetal development.

secondary curvatures Curvature of the lumbar and cervical vertebrae that develops once a child learns to walk.

Curvatures of the Spinal Column

As you probably noticed, the spinal column is structured so that there are two main curvatures.

The primary curvatures (Figure 3-26) form during fetal development in the womb. As the embryo grows and begins to develop a head, the primary curvatures begin to form. This creates two primary curvatures: a thoracic curvature and a sacral curvature. These are found in the thoracic and sacral regions of the spinal column. These curves may also be referred to as kyphotic curvatures, and an exaggerated curvature in these regions is referred to as kyphosis (discussed in greater detail later in this chapter).

Secondary curvatures (Figure 3-26), which include the cervical and lumbar curvatures, form after birth as a person's muscles develop. The cervical curvature develops when an infant begins to hold his or her head upright. The lumbar curvature forms when a toddler begins to stand upright. These curves may also be referred to as lordotic curvatures, and an exaggerated curvature in these regions is referred to as lordosis (discussed in greater detail later in this chapter).

LEARNING OBJECTIVE 3.3.11 Identify cervical, thoracic, lumbar, sacral, and coccygeal vertebrae.

LEARNING OBJECTIVE 3.3.12 Describe the structure of a vertebra.

LEARNING OBJECTIVE 3.3.13 Contrast the structural characteristics of cervical, thoracic, lumbar, sacral, and coccygeal vertebrae.

KEY TERM

bifid Spinous process that splits into two smaller processes so that it resembles a Y-shaped projection from the vertebral arch.

Structure of Vertebrae

Although they are grouped into different regions, vertebrae all have similar major regions and landmarks. The vertebral body is large and round. The vertebral arch is the posterior region of vertebra. It is formed by the following (Figure 3-11):

- Lamina
- Pedicle
- Spinous process
- Transverse process

Even though vertebrae do share the same general structure, there are a few major differences between the different types of vertebrae.

- Cervical vertebrae (Figure 3-27AB). Smallest individual vertebrae that have transverse processes that feature foramina. They also have a **bifid** spinous process, which splits into two smaller processes so that it resembles a Y-shaped projection from the vertebral arch.

- Thoracic vertebrae (Figure 3-28AB). Vertebrae that have a heart-shaped body and a long, downward-facing spinous process. The transverse processes and body feature sites for attachment of a person's ribs.
- Lumbar vertebrae (Figure 3-29AB). Largest individual vertebrae that have a round vertebral body and a short, broad spinous process.
- Sacral vertebrae (Figure 3-29B). Fused vertebral bodies that attach to the ilium of the pelvis.
- Coccygeal vertebrae (Figure 3-29B). Small, fused vertebrae that hang off of the inferior end of the sacrum. Due to their location, they are frequently fractured.

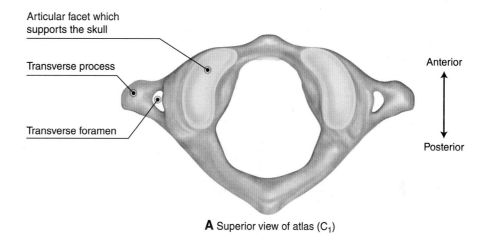

A Superior view of atlas (C$_1$)

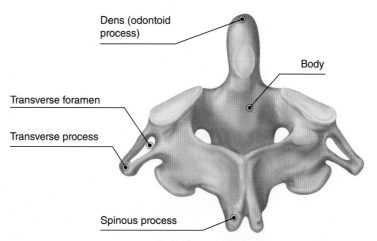

B Posterior-superior view of axis (C$_2$)

FIGURE 3-27AB First and second cervical vertebrae.

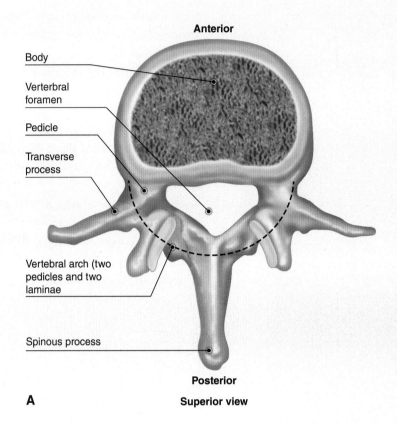

Anterior

Body

Verterbral foramen

Pedicle

Transverse process

Vertebral arch (two pedicles and two laminae)

Spinous process

Posterior

A

Superior view

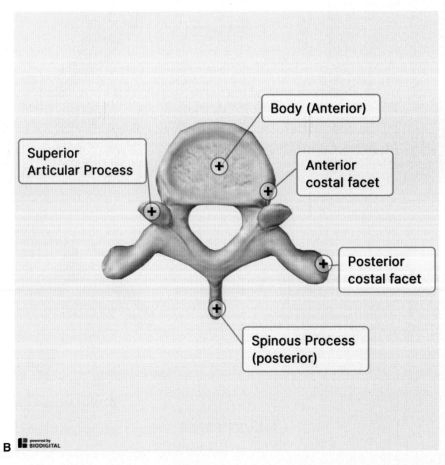

Body (Anterior)

Superior Articular Process

Anterior costal facet

Posterior costal facet

Spinous Process (posterior)

B BIODIGITAL

FIGURE 3-28AB Thoracic vertebra.

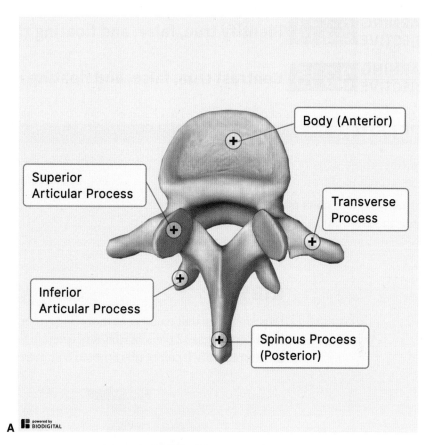

A

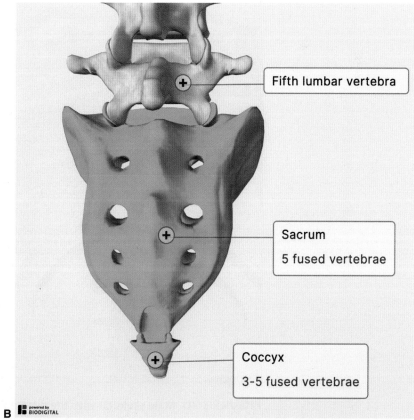

B

FIGURE 3-29AB (A) Superior view of a lumbar vertebra. (B) Posterior view of the sacral and coccygeal vertebrae.

LEARNING OBJECTIVE 3.3.14 Identify true, false, and floating ribs.

LEARNING OBJECTIVE 3.3.15 Contrast true, false, and floating ribs.

KEY TERMS

false ribs Three pairs of ribs inferior to true ribs that attach to sternum indirectly.

floating ribs Two pairs of ribs that do not connect with the sternum.

true rib Seven most superior pairs of ribs that connect directly with sternum.

RIBS

Ribs are bones that connect to thoracic vertebrae and, in some cases, the sternum. Each person has 12 pairs of ribs, and each rib pair is named for their attachment to the sternum. Each pair of ribs is noted below, from superior to inferior (Figure 3-30):

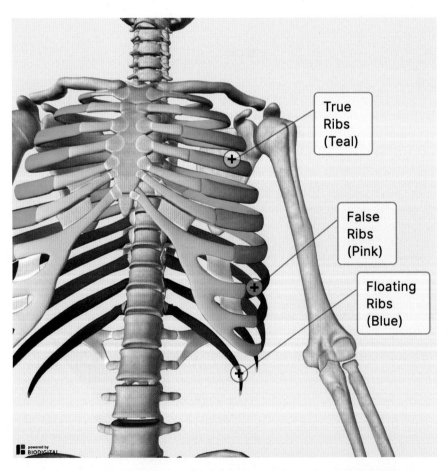

True Ribs (Teal)

False Ribs (Pink)

Floating Ribs (Blue)

FIGURE 3-30 Male skeleton with the different types of ribs highlighted. True ribs (light blue) are the most superior seven rib pairs. False ribs (pink) are found inferior to the true ribs. Floating ribs (dark blue) are the most inferior two rib pairs.

- **True ribs.** Seven most superior pairs of ribs (1–7) that attach directly to the sternum through their own costal cartilages.
- **False ribs.** Three pairs of ribs inferior to the true ribs (8–10) that attach to sternum indirectly. The costal cartilages of false ribs join the costal cartilages of true ribs to attach to the sternum.
- **Floating ribs.** Two pairs of ribs inferior to the false ribs (11–12). Floating ribs do not reach the sternum. They are short and do not reach the anterior thoracic wall. They do not feature costal cartilages.

LEARNING OBJECTIVE 3.3.16 Identify the humerus, radius, ulna, carpal group, metacarpal group, and phalanges.

LEARNING OBJECTIVE 3.3.17 Describe the structure and important landmarks of the bones found in the upper extremities.

KEY TERMS

pronation Rotation of the hand and forearm so that the palm faces downward.

supination Rotation of the forearm and hand so that the palm faces upward.

UPPER EXTREMITIES

In addition to the ribs, the sternum also articulates with the clavicle, which makes up part of the pectoral girdle. The pectoral girdle provides an attachment for the upper limbs (Figure 3-31). The bones of the upper limbs, all of which are part of the appendicular skeleton, include the following:

- Humerus (Figure 3-31). Long bone in the arm. It makes up part of the shoulder joint and elbow joint. Important landmarks and structures of the humerus are the humeral head, the trochlea, and the capitulum. The head of the humerus forms the shoulder joint when it articulates with the scapula. The trochlea and capitulum form the elbow joint when they articulate with the ulna and radius.
- Radius and ulna (Figure 3-31). Long bones that make up the forearm. They also make up part of the elbow joint and wrist joint. Important structures and landmarks include the head of the radius and the olecranon process of the ulna. The head of the radius rotates around the capitulum of the humerus. This permits pronation and supination of the hand. The olecranon process of the ulna articulates with the trochlea of the humerus to form the elbow joint.
- Carpal bones (Figure 3-31). Short bones of the wrist.
- Metacarpal bones (Figure 3-31). Long bones that make up the hand and are located between the wrist and fingers.
- Phalanges (Figure 3-31). Bones that make up the fingers. Even though they are small in length, they are considered long bones because of the characteristics they share with other long bones in the body.

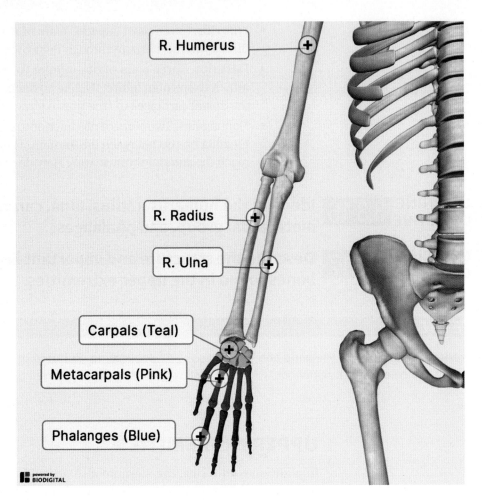

R. Humerus

R. Radius

R. Ulna

Carpals (Teal)

Metacarpals (Pink)

Phalanges (Blue)

powered by
BIODIGITAL

FIGURE 3-31 Bones of the upper extremities, including the carpals (highlighted in light blue), metacarpals (highlighted in pink), and phalanges (highlighted in dark blue).

LEARNING OBJECTIVE 3.3.18 Identify the ilium, ischium, and pubis.

LEARNING OBJECTIVE 3.3.19 Describe the structure and important landmarks of the pelvic bones.

THE PELVIS

In addition to connecting to the upper extremities via the clavicle, the spinal column also connects to the pelvis. The pelvis is comprised of the sacrum and three sets of paired bones (Figure 3-32):

- Ilium. Broad, flat bones that attach to the sacrum.
- Ischium. Small irregular bones that form the inferior part of the pelvis.
- Pubis. Small irregular bones that form the anterior part of the pelvis.

The pelvis itself is a bowl shaped, bony structure formed by the fusion of six bones:

- Two iliac bones
- Two ischial bones
- Two pubic bones

The pelvis as a whole has several important structures and landmarks. Knowing these can help assist you in providing care to patients in different clinical scenarios:

- Iliac crest. Superior margin of the ilium. It is often an important landmark for injections and lumbar punctures.
- Ischial tuberosities. Commonly referred to as "sitting bones."
- Two pubic bones joined by pubic symphysis. Cartilaginous joint that allows for slight movement of the pelvis during childbirth.
- Acetabulum. Depression in the lateral pelvis that enables the pelvis to join with the head of the femur.

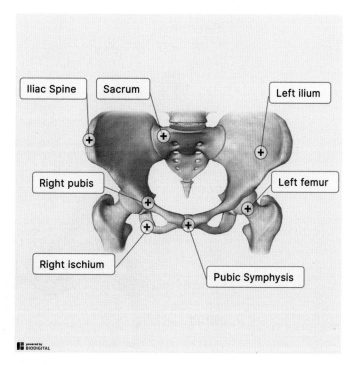

FIGURE 3-32 Male pelvis showing the ilium, pubis, and ischium.

LEARNING OBJECTIVE 3.3.20 **Contrast the male and female pelvis.**

Male versus Female Pelvis

Although the main components of the pelvis do not differ between the sexes, there are some structural differences between the male pelvis and female pelvis. These differences help accommodate changes that occur in the female body during gestation, labor, and childbirth (Figures 3-32 and 3-33 AB). There are three key differences between the male and female pelvis:

- Overall width: The female pelvis is overall wider than the male pelvis. The increased width results in a wider pelvic outlet, allowing the passage of an infant's skull during childbirth.
- Lateral projection: In the female pelvis, the iliac bones project more laterally than in the male pelvis. This provides more space for the growing fetus during gestation.
- Pubic bone angle: The angle between the two pubic bones in the female pelvis is 80–85 degrees, and the male pelvis is roughly 50–60 degrees. The wider angle between the pubic bones reflects the overall wider structure of the female pelvis.

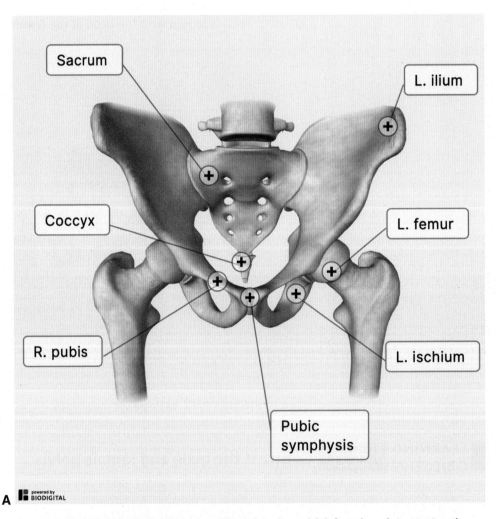

A

FIGURE 3-33AB Differences between the (A) male and (B) female pelvis. Notice the difference in width, angle, and angle between the two pubic bones. (*Continued*)

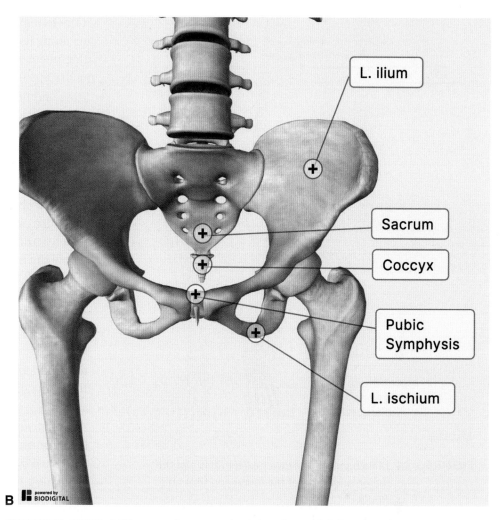

L. ilium

Sacrum

Coccyx

Pubic Symphysis

L. ischium

B

FIGURE 3-33AB Differences between the (A) male and (B) female pelvis. Notice the difference in width, angle, and angle between the two pubic bones.

LEARNING OBJECTIVE **3.3.21** Identify the femur, patella, tibia, fibula, tarsal group, metatarsal group, and phalanges.

LEARNING OBJECTIVE **3.3.22** Describe the structure and important landmarks of bones found in the lower extremities.

LOWER EXTREMITIES

Inferior to the pelvis are the lower extremities. Bones of the lower extremities are part of the appendicular skeleton. These bones serve a variety of purposes and, as such, have specialized structures and landmarks (Figure 3-34).

- Femur (Figure 3-34). Long bone of the thigh that is one of the main weight-bearing bones of the body. The femoral head articulates with the acetabulum of the pelvis to create the hip joint. Just lateral to the femoral head, two projections called trochanters provide attachment sites for muscles that move the thigh. The inferior portion of the bone has condyles, which contribute to the knee joint. The posterior aspect

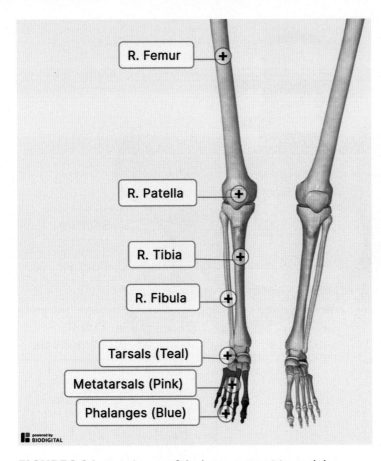

FIGURE 3-34 Main bones of the lower extremities and the major landmarks of the femur and tibia and fibula.

of the femur features a long, raised line along its length. This line is an attachment site for several of the quadriceps muscles.

- Tibia and fibula (3-34). Long bones of the leg that also help bear the weight of the body. They articulate with the femur to make up part of the knee joint and articulate with the tarsal bones to create the ankle joint. The tibia also contains an important structure called the tibial tuberosity, which is the rounded area immediately below the medial and lateral condyles (Figure 3-34). The portion that is typically called the shin is the anterior aspect of the tibia's diaphysis.

- Tarsal bones (Figure 3-34). Short bones of the foot that make up part of the ankle joint. One large tarsal bone, the calcaneus, forms the heel.

- Metatarsal bones (Figure 3-34). Although small in size, they considered long bones. They are located between the tarsal bones and the toes.

- Phalanges (Figure 3-34). The many bones that make up the toes.

- Patella (Figure 3-34). Small bone that forms in the quadriceps tendon that is also known as the kneecap.

UNIT OBJECTIVE 3.4

Describe common pathologies related to the structure and classification of bones.

UNIT INTRODUCTION

Although bones are rigid and perform supportive and protective roles throughout the body, certain pathologies and traumas may cause bones to fracture and break. There are certain areas of bones that may be especially prone to injury based on their shape and function in the body. As a member of the health care team, it will be important for you to understand why bones may break in certain areas as well as common signs and symptoms of bone pathologies.

LEARNING OBJECTIVE **3.4.1** Identify the surgical neck of the femur and humerus.

LEARNING OBJECTIVE **3.4.2** Describe the relationship between the surgical neck of a bone and bone fractures.

KEY TERMS

anatomical neck Bony landmark found between the head and shaft of the bone.

surgical neck Bony landmark in the humerus where breaks often occur.

HUMERUS AND FEMUR FRACTURES

As previously discussed in this chapter, long bones have many different structures and landmarks. Of particular importance are the **anatomical neck** and the **surgical neck**. The anatomical neck is seen in both the femur and the humerus. It is located between the head and shaft of a bone, and it may or may not feature bony landmarks (Figure 3-35AB).

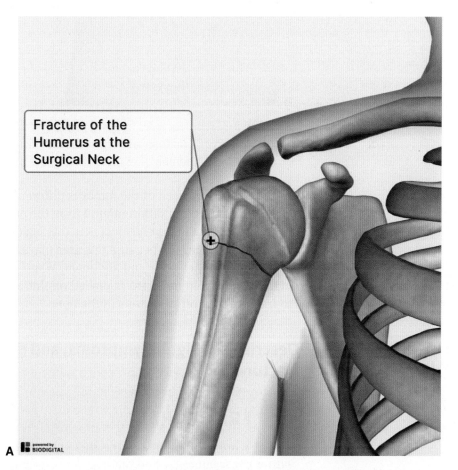

Fracture of the Humerus at the Surgical Neck

A [powered by BIODIGITAL]

FIGURE 3-35AB Fractures in the humerus and the femur. (A) Fracture in the anatomical neck of the humerus. (B) Fracture in the neck of the femur. (*Continued*)

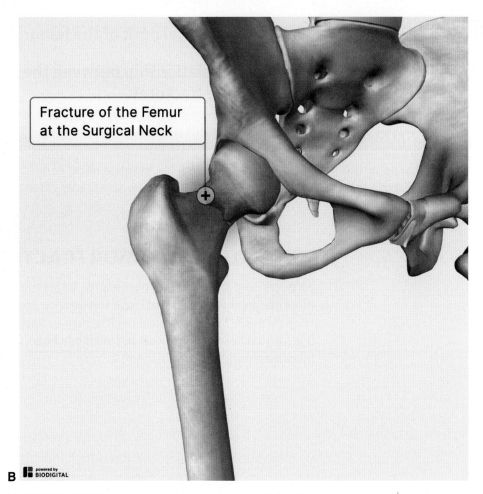

FIGURE 3-35AB Fractures in the humerus and the femur. (A) Fracture in the anatomical neck of the humerus. (B) Fracture in the neck of the femur.

The surgical neck of the femur is different from the anatomical neck. The surgical neck is often differentiated from the anatomical neck in the femur due to the high rate of injury that occurs in this region. Specifically, the femur's surgical neck is a weak spot because this area plays a large role in bearing the weight of the entire upper body and abdomen. When a person falls on the lateral side of the hip, even more stress is placed on this area, which makes it more likely to fracture than other regions of the bone.

LEARNING OBJECTIVE 3.4.3 Describe the signs, symptoms, and diagnosis of a fractured hip.

HIP FRACTURES

The hips are another area of the skeletal system where a high rate of fractures occur. Hip fractures are common in athletes and older adults, particularly older females who more commonly experience decreased bone density and strength due to age-related changes in the body. Technically speaking, a hip fracture is a fracture at the femoral neck; however, it is called a hip fracture because it is close to the hip joint (Figure 3-35B).

Commonly, hip fractures occur after a fall. The patient may complain of a variety of symptoms and display several signs that indicate a hip fracture has occurred:

- Sharp pain in hip
- Unable to bear weight on injured side
- Leg and foot on the injured side often display a lateral or outward rotation
- Bruising and swelling around the injured hip

When a health care provider notes these signs and symptoms, you can expect to assist in carrying out several diagnostic measures to confirm the hip is fractured. These measures can help determine the extent of the injury, which will help determine the appropriate course of treatment:

- The health care provider will note abnormal position of the leg.
- The health care provider will most likely order radiographs of the hip with the suspected injury. This is the most likely way to confirm a hip fracture.
- If the radiographs are inconclusive or if the patient complains of pain high in the hip, additional imaging may be needed to confirm fracture, as fractures high near the hip joint may not be visible on radiographs. In these cases, the health care provider may order magnetic resonance imaging (MRI) or a bone scan to identify a small hairline fracture.

LEARNING OBJECTIVE 3.4.4 Describe the causes of sesamoid bone formation in soft tissue.

KEY TERM

rider's bone Also known as cavalry bone, sesamoid bone that forms in individuals who ride horses often that causes repeated strain on the upper thighs.

SESAMOID BONE FORMATION

Recall that sesamoid bones are bones found within ligaments and tendons. One common example of a sesamoid bone is the patella, also called the kneecap. Occasionally, sesamoid bones may develop in soft tissue as a response to strain. One example of this is known as **rider's bone**, which forms in those who ride horses often. Repeated horseback riding places strain on the upper thigh, causing this sesamoid bone to form.

This strain is not necessarily pathological, but is based on how the joint normally forms and works. For example, without the patella, extension of the knee joint is not very efficient due to the angle of the muscles and the tibia. The patella, however, gives the tendon an attachment that more efficiently transmits forces from the muscle to the tibial tuberosity. In a sense, it acts as a pulley for the tendon that makes the joint move more easily.

Other joints of the body that commonly form sesamoid bones include the metatarsals, metacarpals, feet, and wrists.

UNIT OBJECTIVE 3.5

Describe common pathologies related to the formation and remodeling of bones and bone tissue.

UNIT INTRODUCTION

In addition to understanding common areas of bone that may become injured, it is also important to recognize specific types of bone pathologies. Providing care to patients with bone pathologies requires that you be able to not only recognize the signs and symptoms of different bone pathologies but also that you understand the process through which normal bones heal. Understanding the normal process of bone healing will help you better recognize bone pathologies as well.

LEARNING OBJECTIVE 3.5.1 Identify transverse, linear, oblique, spiral, and comminuted fractures.

LEARNING OBJECTIVE 3.5.2 Describe the six common types of bone fractures and the mechanism that causes them.

LEARNING OBJECTIVE 3.5.3 Contrast the six common types of bone fractures.

KEY TERM

fracture Any type of break in a bone.

TYPES OF FRACTURES

A commonly occurring bone injury is a break in the bone. This is known as a fracture. Fracture refers to any type of break in a bone. There are six main types of fractures that may occur (Figure 3-36):

- Transverse. Most common type of fracture; perpendicular to the length of the bone and are caused by a force striking and bending the bone (Figures 3-36B and 3-37).

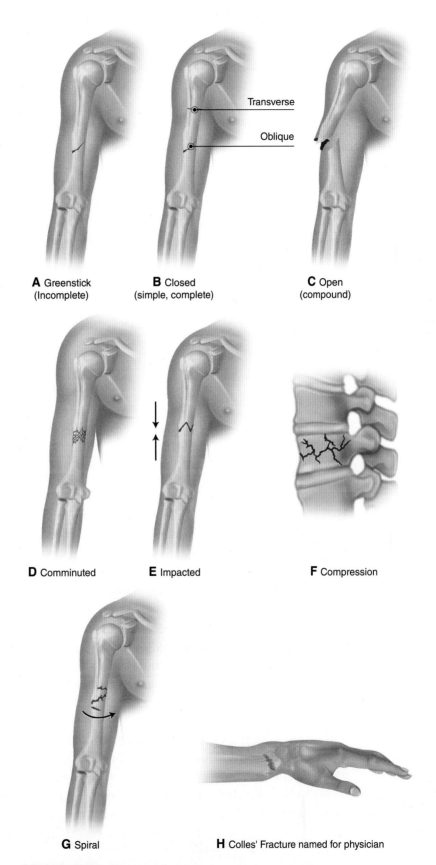

A Greenstick (Incomplete)

B Closed (simple, complete)

Transverse

Oblique

C Open (compound)

D Comminuted

E Impacted

F Compression

G Spiral

H Colles' Fracture named for physician

FIGURE 3-36 Common fractures.

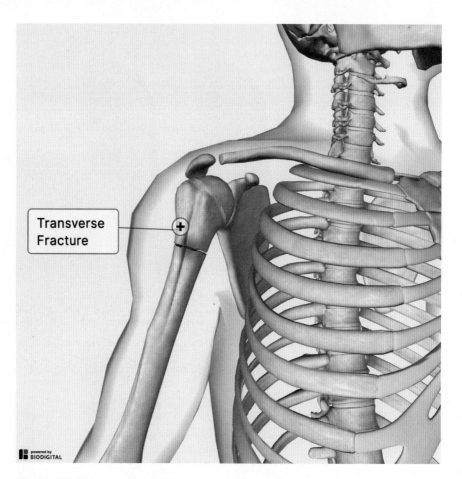

Transverse
Fracture

FIGURE 3-37 Transverse fracture in the upper limb.

- Linear. Break that is a single line; commonly occur as a result of blunt force trauma or hitting the bone directly with a very heavy object.
- Oblique (Figure 3-38). Diagonal to the length of the bone; often result from twisting injuries.
- Spiral (Figure 3-36G). Break in the bone in several places. Similarly to oblique fractures, also occur as a result of twisting bone, but this yields a break that is around the entire bone (Figure 3-36G) rather than a single diagonal break (Figure 3-38). For example, this may occur if someone's foot is firmly planted but their body continues to move.
- Comminuted (Figures 3-36D and 3-39). Several fragments of bone that is often the result of high-impact trauma, such as someone who has been in a motor vehicle accident.
- Greenstick. When a bone bends and snaps (Figure 3-36A) rather than breaking into several pieces; named for its resemblance to a small crack in a tree branch. They are common in children, as their bones still have not fully hardened and have the ability to flex to a very small degree.

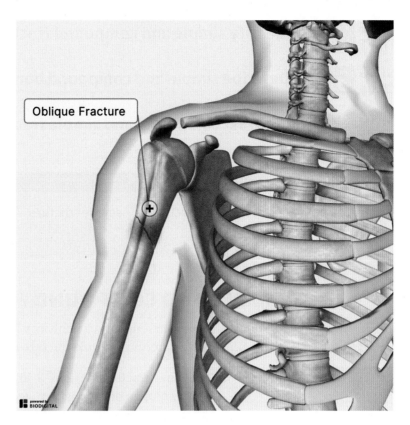

FIGURE 3-38 Oblique fracture in the upper limb.

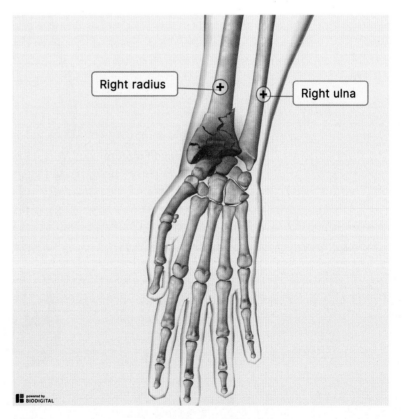

FIGURE 3-39 Comminuted fracture in the wrist.

LEARNING OBJECTIVE 3.5.4 Identify simple and compound fractures.

LEARNING OBJECTIVE 3.5.5 Describe simple and compound bone fractures.

LEARNING OBJECTIVE 3.5.6 Contrast compound and simple fractures.

KEY TERMS

compound fracture Broken bones that puncture the skin and are significantly displaced.

simple fracture Also called closed fractures, breaks in the bone that do not protrude through the skin.

SIMPLE AND COMPOUND FRACTURES

In addition to the different ways a bone may break, bones may also be referred to as compound fractures or simple fractures.

- Compound fractures (Figure 3-40). Also known as open fractures, refer to broken bones that are significantly displaced and that puncture the skin. These may be caused by high-speed collisions. Because the bone protrudes through the skin, they have a high risk of infection and often require surgical correction.

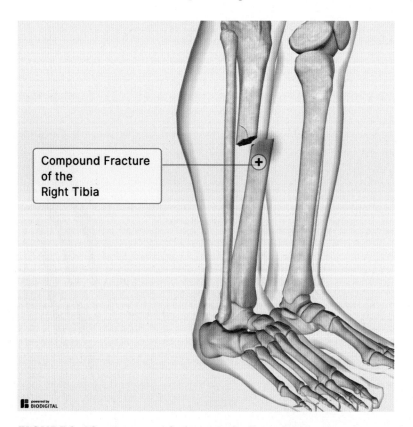

Compound Fracture of the Right Tibia

powered by BIODIGITAL

FIGURE 3-40 Compound fracture in the lower limb.

- **Simple fracture** (Figure 3-37). Also referred to as closed fractures, refer to breaks in the bone that do not protrude through the skin. These are far less likely than compound fractures to cause infection and do not usually require surgery.

LEARNING OBJECTIVE 3.5.7 Explain the four-step process of bone repair and modeling.

KEY TERMS

hematoma Swelling in one area that is filled with blood.

remodeling Process in which osteoblasts and osteoclasts work together to reshape the repair

site of a broken bone so that it resembles original bone before fracture.

BONE REPAIR

After a bone is injured, the body enacts a healing cascade to help repair the broken bone. This process involves four main steps (Figure 3-41ABCD):

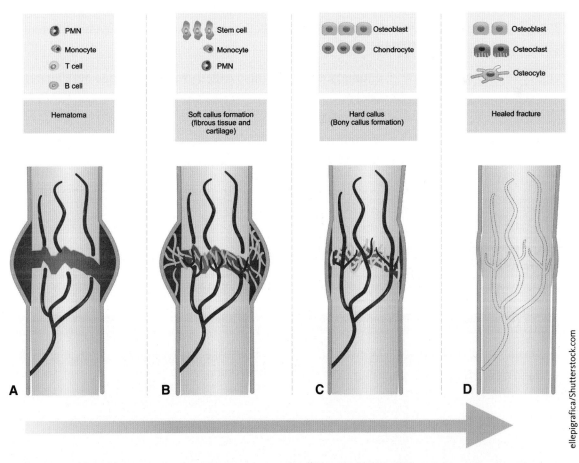

FIGURE 3-41ABCD Four steps of fracture repair. (A) Development of hematoma; (B) soft callus forms; (C) bony callous forms; and (D) woven bone remodeling.

ellepigrafica/Shutterstock.com

- Step 1 (Figure 3-41A): Ruptured blood vessels from the bone begin to form a hematoma around site of fracture that helps to stop bleeding in the area.
- Step 2 (Figure 3-41B): Once clotting begins and a hematoma forms, a soft cartilaginous callus forms around the fractured ends of the bone.
- Step 3 (Figure 3-41C): The soft callus is replaced by a hard, bony callus in a process similar to endochondral ossification (see "Endochondral Ossification" earlier in this chapter for a detailed discussion).
- Step 4 (Figure 3-41D): Newly formed bone is remodeled. In fracture repair, remodeling is a process in which osteoblasts and osteoclasts work together to reshape the repair site so that it resembles the original bone before fracture.

LEARNING OBJECTIVE 3.5.8 Identify common conditions that affect bone formation and growth.

CONDITIONS THAT ALTER BONE REPAIR AND GROWTH

The four-step process of bone repair and the process of bone growth and development mentioned in the last section may be altered by several different conditions that include:

- Pituitary dwarfism (also called growth hormone deficiency)
- Rickets
- Osteomalacia
- Acromegaly
- Gigantism

These conditions are discussed in greater detail in the next sections of this chapter.

LEARNING OBJECTIVE 3.5.9 Describe the signs, symptoms, and diagnosis of pituitary dwarfism.

KEY TERMS

achondroplasia Most common form of dwarfism.

pituitary dwarfism Genetically inherited condition in which the pituitary gland does not release an adequate amount of growth hormone.

Pituitary Dwarfism

Pituitary dwarfism (Figure 3-42) is a genetically inherited condition in which the pituitary gland does not release an adequate amount of growth hormone. This inhibits normal bone development, causing a person to have a smaller adult skeleton (roughly 4 feet tall or shorter). Patients with this condition may either have proportionate or disproportionate dwarfism:

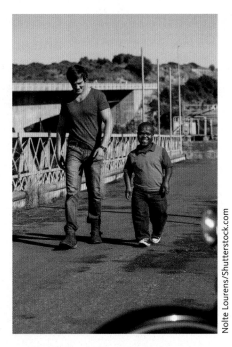

FIGURE 3-42 Person on the right with pituitary dwarfism.

- Proportionate: All parts of the body are small to the same degree. This condition appears at birth or early childhood and causes all growth to be inhibited.
- Disproportionate: Some body parts are small, whereas others are average sized. For example, patients with **achondroplasia**, the most common type of dwarfism, will exhibit an average-sized torso with shorter-than-average limbs. The head may be average sized or slightly larger than normal. This is the result of inhibited bone growth at the epiphyseal plates.

This condition usually presents at birth or early in development when a child does not meet expected growth rates. Common signs and symptoms include below-average growth, immature appearance, and an underdeveloped nose bridge. Diagnosis includes:

- A physical exam that may include measurements of weight, height, and circumference of the skull
- A thorough family history analysis including DNA testing
- Blood tests analyzing growth hormone levels
- X-rays that may reveal skeletal abnormalities
- MRI to identify abnormalities of the hypothalamus or pituitary gland

CLINICAL NOTE	When caring for patients diagnosed with dwarfism, it is best to ask which terminology is preferred, such as *little person*, *person with dwarfism*, or *person of short stature*. Certain terms are considered offensive.

KEY TERMS

acromegaly Condition causing excessive growth in adulthood.

gigantism Growth disorder causing excessive growth in children prior to growth plate closure.

Gigantism and Acromegaly

Gigantism and acromegaly and are both disorders that cause excessive growth due to excess growth hormone. They most commonly arise due to a tumor affecting the pituitary gland.

- **Gigantism** typically affects children prior to growth plate closure. Children with gigantism show exaggerated bone growth and excessive increase in height over a short period of time. Often, children will appear proportional but will experience above-average growth in their epiphyseal plates. This may make them appear very tall and giant-like.

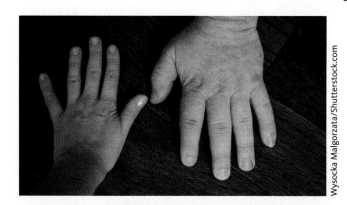

- **Acromegaly** (Figure 3-43) typically affects adults after their growth plates have closed. As such, growth in individuals with this condition occurs slowly. It is not easily recognized early on as in gigantism. Individuals with this condition may also have cardiovascular complications, including an enlarged heart. Patients with acromegaly may begin to have enlarged hands, a deepened voice, and enlarged facial features. Enlarged facial features may occur due to an overgrowth of cartilaginous structures, such as a person's ears and nose. Since this condition causes bones to become enlarged, facial features may become disproportionate, especially the brow and lower jaw.

Wysocka Malgorzata/Shutterstock.com

FIGURE 3-43 Effects of acromegaly compared with an average adult hand. Note the enlarged hands. How acromegaly alters a patient's hand throughout his life.

Rickets

Rickets is a condition caused by prolonged vitamin D deficiency during child-hood. Since vitamin D helps the body absorb and use calcium for bone growth and hardening of the bone (as discussed in Unit 3.1 of this chapter), this deficiency causes the bones to soften and warp into abnormal shapes. Because this occurs in childhood, it affects overall bone growth and development. The osteoid is formed normally, but the bone is not able to mineralize properly.

There are many signs and symptoms that may present in patients with this condition. They include:

- Delayed and/or below-average growth
- Pain in spine
- Bowed legs (Figure 3-44)
- Sternum projection
- Delayed closure of **fontanelles**

When a health care provider suspects that a patient may have rickets, several diagnostic tests may be performed to confirm the diagnosis:

- Radiographs can identify bone abnormalities, such as bowing or bending of long bones
- Blood tests will show below-average levels of vitamin D

Forms of Rickets

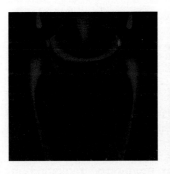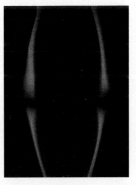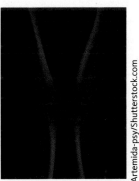

Artemida-psy/Shutterstock.com

FIGURE 3-44 Bowed legs typical in rickets.

LEARNING OBJECTIVE 3.5.13 Identify the condition known as osteomalacia.

LEARNING OBJECTIVE 3.5.14 Describe the signs, symptoms, and diagnosis of osteomalacia.

LEARNING OBJECTIVE 3.5.15 Contrast rickets and osteomalacia.

KEY TERMS

gait How a person walks.

osteomalacia Condition caused by prolonged, severe vitamin D deficiency, which leads to softening and weakening of bones in adulthood.

Osteomalacia

A condition that is similar to rickets is osteomalacia. Also caused by prolonged, severe vitamin D deficiency, osteomalacia causes softness and weakening of the bones. However, this condition occurs in adults rather than in children (as is seen in rickets). As with rickets, this vitamin D deficiency leads to the body's inability to absorb and use calcium. This leads the body to release calcitonin, which is a hormone that stimulates osteoblasts to create new bone matrix. Unlike rickets, this can occur secondary to osteoporosis and causes the bones to be weak and more prone to fractures. This contrasts with rickets, which causes abnormal development of bones.

Signs and symptoms of osteomalacia are similar to those seen in individuals with rickets, with only subtle differences. These include the following:

- Aching pain in the back and lower limbs
- Leg weakness
- Waddling gait
- Weak bones that are more susceptible to fractures, including nontraumatic fractures

When a health care provider suspects osteomalacia based on presenting signs and symptoms, a series of tests can confirm the diagnosis. These include the following:

- Blood and urine tests can be used to determine vitamin D levels in the blood, which will indicate whether the patient is vitamin D deficient.
- Radiographs can identify cracks in bones.
- Bone biopsy can detect osteomalacia.

UNIT OBJECTIVE 3.6

Describe common pathologies related to the spinal column.

UNIT INTRODUCTION

Many of the common bone pathologies we just discussed influence the normal development of bones throughout the body including the spinal column. Specifically, several pathologies may influence the normal curvatures of the spine and have serious effects that relate to a patient's overall health. Every member of the health care team should know and understand the signs, symptoms, and diagnostic procedures to help provide care to patients who have these conditions.

LEARNING OBJECTIVE 3.6.1 Identify common pathologies related to the bones of the spinal column.

KEY TERMS

kyphosis (Exaggeration of the primary curvature of the thoracic spine.)

lordosis (Exaggeration in the curvature of the lumbar spine.)

scoliosis Lateral bending of the spinal column caused by birth defect or other conditions.

COMMON SKELETAL SYSTEM PATHOLOGIES

As with other body systems, the skeletal system may also experience pathologic conditions. Pathologies affecting the skeletal system may be the result of a variety of factors, including genetics, age, posture, or environmental factors. Some of the most common pathologies affecting the skeletal system involve abnormalities in the spinal column. Specifically, these pathologies may cause abnormal curvatures of the spinal column (Figure 3-45ABC). These conditions include:

- Scoliosis
- Lordosis
- Kyphosis

Although these conditions all change the spinal column and may be diagnosed using similar tools, such as radiographs, it is important to understand the differences between these conditions to provide excellent patient care.

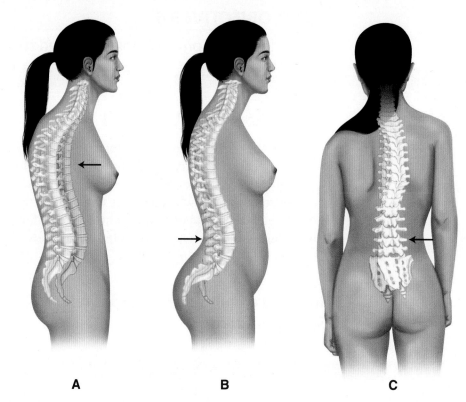

A   **B**   **C**

FIGURE 3-45ABC Differences of how (A) kyphosis, (B) lordosis, and (C) scoliosis
impact the curvatures of the spinal column.

LEARNING OBJECTIVE 3.6.2 Identify scoliosis of the spinal column.

LEARNING OBJECTIVE 3.6.3 Describe the signs, symptoms, and diagnosis of scoliosis.

Scoliosis

Scoliosis refers to a lateral bending in the coronal plane of the spinal column
(Figure 3-46). It can be caused by birth defects in the shape of the spinal column
or the presence of other conditions, such as muscular dystrophy or cerebral
palsy. Generally, the condition becomes more pronounced during childhood
and adolescence. As such, screening for scoliosis is commonly performed in
public schools throughout the United States during late elementary and early
middle school.

The severity of scoliosis (i.e., the degree of bending found in the spine)
may vary from person to person. However, a person with scoliosis commonly
presents with the following signs and symptoms:

- Uneven shoulders in which one shoulder appears higher than the
  other (Figure 3-46)
- One scapula protruding more prominently than the other scapula

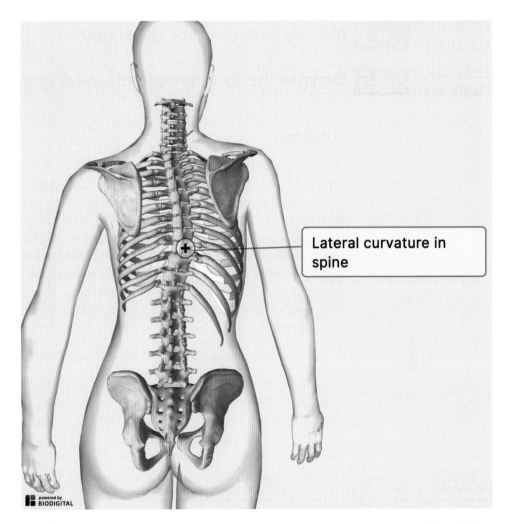

Lateral curvature in spine

FIGURE 3-46 Curvature of the spinal column that appears in patients with scoliosis.

- Pelvis may be tilted to one side
- Uneven waist in which one hip appears to be higher than the other

Once a health care provider suspects scoliosis may be present, several measures can be taken to confirm the diagnosis. Diagnostics include the following:

- Physical examination, which will confirm the previously mentioned signs and symptoms.
- Radiograph, which will reveal the curvature and help determine the degree and location of abnormal curvatures.
- Magnetic resonance imaging (MRI), which may be required to provide better visualization of the disease's progression and impact on the spinal column.

Clear visualization of the curvature is important for determining the appropriate treatment of the condition.

LEARNING OBJECTIVE 3.6.4 **Identify lordosis of the spinal column.**

LEARNING OBJECTIVE 3.6.5 **Describe the signs, symptoms, and diagnosis of lordosis.**

Lordosis

Lordosis (Figure 3-47) refers to an exaggeration in the curvature of the lumbar spine. As you may recall from Unit 3.3 of this chapter, the secondary curvature of the spine develops as a person's muscles develop. Thus, this condition is primarily caused by musculature that is very tight and pulls the lumbar vertebrae into a more exaggerated curvature. Frequently, this is a result of poor posture or excessive weight. It is difficult for the body to carry extra weight near the abdomen, which may be seen in patients who are overweight and obese. These patients may tend to lean back while standing. Eventually, the body adapts to this position and the musculature tightens to compensate.

A person with lordosis may present with the following signs and symptoms:

- Lumbar spine features deep curve
- Protruded abdomen due to exaggerated curve
- Pelvis tilts anteriorly

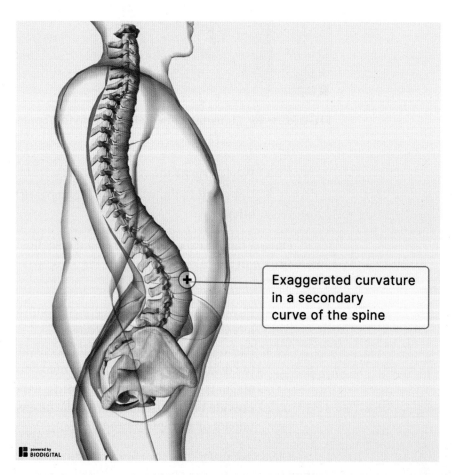

Exaggerated curvature in a secondary curve of the spine

FIGURE 3-47 Curvature of the spinal column that appears in patients with lordosis.

Diagnosis of this condition involves physical examinations to determine what signs and symptoms are present. The patient will also likely undergo radiographs to visualize the spine and determine the severity of the disease. Since this condition occurs due to abnormally tight musculature, it can be treated through physical therapy that restores normal muscle function and returns spinal curvature to a normal state.

LEARNING OBJECTIVE 3.6.6 Identify kyphosis of the spinal column.

LEARNING OBJECTIVE 3.6.7 Describe the signs, symptoms, and diagnosis of kyphosis.

Kyphosis

Kyphosis (Figure 3-48) is an exaggeration of the primary curvature of the thoracic spine. Unlike the musculature causes of lordosis, kyphosis occurs when thoracic vertebrae change and become more wedge shaped.

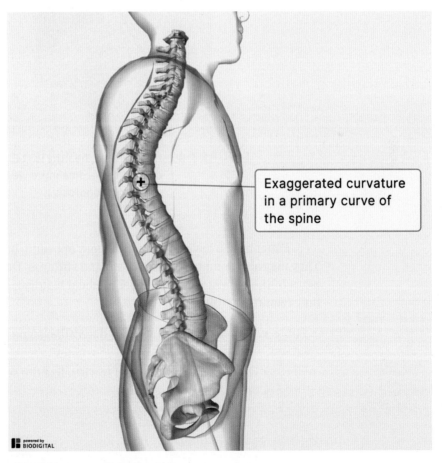

Exaggerated curvature in a primary curve of the spine

FIGURE 3-48 Curvature of the spinal column that appears in patients with kyphosis.

Kyphosis that occurs in adults is often the result of underlying pathologies that degrade bone structure and disc structure, such as osteoporosis and other osteodegenerative diseases (Figure 3-49). When it occurs in children, it is often due to vertebrae that have developed abnormally.

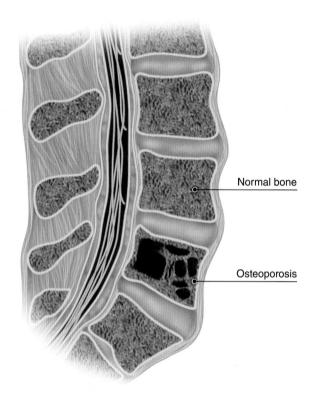

Normal bone

Osteoporosis

FIGURE 3-49 How normal, healthy vertebrae may change to become more wedge shaped due to osteoporosis.

Patients who have this condition may appear to have a "hump" (Figure 3-50). They may also complain of back pain and stiffness. Depending on the characteristics of the patient (age, sex, past medical history), diagnosis of the condition may require the following:

- Physical examination to determine signs and symptoms present
- Radiograph and/or MRI to visualize the spine and its condition
- Bone density test

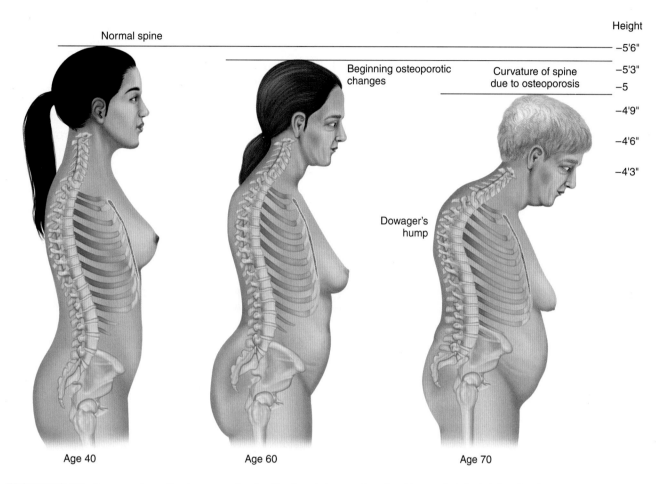

Height
−5'6"
−5'3"
−5
−4'9"
−4'6"
−4'3"

Normal spine

Beginning osteoporotic changes

Curvature of spine due to osteoporosis

Dowager's hump

Age 40   Age 60   Age 70

FIGURE 3-50 Progression of osteoporosis. On the far right, notice the disease has led to kyphosis.

LEARNING OBJECTIVE **3.6.8** Contrast the conditions of scoliosis, lordosis, and kyphosis.

DIFFERENCES BETWEEN COMMON SPINAL CONDITIONS

As previously mentioned, scoliosis, lordosis, and kyphosis are all conditions of abnormal bending or curvature in the spine; however, they differ in type and place of curvature, causes, typical appearance, and diagnostic methods (Table 3-1). In scoliosis, the curvature is lateral, whereas lordosis and kyphosis involve exaggerated anterior and posterior sagittal curvature, respectively. The bending in scoliosis can occur throughout the spinal column, affecting the shoulders, scapulae, and pelvis. Lordosis occurs only in the lumbar spine, and kyphosis occurs only in the thoracic spine.

Scoliosis, lordosis, and kyphosis differ widely in their causes (Table 3-1). Scoliosis is caused mainly by birth defects or other underlying conditions. Lordosis occurs as a result of poor posture or excessive weight. Kyphosis usually occurs late in life as a result of osteodegenerative disease.

The typical appearance of each condition is a result of the curvature. Common signs of scoliosis include lateral unevenness in the shoulders, scapulae, or pelvis. The exaggerated anterior curvature of lordosis results in a protruded abdomen and anteriorly tilted pelvis, while the posterior curvature of kyphosis produces a "hump" in the upper back. Physical examination and radiograph are helpful in diagnosing all three conditions. Diagnosis of kyphosis may also benefit from a bone density test.

Table 3-1 Comparison of Scoliosis, Lordosis, and Kyphosis

	SCOLIOSIS	LORDOSIS	KYPHOSIS
Description of abnormality	Lateral bending in the coronal plane of the spinal column	Exaggeration of the curvature of the lumbar spine	Exaggeration of the primary curvature of the thoracic spine
Areas impacted	Spinal column	Lumbar spine	Thoracic spine
Causes and implications	Birth defects in the shape of the spinal column; muscular dystrophy; cerebral palsy	Tight musculature as a result of poor posture or excessive weight	Abnormal development of vertebrae; underlying pathologies that degrade bone structure and disc structure
Typical appearance	Uneven shoulders; greater protrusion of one scapula; tilted pelvis; uneven waist	Deeply curved lumbar spine; protruded abdomen; anteriorly tilted pelvis	"Hump" in the upper back
Diagnostic methods	Physical examination; radiograph; magnetic resonance imaging (MRI)	Physical examinations; radiograph	Physical examinations; radiograph; MRI; bone density test

Chapter 4

Joints of the Human Body

Chapter Introduction

In this chapter, we learn about the different joints and their function in the human body. Joints, also known as articulations, are places where bones or bone and cartilage come together to form a connection. Every joint is constructed differently to allow for different degrees and types of skeletal movement. Joints hold the skeleton together and give it mobility. We discuss the range of motion and different functions of the three types of joints.

UNIT OBJECTIVE 4.1

Describe articulations that are synarthroses, amphiarthroses, and diarthroses.

UNIT INTRODUCTION

The functional classification of joints is based on the amount of movement allowed by the joint. There are three functional classifications of joints: synarthroses, amphiarthroses, and diarthroses. This unit discusses the joints that are found in each of these three classifications, as well as the movement that is permitted by each functional classification of joints.

LEARNING OBJECTIVE 4.1.1 Identify synarthrotic joints in the body.

KEY TERMS

alveolus Bony socket for the root of a tooth.

articulating bones Bones that move around a connecting joint.

cranial plates Bones of the skull.

gomphosis Fibrous joint that holds the teeth in their sockets and is found on the maxilla and mandible.

interosseous membrane Broad, thick, and dense fibrous tissue between many bones in the body.

ligament Fibrous connective tissue that supports and holds the bones and internal organs in a stable position.

mandible Lower jaw.

maxilla Upper jaw.

periodontal ligament Group of specialized connective fibers that attach a tooth to the alveolar bone.

pronate To rotate the hand so that the palm is facing downward or to turn the sole of the foot outward.

supinate To hold a hand, foot, or limb so that the palm or sole is facing upward or outward.

sutures Immovable joints between skull bones.

syndesmoses Fibrous joint in which connective tissue joins the bones such as fibula and tibia.

synostoses Fusion of two bones.

SYNARTHROTIC JOINTS OF THE BODY

Synarthrotic joints are either slightly movable or immovable. Generally, synarthrotic joints are fibrous. The immobile nature of these joints forms a strong union between the articulating bones they connect. Because of this strength, synarthrotic joints are important at locations where bones provide protection for internal organs. An example is the manubriosternal joint. This cartilaginous joint unites the manubrium and the body of the sternum for protection of the heart. Let's take a moment and discuss the types of synarthrotic joints.

There are three types of synarthrotic joints: the sutures, gomphosis, and syndesmoses. The word *sutures* literally means "seams." Suture joints are only found in the skull (Figure 4-1). All of the bones in the skull, except the mandible, are connected with suture joints. These joints contain short, interlocking, and very rigid fibrous connective tissue that prevents the movement of the cranial plates and protects the brain. Initially, the fibrous nature of the suture joints allows the skull to expand as the brain grows during youth. As aging occurs, the fibers harden and the skull bones harden into a single unit. At this point, they are called synostoses.

The second type of synarthrotic joint is gomphosis, also known as a peg-and-socket joint. These are joints in which a conical process fits into a socket and is held in place by ligaments. The only place gomphosis exist in the body

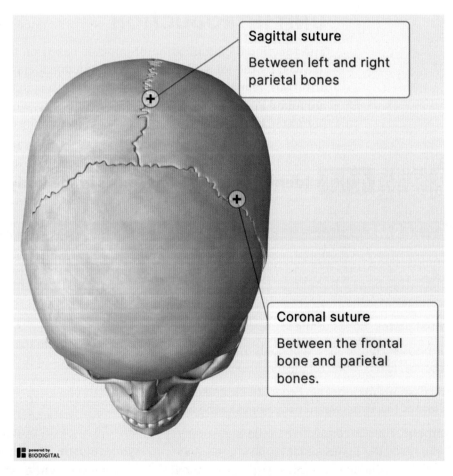

Sagittal suture

Between left and right parietal bones

Coronal suture

Between the frontal bone and parietal bones.

FIGURE 4-1 The sutures found between cranial bones.

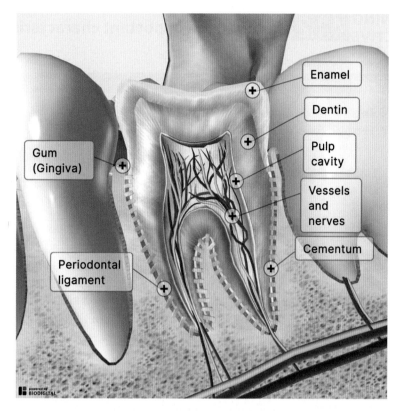

FIGURE 4-2 Cross section of the tooth showing a gomphosis joint.

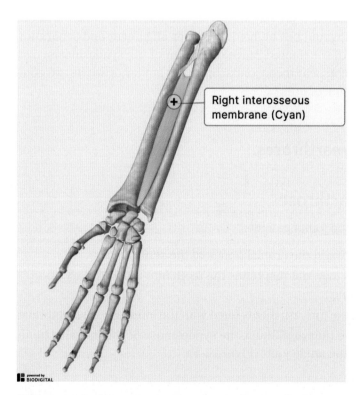

FIGURE 4-3 The interosseous membrane between the radius and ulna is a type on synarthrotic joint.

is in the mouth, where teeth roots are held into the **alveolus** (Figure 4-2). The teeth are held in place by the **periodontal ligament**. These fibrous joints bind the teeth into the bony sockets of the **maxilla** and mandible.

Lastly, a syndesmosis is a joint that is slightly moveable. At a syndesmosis, the bones are more widely separated but are held together by a strap of fibrous connective tissue called a **ligament** or a wide sheet of connective tissue called an **interosseous membrane**. The amount of movement at a syndesmosis is dependent on the length of the connecting fibers, which can vary. Short fibers allow for little or no movement, while longer fibers allow for more movement. An example of a fibrous joint with short connecting fibers is the joint that binds the tibia and fibula. An example of a fibrous joint with longer connecting fibers is found where the radius articulates with the ulna (Figure 4-3). Because of syndesmosis, these bones move as one when we **pronate** or **supinate** the forearm or rotate the lower leg.

KEY TERM

fibrous joints Fixed or immobile joints that are
connected by dense, tough connective tissue.

Characteristics of a Synarthrosis

An important characteristic of a synarthrosis is that the **fibrous joints** do not
have a cavity between them and the adjacent bones are directly connected by
fibrous connective tissue. The fibrous connective tissue between the suture
bones is what prevents movement or provides for very limited movement. The
immobility of the sutures in the skull is essential for the protection of internal
organs such as the brain. Without the fibrous joints the plates of the skull would
be malleable, moving over each other slightly and putting the brain at risk for
injury.

Gomphosis allows for minimal movement of the teeth when chewing. This
movement lessens the impact between the upper and lower teeth during biting,
allowing the pressure created while chewing to be evenly distributed among
all teeth. This limited movement is also what allows braces to do their work—
they use this range of movement to push teeth into new positions. Syndesmosis
provides strength and stability, preventing the separation of the bones. Without
syndesmosis the joints would not be held in proper alignment and separation
would occur. Because of the limited range of motion of the syndesmosis, ligament injuries are common near these joints. Sprained ankles or wrists are common examples of this type of injury.

Examples of Synarthroses

Examples of synarthrotic joints include:

- Sutures between the cranial bones of the skull.
- The fibrous material that binds the teeth into the maxillary bone
  and mandible.
- The gap in the forearm that is filled with the interosseous membrane.
- Between the tibia and fibula, the syndesmosis locks the talus bone
  in place at the ankle joint (Figure 4-4).

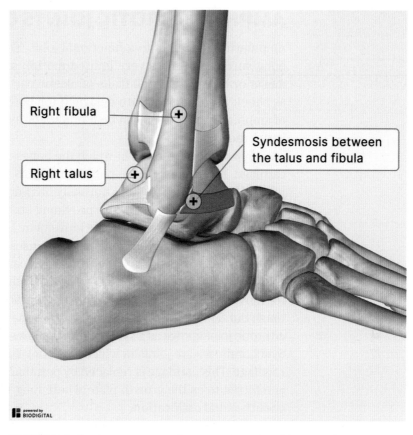

Right fibula ⊕

Right talus ⊕

Syndesmosis between the talus and fibula

⊕

powered by
BIODIGITAL

FIGURE 4-4 The connection between the tibia, fibula, and talus bones is a type of syndesmosis. The short fibers of the syndesmosis allow for a limited range of motion.

LEARNING OBJECTIVE 4.1.4 Identify amphiarthrotic joints in the body.

KEY TERMS

cartilaginous joints Joints connected by fibrocartilage or hyaline cartilage that allow for movement.

endochondral ossification Process through which bone is created from a cartilage model.

hyaline cartilage Type of connective tissue that is to some degree flexible and found in areas of the body, such as the nose, ears, and ribs.

relaxin Hormone; in pregnant women, the placenta secretes relaxin and relaxes the pelvic ligaments.

symphyses Fibrocartilaginous joint fusion between two bones.

symphysis pubis Cartilaginous joint that joins the left and right superior rami of the pubic bone.

synchondrosis Slightly moveable joint between bones that is composed of hyaline cartilage.

AMPHIARTHROTIC JOINTS OF THE BODY

Amphiarthrosis refers to a functional joint. This type of articulation between bony surfaces permits very limited motion and is connected by either ligaments or broad, flattened disks of elastic cartilage. Amphiarthrotic joints act as shock absorbers and are designed for both strength and flexibility. Types of amphiarthrotic joints can be found in the **symphysis pubis** and between the vertebrae.

Symphyses are joints in which the bones are connected by a disk of fibro-cartilage. An example is the pubic symphysis where the two pelvic bones are joined (Figure 4-5). This joint normally has very limited mobility, which allows the pelvis to bear weight while providing stability to the body. However, the fibrocartilage does allow for some movement. During pregnancy and childbirth, increased levels of the hormone **relaxin** causes increased mobility of the pelvic bones, making it easier for the mother to carry and deliver her baby. These **cartilaginous joints** also unite the bodies of the adjacent vertebrae, providing for movement. Cartilaginous joints are characterized by a lack of cavity. The tough but flexible cartilage lies adjacent to the bones uniting them. The amphiarthrotic joint known as a **synchondrosis** allows for the growth of the long bones. Synchondroses are joints in which two bony surfaces are connected by **hyaline cartilage**. This cartilage is replaced by permanent bone later in life. This is what is referred to as the growth plate where long bones develop longitudinally by **endochondral ossification**.

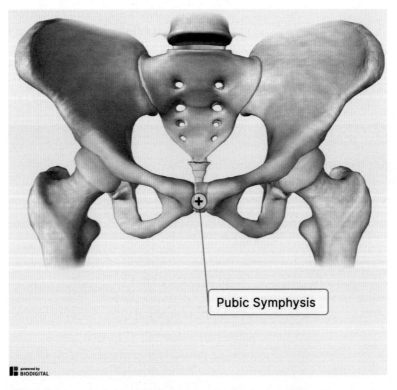

Pubic Symphysis

FIGURE 4-5 The pubic symphysis is where the right and left sides of the pelvis connect anteriorly. This joint only provides for very limited movement.

LEARNING OBJECTIVE **4.1.5** **Describe the important characteristics of an amphiarthrosis.**

KEY TERM

fibrocartilage Type of durable cartilage with many fibers and very little extracellular matrix found in the intervertebral discs, the menisci of the knee, and the pubic symphysis; acts as a shock absorber and resists compression.

Characteristics of an Amphiarthrosis

Amphiarthrotic joints are classified as cartilaginous joints and are slightly moveable, providing for very little range of movement. The amphiarthrosis contains an interosseous joint space that is occupied by **fibrocartilage** or hyaline cartilage. The cartilage that fills the joint space is surrounded by ligaments providing stability for the joint. Their structure is mainly cartilaginous, and the bony surfaces of the joint are generally flat or concave. These cartilaginous joints are connected by fibrocartilage or hyaline cartilage. These two types of joints are synchondrosis and symphysis. A synchondrosis is a joint where the bones are joined or united by hyaline cartilage (Figure 4-6). Fibrocartilage joins the bones in a symphysial joint (Figure 4-7).

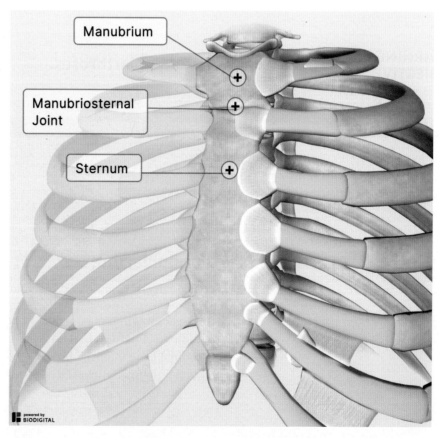

FIGURE 4-6 The joint between the manubrium and sternum is a type of synchondrosis.

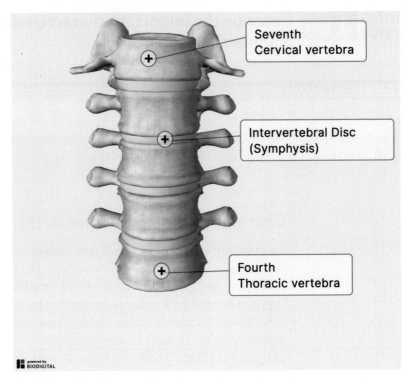

FIGURE 4-7 Another type of symphysis joint are the intervertebral disks found between the vertebrae of the spinal column.

LEARNING OBJECTIVE 4.1.6 **List examples of amphiarthroses.**

KEY TERM

epiphyseal line Junction line of long bone end part (epiphysis) and central part of the long bone (diaphysis), where growth in length occurs.

Examples of Amphiarthroses

Synchondrosis consisting of hyaline cartilage include:

- Epiphyseal growth plate—a disk of cartilage that is organized into a physiological pattern that as it matures is responsible for the longitudinal growth of the bones (Figure 4-8ABC). Once growth is completed, the plate turns into the **epiphyseal line**.

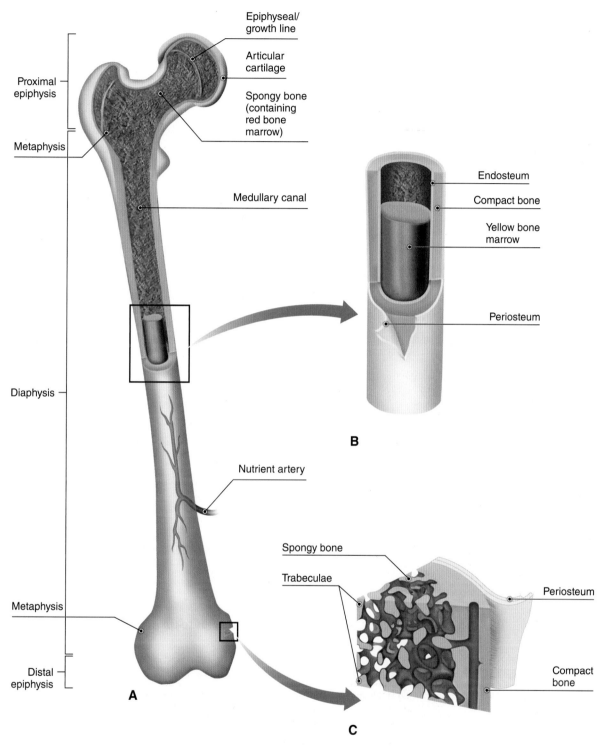

Proximal
epiphysis

Metaphysis

Diaphysis

Metaphysis

Distal
epiphysis

A

Epiphyseal/
growth line

Articular
cartilage

Spongy bone
(containing
red bone
marrow)

Medullary canal

Nutrient artery

Endosteum

Compact bone

Yellow bone
marrow

Periosteum

B

Spongy bone

Trabeculae

Periosteum

Compact
bone

C

FIGURE 4-8ABC The epiphyseal growth plate is where the bone lengthens as it grows. Due to the presence of cartilage, the epiphyseal growth plate is a type of synchondrosis.

- Manubriosternal junction—the articulation between the upper two parts of the sternum, the manubrium and sternal body.
- Costal cartilage—segments of cartilage that connect the sternum to the ribs (Figure 4-9).

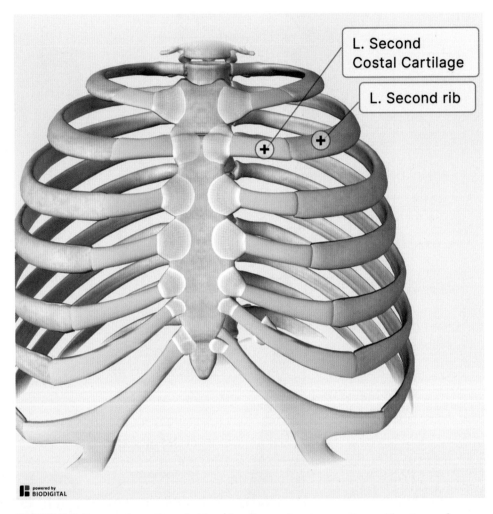

FIGURE 4-9 Costal cartilage linking the ribs to the sternum is another type of synchondrosis.

Symphyses consisting of fibrocartilage include:

- Intervertebral disk—a layer of cartilage that separates the vertebrae in the spine.
- Pubic symphysis—a cartilaginous joint that is located between the left and right pubic bones near the midline of the body.
- Temporomandibular joint—the hinge joint between the temporal bone and the lower jaw (Figure 4-10).

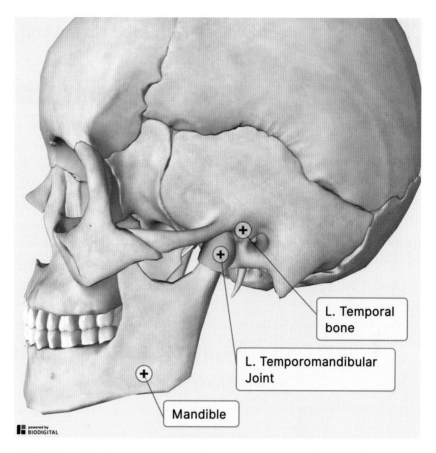

FIGURE 4-10 The temporomandibular joint contains fibrocartilage and is a type of symphysis joint.

CLINICAL TIP	The manubriosternal joint is also known as the angle of Louis. The angle of Louis is an important landmark formed between the manubrium and the body of the sternum. This landmark is used to identify the location of the following:

- The intervertebral disk between T-4 and T-5 in the spine, which is at the exact same level as the angle of Louis
- The second rib, which is important when counting ribs and identifying cardiac landmarks, articulates at the angle of Louis
- The aortic arch (the curved part of the aorta between the ascending and descending aorta)
- The point where the trachea divides into the bronchi
- Cardiac plexus nerves that lie behind the concavity of the aortic arch
- Division of the pulmonary trunk into the right and left pulmonary branches
- Left recurrent laryngeal, which contains the vagus nerve and is located left of the aortic arch
- The ligament arteriosum, which connects the aortic arch to the pulmonary trunk
- The thoracic duct that empties into the left subclavian vein

**LEARNING
OBJECTIVE** 4.1.7 **Identify diarthrotic joints in the body.**

KEY TERMS

ball-and-socket joint Spheroidal joint that allows for extension, flexion, abduction, and internal and external rotation.

ellipsoidal joint Joint shaped like a ball and socket that can rotate on two axes but does not allow for rotation.

gliding joint Also known as a plane or planar joint, allows the bones to glide past one another in any direction along the plane of a joint;

directions include left and right, up and down, and diagonally.

hinge joint Joint formed from two or more bones where the bones can only move along one axis to flex or extend.

pivot joint Type of joint that permits rotation around a single axis.

saddle joint Joint that allows for abduction, adduction, flexion, and extension.

DIARTHROTIC JOINTS IN THE BODY

Diarthrotic joints in the body include:

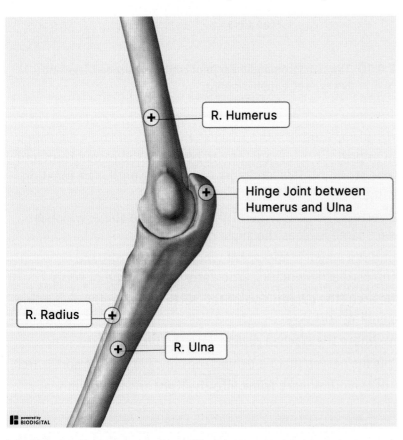

FIGURE 4-11 The elbow, which connects the humerus and ulna, is a type of synovial hinge joint.

- **Hinge joint**—Joint formed from two or more bones where the bones can only move along one axis to flex or extend (Figure 4-11).
- **Pivot joint**—Type of joint that permits rotation around a single axis (Figure 4-12).
- **Gliding joint**—Also known as a plane or planar joint, this joint allows the bones to glide past one another in any direction along the plane of a joint. The directions include left and right, up and down, and diagonally (Figure 4-13).
- **Ellipsoidal joint**—Joint shaped like a ball and socket that can rotate on two axes but does not allow for rotation (Figure 4-14).
- **Saddle joint**—Joint that allows for flexion, extension, abduction, and adduction (Figure 4-15).

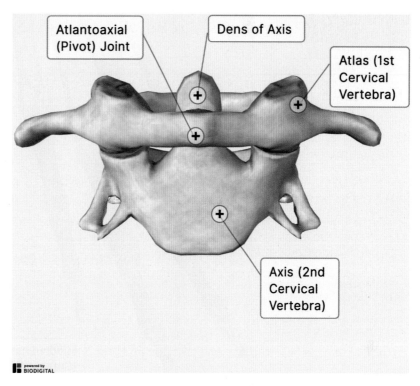

FIGURE 4-12 The pivot joint between the atlas (C-1) and axis (C-2) is a type of synovial pivot joint.

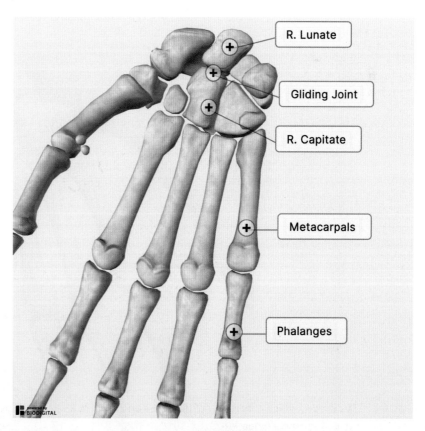

FIGURE 4-13 The joints found between the carpal bones of the wrist and tarsal bones of the ankle are gliding joints.

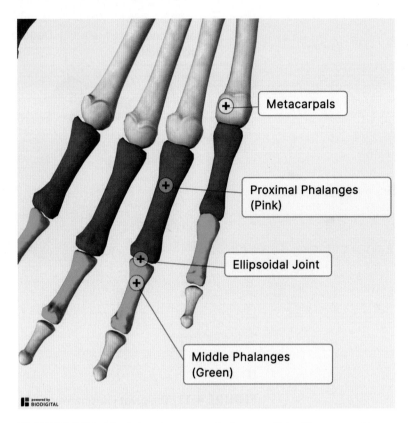

FIGURE 4-14 The joints between the bones of the fingers and toes are types of ellipsoidal joints.

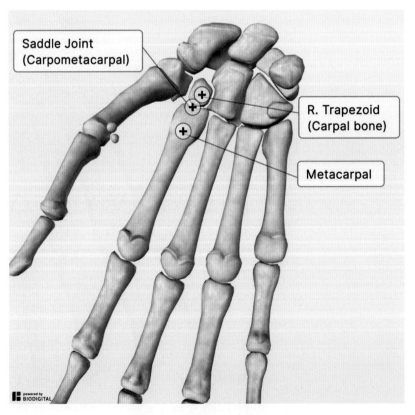

FIGURE 4-15 The joints between the carpal bones of the wrist and metacarpal bones of the hand are saddle joints.

- Ball-and-socket joint—Spheroidal joint that allows for flexion, extension, abduction, and internal and external rotation (Figure 4-16).

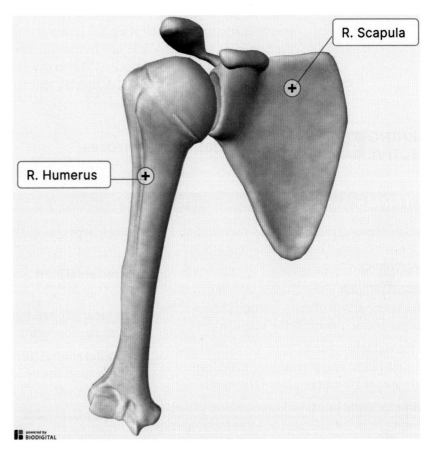

R. Scapula

R. Humerus

powered by
BIODIGITAL

FIGURE 4-16 The joint formed by the humerus and scapula of the shoulder is a ball-and-socket joint.

LEARNING OBJECTIVE 4.1.8 **Describe the important characteristics of a diarthrosis.**

KEY TERMS

axes Imaginary lines about which parts of the body rotate; in anatomy, an axis is termed as the three anatomical planes, namely frontal, transverse, and sagittal.

biaxial Allows movement within two principal axes; the wrist and ankles are examples.

multiaxial Allows movement along all the three axes; the hip joint is an example.

nonaxial Allows for gliding movement between bones.

synovial fluid Viscous fluid found in the cavities of the joints that permits smooth movement and provides nourishment to the joints.

synovial joints Diarthrosis joint, a connection between two existing bones that consists of fluid-filled cartilage-lined cavity; common joint in mammals.

uniaxial Allows movement in a single plane or axis; the elbow is an example.

Characteristics of a Diarthrosis

Diarthrotic joints are freely movable synovial joints. These joints provide for the majority of the movement in the body. All diarthrotic joints are synovial joints. Synovial joints are surrounded by a capsule filled with synovial fluid, which prevents friction by lubricating the joints and permitting smooth movement of the bones. Diarthrotic joints are further divided into categories that are based on the number of axes of motion. The axes of motion that describe diarthrotic joints include nonaxial, uniaxial, biaxial, and multiaxial joints.

LEARNING OBJECTIVE 4.1.9   **List examples of diarthroses.**

KEY TERMS

acetabulofemoral joint Ball-and-socket joint of the hip, located between the femur and acetabulum.

acromioclavicular joint Gliding joint located at the upper portion of the shoulder, between the clavicle and acromion of the scapula.

atlantoaxial joint Pivotal joint formed between the first (atlas) and second (axis) cervical vertebrae in the upper part of the neck.

carpometacarpal joint Saddle joint that allows movement of the thumb; connects the trapezium to the first metacarpal bone.

ginglymus joint Hinge joint; another name for the elbow joint.

glenohumeral joint Ball-and-socket joint between the scapula and humerus.

intercarpal joint Gliding joint that allows for movement of the wrist.

intertarsal joint Joints between the tarsal bones of the foot.

metacarpophalangeal joint Ellipsoidal joints that allow movement of the fingers.

patellofemoral joint One of the joints that form the knee, for which the hinge joint allows for movement.

tibiofemoral joint The synovial joint between the femur, tibia, and patella bones; another name for the knee joint.

zygapophyseal joint Apophyseal joint between the superior and inferior articular process of adjacent vertebrae; hingelike joints link the vertebrae together.

Examples of Diarthroses

Examples of diarthrosis include:

- Acetabulofemoral joint: Ball-and-socket joint of the hip, located between the femur and acetabulum.
- Acromioclavicular joint: Gliding joint at the top of the shoulder, located between the clavicle and acromion of the scapula.
- Atlantoaxial joint: Pivot joint located in the upper part of the neck between the first and second cervical vertebrae known as the atlas and the axis.
- Carpometacarpal joint: Saddle joint that allows movement of the thumb; it connects the trapezium to the first metacarpal bone.

- **Ginglymus joint**: Hinge joint; another name for the elbow joint.
- **Glenohumeral joint**: Ball-and-socket joint between the scapula and humerus.
- **Intercarpal joint**: Gliding joint that allows for movement of the wrist.
- **Intertarsal joint**: Gliding joints, located between of the tarsal bones of the foot.
- **Metacarpophalangeal Joint**: Ellipsoidal joints that allow movement of the fingers.
- **Patellofemoral** and **tibiofemoral joints**: Form the knee, for which the hinge joint allows for movement.
- **Zygapophyseal joint**: Hingelike joints between the superior and inferior articular processes of adjacent vertebrae that link the vertebrae together.

UNIT OBJECTIVE 4.2

Describe the structure, types, and movements of synovial joints (diarthroses).

UNIT INTRODUCTION

Synovial joints, also known as diarthroses, are joints in which the articulating bones are separated by a joint cavity containing fluid. Synovial joints are the most common and movable type of joints in a mammal, allowing for a wide range of movement for the bones in the body.

LEARNING OBJECTIVE 4.2.1 Identify synovial joints.

KEY TERMS

acromioclavicular joint Gliding joint located at the upper portion of the shoulder, between the clavicle and acromion of the scapula.

bursae Small sacs filled with lubricating fluid to reduce friction in the moving body joints.

sternoclavicular joint Gliding-type joint between the sternum and the clavicle.

temporomandibular joint Joint formed by the temporal bone and mandible often referred to as the jaw joint.

tendon A tough fibrous connective tissue that connects muscle to bone to withstand tension.

SYNARTHROTIC JOINTS OF THE BODY

Synovial joints are the most common and most movable type of joints in the body. Synovial joints are diarthrotic joints that have a fluid-filled joint cavity known as a synovial cavity. The fluid is contained in a fibrous capsule. A synovial joint is surrounded by muscle and has accessory ligaments made up of dense connective tissue. This connective tissue is called a **tendon** and serves to protect the joint from strain when extreme movements occur that may damage the joint. Some synovial joints contain menisci. Menisci are tough firbous tissues that serve to absorb shock. In humans, menisci are found in the knee, wrist, **acromioclavicular joint**, **sternoclavicular joint**, and **temporomandibular joint**. Synovial joints also include articular nerves and an abundant supply of blood vessels. Lastly, the joints also contain **bursae**, which are lined by the synovial membrane (Figure 4-17).

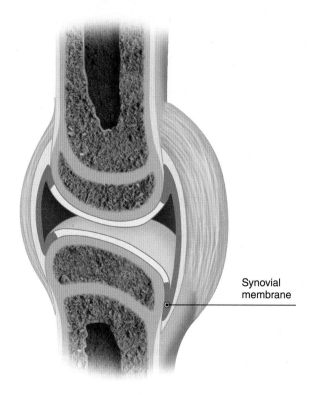

Synovial
membrane

FIGURE 4-17 The synovial membrane produces synovial fluid that helps lubricate the movements of synovial joints.

LEARNING OBJECTIVE 4.2.2 List the parts of a synovial joint.

KEY TERMS

articular capsule Double-layered capsule that surrounds the synovial joint.

articular cartilage Hyaline cartilage covering bone ends at movable joints.

articular cavity Joint cavity bounded by the synovial membrane and articular cartilage of all synovial joints; normally only contains synovial fluid.

synovial fluid Viscous fluid found in the cavities of the joints that permits smooth movement and provides nourishment to the joints.

synovial membrane Connective tissue that lines the inner surface of capsules of synovial joints.

Parts of a Synovial Joint

The key structures of a synovial joint include:

- **Articular capsule**: Made up of an outer layer of fibrous connective tissue that attaches to each bone and surrounds the bones' articulating surface, allowing for the bones of the joint to articulate with each other within the synovial joint cavity.
- **Articular cartilage**: The articulating surfaces are covered with hyaline cartilage. The purpose of the cartilage is to absorb shock and minimize the friction between the joints upon movement.
- **Articular cavity**: The joint cavity is the space between bones that is filled with a small amount of synovial fluid. This cavity is unique to synovial joints.
- **Synovial fluid**: The inner layer of the articular capsule is made up of the **synovial membrane**. The cells of the synovial membrane secrete a thick material called synovial fluid. This lubricating fluid moves into the cartilage when the joint is resting and out of the cartilage when it is active. This fluid lubricates the joints, allows for smooth movement, and provides nourishment to the articular cartilage.

LEARNING OBJECTIVE **4.2.3** **Describe the functions of synovial joints.**

KEY TERMS

abduction Movement away from the midline of the body.

adduction Movement toward the midline of the body.

circumduction Movement of the distal end of a limb in a circular motion.

depression Downward movement of body structures.

dorsiflexion Bending at the ankle such that the toes are lifted toward the shin.

elevation Upward movement of body structures.

eversion Act of turning the feet outwards or inside out.

extension Straightening movement that increases the angle between the bones of the joint.

excursion Range of motion regularly repeated.

flexion Bending of the joint decreasing the angle of the bones at the joint.

hyperextension Continuation of the extension movement beyond the natural anatomical position.

inferior rotation Rotation downward.

inversion Movement of the soles of the feet inward toward the midline of the body.

lateral rotation Movement away from the body.

medial rotation Movement toward the midline of the body.

opposition Rotation of the thumb touching each of the fingers of the same hand.

plantarflexion Bending at the ankle when the heel is lifted, flexing the foot or toes downward.

pronation Rotation of the hand and forearm so that the palm faces downward.

protraction Movement of a body part in an anterior direction.

reposition Movement of the thumb and fingers away from each other.

retraction Drawn backward movement of the body.

rotation Movement around a single longitudinal axis.

superior rotation Rotation upward.

supination Rotation of the forearm and hand so that the palm faces upward.

synovial joints Diarthrosis joint, a connection between two existing bones that consists of fluid-filled cartilage-lined cavity; common joint in mammals.

Functions of Synovial Joints

Synovial joints are the most common type of freely moving joints in the body. The function of the synovial joints is to provide movement and stability in the body; examples of these types of body motions include:

- **Superior rotation:** rotation upward
- **Inferior rotation:** rotation downward
- **Medial rotation:** movement toward the midline of the body
- **Lateral rotation:** movement away from the body
- **Elevation:** upward movement of body structures (Figure 4-18)
- **Depression:** downward movement of body structures (Figure 4-18)
- **Rotation:** movement around a single longitudinal axis
- **Abduction:** movement away from the midline of the body (Figure 4-19)
- **Adduction:** movement toward the midline of the body (Figure 4-19)
- **Excursion:** a range of motion regularly repeated
- **Retraction:** movement of the body part in the posterior direction (Figure 4-20)

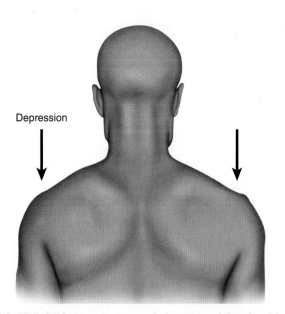
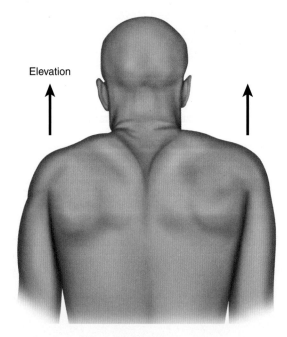

FIGURE 4-18 Depression and elevation of the shoulders.

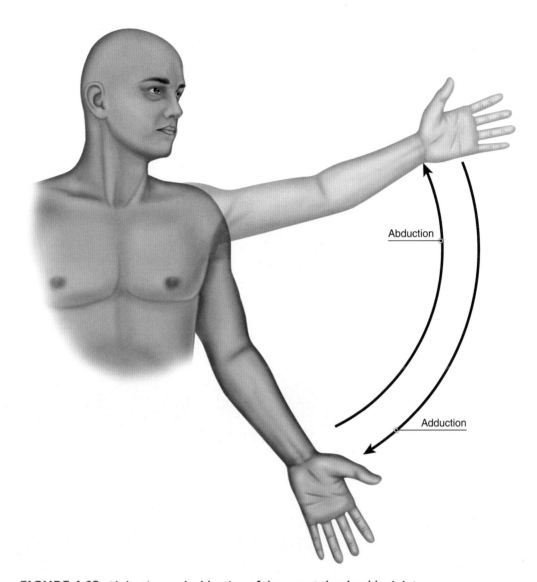

FIGURE 4-19 Abduction and adduction of the arm at the shoulder joint.

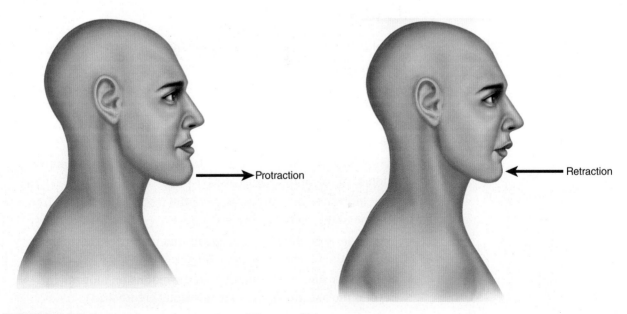

FIGURE 4-20 Protraction and retraction of the mandible.

- **Protraction:** movement of a body part in an anterior direction (Figure 4-20)
- **Reposition:** movement of the thumb and fingers away from each other
- **Circumduction:** movement of the distal end of a limb in a circular motion (Figure 4-21)

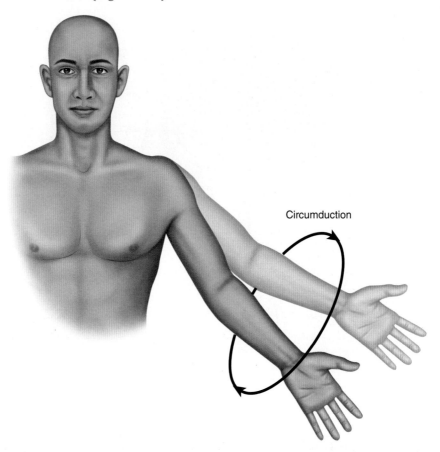

Circumduction

FIGURE 4-21 Circumduction of the arm at the ball and socket shoulder joint allows the arm to move in a circular motion.

- **Supination:** rotation of the forearm and hand so that the palm faces upward (Figure 4-22)
- **Pronation:** rotation of the hand and forearm so that the palm faces downward (Figure 4-22)
- **Opposition:** rotation of the thumb touching each of the fingers of the same hand
- **Inversion:** movement of the soles of the feet inward toward the midline of the body (Figure 4-23)
- **Eversion:** movement of the soles of the feet outward away from the midline of the body (Figure 4-23)
- **Extension:** straightening movement that increases the angle between the bones of the joint (Figure 4-24)
- **Hyperextension:** a continuation of the extension movement beyond the natural anatomical position (Figure 4-24)

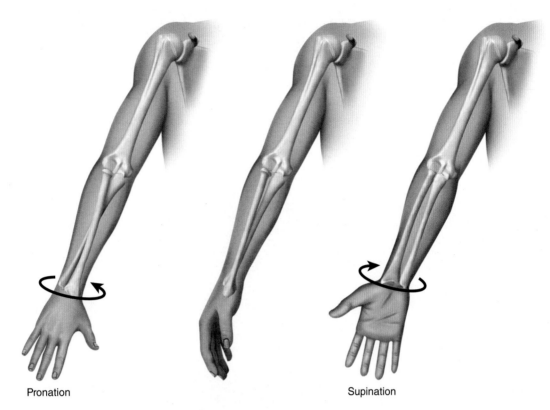

Pronation

Supination

FIGURE 4-22 Rotating the hand and forearm so the palm faces downward is an example of pronation. Rotating the hand and forearm so the palm faces upward is an example of supination.

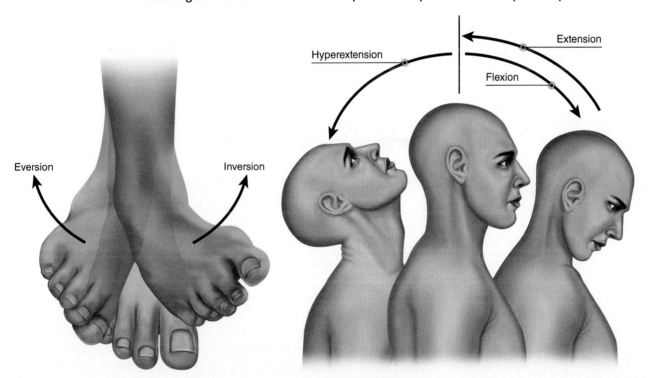

Eversion

Inversion

Hyperextension

Extension

Flexion

FIGURE 4-23 Moving the soles of the feet away from the midline of the body is an example of eversion. Moving the soles of the feet toward the midline of the body is an example of inversion.

FIGURE 4-24 Moving the head backward in an unnatural position is an example of hyperextension. Moving the head down toward the chest is an example of a flexion movement. Moving the head from that downward position back to its natural position is an example of extension.

- **Flexion**: bending of the joint decreasing the angle of the bones at the joint (Figure 4-24)
- **Dorsiflexion**: bending at the ankle such that toes are lifted toward the shin (Figure 4-25)
- **Plantarflexion**: bending at the ankle when the heel is lifted flexing the foot or toes downward (Figure 4-25)

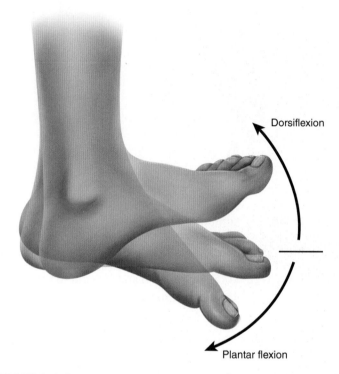

Dorsiflexion

Plantar flexion

FIGURE 4-25 Flexing the foot upward toward the tibia of the lower leg is dorsiflexion. Flexing the foot downward toward the ground is plantar flexion.

LEARNING OBJECTIVE 4.2.4 Identify the six types of synovial joints.

The Six Types of Synovial Joints

There are six types of synovial joints that provide for different types of movement and range of motion. These joints are subdivided based on the shapes of the articulatory surfaces of the bones that form each joint. These joints include:

- Pivot (Figure 4-26)
- Hinge (Figure 4-27)
- Saddle (Figure 4-28)
- Gliding (also known as a plane joint) (Figure 4-29)
- Ellipsoidal (also known as a condyloid joint) (Figure 4-30)
- Ball and socket (also known as a universal joint) (Figure 4-31)

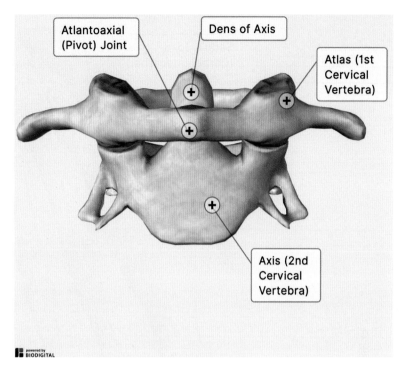

FIGURE 4-26 The pivot joint between the atlas (C-1) and axis (C-2) is a type of synovial pivot joint.

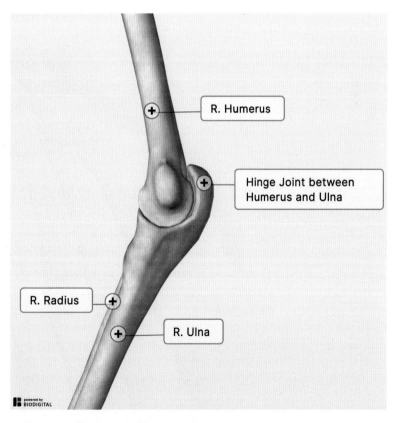

FIGURE 4-27 The elbow, which connects the humerus and ulna, is a type of synovial hinge joint.

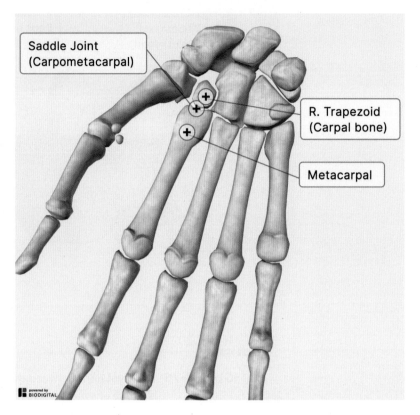

FIGURE 4-28 The joints between the carpal bones of the wrist and metacarpal bones of the hand are saddle joints.

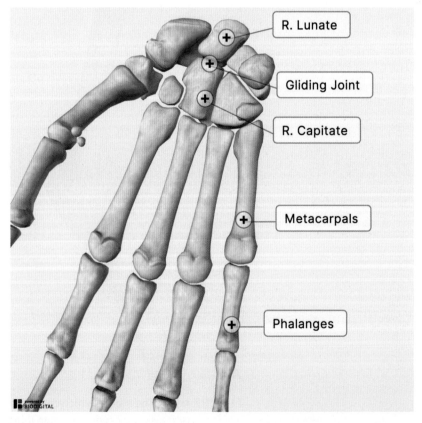

FIGURE 4-29 The joints found between the carpal bones of the wrist and tarsal bones of the ankle are gliding joints.

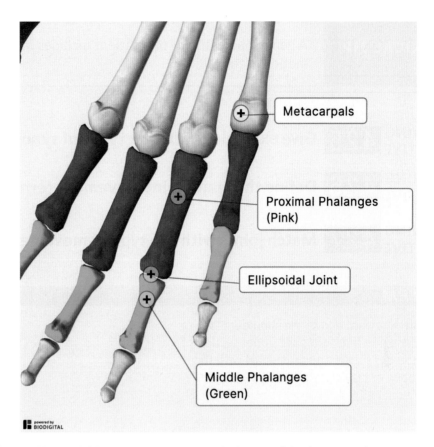

FIGURE 4-30 The joints between the bones of the fingers and toes are types of ellipsoidal joints.

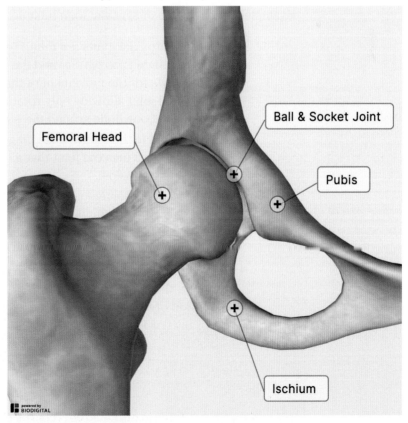

FIGURE 4-31 The joint formed by the femoral head and acetabulum of the pelvis form a ball-and-socket joint.

<table>
<tr><td>**CLINICAL TIP**</td><td>A general assessment of a patient includes observing the range of motion in the joints.</td></tr>
</table>

LEARNING OBJECTIVE 4.2.5 Give examples of the six types of synovial joints.

LEARNING OBJECTIVE 4.2.6 Define the major joint movement terms.

LEARNING OBJECTIVE 4.2.7 Match joints with the type of movements they facilitate.

KEY TERM

acromion Outward end of the shoulder blade or scapular spine that forms the upper section of the shoulder socket and articulates with the collarbone or clavicle.

Examples of the Six Types of Synovial Joints and the Types of Movement They Permit

Examples for each type of synovial joint include:

- Pivot: Atlantoaxial joints are found between the atlas and axis bones (C1 and C2 vertebrae) and the proximal radioulnar joint, which allows for the movement of the forearms. This type of joint is a uniaxial joint allowing only rotational movement around a single axis of one bone around the other.
- Hinge: Found in the elbow, knee, fingers, ankles, and toes. This type of joint is a uniaxial joint that allows for movements such as flexion and extension.
- Saddle: First carpometacarpal joint (thumb) and sternoclavicular joints. This type of joint is a biaxial joint allowing for movements that include flexion, extension, adduction, abduction, and circumduction.
- Gliding: Intercarpal joints of the wrist, intertarsal joints of the foot, the acromioclavicular joint between the clavicle and acromion of the scapula, and the zygapophyseal joints located

between the superior and inferior adjunct vertebrae. This type of joint is a multiaxial joint allowing for multiple movements and is located where bones meet at a flat or slightly curved articulate surface. The joint allows for movement of the bones past one another in any direction along the plane of the joint.

- Ellipsoidal: Joints between the metacarpal and phalanges (knuckles) and the wrist. This type of joint is a biaxial joint allowing for two planes of movement that includes flexion, extension, adduction, abduction, and circumduction.

- Ball and socket: Shoulder and hip. This joint provides for the greatest range of motion and is a multiaxial joint allowing movements that include flexion, extension, adduction, abduction, and internal and external rotation.

Different joints are able to move along a different range of motion:

- Wrist: ellipsoidal
- Elbow: hinge movement
- Thumb: saddle movement
- Vertebrae: gliding movement
- Shoulder: ball-and-socket movement
- Atlas and axis bones: pivot movement

LEARNING OBJECTIVE 4.2.8 Identify bursae associated with skeletal articulations.

BURSAE ASSOCIATED WITH SKELETAL ARTICULATIONS

There are four types of bursae found in the body. The bursae associated with skeletal articulations include (Figure 4-32):

- Subcutaneous bursa
- Submuscular bursa
- Subtendinous bursa

The fourth type of bursa is an adventitious, or accidental bursa. This bursa arises from the repeated friction or stresses over bony protrusions. A bunion is a common form of an adventitious bursa.

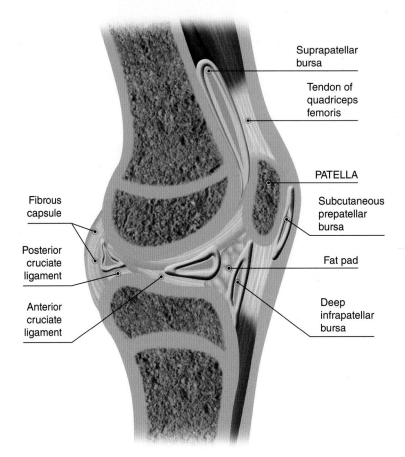

FIGURE 4-32 Bursae provide shock absorption for many skeletal joints.

Describe the function and types of bursae.

KEY TERMS

subcutaneous bursa Under the skin.
submuscular bursa Under the muscles.

subtendinous bursa Found between a tendon and a bone.

Function and Types of Bursae

There are approximately 160 bursae present in different synovial joints throughout the body. Bursae are found between a bone and a tendon or muscle and act as lubricated cushions. The bursae are located at different points of friction between bone and soft tissue; their presence lessens the friction that occurs. The locations for which bursa are found include:

- **Subcutaneous bursa:** located between the skin and underlying bone, allowing the skin to move smoothly over the bone
- **Submuscular bursa:** located between the muscle and the underlying bone or between adjacent muscles
- **Subtendinous bursa:** found between a tendon and a bone

LEARNING OBJECTIVE 4.2.10 Identify the major structural components of the knee joint.

LEARNING OBJECTIVE 4.2.11 Describe how the structure of the knee joint relates to its function and the movements it facilitates.

KEY TERMS

anterior cruciate ligament (ACL) One of the major ligaments in the human knee; provides rotational stability for the knee; it is also the most frequently injured ligament of the knee.

arcuate popliteal ligament Y-shaped extracapsular ligament that attaches to the posterior portion of the head of the fibula.

condyles Rounded prominence at the point where two bones meet.

femur Long bone of the upper leg; longest bone in the body.

lateral (fibular) collateral ligament Ligament located on the lateral side of the knee, stretching from the femur to the fibula. Because it does not fuse with the capsular ligament or the lateral meniscus, it is more flexible.

medial collateral (tibial) ligament Ligament found on the medial side of the knee; its primary function is to resist the outward turning of the knee.

menisci Fibrous cartilage within a joint, especially the knee.

oblique popliteal ligament Ligament that originates at the tibia and connects to the femur, crossing in back of the knee joint; provides a reinforcing structure, acting as a stabilizing force for the posterior of the knee.

patella Small sesamoid bone commonly called the kneecap.

patellofemoral joint

posterior cruciate ligament (PCL) One of the major ligaments in the human knee, connecting the posterior intercondylar area of the tibia to the medial condyle of the femur.

tibia Anterior long bone in the lower leg that articulates with the femur, fibula, and talus.

tibiofemoral joint The synovial joint between the femur, tibia, and patella bones; another name for the knee joint.

STRUCTURAL COMPONENTS OF THE KNEE JOINT

The knee is the largest joint in the body, connecting the thigh to the leg. Although there is only one joint cavity, the knee consists of two joints: the **tibiofemoral joint**, between the **femur** and **tibia**, and the **patellofemoral joint**, between the femur and **patella**.

This tibiofemoral joint is formed by the meeting of the **condyles** on the distal end of the femur and the concave condyles on the proximal end of the tibia. The articulating surfaces of the knee are covered with hyaline cartilage, and there are two crescent-shaped pieces of fibrocartilage (called **menisci**) located on the articular surfaces of the tibia. This joint is primarily a hinge joint, allowing flexion and extension. A knee joint can only move along one axis to either flex or extend. However, small rotation of the knee is possible when it is partially flexed or extended (Figure 4-31).

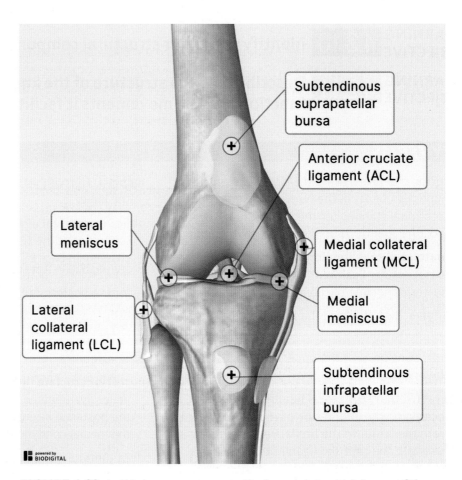

FIGURE 4-33 In this image, we can see the knee joint, which is one of the most complex joints in the body.

The patellofemoral joint is the area in which the patella articulates with the femur. The fibrous capsule that surrounds the articular surfaces of the patella contain the inner synovial membrane and provides physical stability. The synovial membrane surrounding the knee joint provides nourishment to the cartilage and protection and support of the joint. Several synovial pouches, known as bursae, surround the knee joint, serving as gliding surfaces that reduce the friction of the tendons that are attached to the bones and muscles. The muscles of the quadriceps that are connected to the knee by tendons are responsible for performing the movement of the knee joint.

The stability of the knee is maintained by ligaments. The extracapsular ligaments stabilize and strengthen the capsule of the knee joint. Extracapsular ligaments include:

- **Medial collateral (tibial) ligament**: resists outward turning forces of the knee
- **Lateral (fibular) collateral ligament**: maintains the stability of the knee by preventing side-to-side motion during movement
- **Arcuate popliteal ligament** and **oblique popliteal ligament**: act as stabilizing structures for the knee's posterior

Intracapsular ligaments cross each other, forming an X between the femoral condyles. These ligaments prevent displacement of the articular surfaces and secure the articulating bones when standing. Intracapsular ligaments include:

- **Anterior cruciate ligament (ACL)**: resists anterior motion and extreme extension
- **Posterior cruciate ligament (PCL)**: resists extreme flexion

These joints and ligaments work together to perform one of the most essential functions of the body: carrying the weight of the body during movement.

LEARNING OBJECTIVE 4.2.12 Identify the structural components of the shoulder joint.

LEARNING OBJECTIVE 4.2.13 Describe how the structure of the shoulder joint relates to its function and the movements it facilitates.

KEY TERMS

clavicle Bone of the shoulder connecting the scapula and the sternum; also called the collarbone.

coracohumeral ligament Broad ligament that strengthens the upper part of the capsule of the shoulder joint.

glenohumeral ligament Three ligaments on the anterior position of the shoulder joint.

humerus Long bone of the upper arm extending from the shoulder to the elbow.

scapula Triangular-shaped bone in the back that articulates with the posterior rib cage, humerus, and clavicle.

scapulothoracic joint An articulation between anterior scapula and posterior thoracic rib.

STRUCTURAL COMPONENTS OF THE SHOULDER JOINT

The shoulder joint is the most mobile joint of the human body, and therefore the least stable. Structurally, it is a ball-and-socket joint. Movement of the shoulder includes the extension, flexion, abduction, adduction, internal and external rotation, and circumduction.

The structural components of the shoulder consist of three bones: scapula, clavicle, and humerus. The shoulder contains four joints, which include the glenohumeral, acromioclavicular, sternoclavicular, and the scapulothoracic. The glenoid in the scapula forms the socket for the head of the humerus, which is known as the glenohumeral joint. This joint has a labrum, which is a fibrous ring of cartilage attached to the rim of the socket, resulting in a deepening of the socket and an increase in the stability of the joint. The acromioclavicular joint is where the acromion on the scapula link to form a joint with a gliding motion. The sternoclavicular joint is also a gliding-type joint found between the sternum and the clavicle. The scapulothoracic joint is where the scapula meets the back of the thoracic cage.

The shoulder joints are encapsulated in synovial fluid that lubricates the joints and provides nourishment. Bursa is also found in the shoulder region, which help the muscles, tendons, and other joint structures of the shoulder slide freely. There is a network of tendons and muscles that extends from the scapula to the top of the humerus known as the rotator cuff. The primary function of the rotator cuff is to keep the humerus centered in the glenoid during movement, as well as help lift and rotate the shoulder in different directions. There are only two main ligaments within the shoulder joint; this contributes to the large range of motion possible in the shoulder. These ligaments are the coracohumeral ligament, which helps support the weight of the upper limb, and the glenohumeral ligament, which weakly strengthen the front of the shoulder capsule.

UNIT OBJECTIVE 4.3

Describe common pathologies affecting the articulations of the skeletal system.

UNIT INTRODUCTION

Because of the flexibility they provide, joints and the bones and other structures that surround them may be easily injured. Although bones are most frequently injured due to traumatic injury (such as a break or a fracture), joints, cartilage, and ligaments often experience injury as a result of friction caused by overuse and inflammatory conditions. Genetics also often play a role.

LEARNING OBJECTIVE **4.3.1** **Identify common pathologies affecting skeletal articulations.**

KEY TERMS

autoimmune disorders Disorders in which the immune system mistakenly attacks the body.

bisphosphonates Group of drugs used to limit the loss of bone density.

degenerative Progressive, often irreversible deterioration.

uric acid A breakdown or a waste product generated from the metabolism (nitrogenous) of purine nucleotides; a normal component of urine.

COMMON PATHOLOGIES AFFECTING SKELETAL ARTICULATIONS

Some of the most common pathologies that affect the skeletal articulations are bursitis, Paget's disease, osteoarthritis, osteogenesis imperfecta, osteoporosis, gout, osteomalacia, rheumatoid arthritis, and rickets.

Bursitis

Bursitis is the inflammation of the bursae (Figure 4-34). It is most commonly caused by repetitive movement of the joint, but can also be caused by trauma, inflammatory conditions, and autoimmune disorders. The most common symptom of bursitis is joint pain and stiffness that worsens during repetitive activity. Treatment usually involves rest, ice, elevation of the affected joint, and anti-inflammatory medicine.

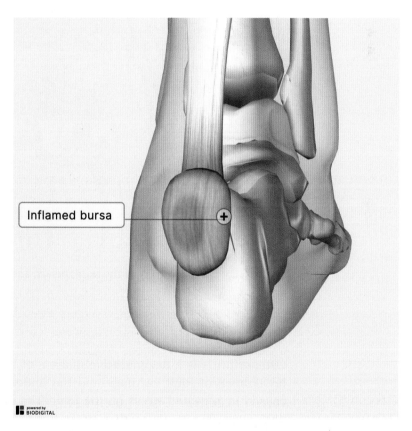

Inflamed bursa

FIGURE 4-34 Bursitis is an inflammation of the bursa found in many joints.

Paget's Disease

Paget's disease is the abnormal remodeling of bone (Figure 4-35). This remodeling causes the bone to weaken and may result in pain, deformity, fracture, or arthritis. Paget's disease is frequently asymptomatic; the most common symptom that does occur is bone pain. While the exact cause is unknown, the disease is thought to have genetic or viral origins. Paget's disease is most frequently treated using medication—both to reduce the pain felt and to prevent further deterioration of the bone. Surgery may be used to repair fractures, replace joints, or realign bone that is deformed near weight-bearing joints.

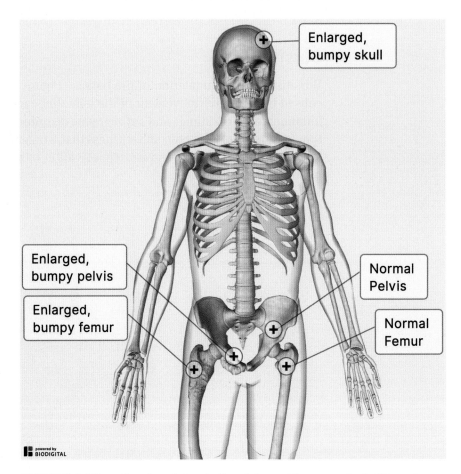

Enlarged, bumpy skull

Enlarged, bumpy pelvis

Enlarged, bumpy femur

Normal Pelvis

Normal Femur

FIGURE 4-35 Deformity of the skull, pelvis, and femur typical of Paget's disease.

Osteoarthritis

Osteoarthritis is a degenerative disease of the joints that results from the breakdown of joint cartilage and the underlying bone (Figure 4-36). It is caused by repeated stress on the joint. The most frequent symptom is joint pain and stiffness, although joint swelling, decreased range of motion, and numbness of the arms and legs also occur. The goal of treatment is to decrease the stress placed on the joints and to manage pain. Exercise and weight loss is recommended for overweight people with osteoarthritis. Common over-the-counter medications, such as NSAIDs or acetaminophen, are used to manage pain. Joint replacement surgery, most commonly for hips or knees, is also a treatment.

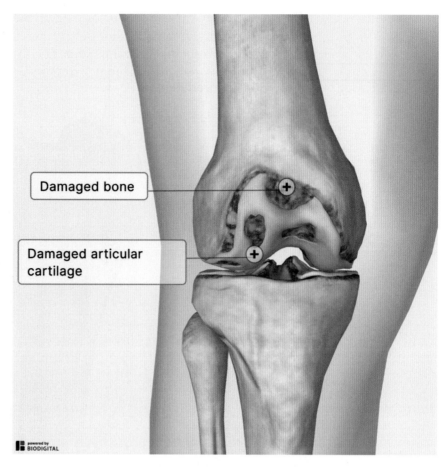

Damaged bone

Damaged articular cartilage

powered by BIODIGITAL

FIGURE 4-36 Loss of joint space; destruction of cartilage and bone; and an inflamed, thickened synovial membrane is seen in this example of osteoarthritis.

Osteogenesis Imperfecta

Osteogenesis imperfecta is a genetic fragile bone disorder, due to a problem with the connective tissue and a lack of collagen. It is also known as brittle bone disease. Easily broken bones are the most prominent symptom. While there is no cure, maintaining a healthy lifestyle, including a balanced diet, exercise, and not smoking, can reduce the likelihood of fractures occurring. Treatment includes treating fractures as they occur, pain medication, and physical therapy. Metal rods may also be surgically placed through long bones to strengthen them.

Osteoporosis

Osteoporosis is a disease that results in weak and brittle bones (Figure 4-37). There are generally no symptoms until fractures occur. Maintaining proper nutrition from childhood through adulthood, especially good dietary sources of calcium and vitamin D; exercise; not smoking; and moderating alcohol consumption can help prevent osteoporosis from developing. Osteoporosis can be managed with lifestyle changes and taking **bisphosphonates** to prevent further loss of bone density.

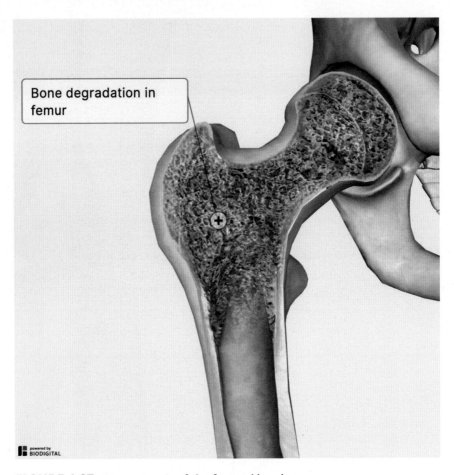

Bone degradation in femur

FIGURE 4-37 Osteoporosis of the femoral head.

Gout

Gout is a type of inflammatory arthritis. It is caused by a deposition of **uric acid** crystals in the joints, skin, and kidneys (Figure 4-38). The most common symptom is a red, tender, inflamed joint, and the joint at the base of the big toe is the most common place for symptoms of gout to occur. NSAIDs are frequently used to treat the symptoms of gout; after the initial attack has subsided, lifestyle changes can lower the levels of uric acid.

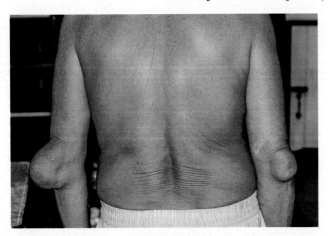

FIGURE 4-38 Swelling and inflammation of the elbow joint caused by gout.

Osteomalacia

Osteomalacia is the softening of the bones in adults that is caused by a vitamin D or calcium deficiency. Symptoms include body pain, muscle weakness, and fragile bones. Osteomalacia responds well to oral daily intake of vitamin D3.

Rheumatoid Arthritis

Rheumatoid arthritis (RA) is an autoimmune disorder that affects the connective tissue in the joints. It results in swollen, painful joints (Figure 4-39). In RA, the body's immune system attacks the joints. There is no cure for RA. The goal of treatment is to minimize pain and prevent bone deformity. Antirheumatic drugs are used to slow the progression of the RA so as to prolong day-to-day functioning of the client.

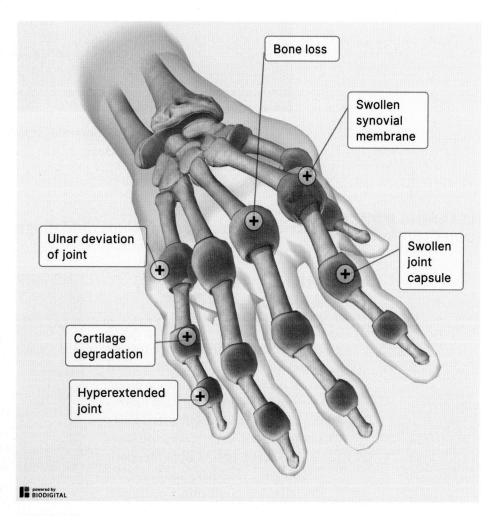

FIGURE 4-39 Autoimmune destruction and deformity in the joints of the hand.

Rickets

Rickets is a childhood disorder that causes the bones to soften, making them prone to fractures and deformities (Figure 4-40). It is caused by a lack of vitamin D, phosphate, or calcium. Symptoms include bone tenderness, bone fractures, and bowed legs or knocked knees. If diagnosed early enough, administration of vitamin D and calcium is used. Surgery to remove bone abnormalities may be necessary in cases that are not diagnosed early.

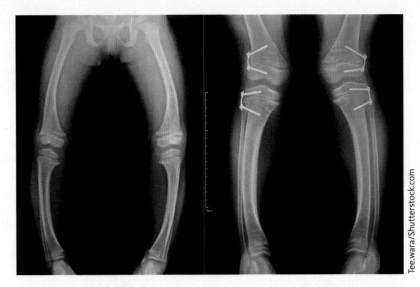

FIGURE 4-40 X-ray showing the bowed legs typically found in children with Rickets.

LEARNING OBJECTIVE 4.3.2 Describe the signs, symptoms, and diagnosis of scurvy.

SIGNS, SYMPTOMS, AND DIAGNOSIS OF SCURVY

Scurvy is a disorder that occurs due to lack of vitamin C and is diagnosed based on a client's diet history, physical symptoms, and resolution following vitamin C administration. Early symptoms of scurvy include malaise, lethargy, loss of appetite, poor weight gain, diarrhea, and fever. As the clinical condition continues, the client will develop shortness of breath, bone pain, anemia, soft bleeding gum tissue, loose teeth, poor wound healing, and emotional changes (Figure 4-41). In early childhood, scurvy can cause musculoskeletal problems.

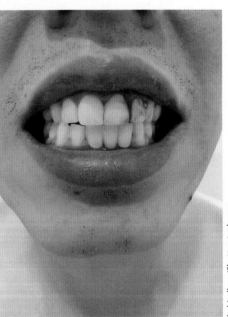

FIGURE 4-41 Bleeding of the gums that is often seen in patients with scurvy.

LEARNING OBJECTIVE 4.3.3 Describe the signs, symptoms, and diagnosis of Marfan syndrome.

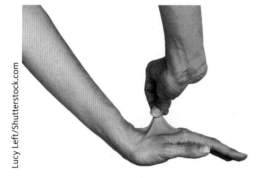

FIGURE 4-42 Due to connective tissue mutations, those with Marfan syndrome often have flexible joints and stretchy skin.

SIGNS, SYMPTOMS, AND DIAGNOSIS OF MARFAN SYNDROME

Marfan syndrome is caused by a genetic mutation for which the structure of the connective tissue is affected (Figure 4-42). The progression of the disease varies from one individual to another, but will typically advance over time.

Clinical features of the disease include:

- Tall, thin, body stature
- **Arachnodactyly**
- Heart murmurs
- **Scoliosis** or **kyphosis** (Figures 4-43 and 4-44)
- Sunken or protruding chest

- **Ligamentous laxity**
- Flat feet
- Widening or bulging of the **dural sac**
- Elongated narrow face
- Crowded teeth as a result of a high palate

The symptoms that occur from Marfan syndrome are related to the structures in the human body that have been affected by the disease. Symptoms may include:

- Joint, bone, and muscle pain
- Stretch marks on the skin
- Nearsightedness, farsightedness, detached retina, glaucoma, cataracts
- Angina
- Shortness of breath
- Heart palpitations
- Fatigue

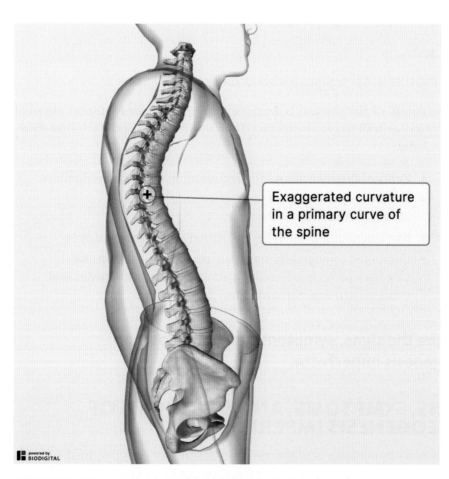

Exaggerated curvature in a primary curve of the spine

FIGURE 4-43 Excessive curvature of the spinal column results in a hunch-back appearance.

Lucy Lefr/Shutterstock.com

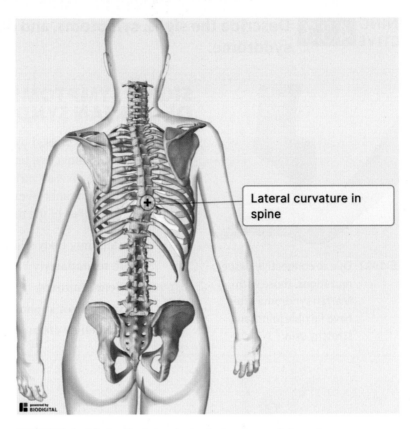

FIGURE 4-44 Scoliosis is a lateral curvature of the spine.

Diagnosis of the disease is based on an external and internal physical examination, as well as genetic testing. Diagnostic testing of the internal structures includes:

- Echocardiogram: allows for visualization of cardiac structures
- Electrocardiogram: provides information on the electroconductivity of the heart
- Eye examination: includes evaluation of the lenses of eyes
- Computed tomography, magnetic resonance imaging, and/or x-rays: provide information about cardiac, orthopedic, and connective tissue abnormalities

LEARNING OBJECTIVE 4.3.4 Describe the signs, symptoms, and diagnosis of osteogenesis imperfecta.

SIGNS, SYMPTOMS, AND DIAGNOSIS OF OSTEOGENESIS IMPERFECTA

Osteogenesis imperfecta is a genetic disorder that occurs due to the body's inability to produce strong bones. The symptoms of osteogenesis imperfecta vary significantly from person to person and are based on its type. However, all four types of osteogenesis imperfecta have some degree of bone fragility, fracturing, and bone deformity. Its diagnosis is based on the clinical presentation, collagen analysis of the skin, and DNA sequencing.

Common signs and symptoms included in the types of the disease include:

- Fatigue
- Bone pain
- Brittle teeth
- Short stature
- Cardiac issues
- Bone deformity
- Muscle weakness
- Low bone density
- Blue or purple sclera
- Triangular-shaped face
- Curved spine with bowed legs
- Skin hyperlaxity; easy bruising
- Loose joints, ligament laxity, and muscle weakness
- Skin, blood vessels, and internal organs that may be fragile
- Vision problems including myopia and risk for retinal detachment
- Late-closing fontanels; head circumference greater than average
- Hearing loss that may begin in the early 20s; by middle age it is present in more than half the people with osteogenesis imperfecta
- Respiratory problems including asthma; problems may be aggravated by chest wall deformity and spine deformity

LEARNING OBJECTIVE 4.3.5 **Contrast the signs, symptoms, and diagnosis of osteogenesis imperfecta and Marfan syndrome.**

KEY TERMS

arachnodactyly Condition in which the fingers and toes are abnormally long and slender and the thumb is pulled in toward the palm.

dural sac Membranous sheath that surrounds the spinal cord and the cauda equina.

fontanels Soft, membranous gaps between the cranial bones of an infant.

kyphosis Exaggeration of the primary curvature of the thoracic spine.

ligamentous laxity Loose ligaments.

myopia Nearsightedness.

sclera Opaque, the fibrous, protective outer layer of the human eye; also known as the white of the eye.

scoliosis Lateral bending of the spinal column caused by birth defects or other conditions.

COMPARING OSTEOGENESIS IMPERFECTA AND MARFAN SYNDROME

Although both diseases are heritable disorders, the signs and symptoms of Marfan syndrome are based on abnormal connective tissue. Signs and symptoms of osteogenesis imperfecta are based on abnormal bone formation. In both osteogenesis imperfecta and Marfan syndrome, the collagen in the connective tissue is abnormal. However, in osteogenesis imperfecta, it is the Type I collagen, which makes up bones and scar tissue, that is abnormal, while in Marfan syndrome, the fibrillin and elastin, which make up the ligaments and is present in the lungs, are abnormal.

Patients with osteogenesis imperfecta are usually short in height. Osteogenesis imperfecta commonly causes bones to fracture, blue sclera, and hearing loss. There are also frequently neurological abnormalities involving the central nervous system, which result from the incorrect formation of the skeletal structures that surround it. Neurological complications pose the greatest threat for patients with osteogenesis imperfecta, as these complications can adversely affect life expectancy.

Patients with Marfan syndrome are usually tall in height, with long arms, legs, fingers, and toes. Marfan syndrome commonly causes hypermobile joints, aortic dissection, and mitral-valve abnormalities. The heart abnormalities are the most serious, as they pose a risk for mitral-valve prolapse and aortic aneurism.

While both osteogenesis imperfecta and Marfan syndrome have severe forms that can cause life-threatening complications, they are generally diseases that can be managed and do not affect life expectancy. With osteogenesis imperfecta, maintaining a healthy lifestyle and avoiding smoking can help prevent broken bones. Treatment involves treating broken bones, physical therapy, braces, and surgery that strengthens long bones by placing rods in them. With Marfan syndrome, strenuous exercise is to be avoided. Treatment frequently includes taking beta blockers, calcium channel blockers, or ACE inhibitors. For significant heart issues, surgery is sometimes required to repair the aorta or replace the heart valve.

Chapter 5

The Muscular System

Chapter Introduction

Muscles make up between 40% and 50% of our body weight. We often think of muscles producing movement, but muscles also help to keep us alive. There are at least 650 muscles in the human body that help us move and keep our hearts beating and our lungs expanding and contracting. Muscles move our eyes, help to control digestion, regulate blood flow, and produce heat. The human body would not be able to survive without muscles.

UNIT OBJECTIVE 5.1

Describe the role the muscular system plays in human physiology.

UNIT INTRODUCTION

Muscles play an important role in human physiology. In addition to providing movement, muscles work to maintain homeostasis in many body systems including blood pressure and temperature regulation, breathing, and the cellular metabolism of glucose. In this unit, we explore the role the muscular system plays in human physiology.

LEARNING OBJECTIVE 5.1.1 Describe the overall structure of the muscular system.

KEY TERMS

contractile proteins Proteins located in muscle cells that assist in muscle contraction.

muscle tissue One of four primary tissue types, contracts and creates a force resulting in movement.

STRUCTURE OF THE MUSCULAR SYSTEM

Muscles are the important organs of movement of the body and are designed to move structures by contracting. Muscles are made of protein and if we were to examine a skeletal muscle under a microscope, we would see that it is composed of cells containing tiny protein fibers or filaments. These contractile proteins are arranged in structural units containing overlapping proteins. When a muscle receives a command from the nervous system to contract, protein filaments inside of muscle cells slide past each other, causing muscles cells to shorten in length.

Muscle cells are called myocytes and contain many of the structures of other eukaryotic cells. For example, in addition to protein filaments, skeletal muscle cells contain many nuclei, cytosol, cell membrane, mitochondria, and a specialized structure called the sarcoplasmic reticulum.

Muscle tissue is connected to or embedded within organ structures to provide mobility of structures and substances.

LEARNING OBJECTIVE 5.1.2 Identify the general functions of the muscular system.

LEARNING OBJECTIVE 5.1.3 Describe the general functions of the muscular system.

KEY TERMS

intrathoracic pressure Gas pressure inside of the thoracic cavity.

ventilation Movement of air into and out of the lungs.

GENERAL FUNCTIONS OF THE MUSCULAR SYSTEM

The general functions of the muscular system include movement, posture and stability, ventilation, blood flow, vision, temperature regulation, urination, organ protection, childbirth, and glucose regulation.

Movement. Skeletal muscles attach to bones and give our bodies mobility. Most skeletal muscles are under conscious control, allowing us to move at will. Smooth muscle helps to move food through the digestive tract. Food moves faster in the upper digestive tract while it is broken down by mastication and enzymes and transported by the esophagus to the stomach and small intestine where it is further broken down and absorbed. Skeletal muscles surrounding the eye allow it to move and track objects.

Posture and stability. Some skeletal muscles are controlled unconsciously. These muscles help to stabilize joints and assist in maintaining posture.

Ventilation. Muscles assist the respiratory system by supporting ventilation. The diaphragm is a dome-shaped muscle located at the base of the thoracic cavity. The diaphragm contracts, causing expansion of the thoracic cavity, which changes intrathoracic pressure and promotes air movement into the lungs.

Blood flow. Cardiac muscle in the heart helps to move blood between the heart's chambers and out of the heart to the lungs and arteries. Smooth muscle can constrict and dilate blood vessels, which helps to move blood by maintaining blood pressure.

Vision. Tiny muscles inside of the eye help to regulate the amount of light entering the eye by controlling dilation and constriction of the pupil.

Temperature regulation. Muscles generate heat when contracting. When body temperature drops, muscles shiver to produce heat and constrict blood vessels to conserve heat. Muscle contraction accounts for most of the heat produced by the body.

Urination. Smooth muscle in the ureters and urinary bladder and skeletal muscle in the urethra work to conserve and eliminate urine.

Organ protection. Skeletal muscles surrounding the body cavities work to absorb shock and provide a barrier of protection for internal organs. Muscles also protect bones from external forces.

Labor and delivery. Smooth muscle in the uterus responds to hormonal changes and produces powerful contractions during labor and delivery.

Blood glucose regulation. Muscles use glucose for fuel and help to maintain normal ranges of blood glucose by lowering blood glucose levels during periods of muscular contraction.

LEARNING OBJECTIVE 5.1.4 Identify skeletal, smooth, and cardiac muscle.

KEY TERMS

cardiac muscle Type of striated muscle tissue found in the heart.

smooth muscle One of three types of muscle tissues characterized by the lack of striations and involuntary control.

TYPES OF MUSCLE TISSUE

The muscular system consists of three types of muscles. Skeletal muscles attach to bones and produce movement and heat (see Figure 5-1). **Cardiac muscle** (see Figure 5-2) moves blood between the chambers of the heart and out to the lungs and body. **Smooth muscle** (see Figure 5-3) lines organs and blood vessels and helps to transport substances and regulate blood pressure.

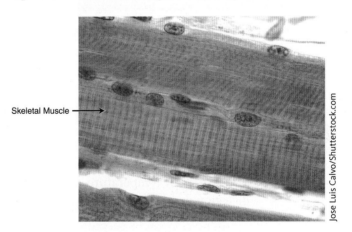

Skeletal Muscle →

Jose Luis Calvo/Shutterstock.com

FIGURE 5-1 Skeletal muscle attaches to bones to produce movement.

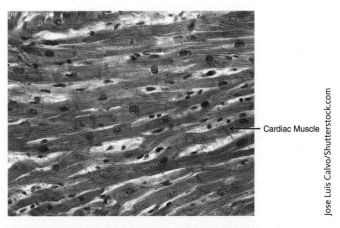

← Cardiac Muscle

Jose Luis Calvo/Shutterstock.com

FIGURE 5-2 Cardiac muscle is only found in the heart and contracts to allow the heart to pump blood.

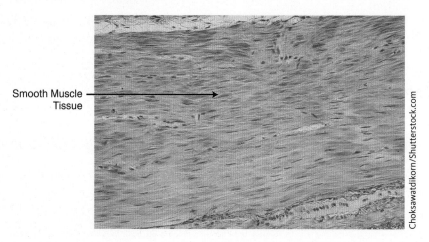

Smooth Muscle Tissue

Choksawatdikorn/Shutterstock.com

FIGURE 5-3 Smooth muscle lines blood vessels and hollow organs.

List the ways that the muscular system contributes to overall homeostasis.

KEY TERMS

blood pressure Fluid (hydrostatic) pressure in the vascular system.

homeostasis A dynamic equilibrium that keeps the internal state of the body balanced.

MUSCLES AND HOMEOSTASIS

Muscles play an important role in maintaining the body's homeostasis. The muscular system contributes to the body's homeostasis by helping to regulate blood pressure, body temperature, ventilation, blood flow, light entering the eye, and digestion and to protect the body through the action of reflexes.

Explain how the muscular system contributes to overall homeostasis.

KEY TERMS

negative feedback When a product of the stimulus leads to the decrease or inhibition of the original stimulus that caused the original increase in the product.

vasoconstriction Narrowing of blood vessels.

HOW THE MUSCULAR SYSTEM CONTRIBUTES TO HOMEOSTASIS

Functions of the muscular system contribute to the body's homeostasis. Homeostasis relies on feedback mechanisms and most of the body's homeostasis systems exhibit negative feedback. In negative feedback, the stimulus and response have opposite effects. For example, a thermostat will exhibit negative feedback by switching on the furnace when the room temperature drops below the set point.

Below are some examples of negative feedback in the muscular system.

Vasoconstriction of blood vessels. Smooth muscle in arteries can constrict in order to maintain blood pressure. The stimulus of decreasing blood pressure results in the response of increasing blood pressure by vasoconstriction of blood vessels. Blood vessels can also constrict in response to blood loss when the vessels are damaged. The stimulus of blood loss promotes vasoconstriction to elicit the response of decreasing blood loss.

Maintaining body temperature. Muscles play an important role in maintaining normal body temperature. For example, muscles respond to a decrease in body temperature by shivering. The stimulus of decreasing body temperature promotes the response of increasing body temperature.

Protection. Skeletal muscles help to protect the body from dangerous stimuli by rapidly contracting to withdraw a limb from a painful stimulus. The stimulus of pain or tissue damage promotes the withdrawal response to decrease the pain or tissue damage.

Regulation of light entering the eye. Smooth muscle surrounding the pupil of the eye helps to regulate light entering the eye by constricting or dilating the pupils. For example, the stimulus of too much light entering the eye promotes the response of constricting the pupil to allow less light into the eye.

Regulation of digestion. Smooth muscle in the digestive tract helps to regulate digestion by moving substances through the digestive tract. For example, movement of substances (chyme) out of the stomach promotes decreased constriction of the stomach in order to slow the movement of substances into the small intestine.

UNIT OBJECTIVE 5.2

Describe the structure and function of skeletal muscle.

UNIT INTRODUCTION

Although all muscles in the human body contract, they can have different structural characteristics depending on the type of contraction needed. For example, muscles performing strong contractions for lifting loads will have a different structure than muscles performing slow, wavelike contractions for moving substances through the digestive tract. In this unit, we explore the structure and function of skeletal muscle tissue.

LEARNING OBJECTIVE 5.2.1 **Identify the important structural characteristics of skeletal muscle tissue.**

KEY TERMS

heme Iron-containing portion of hemoglobin.

myoglobin Reddish-colored molecule found in muscle tissue that carries oxygen.

nuclei Portions of cells that contain DNA.

protein filaments Contractile proteins in muscle tissue.

STRUCTURE OF SKELETAL MUSCLE TISSUE

The general structure of skeletal muscle consists of bundles of contractile protein filaments organized in structural units throughout the length of a muscle. Skeletal muscle cells are called myocytes. These elongated cells extend and interconnect throughout the long axis of a muscle. Myocytes contain overlapping contractile **protein filaments** that form contractile units. As the protein filaments slide past each other, the contractile units shorten, which cause the myocytes and subsequent muscle to shorten. Myocytes in skeletal muscle contain many **nuclei** (multinucleated) along with protein filaments (see Figure 5-4). Myocytes also contain a red oxygen-containing **heme** molecule called **myoglobin**.

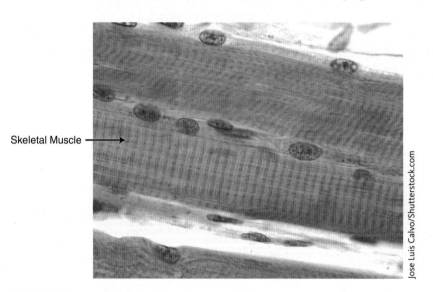

Skeletal Muscle →

Jose Luis Calvo/Shutterstock.com

FIGURE 5-4 Skeletal muscle tissue contains multiple nuclei and striations.

LEARNING OBJECTIVE 5.2.2 **Identify the levels of organization found in skeletal muscle.**

SKELETAL MUSCLE ORGANIZATION

Skeletal muscles contain multiple levels of organization. Muscle cells consist of groups of myofibrils containing protein filaments. These groups of myofibrils are covered by a membrane and combine to form bundles, which are also covered by a membrane. The bundles then combine to form the muscle which is covered by fascia.

Skeletal muscle can be organized by arrangement of fascicles, which include fusiform, unipennate, bipennate, and multipennate arrangements. Skeletal muscles can also be organized according to their structure beginning with muscle cells and progressing to bundles of cells forming structures called fascicles which combine to form the muscle.

LEARNING OBJECTIVE 5.2.3 Describe the levels of organization found in skeletal muscles.

KEY TERMS

bipennate Feather-like arrangement of fascicles in muscle tissue attaching to a central structure.

fascicles Small bundles of muscle fibers.

fusiform Shape of a muscle that is wider in the middle and narrower on each end.

multipennate Arrangement of muscle fibers consisting of multiple feather-like structures connecting to a central structure.

myocytes Muscle cells.

myofibrils Contractile proteins found in skeletal muscle tissue.

myoglobin Reddish-colored molecule found in muscle tissue that carries oxygen.

pennate Feather-like arrangement of muscle fibers in which many fibers connect in an oblique fashion to a central tendon.

sarcoplasm Fluid portion of a muscle cell (myocyte).

sarcoplasmic reticulum Network of membranous channels surrounding a muscle cell.

unipennate Arrangement of muscle fascicles in which fascicles connect to one side of a tendon.

LEVELS OF ORGANIZATION OF SKELETAL MUSCLE

Muscle Structure

Muscles consist of contractile cells called myocytes. Myocytes are long cylindrical cells that contain structures called myofibrils, which contain bundles of contractile proteins. Myocytes in skeletal muscle contain multiple nuclei, while cardiac and smooth muscle myocytes contain a single nucleus. Myocytes contain a cytoplasm known as the sarcoplasm, which contains a reddish pigment called myoglobin. The myofibrils contain contractile units that repeat throughout the length of the cell. The contractile units are called sarcomeres and consist of overlapping contractile proteins. Myocytes are covered by a membrane called a sarcolemma. Surrounding the outer portion of myofibrils is a structure consisting of a network of membranous channels called the sarcoplasmic reticulum. Myofibrils bundle together to form fascicles, which also form bundles covered by membranes.

Muscle Fascicles

Skeletal muscles can be organized by the orientation of fascicles. Muscles that are wider in the middle and thinner at each end are called fusiform muscles. The biceps brachii is an example of a fusiform muscle. The force a fusiform muscle produces is proportional to the diameter at its widest point.

Pennate muscles contain muscle fascicles attached to a central tendon in an oblique fashion much like a feather. There are three types of pennate muscles, including unipennate, bipennate, and multipennate. Unipennate muscles contain fascicles only on one side of the tendon. The semimembranosus muscle of the hamstring group is an example of a unipennate muscle. Bipennate muscles contain fascicles that attach to a central tendon from both sides. The rectus femoris muscle of the quadriceps group is an example of a bipennate muscle. Multipennate muscles have a structure similar to multiple feathers converging at a single point. The deltoid muscle of the shoulder is an example of a multipennate muscle.

LEARNING OBJECTIVE 5.2.4 Define the following muscle terms: epimysium, perimysium, endomysium, muscle fascicle, muscle fiber, myofibril, transverse tubule, sarcolemma, and sarcomere.

KEY TERMS

endomysium Thin, loose connective tissue membrane surrounding muscle cells.

epimysium Thin connective tissue membrane surrounding a muscle.

fascicles Small bundles of muscle fibers.

fibers Muscle cells containing strands of contractile proteins.

perimysium Membrane covering a muscle fascicle.

phospholipid bilayer Cell membrane consisting of an arrangement of two layers of phospholipids.

sarcolemma Membrane covering muscle cells (myocytes).

t-tubules Membranous tubular channels that result from the enfolding of the sarcolemma extending into the sarcoplasm of muscle cells.

SKELETAL MUSCLE STRUCTURE

Skeletal muscle consists of bundles of muscle cells called muscle fibers (see Figure 5-5). Skeletal muscle cells contain overlapping contractile protein filaments arranged in contractile units called sarcomeres. These overlapping filaments produce dark and light bands called striations. The cell membrane of a muscle cell is called the sarcolemma and is similar to other human body cells in that it consists of a phospholipid bilayer. The sarcolemma extends into the cytoplasm of the cell, forming membranous tubular channels. These invaginations are called t-tubules and help to carry substances needed for muscle contraction.

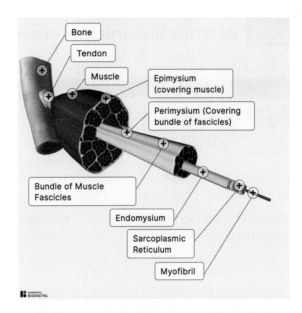

FIGURE 5-5 Skeletal muscle consists of bundle of fibers and cells.

Skeletal muscle cells are surrounded by a thin, loose connective tissue membrane called the **endomysium** (see Figure 5-6). Skeletal muscle cells are grouped together to form larger structures called **fascicles**. Each fascicle is covered by a connective tissue sheath called the **perimysium**. The entire muscle consists of groups of fascicles and is covered by a fibrous sheath called the **epimysium**.

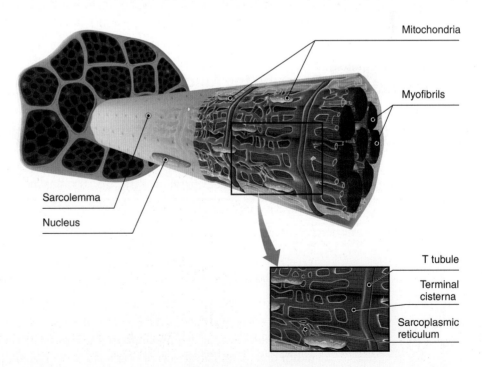

FIGURE 5-6 Skeletal muscle structure. Skeletal muscle cells are surrounded by a network of membranous channels.

LEARNING OBJECTIVE 5.2.5 **Describe the structure of a neuromuscular junction.**

KEY TERMS

axon terminal Portion of a neuron located at the end of an axon that releases neurotransmitter into the synaptic cleft.

motor end plate Specialized area in muscle tissue where neurons connect.

motor neuron Neuron that connects to and sends impulses to muscle tissue.

neuromuscular junction Areas between motor neurons and the point of attachment to muscles.

neurotransmitter Molecule secreted by neurons that produces changes in other neurons or organs.

synaptic cleft Fluid-filled space located between a neuron and another neuron or organ.

THE NEUROMUSCULAR JUNCTION

The nervous system controls skeletal muscle function. The nervous system connects to skeletal muscle at the neuromuscular junction. The nervous system sends a message to a muscle to contract by way of a nervous system cell called a **motor neuron**. The motor neuron contains a long process called an axon that extends to the muscle and contains a structure called the **axon terminal** at its end. The axon terminal releases a chemical called a **neurotransmitter** that tells the muscle to contract. There is a small fluid-filled separation between the axon terminal and the muscle called a **synaptic cleft**. The muscle has a specialized enfolded structure at this area called the **motor end plate**. The motor neuron's axon terminal, synaptic cleft, and motor end plate are collectively called the **neuromuscular junction**.

LEARNING OBJECTIVE 5.2.6 **Describe the function of a neuromuscular junction.**

KEY TERMS

neurons Cells found in nervous tissue that detect stimuli, process information, and transmit electrical impulses from one area of the body to another.

synapses Specialized site of communication between the axon terminal bud of one neuron and a receptor found on another neuron, gland, or muscle.

Function of the Neuromuscular Junction

The nervous system controls the action of muscles. Nervous system cells called **neurons** send messages in the form of chemical packets, or neurotransmitters, to muscle cells. A neuron connects to a muscle cell at a specialized region called the motor end plate. The action of sending a neurotransmitter from the neuron to the motor end plate is called a synapse. The neuromuscular junction (see Figure 5-7) is the area where **synapses** occur between the neuron and muscle cell.

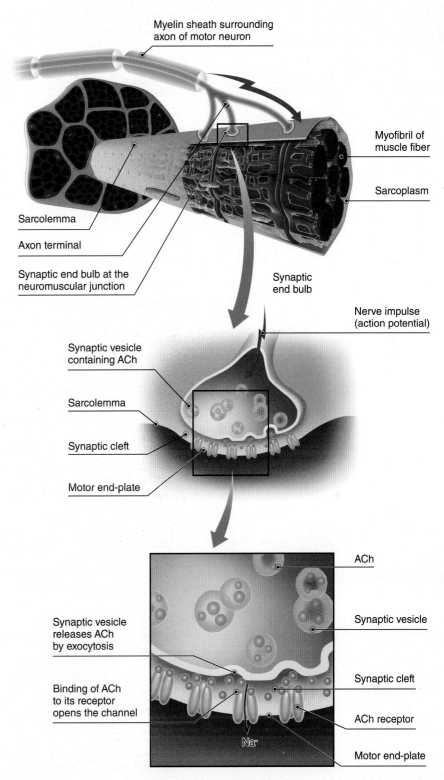

Myelin sheath surrounding axon of motor neuron

Myofibril of muscle fiber

Sarcoplasm

Sarcolemma

Axon terminal

Synaptic end bulb at the neuromuscular junction

Synaptic end bulb

Nerve impulse (action potential)

Synaptic vesicle containing ACh

Sarcolemma

Synaptic cleft

Motor end-plate

ACh

Synaptic vesicle

Synaptic cleft

ACh receptor

Motor end-plate

Synaptic vesicle releases ACh by exocytosis

Binding of ACh to its receptor opens the channel

Na+

FIGURE 5-7 The neuromuscular junction consists of a motor neuron's connection to the motor end plate of a muscle fiber.

LEARNING OBJECTIVE 5.2.7 Identify the structure of a sarcomere and myofibril.

LEARNING OBJECTIVE 5.2.8 Describe the structure and physical characteristics of a sarcomere and myofibril.

KEY TERMS

myofibrils Contractile proteins found in skeletal muscle tissue.

sarcomere Arrangement of contractile protein filaments forming a contractile unit in muscle tissue.

THE SARCOMERE AND MYOFIBRIL

Most of the volume of muscle cells consists of long tubular structures that run the length of the cells called **myofibrils**. Myofibrils consist of chains of contractile units called **sarcomeres**. The sarcomere is considered the functional unit of muscle since it is the smallest structural unit that is capable of performing muscle contraction. Each **sarcomere** consists of overlapping protein filaments. The filaments consist of thick and thin proteins that can make connections called cross-bridges. Muscle fibers contain thousands of sarcomeres. For example, it is estimated the biceps brachii muscle can contain 100,000 sarcomeres. In sarcomeres, the overlapping contractile protein filaments form regions of dark and light bands that give skeletal (and cardiac) muscle its striated appearance. The thin protein filaments are anchored at each end of a sarcomere to a structure called a Z-disk. Z-disks mark the beginning and end of a sarcomere.

LEARNING OBJECTIVE 5.2.9 Identify the structure of an actin molecule.

LEARNING OBJECTIVE 5.2.10 Describe the structure and function of actin.

KEY TERMS

actin Double-helix contractile protein found in muscle tissue.

globular proteins Protein structures containing small protein chains and large globular proteins.

THE CONTRACTILE PROTEIN ACTIN

The contractile proteins include actin and myosin. **Actin**, the thin filament, consists of two strands of **globular proteins** twisted together to form a helix. Actin forms a surrounding network around the other contractile protein, myosin, which can bind to and move actin.

Actin contains binding sites for myosin. The myosin binding sites are covered by a protein complex called the troponin–tropomyosin complex. During muscle contraction, the troponin–tropomyosin complex moves, exposing the myosin binding sites and allowing myosin to bind to actin, forming cross-bridges. Myosin can then pull actin along, causing shortening of the sarcomere.

LEARNING OBJECTIVE 5.2.11 Identify the structure of a myosin molecule.

LEARNING OBJECTIVE 5.2.12 Describe the structure and function of myosin.

KEY TERMS

globular protein chains Protein structures containing small protein chains and large globular proteins.

myosin Thick protein filament containing globular protein heads found in muscle tissue.

THE CONTRACTILE PROTEIN MYOSIN

Myosin, the thick filament, is a large protein molecule consisting of two heavy and two light globular protein chains (see Figure 5-8). The heavy chains form a globular head and twist around each other to form a smaller tail, while the light chains twist around the neck of the molecule.

Actin, the thin filament, overlaps myosin, forming contractile units called sarcomeres (see Figure 5-8). Actin contains binding sites for myosin. During muscle contraction, myosin binding sites on actin are exposed, allowing myosin to bind with actin. Myosin uses the energy from ATP to form cross-bridges with actin and move actin, causing shortening of the sarcomere and subsequent muscle contraction.

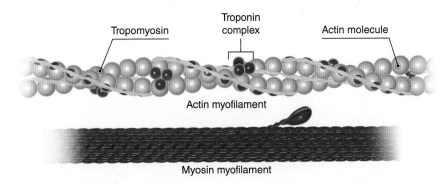

Tropomyosin   Troponin complex   Actin molecule

Actin myofilament

Myosin myofilament

FIGURE 5-8 The contractile proteins actin and myosin.

LEARNING OBJECTIVE 5.2.13 **Contrast the structure and function of actin and myosin.**

helix protein Protein structure in the shape of a helix.

hydrolyze Catabolic chemical reaction in which water is removed and a larger molecule is split into smaller molecules.

troponin–tropomyosin complex Structure containing troponin and tropomyosin that is capable of undergoing a conformational change in response to the binding of calcium to troponin.

COMPARING ACTIN AND MYOSIN

Actin, the thin filament, consists of a helix protein that forms a surrounding network around myosin in the sarcomere. Actin is surrounded by another protein complex called the troponin–tropomyosin complex. Myosin, the thick filament, contains globular proteins that hydrolyze ATP and form cross-bridges with actin.

Although actin and myosin are both considered contractile proteins, they contain structural and functional differences. Actin consists of a double-helix protein structure, whereas myosin contains large globular proteins. Actin contains myosin binding sites that are covered by the troponin–tropomyosin complex, which responds to calcium. Myosin has ATPase activity whereas actin does not. Because of the ability to use ATP, myosin can pull actin along, causing sarcomere shortening and contraction of the muscle. Actin's role during muscle contraction is to form a static supportive network that surrounds myosin.

LEARNING OBJECTIVE 5.2.14 **Define the following terms related to sarcomere structure and function: M-line, Z-line, A-band, I-band, H-zone, troponin, and tropomyosin.**

A-bands Dark regions in sarcomeres where the contractile proteins, actin and myosin, overlap.

H-zone Portion of a sarcomere at the center of an A-band consisting of myosin filaments.

I-Bands Regions of the sarcomere containing only actin filaments.

M-line Portion of the sarcomere where myosin filaments attach.

sarcomere Arrangement of contractile protein filaments forming a contractile unit in muscle tissue.

tropomyosin Double-stranded helical protein located in muscle cells.

troponin Protein complex consisting of three units that function to cover the myosin binding site on actin.

Z-disks Portion of the sarcomere where actin filaments attach, marking the ends of a sarcomere.

THE SARCOMERE

The sarcomere is the contractile unit in muscle tissue (see Figure 5-9). Myofibrils consist of chains of sarcomeres along the length of a muscle. Sarcomeres consist of the overlapping contractile proteins, actin and myosin, that form regions within the sarcomere.

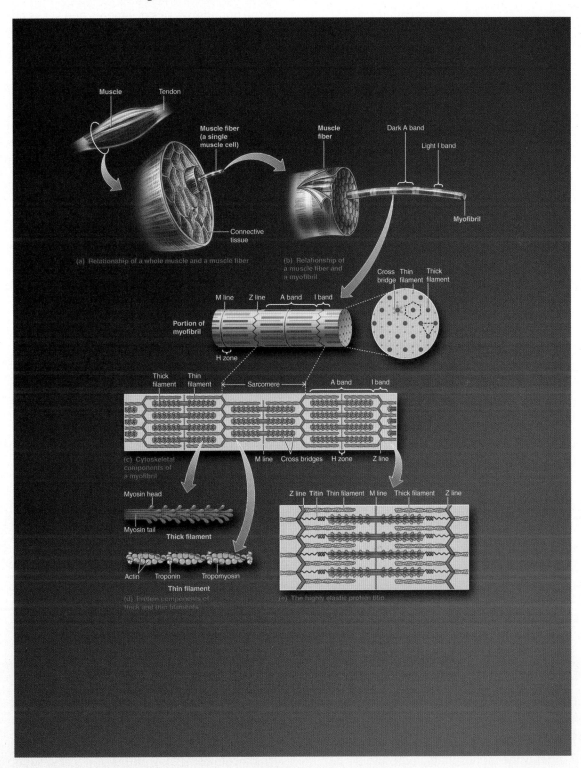

FIGURE 5-9 Organization of muscle structure.

Actin, the thin filament, consists of a double-helix protein structure. Another protein complex wraps around the actin molecule. This complex consists of troponin and tropomyosin. **Tropomyosin** is a fibrous protein that wraps around the length of the actin molecule. **Troponin** consists of three polypeptide subunits that attach to tropomyosin and cover a myosin binding site on actin.

Sarcomeres are defined at the beginning and end by structures forming dark lines called **Z-disks**. Z-disks are the boundaries of sarcomeres and act as connection points for actin. Sarcomeres also contain light and dark bands formed by the overlapping of actin and myosin. These include **A-bands** and **I-bands**.

A-bands are dark regions where actin and myosin overlap. These dark regions are variable and can increase in size during muscle contraction as more actin and myosin overlap (see Figure 5-10). Lighter regions called I-bands are formed by actin only. These regions can decrease in size during muscle contraction. At the center of an A-band is a region consisting only of myosin called the **H-zone**. Myosin connects to the sarcomere at a region called the **M-line**. M-lines are located at the center of a sarcomere.

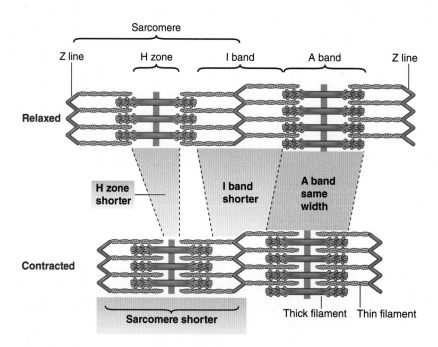

FIGURE 5-10 Sarcomere shortening.

LEARNING OBJECTIVE `5.2.15` **Explain the sequence of events that are collectively known as the sliding filament theory of muscle contraction.**

KEY TERMS

acetylcholine Neurotransmitter secreted by motor neurons that promotes contraction of skeletal muscle.

ADP Adenosine diphosphate; molecule consisting of the amino acid adenosine and two phosphates; an additional phosphate can be added to form adenosine triphosphate.

ATP Adenosine triphosphate; energy-storing molecule consisting of the amino acid adenosine and three phosphate molecules.

cisternae Tiny membranous channels located around muscle cells that combine to form the sarcoplasmic reticulum.

cross-bridge Connections in muscle tissue formed by the binding of myosin to actin.

cross-bridge cycling Cycle in which myosin attaches to actin, moves actin, then releases from actin while powered by ATP.

depolarizes Process of depolarization such as in a cell membrane becoming less polarized.

ligand-gated transport proteins Transport proteins that are activated by other molecules that bind to them.

membrane potential Electrical charge of a membrane.

polarized Pertaining to a difference in electrical potential on either side of a membrane.

power stroke Portion of the sliding filament model of muscle contraction in which a myosin molecule moves an actin molecule while powered by ATP.

sliding filament theory Theory explaining the physiology of skeletal muscle contraction.

voltage-gated calcium channels Transport proteins located in muscle tissue, particularly in the sarcoplasmic reticulum, that open in response to depolarization and release calcium into the cell.

THE SLIDING FILAMENT THEORY OF MUSCLE CONTRACTION

The essence of the sliding filament theory of muscle contraction is the action of actin and myosin sliding past each other (see Figure 5-11). When this happens, the sarcomere shortens and the muscle contracts. The process begins when an impulse travels from a motor neuron to a muscle fiber.

Motor Neuron Sends Message to Muscle to Contract

A motor neuron releases a message in the form of the neurotransmitter acetylcholine to the muscle fiber to tell it to contract. The neurotransmitter travels across an area between the neuron and muscle called the synaptic cleft to a specialized area of the muscle fiber called the motor end plate. The sarcolemma is enfolded at the motor end plate in order to increase the surface area.

Muscle Cell Depolarizes

Muscle cells exist in a polarized state in which there is a difference in voltage between the inside and outside of the cell. In muscle cells, the voltage on the inside of the cell is negative with respect to the outside. This difference is maintained by electrolyte channels located within the cell membranes of myocytes. This electrical state of muscle tissue is known as resting membrane potential. The resting membrane potential of muscle tissue ranges from about −70 mV to −90 mV.

When acetylcholine reaches the motor end plate, it attaches to receptors on ligand-gated transport proteins. These transport proteins respond by opening to allow the movement of sodium inside of the cell. Since sodium is a positive

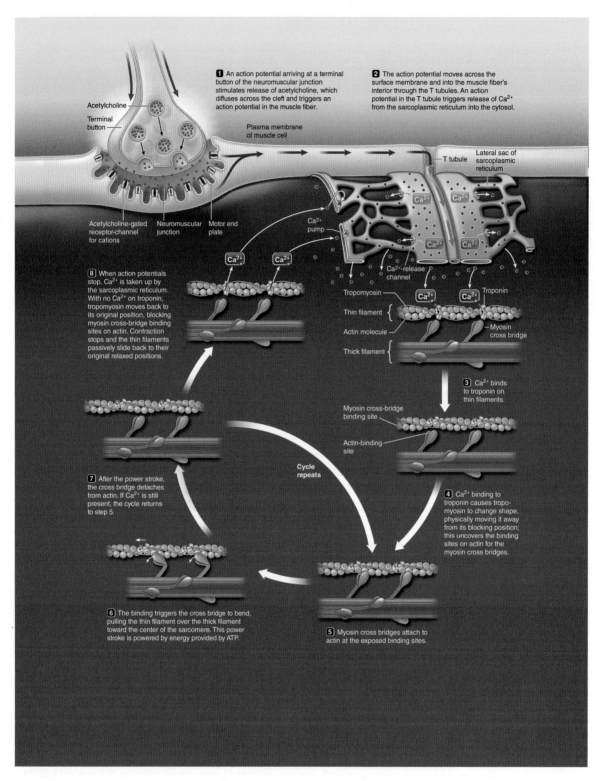

FIGURE 5-11 Events of skeletal muscle contraction.

electrolyte, the movement of sodium inside of the cell causes the membrane potential to change. The membrane potential becomes less negative. Since the muscle cell began in a polarized state, the movement of sodium to the inside of the cell causes the cell to depolarize. We say the muscle cell **depolarizes**.

Release of Calcium by the Sarcoplasmic Reticulum

The sarcolemma surrounding the muscle cell contains tube-like structures called t-tubules. The t-tubules reach into the muscle fiber and encircle the sarcomere. Since the t-tubule connects to the outside of the cell, it contains extracellular fluid. A specialized type of endoplasmic reticulum called the sarcoplasmic reticulum is located between the t-tubules. The sarcoplasmic reticulum consists of a network of membranous channels called **cisternae.**

The sarcoplasmic reticulum contains active calcium transport proteins that create and maintain a high concentration gradient. The concentration of calcium inside the sarcoplasmic reticulum is 2000 times greater than inside the muscle cell.

The sarcoplasmic reticulum also contains **voltage-gated calcium channels** in the terminal cisternae that respond to depolarization. These channels remain closed when the muscle is at rest. When the muscle cells depolarize in response to the release of acetylcholine and subsequent opening of sodium channels at the motor end plate, the voltage-gated channels open to allow calcium out of the sarcoplasmic reticulum and into the cell. This process is called excitation–contraction coupling.

Calcium Binds to the Troponin on the Actin

The calcium released by the sarcoplasmic reticulum rushes into the sarcoplasm of the muscle cell. The troponin on the troponin–tropomyosin complex wrapped around actin is responsive to calcium. The troponin–tropomyosin complex normally covers the myosin binding site on actin. When calcium enters the sarcoplasm, it attaches to the troponin portion. This causes a change in the position of troponin, exposing the myosin binding site on the actin. Myosin now binds with actin, forming a **cross-bridge.**

Sarcomere Shortening

Myosin can now move the actin, causing the two filaments to slide past each other. Myosin releases from actin at the end of one cycle of movement (**cross-bridge cycling**) and returns to its original position. It is now free to repeat the cycle and bind with another site on the actin. One cycle consists of cross-bridge formation, movement, release, and myosin's return to its original position. When nervous system stimulation stops, muscle cells return to their original polarized state and the voltage-gated calcium channels in the sarcoplasmic reticulum close. Calcium releases from troponin, causing troponin to move and cover the myosin binding site. Calcium is pumped from the sarcoplasm to the sarcoplasmic reticulum. The sarcomere then lengthens as the muscle relaxes.

One **ATP** molecule provides the energy needed for one cross-bridge cycle. ATP binds to the myosin head, which can use ATP for energy (ATPase activity). The ATP releases energy and breaks into **ADP** and a phosphate molecule. Once calcium attaches to troponin and exposes the binding site, the myosin moves and binds to actin while releasing the phosphate and extracting the energy from the phosphate bond. ADP is released from the myosin head when myosin moves actin. Another ATP must again bind to the myosin head to allow for release of the myosin head from actin. The myosin head releases from actin and resumes its resting position with the ADP and phosphate still attached.

Movement of the myosin head while it is attached to actin is called the **power stroke**, while movement of the myosin head back to its original position is called the recovery stroke. Resting muscles store energy from ATP in the myosin heads while they wait for another contraction.

LEARNING OBJECTIVE 5.2.16 List the energy sources available to skeletal muscles.

KEY TERMS

citric acid cycle System of reactions located in the mitochondrion that convert acetyl-coenzyme A into ATP, FADH2, and NADH for providing energy to the body.

creatine phosphate Energy-storing molecule located around muscle tissue that can lend its phosphate for phosphorylation of ADP to make ATP.

glycolysis Metabolic process in which one molecule of glucose is converted to two molecules of pyruvic acid while producing a net gain of two molecules of ATP.

phosphorylation Chemical process by which a phosphate molecule is added to adenosine diphosphate to produce one molecule of adenosine triphosphate.

SKELETAL MUSCLE ENERGY SOURCES

Skeletal muscles are powered by ATP. Sources of ATP include chemical pathways of cellular metabolism. These include **glycolysis**, the **citric acid cycle**, electron transport chain, and **creatine phosphate**. Glycolysis occurs in the cytoplasm, while the citric acid cycle and electron transport chain occur in the mitochondria of muscle cells. Glycolysis produces ATP and products that can enter the citric acid cycle and electron transport chain. Glycolysis can supply energy during intense activity lasting a few minutes under anaerobic conditions. The citric acid cycle and electron transport chain work together to supply the majority of ATP for the body's needs under aerobic conditions (if oxygen is present). Muscle contains the protein myoglobin, which can bind with oxygen providing a supply of oxygen to muscle tissue. Creatine phosphate stored around muscle tissue can lend its phosphate for **phosphorylation** of ADP under anaerobic conditions for about 15 seconds of muscle contraction during intense activity. In phosphorylation, a phosphate is added to ADP to produce ATP.

UNIT OBJECTIVE 5.3

Describe how muscles respond to stimulation.

UNIT INTRODUCTION

Muscle contraction is controlled by the nervous system. Muscles contract in response to nervous system impulses traveling through nerves. The nerves release neurotransmitters that promote changes in the electrical state of muscle tissue, causing muscle contraction. In this unit, we explore how muscles respond to stimulation.

LEARNING OBJECTIVE 5.3.1 **Describe neural control of macroscopic muscle contraction.**

cerebellum Portion of the brain located in the posterior region and inferior to the cerebrum. Processes fine motor movements, balance, coordination, and proprioception.

frontal lobes Anterior portion of the cerebrum that processes motor information and higher-level

brain functions such as concentration, planning, problem solving, and personality.

primary motor cortex Area of the frontal lobe that contains neurons that lead to physical movements.

proprioception Sense of the position of a joint.

NERVOUS SYSTEM CONTROL OF MUSCLE CONTRACTION

Muscles respond to stimulation from the nervous system by depolarizing from their resting membrane potentials. The depolarization travels across muscle cells, causing cross-bridge formation and sarcomere shortening resulting in muscle contraction. The nervous system cell that connects to muscle tissue is known as a motor neuron. Motor neurons can connect to just a few muscle fibers or many muscle fibers depending on the specificity of the movement. Each motor neuron and the muscle fibers it connects to is called a motor unit.

Muscle contraction is regulated by a combination of information processed in parts of the brain and stretch information from sensory receptors in muscle tissue. Areas of the brain involved in muscle contraction include areas of the frontal lobes called the primary motor cortex. The cerebellum also plays a role in muscle contraction by helping to regulate coordination, fine muscle movements, and proprioception.

LEARNING OBJECTIVE 5.3.2 **Describe neural control of microscopic muscle contraction.**

NEURAL REGULATION OF MUSCLE CONTRACTION

Muscle contraction is regulated and fine-tuned by the nervous system. Portions of the brain that process muscle contraction send impulses to the spinal cord, which relay these impulses to muscles by way of nerves. Sensory receptors in muscle tissue feedback information to the brain regarding stretch, loading, and joint position so the brain can work to fine-tune muscle contraction.

For example, nervous system cells called alpha motor neurons extend from the spinal cord to muscles. These neurons carry impulses to muscles, telling them to contract. Muscle contraction is fine-tuned by stretch receptors in muscle tissue. These stretch receptors sense changes in muscle length and send impulses to the spinal cord to help regulate muscle contraction.

Stretch receptors known as muscle spindles sense changes in muscle length while performing deep tendon reflexes such as the knee jerk reflex. Reflexes can be used to identify nervous system dysfunction. For example, exaggerated reflexes indicate problems with the brain or spinal cord, while diminished or absent reflexes indicate problems with the nerves, bringing impulses to the muscles.

LEARNING OBJECTIVE 5.3.3 Define resting membrane potential.

LEARNING OBJECTIVE 5.3.4 Explain the resting potential of a muscle cell.

KEY TERMS

ions Chemical compound possessing an overall charge that is less than or greater than zero.

polarized Pertaining to a difference in electrical potential on either side of a membrane.

resting membrane potential Electrically polarized state of muscle and nerve cells during an absence of stimulation.

sodium-potassium pump Type of transport protein located in cell membranes that requires energy (ATP) to move three sodium ions outside and two potassium ions into a cell.

RESTING MEMBRANE POTENTIAL OF MUSCLE TISSUE

Muscle tissue exists in a polarized state known as resting membrane potential. In muscle cells, resting membrane potential is between –70mV and –90mV.

The resting membrane potential of muscle cells is created and maintained by the movement of ions in and out of the cells. Muscle cells exist in an environment in which there are a greater number of positive charges outside of the cells than inside. This results in a negative charge inside of the cell as compared to the outside (see Figure 5-12).

Sodium is the main extracellular electrolyte. Sodium has a positive charge and is at a higher concentration outside of muscle cells than inside. The sodium gradient is maintained by the sodium-potassium pump located in muscle tissue cells (see Figure 5-13). The sodium-potassium pump also maintains a potassium gradient in which more potassium is located inside of muscle cells than outside. Muscle cells contain additional passive protein channels that leak sodium and potassium into and out of the cell. Some sodium leaks into the cell and some potassium leaks out of the cell. There is a greater membrane permeability to potassium, so more potassium exits the cell than enters. Chloride ions also play a role in resting membrane potential as a small amount of negatively charged chloride ions move into muscle cells. The combined effect of both the active and passive protein channels produces the resting membrane potential of muscle cells, which is about –70 mV to –90 mV.

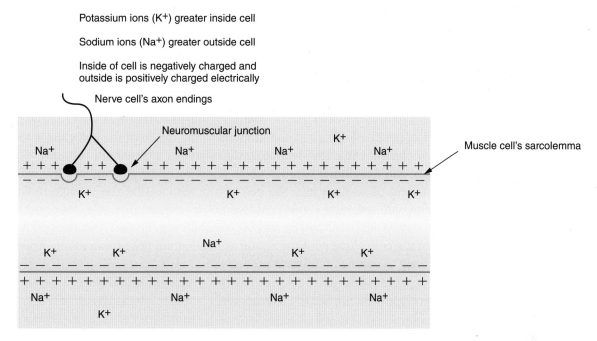

Potassium ions (K⁺) greater inside cell

Sodium ions (Na⁺) greater outside cell

Inside of cell is negatively charged and outside is positively charged electrically

Nerve cell's axon endings

Neuromuscular junction

Muscle cell's sarcolemma

FIGURE 5-12 Electrical factors affecting skeletal muscle.

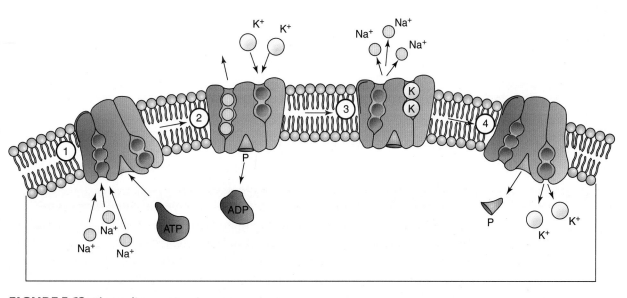

FIGURE 5-13 The sodium-potassium pump.

LEARNING OBJECTIVE 5.3.5 Explain the creation, transmission, and physiologic effect of an action potential.

KEY TERM

action potential Rapid change in voltage generated by muscle and nervous tissue.

ACTION POTENTIALS

Action potentials are created in muscle cells in response to stimulation by the nervous system. Neurons secrete the neurotransmitter acetylcholine, which travels across the synaptic cleft to the motor end plate on muscle tissue. Acetylcholine then attaches to ligand-gated transport proteins that open to allow sodium to flow down its concentration gradient to inside of the cell. The movement of positively charged sodium ions to the inside of the cell causes the cell to depolarize. Once the depolarization reaches a threshold (around –50mV), voltage-gated sodium channels open, allowing more sodium into the cell. The movement of sodium into the cell continues causing the voltage to rapidly change until reaching +30 mV. At this point, sodium channels close and potassium moves out of the cell by way of leak channels. The movement of potassium out of the cell, along with the action of the sodium-potassium pump, brings the cell back to resting membrane potential.

CLINICAL TIP	The electrical activity of muscles can be measured by a test called an EMG (electromyography). EMG can help to determine muscle function and disease.

LEARNING OBJECTIVE 5.3.6 Identify the structure of a motor unit.

LEARNING OBJECTIVE 5.3.7 Describe the characteristics of a motor unit.

LEARNING OBJECTIVE 5.3.8 Describe the function of a motor unit.

KEY TERMS

axons Long processes extending from the cell bodies of neurons; can be myelinated or unmyelinated.

axon terminal Portion of a neuron located at the end of an axon that releases neurotransmitter into the synaptic cleft.

muscle fibers Long, cylindrical cells that make up skeletal muscle tissue.

THE MOTOR UNIT

Axons of motor neurons connect to muscle fibers by way of the motor neuron's **axon terminal**. A motor unit consists of a motor neuron's axon terminal and the muscle fibers the axon terminal connects to (see Figure 5-14).

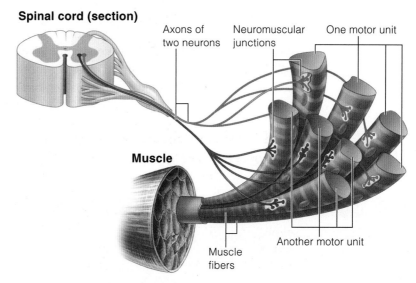

Spinal cord (section)

Axons of two neurons   Neuromuscular junctions   One motor unit

Muscle

Muscle fibers   Another motor unit

FIGURE 5-14 Skeletal muscle motor unit.

Characteristics and Structure of Motor Units

Activation of a motor unit will result in contraction of all the connected muscle fibers. **Axons** can innervate few or many muscle fibers. For example, larger muscles in the thigh have arrangements in which one motor neuron connects to many **muscle fibers**, whereas muscles that control eye movement may have as few as 10 muscle fibers connected to one motor neuron. The number of connections depends on the accuracy of movement needed. In muscles that produce large, less accurate movements, one neuron will connect with many muscle fibers. In muscles that produce smaller, more accurate movements, one neuron will connect with fewer muscle fibers.

LEARNING OBJECTIVE 5.3.9 Describe resting membrane potential.

KEY TERMS

electrolytes Minerals, typically salts, that carry a charge and are responsible for many essential processes in the body.

membrane permeability Property of a membrane that allows substances to pass through.

resting membrane potential Electrically polarized state of muscle and nerve cells during an absence of stimulation.

RESTING MEMBRANE POTENTIAL DETAIL

The **resting membrane potential** is established by the concentration gradients of **electrolytes** and is maintained by the sodium-potassium pump and the cell's electrolyte **membrane permeability**. For example, the sodium-potassium pump moves three sodium ions outside of the cell while moving two potassium ions inside. The resultant gradient creates a negative charge inside of the cell as compared to outside. The cell membrane also contains passive sodium and potassium protein leak channels. These channels transport more potassium out of the cell than sodium into the cell, which results in a net loss of positive charges from the cell.

LEARNING OBJECTIVE 5.3.10 Define recruitment, inhibitory post-synaptic potentials, and excitatory post-synaptic potentials.

KEY TERMS

excitatory neurotransmitter Neurotransmitter that promotes the opening of sodium channels on adjacent tissue.

inhibitory neurotransmitter Neurotransmitter that inhibits the generation of an action potential in a post-synaptic neuron by promoting the opening of potassium and chloride gates.

excitatory post-synaptic potentials Secretion of neurotransmitters that promote depolarization of the post-synaptic membranes of tissues.

inhibitory post-synaptic potentials Potential that inhibits the generation of an action potential in a post-synaptic neuron.

recruitment Action of additional firing of motor units.

NEUROTRANSMITTER FUNCTION AT THE SYNAPTIC CLEFT

The strength of a muscle contraction depends on the number of motor units activated. Activation of greater numbers of motor units will produce stronger contractions. **Recruitment** is the activation of more motor units to produce stronger contractions.

Inhibitory post-synaptic potentials consist of the release of an **inhibitory neurotransmitter** from a presynaptic neuron that travels across the synaptic cleft to inhibit the generation of an action potential in the post-synaptic neuron or muscle.

Excitatory post-synaptic potentials consist of the release of an **excitatory neurotransmitter** from a pre-synaptic neuron that travels across a synaptic cleft to a post-synaptic neuron or muscle tissue. These neurotransmitters promote the generation of action potentials on the post-synaptic neuron or muscle.

LEARNING OBJECTIVE 5.3.11 Explain the role of recruitment, inhibitory post-synaptic potentials, and excitatory post-synaptic potentials in muscle contraction.

KEY TERMS

concentration gradient Difference in concentration between two sides of a membrane.

depolarization Change in voltage from a negative resting membrane potential toward a positive state from the movement of sodium ions inside of a cell.

POST-SYNAPTIC POTENTIALS

Activation of one motor unit will result in contraction of all the connected muscle fibers, producing a weak muscle contraction. In many cases, more motor units are needed to produce a contraction with enough force to accomplish a given task. In this case, more motor units will activate in order to produce a stronger contraction. Recruitment is the activation of additional motor units in order to produce a stronger contraction. Recruitment occurs with the activation of smaller motor units first, followed by activation of larger motor units.

In the case of muscle contraction, the action potential generated by a motor neuron causes the release of the neurotransmitter acetylcholine from the axon terminal. Acetylcholine promotes opening of ligand-gated sodium channels, allowing the movement of sodium down its concentration gradient into the muscle cell and the cell depolarizes. Synaptic potentials of this type that promote depolarization are called excitatory post-synaptic potentials.

Neurotransmitters promoting the opening of chloride and potassium channels will work to hyperpolarize the cell. The opening of chloride channels causes the movement of chloride into the cell, resulting in greater negative membrane potential. Likewise, opening potassium channels promotes the movement of potassium out of the cell as potassium follows its concentration gradient, which adds to the increased membrane negative potential. Since this action makes it more difficult for the cell to depolarize and generate an action potential, these are known as inhibitory post-synaptic potentials. Both excitatory and inhibitory post-synaptic potentials work together to regulate the activation of muscle cells.

LEARNING OBJECTIVE 5.3.12 Explain the all-or-none rule of muscle contraction.

KEY TERMS

all-or-none rule Contraction of a muscle fiber once the threshold for voltage is reached.

stimulus Substance or event invoking a change in a system.

threshold Voltage in muscle or nervous tissue that results in the generation of an action potential when reached.

THE ALL-OR-NONE RULE OF MUSCLE CONTRACTION

Muscle fibers never partially contract. Once a muscle fiber's stimulus reaches a threshold, the entire muscle fiber contracts. This is known as the all-or-none rule of muscle contraction. The force created by muscle fiber contraction will not increase with an additional stimulus once the threshold has been reached. Muscles at rest have a membrane potential of between –70 mV to –90 mV. Stimulation of the muscle by excitatory neurotransmitters causes the membrane potential to become less negative. When the membrane reaches about –50 mV, voltage-gated sodium gates open, allowing more positively charged sodium into the cell until it reaches +30 mV. The cell must reach –50 mV in order to generate an action potential and subsequently contract. The –50 mV voltage is known as the **threshold** for muscle contraction.

LEARNING OBJECTIVE 5.3.13 Describe a muscle twitch.

KEY TERMS

muscle twitch Single contraction of a muscle fiber.

myosin binding site Area on the thin actin filament where myosin can bind to form a cross-bridge.

THE MUSCLE TWITCH

A single impulse from a motor neuron will result in a single contraction of a muscle fiber. The contraction lasts for only a few milliseconds and is called a **muscle twitch**. The muscle twitch consists of three phases: latent, contraction, and relaxation.

The latent period is characterized by the time between action potential generation in the muscle and muscle contraction. The latent period is about 1–2 milliseconds in duration. During this time, calcium is released by the sarcoplasmic reticulum and enters the muscle cell. Calcium attaches to the troponin, causing it to move and expose the myosin binding site on actin allowing for cross-bridge formation. Also during the latent phase, active transport proteins move calcium back into the sarcoplasmic reticulum. The troponin moves back into position blocking the **myosin binding site** on the actin and the muscle lengthens. A muscle twitch can last up to 100 milliseconds.

The next phase is the contraction (shortening) phase. During this phase, cross-bridge cycling occurs as myosin pulls actin, causing actin and myosin to slide past each other. The sarcomere shortens and muscle contraction occurs.

The relaxation phase is characterized by the release of myosin from actin (see Figure 5-15).

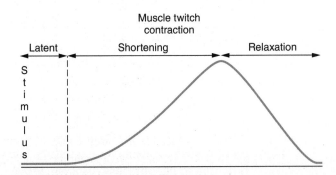

FIGURE 5-15 Muscle twitch.

LEARNING OBJECTIVE 5.3.14 Describe a sustained muscle contraction.

THE SUSTAINED MUSCLE CONTRACTION

There is no **refractory period** in muscle fibers. For example, continuous stimulation of a muscle by a high rate of action potentials would result in a gradual increase in the number of motor units contracting with no relaxation. Eventually, the muscle would exhibit a sustained or **tetanic contraction**. Tetanic contractions occur with postural muscles and when continually holding a weight. Weak tetanic contractions occur to produce **muscle tone**. For example, many muscles contract unconsciously in order to maintain different postures such as sitting or standing. These muscles exhibit tetanic or continuous contractions in order to stabilize joints. It would be impossible to consciously contract all of the muscles needed to maintain these postures.

The disease tetanus can cause tetanic contractions. Tetanus is caused by a bacterium that blocks inhibitory neurotransmitters in the synaptic cleft that work to control muscle contraction. The result is the sustained tetanic contractions seen in the disease.

LEARNING OBJECTIVE 5.3.15 Distinguish between a muscle twitch and sustained contraction.

COMPARING MUSCLE TWITCHES AND SUSTAINED CONTRACTIONS

A muscle twitch is the single contraction of a muscle fiber that includes a **relaxation phase** resulting from a single motor unit impulse. For example, while lifting a weight, many muscle fibers will perform muscle twitches. If all of the muscle fibers contracted together, the result would be a jerky contraction of the entire muscle. So, muscle fibers contract and relax at different time periods. This is known as asynchronous contraction of muscle fibers. During asynchronous contraction, one fiber contracts and relaxes while another fiber contracts before the first relaxes. The asynchronous contraction of muscle fibers produces a smooth continuous movement.

Some muscles produce sustained contractions. During sustained contractions, there is continuous stimulation from the nervous system. The muscle contracts continuously with no relaxation phase. Sustained contractions occur with continual motor neuron impulses and do not include a relaxation phase. In skeletal muscle, tetanic contractions are examples of sustained contractions. Smooth muscle will also produce sustained contractions. For example, sustained contractions occur in smooth muscle lining the digestive tract to help transport substances through it.

LEARNING OBJECTIVE 5.3.16 Describe the characteristics of fast-twitch muscle fibers.

LEARNING OBJECTIVE 5.3.17 Describe the characteristics of slow-twitch muscle fibers.

LEARNING OBJECTIVE 5.3.18 Distinguish between fast- and slow-twitch muscle fibers.

KEY TERMS

fast-twitch fibers Small groups of muscle fibers that can generate a high degree of force for a short duration.

intermediate fibers Muscle fibers exhibiting characteristics of both fast- and slow-twitch fibers.

slow-twitch fibers Type of muscle fiber capable of producing low force over long durations while relying on aerobic sources of energy.

TYPES OF MUSCLE FIBERS

There are three types of skeletal muscle fibers: fast-twitch (Type II), slow-twitch (Type I), and intermediate (Type IIa).

Fast-twitch fibers generate high force for brief periods of time. Slow-twitch fibers generate lower amounts of force but can do so for longer periods of time. Intermediate fibers have some characteristics of both fast- and slow-twitch fibers.

Fast-twitch fibers are the predominant fibers in the body and contain a large number of myofibrils. They respond quickly to stimuli, generate a high force for short periods of time, and rely on anaerobic sources of ATP. They have a large diameter due to the large number of myofibrils. Their activity is fueled by ATP generated from anaerobic metabolism (see Figure 5-16AB).

Slow-twitch fibers respond much more slowly to stimuli than fast-twitch fibers. They are smaller in diameter and contain many mitochondria. They can sustain long contractions and obtain their ATP from aerobic metabolism.

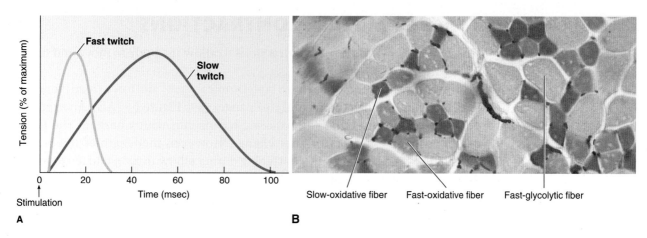

FIGURE 5-16AB Muscle fiber types.

Slow-twitch fibers are surrounded by capillary networks that supply oxygenated blood for use in the aerobic energy systems. They contain a red pigment called myoglobin. Myoglobin can bind oxygen (like hemoglobin) and provide a substantial oxygen reserve. Because of the reddish color of myoglobin, these fibers are often called red muscle fibers.

Intermediate fibers resemble fast-twitch fibers because they contain small amounts of myoglobin. They also have a capillary network surrounding them and do not fatigue as readily as fast-twitch fibers. They contain more mitochondria than fast-twitch fibers but not as many as slow-twitch fibers. The speed of contraction and endurance also lie between fast- and slow-twitch fibers.

Muscles containing a predominance of slow fibers are sometimes referred to as red muscles. Examples of these muscles include some muscles in the back and areas of the legs. Muscles containing a predominance of fast fibers are referred to as white muscles. Due to the accuracy and speed of muscle contraction required, there are no slow-twitch fibers in the eye muscles or muscles of the hands.

Athletic activities can predominantly rely on different muscle fibers. Activities requiring a short burst of muscular power rely more on fast-twitch fibers, whereas activities requiring less power over longer durations relay more on slow-twitch fibers. For example, sprinting, powerlifting, and jumping would activate more fast-twitch fibers. Activities such as running, bicycling, or swimming long distances would activate more slow-twitch fibers.

LEARNING OBJECTIVE 5.3.19 **Explain how different types of muscle contraction allow the body to move and maintain posture.**

KEY TERMS

concentric contractions Contractions in which a muscle shortens while moving a load.

eccentric contractions Muscle contraction in which a muscle lengthens while supporting a load.

isometric contractions Muscle contraction characterized by the length of the contracting muscle not changing while the load the muscle pulls or pushes can change.

isotonic contractions Muscle contraction characterized by the length of the contracting muscle changing while the load the muscle pulls or pushes does not change.

TYPES OF MUSCLE CONTRACTIONS

Muscles perform a variety of contractions to allow the body to move and maintain posture.

In **isotonic contractions** (iso = equal, tonic = tone), the force (load) remains the same but the length of the muscle changes (see Figure 5-17AB). An example of an isotonic contraction is the classic biceps curl with a barbell. The force exhibited by the barbell does not change. However, the length of the biceps brachii muscle can change by shortening during elbow flexion and lengthening during extension. Isotonic exercises are used in many gym settings in which participants use barbells and weight equipment.

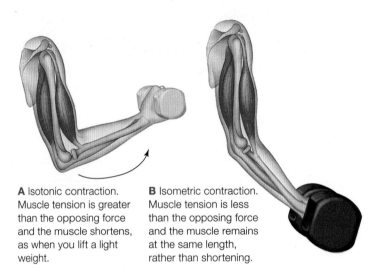

A Isotonic contraction. Muscle tension is greater than the opposing force and the muscle shortens, as when you lift a light weight.

B Isometric contraction. Muscle tension is less than the opposing force and the muscle remains at the same length, rather than shortening.

FIGURE 5-17AB Isotonic (A) and isometric (B) contractions.

In **isometric contractions** (iso = equal, metric = length) the force can change but the length of the muscle remains the same (see Figure 5-17AB). In isometric contractions, there is no movement of the joint since the muscle length does not change. An example of an isometric contraction would be to push against an object that cannot be moved, such as a wall. The push or force can change, but there is no joint movement. The muscular system helps to maintain posture through isometric contractions.

Concentric contractions are characterized by muscles shortening against a load. For example, the biceps brachii muscle shortens when bending the elbow while performing a biceps curl. We say the biceps brachii is performing a concentric isotonic contraction.

Eccentric contractions are characterized by muscles lengthening against a load. For example, during the second part of a biceps brachii curl exercise, where the elbow is straightened while lowering the weight, the biceps brachii muscle elongates. We say the biceps brachii is performing an eccentric isotonic contraction.

CLINICAL TIP

Physical therapy can involve rehabilitation of damaged muscle tissue by having patients perform isometric and isotonic contractions. In many cases, isometric exercises are performed before isotonic exercises due to the ability to exercise at different joint angles without overloading the muscle.

     Muscles are more prone to injury while performing eccentric contractions versus concentric contractions. Physical therapists and personal trainers will sometimes prescribe an eccentric training regimen in order to reduce injuries.

LEARNING OBJECTIVE | **5.3.20** | **Explain oxygen debt.**

KEY TERMS

glycolysis Metabolic process in which one molecule of glucose is converted to two molecules of pyruvic acid while producing a net gain of two molecules of ATP.

lactic acid By-product of glycolysis resulting from the production of pyruvic acid.

oxygen debt Use of oxygen in the conversion of lactic acid to pyruvic acid and glucose.

phosphocreatine Molecule that can lend a phosphate molecule to ADP to produce ATP.

pyruvic acid Product of glycolysis.

OXYGEN DEBT

Muscles use ATP as an energy source for contraction. ATP can come from aerobic and anaerobic metabolism. Lactic acid is produced when the muscular system uses anaerobic metabolism systems to supply ATP, such as anaerobic glycolysis and the phosphocreatine system. Lactic acid then needs to be converted back to pyruvic acid and glucose. Since oxygen is needed for this process, we say that intense muscle activity results in oxygen debt.

     You may have noticed that your breathing rate remains elevated after a period of strenuous activity. Breathing rate increases while the body is experiencing oxygen debt, as lactic acid is converted back to glucose.

CLINICAL TIP

Lactic acid can build up in the muscles when performing intense activity, such as in sports. The buildup of lactic acid can limit (inhibit) the anaerobic energy system and reduce performance. Athletic trainers will sometimes instruct athletes to perform low-level repetitive exercise in order to help to eliminate lactic acid in the muscles. When exercising at intense levels, the "burn" felt results from lactic acid buildup.

KEY TERMS

lactic acid By-product of glycolysis resulting from the production of pyruvic acid.

pH Exponential (logarithmic) scale measuring the acidity or alkalinity of a substance.

MUSCLE FATIGUE

Muscle fatigue occurs when there is no contraction in response to stimulation from the nervous system. Muscle fatigue can result from periods of intense activity. A number of factors contribute to muscle fatigue, including decreased ATP reserves, lowered **pH** due to **lactic acid** buildup from anaerobic glycolysis, and electrolyte imbalances affecting calcium release from the sarcoplasmic reticulum.

Muscle fatigue can also occur when the nervous system fails to stimulate motor neurons to muscle tissue. Psychologically based muscle fatigue results from pain or discomfort from strenuous exercise or from decreased motivation for performing an activity. For example, pain from intense athletic competition could produce neurologically based muscle fatigue. Likewise, decreased motivation from performing a repetitive task could also produce fatigue.

UNIT OBJECTIVE 5.4

Describe the structure and function of smooth muscle.

UNIT INTRODUCTION

Smooth muscle is a special type of muscle found lining the organs (except for the heart) and blood vessels. Smooth muscle contains many of the structures of skeletal and cardiac muscle and is under involuntary control. Smooth muscle is capable of maintaining contractions for long periods and can produce wave-like contractions needed to move substances through the body. In this unit, we examine the characteristics and function of smooth muscle.

KEY TERMS

calmodulin Calcium-binding protein found in smooth muscle.

striated Light and dark areas in muscle tissue formed by overlapping contractile protein filaments.

STRUCTURE OF SMOOTH MUSCLE

Smooth muscle is found throughout the body in organs, blood vessels, and tube-like structures. Smooth muscle consists of long, spindle-shaped single nucleated cells containing actin and myosin. Smooth muscle is not **striated** since actin and myosin are not arranged in sarcomeres but are scattered about the muscle (see Figure 5-18ABC). Unlike the more cordlike appearance of skeletal muscle, smooth muscle is arranged in sheet like layers. Smooth muscle contains a calcium-binding protein called **calmodulin**, has no t-tubules, and the myosin has a larger number of globular protein heads. The fibers in smooth muscle are smaller than in skeletal muscle.

A Skeletal muscle

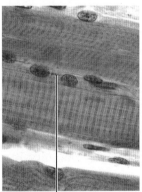

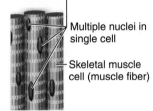

Multiple nuclei in single cell

Skeletal muscle cell (muscle fiber)

Classification: Striated muscle, voluntary muscle

Description: Bundles of long, thick, cylindrical, striated, contractile, multinucleate cells that extend the length of the muscle

Typical location: Attached to bones of skeleton

Function: Movement of body in relation to external environment

B Cardiac muscle

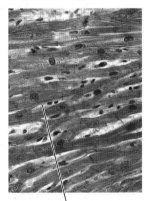

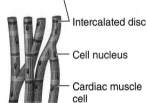

Intercalated disc

Cell nucleus

Cardiac muscle cell

Classification: Striated muscle, involuntary muscle

Description: Interlinked network of short, slender, cylindrical, striated, branched, contractile cells connected cell to cell by intercalated discs

Location: Wall of heart

Function: Pumping of blood out of heart

C Smooth muscle

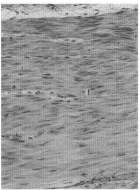

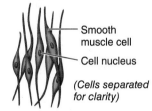

Smooth muscle cell

Cell nucleus

(Cells separated for clarity)

Classification: Unstriated muscle, involuntary muscle

Description: Loose network of short, slender, spindle-shaped, unstriated, contractile cells that are arranged in sheets

Typical location: Walls of hollow organs and tubes, such as stomach and blood vessels

Function: Movement of contents within hollow organs

FIGURE 5-18ABC Muscle tissue types.

LEARNING OBJECTIVE 5.4.2 **Contrast the structural characteristics of skeletal muscle tissue and smooth muscle tissue.**

KEY TERMS

autonomic nervous system Division of the peripheral nervous system that regulates organ function; composed of the sympathetic

pacesetter cells Cells located in the digestive system that undergo spontaneous depolarization and promote smooth muscle contraction.

somatic nervous system Portion of the nervous system innervating the skin, muscles, and viscera.

varicosities Small eminences on axons of neurons innervating smooth muscle that release neurotransmitters.

COMPARING SKELETAL AND SMOOTH MUSCLE STRUCTURE

Unlike skeletal muscle's innervation by the somatic nervous system, smooth muscle is controlled by the autonomic nervous system (involuntary).

Smooth muscle contraction differs from skeletal or cardiac muscle contraction. After release from the sarcoplasmic reticulum, calcium binds to a protein called calmodulin, which allows for the formation of cross-bridges. Because of the structure of smooth muscle, length and tension are not related. When smooth muscle is stretched, it adapts to its new resting length and can continue to contract.

Smooth muscle contraction is involuntary, requires very little energy, and can perform sustained contractions in the absence of calcium. The axons of motor neurons have a unique structure and travel through smooth muscle. Unlike the neuromuscular junctions in skeletal muscle, axons innervating smooth muscle contain small neurotransmitter-releasing bumps called varicosities. Smooth muscle in hollow organs also contains cells that can spontaneously generate action potentials called pacesetter cells.

LEARNING OBJECTIVE 5.4.3 Describe the general function of smooth muscle.

FUNCTION OF SMOOTH MUSCLE

Smooth muscle generally works to regulate the movement of structures and substances through the body. Examples include the regulation of the diameters of arteries and veins to control blood flow, movement of substances through the digestive and urinary tracts, regulation of light entering the eye, movement of hair follicles in the skin in response to cold temperatures, and air flow regulation in the respiratory system. With the exception of the heart, smooth muscle is found lining hollow organs of the body.

LEARNING OBJECTIVE 5.4.4 Identify the structure of multi-unit smooth muscle tissue.

LEARNING OBJECTIVE 5.4.5 Explain the function of multi-unit smooth muscle tissue.

arrector pili muscles Small smooth muscles located in the integument that can move hair follicles.

multi-unit Arrangement of smooth muscle characterized by interconnected motor units.

visceral Pertaining to the organs of the body.

MULTI-UNIT SMOOTH MUSCLE

Smooth muscle cells are classified as **multi-unit** or **visceral**. Multi-unit smooth muscle is organized into motor units that are not dependent on each other. The nervous system must stimulate each motor unit separately. Multi-unit smooth muscle is controlled by the autonomic nervous system and, like skeletal muscle, can perform graded contractions in which motor units are recruited to perform stronger contractions.

Multi-unit smooth muscle is located in blood vessels for vasoconstricting and vasodilating arteries. Multi-unit smooth muscle is also found in the **arrector pili muscles** in the integument, surrounding the pupil, and in the bronchioles.

CLINICAL TIP | Multi-unit smooth muscle function can be observed by testing the pupillary reflex. This test is performed by shining a light in one eye and observing the pupils constrict in the same and opposite eyes. The pupillary reflex examines the pathways of two cranial nerves as well as the function of the muscles in the eye.

LEARNING OBJECTIVE 5.4.6 Identify visceral smooth muscle tissue.

LEARNING OBJECTIVE 5.4.7 Explain the function of visceral smooth muscle tissue.

gap junctions Hollow, water-filled cylinders that allow things like nutrients and ions to pass between neighboring cells; most commonly found in cardiac cells and embryonic cells.

peristalsis Process of smooth muscle contraction along the GI tract that forces material to move further along the tract.

visceral smooth muscle Type of smooth muscle characterized by sheetlike layers that contract as a unit.

VISCERAL SMOOTH MUSCLE

Visceral smooth muscle cells contract as a unit, do not connect directly with motor neurons, and are arranged in layers. **Gap junctions** connect layers of smooth muscle so that one area can influence others when contracting. This can produce a wavelike contraction called **peristalsis**.

Visceral smooth muscle helps to move substances through organs and passages. For example, peristaltic contractions in the digestive tract move food from one portion of the tract to another to allow for digestion and absorption of nutrients.

LEARNING OBJECTIVE 5.4.8 **Contrast the structure and function of multi-unit smooth muscle tissue and visceral smooth muscle tissue.**

KEY TERM

autonomic nervous system neurons Nervous system cells (neurons) belonging to the autonomic nervous system.

COMPARING MULTI-UNIT AND VISCERAL SMOOTH MUSCLE

Multi-unit smooth muscle is organized like skeletal muscle, with motor units innervated by autonomic nervous system neurons. Visceral smooth muscle is arranged in layers connected by gap junctions that allow one area of muscle to influence another (see Figure 5-19AB). Multi-unit smooth muscle, like skeletal muscle, can exhibit recruitment of motor units when stronger contractions are

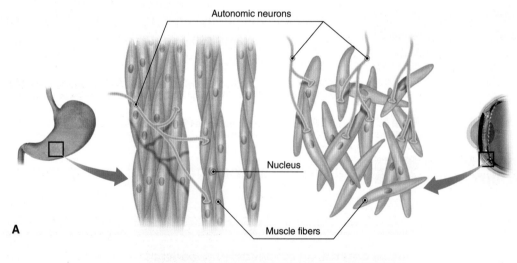

A

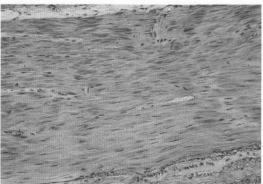

B

FIGURE 5-19AB Visceral and multi-unit smooth muscle.

needed. Since visceral smooth muscle does not have motor units, it does not exhibit recruitment. Because visceral smooth muscle fibers are connected by gap junctions, they contract together as a single unit. Multi-unit smooth muscle responds to nervous system impulses while visceral smooth muscle can also respond to hormonal stimulation.

LEARNING OBJECTIVE 5.4.9 Identify locations where multi-unit smooth muscle tissue can be found.

LEARNING OBJECTIVE 5.4.10 Identify locations where visceral smooth muscle tissue can be found.

WHERE MULTI-UNIT AND VISCERAL SMOOTH MUSCLE ARE FOUND IN THE BODY

Multi-unit smooth muscle can be found surrounding the pupils of the eyes, in the arrector pili muscles of the skin, in large air passages of the respiratory system, and in large arteries.

Visceral (single-unit) smooth muscle is the most common type of smooth muscle in the body. It is found in the walls of hollow organs (except the heart) such as the bronchioles, digestive tract, and blood vessels.

LEARNING OBJECTIVE 5.4.11 Compare the mechanisms of contraction found in skeletal muscle and smooth muscle.

KEY TERMS

alimentary canal The long muscular tube of the digestive system that transports ingested materials from the mouth to anus; site of mechanical and chemical digestion.

hormones Chemical substances, secreted by endocrine glands, that target another tissue in the body.

COMPARING SMOOTH MUSCLE AND SKELETAL MUSCLE CONTRACTION

Skeletal muscle contractions occur from impulses sent from voluntary motor neurons, whereas smooth muscle is under the control of the autonomic nervous system and **hormones**. Both smooth and skeletal muscles can respond to stretch; however, the mechanisms are different. Smooth muscle can directly respond to stretch while skeletal muscle relies on activation of stretch receptors (muscle spindles) that send impulses to the central nervous system to activate motor neurons, which promote muscle contraction.

Skeletal muscle can produce fast or slow contractions, while smooth muscle only contracts slowly. Skeletal muscle uses more energy than smooth muscle and has a different calcium-regulating mechanism than smooth muscle. Calcium connects to troponin in skeletal muscle while calmodulin binds with calcium in smooth muscle to active myosin kinase, which transfers phosphate from ATP to myosin cross-bridges.

Smooth muscle contraction is influenced by the presence of gap junctions connecting groups of smooth muscle cells. Gap junctions allow for synchronous contraction of motor units, whereas skeletal motor units contract independently. Smooth muscle in portions of the alimentary canal contains pacesetter cells that help to regulate the rate of contraction for an entire sheet of smooth muscle. Pacesetter cells can exhibit spontaneous depolarization but will also respond to autonomic nervous system and hormonal stimulation.

UNIT OBJECTIVE 5.5

Describe the structure and function of cardiac muscle.

UNIT INTRODUCTION

The heart beats over three billion times in an average lifetime and all of these heartbeats are performed by cardiac muscle. Cardiac muscle is only found in the heart and contains specific structures to allow the chambers of the heart to efficiently contract throughout the lifespan. This unit examines the structure and function of cardiac muscle.

LEARNING OBJECTIVE 5.5.1 Identify the structure and functions of cardiac muscle.

LEARNING OBJECTIVE 5.5.2 Describe the structure and functions of cardiac muscle.

KEY TERMS

cardiac muscle cells Tissue cells of cardiac muscle.

glycogen Molecule that is the storage form of glucose.

lipids Class of molecules containing fats.

mitochondria Organelle of the cell that produces energy by way of aerobic metabolism.

pacemaker cells Cells in the heart that produce action potentials that govern the rhythm of the heart.

terminal cisternae Tubular channel located in the sarcoplasmic reticulum.

tetanic contraction Muscle contraction in which motor units completely contract without relaxing.

CARDIAC MUSCLE

Cardiac muscle cells are striated and contain one or two nuclei. They have a different arrangement of t-tubules (see Figure 5-20AB). The sarcoplasmic reticulum does not have a terminal cisternae. Cardiac muscle fibers are powered by aerobic metabolism and contain energy reserves in the form of glycogen and lipids. Cardiac muscle cells contain large numbers of mitochondria to utilize aerobic energy systems.

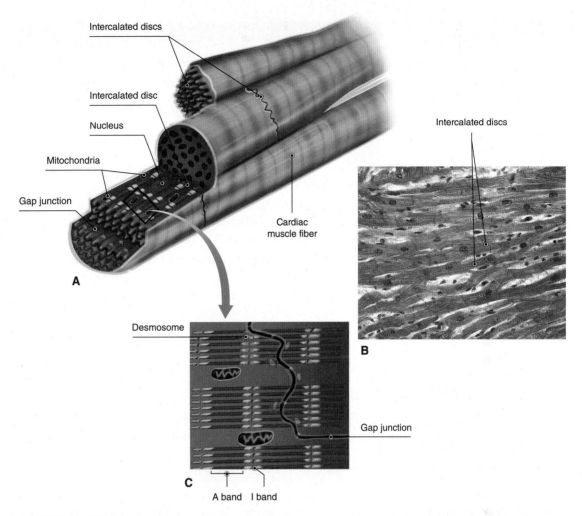

FIGURE 5-20ABC Cardiac muscle.

Cardiac muscle can contract without a stimulus from the nervous system. Cardiac muscle contains self-generating action potential cells called **pacemaker cells**. The pacemaker cells can respond to the nervous system by changing the rate and force of contraction of cardiac muscle cells. Cardiac muscle cannot undergo **tetanic contractions** due to the structure of the cell membrane.

Cardiac muscle is only found in the heart and works to contract the hollow chambers of the heart in order to move blood between chambers and out of the heart to the lungs and body.

CLINICAL TIP | The electrical impulses generated by the nodes in the heart can be measured by way of an ECG (electrocardiogram) test. ECGs can help to determine abnormal heart rhythms.

LEARNING OBJECTIVE 5.5.3 Compare the structure of skeletal, smooth, and cardiac muscle tissue.

extracellular fluid (ECF) Fluid located outside of cells.

multinucleated cells Cells containing more than one nucleus such as in skeletal muscle cells.

SKELETAL, SMOOTH, AND CARDIAC MUSCLE STRUCTURE

Skeletal muscle is striated and consists of long, multinucleated cells. Cardiac muscle cells are also striated, contain one or two nuclei and form branching chains of cells. Smooth muscle cells are not striated, contain one nucleus and are exists in single unit (visceral) or multi-unit arrangements.

Skeletal muscle fibers are arranged in bundles containing epimysium, perimysium, and endomysium coverings. Cardiac and smooth muscle fibers only contain an endomysium covering. Both skeletal and cardiac muscles use calcium to expose myosin binding sites on actin through binding calcium with troponin. Smooth muscle uses calmodulin to bind to calcium to form myosin cross-bridges. Calcium comes from the sarcoplasmic reticulum in skeletal and cardiac muscle, whereas smooth muscle uses calcium from extracellular fluid (ECF) (see Table 5-1).

Table 5-1 Comparison of Muscle Types

CHARACTERISTIC	SKELETAL MUSCLE	MULTIUNIT SMOOTH MUSCLE	SINGLE-UNIT SMOOTH MUSCLE	CARDIAC MUSCLE
Mechanism of contraction	Sliding filament mechanism	Sliding filament mechanism	Sliding filament mechanism	Sliding filament mechanism
Innervation	Somatic nervous system	Autonomic nervous system	Autonomic nervous system	Autonomic nervous system
Level of control	Under voluntary control; also subject to subconscious regulation	Under involuntary control	Under involuntary control	Under involuntary control
Initiation of contraction	Neurogenic	Neurogenic	Myogenic (pacemaker potentials and slow-wave potentials)	Myogenic (pacemaker potentials)
Role of nervous stimulation	Initiates contraction; accomplishes gradation	Initiates contraction; contributes to gradation	Modifies contraction; can excite or inhibit; contributes to gradation	Modifies contraction; can excite or inhibit; contributes to gradation
Modification by hormones	No	Yes	Yes	Yes
Presence of myosin and actin filaments	Yes	Yes	Yes	Yes
Presence of troponin and tropomyosin	Yes	Tropomyosin only	Tropomyosin only	Yes
Presence of t-tubules	Yes	No	No	Yes
Development of sarcoplasmic reticulum	Well developed	Poorly developed	Poorly developed	Moderately developed

(Continued)

CHARACTERISTIC	SKELETAL MUSCLE	MULTIUNIT SMOOTH MUSCLE	SINGLE-UNIT SMOOTH MUSCLE	CARDIAC MUSCLE
Source of increased cytosolic ca²⁺	Sarcoplasmic reticulum	ECF and sarcoplasmic reticulum	ECF and sarcoplasmic reticulum	ECF and sarcoplasmic reticulum
Mechanism of ca²⁺ action to permit cross-bridge binding	Physically repositions troponin-tropomyosin complex in thin filaments to uncover actin cross-bridge binding sites	Chemically brings about phosphorylation of myosin cross bridges in thick filaments so that they can bind with actin	Chemically brings about phosphorylation of myosin cross bridges in thick filaments so that they can bind with actin	Physically repositions troponin-tropomyosin complex in thin filaments to uncover actin cross-bridge binding sites
Presence of gap junctions	No	Yes (very few)	Yes	Yes
Speed of contraction	Fast or slow, depending on type of fiber	Very slow	Very slow	Slow
Means by which gradation is accomplished	Varying number of motor units contracting (motor unit recruitment) and frequency at which they are stimulated (twitch summation)	Varying number of muscle fibers contracting and varying cytosolic ca²⁺ concentration in each fiber by autonomic and hormonal influences	Varying cytosolic ca²⁺ concentration through myogenic activity and influences of the autonomic nervous system, mechanical stretch, hormones, and local metabolites	Varying length of fibers (extent of filling of heart chambers) and varying cytosolic ca²⁺ concentration through autonomic, hormonal, and local metabolite influences
Clear-cut length-tension relationship	Yes	No	No	Yes

LEARNING OBJECTIVE 5.5.4   **Identify the intercalated disks and gap junctions of cardiac muscle.**

KEY TERM

intercalated disks Specialized cell junctions found in cardiac muscle.

INTERCALATED DISKS

Cardiac muscle cells connect with one another by specialized cell junctions called **intercalated disks** that allow the flow of chemicals between cells and help to maintain the structure of the muscle. Intercalated disks contain cell junctions called desmosomes, which contain protein filaments extending from thick, flattened structures called plaques. Thin protein filaments extend from a plaque from one cell to an adjacent cell while thick protein filaments extend from the plaque to the inner cytoplasm of the cell.

Intercalated disks also contain gap junctions that consist of hollow cylindrical protein structures that extend between adjacent cells that are in close proximity to one another. Gap junctions allow for the movement of substances such as electrolytes between adjacent cells.

LEARNING OBJECTIVE 5.5.5 Explain the role that intercalated disks and gap junctions play in signal transduction.

KEY TERMS

desmosomes Junctions that are scattered throughout the cell membrane and act as anchors to prevent cells from being pulled apart due to mechanical stress.

syncytia Group of motor units in muscle that contract together.

SIGNAL TRANSDUCTION IN CARDIAC MUSCLE

Intercalated disks contain gap junctions (hollow protein channels) that allow the movement of ions from one cell to another during depolarization. This allows adjacent fibers to pull together in a more coordinated contraction. Instead of motor units working separately in skeletal muscle, intercalated disks allow cardiac muscle to contract in large uniform segments called syncytia. Intercalated disks also contain desmosomes that work to anchor the ends of the muscle fiber together during contractions.

UNIT OBJECTIVE 5.6

Explain the structural characteristics and functions of muscles and muscle groups.

UNIT INTRODUCTION

Muscles attach to bones to perform movements of the body by working together and using leverage to efficiently move limbs and external objects. Muscles attach to bones by way of dense connective tissue, tubular structures called tendons, or flat structures called aponeuroses. The many muscles of the body can be organized according to location or function. This unit examines functions of muscles, and how muscles are structured and organized into groups.

LEARNING OBJECTIVE 5.6.1 Explain how skeletal muscle attachments, locations, and grouping allow different body movements.

KEY TERMS

atlanto-occipital joint Joint formed between the occipital bone of the skull and the first cervical vertebra.

fulcrum In a lever, the fulcrum is the pivot point in which a load is attached to a structure on each side.

pull With respect to levers, the pull is the load.

temporomandibular joint Joint formed by the temporal bone and mandible often referred to as the jaw joint.

SKELETAL MUSCLES AND BODY MOVEMENTS

Muscles are grouped so that one group will produce a movement, while another group works to oppose that movement. For example, when performing the first part of a biceps curl exercise, muscles on the anterior side of the arm contract to lift the weight, while muscles on the posterior side work to oppose the lifting action to help to stabilize the elbow joint.

Muscle tissue extends over bones that act as pulleys and levers. There are three types of lever arrangements in the muscular system (Figure 5-21ABC).

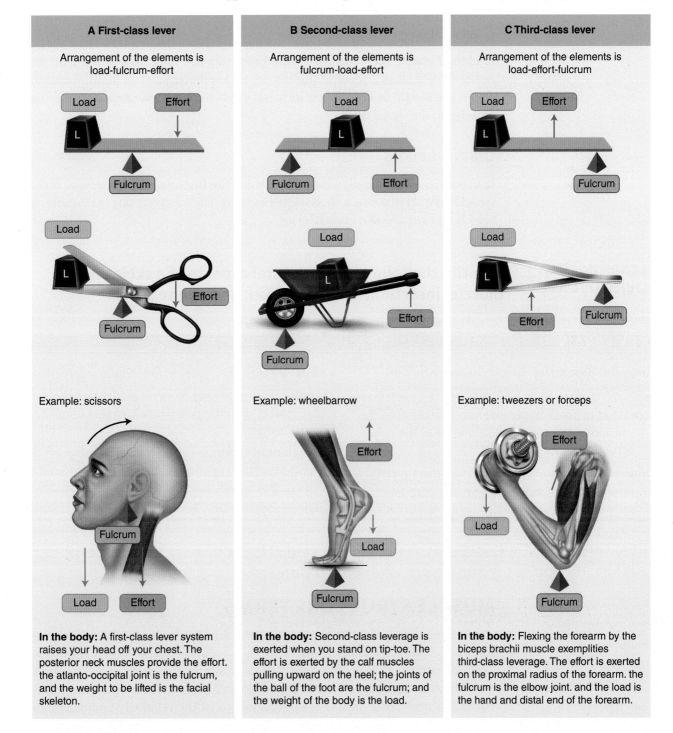

A First-class lever

Arrangement of the elements is load-fulcrum-effort

Example: scissors

In the body: A first-class lever system raises your head off your chest. The posterior neck muscles provide the effort. the atlanto-occipital joint is the fulcrum, and the weight to be lifted is the facial skeleton.

B Second-class lever

Arrangement of the elements is fulcrum-load-effort

Example: wheelbarrow

In the body: Second-class leverage is exerted when you stand on tip-toe. The effort is exerted by the calf muscles pulling upward on the heel; the joints of the ball of the foot are the fulcrum; and the weight of the body is the load.

C Third-class lever

Arrangement of the elements is load-effort-fulcrum

Example: tweezers or forceps

In the body: Flexing the forearm by the biceps brachii muscle exemplifies third-class leverage. The effort is exerted on the proximal radius of the forearm. the fulcrum is the elbow joint. and the load is the hand and distal end of the forearm.

FIGURE 5-21ABC Muscles connect to bones and work as levers.

Muscles exert a force called a pull on a weight and the lever contains a pivot point called a **fulcrum**.

Class 1 Levers

In class 1 levers, the fulcrum is located between the pull and the weight. An example of a class 1 lever is the **atlanto-occipital joint** in the spine. The joint acts as a fulcrum while the posterior back muscles exert a **pull** on the skull. The joint lies between the muscles and the skull.

Class 2 Levers

In class 2 levers, the weight is located between the fulcrum and the pull. An example of a class 2 lever is the **temporomandibular joint**. When the mouth opens, the weight or mandible is located between the fulcrum and the pull from muscles in the throat.

Class 3 Levers

In class 3 levers, the pull is located between the fulcrum and the weight. Most muscles are arranged in a class 3 lever system. The biceps acting on the elbow joint is an example of a class 3 lever.

LEARNING OBJECTIVE 5.6.2 Identify the following structural aspects of a skeletal muscle: insertion, origin, tendon, and aponeurosis.

KEY TERMS

bicipital tuberosity Broad eminence on the anterior portion of the radius bone.

coracoid process Bony extension on the anterior portion of the scapula just inferior to the acromion process.

insertions Point of a muscle attachment on the relatively more moveable end of a joint.

origins Muscle attachment on the relatively immoveable end of a joint.

radius Tubular bone located in the lateral forearm.

scapula Triangular-shaped bone in the back that articulates with the posterior rib cage, humerus, and clavicle.

supraglenoid tubercle Small rounded eminence located on the superior portion of the glenoid cavity that serves as an attachment point for the biceps brachii muscle.

MUSCLE STRUCTURE TERMS

Tendons consisting of dense connective tissue attach muscles to bones. Contracting muscles pull on tendons to elicit specific movements. Some muscles attach to bones or cartilage by way of a broad, flat, sheet like tendon called an aponeurosis.

Muscles connect to bones at specific locations called **origins** and **insertions**. The origin of a muscle is the connection at the relatively immovable or fixed end of a joint (see Figure 5-22). The insertion is the muscle attachment at the more moveable end of a joint. For example, the biceps brachii muscle's origin is on the **coracoid process** and **supraglenoid tubercle** of the **scapula** while its insertion is at the **bicipital tuberosity** of the **radius**.

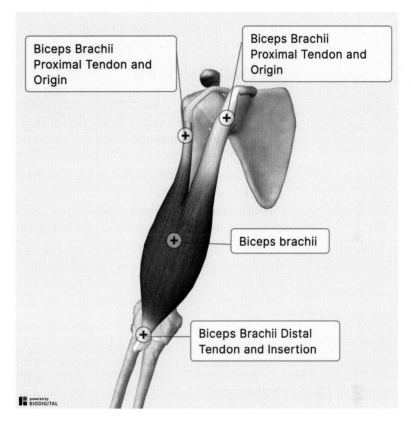

FIGURE 5-22 Muscle: tendons, origins, and insertions.

CLINICAL TIP	Tendonitis is a painful condition characterized by inflammation of a tendon. Tendonitis is usually caused by overuse of a muscle and joint complex.

LEARNING OBJECTIVE 5.6.3 Identify the location of the two aponeuroses present in the human body.

KEY TERMS

abdominal aponeurosis Flat, sheetlike tendinous structure located at the anterior abdominal wall and formed by the tendons of three abdominal muscles: internal obliques, external obliques, and transversus abdominis.

dense connective tissue Type of fibrous connective tissue found in ligaments and tendons.

epicranial aponeurosis Flat, broad area of fibrous connective tissue located on the superior portion of the skull.

gala aponeurotica Alternative name for the epicranial aponeurosis.

APONEUROSES

An aponeurosis is a broad, flat sheet of fibrous connective tissue that either interconnects muscles, surrounds muscles, or connects muscles to bones (see Figure 5-23).

The **epicranial aponeurosis** is located on the superior portion of the skull. It consists of a broad layer of **dense connective tissue** that connects with the frontalis and occipitalis muscles. The epicranial aponeurosis is sometimes called the **gala aponeurotica**.

The **abdominal aponeurosis** is located at the anterior abdominal wall and is formed by the tendons of three abdominal muscles (internal obliques, external obliques, transversus abdominis) (see Figure 5-24). The aponeurosis encases the fourth abdominal muscle (rectus abdominis). The muscles combine anteriorly to form the linea alba (white line), which is a fibrous structure that extends from the xiphoid process of the sternum to the pubic symphysis.

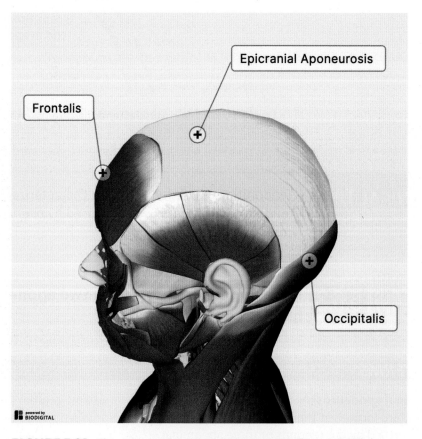

FIGURE 5-23 The epicranial aponeurosis is a broad layer of dense connective tissue on the superior portion of the skull.

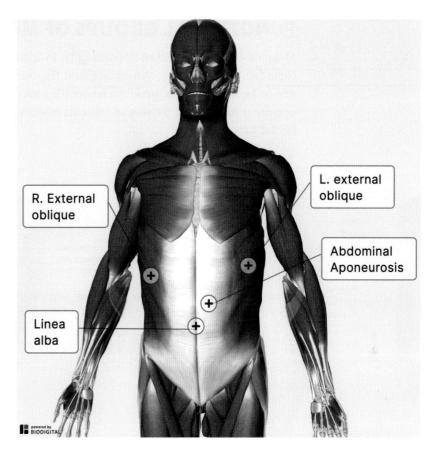

FIGURE 5-24 The abdominal aponeurosis is a flattened layer of dense connective tissue formed by the tendons of the external obliques, internal obliques, and transversus abdominis muscles.

LEARNING OBJECTIVE 5.6.4 Define prime mover, synergist, agonist, and antagonist.

KEY TERMS

agonist muscles Muscles performing a specific movement.

antagonist muscles Muscles opposing a specific joint movement.

fixator Muscle that assists in holding a joint immobile, such as in maintaining posture.

prime movers Muscle most responsible for a specific joint movement.

synergist muscles Muscles that work together to perform a specific movement.

FUNCTIONAL GROUPS OF MUSCLES

Muscles can be organized according to four functional groups: prime movers (agonists), antagonists, synergists, and fixators (see Figure 5-25). **Prime movers**, or **agonist muscles**, produce a specific movement, while **antagonist muscles** oppose a movement. **Synergist muscles** assist prime movers and **fixators** work to stabilize joints.

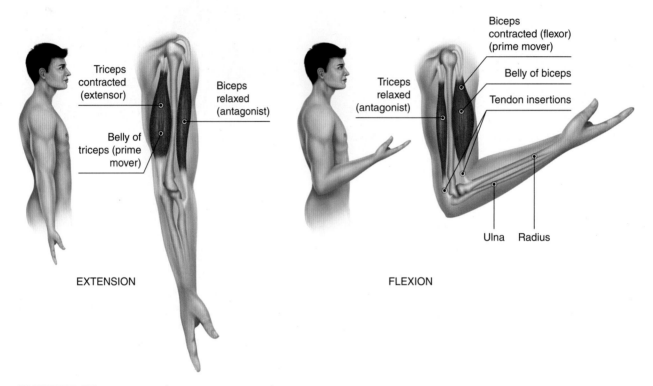

Triceps contracted (extensor)

Biceps relaxed (antagonist)

Belly of triceps (prime mover)

EXTENSION

Biceps contracted (flexor) (prime mover)

Triceps relaxed (antagonist)

Belly of biceps

Tendon insertions

Ulna   Radius

FLEXION

FIGURE 5-25 Agonist and prime mover muscles.

For example, the biceps brachii and brachialis muscles work together during the lifting portion of the biceps curl exercise. Since the brachialis contributes most of the force to lift the weight, it is considered the prime mover. The biceps brachii muscle assists the brachialis and is considered a synergist muscle. The triceps muscle is considered an antagonist during the lifting portion of the biceps curl exercise because it opposes the movement.

It is important to know that the functional group can change depending on the movement. For example, in performing an activity in which the elbow is flexed to pull on an object, the biceps is the agonist while the triceps is the antagonist. However, performing an activity in which the elbow is flexed to push on an object, the triceps is not the agonist, while the biceps brachii is an antagonist.

Some muscles work to hold bones in place. These muscles are called fixators or stabilizers. For example, muscles work to stabilize the scapula while moving the arm.

LEARNING OBJECTIVE 5.6.5 Identify the muscles involved in eye movement.

EXTRINSIC MUSCLES OF THE EYE

There are six extrinsic eye muscles that move the eyeball: the **superior rectus**, **inferior rectus**, **medial rectus**, **lateral rectus**, **superior oblique**, and **inferior oblique** muscles (see Figures 5-26 and 5-27). The four rectus muscles originate on the posterior surface of the bony orbit and extend to the surface of the eyeball. The superior oblique attaches to the medial surface of the orbit. Its tendon passes through a fibrocartilaginous pulley called the **trochlea** and attaches to the superolateral surface of the eyeball. The inferior oblique extends from the medial wall of the orbit to its attachment on the inferolateral aspect of the eyeball.

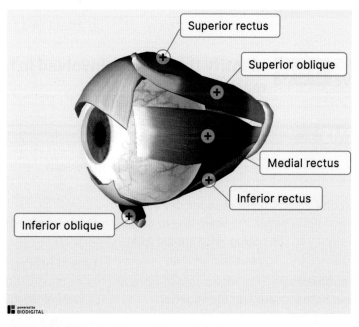

FIGURE 5-26 Medial view of eye muscles.

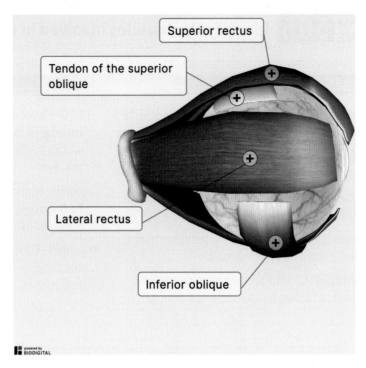

FIGURE 5-27 Lateral view of eye muscles.

CLINICAL TIP	The extrinsic eye muscles can be examined by performing the H in space test. An examiner will trace the outline of the letter *H* in front of a patient while the patient follows the movements with his or her eyes. The examiner looks for the ability of the patient to track the object with his or her pupils. This test examines the eye muscles along with the cranial nerves that innervate them.

LEARNING OBJECTIVE **5.6.6** **Identify the muscles involved in facial expression and mastication.**

KEY TERMS

Buccinator Muscle located in the cheek that compresses the cheek against the teeth.

cerebrovascular accident The sudden death of neurons and neuroglia in the brain due to a lack of blood supply to the region. Also known as a stroke.

epicranial aponeurosis Flat, broad area of fibrous connective tissue located on the superior portion of the skull.

frontalis Muscle located in the anterior portion of the skull that attaches to the epicranial aponeurosis.

lacrimal glands Gland near the eye that produces tears.

lateral pterygoid Muscle contributing to chewing or mastication located lateral to the medial pterygoid muscle.

mandible Lower jaw.

masseter Chewing (mastication) muscle located in the cheek area that works to close the jaw.

mastication Chewing.

medial pterygoid One of the muscles of mastication located in the deep lateral portion of the jaw.

occipitalis Muscle located on the posterior portion of the skull that attaches to the epicranial aponeurosis.

orbicularis oculi Circular muscle surrounding the eye and causing the action of blinking the eye.

orbicularis oris Circular muscle surrounding the mouth and causing the action of puckering the lips.

platysma Superficial muscle of the neck that produces frowning.

sphincters Type of muscle with a circular shape that functions to constrict and dilate an area of the body.

temporalis Muscle located on the lateral portion of the skull.

zygomaticus Muscle of facial expression that moves the ends up the mouth superior as if in smiling.

MUSCLES OF FACIAL EXPRESSION AND MASTICATION

Located on top of the head is a broad flat tendon called the **epicranial aponeurosis** (see Figure 5-28). There are two muscles attached to this aponeurosis. The anterior muscle is called the **frontalis** and works to lift the eyebrows. The posterior muscle is called the **occipitalis** and works as a weak head extensor (see Table 5-2). During times of increased stress, chronic contraction of the occipitalis muscle can cause tension headaches.

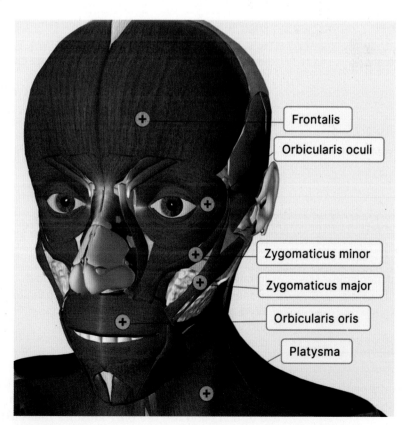

FIGURE 5-28 Muscles of facial expression.

Table 5-2 Muscles of Facial Expression and Mastication

MUSCLE	ORIGIN	INSERTION	ACTION
frontalis	Fibers of superior facial muscles	Epicranial aponeurosis	Wrinkles forehead
occipitalis	Nuchal line and mastoid process of temporal bone	Epicranial aponeurosis	Stabilizes epicranial aponeurosis
orbicularis oculi	Anterior surface of orbital margin	Lateral palpebrae raphae	Closes the eye
orbicularis oris	Anterior surface of maxilla and mandible Modiolus at angle of mouth	Membrane of margin of lips and raphe at modiolus	Purses and puckers lips
zygomaticus	Anterior surface of zygomatic bone	Modiolis at angle of mouth	Elevates the corners of the mouth
buccinator	External alveolar margins of maxilla and mandible bones	Thick layer of connective tissue in the cheek	Pulls cheeks inward against teeth
zygomaticus	Anterior surface of zygomatic bone	Modiolis at angle of mouth	Elevates the corners of the mouth
platysma	Inner portion of the skin in the lower cervical and upper thoracic regions	Inferior border of mandible and inner portion of skin over the lower portion of the mouth	Depresses skin over lower portion of face
masseter	zygomatic arch	Angle and ramus of mandible	Elevates mandible
temporalis	Temporal fossa	Anterior and medial portions of the coronoid process of the mandible	Elevates mandible
medial pterygoid	Medial portion of lateral pterygoid plate and fossa between medial and lateral plates along with the tuberosity of maxilla and pyramidal process of palatine bone	Medial portion of angle of mandible	Elevates mandible
lateral pterygoid	Infratemporal surface of sphenoid bone along with lateral surface of lateral pterygoid plate	Below condyloid process of mandible	Elevates mandible

There are two circular muscles called **sphincters**. The **orbicularis oculi** encircle the eyes. They compress the **lacrimal glands**, which aid in the drainage of tears and are the only muscles that close the eyes. The **orbicularis oris** encircles the mouth and causes the lips to pucker (see Table 5-2).

The **buccinator** is located in the cheek. It compresses the cheek against the teeth and pulls back the angle of the mouth (see Table 5-2). The **zygomaticus** muscle has major and minor divisions and attaches to the orbicularis oris and zygomatic bone (see Table 5-2). It raises the lateral ends of the mouth when smiling. The **platysma** is a very thin and superficial muscle located under the chin. It causes the action of frowning when contracted.

CLINICAL TIP	A sign of a **cerebrovascular accident** (stroke) is the flaccidity of the muscles of facial expression causing drooping on one side of the face. This results from brain damage causing a lack of nervous system impulses from the brain to the facial muscles.

The muscles of **mastication** (chewing) include the **masseter**, **temporalis**, and **medial** and **lateral pterygoids** (Figures 5-29 and 5-30) (see Table 5-2). The masseter muscles attach to the **mandible** and allow for closing the jaw. The temporalis is located in the lateral skull and attaches to the temporal bone. The temporalis aids in closing the jaw. You can feel your temporalis muscle contract when touching the sides of your head when clenching your jaw. The medial and lateral pterygoids are deep muscles in the jaw. These can elevate, depress, protract, and cause lateral movement of the mandible.

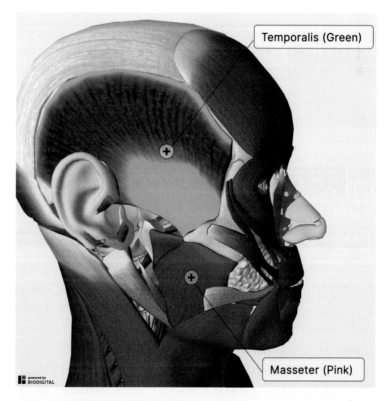

Temporalis (Green)

Masseter (Pink)

powered by BIODIGITAL

FIGURE 5-29 Muscles of mastication: masseter and temporalis muscles.

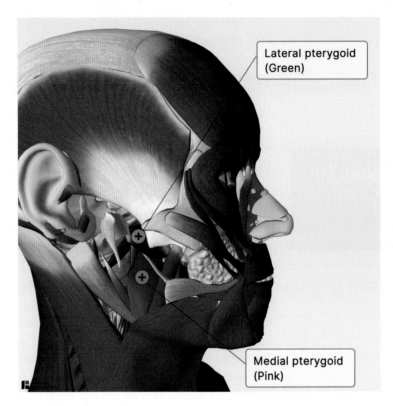

FIGURE 5-30 Muscles of mastication: medial and lateral pterygoids.

CLINICAL TIP	The muscles of mastication are often involved in temporomandibular joint (TMJ) disorder. Sometimes, patients with TMJ disorder suffer from headaches resulting from spasms of the temporalis muscle or pain emanating from the pterygoids or masseter muscles.

LEARNING OBJECTIVE 5.6.7 Identify the muscles of the upper arm and shoulder.

KEY TERMS

biceps brachii Muscle in the upper arm attaching to the scapula and humerus.

brachialis Muscle in the upper arm that attaches to the humerus and extends to the radius.

brachioradialis Muscle in the forearm that attaches to the humerus and extends to the radius.

coracobrachialis Muscle in the upper arm extending from the coracoid process of the scapula to the humerus.

deltoid Superficial muscle of the shoulder.

humerus Long bone of the upper arm extending from the shoulder to the elbow.

latissimus dorsi Large muscle in the back that extends to the intertubercular groove of the humerus.

levator scapula Muscle in the back connected to the superior portion of the scapula and extending to the skull that functions to elevate the scapula.

pectoral girdle Clavicle and scapula bones.

pectoralis major Superficial muscle in the anterior thorax connecting to the ribcage, clavicle, and humerus.

pectoralis minor Deep muscle in the anterior thorax connecting to the rib cage and scapula.

rhomboid major Deep muscle of the back that attaches to the medial border of the scapula and extends to the spine.

rhomboid minor Deep muscle of the back located just superior to the rhomboid major muscle.

scapula Triangular-shaped bone in the back that articulates with the posterior rib cage, humerus, and clavicle.

serratus anterior Muscle located on the lateral rib cage and extending to the anterior portion of the scapula.

supraspinatus One of four rotator cuff muscles that attaches to the scapula and extending to the humerus that functions to externally rotate the humerus.

teres major Shoulder muscle that attaches to the lateral portion of the scapula and extends to the humerus.

trapezius Superficial muscle of the back that extends from the occipital bone to the 12th thoracic vertebra and laterally to the spine of the scapulae.

triceps Muscle located on the back of the upper arm with three heads that work to extend the elbow.

MUSCLES OF THE UPPER ARM AND SHOULDER

The shoulder consists of the **humerus** and **scapula**. The arm and scapula work together to allow the arm to move. The following muscles of the **pectoral girdle** work to move the scapula in concert with the arm (see Figures 5-31 and 5-32).

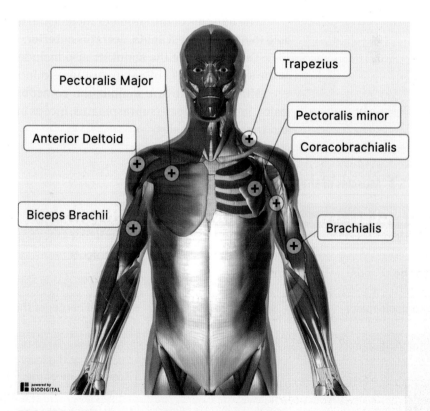

FIGURE 5-31 Anterior muscles of the shoulder and arm.

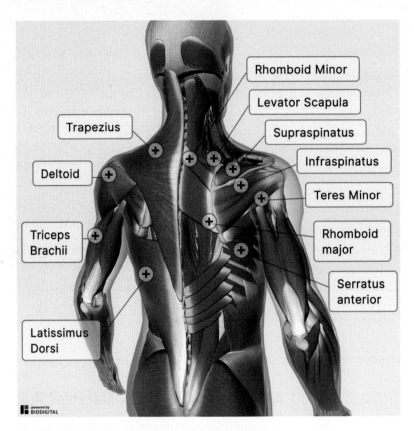

FIGURE 5-32 Posterior muscles of the shoulder and arm.

The muscles of the shoulder include the **trapezius, rhomboid major, rhomboid minor, levator scapula, serratus anterior, pectoralis minor,** and **deltoid.**

The muscles of the shoulder also include the rotator cuff, which consists of the supraspinatus, infraspinatus, teres minor and subscapularis muscles.

Muscles of the arm include the **coracobrachialis, pectoralis major, teres major, latissimus dorsi, supraspinatus, biceps brachii, brachialis, brachioradialis,** and **triceps** (see Table 5-3).

Table 5-3 Muscles of the Upper Arm and Shoulder

MUSCLE	ORIGIN	INSERTION	ACTION
trapezius	Occipital bone, spines of C7, and all thoracic vertebrae	Spine and acromion of scapula	Extends head; elevates, depresses, rotates, and retracts scapula
rhomboid major	Spinous processes of T2–T5 vertebrae	Medial border of the scapula	Retracts the scapula
rhomboid minor	Spinous processes of C7–T1 vertebrae	Medial border of the scapula at the level of the spine of the scapula	Retracts the scapula

(Continued)

MUSCLE	ORIGIN	INSERTION	ACTION
levator scapula	Transverse processes of C1–C4	Superior portion of medial border of scapula	Elevates the medial border of the scapula
serratus anterior	Upper eight ribs	Anterior aspect of medial border of scapula	Protracts and rotates scapula
pectoralis minor	Ribs 3, 4, and 5	Coracoid process of scapula	Draws scapula anterior and inferior
deltoid	Lateral third of clavicle, acromion process, and spine of scapula	Deltoid tuberosity of humerus	Abducts the humerus, anterior portion flexes and internally rotates humerus, posterior portion extends and externally rotates humerus
supraspinatus	Supraspinous fossa of scapula	Greater tubercle of the humerus	Abducts and stabilizes humerus
infraspinatus	Infraspinous fossa	Greater tubercle of the humerus	Laterally rotates humerus
teres minor	Lateral border of the scapula	Greater tubercle of the humerus	Laterally rotates humerus
teres major	Lower third of lateral border of the scapula	Bicipital groove of humerus	Medially rotates the humerus
subscapularis	Medial portion of subscapular fossa	Lesser tuberosity of the humerus and upper portion of bicipital groove	Internally rotates the humerus
coracobrachialis	Coracoid process of the scapula	Upper one half of medial border of the humerus	Flexes the humerus
triceps brachii	Axillary border of scapula, posterior humerus	Olecranon process of the ulna	Extends forearm, stabilizes shoulder
biceps brachii	Coracoid process, intertubercular groove of the humerus	Radial tuberosity	Flexes arm and forearm, supinates hand
brachialis	Distal anterior humerus	Coronoid process of ulna	Flexes forearm
latissimus dorsi	Lower vertebrae, iliac crest	Intertubercular groove of humerus	Extends, adducts, and medially rotates arm
pectoralis major	Clavicle, sternum, costal cartilages	Greater tubercle of humerus	Flexes, adducts, and medially rotates arm
Brachioradialis	Distal humerus	Styloid process of radius	Flexes forearm

LEARNING OBJECTIVE 5.6.8 Identify the muscles of the forearm.

KEY TERMS

acromion process Large process extending off the superior portion of the scapula.

anaconeus Small muscle of the elbow that attaches to the humerus and ulna.

brachialis Muscle in the upper arm that attaches to the humerus and extends to the radius.

extensor carpi radialis brevis Muscle in the posterior forearm that attaches to the humerus and extends to the radius.

extensor carpi radialis longus Muscle in the posterior forearm that attaches to the humerus and extends to the radius.

extensor carpi ulnaris Muscle on the posterior forearm that attaches to the humerus and extends to the ulna.

extensor digiti minimi Muscle located in the posterior hand region that moves the fingers or digits into extension.

extensor digitorum Muscle in the posterior forearm that moves the fingers or digits into extension.

flexor carpi radialis Muscle on the anterior portion of the forearm extending from the radius to the carpals.

flexor carpi ulnaris Muscle located in the anterior forearm extending from the humerus to the ulna.

flexor digitorum profundus Muscle in the anterior forearm that produces flexion of the toes.

flexor digitorum superficialis Muscle in the anterior forearm that produces flexion of the toes.

palmaris longus Muscle located in the anterior forearm that connects to the flexor retinaculum and is absent in about 14% of the population.

pronator quadratus Muscle located in the distal forearm between the ulna and radius that works to pronate the forearm and wrist.

pronator teres Muscle located in the proximal forearm between the humerus, ulna, and radius that works to pronate the forearm and wrist.

Supinator Muscle in the posterior portion of the forearm that functions to supinate the forearm.

MUSCLES OF THE FOREARM

Muscles of the forearm include the supinator, pronator teres, pronator quadratus, flexor carpi radialis, flexor carpi ulnaris, palmaris longus, flexor digitorum superficialis, flexor digitorum profundus, extensor carpi radialis longus, extensor carpi radialis brevis, extensor carpi ulnaris, extensor digitorum, extensor digiti minimi, and anaconeus (see Figures 5-33, 5-34, 5-35, and 5-36) (see Table 5-4).

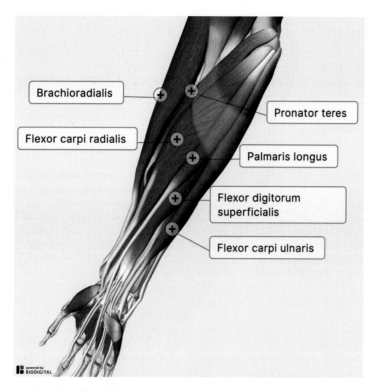

FIGURE 5-33 Anterior muscles of the forearm (superficial).

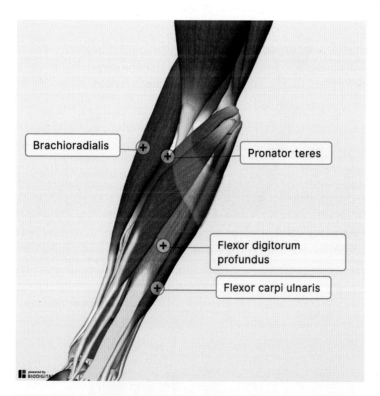

FIGURE 5-34 Anterior muscles of the forearm (Deep). Flexor carpi radialis and flexor digitorum superficialis muscles removed to show the flexor digitorum profundus muscle.

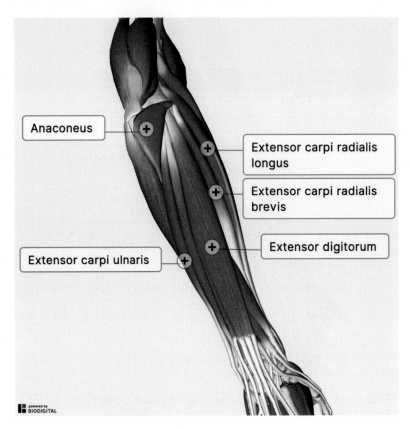

FIGURE 5-35 Posterior muscles of the forearm (Superficial).

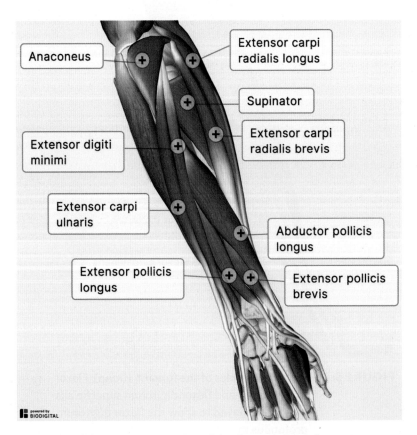

FIGURE 5-36 Posterior muscles of the forearm (Deep).

Table 5-4 Muscles of the Forearm

MUSCLE	ORIGIN	INSERTION	ACTION
supinator	Lateral proximal portion of the ulna, lateral epicondyle, lateral collateral ligament of the elbow, and annular ligament	Proximal lateral portion of the radius	Supinates forearm when elbow is extended
pronator teres	Medial epicondyle of humerus	Lateral radius	Pronates and flexes forearm
flexor carpi radialis	Medial epicondyle of humerus	Base of 2nd and 3d metacarpals	Flexes wrist, abducts hand
flexor carpi ulnaris	Medial epicondyle of humerus, olecranon process	Base of 5th metacarpal, pisiform, and hamate	Flexes wrist, adducts hand
palmaris longus	Medial epicondyle of humerus	Palmar aponeurosis	Flexes wrist
flexor digitorum superficialis	Medial epicondyle of humerus and medial collateral ligament of the elbow Medial border of coronoid process of ulna and lateral and middle potions of shaft of radius	Middle phalanges of medial four digits	Flexes proximal interphalangeal and metacarpophalangeal joints
flexor digitorum profundus	Medial olecranon, proximal three quarters of anterior and medial surface of ulna	Distal phalanges of medial four fingers	Flexes distal interphalangeal, proximal interphalangeal, and metacarpophalangeal joints
extensor carpi radialis longus	Lateral epicondyle of humerus	Second and third metacarpals	Extends and abducts wrist
extensor carpi radialis brevis	Lateral epicondyle of humerus	Posterior base of third metacarpal	Extends and abducts hand
extensor carpi ulnaris	Lateral epicondyle of humerus	Metacarpal V	Extends and adducts wrist
extensor digitorum	Lateral epicondyle of the humerus	posterior surfaces of distal phalanges of digits 2–5	Extends fingers and wrist, abducts fingers
extensor digiti minimi	Lateral epicondyle of humerus	metacarpophalangeal joint of fourth digit	Extends fourth digit
anaconeus	Lateral epicondyle of humerus	Lateral portion of olecranon process of ulna	Extends and pronates the ulna

LEARNING OBJECTIVE 5.6.9 Identify the muscles of the rotator cuff.

LEARNING OBJECTIVE 5.6.10 Describe the function of the rotator cuff.

KEY TERMS

external rotation Outward or lateral rotation.

greater tubercle of the humerus Bony prominence located on the lateral humerus.

infraspinatus One of the rotator cuff muscles connected to the scapula and extending to the humerus; produces external rotation of the shoulder.

internal rotation Inward or medial rotation of a joint.

lesser tubercle of the humerus Small bony eminence located on the proximal portion of the humerus anterior and medial to the greater tubercle of the humerus.

scapula Triangular-shaped bone in the back that articulates with the posterior rib cage, humerus, and clavicle.

subscapularis One of four rotator cuff muscles located on the anterior portion of the scapula and extending to the humerus.

suprascapular fossa Groove located on the scapula just superior to the spine of the scapula.

supraspinatus One of four rotator cuff muscles that attaches to the scapula and extending to the humerus that functions to externally rotate the humerus.

teres minor One of four rotator cuff muscles that attaches to the lateral portion of the scapula and extends to the humerus; functions to externally rotate the humerus.

THE ROTATOR CUFF

The rotator cuff consists of four muscles, three of which rotate the humerus externally while one rotates the humerus internally (see Figures 5-37 and 5-38). The first letter of each muscle can be taken to spell the acronym *SITS*, which stands for **supraspinatus, infraspinatus, teres minor,** and **subscapularis.**

The supraspinatus attaches to the superior portion of the scapula at the suprascapular fossa and extends to the greater tubercle of the humerus. It abducts as well as moves the arm into **external rotation.**

The infraspinatus attaches to the posterior portion of the **scapula** at the subscapular fossa and extends to the **greater tubercle of the humerus.** It externally rotates the arm.

The subscapularis attaches on the anterior surface of the scapula and extends to the **lesser tubercle of the humerus.** It is the only rotator cuff muscle that provides **internal rotation.**

The teres minor attaches to the lateral border of the scapula and extends to the greater tubercle of the humerus. It externally rotates the arm.

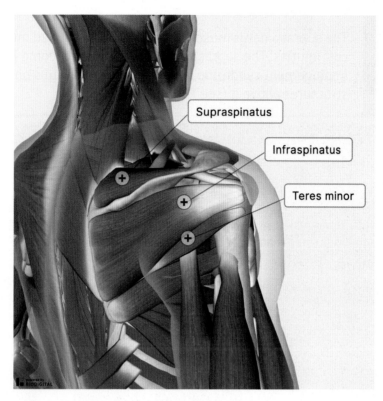

FIGURE 5-37 Rotator cuff muscles.

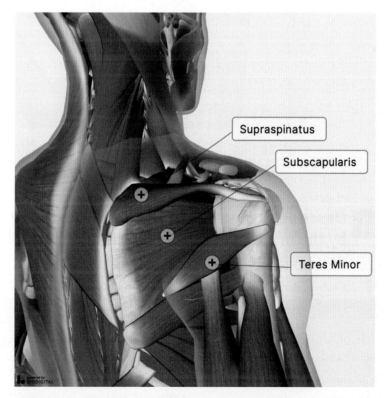

FIGURE 5-38 Rotator cuff muscles. The infraspinatus and scapula have been removed to view the subscapularis muscles.

CLINICAL TIP   The supraspinatus muscle is a frequently involved muscle in rotator cuff injuries. The supraspinatus tendon can become inflamed in impingement syndrome in which the tendon rubs on the bony structures above it (see Figure 5-39).

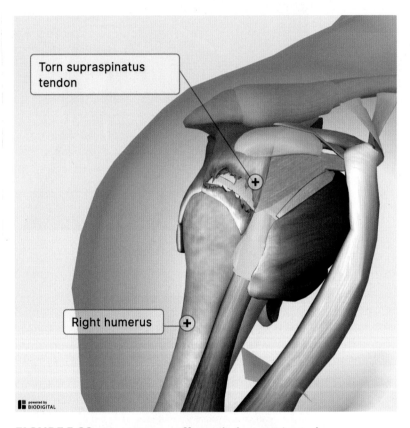

Torn supraspinatus tendon

Right humerus

powered by BIODIGITAL

FIGURE 5-39   Torn rotator cuff muscle (supraspinatus).

LEARNING OBJECTIVE 5.6.11 **Describe the location and the types of movement created by the muscles of the shoulder, upper arm, lower arm, wrist, and hand.**

KEY TERMS

anaconeus Small muscle of the elbow that attaches to the humerus and ulna.

biceps brachii Muscle in the upper arm attaching to the scapula and humerus.

brachioradialis Muscle in the forearm that attaches to the humerus and extends to the radius.

coracobrachialis Muscle in the upper arm extending from the coracoid process of the scapula to the humerus.

coracoid process Bony extension on the anterior portion of the scapula just inferior to the acromion process.

coronoid process Bony triangular process located on the ulna.

costal cartilages Areas of hyaline cartilage extending from the anterior portion of the ribs to the sternum.

deltoid Superficial muscle of the shoulder.

extensor carpi radialis brevis Muscle in the posterior forearm that attaches to the humerus and extends to the radius.

extensor carpi radialis longus Muscle in the posterior forearm that attaches to the humerus and extends to the radius.

extensor carpi ulnaris Muscle on the posterior forearm that attaches to the humerus and extends to the ulna.

extensor digiti minimi Muscle located in the posterior hand region that moves the fingers or digits into extension.

extensor digitorum Muscle in the posterior forearm that moves the fingers or digits into extension.

flexor carpi radialis longus Muscle located in the anterior forearm extending from the humerus to the radius.

flexor carpi ulnaris Muscle located in the anterior forearm extending from the humerus to the ulna.

flexor digitorum profundus Muscle in the anterior forearm that produces flexion of the toes.

flexor digitorum superficialis Muscle in the anterior forearm that produces flexion of the toes.

flexor retinaculum Band of connective tissue in the wrist that forms the carpal tunnel.

greater tubercle of humerus Bony prominence located on the lateral humerus.

intertubercular groove Groove between the greater and lesser tubercle of the humerus.

iliac crest Superior portion of the ilium of the coxal bone.

lateral epicondyle Small, bony protuberance located on the distal lateral portion of the humerus and femur.

latissimus dorsi Large muscle in the back that extends to the intertubercular groove of the humerus.

levator scapula Muscle in the back connected to the superior portion of the scapula and extending to the skull that functions to elevate the scapula.

medial epicondyle Small, bony protuberance located in the distal medial portion of the humerus and femur.

olecranon process Bony protuberance on the proximal portion of the ulna commonly referred to as the elbow.

palmaris longus Muscle located in the anterior forearm that connects to the flexor retinaculum and is absent in about 14% of the population.

pectoralis major Superficial muscle in the anterior thorax connecting to the ribcage, clavicle, and humerus.

pectoralis minor Deep muscle in the anterior thorax connecting to the rib cage and scapula.

pronator quadratus Muscle located in the distal forearm between the ulna and radius that works to pronate the forearm and wrist.

pronator teres Muscle located in the proximal forearm between the humerus, ulna, and radius that works to pronate the forearm and wrist.

rhomboid major Deep muscle of the back that attaches to the medial border of the scapula and extends to the spine.

rhomboid minor Deep muscle of the back located just superior to the rhomboid major muscle.

serratus anterior Muscle located on the lateral rib cage and extending to the anterior portion of the scapula.

styloid process Sharp, pointed process located on several bones of the body.

supinator Muscle in the posterior portion of the forearm that functions to supinate the forearm.

supracondylar ridge of the humerus Roughed area on the distal, medial portion of the humerus.

supraspinatus One of four rotator cuff muscles that attaches to the scapula and extending to the humerus that functions to externally rotate the humerus.

teres major Shoulder muscle that attaches to the lateral portion of the scapula and extends to the humerus.

trapezius Superficial muscle of the back that extends from the occipital bone to the 12th thoracic vertebra and laterally to the spine of the scapulae.

triceps brachii Muscle located on the back of the upper arm with three heads that work to extend the elbow.

MUSCLES OF THE SHOULDER, UPPER ARM, LOWER ARM, WRIST, AND HAND

Muscles of the Shoulder

The trapezius muscle has upper, middle, and lower divisions. The trapezius attaches to the thoracic and cervical vertebrae and extends upward to the occipital bone and laterally to the scapula. The upper portion raises the shoulder and scapula. The middle portion pulls the scapula toward the vertebral column and the lower portion pulls the scapula downward.

There are two rhomboid muscles that attach to the medial border of the scapula and extend to the spine. They work to pull the scapula upward and medially. The larger rhomboid major is the inferior muscle of the two. The smaller rhomboid minor is superior to the major.

The levator scapula is a long, thin muscle that attaches to the superior border of the scapula and extends upward to the occipital bone. As its name implies, the levator scapula works to elevate the scapula.

The serratus anterior attaches to the anterior surface of the scapula and extends to the ribs. The serratus anterior works to hold or stabilize the scapula against the rib cage.

The pectoralis minor muscle is located deep to the major. It attaches to the upper ribs and extends to the coracoid process of the scapula. It works to pull the scapula anterior and inferior. The pectoralis minor is also an accessory muscle of inspiration.

The deltoid is located on top of the humeral head. It attaches to the spine of the scapula and acromion process and extends to the deltoid tuberosity of the humerus. The deltoid works to flex, abduct, and extend the arm.

Muscles of the Upper Arm

The arm can perform a variety of movements, which include flexion, extension, adduction, abduction, and internal and external rotation as well as combinations of these movements. The arm flexors include the coracobrachialis, pectoralis major, and deltoid.

The coracobrachialis attaches to the coracoid process of the scapula and extends to the shaft of the humerus. It runs deep to the deltoid and biceps muscles. The pectoralis major attaches to the clavicle, sternum, and costal cartilages of the ribs and extends to the intertubercular groove of the humerus.

The arm extensors include the **teres major** and **latissimus dorsi**. The teres major attaches to the lateral border of the scapula and extends to the **intertubercular groove** of the humerus. The latissimus dorsi attaches to the lower thoracic area to the **iliac crest** and extends to the intertubercular groove of the humerus.

The muscles that move the arm laterally away from the body (abduction) include the supraspinatus and deltoid. The supraspinatus attaches on the posterior surface of the scapula above the spine of the scapula and extends to the **greater tubercle of the humerus**.

The supraspinatus attaches to the superior portion of the scapula at the **suprascapular fossa** and extends to the greater tubercle of the humerus. It abducts as well as externally rotates the arm.

The muscles that move the arm into flexion include the **biceps brachii**, **brachioradialis**, and **brachialis**.

The biceps brachii attaches to the scapula and inserts into the radial tuberosity. This muscle has two tendons at its proximal region. It works to flex the elbow. The long tendon (long head) originates on the supraglenoid tubercle of the scapula and the short head originates on the tip of the coracoid process of the scapula.

The brachialis lies deep to the biceps brachii and extends to the ulna. The brachialis originates on the anterior lower portion of the humerus and inserts into the **coronoid process** of the ulna.

The brachioradialis originates on the upper two-thirds of the lateral **supracondylar ridge of the humerus** and inserts on the **styloid process** of the radius.

There is only one muscle that functions in elbow extension. This muscle is the **triceps brachii**. This muscle is a large three-headed muscle. The long head originates on the infraglenoid tubercle of the scapula. The lateral head originates on the posterolateral humerus and the medial head originates on the posteromedial surface of the inferior humerus. The triceps brachii inserts on the **olecranon process** of the ulna. It is the only muscle on the posterior side of the arm.

Muscles of the Lower Arm, Wrist, and Hand

The muscles that rotate the forearm include the **supinator**, **pronator teres**, and **pronator quadratus**.

The supinator attaches to the ulna and extends to the lateral aspect of the humerus. It works to rotate the wrist into supination.

The pronator teres attaches to the humerus and ulna and extends to the radius. It works to rotate the wrist into pronation.

The pronator quadratus attaches to the distal ulna and radius. It also works to pronate the wrist.

The flexors of the hand and wrist include the **flexor carpi radialis longus**, **flexor carpi ulnaris**, **palmaris longus**, **flexor digitorum superficialis**, and **flexor digitorum profundus**.

The flexor carpi radialis longus attaches to a flexor tendon on the **medial epicondyle** of the humerus and extends to the base of the second and third metacarpals. The **flexor carpi ulnaris** also attaches to the medial epicondyle and extends to the metacarpals. The **palmaris longus** muscle lies between the flexor carpi radialis longus and flexor carpi ulnaris and extends to the **flexor retinaculum** of the wrist (see Table 5-6). The palmaris longus begins as a common flexor tendon extending from the medial epicondyle of the humerus and inserts in the flexor retinaculum. The palmaris longus muscle is only present in about 13% of the population. The group of wrist flexors attach on the medial epicondyle.

The **flexor digitorum superficialis** lies deep to the flexor carpi radialis longus and flexor carpi ulnaris and extends to the proximal phalanges. The flexor digitorum profundus lies deep to the flexor digitorum superficialis and extends to the distal phalanges.

Some muscles extend through the flexor retinaculum and can contribute to carpal tunnel syndrome, which is an inflammation of the median nerve. Some cases of carpal tunnel are caused by inflammation of the tendons of these muscles. These include:

- Flexor carpi radialis longus and brevis
- Flexor digitorum profundus
- Flexor digitorum superficialis

The wrist and hand extensors are located on the posterior portion of the forearm. The wrist extensors have a common origin on the **lateral epicondyle**.

The wrist and hand extensors include the **extensor carpi radialis longus, extensor carpi radialis brevis, extensor carpi ulnaris, extensor digitorum**, and **extensor digiti minimi** (see Table 5-5).

Table 5-5 Tennis and Golfer's Elbow

DISORDER	DESCRIPTION	AREA AFFECTED	SYMPTOMS
Tennis elbow	Inflammation of the wrist extensor tendons	Area around origin of wrist extensors at lateral epicondyle of humerus	Pain and swelling in the lateral forearm and elbow
Golfer's elbow	Inflammation of the wrist flexor tendons	Area around origin of wrist flexors at medial epicondyle of the humerus	Pain and swelling in the medial forearm and elbow

CLINICAL TIP Tendonitis in the wrist extensors where they insert at the lateral epicondyle is known as tennis elbow or lateral epicondylitis (see Figure 5-40). Sometimes tendonitis can develop where the wrist flexors insert at the medial epicondyle of the humerus known as golfer's elbow (see Figure 5-41).

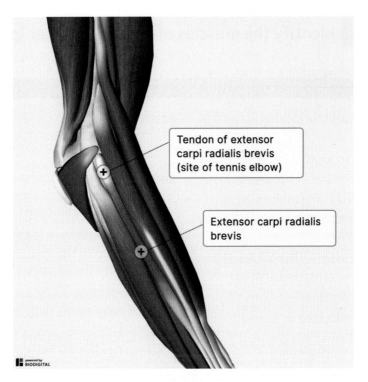

FIGURE 5-40 Tendon of the extensor carpi radialis brevis is most commonly inflamed in tennis elbow.

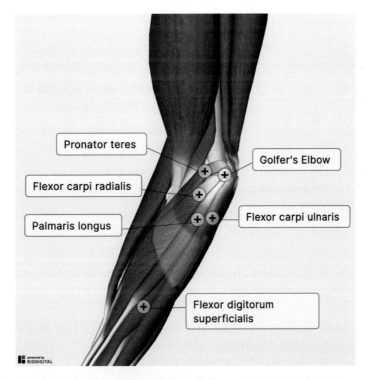

FIGURE 5-41 In golfer's elbow, inflammation occurs at the medial epicondyle and involves the tendons of the pronator teres, flexor carpi radialis, flexor carpi ulnaris, flexor digitorum superficialis, and palmaris longus muscles.

LEARNING OBJECTIVE 5.6.12 **Identify the muscles of buttocks, upper leg, and lower leg.**

KEY TERMS

abductor digiti minimi Muscle located in the first layer of the foot.

abductor hallucis Muscle located in the first layer of the foot that is connected to the big toe.

adductor brevis Muscle located in the medial thigh region that performs adduction of the hip; part of the adductor group of muscles.

adductor hallucis Muscle in the third layer of the foot that maintains the transverse arch of the foot; part of the adductor group of muscles.

adductor longus Muscle located in the medial thigh region that performs adduction of the hip; part of the adductor group of muscles.

adductor magnus Muscle located in the medial thigh region that performs adduction of the hip; part of the adductor group of muscles.

biceps femoris Muscle in the posterior portion of the leg and part of the hamstring group.

dorsal interossei Small muscles located on the back or dorsal region of the hand.

extensor digitorum brevis

extensor digitorum longus Muscle in the lower leg located deep to the tibialis anterior and works to dorsiflex the ankle.

extensor hallucis longus Deep muscle of the lower leg that works to extend the big toe.

fibularis tertius One of the fibularis group of muscles located in the lateral portion of the lower leg.

flexor digiti minimi brevis Muscle located in the third layer of foot muscles producing flexion of the toes.

flexor digitorum brevis Muscle located in the first layer of foot muscles producing flexion of the toes.

flexor digitorum longus Muscle in the posterior leg that produces flexion of the toes.

flexor hallucis brevis Muscle in the lower leg that flexes the big toe.

gastrocnemius Muscle on the posterior portion of the lower leg that crosses both the knee and ankle joint.

gluteus maximus Large muscle in the posterior pelvis region that attaches to the femur and produces flexion of the leg.

gluteus medius Muscle located in the posterior pelvis deep to the gluteus maximus that works to stabilize the sacroiliac joint.

gluteus minimus Muscle located in the posterior pelvis deep to the gluteus medius.

gracilis Muscle located in the medial thigh that works to produce hip adduction.

hamstring One muscle of a group of muscles located in the posterior thigh.

inferior gemellus Deep muscle of the posterior pelvis that functions as an external rotator of the hip.

lumbricales Deep muscles of the hand that flex the hand and extend the fingers.

obturator externus Deep posterior pelvic muscle that produces external rotation of the hip.

obturator internus Deep posterior pelvic muscle that produces external rotation of the hip.

pectineus Muscle located on the medial portion of the thigh that works to adduct the hip.

piriformis Deep posterior pelvic muscle in close proximity to the sciatic nerve that produces external rotation of the hip.

plantar interossei Small muscles between the toes located in the fourth layer of the foot muscles.

popliteus Muscle located on the posterior portion of the knee.

quadratus femoris Muscle located on the posterior portion of the hip joint that works to produce external rotation of the hip.

quadratus plantus Muscle of the second layer of foot muscles.

---

quadriceps Group of four muscles on the anterior thigh that includes the rectus femoris, vastus medialis, vastus lateralis, and vastus intermedius.

rectus femoris One of the quadriceps muscles located in the anterior thigh.

sartorius Superficial muscle of the thigh attached to the ilium and extending to the medial knee.

semimembranosus One of three hamstring muscles located on the medial portion of the posterior thigh.

semitendinosus One of three hamstring muscles located on the medial portion of the posterior thigh and superficial to the semimembranosus.

soleus Muscle located on the posterior lower leg just deep to the gastrocnemius muscle.

superior gemellus Deep muscle of the pelvis that functions to externally rotate the hip.

tibialis anterior Muscle located in the anterior portion of the lower leg just lateral to the tibia that works to dorsiflex the ankle.

tibialis posterior Deep muscle located deep to the soleus muscle that works to stabilize the lower leg.

vastus intermedius One of four quadriceps muscles located in the anterior thigh just deep to the rectus femoris muscle that works to extend the knee joint.

vastus lateralis One of four quadriceps muscles located in the lateral thigh that works to extend the knee joint.

vastus medialis One of four quadriceps muscles located in the medial thigh that works to extend the knee joint.

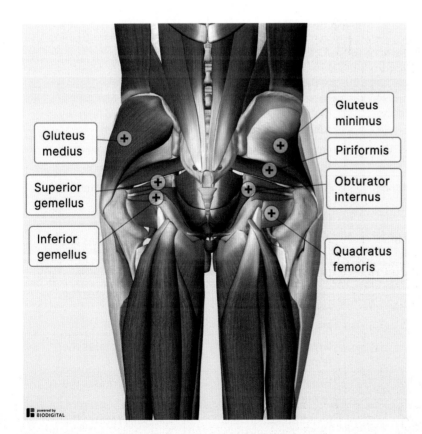

FIGURE 5-42 Deep muscles of the posterior pelvis.

MUSCLES OF THE PELVIS, UPPER LEG, AND LOWER LEG

Muscles of the Pelvis

The muscles of the buttocks include the **gluteus maximus, gluteus medius, gluteus minimus, piriformis, obturator internus, obturator externus, superior** and **inferior gemellus,** and **quadratus femoris** (see Figure 5-42). The psoas major muscles are located deep in the pelvic region. Each psoas major muscle originates on the lumbar spine and extends inferior. The psoas major muscles combine with the iliacus muscles to form a common tendon that inserts on the lesser trochanter of the femur (see Figure 5-43) (see Table 5-6).

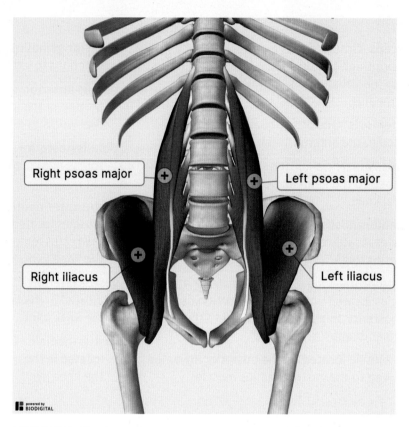

FIGURE 5-43 The Iliopsoas muscles consist of the iliacus and psoas major muscles.

Table 5.6 Muscles of the Pelvis

MUSCLE	ORIGIN	INSERTION	ACTION
gluteus maximus	Ilium, Sacrum, Coccyx	Iliotibial tract, gluteal tuberosity of femur	Extends and laterally rotates thigh
gluteus medius	Ilium	Greater trochanter of the femur	Abducts and medially rotates thigh
gluteus minimus	Lateral portion of ilium	Anterior surface of greater trochanter of femur	Abducts and medially rotates hip
piriformis	Anterior portion of sacrum	Anterior part of medial aspect of greater trochanter of femur	Laterally rotates and stabilizes hip
obturator externus	Outer border of obturator foramen	Trochanteric fossa on medial surface of greater trochanter	Laterally rotates the hip
superior gemellus	Ischial spine	Greater trochanter of femur	Laterally rotates the hip
inferior gemellus	Ischial tuberosity	Greater trochanter of femur	Laterally rotates the hip
quadratus femorus	Ischial tuberosity	Quadrate tubercle of femur extending to the lesser trochanter	Laterally rotates the hip

Muscles of the Upper Leg

Muscles on the proximal medial portion of the thigh include the **adductor longus**, **adductor brevis**, **adductor magnus**, **pectineus**, and **gracilis** (see Figure 5-44) (see Table 5-7).

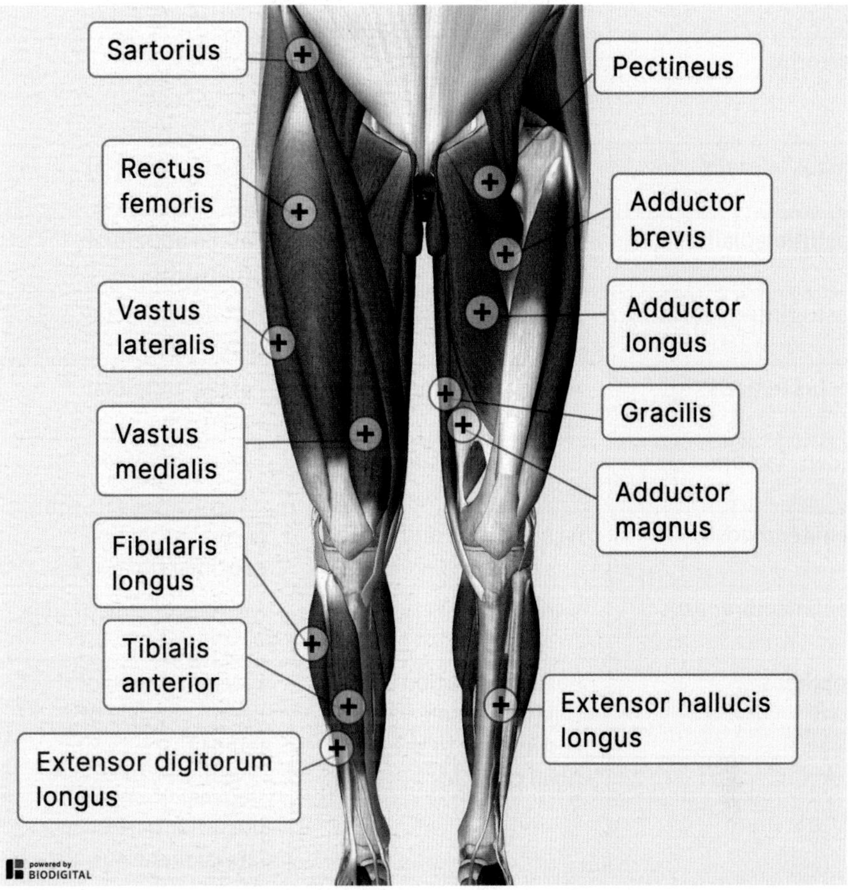

FIGURE 5-44 Anterior leg muscles. The vastus medialis, rectus femoris, and extensor digitorum longus muscles have been removed on the left side to view the deep muscles.

Table 5-7 Muscle of the Upper Leg

MUSCLE	ORIGIN	INSERTION	ACTION
Adductor longus	inferior and medial portion of the pubis	Lower two-thirds of medial linea aspera	Adducts and medially rotates hip
Adductor brevis	Inferior ramus and body of pubis	Upper third of linea aspera	Adducts hip
Adductor magnus	Adductor portion: ischiopubic ramus Hamstring portion: lower outer portion of posterior surface of ischial tuberosity	Adductor portion: lower gluteal line and linea aspera Hamstring portion: adductor tubercle	Adductor portion: adducts and medially rotates hip Hamstring portion: extends hip

(Continued)

MUSCLE	ORIGIN	INSERTION	ACTION
pectineus	Lateral portion of pubis	Inferior to the lesser trochanter of the femur	Flexes, adducts, and medially rotates hip
gracilis	Pubis	Medial tibia	Adducts thigh, flexes and medially rotates leg
sartorius	Anterior superior iliac spine	Tibia	Flexes, abducts, and laterally rotates thigh; flexes lower leg
vastus lateralis	Linea aspera	Patella and tibial tuberosity	Extends lower leg, stabilizes knee
vastus medialis	Linea aspera	Patella and tibial tuberosity	Extends lower leg
vastus intermedius	Proximal femur	Patella and tibial tuberosity	Extends lower leg
rectus femoris	Anterior inferior iliac spine	Patella and tibial tuberosity	Extends knee, flexes thigh
biceps femoris	Ischial tuberosity and femur	Tibia and fibula	Extends thigh, flexes lower leg
semitendinosus	Ischial tuberosity	Medial aspect of proximal tibia	Extends thigh, flexes lower leg
semimembranosus	Ischial tuberosity	Medial condyle of tibia	Extends thigh, flexes lower leg
popliteus	Posterior portion of tibia above soleal line and inferior to the tibial condyles	Lateral portion of lateral condyle of femur Capsule of knee to posterior part of lateral meniscus	Laterally rotates femur on tibia

The large muscles on the anterior portion of the thigh include the sartorius and quadriceps group. The quadriceps group consists of four muscles: rectus femoris, vastus medialis, vastus lateralis, and vastus intermedius (see Figure 5-44).

The posterior thigh muscles include the hamstring group. The hamstrings consist of three muscles which include the biceps femoris, semimembranosus, and semitendinosus. The popliteus is located in the posterior portion of the knee (see Figure 5-45).

Muscles of the Lower Leg and Foot

The muscles of the anterior portion of the leg include the tibialis anterior, extensor hallucis longus, extensor digitorum longus, and fibularis tertius (see Figure 5-46). Muscles on the posterior portion of the leg include the gastrocnemius, soleus, flexor digitorum longus, and tibialis posterior (see Figure 5-46) (see Table 5-8).

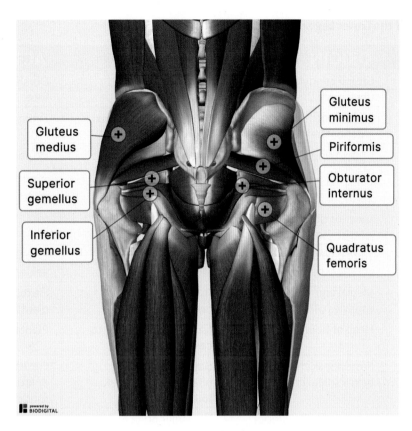

FIGURE 5-45 Posterior leg muscles. The gluteus maximus, semitendinosus, and gastrocnemius have been removed on the right side of the diagram to view the deep muscles.

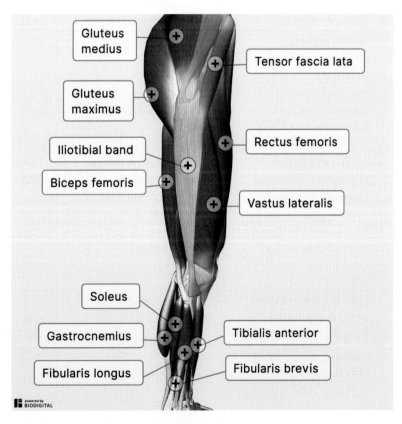

FIGURE 5-46 Lateral hip, thigh, and leg muscles.

Table 5-8 Muscles of the Lower Leg and Foot

MUSCLE	ORIGIN	INSERTION	ACTION
tibialis anterior	Lateral condyle and tibial shaft	First cuneiform and first metatarsals	Dorsiflexes and inverts foot
extensor hallucis longus	Middle portion of anterior shaft of fibula	Base of distal phalanx of great toe	Extends big toe and foot, inverts ankle
extensor digitorum longus	Upper two-thirds of anterior shaft of fibula, interosseous membrane, and superior tibiofibular joint	Lateral four toes	Extends toes and ankle
fibularis tertius	Third quarter of anterior shaft of fibula	Shaft and base of 5th metatarsal	Extends and everts te ankle
gastrocnemius	Medial and lateral condyles of femur	Achilles tendon and calcaneal tendon	Flexes lower leg, plantarflexes foot
soleus	Head of fibula and tibia	Calcaneal tendon onto calcaneus	Plantarflexes foot
flexor digitorum longus	Posterior shaft of tibia below soleal line	Base of distal phalanges of lateral four toes	Flexes distal phalanges of lateral four toes and foot at ankle
tibialis posterior	Upper half of posterior portion of tibia and upper half of fibula between	Navicular bone and tarsal bones	Plantarflexes and inverts ankle
extensor digitorum brevis	Superior surface of anterior calcaneus	Proximal phalanx of big toe and toes 2, 3, and 4	Extends toes during ankle dorsiflexion
flexor digitorum brevis	Medial process of posterior calcaneal tuberosity	Four lateral toes	Flexes four lateral toes
abductor hallucis	Medial process of posterior calcaneal tuberosity and flexor retinaculum	Medial portion of base of proximal phalanx of big toe	Flexes and abducts big toe
abductor digiti minimi	Medial and lateral processes of posterior calcaneal tuberosity	Lateral portion of base of proximal phalanx of fifth toe and fifth metatarsal	Flexes and abducts fifth toe
quadratus plantus	Lateral head-tuberosity of calcaneus, medial head-medial side of calcaneus	Lateral border long flexor tendons	Flexes toes
lumbricales	Lateral 3: four tendons of flexor digitorum longus Medial 1: medial aspect of first tendon	Dorsal extensor expansion	Extends toes at interphalangeal joints and flexes metatarsal phalangeal joints

(Continued)

MUSCLE	ORIGIN	INSERTION	ACTION
adductor hallucis	Oblique head: base of 2, 3, 4 metatarsals Transverse head: plantar metatarsal ligaments and deep transverse ligament	Lateral side of base of proximal phalanx of big toe and lateral sesamoid	Adducts and flexes metatarsophalangeal joint of big toe
flexor digiti minimi brevis	Base of fifth metatarsal and portion of fibularis longus	Lateral side of base of proximal phalanx of little toe	Flexes metatarsophalangeal joint of little toe
flexor hallucis brevis	Cuboid and lateral cuneiform	Base of proximal phalanx of big toe	Flexes metatarsophalangeal joint of big toe
dorsal interossei	Metatarsals	Bases of proximal phalanges	Abducts toes 2, 3, and 4
plantar interossei	Shafts of metatarsals 3, 4, and 5	Medial portion of bases of proximal phalanges	Abducts toes 3, 4, and 5

The top of the foot is known as the dorsum of the foot. The only muscle located exclusively on the dorsum of the foot is the **extensor digitorum brevis** (see Figure 5-47).

The bottom or sole of the foot is known as the plantar region of the foot. This area contains four layers of muscles (see Figures 5-48, 5-49, 5-50, and 5-51).

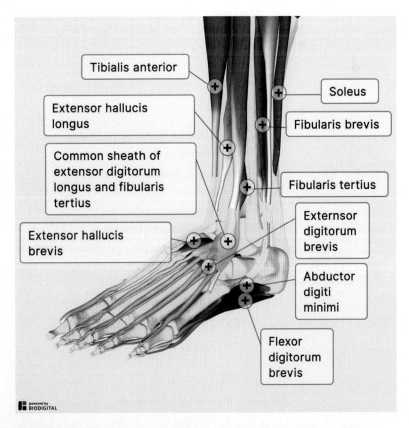

FIGURE 5-47 Muscles of the dorsum of the foot and lateral leg.

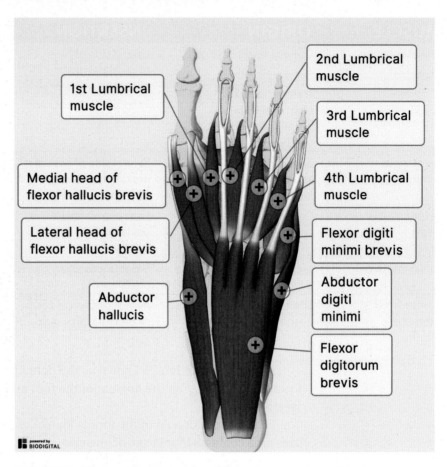

FIGURE 5-48 Superficial muscles of the plantar region of the foot.

The layers from superficial to deep include:
Layer 1:

- **Flexor digitorum brevis**
- **Abductor hallucis**
- **Abductor digiti minimi**

Layer 2:

- **Quadratus plantus**
- **Lumbricales**

Layer 3:

- **Adductor hallucis**
- **Flexor digiti minimi brevis**
- **Flexor hallucis brevis**

Layer 4:

- **Dorsal interossei**
- **Plantar interossei**

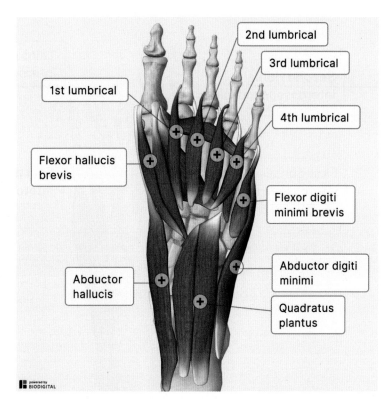

FIGURE 5-49 Muscles of the plantar region of the foot. Deep layer 2 showing quadratus plantus muscle.

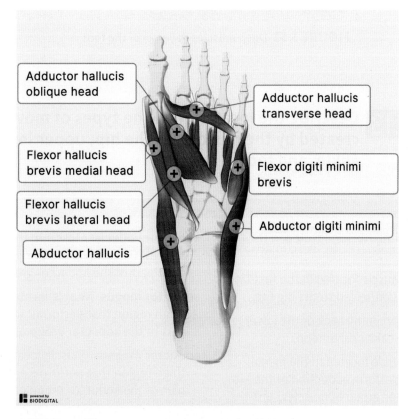

FIGURE 5-50 Deep muscles (layer 3) of the foot.

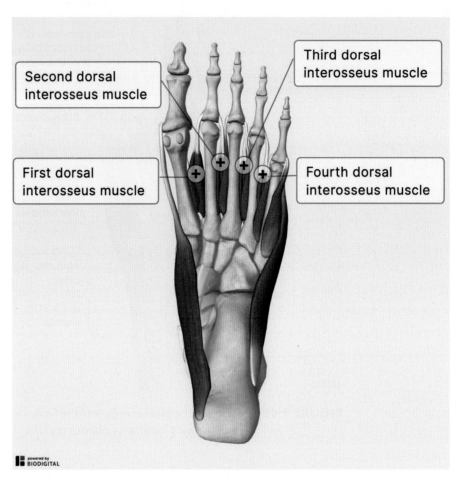

Second dorsal interosseus muscle

Third dorsal interosseus muscle

First dorsal interosseus muscle

Fourth dorsal interosseus muscle

powered by BIODIGITAL

FIGURE 5-51 Deep muscles (layer 4) of the foot.

LEARNING OBJECTIVE 5.6.13 **Describe the location and the types of movement created by the muscles of the hip, upper leg, lower leg, ankle, and foot.**

KEY TERMS

abductor digiti minimi Muscle located in the first layer of the foot.

abductor hallucis Muscle located in the first layer of the foot that is connected to the big toe.

Achilles Large tendon in the back of the lower leg, also known as the calcaneal tendon.

adductor brevis Muscle located in the medial thigh region that perform adduction of the hip; part of the adductor group of muscles.

adductor hallucis Muscle in the third layer of the foot that maintains the transverse arch of the foot; part of the adductor group of muscles.

adductor longus Muscle located in the medial thigh region that performs adduction of the hip; part of the adductor group of muscles.

adductor magnus Muscle located in the medial thigh region that performs adduction of the hip; part of the adductor group of muscles.

anterior superior iliac spine Bony landmark located on the anterior portion of the ilium of the pelvis.

aponeurosis of the sacrospinalis Flat, broad, tendinous structure that attaches to the sacrospinalis muscles.

biceps femoris Muscle in the posterior portion of the leg and part of the hamstring group.

coccyx Small bone attached to the inferior portion of the sacrum.

dorsal interossei Small muscles located on the back or dorsal region of the hand.

dorsiflex Movement of the ankle in which the toes are extended upward as if walking on the heels.

dorsum Pertaining to the back or posterior region of the body.

evert To move the ankle so the sole of the foot is pointing away from the midline of the body.

extensor digitorum brevis Muscle in the posterior forearm that moves the fingers or digits into extension.

extensor digitorum longus Muscle in the lower leg located deep to the tibialis anterior and works to dorsiflex the ankle.

extensor hallucis longus Deep muscle of the lower leg that works to extend the big toe.

femur Long bone of the upper leg; longest bone in the body.

fibula Bone in the lateral portion of the lower leg.

fibularis tertius One of the fibularis group of muscles located in the lateral portion of the lower leg.

fifth metatarsal Most lateral metatarsal bone in the foot.

first metatarsal Most medial metatarsal bone in the foot.

flexor digiti minimi brevis Muscle located in the third layer of foot muscles producing flexion of the toes.

flexor digitorum brevis Muscle located in the first layer of foot muscles producing flexion of the toes.

flexor digitorum longus Muscle in the posterior leg that produces flexion of the toes.

flexor hallucis brevis Muscle in the lower leg that flexes the big toe.

gastrocnemius Muscle on the posterior portion of the lower leg that crosses both the knee and ankle joint.

gluteus maximus Large muscle in the posterior pelvis region that attaches to the femur and produces flexion of the leg.

gluteus medius Muscle located in the posterior pelvis deep to the gluteus maximus that works to stabilize the sacroiliac joint.

gluteus minimus Muscle located in the posterior pelvis deep to the gluteus medius.

gracilis Muscle located in the medial thigh that works to produce hip adduction.

greater trochanter of the femur Large bony prominence located on the lateral femur.

hamstring One muscle of a group of muscles located in the posterior thigh.

iliac crest Superior portion of the ilium of the coxal bone.

iliacus Deep pelvic muscle connecting to the ilium and extending to the femur causing hip flexion.

iliopsoas Combination of two muscles, the iliacus and psoas major, that extend from the pelvis to the femur.

iliotibial band Broad band of fibrous connective tissue located on the lateral portion of the thigh.

ilium Most superior portion of the coxal bone.

inferior gemellus Deep muscle of the posterior pelvis that functions as an external rotator of the hip.

interosseous membrane Broad, thick, and dense fibrous tissue between many bones in the body.

ischial tuberosity Broad eminence of bone located on the posterior portion of the ischium.

lateral condyle of the tibia Large rounded process on the proximal portion of the tibia on the lateral side.

lesser trochanter of the femur Bony eminence on the proximal portion of the lateral femur just inferior to the greater trochanter.

linea aspera Protruding ridge of bone located on the posterior portion of the femur.

lumbricales Deep muscles of the hand that flex the hand and extend the fingers.

medial condyle of tibia Large, rounded process on the proximal medial portion of the tibia.

medial cuneiform One of three cuneiform bones of the foot located just anterior to the navicular bone.

metatarsals Bones of the foot located just anterior to the tarsal bones and posterior to the phalanges.

obturator externus Deep posterior pelvic muscle that produces external rotation of the hip.

obturator internus Deep posterior pelvic muscle that produces external rotation of the hip.

patella Small sesamoid bone commonly called the kneecap.

patellar tendon Dense connective tissue structure that anchors the distal patella to the tibial tuberosity of the tibia.

pectineus Muscle located on the medial portion of the thigh that works to adduct the hip.

phalanges Fingers or toes.

piriformis Deep posterior pelvic muscle in close proximity to the sciatic nerve that produces external rotation of the hip.

plantar aponeurosis (Band of fibrous connective tissue located at the sole of the foot.)

plantar interossei Small muscles between the toes located in the fourth layer of the foot muscles.

plantarflex Bending at the ankle when the heel is lifted, flexing the foot or toes downward.

popliteus Muscle located on the posterior portion of the knee.

pronation Rotation of the hand and forearm so that the palm faces downward.

psoas major Deep muscle of the abdominopelvic region that attaches to the lumbar spine and extends to the femur.

pubic bone One of three fused coxal bones located on the anterior–inferior portion of the coxal bone.

quadratus femoris Muscle located on the posterior portion of the hip joint that works to produce external rotation of the hip.

quadratus plantus Muscle of the second layer of foot muscles.

quadriceps Group of four muscles on the anterior thigh that includes the rectus femoris, vastus medialis, vastus lateralis, and vastus intermedius.

rectus femoris One of the quadriceps muscles located in the anterior thigh.

sacrum Triangular bone located just below the spine that articulates with the lowest lumbar spinal segment and both coxal bones.

sartorius Superficial muscle of the thigh attached to the ilium and extending to the medial knee.

semimembranosus One of three hamstring muscles located on the medial portion of the posterior thigh.

semitendinosus One of three hamstring muscles located on the medial portion of the posterior thigh and superficial to the semimembranosus.

soleus Muscle located on the posterior lower leg just deep to the gastrocnemius muscle.

superior gemellus Deep muscle of the pelvis that functions to externally rotate the hip.

tensor fascia latae Muscle located on the superior and lateral side of the thigh.

tibia Anterior long bone in the lower leg that articulates with the femur, fibula, and talus.

tibial tuberosity Broad eminence located on the anterior proximal portion of the tibia that serves as an attachment point of the patellar tendon.

tibialis anterior Muscle located in the anterior portion of the lower leg just lateral to the tibia that works to dorsiflex the ankle.

tibialis posterior Deep muscle located deep to the soleus muscle that works to stabilize the lower leg.

vastus intermedius One of four quadriceps muscles located in the anterior thigh just deep to the rectus femoris muscle that works to extend the knee joint.

vastus lateralis One of four quadriceps muscles located in the lateral thigh that works to extend the knee joint.

vastus medialis One of four quadriceps muscles located in the medial thigh that works to extend the knee joint.

PELVIC, LOWER EXTREMITY, AND FOOT MUSCLE FUNCTIONS

Muscles of the Thigh

Muscles that move the thigh connect to the pelvis and **femur**. The anterior muscles include the **iliopsoas** and **iliacus** and the posterior muscles include the **gluteus maximus**, **gluteus medius**, **gluteus minimus**, and **tensor fascia latae** (see Figures 5-43, 5-44, and 5-45).

The psoas portion of the iliopsoas muscle includes two divisions. The **psoas major** attaches to the lower lumbar vertebra and extends to the **lesser trochanter of the femur**. The psoas minor muscle is smaller and inserts on the **pubic bone**. The Iliacus muscle attaches to the **ilium** and extends to the lesser trochanter of the femur. Since both the psoas major and iliacus share a common insertion, they are often referred to as the iliopsoas. The iliopsoas works to flex the hip (see Figure 5-43).

The gluteus maximus is one of the strongest and largest muscles of the body. It attaches to the **iliac crest**, **sacrum**, **coccyx**, and the **aponeurosis of the sacrospinalis**. It extends to the **linea aspera** of the femur and the **iliotibial band**. It works to produce hip extension (see Figure 5-46).

The gluteus medius lies deep to the gluteus maximus. It attaches to the ilium and extends to the greater trochanter of the femur. It works to produce hip abduction and extension.

The gluteus minimus lies deep to the gluteus medius. It is the smallest gluteal muscle.

The tensor fascia latae is located on the lateral aspect of the thigh. It attaches to the iliac crest and extends to a band of dense connective tissue called the iliotibial tract or band. The iliotibial band extends down the lateral aspect of the femur to the **tibia**. Tendonitis can develop in this tendon in a condition known as iliotibial band syndrome (see Figure 5-46).

Deep muscles in the posterior pelvic area include the **piriformis**, **obturator internus**, **obturator externus**, **superior** and **inferior gemellus**, and **quadratus femoris** muscles. All these muscles work to externally rotate and abduct the hip (see Figure 5-46).

Muscles on the proximal medial aspect of the thigh include the **adductor longus**, **adductor brevis**, **adductor magnus**, **pectineus**, and **gracilis**. These muscles attach to the pubic bone and extend down the thigh to various insertion points on the femur. They work to adduct the hip (Figure 5-44).

The large muscles on the anterior portion of the thigh include the sartorius and quadriceps group.

The sartorius (tailor's muscle) attaches to the anterior superior iliac spine and extends from lateral to medial across the thigh to insert on the medial aspect of the upper tibia. This muscle has multiple actions including flexion, abduction, and external rotation of the hip (Figure 5-44).

The quadriceps group consists of the rectus femoris, vastus medialis, vastus lateralis, and vastus intermedius (Figure 5-44). The quadriceps muscles work together to produce knee extension. The rectus femoris is located in the middle of the thigh. It attaches to the anterior superior iliac spine and extends inferiorly to the patella. The vastus medialis is located in the medial aspect of the thigh. It attaches to the linea aspera of the femur and extends to the patella. The vastus lateralis is located in the lateral aspect of the thigh. It attaches to the greater trochanter of the femur and extends to the patella. The vastus intermedius lies deep to the rectus femoris. It attaches to the femur and extends to the patella. The quadriceps muscles have a common insertion point on the patellar tendon. The patellar tendon inserts on the tibial tuberosity.

The posterior thigh muscles include the hamstring group (see Figure 5-45). The hamstrings consist of three muscles that include the biceps femoris, semimembranosus, and semitendinosus. The hamstrings work to produce knee flexion. The biceps femoris is a two-headed muscle. The long head attaches to the ischial tuberosity and the short head attaches to the linea aspera and lateral supracondylar line of the femur. The muscle then extends inferiorly to attach to the head of the fibula. The semimembranosus attaches to the ischial tuberosity and extends inferiorly to attach to the medial condyle of the tibia and lateral condyle of the femur. The semitendinosus attaches to the ischial tuberosity and extends inferiorly to attach to the medial aspect of the upper tibia.

Muscles of the Lower Leg (see Figures 5-46 and 5-47)

Located in the posterior portion of the knee is the popliteus muscle. If the femur is fixed the popliteus works to internally rotate the tibia. If the tibia is fixed it works to externally rotate the femur.

The muscles of the anterior portion of the leg work to dorsiflex the foot. These include the tibialis anterior, extensor hallucis longus, extensor digitorum longus, and fibularis tertius. The tibialis anterior is located just lateral to the tibia. It attaches to the lateral condyle of the tibia, the lateral aspect of the proximal portion of the tibia, and the interosseous membrane that connects the tibia and fibula. It extends downward to attach to the medial cuneiform and first metatarsal.

The extensor hallucis longus lies deep to the tibialis anterior. It attaches to the anterior aspect of the fibula and interosseous membrane and extends downward to attach to the first distal phalanx. Besides being a synergist for dorsiflexion of the foot, it also extends the big toe.

The extensor digitorum longus also lies deep to the tibialis anterior. It attaches to the lateral condyle of the tibia, shaft of the fibula, and interosseous membrane. It works as a synergist in dorsiflexion of the foot and extends the toes. It also works to tighten the plantar aponeurosis.

The fibularis tertius is part of the fibularis group that includes the fibularis longus and fibularis brevis. This muscle works to dorsiflex and evert the foot. It attaches to the medial surface of the lower portion of the fibula and extends to the fifth metatarsal. The fibularis group works together to evert the foot.

The muscles of the posterior leg work to plantarflex the foot. These include the gastrocnemius, soleus, flexor digitorum longus, and tibialis posterior.

The gastrocnemius is a two-headed muscle that crosses both the knee and ankle joints. Its action in the knee is to help with knee flexion. It also works to produce ankle plantarflexion. It attaches to the femoral condyles and posterior surface of the distal femur and extends downward to attach to the calcaneus. The soleus lies deep to the gastrocnemius. It attaches to the posterior aspect of the proximal fibula and tibia and extends downward to attach to the calcaneus. The soleus only crosses the ankle joint and produces ankle plantarflexion.

The gastrocnemius and soleus both insert on the large Achilles (calcaneal) tendon and are known collectively as the triceps surae.

The tibialis posterior is also a deep muscle of the posterior leg. It attaches to the posterior proximal surface of the tibia and fibula and extend downward to attach to the navicular, medial cuneiform, and second to fourth metarasals. It works to produce plantarflexion and helps to control pronation of the foot while walking.

The flexor digitorum longus is a deep muscle of the posterior leg. It attaches to the posterior surface of the tibia and extends downward to attach to the second through fifth distal phalanges. It works to flex the toes and stabilizes the metatarsal heads.

The peroneus (fibularis) longus is located on the lateral aspect of the lower leg. It attaches to the tibia and fibula and extends to the medial cuneiform and first metatarsal.

The flexor hallucis longus is a deep muscle on the lateral aspect of the leg. It attaches to the distal portion of the fibula and interosseous membrane and extends to attach to the big toe. It works to flex the big toe.

Muscles of the Foot (see Figures 5-47, 5-48, 5-49, 5-50, and 5-51)

The top of the foot is known as the dorsum of the foot. The only muscle located exclusively on the dorsum of the foot is the extensor digitorum brevis. This muscle attaches to the calcaneus and extensor retinaculum of the ankle and extends to the big toe and tendons of the extensor digitorum longus. It works to produce extension of the toes.

The bottom or sole of the foot is known as the plantar region of the foot. This area contains four layers of muscles.

The layers from superficial to deep include:

Layer 1:

- **Flexor digitorum brevis:** Flexes the toes.
- **Abductor hallucis:** Abducts the great toe.
- **Abductor digiti minimi:** Abducts and flexes the great toe.

Layer 2:

- **Quadratus plantus:** Works with the flexor digitorum longus to assist in toe flexion.
- **Lumbricales:** Flex toes at metatarsophalangeal joints and extends toes at interphalangeal joints.

Layer 3:

- **Adductor hallucis:** Maintains transverse arch of the foot.
- **Flexor digiti minimi brevis:** Flexes little toe.
- **Flexor hallucis brevis:** Flexes great toe.

Layer 4:

- **Dorsal interossei:** Abducts toes.
- **Plantar interossei:** Adducts toes.

| **CLINICAL TIP** | Giving intramuscular injections is an important clinical skill. An important site for injections is the gluteus medius muscle. It is important to know the location of this muscle to avoid injecting substances into the sciatic nerve. |

| **CLINICAL TIP** | The biceps femoris muscle is the most commonly injured hamstring muscle. This is likely due to the increased force in the muscle during knee extension while the muscle is eccentrically contracting. |

LEARNING OBJECTIVE 5.6.14 Identify the muscles of the neck and back.

LEARNING OBJECTIVE 5.6.15 Identify the nine muscles that compose the erector spinae.

LEARNING OBJECTIVE 5.6.16 Describe the location and the types of movement created by the muscles of the neck and back.

KEY TERMS

clavicle Bone of the shoulder connecting the scapula and the sternum; also called the collarbone.

digastric Muscle in the region of the neck.

erector spinae group Group of back muscles that function in extension of the trunk that consist

of the spinalis, longissimus, iliocostalis, and semispinalis muscles.

hyoid bone U-shaped bone in the anterior portion of the neck just inferior to the mandible.

iliocostalis Muscle in the back; part of the erector spinae group of back muscles.

longissimus Muscle located in the back that is part of the erector spinae group of muscles.

mastoid process Bony protuberance off of the temporal bone.

mylohyoid Muscle in the anterior cervical region connecting to the hyoid bone.

occipital bone One of the bones of the skull located in the posterior inferior region of the skull.

omohyoid Muscle located in the anterior cervical region connecting to the hyoid bone.

platysma Superficial muscle of the neck that produces frowning.

semispinalis capitis Muscle located in the posterior cervical region connecting to the skull.

semispinalis muscles Muscles located in the back that are part of the erector spinae group.

spinalis Muscles of the back that are part of the erector spinae group.

splenius capitis Muscle located in the upper posterior portion of the cervical area connecting to the occipital bone.

sternocleidomastoid Muscle located in the lateral cervical region extending from the mastoid process to the clavicle and sternum.

sternohyoid Muscle located in the anterior portion of the cervical region attaching to the sternum and hyoid bones.

sternothyroid Muscle located in the anterior portion of the cervical region attaching to the sternum and thyroid cartilage.

sternum Bone located in the anterior portion of the thorax that has three divisions (manubrium, body, xiphoid process) and connects to the ribs and clavicles.

stylohyoid Muscle in the anterior portion of the cervical region attaching to the styloid process of the temporal bone and hyoid bone.

temporal bone One of the bones of the skull located on the lateral sides.

thyrohyoid Muscle located in the anterior cervical region connecting to the thyroid cartilage and hyoid bone.

MUSCLES OF THE NECK AND BACK
Muscles of the Neck (see Figures 5-52, 5-53, and 5-54)

Muscles of the neck include the platysma, sternocleidomastoid, splenius capitis, semispinalis capitis, digastric, stylohyoid, mylohyoid, sternothyroid, omohyoid, thyrohyoid, and sternohyoid (see Table 5-9).

There are a number of muscles attached to the vertebral column that move the head. The sternocleidomastoid attaches to the mastoid process of the temporal bone as well as the clavicle and sternum. It produces contralateral rotation when one muscle contracts and neck flexion when both muscles contract.

The splenius capitis is located in the posterior portion of the neck. It helps bring the head into an upright position (head extension). It also causes ipsilateral rotation and lateral flexion when one muscle contracts.

The semispinalis capitis also produces head extension as well as lateral flexion and rotation. It connects to the occipital bone and vertebra of the cervical and thoracic spines.

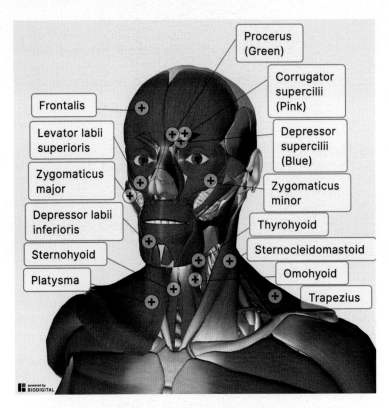

FIGURE 5-52 Superficial muscles of the anterior neck and head.

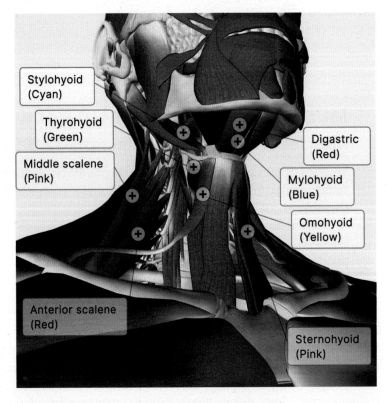

FIGURE 5-53 Deep muscles of the anterior neck.

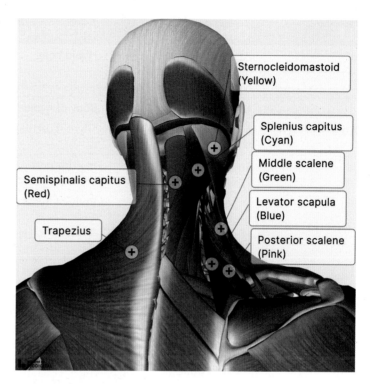

FIGURE 5-54 Posterior neck muscles.

Table 5-9 **Muscles of the Neck**

MUSCLE	ORIGIN	INSERTION	ACTION
platysma	Inner portion of the skin in the lower cervical and upper thoracic regions	Inferior border of mandible and inner portion of skin over the lower portion of the mouth	Depresses skin over lower portion of face
sternocleidomastoid	Manubrium, clavicle	Mastoid process	Singly, rotates head to opposite shoulder; together, flexes head
splenius capitus	Lower ligament nuchae, spinous processes, and supraspinous ligaments T1–3	Lateral occiput between superior and inferior nuchal lines	Extends and rotates cervical spine
semispinalis capitus	Articular processes of C4–6 and transverse processes of C7–T1	Occipital bone	Extension of the cervical spine
digastric	Medial portion of mastoid process of temporal bone	Hyoid bone	Elevates hyoid bone and assists in swallowing

MUSCLE	ORIGIN	INSERTION	ACTION
stylohyoid	Base of styloid process of temporal bone	Hyoid bone	Elevates and retracts hyoid bone, elevates larynx
mylohyoid	Mandible	Body of hyoid bone	Elevates hyoid bone
sternothyroid	Medial posterior portion of manubrium	Thyroid cartilage	Depresses larynx
thyrohyoid	Thyroid cartilage	Inferior portion of the body of hyoid bone	Elevates larynx
sternohyoid	Superior lateral posterior portion of manubrium of sternum	Body of hyoid bone	Depresses hyoid bone
omohyoid	Suprascapular ligament and scapula	Body of hyoid bone	Depresses hyoid bone

Muscles in the anterior portion of the neck include the platysma, a superficial muscle, and a number of deep muscles that depress the mandible and move the **hyoid bone**.

The digastric muscle attaches to the temporal bone and extends to the hyoid bone. It works to depress the mandible (open the mouth).

The mylohyoid attaches to the mandible and extends to the hyoid bone. It works to elevate the hyoid bone and depress the mandible.

The stylohyoid attaches to the styloid process of the temporal bone and extends to the hyoid bone. It works to elevate and retract the hyoid bone.

The sternohyoid attaches to the sternum and clavicle and extends to the hyoid bone. It works to depress the hyoid bone.

The omohyoid attaches to the superior border of the scapula and extends to the hyoid bone. It works to depress the hyoid bone.

The thyrohyoid attaches to the thyroid cartilage of the larynx and extends to the hyoid bone. It works to depress the hyoid and elevate the larynx.

CLINICAL TIP	Weakness of the sternocleidomastoid muscle can indicate a problem with cranial nerve XI, also known as the accessory nerve.

Muscles of the Back

Muscles of the back include the **erector spinae group** (see Figure 5-55). The erector spinae group of muscles consists of deep back muscles running up and down the spine. These consist of the spinalis, longissimus, iliocostalis, and semispinalis muscles. They are located in the cervical, thoracic, and lumbar areas of the spine. The names of these muscles provide clues to their locations. For example, the **spinalis** muscles are located medially, attaching directly to the

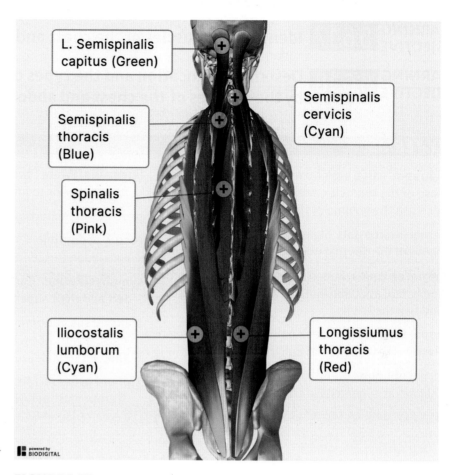

FIGURE 5-55 Erector spinae muscles.

spinal segments. The **iliocostalis** muscles attach to the ribs (iliocostalis thoracis) (costal = ribs). The **longissimus** muscles have long fibers and the **semispinalis muscles** run just lateral to the spinal segments (see Table 5-10).

Table 5-10 Muscles of the back.

MUSCLE	ORIGIN	INSERTION	ACTION
spinalis	Spinal segments of cervical, thoracic and lumbar vertebrae	Spinal segments of cervical, thoracic, and lumbar vertebrae	Extends and laterally flexes spine
iliocostalis	Iliac crest, sacrum, lumbar vertebrae	Ribs, cervical transverse processes	Extends and laterally flexes spine
longissimus	Transverse processes of vertebrae	Transverse processes of vertebrae above origins	Extends spine
seimispinalis	Transverse processes of vertebrae	Spinous processes and occipital bone (for semispinalis cervicis)	Extends and laterally flexes spine

Identify the muscles of the chest and abdomen.

Describe the location and the types of movement created by the muscles of the chest and abdomen.

KEY TERMS

diaphragm Large skeletal muscle located at the base of the thoracic cavity that contracts to increase the volume of the thoracic cavity.

external intercostals Superficial muscles located between the ribs that work to spread apart the ribs.

external obliques Superficial muscles located on the lateral abdominal region that work to rotate and flex the trunk.

internal intercostals Deep muscles locate between the ribs that function to pull the ribs together.

internal obliques Deep muscles of the abdomen that act as synergists in trunk flexion.

linea alba White fibrous structure that extends from superior to inferior in the abdomen.

protracting Extension of a part of the body.

rectus abdominis One of the abdominal muscles located in the center of the abdomen.

symphysis pubis Cartilaginous joint that joins the left and right superior rami of the pubic bone.

transversus abdominis Deepest abdominal muscle with fibers running anterior to posterior that act to stabilize the trunk.

xiphoid process Most inferior portion of the sternum just below the body of the sternum.

MUSCLES OF THE CHEST AND ABDOMEN (SEE FIGURES 5-56 AND 5-57)

Muscles of the Chest

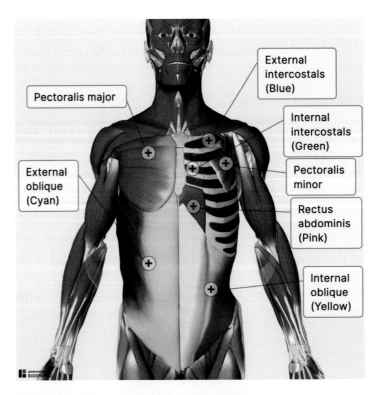

FIGURE 5-56 Muscles of the chest and abdomen.

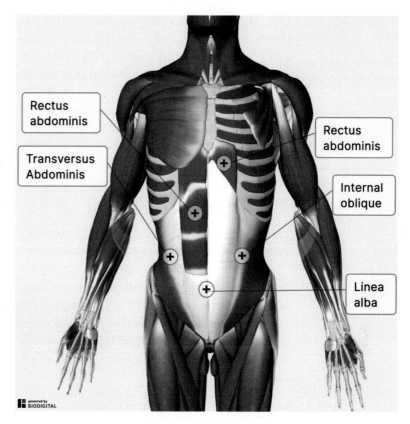

Rectus
abdominis

Transversus
Abdominis

Rectus
abdominis

Internal
oblique

Linea
alba

FIGURE 5-57 Deep muscles of the abdomen.

The muscles of the chest include the **internal intercostals**, **external intercostals**, and **diaphragm** (see Table 5-11).

The external and internal intercostal muscles assist with breathing. The external intercostals attach to the inferior portions of ribs 1–11 and extend to the superior portions of each lower rib. These muscles work to expand the thoracic cavity during inhalation by elevating and **protracting** (spreading) the

Table 5-11 Muscles of the Chest

MUSCLE	ORIGIN	INSERTION	ACTION
internal intercostals	Inferior border of ribs as far back as posterior angles	Superior border of ribs below, passing obliquely downward and backward	Elevates ribs
external intercostals	Inferior border of ribs as far back as posterior angles	Superior border of ribs below, passing obliquely downward and backward	Elevates ribs
diaphragm	Lumbar vertebrae, lower six ribs, posterior portion of xiphoid process of sternum	Central tendon	Expands thoracic cavity

ribs. The internal intercostals attach to the superior portions of ribs 1–12 and the sternum and extend to the inferior portions of each lower rib. These muscles work to elevate the rib cage during inhalation. During exhalation, the internal intercostals work to compress the thoracic cavity by depressing and retracting the ribs.

The diaphragm is the primary muscle of inhalation. It expands the thoracic cavity by contracting and pulling downward. The diaphragm attaches to the sternum, ribs, and lumbar vertebrae and extends to the central tendon of the diaphragm.

Muscles of the Abdomen

The muscles of the abdomen include the **rectus abdominis**, **external obliques**, **internal obliques**, and **transversus abdominis** (see Table 5-12).

The contents of the abdomen are protected by a band of muscles. There are three layers of abdominal muscles that include four muscles. The first layer consists of the rectus abdominus, which lies in the anterior and medial aspect of the abdomen and the external oblique, which is located on the sides of the abdomen. The second layer consists of the internal obliques, which lie deep to the external obliques, and the third layer consists of the transverse abdominus.

Some of the abdominal muscles attach to a broad dense band of connective tissue known as the **linea alba**. The linea alba extends from the **xiphoid process** to the **symphysis pubis**.

The abdominal muscles aid in trunk flexion. They also compress the contents of the abdominal cavity, increase intra-abdominal pressure, and help to transmit force through the trunk to protect the spine and contents of the abdominal cavity.

Table 5-12 Muscles of the Abdomen

MUSCLE	ORIGIN	INSERTION	ACTION
rectus abdominis	Pubic crest and pubic symphysis	Ribs 5–7 and xiphoid process	Flexes trunk
internal oblique	Lumbodorsal fascia	Lower four ribs	Flexes and rotates trunk
external oblique	Lower eight ribs	Iliac crest and linea alba	Flexes and rotates at waist
transverse abdominis	Iliac crest, cartilages of lowest ribs	Linea alba and pubic crest	Compresses abdominal wall

UNIT OBJECTIVE 5.7

Describe common pathologies affecting skeletal muscle.

UNIT INTRODUCTION

Like any of the tissues of the body, muscle tissue can be affected by disease or injury. Some injuries occur from trauma to muscle tissue whereas others are genetic in origin. This unit examines some of the more common pathologies affecting skeletal muscle.

LEARNING OBJECTIVE 5.7.1 **Identify common disorders affecting skeletal muscle tissue.**

KEY TERMS

electrolyte imbalance Abnormalities of concentration of electrolytes such as sodium, potassium, and calcium.

involuntary contraction Muscle contraction produced without volition or intention.

myalgia Muscle pain.

myositis Inflammation of muscle tissue.

COMMON SKELETAL MUSCLE DISORDERS

Muscle Strain

Muscle strains involve a partial or complete tearing of muscle fibers. Muscle strains are commonly called muscle pulls and are caused by muscles exposed to forces greater than they can handle. Muscle strains can cause inflammation and muscle pain (**myalgia**). Muscle strains can be graded as first-, second-, and third-degree strains.

In first-degree strains, a few muscle fibers are torn, resulting in pain, tightness, or cramping. The torn muscle can usually perform a full range of motion in first-degree strains. Second-degree strains are characterized by tearing of more muscle fibers with potential bruising and limited range of motion. Third-degree strains are characterized by a complete tear of the muscle and will exhibit severe pain, swelling, and loss of motion.

Muscle Cramps

Muscle cramps are characterized by a continuous, **involuntary contraction** of a muscle that results in pain. Cramps can occur from a variety of causes, including fluid and **electrolyte imbalance** such as dehydration or potassium imbalances in the blood. Other causes include poor circulation and accumulation of lactic acid from exercise. Some medications such as diuretics used to treat hypertension can produce muscle cramps.

CLINICAL TIP	Muscle cramps can be a sign of dehydration.

Myositis

Myositis is an inflammation of muscle tissue. Myositis can have many causes, including autoimmune disorders; genetics; viruses such as colds, flu, and polio; and medications. In some cases, diseases that produce inflammation of other body tissues also affect muscles. Examples of these include autoimmune disorders such as polymyositis, dermatomyositis, lupus erythematosus, rheumatoid arthritis, and scleroderma. These autoimmune disorders produce antibodies that attack muscle tissue, causing inflammation. Medications that can cause myositis include statins used for lowering cholesterol, colchicine, which is used to treat gout; alcohol; and hydroxychloroquine, which is used to treat malaria in tropical climates. Symptoms of myositis include muscle weakness, pain, and fatigue.

LEARNING OBJECTIVE 5.7.2 Describe the signs, symptoms, and diagnosis of muscular dystrophy.

KEY TERMS

Becker MD Type of muscular dystrophy characterized by low levels of dystrophin protein in muscle cells.

creatine kinase Enzyme found in muscle tissue that is released into the blood when muscles become damaged.

Duchenne MD Most common type of muscular dystrophy affecting young boys between the ages of 3 and 5 years old characterized by the absence of the muscle dystrophin protein.

dystrophin Type of structural protein in muscle tissue that helps to provide strength to muscle fibers.

electromyography Medical test measuring the electrical activity in muscle and nerve tissues.

Facioscapulohumeral MD Form of muscular dystrophy in teenage boys that affects the muscles of the shoulder, chest, face, arms, and legs.

muscular dystrophy Genetic disorder that includes several variants, with Duchenne muscular dystrophy being the most common form; characterized by the lack of the muscle protein dystrophin, which results in muscle weakness.

myotonic MD Type of muscular dystrophy that can affect adults, causing muscle spasms, heart problems, endocrine problems, and cataracts.

swanlike neck Long, thin neck resulting from a form of muscular dystrophy called myotonic MD.

waddling gait Type of shuffling gait exhibited by people suffering from muscular dystrophy.

MUSCULAR DYSTROPHY

Muscular Dystrophy (MD) is not one disease but consists of a group of more than 30 genetic diseases. MD primarily affects skeletal muscles and causes progressive weakness and degeneration. MD is usually seen in early childhood but can also affect adults. The degree and rate of dysfunction varies with the type of MD.

The most common form of MD is called **Duchenne MD**, which primarily affects young boys between 3 and 5 years old (see Figure 5-58). Duchenne MD is caused by the absence of the protein **dystrophin**. Dystrophin is a structural muscle protein that helps to maintain the strength of the muscle fiber. MD tends to progress so that patients will be wheelchair-bound by age 12 and will eventually need to be placed on a ventilator. Until recently, children with Duchenne MD did not survive beyond about 12 years. At present, with recent medical advances, life expectancy has reached to adulthood and middle age, with some patients living into their 50s.

Becker MD is less severe than Duchenne MD and is characterized by faulty or lower levels of dystrophin. Other forms of MD include **facioscapulohumeral MD**, which affects teenage boys, is less severe, progresses slowly, and is limited to affecting the muscles of the shoulder, chest, face, arms, and legs. **Myotonic MD** affects adults and causes muscle spasms, cardiac problems, cataracts, and endocrine problems. Myotonic MD produces a characteristic thin, long face; **swanlike neck**; and drooping eyelids.

Signs and symptoms of MD include muscle weakness such as difficulty in standing up, running, jumping, and speech. Patients with MD can develop a **waddling gait**. With Duchenne MD, the symptoms may progress so that the patient will be unable to walk, swallow, or breath.

A number of tests can help to diagnose MD. These include **electromyography** to measure muscle function, enzyme testing for elevation of the **creatine kinase** enzyme indicating muscle damage, genetic testing looking for gene mutations that can cause MD, and muscle biopsy examining dystrophin.

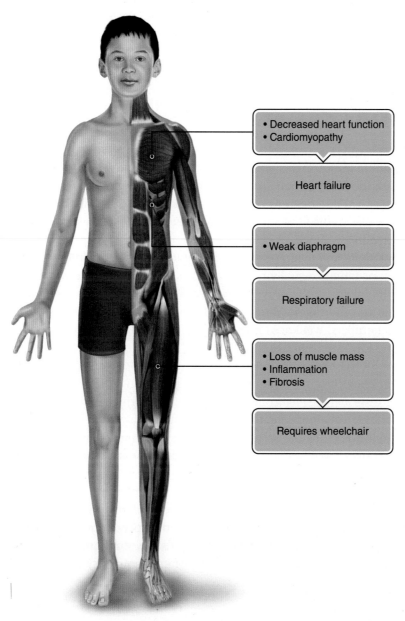

- Decreased heart function
- Cardiomyopathy

Heart failure

- Weak diaphragm

Respiratory failure

- Loss of muscle mass
- Inflammation
- Fibrosis

Requires wheelchair

FIGURE 5-58 Duchenne's muscular dystrophy is most common in boys.

LEARNING OBJECTIVE 5.7.3 Describe the signs, symptoms, and diagnosis of myasthenia gravis.

MYASTHENIA GRAVIS

Myasthenia gravis (MG) is a neurological disease that affects the acetylcholine receptors in muscle tissue. MG is an autoimmune disorder in which antibodies destroy or block the acetylcholine receptors at the motor end plate in muscle tissue. MG causes varying degrees of muscle weakness and usually begins by affecting the muscles of the eyes and then progresses to the muscles of the face and muscles used in swallowing.

The initial signs and symptoms of MG include muscle weakness in the absence of pain or fatigue, usually beginning with eye muscles. The weakness gets worse with activity and improves with rest. The weakness can then progress and extend to other skeletal muscles of the neck and jaw. MG can also present with generalized weakness involving the face and neck and spreading to the upper and lower extremities.

Diagnosis of MG begins with a physical and neurological examination. The doctor will check eye movement, reflexes, sensation, coordination, and strength. Other tests include electromyography (EMG) in which repeated stimulation causes muscle weakness and an edrophonium test in which injections of edrophonium chloride block the breakdown of acetylcholine, resulting in more acetylcholine at the neuromuscular junction. The edrophonium test temporarily relieves the symptoms of MG.

Patients with MG may present with an enlarged or tumorous thymus gland. In some cases, computed tomography (CT) can identify abnormalities of the thymus. The thymus gland may be involved in producing antibodies that block the acetylcholine receptors in muscle tissue. Pulmonary function testing can also be performed to indicate whether respiratory failure may occur.

UNIT OBJECTIVE 5.8

Describe common pathologies affecting how muscles respond to stimulation.

UNIT INTRODUCTION

Some pathologies affect how muscles respond to stimulation from the nervous system. These diseases can affect motor neurons or the neuromuscular junction. This unit examines pathologies affecting the link between the nervous system and muscles.

LEARNING OBJECTIVE 5.8.1 Identify common disorders affecting muscle stimulation and response.

KEY TERMS

amyotrophic lateral sclerosis A chronic, progressive neurological disease that affects the motor neurons of the brain and spinal cord. Also known as Lou Gehrig's disease.

anterior horn Anterior portions of the gray matter of the spinal cord.

antibodies Immune system proteins produced in response to a specific antigen that non-self cells for destruction.

cranial nerves Sensory and motor neurons that primarily control and detect stimuli of the head and neck but do not arise from the spinal cord.

Lambert-Eaton syndrome Autoimmune disease in which antibodies attack the neuromuscular junction.

DISORDERS AFFECTING MUSCLE STIMULATION AND RESPONSE

Disorders affecting muscle stimulation and response include **amyotrophic lateral sclerosis** and **Lambert-Eaton syndrome**.

Amyotrophic lateral sclerosis (ALS) is a motor neuron disease of unknown cause that affects motor neurons in the **anterior horn** of the spinal cord and the nuclei of **cranial nerves**. It affects adults between 40 and 60 years old and has a survival range of 3–5 years.

ALS affects the function of motor neurons causing them to degenerate, resulting in loss of voluntary motor function that can eventually affect the ability to move, speak, eat, and breathe. Loss of breathing begins with loss of function of the accessory muscles of respiration with eventual degeneration of the phrenic nerves to the diaphragm. Loss of motor input to the diaphragm results in atrophy of diaphragm skeletal muscle tissue and loss of function.

Lambert-Eaton syndrome (LEMS) is an autoimmune disease in which antibodies attack the neuromuscular junction, specifically the calcium channels that affect release of the neurotransmitter acetylcholine. LEMS causes weakness in the extremities and can affect muscles of the mouth and throat involved in talking, swallowing, and chewing. LEMS can result from the body's production of antibodies in response to certain types of lung cancer.

LEARNING OBJECTIVE 5.8.2 Describe the signs, symptoms, and diagnosis of tetanus.

KEY TERMS

Clostridium tetani Bacterium that produces the tetanus toxin.

hypertension High blood pressure as indicated by a systolic pressure greater than 130/80 mm Hg.

lockjaw Result of the disease tetanus in which the muscles of the jaw contract.

opisthotonos Type of severe tetanic contraction that occurs from untreated tetanus in which the back muscles spasm and bend into extension.

serum antitoxin blood test Medical test used to diagnose tetanus.

tachycardia Heart rate greater than 100 beats per minute.

tetanospasmin toxin Toxin produced by the bacterium *Clostridium tetani* that produces tetanus.

tetanus Muscular disorder characterized by muscle spasms resulting from the tetanospasm toxin produced by the bacterium *Clostridium tetani*.

trismus Spasm of the jaw muscles, commonly referred to as lockjaw, that results from tetanus.

TETANUS

Tetanus is an infection caused by the bacterium Clostridium tetani and is sometimes referred to as "lockjaw." Tetanus is characterized by muscle spasms beginning in the jaw (trismus) and progressing to other muscles of the body including the face, back, and extremities (see Figure 5-59AB). The spasms begin periodically and increase in intensity and frequency. Patients with generalized tetanus can exhibit an arched-back posture from back muscle spasms called opisthotonos. Facial muscles can be affected and can produce a sardonic smile (risus sardonicus) and spasms of the muscles of mastication. The muscle spasms are painful and can be severe enough to fracture bones. Tetanus can also produce an elevated heart rate (tachycardia), fever, hypertension, and sweating.

The tetanus bacteria are usually found in soil, dust, and feces and can enter the body through a cut or wound. The incubation period for the bacteria is 3–14 days. The bacteria produce the tetanospasmin toxin that blocks signals from the nervous system to muscles at the neuromuscular junction.

Diagnosis of tetanus includes a physical examination and history of immunizations and wounds. Doctors will check for muscle spasms, particularly in the jaw and face; fever; hypertension; and tachycardia. A serum antitoxin blood test may be performed.

Patients with tetanus will be treated with antibiotics along with a tetanus antitoxin. Other medications affecting contraction of involuntary muscles for breathing and the heart, such as beta-adrenergic antagonists (beta blockers), may also be used.

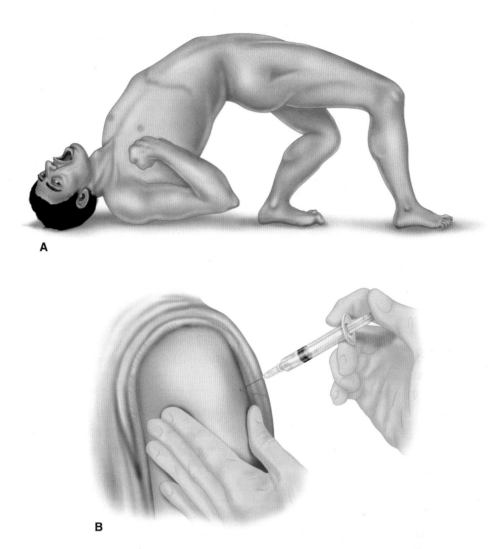

A

B

FIGURE 5-59AB Tetanus causes powerful back spasms called opisthotonos.

| **CLINICAL TIP** | The tetanus vaccine (Tdap) is given during childhood, with booster vaccines recommended every 10 years during adulthood. |

LEARNING OBJECTIVE **5.8.3** **Describe how botulinum toxin affects neuromuscular signal transmission.**

KEY TERMS

alpha motor neurons Large motor neurons of the brainstem and spinal cord that extend to skeletal muscle.

Botulinum toxin Substance produced from the bacterium *Clostridium botulinum* that paralyzes muscles.

Clostridium botulinum Bacterium that produces the botulinum toxin.

hyperhidrosis Condition in which patient experiences excessive sweating.

neuralgia Nerve pain.

BOTULINUM TOXIN

Botulinum toxin is a poisonous substance produced by the bacterium **Clostridium botulinum**. Botulinum toxin produces the condition known as botulism, which is a potentially fatal disease. Botulism causes muscle paralysis that usually begins in the muscles supplied by the cranial nerves, causing double vision, problems with chewing and swallowing, and flaccidity of the facial muscles. The disease then spreads to the extremities, chest, and abdomen, affecting both skeletal and smooth muscle tissue. Patients with botulism will experience progressive muscle paralysis that can eventually affect the respiratory muscles, causing loss of gas exchange and respiratory function.

Botulism toxin can also be used as a treatment for muscular disorders that produce muscle spasm such as headaches, **hyperhidrosis** (excessive sweating), overactive bladder, teeth grinding, **neuralgia**, eye twitching, and overactive bladder. The toxin is also used for cosmetic treatments involving treating muscles that cause wrinkles.

Botulinum toxin affects the neuromuscular junction by blocking the secretion of acetylcholine from **alpha motor neurons**, resulting in the inhibition of muscle contraction. The toxin takes 24–72 hours to elicit an effect lasting up to 8–12 weeks.

CLINICAL TIP	Botox injections are used in cosmetic procedures to reduce facial wrinkles, especially around the forehead and eyes. Physicians will inject multiple sites on each side of the forehead and eyes. The amount of toxin injected paralyzes the muscles that cause wrinkles.

UNIT OBJECTIVE 5.9

Describe common pathologies affecting smooth muscle.

UNIT INTRODUCTION

Although less common than skeletal muscle disorders, smooth muscle disorders can produce serious effects on the viscera of the body. This unit examines some pathologies affecting smooth muscle.

LEARNING OBJECTIVE 5.9.1   Identify common disorders affecting smooth muscle tissue.

KEY TERMS

alimentary canal The long muscular tube of the digestive system that transports ingested materials from the mouth to anus; site of mechanical and chemical digestion.

hypotonic bladder Loss of smooth muscle tone in the urinary bladder.

hypoperistalsis Wavelike smooth muscle contraction that is weaker than normal.

multisystemic smooth muscle dysfunction syndrome Disorder affecting smooth muscle throughout the body.

SMOOTH MUSCLE DISORDERS

Multisystemic smooth muscle dysfunction syndrome affects smooth muscle throughout the body and can result in abnormal responses to light by the pupils, blood vessel constriction problems, **hypotonic bladder**, and **hypoperistalsis** of the **alimentary canal**, which affects food digestion. This syndrome is a genetic condition caused by a rare gene mutation. Multisystemic smooth muscle dysfunction syndrome has no cure, and treatment is provided for the effects of the disease.

Dysphagia, or difficulty swallowing, can result from abnormal functioning of the smooth muscles involved in swallowing.

LEARNING OBJECTIVE 5.9.2 Describe the signs, symptoms, and diagnosis of dysphagia.

KEY TERMS

barium contrast Thick solution of barium sulfate used to enhance x-ray images, particularly of the digestive tract.

congestive heart failure Type of heart disease characterized by damage to heart muscle resulting in the inability of the heart to pump blood.

dysphagia Inability to swallow normally.

endoscopy Medical procedure incorporating the use of a device called an endoscope for visualizing internal anatomical structures.

esophageal dysphagia Type of swallowing abnormality that affects the esophagus.

esophageal sphincter Sphincters that close the esophagus when food is not being swallowed; the upper esophageal sphincter surrounds the upper part of the esophagus, and the lower esophageal sphincter surrounds the lower part of the esophagus at the junction between the esophagus and stomach.

oropharyngeal dysphagia Type of swallowing disorder affecting the smooth muscles of the oropharynx.

Dysphagia

Dysphagia, or difficulty in swallowing, comes in two types. Oropharyngeal dysphagia results from neuromuscular dysfunction affecting the pharyngeal and upper esophageal smooth muscles. Since cranial nerves send impulses to these muscles, this type of dysphagia often results from damage to the brain or cranial nerves. Esophageal dysphagia can result from inflammation of the esophageal lining from gastric reflux, esophageal tumors, tumors in the thoracic cavity, an enlarged heart from congestive heart failure, and neuromuscular disorders involving the nerves and esophageal muscles (see Figure 5-60).

The primary sign and symptom of dysphagia is the feeling that swallowed substances do not move from the esophagus to the stomach. Other signs and symptoms include choking, coughing, and aspiration pneumonia, which occurs from substances moving into the respiratory tract. Patients with dysphagia may also exhibit a hoarse or husky voice and substances may lodge in the esophagus, requiring endoscopy to remove them.

Diagnosis of dysphagia begins with a history to help to determine whether oropharyngeal or esophageal dysphagia is present. A swallowing function test

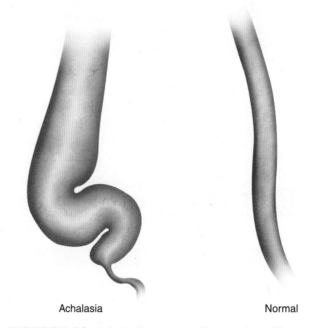

Achalasia   Normal

FIGURE 5-60 Achalasia is a rare disease that affects
the ability of the esophageal muscles
to contract, which results in difficulty
swallowing, or dysphagia. This x-ray
shows a patient with achalasia who
suffers from dysphagia.

may be performed in which foods of varying consistency and containing **barium
contrast** are given to the patient. The patient's attempts to swallow the foods are
monitored by x-ray and help to determine whether the foods can pass through
the upper **esophageal sphincter.**

Nasal endoscopy can be employed to stimulate the back of the throat with
air to test muscle response. **Endoscopy** of the esophagus can also be used to
inspect the esophageal lining and biopsy samples taken. Imaging including CT
or MRI can be used if tumors of the brain and neck are present. Dysphagia is
a common finding in brain tumor patients, especially those with tumors in the
more inferior portions of the brain and brainstem, which contain nerves that
control and coordinate swallowing.

UNIT OBJECTIVE 5.10

Describe common pathologies affecting cardiac muscle.

UNIT INTRODUCTION

Disorder of cardiac muscle can range from the production of abnormal heart
beats to complete failure of the heart. This unit examines some of the common
pathologies affecting cardiac muscle.

LEARNING OBJECTIVE 5.10.1 Identify common disorders affecting cardiac muscle tissue.

arrhythmias Abnormal heart rhythms.

cardiomyopathy Disease characterized by damage to heart muscle tissue.

ischemic heart disease Disease of heart tissue resulting from a lack of blood flow to heart muscle.

nodal tissue Tissue capable of producing action potentials.

CARDIAC MUSCLE DISORDERS

Common disorders affecting cardiac muscle include **cardiomyopathy**, **arrhythmias**, and **ischemic heart disease**.

Cardiomyopathy is a condition characterized by diseased cardiac muscle that affects its function. Arrhythmias are abnormal heartbeats that can be caused by damage to the **nodal tissue** or conduction pathways found in cardiac muscle. Arrhythmias can range from abnormally slow or fast heart rates to more serious abnormalities that result in the inability of the heart to move blood. Some arrhythmias can be severe enough to cause death.

In ischemic heart disease, cardiac muscle becomes damaged by poor blood flow. Ischemic heart disease can cause extensive damage to heart muscle, resulting in a condition known as congestive heart failure in which the heart loses its capability to pump blood.

LEARNING OBJECTIVE 5.10.2 Describe the signs, symptoms, and diagnosis of cardiomyopathy.

KEY TERMS

angina Chest pain occurring from ischemia of heart muscle.

arrhythmogenic right-ventricular dysplasia Type of cardiomyopathy that occurs in the right ventricle and causes arrhythmias.

BNP B-type natriuretic peptide; produced by the heart and tends to rise with heart damage.

cardiomyopathy Disease characterized by damage to heart muscle tissue.

congenital heart disease Form of heart disease that is inherited.

coronary artery disease Narrowing of the inner lumen of coronary arteries usually from atherosclerotic plaquing.

CT Computed tomography. Imaging study in which x-rays are used to produce a three-dimensional image.

Dilated cardiomyopathy Type of heart disease in which the ventricles become enlarged and are unable to adequately move blood.

ECG Electrocardiogram; test that measures electrical impulses generated by the heart.

echocardiogram Imaging test using highfrequency sound waves (ultrasound).

edema Localized area of excess fluid.

heart valve disease Disease affecting one or more of the four valves of the heart.

hypertension High blood pressure as indicated by a systolic pressure greater than 130/80 mm Hg.

hypertrophic cardiomyopathy Type of heart disease characterized by thickening of the muscular walls of the heart.

palpitations Heartbeats that are fast, strong, or irregular that can be felt.

restrictive cardiomyopathy Type of cardiomyopathy characterized by stiffness of the heart's muscular walls.

Cardiomyopathy

Cardiomyopathy is characterized by genetic or nongenetic diseased cardiac muscle. In cardiomyopathy there is no underlying **coronary artery disease**, **hypertension**, **heart valve disease**, or **congenital heart disease**.

There are several types of cardiomyopathy, including:

- **Hypertrophic cardiomyopathy** is a genetic disorder associated with the sudden death of athletes and fit adults (see Figure 5-61).
- **Dilated cardiomyopathy** is a condition that can result from genetic or nongenetic causes such as viral myocarditis, alcoholism, and nutritional deficiencies (Figure 5-61). This condition is often associated with other genetic disorders such as Duchenne and Becker muscular dystrophies.
- **Restrictive cardiomyopathy** is characterized by stiffness of cardiac muscle and can affect filling of the chambers of the heart.
- **Arrhythmogenic right-ventricular dysplasia** (ARVD) is a type of cardiomyopathy that usually affects young adults and is characterized by replacement of normal cardiac muscle in the right ventricle with scar tissue.

Symptoms of cardiomyopathy include shortness of breath, **palpitations**, fatigue, chest pain (**angina**), and **edema** from fluid retention.

Diagnosis of cardiomyopathy usually begins with a physical examination and testing. Tests can include:

- Chest x-ray to look for an enlarged heart.
- **ECG** (electrocardiogram), which measures electrical activity of the heart to detect abnormal heart rhythms.
- **Echocardiogram**, which uses images produced by ultrasound to examine the heart valves.
- Cardiac muscle biopsy performed by using a catheter to examine the quality of heart muscle.
- Stress test involving a treadmill to monitor heart rhythm, blood pressure, and breathing during physical exertion.
- Computed tomography (**CT**) scans of the heart to help determine abnormalities of heart structures.
- Blood testing including a B-type natriuretic peptide (**BNP**) test. BNP is produced by the heart and tends to rise with heart damage.
- Genetic testing to determine whether there is a genetic component to the cardiomyopathy.

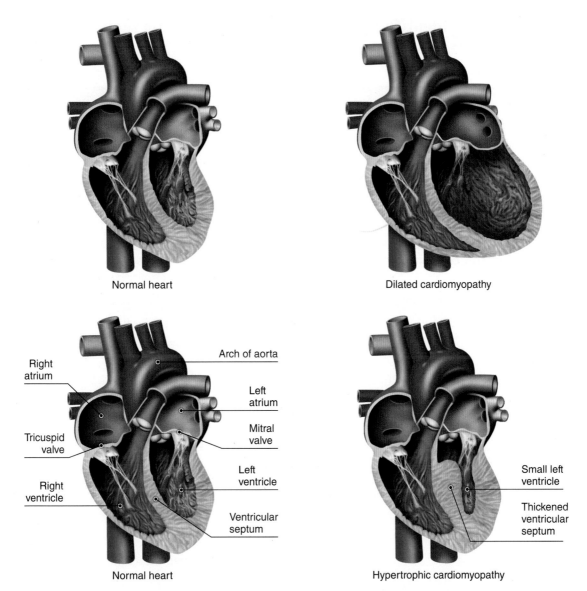

Normal heart

Dilated cardiomyopathy

Normal heart

Hypertrophic cardiomyopathy

FIGURE 5-61 Dilated versus hypertrophic cardiomyopathy. In dilated cardiomyopathy, the main pumping chamber of the heart (left ventricle) becomes enlarged, which decreases the ability of the heart to pump blood. In hypertrophic cardiomyopathy, the walls of the left ventricle become thickened, causing stiffness and decreased ability to pump blood.

UNIT OBJECTIVE 5.11

Describe common pathologies affecting individual muscles, muscle groups, and movement.

UNIT INTRODUCTION

Sometimes, muscles become injured. Muscle injuries can result when forces applied to muscles exceed their abilities to handle it. Other injuries occur from diseases that affect muscle tissue. This unit examines common pathologies affecting muscles.

LEARNING OBJECTIVE 5.11.1　Identify common pathologies affecting skeletal muscles, muscle groups, and movement.

KEY TERMS

acupuncture Healing modality characterized by the insertion of needles or manipulation of points along lines known as meridians running throughout the body.

anticonvulsants Drug used to prevent brain seizures from epilepsy or other brain disorders.

antidepressants Drug used to prevent depression and other brain disorders including anxiety, pain, and addictions.

chiropractic Healing modality characterized by manipulation of joints and soft tissues of the body.

cognitive-behavioral therapy Type of psychotherapy that works to change negative behaviors.

duloxetine Antidepressant medication used to treat nerve pain, depression, and anxiety.

fascia Band of connective tissue that separates or surrounds anatomical structures.

fibromyalgia Diffuse pain syndrome extending throughout the body and producing sleep disturbances and cognitive problems along with muscle pain.

golfer's elbow Also known as medial epicondylitis and characterized by inflammation of the wrist flexor tendons near their insertion at the medial epicondyle of the humerus bone.

jumper's knee Disorder characterized by inflammation of the patellar tendon usually caused by jumping.

milnacipran Medication used to treat fibromyalgia and nerve pain and functioning as a selective serotonin and norepinephrine reuptake inhibitor.

multidisciplinary approach Treatment approach characterized by a combination of different healing modalities.

myofascial pain syndrome Muscular pain syndrome characterized by the presence of painful areas called trigger points in muscle tissue.

palpation Act of examining by touching.

pitcher's shoulder Type of shoulder tendinitis that occurs from throwing a ball.

pregabalin Medication used to treat fibromyalgia.

spray and stretch Type of therapy used to treat muscles in which a coolant is sprayed on a muscle just before manually stretching it.

swimmer's shoulder Syndrome of the shoulder resulting from the action of swimming causing overuse of the muscles, tendons, and bursae of the shoulder.

tennis elbow Tendinitis of the wrist extensor tendons near their attachment at the lateral epicondyle of the humerus; also known as lateral epicondylitis.

trigger points Localized, painful areas in muscles that refer pain to other areas of the body.

trigger point injection Medical procedure in which a medication such as a steroid or anesthetic is injected into a trigger point.

PATHOLOGIES AFFECTING MUSCLES
Fibromyalgia

Fibromyalgia is a chronic widespread pain syndrome that produces painful, tender areas throughout the body. The cause of fibromyalgia is unknown and may result from a combination of genetic and environmental factors. Patients with fibromyalgia experience pain in multiple areas of the body, fatigue, sleep disturbances, increased sensitivity to pain, and cognitive problems. Fibromyalgia occurs more in women than in men and is often associated with anxiety and depression. Stress often exacerbates symptoms of fibromyalgia. There is no cure, but a **multidisciplinary approach** to treatment may provide the best effect. Treatments including aerobic exercise, **cognitive-behavioral therapy**, physical therapy, and medications, along with complementary therapies such as **chiropractic**, **acupuncture**, and herbal and nutritional supplements. Medications approved by the Food and Drug Administration for the treatment of fibromyalgia include the **antidepressants duloxetine** and **milnacipran** and **pregabalin**, an antiseizure medication.

Myofascial Pain Syndrome

Myofascial pain syndrome (MPS) is a chronic disorder characterized by multiple tender points in muscle or **fascia** called **trigger points**. Deep **palpation** of trigger points causes pain referral to other areas of the body. Patients with MPS can also experience muscle soreness and stiffness, sleep disturbances, muscle weakness, and increased pain with stretching muscles. Diagnosis of MPS relies on the presence of trigger points as stimulated through deep palpation by a physician. Treatments include medications (muscle relaxants, nonsteroidal anti-inflammatories, analgesics, antidepressants, **anticonvulsants**, and Botox injections), dry needling of trigger points, **trigger point injections**, physical therapy, massage therapy, and a neuromuscular technique called **spray and stretch**.

Tendonitis

Tendonitis can occur in any of the tendons in the body and is characterized by chronic inflammation usually located near the point where the tendon attaches to bone. Some common names for tendonitis include **golfer's elbow**, **tennis elbow**, **pitcher's shoulder**, **jumper's knee**, and **swimmer's shoulder**. Tendonitis can occur from a single strenuous event, overuse, or inflammatory arthritis. Symptoms of tendonitis include localized pain and swelling. Treatment includes anti-inflammatory medication, physical therapy, and surgery for more severe cases.

Rotator Cuff Injuries

Rotator cuff injuries consist of strains of the rotator cuff muscles of the shoulder. The most commonly injured muscle is the supraspinatus muscle, which tends to impinge on the surrounding bony structures. Treatment in the early stages includes anti-inflammatories, physical therapy, and stretching. Surgery to reattach the tendon may be necessary for more severe injuries.

LEARNING OBJECTIVE 5.11.2 Explain how a tear of the patellar tendon affects the patella's physical location and movement of the entire leg.

KEY TERMS

patella alta X-ray sign in which the patella is located in a superior position resulting from rupture of the patellar ligament.

patellar tendon Dense connective tissue structure that anchors the distal patella to the tibial tuberosity of the tibia.

quadriceps Group of four muscles on the anterior thigh that includes the rectus femoris, vastus medialis, vastus lateralis, and vastus intermedius.

Patellar Tendon Tear

The patellar tendon anchors the distal patella to the tibia at the tibial tuberosity and biomechanically works with the quadriceps muscles of the thigh. Complete rupture of the patellar tendon usually occurs from a fall or jumping and would cause the patella to migrate to a superior position, causing an increased distance between the tibial tuberosity and lower margin of the patella. This can be seen on x-ray and is referred to as patella alta (Figure 5-62). Patients with this injury would experience problems with performing leg extension and have difficulty bearing weight on the affected leg such as in standing.

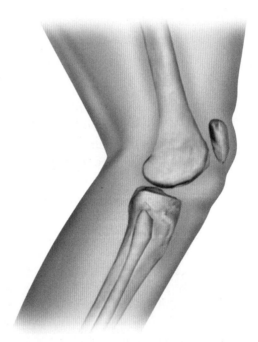

FIGURE 5-62 X-ray showing patella alta. Notice the patella is in a more superior position than normal.

Chapter 6

Nervous System

Chapter Introduction

The human nervous system is a complex body system that incorporates many unique cell types and organ structures to regulate and control the body. In this chapter, we discuss the overall organization of the nervous system, including the types of cells and how those cells work together. We also discuss the basic functional properties of neurons and the regions of the brain and spinal cord. Special attention is paid to the sensory systems as well as disorders of the nervous system.

UNIT OBJECTIVE 6.1

Describe the general functions of the nervous system.

UNIT INTRODUCTION

Imagine a world without any form of communication. Everything and everybody working independently; each doing all jobs necessary for survival. Finding food, building shelter, protection from predation, and many other tasks would need to be performed by every individual. Society allows for specialization of jobs, and communication makes sure we balance the needs of the society. Your body is a society of organs working together for collective survival. The nervous system is one way (the other being via hormones) the body can regulate each organ to maintain balance in society—to maintain body homeostasis.

LEARNING OBJECTIVE 6.1.1 Identify the different functions of the nervous system.

THE ROLE OF THE NERVOUS SYSTEM

Our body's organs depend on each other to ensure our survival. The nervous system integrates the current state of the body and coordinates organ function. In addition, the nervous system allows us to interact with the outside world. Our senses bring in information about light, touch, and sound, for example, which is then processed in the brain. Exploring the effect of neurological disorders will demonstrate the importance of the nervous system in how we experience the world. But the nervous system also determines how we then influence the

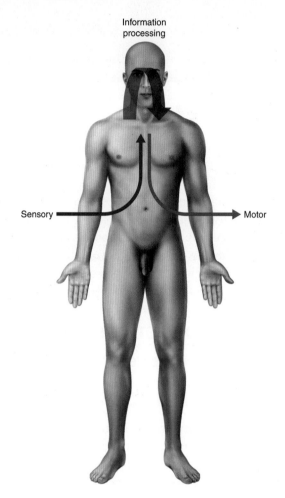

FIGURE 6-1 Sensory input, motor output, and neuron processing are the three functions of the nervous system.

world—controlling our muscles and behaviors. Thus, the nervous system can be broken down into having three broad functions (Figure 6-1):

1. taking in information from the outside world (and inner body),
2. processing information, and
3. causing action (via muscles or organs/glands)

LEARNING OBJECTIVE 6.1.2 Identify the two general classes of cells found in the nervous system.

KEY TERMS

glia Support cells of the nervous system that directly and indirectly help all neurons to function properly.

neurons Cells found in nervous tissue that detect stimuli, process information, and transmit electrical impulses from one area of the body to another.

NERVOUS SYSTEM BASICS

As we discuss the nervous system in this chapter, keep in mind that all the amazing abilities are through two types of cells: neurons and glia (Figure 6-2). **Neurons**, or nerve cells, are cells of the nervous system specialized for rapidly communicating information over long distances. We see that in addition to their speed, another advantage neurons have is the ability to target individual cells. This allows you to move one finger at a time and identify the precise location someone touches your hand without seeing. **Glia**, or glial cells, are support cells in the nervous system. They help supply nutrients to neurons, make neurons more efficient, and can even directly alter neuron communication.

The nervous system can be broken up into three functions based on how neurons connect (Figure 6-1). Neurons in the sensory system are activated by something other than a neuron. This may be light or sound or may be the current state of an organ. Neurons in the motor system output onto something other than a neuron. This may lead to contraction of muscle or changing the function of an organ. All other neurons in the nervous system communicate only with other neurons.

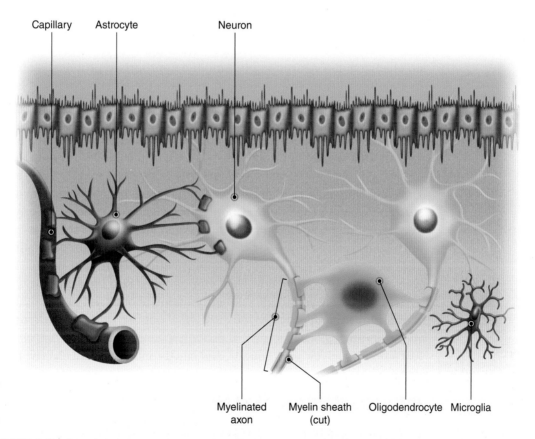

FIGURE 6-2 The nervous system is composed of neurons, specialized for long-distance communication, and glia, a collection of nervous system cells that supports the function of neurons.

LEARNING
OBJECTIVE **6.1.3** List the functions of sensory receptors.

LEARNING
OBJECTIVE **6.1.4** Explain how the nervous system responds to stimuli.

KEY TERMS

motor system Division of the nervous system involved in stimulating muscle contraction or regulating organ function.

sensory receptors Specialized proteins that change a sensory stimulus and convert it into a neuronal signal.

sensory system Division of the nervous system involved in detecting stimuli from outside.

SENSORY INPUT

Various parts of our body, such as the eyes, ears, and skin, are able to detect stimuli in our surrounding world. This is due to specialized sensory receptors that exist in each part. These receptors detect and convert environmental stimuli, such as light or temperature, into a language that neurons can understand (discussed in Unit 6.9). Shining a flashlight onto most neurons will cause no change, but a neuron expressing the appropriate proteins is able to alter its function in response to light. In this way, the world around us is merely a representation made by what our sensory receptors are capable of detecting.

In addition to requiring information about the world around us, our body also needs to know information about the world inside us—our organs. Despite the fact that we are not consciously aware of our blood pressure, electrolyte levels, and other important vital signs, our body is constantly monitoring them and constantly making changes to keep them in a normal range. Imagine being sick and going to the doctor. Upon your arrival, someone will likely measure your heart rate, respiration rate, and oxygen levels. If the doctor is concerned, lab testing, such as blood sugar and electrolyte levels, might be required. These vital signs provide the doctor with information about your health. Your body also cares about your health. This information is also measured by the sensory system, providing your body with information about itself just as other parts of the sensory system provides information about the world around you. Sensory receptors are regions of a cell that contain specialized proteins that change physical stimuli, such as light, sounds, and smells, into neuronal electrical activity.

NEURON PROCESSING

An overly simplistic perspective is to break down the nervous system into inputs, outputs, and everything in between. But the processing that goes on between sensory input and motor output is what makes human cognition different from other animals. When neurons communicate with other neurons, they do not do so in a one-to-one fashion. As many as 10,000 neurons may work together to activate a single neuron. And that single neuron will influence as many as 10,000 different neurons. It is the neuron's ability to simultaneously integrate so many inputs and affect so many outputs that allows for complex cognitive abilities such as language and thought.

SKELETAL MUSCLE, ORGAN, AND GLAND REGULATION

The opposite of sensory input is the output onto skeletal muscle, organs, and glands. Neurons in the motor system control our behavior by receiving input from other neurons and ending on muscles or organs. It is through the motor system that we participate in the world; the motor system influences the outside world (by muscle contraction) and the inside world (by altering organ function).

UNIT OBJECTIVE 6.2

Describe the cells of the nervous system and their function.

UNIT INTRODUCTION

The basic unit of life is a cell. There are two major cell types that make up the nervous system, neurons and glial cells. In this unit we discuss the parts of neurons that aid in their functions and are introduced to the various types of glial cells and the role each plays in support of neuron function.

LEARNING OBJECTIVE 6.2.1 Identify the parts of a neuron.

LEARNING OBJECTIVE 6.2.2 Describe the function of the dendrite, soma, axon, myelin, nodes of Ranvier, and axon terminal bud.

KEY TERMS

axon Sing, long extension of the cell membrane of a neuron; carries outgoing signals to other cells.

axon terminal buds Specialized region of the neuron that releases neurotransmitters and serves as the output zone.

dendrites Specialized regions of the neuron that have neurotransmitter receptors and serve as the input zone.

myelin Wrapping of glial cell membrane around an axon that acts to speed up conduction of action potentials.

neuron Cells found in nervous tissue that detect stimuli, process information, and transmit electrical impulses from one area of the body to another.

nodes of Ranvier Small spaces in between areas of myelination on an axon; nerve impulse jumps from node to node.

soma Cell body of a neuron containing the nucleus and other cell organelles.

synapse Specialized site of communication between the axon terminal bud of one neuron and a receptor found on another neuron, gland, or muscle.

NEURONS ARE SPECIALIZED TO COMMUNICATE

Any cell in our body that performs a particular task will optimize its shape and function to best perform that task. In oral communication between two people, one person speaks using their mouth and another listens using their ears. A **neuron** (Figure 6-3AB) also specializes its parts, with an area optimized for receiving information from another cell (listening), another area optimized for sending information to another cell (speaking), and a third area for passing information between the two areas within the same neuron.

The Soma

The **soma** of a neuron is the cell body of the neuron. This is the part of the neuron that contains the parts of a prototypic cell. The main organelles, such as the nucleus, endoplasmic reticulum, and mitochondria are in this region. While neurons cannot divide to form new neurons, a neuron requires constant production of new proteins. The nucleus contains the genetic information with the instructions for their production. A neuron has only one soma, with a single axon coming off it at one end and typically numerous dendrites attached to the other end.

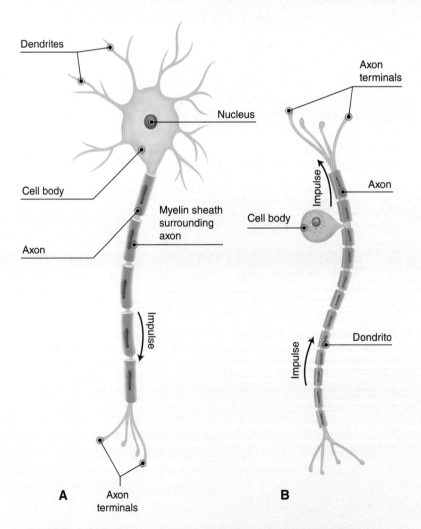

FIGURE 6-3AB Every neuron has the same basic parts: a soma, dendrites, axon terminal buds, and an axon.

The Dendrites

The **dendrites** are parts of the neuron specialized for receiving information. They are highly branched to allow thousands of other neurons to simultaneously interact with a single neuron's dendrites. This connection, termed a *synapse*, uses chemicals to transmit information between the two cells. The dendrites contain large numbers of receptors capable of binding to these chemicals, which influences the function of the neuron. The dendrites consolidate the inputs onto the neuron's soma before sending a single signal down the axon.

The Axon

As opposed to the numerous dendrites, each neuron only has a single **axon** attached to the soma. This extension allows for rapid transmission of information within a single neuron across great distances in the body. The longest neurons in the body are in the sciatic nerve, which reaches from the base of the spine to the tip of the toes. This distance is mostly spanned by the axon.

Axons use an electrical signal, termed an action potential, to rapidly transmit information from one end of the neuron to the other. Proteins that modify the electrical properties of the neuron are found in the axon to generate the action potential. Many neurons have a layer of insulation, or **myelin**, surrounding the axon that improves the efficiency of electrical communication. The myelin is composed of oligodendrocytes or Schwann cells, which wrap their cell membranes around the axon. There are regular spaces in the myelin, termed **nodes of Ranvier**, that allow the neuron cell membrane to interact with the extracellular fluid (Figure 6-4ABC).

The Axon Terminal Buds

Although a neuron has a single axon taking information to a single area of the body, that neuron may influence the functions of thousands of other cells in the region. Axons end in **axon terminal buds**. An axon terminal bud joins with a dendrite of another cell to make a synapse. We often think of neurons making synapses with other neurons, but they also synapse with glands and organs. Chemicals released from axon terminal buds of one neuron can bind to receptors on the dendrites of another neuron. In this way, the neuron uses the axon terminal buds to speak to other cells.

The Synapse

Neurons are cells specialized for communication. The axon transmits information within a neuron. But a **synapse** is the site of communication between two (or more) neurons and often other structures such as glands, muscles, and other organs. A typical synapse involves the chemicals released from an axon terminal bud activating receptors on the dendrites of another neuron.

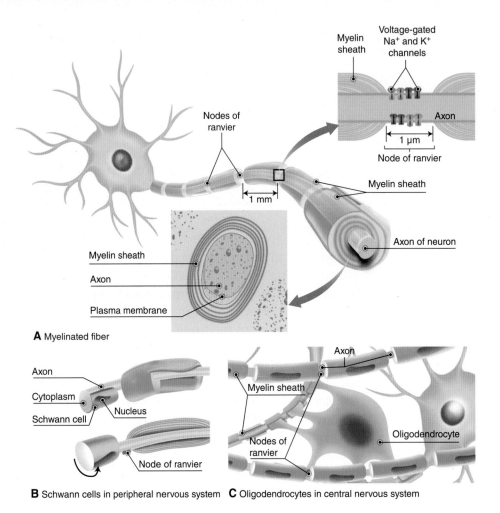

A Myelinated fiber

B Schwann cells in peripheral nervous system   C Oligodendrocytes in central nervous system

FIGURE 6-4ABC Nodes of Ranvier are gaps in the glial wrapping. Action potentials occur here.

LEARNING OBJECTIVE 6.2.3 Describe the relationship between myelination, the nodes of Ranvier, and the speed of signal conduction.

THE EFFECT OF MYELIN

As we discussed, myelin is a layer of glial cell membrane wrapped around the axon cell membrane with regular gaps known as nodes of Ranvier. But, not all axons in the body are wrapped in myelin. These differences relate to the function of the neurons. Axons use an electrical signal to transmit information. Myelinated axons, because of the effectively thicker cell membrane formed by the layers of myelin, retain the electrical signal within the neuron, similar to how a coat improves your own ability to retain body heat on a cold day. This makes body heat difficult to dissipate away from your body. Action potentials occur at each node and then spread down the axon in all directions. A small portion of this charge can be lost across an axon's cell membrane out of the neuron. Axons with myelin are better able to keep the charge inside. The main result is the signaling down myelinated axons is up to 200 times faster than unmyelinated axons. For example, the axons of neurons that encode burning pain do not have myelin and transmit action potentials more slowly than the quick, sharp pain encoded by fully myelinated pain neurons.

LEARNING OBJECTIVE 6.2.4 Identify gray matter in the central nervous system.

LEARNING OBJECTIVE 6.2.5 Describe the structure and structural characteristics of gray matter.

LEARNING OBJECTIVE 6.2.6 Describe the function of gray matter.

GRAY MATTER

Continuing the analogy from the previous section, as we travel along the highway we have not accomplished our goal—we have not visited our family. The **gray matter** of the brain and spinal cord contains synapses and cell bodies of neurons. This is where the dendrites of one neuron can communicate with the axon terminal buds of another (or typically many other) neuron(s). The gray matter represents the goal of traveling, which is visiting our family. It is in the gray matter that neurons actually communicate with one another. Despite traveling alongside another neuron, no communication between neurons is occurring in the white matter between axons.

The gray matter forms the internal butterfly-shaped structure of the spinal cord and the outer rim of the brain. In the spinal cord, these regions are the dorsal gray horn and the ventral gray horn. Damage to these areas will cause a disruption in signaling for the nerves entering and leaving the spinal cord to various body parts. In the brain, the outermost rim has the gray matter and is the site of connections between neurons. The gray matter is where the cell bodies, or soma, are located. The processing that occurs in these regions depends on the information being encoded by the neurons making connections.

LEARNING OBJECTIVE 6.2.7 Identify white matter in the central nervous system.

LEARNING OBJECTIVE 6.2.8 Describe the structure and structural characteristics of white matter.

LEARNING OBJECTIVE 6.2.9 Describe the function of white matter.

WHITE MATTER

Neurons are specialized for communication in two ways. The dendrites of one neuron and the axon terminal buds of another neuron contain special proteins to transmit information between them at the synapse. The axon of a single neuron contains other proteins that create an electrical signal to move rapidly from one region of the body to another within a single cell. In synchrony with these functions, the nervous system is organized such that synapses tend to be in the same region and axon pathways tend to aggregate together as they travel between regions of the body. In the brain and spinal cord (which together are the central nervous system), we can visually distinguish these areas by their colors (Figure 6-5). **White matter** consists of brain and spinal cord regions primarily containing axons and almost devoid of synapses. The areas are white due to the high

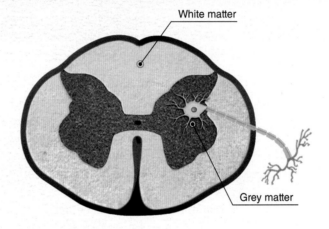

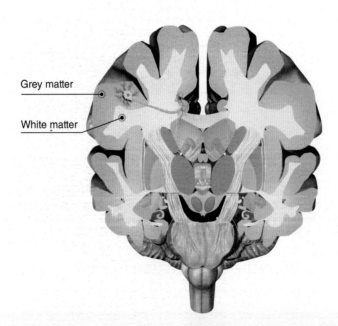

FIGURE 6-5 White matter and gray matter are distinct in the nervous system. Note that the white matter is internal and the gray matter is toward the outside of the brain, whereas the gray matter is internal and the white matter is toward the outside of the spinal cord.

fat content found in the glial cell membranes that make up the myelin covering the axons. Gray matter consists of brain and spinal cord regions primarily containing synapses between neurons. This area is darker in color because it lacks myelin.

When traveling to different body regions, our neurons will group together. Think of traveling several hundred miles by automobile to visit a family member. You will likely start your journey using large highways alongside of others who are moving in the same general location (north, for example), even if not ultimately heading to the same final destination. As you get closer to your family, you will leave the larger highway. The highway can be thought of as axon pathways. Axons originating, for example, from a lower region of the spinal cord to the brain will eventually be grouped with neurons from a higher region on their shared journey toward the brain. These axons become grouped together because they have the same overall destination (the brain) despite their specific final destination being different (as they represent different body parts). This analogy holds true as axons travel between distant areas of the brain as well.

The outer regions of the spinal cord contain white matter. Axons are grouped together based on the type of information they are encoding as well as their destination. White matter pathways can be broadly classified as ascending, sending information to the brain, or descending, information leaving the brain. In the brain, however, white matter is found in the more internal regions. White matter in the brain can be connecting different brain regions or containing information entering from or leaving the spinal cord.

LEARNING OBJECTIVE 6.2.10 Contrast the structure and function of gray matter and white matter.

COMPARING WHITE MATTER AND GRAY MATTER

If we look closely at Figure 6-5, the locations of white and gray matter in the brain and spinal cord are different. In the brain, the gray matter forms an outer layer and the white matter is at the center. However, in the spinal cord, white matter is the outer layer and gray matter is at the center. Despite the anatomical differences, the properties of each area remain the same. In the spinal cord, the gray matter is the site of processing for spinal reflexes. The patellar reflex, for example, is initiated by striking the patellar ligament, causing it and the quadriceps muscle to stretch. A sensory neuron detects this stretch and sends a signal into the spinal cord. That neuron then makes a direct connection in the gray matter onto a motor neuron, which contracts the quadriceps to compensate for the stretch. Other neurons in the gray matter are also activated by that sensory neuron. They send that information up to the brain (in white matter). It is those signals that allow you to feel the tap of the hammer striking the tendon. In the brain, white matter pathways end in gray matter in the outer regions. Again, this is the site of connection between neurons, where processing and thinking can occur.

LEARNING OBJECTIVE 6.2.11 Identify the following types of neuroglia in the CNS: oligodendrocytes, microglia, astrocytes, and ependymal cells.

LEARNING OBJECTIVE 6.2.12 Describe the function of each type of neuroglia found in the CNS.

GLIAL CELLS

Due to their larger size and easily measured electrical properties, for decades neuroscientists focused much of their work on neurons. As a result, the "other" cells of the nervous system were lumped together as glial cells (or glia) simply because they were not neurons. There are numerous types and subtypes of glial cells, some of which share common developmental origins and others are less related. In this section, we discuss the primary glial cells of the central nervous system and their respective roles in supporting neuron function.

Glia of the Central Nervous System

The central nervous system (CNS), consisting of the brain and spinal cord, is a very sensitive system. Thus, it is provided with many protections such as limited access by the blood and specialized circulation regulated by specialized glial cells. The main glial cells in the CNS are the astrocytes, ependymal cells, microglia, and oligodendrocytes (Figure 6-6). These cells participate in a variety of functions that support and protect the CNS neurons.

Astrocytes Astrocytes are the most numerous glial cell in the brain and are named because of their star-like shape. These glial cells found only in the CNS perform numerous important functions. One such function involves feeding neurons. The brain is a metabolically demanding organ, using an estimated 20% of the body's daily calorie intake. Thus, it is highly vascularized, with blood vessels pervasive throughout the brain. However, unlike other body regions, the capillaries in the brain do not easily empty their contents in the surroundings as a method of protection. To regulate access to the brain, astrocytes act as an intermediate for all contents of the blood; in order to reach a brain neuron, the blood contents (such as glucose, oxygen, or a drug) must first enter an astrocyte and then be shuttled into the neuron. This is one reason treating brain diseases is very difficult. In addition to finding an effective medication, one must formulate it in a way that the astrocytes will deliver it to the neurons.

Astrocytes also modify neuron function by altering chemical communication at the synapse. In addition to dendrites and axon terminal buds, astrocytes extend processes (typically across many synapses) that can alter the communication at each synapse. They can respond to neurotransmitters released by axons, alter the activity of those neurotransmitters, and even release their own neurotransmitters. By changing the chemicals present in the synapse, the astrocytes are modifying communication between neurons.

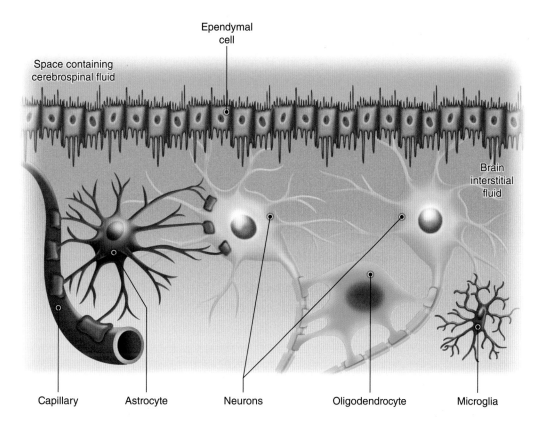

Space containing
cerebrospinal fluid

Ependymal
cell

Brain
interstitial
fluid

Capillary   Astrocyte   Neurons   Oligodendrocyte   Microglia

FIGURE 6-6 Astrocytes, ependymal cells, microglia, and oligodendrocytes are the glia found in the central nervous system.

Ependymal Cells As we discussed in an earlier section, the CNS creates a barrier to carefully regulate which blood components have access. Thus, an alternative CNS-specific circulatory system exists to replace the blood vessel–based circulation. Cerebral spinal fluid (CSF) is a fluid produced in the ventricles of the brain that surrounds the brain and spinal cord. It serves as the major waste collection system from cells in the CNS as well as provides a layer of protection around the brain to cushion from sudden head movements. The **ependymal cells** line the ventricles of the brain and central canal of the spinal cord. In the ventricle of the brain they filter blood plasma to produce the CSF, and in all regions of the CNS their highly ciliated membranes help to move the CSF.

Microglia Surrounding the brain is a thin protective barrier formed by astrocytes known as the blood–brain barrier. This barrier prevents blood cells (red blood cells, white blood cells, and platelets) and many other molecules from entering the brain tissue, which is extremely important. With the exception of the CNS, the human body is protected from disease by the white blood cells that make up the immune system. Since these cells cannot enter the brain tissue, the CNS needs its own "immune system," which is composed of microglia. **Microglia** are cells of the CNS that perform immune and protective functions. These small cells are constantly exploring the brain and spinal cord looking for damaged or infected tissues. Upon finding an area of concern, they become activated and initiate a response. This may be engulfing and digesting a foreign particulate that managed to gain access or by secreting chemicals to protect from damage or promote repair.

Oligodendrocytes Oligodendrocytes are the myelinating cells of the CNS. These cells wrap their cell membrane around the axon of a neuron in the brain or spinal cord. Before wrapping they squeeze the cytoplasm, nucleus, and other important organelles to one side of the cell so the myelin consists of mostly lipids and very little water. Though both oligodendrocytes and Schwann cells myelinate axons, the manner in which they do so differs. A single oligodendrocyte extends multiple processes, each wrapping around an axon. Thus, one oligodendrocyte will contact and myelinate multiple axons. This is different than Schwann cells, which only wrap their membrane around a single axon.

LEARNING OBJECTIVE	6.2.13	Identify the following types of neuroglia in the PNS: Schwann cells and satellite cells.
LEARNING OBJECTIVE	6.2.14	Describe the neuroglia found in the peripheral nervous system and each type's function.

KEY TERMS

satellite cells Glial cell of the PNS that supports the PNS neuron.

Schwann cells Specialized neuroglial cells that myelinate neurons outside of the brain and spinal cord.

Glia of the Peripheral Nervous System

The peripheral nervous system (PNS) consists of the nerves leaving the spinal cord and making connections with the organs, muscles, and sensory structures in the extremities. The PNS is not as sensitive as the CNS and has direct access to the blood supply. The glia in the PNS consist of Schwann cells and satellite cells (Figure 6-7).

Schwann Cells Named after the physiologist who discovered them, Schwann cells are the myelinating cells of the PNS. Like the oligodendrocytes in the CNS, the Schwann cells wrap their cell membrane around the axons of sensory and motor neurons of the PNS. The ability for PNS neurons to regenerate, which CNS neurons typically are unable, is thought to be related to Schwann cell function. Following injury to a nerve, the Schwann cells may aid in digestion of the axon. The myelin remains, forming a tube that the regenerating nerve uses for guidance.

Satellite Cells Satellite cells are non-myelinating glial cells of the PNS that are similar in function to the astrocytes of the CNS. These cells sit on top of the soma of PNS neurons to support and modify their function by supplying nutrients as well as releasing neuroactive chemicals. They also respond rapidly to nerve damage and participate in the pain response.

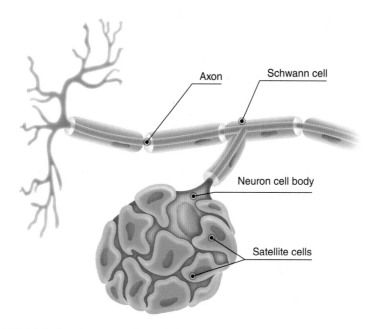

FIGURE 6-7 Schwann cells and satellite cells are the glia found in the peripheral nervous system.

LEARNING OBJECTIVE 6.2.15 Contrast the structure and functions of oligodendrocytes and Schwann cells.

Comparing Schwann Cells and Oligodendrocytes

Despite both oligodendrocytes and Schwann cells both being involved in myelinating axons, the manner in which they do is different. A single oligodendrocyte will extend multiple processes to myelinate many regions of up to 50 different neurons. A single Schwann cell, however, will wrap its entire cell membrane around a single region of an axon. Oligodendrocytes are only found in the CNS, while Schwann cells are only in the PNS. Both glial cell types impact the neurons they myelinate in the same way by increasing the speed of signaling.

UNIT OBJECTIVE 6.3

Describe the structural components of a synapse and the process of signal transduction.

UNIT INTRODUCTION

Neurons are specialized cells that communicate in two ways. First, an electrical signal is transmitted down an axon, within a single neuron, in the form of an action potential. We discuss later in this unit how this is mediated. Second, a neuron communicates with other cells by releasing chemicals at a synapse. We also discuss the composition of a synapse and the way in which activity there is regulated.

LEARNING OBJECTIVE 6.3.1 Identify synapses in the nervous system.

LEARNING OBJECTIVE 6.3.2 Identify presynaptic and post-synaptic neurons.

LEARNING OBJECTIVE 6.3.3 Describe the anatomy of a synapse.

KEY TERMS

neurotransmitter Molecule secreted by neurons that produces changes in other neurons or organs.

post-synaptic neuron Neuron at a synapse that has receptors on dendrites being activated by neurotransmitters.

presynaptic neuron Neuron at a synapse that releases neurotransmitters from the axon terminal buds.

SYNAPSES

As we have discussed in the previous section, neurons communicate with other cells at specialized junctions termed *synapses* (Figure 6-8A). Synapses are where axon terminal buds of one neuron abut the dendrites of another

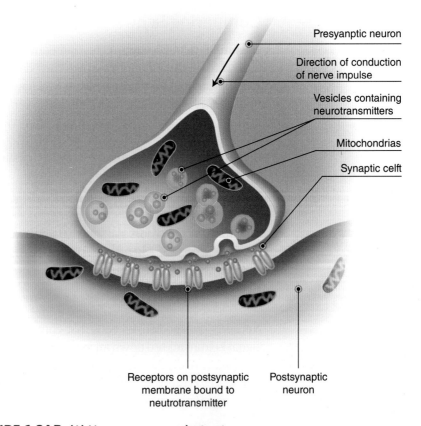

Presyanptic neuron

Direction of conduction of nerve impulse

Vesicles containing neurotransmitters

Mitochondrias

Synaptic celft

Receptors on postsynaptic membrane bound to neutrotransmitter

Postsynaptic neuron

FIGURE 6-8AB (A) Neurons communicate at synapses.

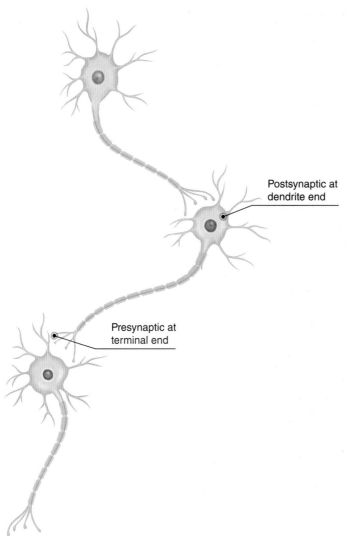

Postsynaptic at
dendrite end

Presynaptic at
terminal end

FIGURE 6-8 AB (B) One neuron can act as both a
presynaptic and post-synaptic neuron.

neuron (often with astrocytes mediating that signaling). This occurs most often in the gray matter of the brain and spinal cord, as well as where neurons terminate on muscles and other organs (with the difference being the organs do not have dendrites, as the target cells are not neurons). Axon terminal buds release chemicals, termed **neurotransmitters**, which act on receptor proteins embedded in the membrane of the dendrites. In this way, information is passed from a neuron to another neuron or receiving cell at the synapse.

The flow of information is unidirectional; axon terminal buds only release neurotransmitters (not respond to them) and dendrites only respond to neurotransmitters (and do not release them). Therefore, we can describe the structures of a neuron based on their relative positions. The neuron containing the axon terminal buds, on the releasing side of the synapse, is referred to as the **presynaptic neuron**. The neuron containing the dendrites, on the receiving side of the synapse, is referred to as the **post-synaptic neuron**. These terms, however, are relative to a synapse being discussed and not the neuron itself. A comparison can be made to the terms "greater than" and "less than" that are used when comparing numbers. Just as we cannot simply refer to 4 as being "less than," we cannot simply refer to a neuron as "presynaptic" (Figure 6-8B). The number 4 is both less than 5 but also greater than 3. Since neurons consist of both axon terminal buds and dendrites, a single neuron acts as both a presynaptic neuron and post-synaptic neuron. It functions as a post-synaptic partner at its dendrites and sends that information via the axon to the axon terminal buds, where it then acts as a presynaptic neuron when signaling the next neuron or cell.

LEARNING OBJECTIVE 6.3.4 Identify common neurotransmitters.

LEARNING OBJECTIVE 6.3.5 List common neurotransmitters of the central and peripheral nervous systems.

NEUROTRANSMITTERS

Neurons communicate with other cells using chemicals released from the axon terminal buds at synapses. These chemicals are collectively known as **neurotransmitters**. A neurotransmitter is a definition based on action—it specifically describes a chemical being released from the axon terminal buds at the synapse. Many chemicals that act as neurotransmitters can be released into the bloodstream from endocrine glands (hormones) or neurons (neurohormones). The target cells cannot differentiate the source of a chemical; thus, a cell responds identically when its receptors are activated by either a neurotransmitter or hormone. For example, when activated during exercise, the sympathetic nervous system will release the neurotransmitter epinephrine directly onto the heart (Figure 6-9). Receptors on heart muscle respond, causing an increase in heart rate. However, if you are startled suddenly, your adrenal gland will release the hormone epinephrine (also known as adrenaline) into the bloodstream. When epinephrine reaches the heart, the same receptors that were stimulated by the sympathetic nerve's neurotransmitter will also be activated by the hormone, causing the same increased heart rate. The heart cannot discriminate the source of the chemical.

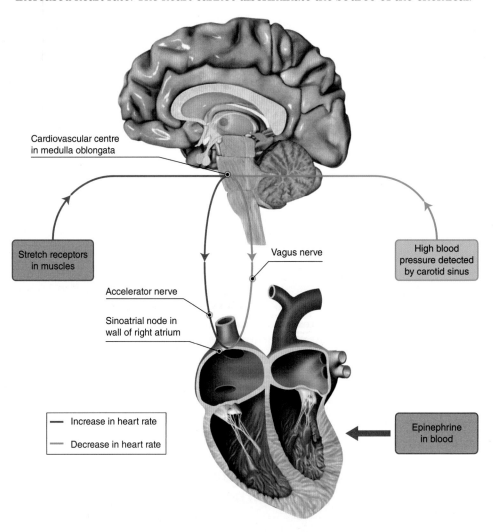

Cardiovascular centre in medulla oblongata

Stretch receptors in muscles

Vagus nerve

High blood pressure detected by carotid sinus

Accelerator nerve

Sinoatrial node in wall of right atrium

— Increase in heart rate
— Decrease in heart rate

Epinephrine in blood

FIGURE 6-9 The effect on a particular organ does not change based on the source of the chemical messenger.

Many different neurotransmitters are used in the central and peripheral nervous systems. They belong to a variety of chemical families, including protein, peptide, amino acid, nucleotide, gas, and others (Table 6-1). The main excitatory neurotransmitter in the adult central nervous system is glutamate. The main inhibitory

Table 6-1 There are a Variety of Types of Neurotransmitters Categorized Based on their Structure. Each Neurotransmitter has Several Receptors it Activates

CLASSES AND EXAMPLES OF NEUROTRANSMITTERS	CHEMICAL STRUCTURE	FUNCTIONS
Choline derivative		
Acetylcholine	Synthesized from choline and acetyl CoA	Major neurotransmitter in PNS*: released from motor nerves that supply skeletal muscle and from parasympathetic nerves that supply smooth muscle, cardiac muscle, and exocrine glands; also acts in CNS**
Biogenic amines (Monoamines)	Amines each derived from a single amino acid	
Norepinephrine	Made from tyrosine; is a catecholamine	Important neurotransmitter in PNS: released from sympathetic nerves that supply smooth muscle, cardiac muscle, and exocrine glands; also acts in CNS in pathways involved with memory, mood, emotions, behavior, sensory perception, sleep, and muscle movements
Dopamine	Made from tyrosine; is a catecholamine	Acts in CNS in many pathways similar to norepinephrine; especially important in "pleasure" pathways and muscle movements
Serotonin	Made from tryptophan; is an indoleamine	Acts in CNS in pathways involving mood, emotions, behavior, appetite, states of consciousness, and muscle movements
Amino acids	Are single amino acids	Most abundant neurotransmitters
Glutamate		Primary excitatory neurotransmitter in CNS; important in pathways involved with memory and learning
Gamma-aminobutyric acid (GABA)		Primary inhibitory neurotransmitter in brain; often acts in same circuits as glutamate
Glycine		Primary inhibitory neurotransmitter in spinal cord and brain stem

*PNS refers to the peripheral nervous system.
**CNS refers to the central nervous system.

neurotransmitter in the adult central nervous system is gamma-aminobutyric acid (GABA). Dopamine is a neurotransmitter often associated with reward (and drug abuse) but is also important in initiating movement and many other functions. Acetylcholine is a neurotransmitter used at the synapses between motor neurons and muscle. Serotonin is associated with mood and the sleep/wake cycle.

CLINICAL TIP	Mood disorders, including depression, bipolar disorder, and anxiety, are not completely understood but are thought to be caused by a dysregulation of serotonin and norepinephrine signaling in the brain. SSRIs and SNRIs are two classes of drugs that act by altering the activity of these neurotransmitters at the synapse. SSRIs (selective serotonin reuptake inhibitors) function by blocking the enzyme that removes serotonin from the synapse. Thus, the normal release of serotonin remains in the synapse longer, increasing its duration of action. SNRIs (serotonin-norepinephrine reuptake inhibitors) also block enzymes that remove neurotransmitters but act on those removing both serotonin and norepinephrine. The action of SNRIs causes released serotonin and norepinephrine to increase their effect on the synapse.

LEARNING OBJECTIVE 6.3.6 Explain how a signal is passed from a presynaptic neuron to a post-synaptic neuron across the synapse.

LEARNING OBJECTIVE 6.3.7 Explain the process of signal termination and how it relates to neurotransmitters present in the synapse.

KEY TERM

vesicles Spheres of cell membrane that contain a high concentration of neurotransmitters in preparation for their release at the synapse from the axon terminal bud.

SYNAPTIC SIGNAL TRANSMISSION AND TERMINATION

Action potentials are electrical signals that travel down the axon toward the axon terminal buds, which we discuss further in upcoming sections. When that electrical signal is detected by proteins in the axon terminal buds, a series of events is initiated resulting in the release of neurotransmitters into the synapse (Figure 6-10). Prior to this, the thousands of neurotransmitter molecules are packaged in small membrane spheres called **vesicles**. The vesicles are tethered extremely close to the cellular membrane of axon terminal buds. When an action potential enters the axon terminal bud, the vesicles fuse with the membrane of

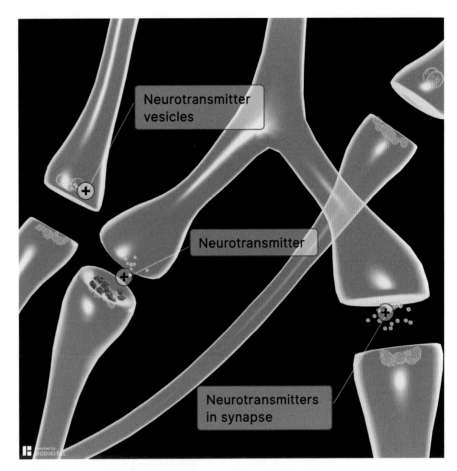

FIGURE 6-10 Neurotransmitters are packaged in vesicles, released from the axon terminal buds of the presynaptic neuron, and bind to receptors on the dendrites of the post-synaptic neuron.

the axon terminal buds, causing the inside of the vesicle to become continuous with the outside of the neuron. This allows for rapid dumping of thousands of neurotransmitter molecules.

Once in the space between two neurons, neurotransmitters spread via diffusion toward the post-synaptic cell. Protein receptors are embedded in the dendrites of the post-synaptic cell. Neurotransmitters, which bind to a receptor on the dendrites, cause a change in the intracellular signaling of the cell. A typical neuron will express a variety of different types of receptors, allowing it to respond to a variety of neurotransmitters. After binding a receptor, the neurotransmitter is typically released unaltered and capable of rebinding to the same receptor.

Neurotransmitter activity and the signal transmission across the synapse can be stopped in one of three ways (Figure 6-11). These three methods of signal termination include removing the neurotransmitter from the synapse, destroying the neurotransmitter, and the neurotransmitter diffusing out of the synapse.

- Removal of neurotransmitter from the synapse: Neurotransmitters can be actively removed from the synapse using pumps. Often these pumps are on the presynaptic neuron but are also found in astrocytes. The removed neurotransmitter is typically recycled as it makes its way back to the releasing neuron to be inserted into a new vesicle for future release.

- Destruction of the neurotransmitter: Neurotransmitters can be broken down by enzymes in the synapse. Because the interaction between neurotransmitters and their protein receptors is extremely specific, chemically altering a neurotransmitter prevents it from binding and ultimately its activity.

- Diffusion of neurotransmitter out of the synapse: Neurotransmitters can simply diffuse out of the synapse. As they are no longer in the area of receptors, they cannot activate them. It is worth noting that these categories are not mutually exclusive and the products of neurotransmitter breakdown often are taken back into presynaptic neurons for recycling or can diffuse out of a synapse.

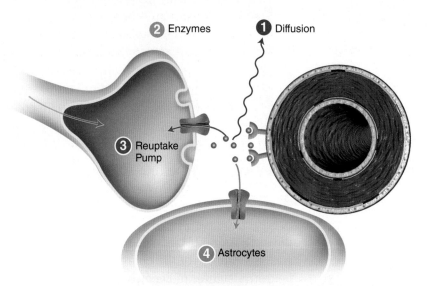

FIGURE 6-11 Neurotransmitters remain active so long as they are available to bind to receptors. Their function is stopped by either reuptake, diffusion out of the synapse, or enzymatic breakdown.

LEARNING OBJECTIVE 6.3.8 Define resting membrane potential.

LEARNING OBJECTIVE 6.3.9 Describe resting membrane potential.

LEARNING OBJECTIVE 6.3.10 Explain the role of electrolytes in the creation of the resting membrane potential.

electrolyte Minerals, typically salts, that carry a charge and are responsible for many essential processes in the body.

membrane potential Electrical charge of a membrane.

resting membrane potential Electrically polarized state of muscle and nerve cells during an bsence of stimulation.

RESTING MEMBRANE POTENTIAL

The cellular membrane of a neuron (and all cells) separate the inner and outer aqueous environments of the cell. The contents of most of the molecules, primarily proteins and **electrolytes**, have an electrical charge. In physics, the term *potential* describes the difference in energy between two regions. **Membrane potential** specifically describes the difference in charge across a cell's membrane. By convention, this is always the charge inside of the cell relative to the charge outside of the cell. **Resting membrane potential** is a description of this charge when the cell is not stimulated. A typical neuron has more positively charged sodium and negatively charged chloride outside of the cell and more positively charged potassium and negatively charged proteins inside the cell. There are ion channels in the membrane that are open even when the cell is inactive, or at rest. These ion channels are selective such that they only allow potassium to cross. Because there is more potassium inside the cell, that positively charged ion will tend to leave cells. As the positively charged potassium leaves, the inside of the membrane becomes more negative (as it just lost a positive charge) and the outside becomes more positive (because it just gained a positive charge). This results in the neuron resting membrane potential being negative.

LEARNING OBJECTIVE 6.3.11 **Define polarization, depolarization, hyperpolarization, and threshold.**

LEARNING OBJECTIVE 6.3.12 **Explain how electrolytes polarize a cell.**

CELL MEMBRANE POLARIZATION

The membranes of neurons have specialized proteins that, when triggered to open, selectively allow particular charged electrolytes to cross the membrane. The direction that the electrolyte flows (into or out of the cell) is dependent on the difference in the concentration gradient, moving from areas of high concentration to areas of low concentration. The resulting effect on the cell's membrane potential depends on both the direction of movement and the charge of the electrolyte. The membrane potential can be made more positive by positive electrolytes entering the cell and/or negatively charged electrolytes leaving the cell (Figure 6-12).

Depolarization

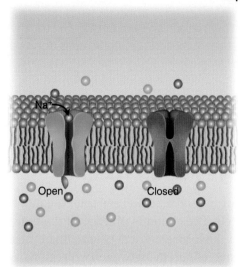 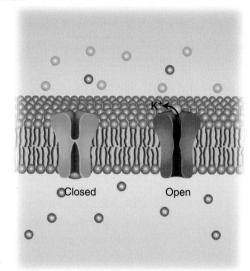

Repolarization

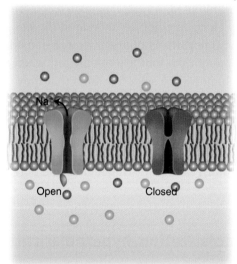 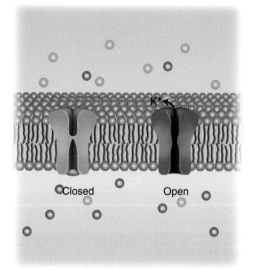

FIGURE 6-12 The direction of movement and charge of the ion determine the effect of an ion flowing across a cell membrane.

KEY TERMS

depolarization Change in voltage from a negative resting membrane potential toward a positive state from the movement of sodium ions inside of a cell.

hyperpolarization Changing the membrane potential of a neuron to make it more negative than at rest.

polarized Pertaining to a difference in electrical potential on either side of a membrane.

repolarization Phase of the action potential in which the neuron is returning back to its negative resting membrane potential.

threshold Voltage in muscle or nervous tissue that results in the generation of an action potential when reached.

Threshold

A neuron should not be constantly active—it must be triggered to fire an action potential. The membrane potential of the neuron is the main determinant of when a neuron fires an action potential. This is because proteins in the membrane change their state based on the membrane potential. When a particular membrane potential is reached, these proteins may open or close, altering the flow of particular ions. Different proteins have different membrane potentials. Threshold is the membrane potential at which action potentials are initiated in the axon of a neuron and is largely determined by the properties of the proteins that allow ions to cross.

Depolarization, Repolarization, and Hyperpolarization

The membrane potential of a neuron is altered to control its activity. Depolarization refers to when the membrane potential becomes more positive (or less negative; Figure 6-13). The membrane potential can be made more positive by both positive electrolytes entering the cell and by negatively charged electrolytes leaving the cell. A neuron undergoing depolarization is moving its membrane potential closer to threshold. This means that depolarization makes neurons more likely to fire an action potential. It is worth noting that the term *depolarization* is used for any positive change in membrane potential. After a negative membrane potential crosses zero, becoming positive, a change in membrane potential causing further positive change is still referred to as a depolarization.

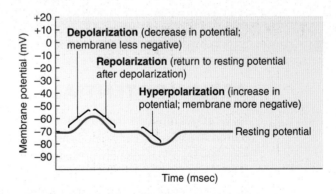

FIGURE 6-13 Depolarization, repolarization, and hyperpolarization.

Following an action potential, the nerve must return to baseline. Repolarization refers to the change in membrane potential after the depolarization phase of an action potential in which the membrane potential returns back to its resting value. In a typical neuron, this is a phase in which the membrane potential becomes increasingly negative, primarily due to the positively charged potassium ion leaving the neuron.

Hyperpolarization refers to when the membrane potential becomes more negative than the original resting membrane potential at the end of an action potential. The cell is becoming more polarized (*hyper*polarized). However, often the term *hyperpolarize* is used to refer to any negative change in membrane potential (regardless of its influence on the action potential). This can occur by negative ions entering the neuron or positive ions leaving the neuron. A hyperpolarized neuron's membrane potential is further from threshold, making it more difficult to fire an action potential. These terms (*depolarization, repolarization,* and *hyperpolarization*) are used because most cells have a negative resting membrane potential and are referred to as **polarized** due to this unequal distribution of charges across the membrane. A cell undergoing depolarization is reducing this difference in charge: making a negative membrane potential move toward zero (become more positive). Remember that by convention, we still refer to a neuron as being depolarized even if its already positive membrane potential becomes more positive. A cell at rest undergoing hyperpolarization, however, is increasing this difference in charge: making the negative membrane potential move away from zero (becoming more negative).

LEARNING OBJECTIVE 6.3.13 Define action potential.

LEARNING OBJECTIVE 6.3.14 List the events leading to the creation of an action potential.

KEY TERMS

action potential Rapid change in voltage generated by muscle and nervous tissue.

voltage-gate ion channels Proteins in the axon that open in response to a change in membrane potential and allow ions to cross the membrane once activated.

ACTION POTENTIAL

Neurons manipulate the electrical properties of their membranes for communication. We have already discussed how axon terminal buds respond to electrical changes by releasing neurotransmitters. This is mediated through proteins that detect changes in membrane potential. The axon contains proteins that respond to electrical stimuli, but to a different end. These proteins, known as **voltage-gated ion channels**, allow particular electrolytes to flow across the membrane and alter the membrane potential of a cell. The coordinated opening of these channels and the resulting electrical changes along the membrane results in an **action potential**, or electrical signal, which will travel down the neuron's axon and cause some type of action (Figure 6-14).

Action Potential Creation

Action potentials are electrical signals in neurons that are described as having an all-or-none response. Once initiated, an action potential will always go to completion. The action potential is driven by sequential opening of voltage-gated sodium and voltage-gated potassium channels. In addition, the term *all-or-none* means that each action potential in a neuron will be of uniform size and shape.

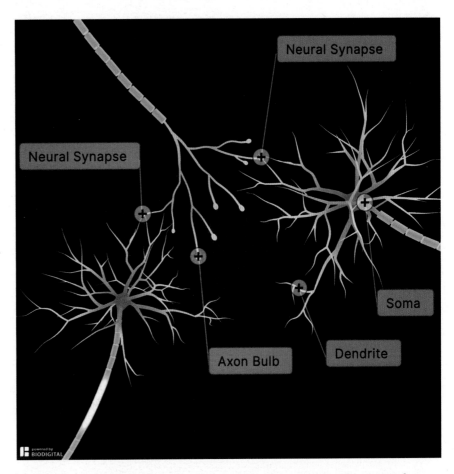

FIGURE 6-14 Neurons use action potentials to transmit information from the soma end of the axon to the axon terminal bud's end of the axon. Note that the release of neurotransmitters from that axon terminal buds is not depicted.

Most neurons use the same basic mechanism to generate an action potential (Figure 6-15):

1. When the membrane potential reaches threshold, the action potential is initiated.

2. The voltage-gated sodium channels open first, allowing sodium to enter the cell. Sodium has a positive charge, so when it enters the negative interior of the cell the result is depolarization of the cell membrane.

3. As more sodium enters, more voltage-gated sodium channels are opened due to the change in membrane potential. This causes a rapid rise in membrane potential.

4. The voltage-gated sodium channels close shortly after being triggered and the voltage-gated potassium channels open. Potassium also has a positive charge, but since it leaves the neuron it causes the opposite effect on charge as sodium entering, repolarizing the neuron.

5. The action potential drops below resting potential due to potassium leaving the axon, resulting in hyperpolarization.

6. As voltage-gated potassium closes, the membrane potential then drifts back to resting potential.

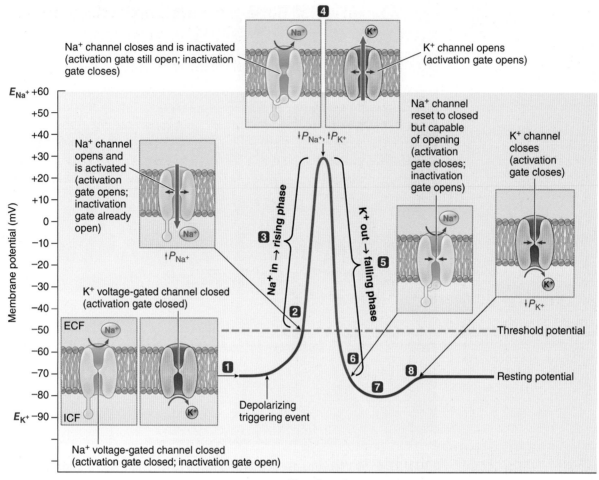

FIGURE 6-15 **Action potentials are local, transient changes in membrane potential.**

1 Resting potential: all voltage-gated channels closed.

2 At threshold, Na⁺ activation gate opens and P_{Na^+} rises.

3 Na⁺ enters cell, causing explosive depolarization to +30 mV, which generates rising phase of action potential.

4 At peak of action potential, Na⁺ inactivation gate closes and P_{Na^+} falls, ending net movement of Na⁺ into cell. At the same time, K⁺ activation gate opens and P_{K^+} rises.

5 K⁺ leaves cell, causing its repolarization to resting potential, which generates falling phase of action potential.

6 On return to resting potential, Na⁺ activation gate closes and inactivation gate opens, resetting channel to respond to another depolarizing triggering event.

7 Further outward movement of K⁺ through still-open K⁺ channel briefly hyperpolarizes membrane, which generates after hyperpolarization.

8 K⁺ activation gate closes, and membrane returns to resting potential.

LEARNING OBJECTIVE 6.3.15 **Explain how an action potential travels down the length of an axon.**

Action Potential Conduction

We discussed above that an action potential is a change in charge in a region of the membrane. However, that local charge can spread, or be conducted, down the axon. The action potential, once generated, propagates down the axon as a wave. When the positively charged sodium enters the axon during the first phase of the action potential, that charge can spread to the nearby negatively charged regions (Figure 6-16). The positive charge in these areas triggers new voltage-gated sodium channels to open, initiating a new action potential.

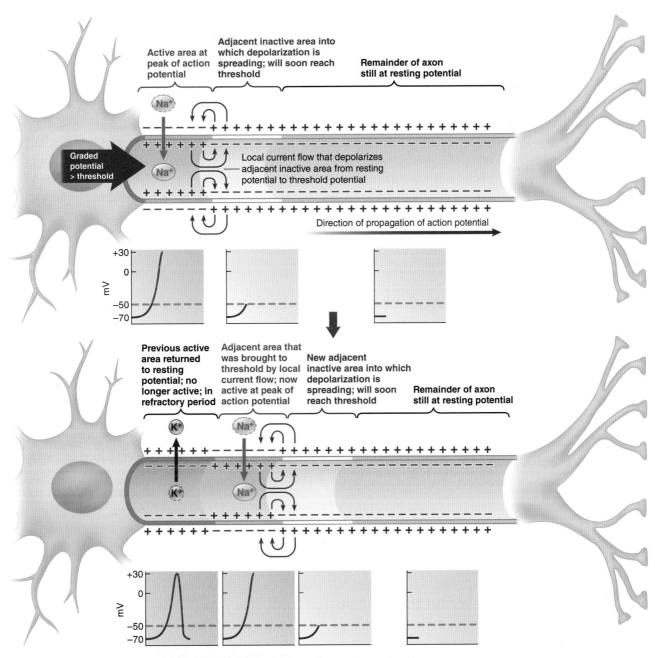

FIGURE 6-16 An action potential in the open region of the axon stimulates a new action potential in neighboring regions.

SIGNAL TRANSDUCTION

We discussed in the second unit that some, but not all, neurons have the cell membrane of specialized glial cells wrapped around the axons. These so-called myelinated axons hold electrical charge within the axon better than unmyelinated axons. Ultimately, the greater the extent of myelination (or the thickness), the faster the action potential is conducted down the axon.

Myelinated Fibers

The myelin on the axon acts in a similar way that the plastic insulation on electrical wires keeps the charge within the wire. You can hold a power cord (to a TV, computer, microwave, etc.) plugged into an outlet without risk of electrocution because the insulation keeps the charge inside the wire. The myelin surrounding the axon keeps the charge that is spreading within an axon during an action potential by making the charge more difficult to cross the membrane (because the myelin effectively thickens the axon membrane). Myelinated neurons concentrate their voltage-gated ion channels only at the gaps between the myelin (nodes of Ranvier). A fraction of the total number of voltage-gated channels can be used, resulting in far greater speed of the action potential spreading down the axon of a myelinated neuron. Thus, an action potential in a myelinated neuron is said to jump from node to node, as no ions are crossing the membrane at the points of the axon covered by myelin.

Unmyelinated Fibers

An unmyelinated axon, on the other hand, does not have as thick of a cell membrane. This results in more electrical charge being lost across the membrane. Unmyelinated axons have a large number of equally spaced, relatively close voltage-gated ion channels. Action potentials still occur as described but will need to be regenerated more often than in the more efficient myelinated axons. Because it takes significantly longer for ion channels to open than for electrical charge to spread within an axon, unmyelinated neurons conduct action potentials at a slower rate than myelinated axons because more voltage-gated channels are involved in the process.

excitatory neuron Presynaptic neuron that makes its post-synaptic partner more likely to fire an action potential.

inhibitory neuron Presynaptic neuron that makes its post-synaptic partner less likely to fire an action potential.

NEURONAL ABILITY TO EXCITE OR INHIBIT

Rather than connecting one-to-one, neurons typically have complex dendrites that make synapses with hundreds to thousands of neurons. This means that a single neuron may have as many as 10,000 inputs and 10,000 outputs. Often a single synaptic neuron is not capable of initiating an action potential in another neuron. It takes the coordinated activity of many presynaptic neurons to depolarize a neuron enough to trigger an action potential.

Not all presynaptic neurons will activate a neuron. In fact, rarely does a single neuron solely determine if an action potential will occur in a post-synaptic neuron. The decision to fire an action potential can be thought of as a community voting on a new law. Everyone can vote yes or no, and if a particular point is reached we will fire an action potential. A presynaptic neuron that votes yes for an action potential is considered excitatory. An **excitatory neuron** is a presynaptic neuron that depolarizes a post-synaptic neuron. Depolarization makes the neuron more likely to fire an action potential by bringing the membrane potential closer to threshold. A presynaptic neuron that votes no for an action potential is considered inhibitory. An **inhibitory neuron** is a presynaptic neuron that hyperpolarizes a post-synaptic neuron. Hyperpolarization makes the neuron less likely to fire an action potential by moving the membrane potential further from threshold.

LEARNING OBJECTIVE 6.3.21 Explain the effects of inhibitory and excitatory neurons on signal transmission.

COMPARING EXCITATORY NEURONS AND INHIBITORY NEURONS

An individual post-synaptic neuron receives constant inputs from many neurons, some of which are excitatory and others inhibitory. But an individual neuron has one potential response, an action potential. A neuron integrates (or brings together the effects) all the active synapses to determine if it will fire an action potential. As we discussed, this is determined by the membrane potential reaching threshold.

Imagine a bucket of water. Now imagine a hole placed in the bottom. The neuron integrates the effects of its inputs much in the same way a bucket of water finds level. The hole can be thought of as inhibitory inputs, lowering the water/membrane potential. Now let us add someone pouring water in the top of the bucket. Adding more water is the excitatory inputs, raising the water/membrane potential. The water does not need to "do" anything to find its level;

likewise, the neuron does not "do" anything to determine its membrane potential. As more water is added or removed, the water level changes in the bucket. The membrane potential is constantly being altered by both excitatory and inhibitory neurons. The neuron will fire an action potential when the membrane potential at the beginning of the axon is at or above threshold.

LEARNING OBJECTIVE 6.3.22 Identify the safety mechanism that prevents a post-synaptic neuron from being continuously stimulated.

POST-SYNAPTIC SAFETY MECHANISMS

All things in moderation—even neuron communication. In order for meaningful communication to take place between two neurons at a synapse, there must be periods of stimulation followed by periods without neurotransmitters. If a synapse was constantly flooded with neurotransmitters, the post-synaptic neuron would face two major problems. First, it would be overstimulated and perhaps exhaust the ion concentration gradients that allow it to function. Depletion of extracellular sodium will prevent any activity of that neuron. But, the neuron also needs to pause between stimulations in order to obtain meaningful information. If the neuron was constantly stimulated it would have no ability to be stimulated again the next time an event occurs. Safety mechanisms are in place to protect against this at the synapse. The enzymes which breakdown neurotransmitters and those that take neurotransmitters back into the synapse can be added to the membrane to increase the rate of clearance of the released neurotransmitters. The presynaptic neuron also has limited neurotransmitters available to be released. Prolonged stimulation of the presynaptic neuron will eventually deplete all potential neurotransmitters to be released. The post-synaptic neuron can also modify its response to prolonged stimulation by removing the neurotransmitter receptors from the membrane. This is one mechanism of the "hangover" effect following the use of drugs of abuse, such as cocaine. Prolonged stimulation of post-synaptic receptors leads to the receptors leaving the membrane. The following day, when the drug is no longer in the body, the presynaptic neuron may release a typical amount of neurotransmitter but the post-synaptic neuron has fewer receptors and responses less robustly.

UNIT OBJECTIVE 6.4

Describe the basic ways in which the nervous system processes information.

UNIT INTRODUCTION

While our brain is a complex organ capable of performing a variety of intricate calculations and behaviors, not all nervous system functions require complicated circuitry. In this unit we discuss how neurons connect with one another into simple circuits. These basic circuits allow for automatic behaviors but also provide simplified models of how neurons communicate with one another in any location.

**LEARNING
OBJECTIVE** 6.4.1 **Identify the components of a neural reflex arc.**

**LEARNING
OBJECTIVE** 6.4.2 **Explain how a neural reflex arc functions.**

KEY TERMS

reflex Involuntary behavior that is processed entirely in the spinal cord.

reflex arc Neurons that create the circuit that starts with a stimulus and ends with reflexive behavior.

NEURAL REFLEX ARC

It is easy to appreciate the brain and the functions it performs, but many vital functions for survival do not involve brain processing at all. A **reflex** is an involuntary behavior that is almost instantaneous in response to a stimulus. This allows for rapid automatic responses to certain stimuli, such as stepping on a sharp tack. A **reflex arc** describes the neurons that create a circuit that begins with the stimulus and ends with the behavior (Figure 6-17).

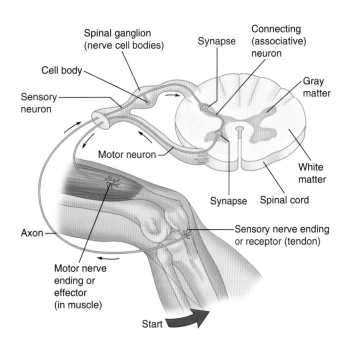

FIGURE 6-17 The simplest reflex consists of a single synapse in the spinal cord.

The simplest reflex arc starts with a sensory neuron being activated by the stimulus. The sensory neuron sends an action potential down its axon and makes a synapse onto a motor neuron. That motor neuron leaves the spinal cord to connect to a muscle or organ. Reflexes offer rapid responses to stimuli that can easily scale with size. A large stimulus will strongly activate a sensory neuron, which will lead to greater stimulation of the motor neuron and will release more neurotransmitters. Most reflexes, however, are not this simple. For example, when stepping on a sharp tack, one must lift the painful foot and simultaneously plant the other foot (to maintain stability). Interneurons are commonly used in reflex arcs to control more complicated responses to stimuli. Once initiated, normal locomotion, such as walking, is processed entirely in the lumbar region of the spinal cord. This complex behavior requires many sensory neurons and interneurons interacting.

LEARNING OBJECTIVE | 6.4.3 | **Identify common reflexes.**

KEY TERMS

crossed extensor reflex Reflex that involves the extension of one leg and the simultaneous retraction of the other.

Golgi tendon reflex Reflex which prevents the muscle from pulling so hard it separates from the bone.

Pupillary light reflex Reflex in which the pupil rapidly constricts in response to a bright light.

stretch reflex Reflex that maintains muscle at a constant length.

withdrawal reflex Reflex in which a limb is rapidly pulled away in response to a painful stimulus.

TYPES OF REFLEXES

While there are many specific examples of reflexes, most can be categorized into four types: stretch reflex, Golgi tendon reflex, crossed extensor reflex, and a withdrawal reflex.

- **Stretch reflex.** The most rapid form of reflex, it allows you to hold a glass steady as someone pours water into it. Despite the glass getting heavier as water is added, the glass remains still. This is because a sensory neuron detects the muscle stretching as the cup gets heavier. That neuron makes a direct connection onto a motor neuron, which causes the muscle to contract an exact amount to compensate for the stretch.

- **Golgi tendon reflex.** Another reflex related to muscle function, it prevents a muscle from contracting so forcefully that it tears itself from the bone. Special receptors are in the tendons connecting the muscle to the bone. When the muscle is at risk for tearing, a sensory neuron is activated, causing the muscle to relax.

- **Crossed extensor reflex.** The previous examples of reflexes have been relatively simple, but this reflex is the extension of one leg when withdrawing the other. Imagine walking barefoot in a dark room and stepping on a tack. Immediately you will pull back the foot in pain. But to remain stable, you must simultaneously plant the other leg. This is made possible via the crossed extensor reflex.

- **Withdrawal reflex**. This is best depicted when rapidly pulling back your hand when touching something hot. The pain-detecting neurons in the hand cause a complex activation of some muscles and inhibition of others to make the hand rapidly pull away from danger.

An additional type of reflex, the **pupillary light reflex**, is the rapid closing of the pupil when a bright light is shined directly into the eye. Emergency room doctors rely on this reflex as a way to assess brainstem function.

LEARNING OBJECTIVE 6.4.4 Explain the Babinski reflex, infant rooting reflex, and gag reflex.

KEY TERMS

Babinski reflex Reflex in infants that involves the big toe flexing and the toes spreading in response to a stroke of the bottom of the foot.

gag reflex Reflex in which the throat contracts in response to an object coming in contact with the back of the mouth.

infant rooting reflex Reflex in which an infant attempts to suckle in response to stroking the cheek.

THE BABINSKI REFLEX, INFANT ROOTING REFLEX, AND GAG REFLEX

Many specific reflexes are clinically relevant and often used in diagnosing infants. The **Babinski reflex** occurs when the sole of the foot is stroked. The big toe then is flexed toward the top of the foot and the rest of the toes are spread. The Babinski reflex typically disappears in children older than 2 years old. When an adult expresses this reflex, it is often an indication of a CNS disorder, such as ALS, multiple sclerosis, or various other brain and spinal cord injuries. The **infant rooting reflex** occurs in response to the cheek or the corner of the mouth being stroked or touched. The infant will turn its head and "root," or suckle, in the direction of the stimulus. The infant rooting reflex lasts approximately 4 months. The **gag reflex** occurs when something touches the roof of the mouth, areas around the tonsils, back of the tongue, and back of the throat. In response to this, the back of the throat contracts attempting to thrust the object out of the mouth. In infants, it is thought that this reflex prevents foods that will not be easily digested from being swallowed. In children and adults, this reflex is only initiated by particularly large objects touching the back of the throat.

LEARNING OBJECTIVE **6.4.5** Explain the role of the spinal cord in the transmission of incoming and outgoing information.

KEY TERMS

dorsal root Region of the spinal cord that sensory neurons enter.

ventral root Region of the spinal cord in which motor neurons exit.

THE SPINAL CORD RECEIVES SENSORY INPUT AND TRANSMITS MOTOR OUTPUT

As we have discussed, the spinal cord segregates the white matter pathways on the outer regions from the gray matter synapses in the inner regions. Likewise, the inputs and outputs of the spinal cord are also specifically organized (Figure 6-18). All sensory information coming into the spinal cord enter the dorsal side via the dorsal root. These neurons may participate in a reflex, making direct connections onto a motor neuron, or synapse onto neurons that ascend the spinal cord to the brain. Likewise, all motor information leaves the spinal cord via the ventral root, making synapses onto muscles or organs.

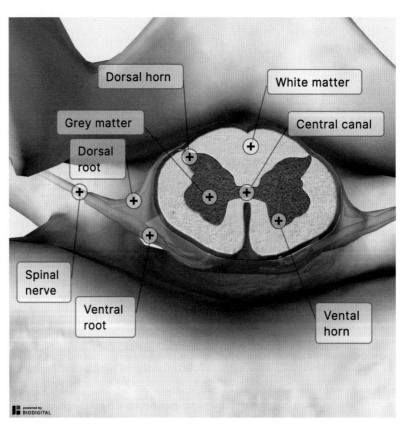

FIGURE 6-18 Spinal cord cross section. Note that the dorsal root and the ventral root leave the spinal cord in separate locations but come together to form a single spinal root.

6.4.6 **Explain the role the brainstem plays in the processing of incoming information.**

THE ROLE OF THE BRAINSTEM IN PROCESSING SENSORY INFORMATION

The brainstem regulates a variety of vital functions such as heart rate, breathing, sleeping, and eating and is critical to maintain body homeostasis. Most of the cranial nerves arise from the brainstem as well. But in order to determine what changes need to be done to the organs via the autonomic nervous system or cranial nerves, the brainstem must have access to the current status of the organs. This is accomplished via sensory portions of the cranial nerves as well as connections to other brain areas, notably the hypothalamus, insular cortex, and amygdala. Additionally, the brainstem serves as a link between the brain and spinal cord. All incoming information headed to the thalamus prior to its ultimate location travels through the brainstem via the ascending pathways, including the spinothalamic tract and dorsal column. Descending motor information also must travel through the brainstem on its route to the spinal cord. There are also numerous areas in the brainstem that themselves are origination points of motor neurons.

6.4.7 **Explain the role the midbrain plays in the processing of incoming information.**

MIDBRAIN PROCESSING OF SENSORY INFORMATION

The midbrain is the topmost region of the brainstem, closest to the brain. It can be broken up into three distinct anatomical and functional regions. The tectum contains regions that receive direct input from both visual and auditory stimuli. This information is used to help make reflexive movements to help align simultaneous auditory and visual stimuli, including driving descending motor neurons onto cervical regions of the spinal cord. For example, if you are walking in a park and hear rustling in the bushes, it is the tectum that helps you turn your head to the exact location without much thought. The tegmentum has several regions—one of which is involved in initiating motor movements and another at regulating the experience of reward. It is this first area that is damaged in Parkinson's disease and the second that is central to the rewarding properties of drugs of abuse and is involved in the development of addiction. The third region of the midbrain is the cerebral peduncles, which are the axons of passing neurons linking the thalamus and cerebellum with the spinal cord. These neurons help to refine motor movements, learn new motor skills, and maintain posture and balance.

LEARNING OBJECTIVE 6.4.8 Explain the role of the cerebral cortex in the processing of incoming information.

THE ROLE OF THE CEREBRAL CORTEX IN PROCESSING SENSORY INFORMATION

The cerebral cortex is what provides us with advanced processing and the higher-order cognitive abilities. We have already discussed that the cerebral cortex is broken up by both its structure (where it is physically located) and its function (the information it processes). All incoming sensory information, prior to reaching the cerebral cortex, first stops in the thalamus. These may be originating from cranial nerves representing primarily (but not only) the special senses (hearing, vision, smell, etc.) or from ascending pathways from the spinal cord representing the general senses (forms of touch). From the thalamus, information is then transmitted to the respective brain lobe. For example, visual information after leaving the eye first stops in the thalamus before being transmitted to the visual cortex of the occipital lobes. Auditory information also goes through the thalamus prior to reaching the auditory cortex of the temporal lobes. Olfactory information also has a specialized processing area in the frontal lobe. Regardless of the sense, the information is processed in a similar fashion: basic features of the system are represented first, then as more processing occurs the neurons begin to represent more complex features of that sense. The parts of the cerebral cortex that do higher-order sensory processing are association areas and are the most developed regions in our brains.

In the early 1900s a German anatomist broke the human cerebral cortex up into distinct areas based on the shapes and sizes of neurons. These 52 so-called **Brodmann areas** have since been shown to have specific functions that are found across individuals. Some of the specific areas have been well studied by early neuroscientists and bear their names. Wernicke's area and Broca's area are two areas of the cerebral cortex involved in language processing. **Broca's area** is a region of the frontal lobe (Brodmann areas 44 and 45) that is involved in the production of speech. In order to properly create speech, Broca's area is directing the muscles of the mouth and larynx but also requires auditory feedback. Hence, it should not be surprising that this region is near the boundary between the frontal (motor) and temporal (hearing) lobes. **Wernicke's area** is a sensory area that allows us to understand spoken and written language. The location of this area is at the junction of the auditory and visual association areas near the boundary of the temporal and occipital lobes (part of Brodmann area 22). The prefrontal cortex is the forwardmost part of the frontal cortex, made up of Brodmann areas 8–14, 24, 25, and 44–47. The prefrontal cortex processes reward, attention, planning, and motivation. These complex executive functions require inputs of all sensory domains, as well as current organ status and previous experience.

UNIT OBJECTIVE 6.5

Describe the components of the central nervous system and their functions.

UNIT INTRODUCTION

The central nervous system, including the brain and spinal cord, is the most complex system we know. Neurons and glia combine and connect in various ways to allow us to think, breathe, and interact with the world around us. In this unit we discuss the major brain and spinal cord anatomy, as well as provide the basic functions of each location.

LEARNING OBJECTIVE 6.5.1 Identify the location of the brain, brainstem, and spinal cord.

LEARNING OBJECTIVE 6.5.2 Explain the relationship between the brain, brainstem, and spinal cord.

THE CENTRAL NERVOUS SYSTEM

The nervous system can be separated into two parts based on their relative locations. The central nervous system is composed of the midline structures of the nervous system, with the peripheral nervous system being the nerve fibers that come from the central nervous system. The spinal cord is a long, thin tube of neural tissue that is enclosed in the vertebral column. The spinal cord leads into the brainstem, with the brain being the topmost neural tissue (Figure 6-19).

The brain is the most complex region of the nervous system, which processes sensory information, directs motor output, and conducts a variety of other complex functions such as memory and emotion. The brainstem is at the interface of the brain and the spinal cord. This region performs many vital involuntary functions, primarily related to organ function. This includes regulating blood pressure, heart rate, respiration rate, and sleeping, as well as being involved in eye movements and balance. The brainstem also contains white matter pathways with axons originating in the spinal cord to the brain, and others back. As we have discussed, the spinal cord contains both ascending and descending neurons as well as the sensory and motor neurons interacting with the peripheral nervous system.

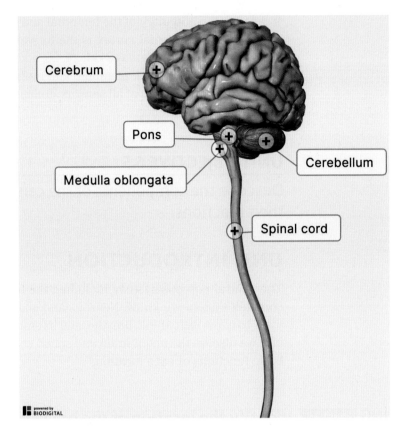

FIGURE 6-19 The central nervous system is made up of the brain and spinal cord.

Identify the location of the midbrain, pons, and medulla oblongata within the brainstem.

Describe the function of the midbrain, pons, and medulla oblongata.

KEY TERMS

medulla oblongata Region of the brainstem that controls respiratory and cardiovascular functions.

midbrain Region of the brainstem that allows for identifying the source of a sound and coordinating body movements.

pons Region of the brainstem regulating breathing, heart rate, blood pressure, hearing, equilibrium, and other functions.

THE BRAINSTEM

The brainstem is the lowest region of the brain and is continuous with the spinal cord. It is critical in regulating a variety of basic cardiovascular and respiratory functions as well as serving a major sensory and motor processing area for the face and neck. It can be broken down into three regions (Figure 6-20). The uppermost region is the midbrain. The midbrain is critical in allowing you to orient your vision toward a sound and is involved in other eye movements. A different region of the midbrain is involved in coordinating body movements. Below the midbrain is the pons. The pons controls critical organ functions. These include breathing, heart rate, blood pressure, hearing, equilibrium, and more. The pons also links the cerebellum with the cerebrum. The medulla oblongata is the lowest part of the brainstem and controls other respiratory and cardiovascular functions. The medulla oblongata also processes vomiting and sneezing. Running along the entire brainstem are axon pathways that send motor information from the brain to the spinal cord as well as sensory information from the spinal cord to the brain.

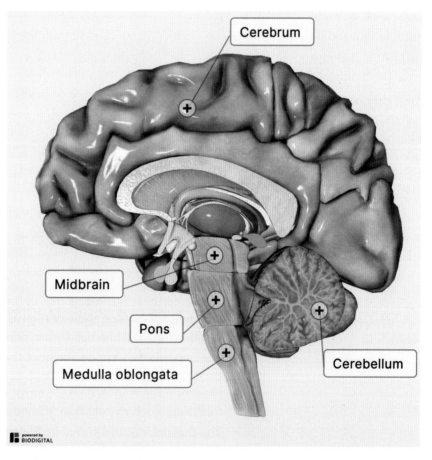

FIGURE 6-20 The brainstem is composed of the midbrain, pons, and medulla.

The brainstem is much more than a connection between the upper brain regions and the spinal cord. It is a critical organizing center for the rest of the body. Damage to this area can be catastrophic. Death often occurs due to the areas involved in heart, lung, and other critical organ functions. Many body system homeostatic processes require the brainstem. But damage to the axon pathways can lead to paralysis. This is because of the spinal cord sending sensory and motor information to the upper brain regions.

LEARNING OBJECTIVE 6.5.5 Identify the location of the cerebellum, thalamus, hypothalamus, cerebrum, and cerebral cortex.

LEARNING OBJECTIVE 6.5.6 Describe the functions of the cerebellum, thalamus, hypothalamus, cerebrum, and cerebral cortex.

KEY TERMS

cerebellum Portion of the brain located in the posterior region and inferior to the cerebrum. Processes fine motor movements, balance, coordination, and proprioception.

cerebrum Largest portion of the brain; located above the brainstem.

cerebral cortex Uppermost layers of the cerebrum involved in sensory, motor, and higher-order processing.

hypothalamus Region of the cerebrum that controls body states such as hunger, thirst, and body temperature and regulates hormone release from the pituitary gland.

thalamus Region of the cerebrum that is the first stop for all sensory information entering the brain prior to going to areas involved in their processing.

THE BRAIN

The brain is the enlarged area of nervous tissue in the head critical for a variety of nervous system functions (Figure 6-21). The brain can be divided into the brainstem, cerebellum, and cerebrum.

- The cerebrum is the largest part of the brain consisting of the left and right hemisphere and some deep brain areas. It controls a variety of functions such as hearing, seeing, personality, emotions, and others.
- The uppermost, wrinkled layer of the cerebrum is the cerebral cortex. The cerebral cortex plays a major role in sensory processing as well as motor control and many other higher-order functions, such as language, planning, and personality.
- The thalamus is an internal brain structure; it cannot be seen without cutting the brain. The thalamus is often thought of as the relay station of the brain. All sensory information coming from the spinal cord goes through the thalamus.

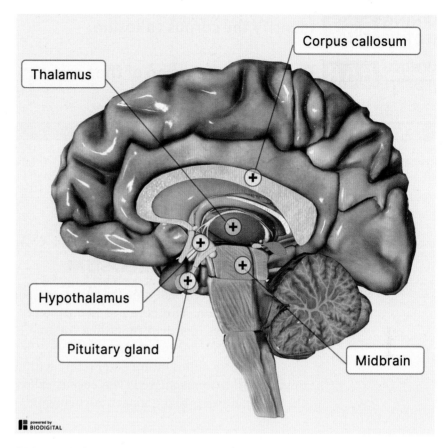

FIGURE 6-21 Major brain regions are the cerebral cortex, cerebellum, brainstem, hypothalamus, and thalamus.

- The **hypothalamus** is another internal brain structure that is below the thalamus. The hypothalamus controls a variety of body states, such as hunger, thirst, body temperature, and others, and regulates hormone release from the pituitary gland.

- The **cerebellum** is tucked between the back of the cerebrum and the brainstem. The cerebellum is involved in motor learning, balance, and posture. The cerebellum cannot initiate movement, but will aid in coordination and precision of the movements. When learning movements for the first time, such as tying a shoelace, you primarily rely on the cerebral cortex to process this information. You were likely unskilled and fumbled often when tying your shoelaces for the first time. After many years of practice, your cerebellum takes over this task and you can smoothly and efficiently tie the laces without much thought.

**LEARNING
OBJECTIVE** 6.5.7 **Identify the corpus callosum.**

**LEARNING
OBJECTIVE** 6.5.8 **Describe the function of the corpus callosum.**

KEY TERMS

corpus callosum Axon pathways that travel between and functionally connect the two cerebral hemispheres.

hemisphere Symmetric halves of the cerebrum that preferentially process the opposite side of the body.

THE CORPUS CALLOSUM

Upon first glance, you'll quickly notice the cerebrum is divided into a left and right portion. The cerebral **hemispheres** are symmetrical areas that perform almost identical functions for one half of the body. We discuss some specialties performed by one hemisphere, but both process all sensory and motor information completely within the respective hemisphere. Some information is shared. The **corpus callosum** is a structure formed by the axon pathways that connect the hemispheres (Figure 6-22). While other

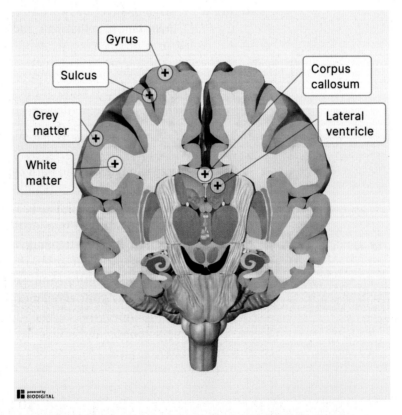

Gyrus

Sulcus

Grey matter

White matter

Corpus callosum

Lateral ventricle

powered by
BIODIGITAL

FIGURE 6-22 Coronal section of a brain showing the corpus callosum connecting the two hemispheres.

connections exist, more than 90% of the connections between the hemispheres are made through the corpus callosum. Some patients with severe epilepsy have the corpus callosum surgically cut to prevent the seizures from spreading between the hemispheres. If you were to meet these individuals on the street, you would not know they had this surgery disconnecting the communication between the two hemispheres. In fact, early scientists who studied these patients in a lab concluded they had no impact on brain processing. Scientists could only detect a difference using specially designed glasses that present different visual stimuli to each hemisphere of the brain. They could then ask each hemisphere (using headphones) what it saw. The left hemisphere could not access visual information processed in the right hemisphere, and vice versa. This emphasizes the extent to which each hemisphere acts independently.

LEARNING OBJECTIVE 6.5.9 **Describe the structure and function of the meninges.**

KEY TERMS

arachnoid matter Middle, spongy layer of the meninges permeated by cerebrospinal fluid.

dura matter Thick, leathery outermost layer of the meninges.

meninges Layers of three membranes that surround and protect the nervous system.

pia matter Innermost thin layer of the meninges that clings tightly to the brain and spinal cord surface.

THE MENINGES

The entire central nervous system is blanketed in membranes that together make up the **meninges** (Figure 6-23AB). This tight covering wraps the brain and spinal cord for protection. There are three distinct layers that make up the meninges. The **pia matter** is the bottom-most thin membrane that tightly adheres to the outer CNS structure. The **dura matter** is the topmost thick, leathery layer that protects the brain and spinal cord. Between these layers is a thin, webby layer of tissue that binds the top and bottom layers of the meninges known as the **arachnoid matter**. A special fluid is infused between the spaces of this membrane to slow down the movements of the brain under the skull. The meninges are infiltrated with many blood vessels to feed the rest of the brain. A subdural hematoma is when these blood vessels break resulting in blood collecting in the space, often following traumatic brain injury. The increased pressure caused by the blood pushing on the brain can be life-threatening.

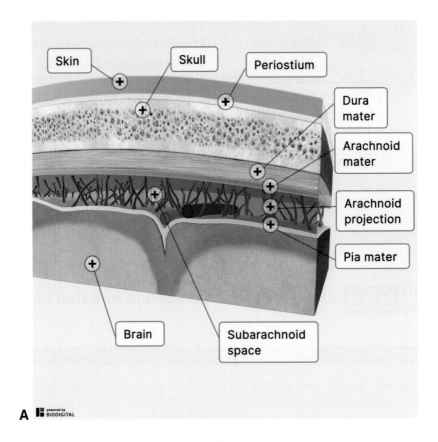

A

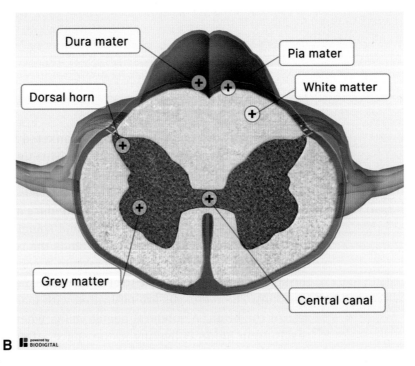

B

FIGURE 6-23AB Meninges are the membranes that cover the (A) brain and (B) spinal cord.

KEY TERMS

cerebral aqueduct One of four fluid-filled cavities
in the brain.

cerebrospinal fluid (CSF) Fluid produced in the
lateral ventricles of the brain that surrounds
the brain and spinal cord to protect and remove
waste products.

fourth ventricle One of four fluid-filled cavities
within the brain.

lateral ventricles C-shaped cavities located in
the center of each cerebral hemisphere in which
cerebrospinal fluid is produced.

third ventricle One of four connected fluid-filled
cavities within the brain.

CEREBROSPINAL FLUID

As we discussed, the brain is wrapped in the meninges and floats in a special
fluid. That fluid is cerebrospinal fluid. Within each hemisphere of the brain are
C-shaped cavities called the lateral ventricles (Figure 6-24). The ependymal cells

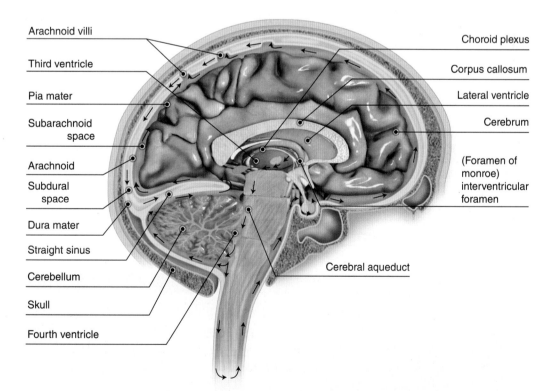

Arachnoid villi
Third ventricle
Pia mater
Subarachnoid space
Arachnoid
Subdural space
Dura mater
Straight sinus
Cerebellum
Skull
Fourth ventricle

Choroid plexus
Corpus callosum
Lateral ventricle
Cerebrum
(Foramen of monroe) interventricular foramen
Cerebral aqueduct

FIGURE 6-24 Cerebrospinal fluid flows from the lateral ventricles through a series of
cavities to bathe the brain and spinal cord between the layers of meninges.

that line the ventricles filter blood, removing all cells and most proteins, to produce the colorless **cerebrospinal fluid (CSF)**. As more cerebrospinal fluid is made, a flow occurs moving out of the lateral ventricles through a series of cavities to under the cerebellum. From the lateral ventricles, the CSF travels into the **third ventricle**, which is a long, thin cavity between the two thalami. The fluid then moves further back into the **cerebral aqueduct**, running through the midbrain of the brainstem, and then into the **fourth ventricle**, the diamond-shaped cavity under the cerebellum. From there the fluid penetrates the middle layer of the meninges, moving in multiple directions to completely surround both the brain and spinal cord. The fluid travels in all directions in the arachnoid matter before collecting in the central canal of the spinal cord. Blood vessels in the meninges reabsorb the CSF back into the bloodstream. The CSF protects the brain from head trauma as well as clears waste from the nervous system cells. The veins of the meninges contain one-way valves that collect cerebrospinal fluid as pressure increases. This mechanism ensures cerebrospinal fluid is constantly bathing the brain.

CLINICAL TIP	The appropriate flow of cerebrospinal fluid around the CNS is critical. This is both because the vital clearance function that the CSF plays and the damage that occurs when flow stops. Because the CSF is continuously made, a blockage will lead to increased pressure because the amount coming into the space is greater than that leaving the space. This results in hydrocephalus, or the buildup of excess fluid in the cavities of the brain. With elevated pressure, the brain tissue gets damaged, resulting in impaired function. While hydrocephalus can occur at any age, it is most common in infants and older adults.

LEARNING OBJECTIVE 6.5.12 Identify the location within the cerebrum of the frontal lobes, parietal lobes, temporal lobes, occipital lobes, and insular lobes.

LEARNING OBJECTIVE 6.5.13 Describe the general functions of each lobe of the cerebrum.

KEY TERMS

frontal lobe Anterior portion of the cerebrum that processes motor information and higherlevel brain functions such as concentration, planning, problem solving, and personality.

insular lobe Region of the cerebrum involved in processing taste and emotions.

occipital lobe Region of the cerebrum that processes visual information.

parietal lobe Region of the cerebrum that processes touch, pain, and temperature information.

temporal lobe Region of the cerebrum that processes auditory information.

THE CEREBRUM

The largest portion of the brain, and the area we generally think of when pondering the amazing functions of the brain, is the cerebrum. The cerebrum can be split into five regions that differ both anatomically (where they are located) and functionally (what they do). Each region is found in both hemispheres (Figure 6-25).

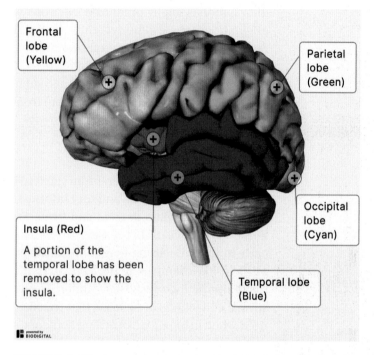

Frontal lobe (Yellow)

Parietal lobe (Green)

Occipital lobe (Cyan)

Insula (Red)

A portion of the temporal lobe has been removed to show the insula.

Temporal lobe (Blue)

powered by
BIODIGITAL

FIGURE 6-25 The cerebrum can be divided into frontal, parietal, temporal, occipital, and insular lobes (inside labeled structure) based on location and function.

Frontal Lobe

The **frontal lobe** is the region of the cerebrum closest to the front. The frontal lobe is involved in motor movements, including a dedicated area for generating speech. There is a strip of cerebral cortex which contains neurons whose activity causes movements in particular body parts. Artificial stimulation of one population of neurons might cause movement of the thumb; stimulation of neurons next to it would cause movement of the index finger, and next to those the middle finger, and so on. A subregion, the prefrontal cortex, is implicated in expression of personality and social behavior. Many complex processes, such as reward, attention, planning, and motivation, happen here.

Parietal Lobe

Behind the frontal cortex, on the top of the cerebrum, is the parietal lobe. The **parietal lobe** processes touch, pain, and temperature information from the skin. As we described for the frontal lobe, a map of the body is represented by activity of neurons in a single strip of cerebral cortex. Stimulation of these neurons does not cause the body part to move; however, it leads to the sensation that the body part is being touched, which is quite disorienting when the person feeling that sensation can see that it is not being touched. Aspects of the parietal lobe also participate in high-level visual processing.

Occipital Lobe

Moving behind the parietal lobe in the rear of the cerebrum is the occipital lobe. The occipital lobe processes visual information. The processing of visual information is highly organized. Neurons will first represent lines of particular orientations (vertical/horizontal/angled). These will connect with neurons that represent shapes (triangles/squares/circles). Higher sets of neurons start to build a generic context, such as a building, desk, or plate. There are even neurons that will respond to particular individuals, such as your grandmother, regardless of what orientation you are viewing them from—the face, the side of head, or even from behind if you know it is that person.

Temporal Lobe

On the outer sides of the cerebrum (next to the ears) is the temporal lobe, which, coincidentally, processes auditory information. The temporal lobe takes the raw sounds that the ears detects and turns provides a context, such as words or music. As with visual processing, this is a highly organized process. The neurons early in the processing may represent particular frequencies of sounds. Interestingly, like the maps of the body in the frontal and parietal lobes, neurons in the temporal lobe represent similar frequencies in nearby neurons. There are special collections of neurons that translate the sounds into words. This area is used when listening or watching someone's mouth make the movements of the word. Damage to this area (Wernicke's aphasia) leads to a patient being unable to understand spoken or written language.

Insula

Tucked into a small fold where the temporal, frontal, and parietal lobes come together is the insular lobe. The function of the insular lobe is not fully understood, but is known to process taste and is involved in emotional processing and self-awareness of body states. One reason the function of the insular lobe is poorly described is its activity changes with a variety of different states, including pain, love, empathy, addiction, and enjoyment of activities. Current perspectives think the insular lobe is creating a sense of overall body awareness—whatever is going on at the time.

LEARNING OBJECTIVE 6.5.14 **Distinguish between the sensory, association, and motor portions of the cerebral cortex.**

KEY TERMS

association cortex Highly developed regions of the cerebral cortex that processes sensory information to a greater extent than the primary areas.

primary motor cortex Area of the frontal lobe that contains neurons that lead to physical movements.

primary sensory cortex First region of a cortical lobe that undergoes sensory processing of the most basic forms of that sense.

AREAS OF THE CEREBRAL CORTEX

Sensory Areas of the Cerebral Cortex

The various areas of the cerebral cortex are interconnected with one another. However, the brain would be far too large for our head to have all regions connected with one another. Instead, the cerebral cortex is organized with a hierarchical structure such that simple information is processed first and as it flows to subsequent regions the information processing becomes more intricate. All sensory information enters the brain first through the thalamus before being sent to the respective lobe of the brain. The first region that each lobe begins the processing of that sense is referred to as the **primary sensory cortex**. These areas process the simplest information from that sense.

Association Areas of the Cerebral Cortex

The primary sensory cortex processes the most basic properties of the sensory stimulus. To extract meaning from these, further processing is done through connections to the so-called **association cortex**. It is the association areas of the brain which are the most developed in humans and allow for complex behaviors. For example, in the visual system, neurons in the primary visual cortex of the occipital lobe may represent edges or contours of objects, but the association areas recognize them as objects such as houses or trees.

Motor Areas of the Cerebral Cortex

A similar organization exists for the motor system, but the layout is reversed. The **primary motor cortex** is the area of the frontal lobe that contains neurons that project to the spinal cord and lead to actions. Artificial activation of neurons in this area will, for example, cause your finger to move. However, most actions are far more complex and involve a complex interplay of several muscles. The association cortex for the motor areas output to the primary motor cortex (as opposed to the opposite for sensory systems). The association areas are involved in planning and executing particular movements. For example, if you want to lift a glass you must coordinate multiple groups of muscles in the hand and arm. To do this action the association areas will initiate the process and connect to the primary motor cortex, which in turn causes the muscles to contract in the required manner.

LEARNING OBJECTIVE 6.5.15 Explain hemisphere dominance.

KEY TERM

hemisphere dominance Concept that some functions are performed better by one cerebral hemisphere than the other.

CEREBRAL HEMISPHERE DOMINANCE

Despite the majority of the functions of each cerebral hemisphere overlapping, some specialization in function does exist on each side. Hemisphere dominance is the concept that some functions are better performed by one side of the brain than the other. The most common example is handedness. Most people are more adept at manipulating objects using their right hand, although some are left-handed. Understanding and production of language also shows hemisphere dominance. Right-handed people typically process language in the left hemisphere. However, the reverse is true for left-handed individuals. In general, the left hemisphere better processes quantitative things, such as time, rules, math, and logic, whereas the right hemisphere better processes more aesthetic-related things, such as emotion, intuition, color, rhythm, and humor.

LEARNING OBJECTIVE 6.5.16 Identify where the storage of memory occurs.

LEARNING OBJECTIVE 6.5.17 Describe the process of memory storage.

KEY TERMS

hippocampus Region of the limbic system involved in memory storage.

long-term memory Maintaining information in the mind on the order of a lifetime.

short-term memory Maintaining information in the mind on the order of minutes.

MEMORY

Our memories of the experiences we have make us who we are. However, memories are a complex phenomenon. Amnesia, a disorder in which you cannot form or access memories, is incredibly disorienting and can potentially have a great impact on the day-to-day life of the sufferer. However, there are also diseases of remembering too much—such as post-traumatic stress disorder, in which a memory of a traumatic event is relived to the detriment of the sufferer. There are even rare disorders in which an individual cannot forget anything and are typically associated with other mental deficits. In general, memories can be categorized into two groups based on the duration they are stored. Short-term memories are those that last on the order of minutes. Long-term memories are memories that may persist for almost the entire life of the individual.

While the exact location and form of memories in the brain is not completely understood, we do know that the hippocampus is a limbic structure that is critical to the formation and retrieval of memories. However, strong evidence exists that memories may be distributed across the cerebral cortex and the hippocampus acts as a gatekeeper of that information. Other brain regions, including the amygdala and cerebellum, are also important in memory storage. The involvement of the amygdala, which processes emotional information, in memory storage is why you can remember the worst days of your life from years ago but not what you had for breakfast even a few days ago.

There are three distinct processes that occur for proper memory. First is encoding of information. This refers to the initial exposure to the information, relating it to past knowledge and experiences and transferring it into the brain. Next, the encoded information must be stored or maintained over time. You are passively aware of tricks to do this, such as repeatedly saying the list items you need to get at the market on your trip there. Your breakfast this morning has been encoded (since you can likely remember it now) but may not be stored (since you likely cannot remember it in a few days). The final critical step in memory is retrieval. This refers to accessing the information when needed.

LEARNING OBJECTIVE	6.5.18	Identify the location of the limbic system and reticular formation.
LEARNING OBJECTIVE	6.5.19	Explain the relationship between the limbic system and human behavior and emotion.
LEARNING OBJECTIVE	6.5.20	Discuss the functions of the limbic system and reticular formation.

KEY TERMS

amygdala Region of the limbic system involved in processing emotion.

limbic system Deep brain region often called the emotional brain that processes emotion, memory, and reward.

nucleus accumbens Region of the limbic system involved in processing reward and reinforcement.

reticular formation Collection of brainstem neurons that are involved in maintaining attention.

THE LIMBIC SYSTEM

Deep in the brain, in a shape similar to the lateral ventricles, is the limbic system (Figure 6-26A). The limbic system is often called the "emotional brain." Two parts of the limbic system are the hippocampus, which encodes memory, and the connected amygdala, which processes emotion. The proximity and interaction between the hippocampus and amygdala should come to no surprise as emotional memories tend to be the strongest. It was once thought that the hippocampus was the site of memory storage, as damage to it leads to amnesia. However, it is now thought that memories are distributed across the brain and the hippocampus acts as an organizing center. The amygdala, in addition to processing emotion, is thought to impact attention. People suffering from depression have disrupted amygdala functioning. It should come as no surprise that one characteristic of depression is reduced ability to sustain attention (and

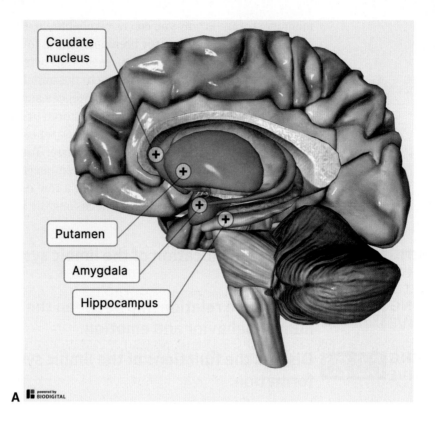

Caudate nucleus

Putamen

Amygdala

Hippocampus

A powered by BIODIGITAL

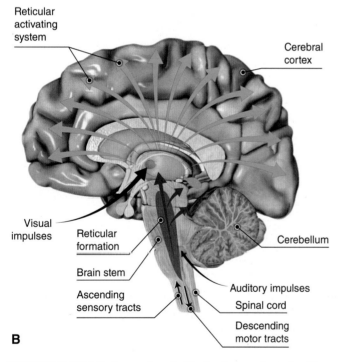

Reticular activating system

Cerebral cortex

Visual impulses

Reticular formation

Brain stem

Ascending sensory tracts

B

Auditory impulses

Cerebellum

Spinal cord

Descending motor tracts

FIGURE 6-26AB Areas deep in the brain have broad-acting effects. (A) The limbic system is made up of the amygdala, hippocampus, and cingulate gyrus. (B) The reticular formation is a collection of areas in the brainstem that send diverging projections throughout the cerebral cortex.

memory deficits). Other parts of the limbic lobe are involved in reward and addiction. One such area is the nucleus accumbens. The **nucleus accumbens** processes reward and reinforcement. Neurons in the nucleus accumbens, and other brain areas, alter their activity as a result of drug taking and the process of addiction. But, the limbic areas also provide a normal sense of satisfaction. A connection between the amygdala and the frontal lobe is thought to provide the achievement you feel when solving a particularly difficult problem. Much of the influence of the limbic system is mediated via hormones and the autonomic nervous system.

THE RETICULAR FORMATION

The **reticular formation** is a collection of neurons throughout the brainstem that project widely to the cerebrum, cerebellum, and spinal cord (Figure 6-26B). The reticular formation has a variety of seemingly distinct functions due to the diversity of areas the neurons project. A major function is its role in maintaining alertness and consciousness, which is thought to occur through interactions with the thalamus and other cortical areas. Also of vital importance is the ability to modulate the subjective experience of pain. There are also areas that interact with the spinal cord and cerebellum that maintain balance and body posture. Another function is to regulate blood pressure by dilating and constricting blood vessels via activation of the autonomic nervous system. The reticular formation is also critical in filtering incoming information to discriminate irrelevant stimuli. Think of your brain as a stage with many distinct things occurring on it. The reticular formation is the spotlight that controls which thing (in our example, a particular stimulus) is the most important to pay attention to at that moment.

LEARNING OBJECTIVE 6.5.21 Describe the structure and functions of the spinal cord.

LEARNING OBJECTIVE 6.5.22 Identify the major neural tracts traveling in the spinal cord.

KEY TERMS

ascending pathways Region of the spinal cord consisting of the axons transmitting sensory information up to the brain.

corticospinal tract Spinal cord pathway containing the axons of neurons controlling skeletal muscle.

descending pathways Region of the spinal cord consisting of the axons transmitting motor information from the brain.

dorsal column Region of the spinal cord containing ascending neurons encoding information about touch.

reticulospinal tract Region of the spinal cord containing the axons of neurons originating in the brainstem (reticular formation).

rubrospinal tract Region of the spinal cord containing the axons of neurons originating in the brainstem (red nucleus of midbrain).

spinocerebellar tract Region of the spinal cord containing the axons of sensory neurons sending information to the cerebellum.

spinothalamic tract Region of the spinal cord containing the axons of sensory neurons sending information to the thalamus.

tectospinal tract Region of the spinal cord containing descending neurons encoding information about head and eye movement.

vestibulospinal tract Region of the spinal cord containing the axons of neurons originating in the brainstem (vestibular nucleus).

MAJOR NEURAL TRACTS OF THE SPINAL CORD

The central nervous system is made up of both the brain and the spinal cord. The spinal cord, however, is more than an area simply connecting the peripheral nerves with the brain. That is one important role, but many of the reflexes we discussed earlier are processed in the spinal cord. The spinal cord can be broken down into inner (gray matter) and outer (white matter) regions, as well as a dorsal (back) and ventral (belly) sides (Figure 6-27). All sensory neurons enter the spinal cord on the dorsal side of the side cord; all motor neurons leave the spinal cord on the ventral side. Within the gray and white matter, the connections and pathways are very well organized. Both white matter and gray matter are

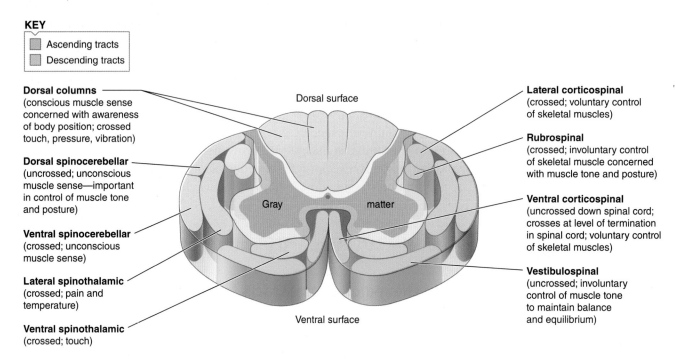

KEY
- Ascending tracts
- Descending tracts

Dorsal columns
(conscious muscle sense concerned with awareness of body position; crossed touch, pressure, vibration)

Dorsal spinocerebellar
(uncrossed; unconscious muscle sense—important in control of muscle tone and posture)

Ventral spinocerebellar
(crossed; unconscious muscle sense)

Lateral spinothalamic
(crossed; pain and temperature)

Ventral spinothalamic
(crossed; touch)

Dorsal surface

Gray   matter

Ventral surface

Lateral corticospinal
(crossed; voluntary control of skeletal muscles)

Rubrospinal
(crossed; involuntary control of skeletal muscle concerned with muscle tone and posture)

Ventral corticospinal
(uncrossed down spinal cord; crosses at level of termination in spinal cord; voluntary control of skeletal muscles)

Vestibulospinal
(uncrossed; involuntary control of muscle tone to maintain balance and equilibrium)

FIGURE 6-27 Common ascending and descending pathways.

organized anatomically, with relatively close areas on the body represented by relatively close neurons. Within the white matter, axons are bundled both on the type of information being represented as well as the destination. Sensory information that goes to the brain is processed via the ascending pathways because they move up to the brain. Motor information traveling from the brain does so via descending pathways. There is a common naming convention of these pathways—the first part describes the origin and the second part the destination.

Ascending Pathways

Ascending pathways bring sensory information to the brain. Three major ascending pathways are the **dorsal column** (breaking convention and being named by its location on the most dorsal portion of the spinal cord), **spinothalamic tract**, and **spinocerebellar tract**. The dorsal column sends sensory information from the skin and joints to the parietal lobe of the brain. Information such as touch, vibration, and a sense of the body in space is transmitted in this pathway. The spinothalamic tract primarily conveys information about temperature and pain, but also some aspects of touch. Like the dorsal column, information sent to the thalamus by the spinothalamic tract is ultimately relayed to the parietal lobe. The spinocerebellar tract also transmits information about the position of the body in space. But instead of sending it to the parietal lobe, as the dorsal column, the spinocerebellar tract sends the information directly to the cerebellum.

Descending Pathways

Five descending pathways send motor information from the brain to the spinal cord. The **corticospinal tract** controls skeletal muscle contractions. Neurons in the motor areas of the frontal lobe send axons into the spinal cord, which then make synapses with neurons that activate the muscles. The other four pathways, the **vestibulospinal**, **tectospinal**, **reticulospinal**, and **rubrospinal tracts**, control organ function and are named based off the brainstem areas they originate. The vestibulospinal tract is named because it originates in the vestibular nuclei of the brainstem and ends on motor neurons on the spinal cord. The vestibular nuclei receive information about the orientation of the head and the vestibulospinal tract causes body movements to maintain body and head positions. The tectospinal tract originates in an area of the midbrain known as the tectum. It allows for body movements that orient to a visual or auditory stimulus. Common examples are turning toward the sound of movement in a bush while walking through the forest or attending to seeing movement in tall grasses out of the corner of your eye. The reticulospinal tract is the primary pathway used by the reticular formation in maintaining body posture. The rubrospinal tract originates in an area of the midbrain that receives input from frontal and cerebellar motor neurons. This pathway influences the corticospinal-mediated muscle movements.

UNIT OBJECTIVE 6.6

Describe the components of the peripheral nervous system and their functions.

UNIT INTRODUCTION

We have already discussed the importance of the central nervous system. However, it cannot perform any of its functions or interact with the environment around us without some help. In this unit we discuss the role of the peripheral nervous system in obtaining information about the world around us; how we control our muscles, organs, and glands; and how we detect the current state of the body.

LEARNING OBJECTIVE 6.6.1   **Identify the major components of the peripheral nervous system.**

KEY TERMS

peripheral nervous system Division of the nervous system that extends off the brain and spinal cord.

somatic nervous system Portion of the nervous system innervating the skin, muscles, and viscera.

THE PERIPHERAL NERVOUS SYSTEM

The **peripheral nervous system** is the collection of sensory and motor neurons that extend from the central nervous system to the skin, muscles, and other organs. Information about the outside world and the current state of the body is brought into the central nervous system by sensory neurons. Motor neurons can change the function of body organs or cause action by contracting skeletal muscle.

The peripheral nervous system is organized into two divisions (Figure 6-28). The **somatic nervous system** controls skeletal muscle and brings in touch sensations from the skin. The somatic nervous system components are primarily under voluntary control. The autonomic nervous system processes the sensory information and regulates the actions of the organs of the body. Most of the autonomic nervous system actions are involuntary.

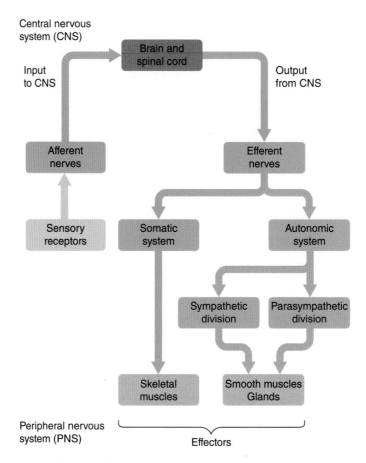

FIGURE 6-28 Nervous system organization.

LEARNING OBJECTIVE **6.6.2** Describe the structure of a peripheral nerve.

KEY TERMS

dorsal root ganglion Enlargement of the dorsal root in which the sensory neuron cell bodies reside.

peripheral nerve Bundle of sensory and motor neurons traveling to a common location outside the vertebral column.

spinal nerve Bundle of sensory and motor neurons traveling to a common area outside the spinal cord but within the vertebral column.

Peripheral Nerve Structure

As we have discussed, the nerves coming off the spinal cord are segregated; sensory neurons only enter the dorsal portion and motor neurons exit the ventral portion. However, before leaving the vertebral column the two populations come together to form a single **spinal nerve** (see Figure 6-18). Once leaving the vertebral column the bundles of sensory and motor neurons will travel to a common location, such as a finger or toe, in the form of a **peripheral nerve**.

Sensory neurons have their cell bodies just outside the spinal cord in a region known as the **dorsal root ganglion**. They extend axons to skin or organs that have dendrites for activation and the same axon continues to synapse in the spinal cord. Motor neurons have their cell bodies in the spinal cord and extend their axons to terminate on skeletal muscle. Autonomic neurons are more complex and require two synapses to reach the target organ. They are discussed more in the following section. Neurons leave the upper and lower regions of the spinal cord. Sympathetic nervous system neurons synapse first close to the spinal cord and then extend a second long neuron to the final organ. For the parasympathetic nervous system, the first neurons are much longer extending to the walls of the organ they innervate and make a synapse on another neuron, which then makes a second synapse in the organ.

LEARNING OBJECTIVE 6.6.3 **Identify the major neurotransmitters utilized in the peripheral nervous system.**

LEARNING OBJECTIVE 6.6.4 **Differentiate between the excitatory and inhibitory neurotransmitters of the PNS.**

Neurotransmitters of the Peripheral Nervous System

The peripheral nervous system allows the central nervous system to communicate with the rest of the body. Sensory information is conveyed via the somatic nervous system. While a variety of neurotransmitters are utilized, the primary neurotransmitter used by sensory neurons entering the spinal cord is glutamate. The peripheral nervous system has two distinct ways to affect the body. The somatic motor neurons communicate with muscles using the neurotransmitter acetylcholine. The autonomic nervous system is more complex and uses both acetylcholine and norepinephrine in modulating organ function. See the section "Neurotransmitters of the Autonomic Nervous System" for greater detail.

LEARNING OBJECTIVE 6.6.5 **Explain how peripheral nerve fibers are classified.**

Classification of Peripheral Nerve Fibers

Peripheral nerves are more than a random bundle of axons traveling back and forth from the spinal cord. As is a common theme in the nervous system, the neurons in a peripheral nerve group together by function as well as destination.

An individual nerve fiber in a peripheral nerve can be classified by its function. Nerve fibers that transmit information about the current state of the body, including external stimuli such as touch or internal organ status, are referred to as sensory neurons. Motor neurons are the nerve fibers that extend from the spinal cord and stimulate the muscles to contract. The autonomic neurons are the nerve fibers that output onto organs. We discuss in later sections that different autonomic neurons have opposite effects on the organs they innervate.

LEARNING OBJECTIVE 6.6.6 List the 12 cranial nerves.

LEARNING OBJECTIVE 6.6.7 Describe the action of each of the 12 cranial nerves.

LEARNING OBJECTIVE 6.6.8 Identify the location of each of the 12 cranial nerves.

KEY TERMS

abducens nerve Cranial nerve VI; controls eye movement.

accessory nerve Cranial nerve XI; controls muscles of head and neck.

cranial nerves Sensory and motor neurons that primarily control and detect stimuli of the head and neck but do not arise from the spinal cord.

facial nerve Cranial nerve VII; motor control and sensory detection of the face.

glossopharyngeal nerve Cranial nerve IX; sensory and motor information of the throat and neck.

hypoglossal nerve Cranial nerve XII; controls motor movements of the tongue.

oculomotor nerve Cranial nerve III; controls movements of the eye.

olfactory nerve Cranial nerve I; contains neurons that detect the sense of smell.

optic nerve Cranial nerve II; visualizes sensory information.

trigeminal nerve Cranial nerve V; sensory and motor information of the jaw and ear.

trochlear nerve Cranial nerve IV; controls movements of the eye.

vagus nerve Cranial nerve X; sensory and motor nerves extending to the visceral organs.

vestibulocochlear nerve Cranial nerve VIII; sensory information of the inner ear structures.

THE CRANIAL NERVES

The spinal nerves are collections of sensory and motor neurons that extend to various parts of the body from the spinal cord. There are many parts of the head that also require peripheral nervous system control. Rather than nerves from the spinal cord needing to move up the neck to interact with the head, cranial nerves serve the same function but project directly from the brain rather than the spinal cord. Cranial nerves control the muscles and various sensory structures of the head (Table 6-2). Unlike spinal nerves, some cranial nerves consist entirely of sensory neurons, others only motor neurons, and some are a mix of both sensory and motor neurons. Each cranial nerve is paired, originating on both sides of the brain.

Table 6-2 Table of Cranial Nerves

NUMBER	NAME	FUNCTION
I	Olfactory	Sensory: smell
II	Optic	Sensory: vision
III	Oculomotor	Motor: movement of the eyeball, regulation of the size of the pupil
IV	Trochlear	Motor: eye movements
V	Trigeminal	Sensory: sensations of head and face, muscle sense Motor: mastication Note: divided into three branches: the ophthalmic branch, the maxillary branch, and the mandibular branch
VI	Abducens	Motor: movement of the eyeball, particularly abduction
VII	Facial	Sensory: taste Motor: facial expressions, secretions of saliva
VIII	Vestibulocochlear	Sensory: balance, hearing Note: divided into two branches: the vestibular branch responsible for balance and the cochlear branch responsible for hearing
IX	Glossopharyngeal	Sensory: taste Motor: swallowing, secretion of saliva
X	Vagus	Sensory: sensation of organs supplied Motor: movement of organs supplied Note: supplies the head, pharynx, bronchus, esophagus, liver, and stomach
XI	Accessory	Motor: shoulder movement, turning of head, voice production
XII	Hypoglossal	Motor: tongue movements

Most of the 12 cranial nerves are named according to their function and numbered according to the relative location (front to back) in which they emerge from the brain (Figure 6-30). They are the olfactory nerve (I), optic nerve (II), oculomotor nerve (III), trochlear nerve (IV), trigeminal nerve (V), abducens nerve (VI), facial nerve (VII), vestibulocochlear nerve (VIII), glossopharyngeal nerve (IX), vagus nerve (X), accessory nerve (XI), and hypoglossal nerve (XII).

The Olfactory Nerve (I)

The olfactory nerve (Figure 6-29) consists of only sensory neurons that process odor information originating from the nose. The olfactory nerve receives information from neurons in the nose specialized to detect odors and project to various areas of the brain responsible for odor processing.

The Optic Nerve (II)

The optic nerve consists of only sensory neurons that process visual information originating from the eye. In the back of the eye several layers of connected neurons form the light-sensitive neuron. Specialized cells in the retina activate

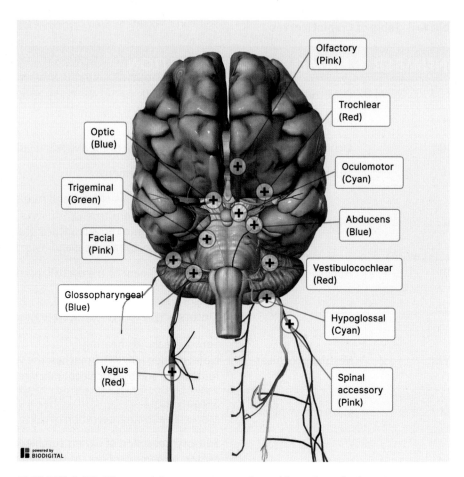

FIGURE 6-29 The cranial nerves are numbered based on the location in which they originate from the brain.

other neurons that are part of a circuit that end in neurons that make up the optic nerve. The optic nerve travels to the thalamus and then sends the visual information to the occipital lobe for visual processing.

The Oculomotor Nerve (III)

As the name suggests, the **oculomotor nerve** controls the movements of the eye (together with other cranial nerves). There are two major types of movements of the eye. The oculomotor nerve controls movements of the eyeball itself, allowing you to look around the room without moving your head. The oculomotor nerve also controls the little muscles contained within the eye that control pupil diameter. Neurons making up the oculomotor nerve originate from the medulla region of the brainstem.

The Trochlear Nerve (IV)

The **trochlear nerve** helps to regulate the movements of the eyeball. Activation of the trochlear nerve leads to downward and inward rotation of the eyeball. Neurons making up the trochlear nerve originate from the midbrain region of the brainstem.

The Trigeminal Nerve (V)

The **trigeminal nerve** is the largest of the cranial nerves and consists of both sensory and motor neurons. It has three major branches that together provide sensory information for most of the face as well as control the muscles of the jaw and ear. The branches are named for the region of the face they connect. The ophthalmic branch innervates the eyes, nose, and forehead regions. The maxillary branch is involved with processing the cheek and upper mouth (maxilla bone). The mandibular branch innervates the jaw (mandible bone) up toward the ear. The neurons that make up the trigeminal nerve originate from the pons and medulla regions of the brainstem.

The Abducens Nerve (VI)

Another cranial nerve that helps to control eye movements is the abducens nerve. The **abducens nerve** consists of only motor neurons that cause outward movements of the eyeball. The abducens allows you to look to the side without moving your head. The neurons that make up the abducens nerve originate from the pons region of the brainstem.

The Facial Nerve (VII)

As the name suggests, the facial nerve controls various aspects of the face. Specifically, the **facial nerve** consists of sensory neurons processing taste and nonauditory sensations from around the ears as well as controls facial expression, some jaw muscles, and glands of the head and neck. The neurons that make up the facial nerve originate from the pons region of the brainstem. There are five branches of the facial nerve. The temporal branch innervates muscles surrounding the eye, leading to wrinkles in the forehead. The zygomatic branch not only innervates muscles surrounding the eye but also allows for the eyes to close. The largest of the five branches, the buccal branch, innervates various cheek, mouth, and eye muscles and is responsible for facial expressions such as smirking, smiling, flaring the nostrils, and others. The marginal mandibular branch innervates muscles of the lower lip and chin, allowing for movements of the mouth and lips. The cervical branch innervates a muscle running along the jaw and neck which when activated can open the mouth or cause a frown.

The Vestibulocochlear Nerve (VIII)

The **vestibulocochlear nerve** consists of only sensory neurons processing sensory information from the inner ear structures. Specialized cells in the cochlea can detect sounds and activate neurons that form part of the vestibulocochlear nerve. The other portion of the vestibulocochlear nerve receives input from the organs of the vestibular system, which is important for maintaining balance. The neurons that make up the vestibulocochlear nerve originate from the pons region of the brainstem.

The Glossopharyngeal Nerve (IX)

The **glossopharyngeal nerve** consists of both motor and sensory information for structures of the throat and neck region. It processes taste from a portion of the tongue and other sensory information from the throat, sinuses, and ear. The glossopharyngeal nerve also controls muscles and glands that aid in swallowing and speech. The neurons that make up the glossopharyngeal nerve originate from the medulla region of the brainstem.

The Vagus Nerve (X)

While the other cranial nerves remain constrained to the head and neck region, the vagus nerve travels to and regulates the function of many abdominal and thoracic organs. The **vagus nerve** consists of both sensory and motor neurons that perform a variety of diverse functions. The best-known function of the vagus nerve is its involvement in sensory and motor processing of the visceral organs, including the heart, lungs, and intestines. In this way, the vagus nerve is acting as part of the parasympathetic nervous system. For example, the vagus nerve (and other parasympathetic neurons) can slow down heart rate by releasing acetylcholine onto the heart. The vagus nerve also controls various muscles of the larynx, pharynx, and tongue and provides sensory information about the ear canal and parts of the throat. The vagus nerve even processes tastes from the very back of the tongue. The neurons that make up the vagus nerve originate from the medulla region of the brainstem.

The Accessory Nerve (XI)

The **accessory nerve** consists of only motor neurons that control the muscles of the neck. The accessory nerve emphasizes the similarity between the spinal nerves and cranial nerves as one portion of the accessory nerve originates from the upper region of the spinal cord. The other neurons originate from the medulla region of the brainstem. Together they form the accessory nerve and project to muscles of the larynx, pharynx, and neck.

The Hypoglossal Nerve (XII)

The **hypoglossal nerve** controls most movements of the tongue. It consists of only motor neurons that project to the majority of muscles that control tongue movements. The neurons that make up the hypoglossal nerve originate from the medulla region of the brainstem.

LEARNING OBJECTIVE 6.6.9 Identify the cervical, thoracic, lumbar, sacral, and coccygeal spinal nerves.

LEARNING OBJECTIVE 6.6.10 Explain how spinal nerves are named.

KEY TERMS

cervical spinal nerves Eight pairs of peripheral nerves that exit from the uppermost region of the spinal cord.

coccygeal spinal nerves One pair of peripheral nerves that exit from the lowermost region of the spinal cord.

lumbar spinal nerves Five pairs of peripheral nerves that exit from the lower-back region of the spinal cord.

sacral spinal nerves Five pairs of peripheral nerves that exit from the lowest region of the spinal cord.

thoracic spinal nerves Twelve pairs of peripheral nerves that exit from the chest region of the spinal cord.

THE SPINAL NERVES

We have already discussed that spinal nerves extend from the spinal cord to various parts of the body. There are 31 pairs of spinal nerves that we can name based on which vertebral column they originate from (Figure 6-30). A shorthand naming convention commonly uses the first letter of the vertebral column they originate from (except from the coccyx) with numbering for the region (top down). The functions of the head and neck are supported by the eight cervical spinal nerves. These are named C1 through C8, despite there only being seven cervical vertebrae. Below these are the 12 thoracic spinal nerves, numbered T1 through T12, which innervate the chest. The lumbar spinal nerves are the next lower five pairs numbered L1 through L5. These nerves control the lower back and front of the legs. Five pairs of sacral spinal nerves (S1 through S5) emerge from two locations of the vertebral column and control the back of the legs and some organ function. The coccygeal spinal nerves are the final pair of spinal nerves emerging from the coccyx (tailbone) and innervating the skin in the area of the coccyx.

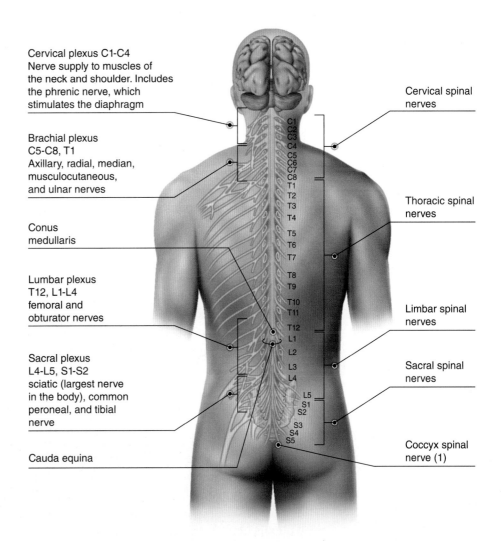

FIGURE 6-30 Spinal nerves are named by the region of the vertebral column from which they emerge.

Describe the general functions of spinal nerves.

KEY TERMS

brachial plexus Network of interconnected nerves formed by four cervical nerves and one thoracic spinal nerve.

cervical plexus Network of interconnected nerves formed by the first 4 cervical nerves.

dermatome Area of the skin of which a particular spinal nerve is influencing.

nerve plexus Branching network of intersecting nerves.

sacral plexus Network of interconnected nerves formed by the lower lumbar and sacral nerves.

Spinal Nerve Functions

All spinal nerves are a mixture of sensory and motor neurons. In general, they represent sensations from the skin and control muscles in the areas of the body that they are near (Figure 6-31). The cervical spinal nerves control muscles of and process sensations from the head, neck, shoulders, arms, and hands. The thoracic spinal nerves control muscles and other organs of the chest and abdominal region as well as process sensory information from the region. The lumbar spinal nerves control muscles of the lower back and front of the legs as well as process sensory information from the region, while sacral spinal nerves control muscles and process sensory information from the back of the legs. The coccygeal spinal neve controls movement and sensation from a portion of the pelvis.

After leaving the spinal cord and vertebral column, the spinal nerves begin to mix with each other before extending to the body parts they ultimately connect. Each spinal nerve will go to a particular body region. A **dermatome** is the skin that a particular spinal nerve is influencing. The branching network of nerves is referred to as a **nerve plexus**. There are five nerve plexuses that loosely correspond to the spinal nerves that make them up. At a nerve plexus, fibers from one spinal nerve, for example, C1, split from the other fibers in C1 to join with a subpopulation of other spinal nerves, for example, C2. Each plexus is quite complex, with several divisions and recombinations with the various spinal nerves that make up the region. The **cervical plexus** is made up of C1 through C4 cervical spinal nerves and innervates the back of the head, neck, and shoulders. The **brachial plexus** is located in the shoulder and is composed of C5 through T1 spinal nerves. The fibers control the arm, hands, and upper back. The lumbar plexus is made up of parts of T12 and L1 through L4 spinal nerves. These innervate the abdomen and parts of the back and legs. The **sacral plexus** is primarily made up of the S1 through S4 spinal nerves, with some contributions by L4 and L5 spinal nerves. The sacral plexus serves the buttocks, genitals, parts of the legs, and the feet. The coccygeal plexus is a small plexus made up of the coccygeal spinal nerve and some of the S5 spinal nerve. The coccygeal plexus only represents the sensory information surrounding the tailbone.

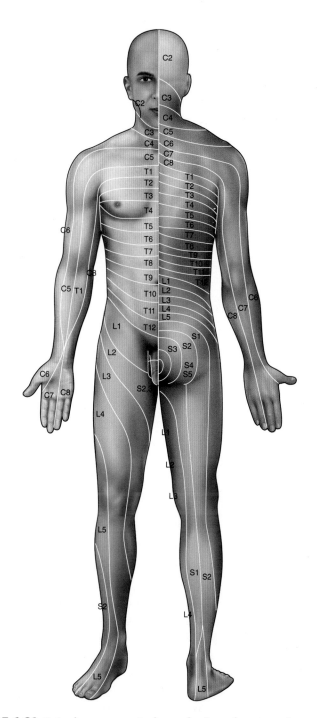

FIGURE 6-31 Spinal nerves control muscles in and represent sensory information from distinct regions of the body.

UNIT OBJECTIVE 6.7

Describe the autonomic nervous system and its functions.

UNIT INTRODUCTION

The nervous system is just one of the many organ systems in the body. All of these systems must work in concert with one another to have a healthy, properly functioning organism. The autonomic nervous system is the division of the peripheral nervous system that regulates organs and organ systems. In this unit we discuss the components and function of the autonomic nervous system and see how they work in balance to maintain optimal body states.

LEARNING OBJECTIVE 6.7.1 Identify the components of the autonomic nervous system.

LEARNING OBJECTIVE 6.7.2 Explain the overall function of the autonomic nervous system.

KEY TERMS

autonomic nervous system Division of the peripheral nervous system that regulates organ function; composed of the sympathetic and parasympathetic nervous systems.

parasympathetic nervous system Portion of the autonomic nervous system (ANS) that promotes digestive and excretory processes.

sympathetic nervous system Region of the autonomic nervous system that activates the fight-or-flight response.

THE AUTONOMIC NERVOUS SYSTEM

Right now as you concentrate on reading this section, your body is performing countless tasks. From breathing to moving blood in your body to digesting your last meal, the internal processes of the body must all be regulated and controlled. The autonomic nervous system is the division of the peripheral nervous system that controls organ and gland function. In contrast to the other peripheral nervous system division, the somatic nervous system, the majority of the autonomic nervous system's functions are involuntary.

The autonomic nervous system has two divisions that work to balance each other's actions (Figure 6-28). Much like a teeter-totter, when one division is activated, the other's activities is inhibited. Each division will control any particular organ, but to opposing effects. The sympathetic nervous system promotes the "flight-or-flight" response by increasing heart rate, respiration, and blood flow to the muscles. The parasympathetic nervous system promotes the "rest-and-digest" response by stimulating digestion, salivation, sexual arousal, urination, and defecation. Note that each division is capable of increasing activity—for example, the sympathetic division increases heart activity and the parasympathetic increases digestive system activity—but the specific organs that each division stimulates do not overlap. The heart rate is only increased by the sympathetic division and the digestive tract is only stimulated by the parasympathetic division. The other side of this is that when a particular organ, for example, the heart, is stimulated by one division, the sympathetic, it will be inhibited by the other division, the parasympathetic.

LEARNING OBJECTIVE **6.7.3** **Describe the origin and characteristics of sympathetic nerves.**

KEY TERMS

postganglionic neuron Second of two autonomic neurons that leave the spinal cord before innervating an organ.

preganglionic neuron First of two autonomic neurons that leave the spinal cord before innervating an organ.

sympathetic chain Structure that runs parallel to the spinal cord and is the site of the preganglionic and postganglionic synapses for the sympathetic nervous system.

THE SYMPATHETIC NERVOUS SYSTEM

The sympathetic and parasympathetic divisions of the autonomic nervous system each use two neurons to extend from the brain or spinal cord to the organs they ultimately affect. The neurons that leave the brain or spinal cord, for both divisions, are referred to as **preganglionic neurons**. The neurons that the preganglionic neurons connect with and which then innervate the organs known as **postganglionic neurons**. Despite a similar architecture, the locations of the synapses between the presynaptic and post-synaptic neurons for each division are in distinct locations. In the sympathetic nervous system, these synapses occur in structures that run parallel to the spinal cord, outside the vertebral column, known as the **sympathetic chain** (Figure 6-32AB). We find the comparable synapses in the parasympathetic division are located closer to the organs they innervate.

LEARNING OBJECTIVE **6.7.4** **Describe the general actions of the sympathetic nervous system.**

Functions of the Sympathetic Nervous System

Imagine that you are out for a hike in the woods. You see ahead of you the bushes shaking. You stop and look closer and see a mountain lion emerge. Your sympathetic nervous system rapidly responds by activating your "fight-or-flight" response. Your body must direct all its available resources to immediate survival and not worry about the long-term maintenance-type functions.

The sympathetic nervous system prepares your body for an emergency situation by rapidly affecting a variety of body systems:

- Cardiovascular: Most notably, your cardiovascular system will change to better serve the muscles of the legs. Blood vessels that lead to skeletal muscles will dilate, increasing blood supply, while simultaneously constricting the vessels that lead to the gastrointestinal organs.

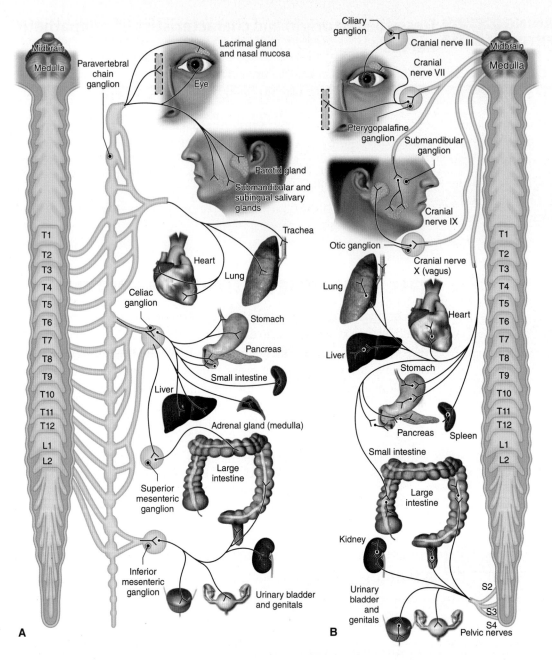

FIGURE 6-32AB The locations of the preganglionic and postganglionic neuron cell bodies differ for the sympathetic and parasympathetic nervous system.

- Respiratory: To maximize oxygen intake, your respiration rate will increase. This allows the blood that is moving to the skeletal muscles to deliver more oxygen.
- Endocrine: Your liver will release stored glucose into the blood. Again, this allows the muscles to remain active by providing an energy source.

- Digestive: The muscles of the digestive tract are inhibited and there are less digestive secretions. During an emergency situation, these processes are less important. All resources are being shifted to the most vital organs to escape.
- Exocrine: The kidneys slow their progress of creating urine and the bladder is inhibited to prevent urination. This, again, allows the body to focus on the vital processes to escape the emergency.
- Sensory: Your pupils will dilate to increase visual acuity by allowing more light into the eye.
- You also begin to sweat to prepare for exercise and heightened alertness.

LEARNING OBJECTIVE 6.7.5 Identify the neurotransmitters associated with the sympathetic nervous system.

Neurotransmitters of the Sympathetic Nervous System

Both divisions of the autonomic nervous system affect the same organs to opposite effects. In order to do this, each division must utilize distinct neurotransmitters in order for the target organ to differentiate the source of the signals. If two brothers were both named John, they would not know who was being called for when they heard their name. In the sympathetic nervous system, all preganglionic release acetylcholine onto the postganglionic neurons in the sympathetic chain. Most postganglionic neurons in the sympathetic nervous system use norepinephrine as a neurotransmitter to alter organ function. Some sympathetic postganglionic neurons use acetylcholine.

LEARNING OBJECTIVE 6.7.6 Describe the origin and characteristics of parasympathetic nerves.

KEY TERM

terminal ganglia Structures in or near an organ that is the site of the preganglionic and postganglionic synapses for the parasympathetic nervous system.

THE PARASYMPATHETIC NERVOUS SYSTEM

While the sympathetic nervous system gets all the hype with "fight-or-flight," in reality prolonged sympathetic activation would not be pleasurable. The body needs a way to relax and recover from the excitement signaled by the sympathetic nervous system. The parasympathetic nervous system serves the purpose of preventing overstimulation by the sympathetic nervous system as well as promoting digestion and other vital body functions.

Like the sympathetic division, the parasympathetic nervous system is organized with preganglionic neurons from the central nervous system projecting to postganglionic neurons, which ultimately impact the organ. But the locations of these neurons are different. The parasympathetic preganglionic neurons originate from the brainstem (in the form of cranial nerves III, VII, IX, and X) and the sacral region of the spinal cord. Rather than projecting to the sympathetic chain, the parasympathetic preganglionic neurons project to areas near, or often on the surface of, the organs they affect. The postganglionic neurons of the parasympathetic nervous system start in these so-called **terminal ganglia** and ultimately project into the organ to influence its function. The postganglionic neurons of the parasympathetic division only travel a short distance in contrast to those of the sympathetic division, which are traveling from the sympathetic chain just outside the vertebral column.

LEARNING OBJECTIVE 6.7.7 **Describe the general actions of the parasympathetic nervous system.**

Functions of the Parasympathetic Nervous System

The parasympathetic nervous system is often relegated to turning off body functions. This is an oversimplification. The parasympathetic nervous system prepares the body to undergo mundane everyday processes. The actions of the parasympathetic nervous system are often referred to as "rest-and-digest" and have the opposing actions on organs of the sympathetic nervous system.

- Digestive: The muscles of the digestive tract and digestive secretions are stimulated. There is also increased blood flow to the digestive system to support muscle function and help with nutrient absorption. Interestingly, salivation, which is involved in the digestive process, is also increased by the parasympathetic nervous system.

- Exocrine: There is an increase in the kidney's filtering of blood to form urine. The bladder will also become more likely to empty.

- Cardiovascular: There is inhibition of the heart and less blood flows to skeletal muscle. As the body is in a restful state, the muscles are not in demand of nutrients.

- Respiration: The respiration rate decreases because the need for oxygen is low.

- The parasympathetic division also promotes sexual arousal and causes the pupils to constrict.

Identify the neurotransmitters associated with the parasympathetic nervous system.

Neurotransmitters of the Parasympathetic Nervous System

The organs of the sympathetic and parasympathetic nervous system must release distinct neurotransmitters from their respective postganglionic neurons in order for the organ to differentiate the signals. But since the locations of the connections between the preganglionic and postganglionic neurons are in different locations, the neurotransmitters of the preganglionic neurons do not need to differ. Like sympathetic preganglionic neurons, the parasympathetic preganglionic neurons use acetylcholine to communicate with the postganglionic neurons. However, in the parasympathetic division, the postganglionic neurons also use acetylcholine to communicate with the organ.

Contrast the sympathetic and parasympathetic divisions of the autonomic nervous system.

COMPARING THE SYMPATHETIC AND PARASYMPATHETIC NERVOUS SYSTEM

The sympathetic nervous system and parasympathetic nervous system together make up the autonomic nervous system. Like good teammates, they have many overlapping similarities and their differences complement each other well. The overarching circuitry is similar. Both systems use a two-neuron pathway to control organs. The sympathetic preganglionic neurons leave from the central areas of the spinal cord while the parasympathetic preganglionic neurons leave from above and below this, in the brainstem and sacral spinal cord. The sympathetic preganglionic neurons travel a relatively short distance to just outside the spinal cord where they synapse onto the postganglionic neurons in the sympathetic chain. The parasympathetic neurons, on the other hand, synapse onto postganglionic neurons in the terminal ganglia near or within the organs they affect. Both divisions release acetylcholine from the preganglionic fibers. The parasympathetic nervous system postganglionic neurons also release acetylcholine on their target organs, but the sympathetic nervous system postganglionic neurons release norepinephrine (Table 6-3).

Of course, the ultimate effect on the body is also balanced. The organs the parasympathetic nervous system activates, the sympathetic nervous system inhibits, and vice versa. For example, the sympathetic nervous system increases heart rate while the parasympathetic nervous system decreases it. The parasympathetic nervous system promotes digestive processes and defecation, while the sympathetic nervous system inhibits these.

Table 6-3 Comparison of Effects of the Autonomic Divisions on Body Systems

ORGAN	EFFECT OF SYMPATHETIC STIMULATION (AND TYPES OF ADRENERGIC RECEPTORS)	EFFECT OF PARASYMPATHETIC STIMULATION
Heart	Increases heart rate and increases force of contraction of the whole heart) (β_1)	Decreases heart rate and decreases force of contraction of the atria only
Most innervated blood vessels	Constricts (α_1)	Dilates vessels supplying the penis and clitoris only
Lungs	Dilates the bronchioles (airways) (β_2) Inhibits mucus secretion (α)	Constricts the bronchioles Stimulates mucus secretion
Digestive tract	Decreases motility (movement) (α_2, β_2) contracts sphincters (to prevent forward movement of contents) (α_1) inhibits digestive secretions (ex2)	Increases motility Relaxes sphincters (to permit forward movement of contents) Stimulates digestive secretions
Urinary bladder	Relaxes (β_2)	Contracts (emptying)
Eye	Dilates the pupil (contracts radial muscle) (α_1) Adjusts the eye for far vision (β_2)	Constricts the pupil (contracts circular muscle) Adjusts the eye for near vision
Liver (glycogen stores)	Glycogenolysis (glucose is released) (β_2)	None
Adipose cells (fat stores)	Lipolysis (fatty acids are released) (β_2)	None
Exocrine glands		
Exocrine Pancreas	Inhibits pancreatic exocrine secretion (α_2)	Stimulates pancreatic exocrine secretion (important for digestion)
Sweat glands	Stimulates secretion by sweat glands; important in cooling the body (α_1; most are cholinergic)	None
Salivary glands	Stimulates a small volume of thick saliva rich in mucus (α_1)	Stimulates a large volume of watery saliva rich in enzymes
Endocrine glands		
Adrenal medulla	Stimulates epinephrine and norepinephrine secretion (cholinergic)	None
Endocrine pancreas	Inhibits insulin secretion; stimulates glucagon secretion (α_2)	Stimulates insulin and glucagon secretion
Genitals	Controls ejaculation (males) and orgasmic contractions (both sexes) (α_1)	controls erection (penis in males and clitoris in females)
Brain activity	Increases alertness (receptors unknown)	None

LEARNING OBJECTIVE 6.7.10 Describe how the functions of the parasympathetic and sympathetic nervous systems regulate a majority of homeostasis.

MAINTAINING HOMEOSTASIS VIA THE AUTONOMIC NERVOUS SYSTEM

Because the divisions of the autonomic nervous system compete for the function of the same organ, it is important to co-regulate their activity to prevent a figurative tug-of-war on an organ. Part of this is simply due to the types of stimuli that promote each response. A stimulation that promotes the sympathetic nervous system is vastly different from that which causes a parasympathetic response. Take, for example, stepping outside from a dark room to a bright sunny day. A signal from your eye will say too much light is coming in and cause the parasympathetic nervous system to constrict the pupil. If the light gets too dim, the signal is no longer present to activate the parasympathetic nervous system and constriction stops. If dim enough, a different signal may activate the sympathetic nervous system and cause the pupil to dilate to allow more light to enter.

Another example is the rapid change in heart rate to modify blood pressure. This takes advantage of the fact that our blood vessels are a series of interconnected tubes set up in what is known as a closed system. When blood pressure drops, the heart will rapidly compensate (on the order of seconds) to increase heart rate via sympathetic activation. As the heart pumps more blood, the pressure in the vessels increases (like making more water flow through a garden hose). To promote this more, a constriction in the diameter of blood vessels is paired with the increase in heart rate. Together, these can rapidly cause blood pressure to increase. When blood pressure is too high, the parasympathetic nervous system will decrease the heart rate and dilate blood vessels. In this way all body systems are maintained in balance, maintaining heart rate, nutrient levels, oxygen levels, and many other autonomic functions.

UNIT OBJECTIVE 6.8

Describe the different sensory functions and how the brain interprets sensory stimuli.

UNIT INTRODUCTION

Sensory systems are our gateway to the world around us. In this unit we are introduced to the types of senses and discuss the general senses, which are primarily detected around the body by receptors in the skin. We will see the importance of receptors tuned to particular stimuli in order for us to detect them.

LEARNING OBJECTIVE 6.8.1 Identify the six general senses.

KEY TERM

general senses Senses that can be detected throughout the body without specialized organs or other structures.

THE SENSES

Our nervous system is a powerful collection of neurons that far exceeds the processing power of the fastest computer. But, like computers, without input to the system, there will be nothing to process. Sensory systems provide information to the central nervous system about the world outside. Sensory systems are categorized as general or special senses. The general senses are termed such because they are encoded by receptors spread throughout the body, as opposed to regional detection by specialized organs of the special senses. The six general senses are touch, pressure, temperature, vibration, pain, and proprioception.

LEARNING OBJECTIVE 6.8.2 Define touch, pressure, temperature, vibration, pain, and proprioception.

KEY TERMS

pain Perception of damaged cells or tissues.

pressure Deeper form of touch requiring a heavy, but nondamaging physical stimulus.

proprioception Sense of the position of a joint.

temperature Ability to detect changes in the amount of heat in the body.

touch Sense of a normal, nondamaging light physical stimulus to the skin.

vibration Ability to detect rapid physical oscillations.

General Senses

The general senses detect various forms of touch and body position from around the body. There are six general senses (Figure 6-33AB). As with most forms of cellular communication, sensory neurons require receptor proteins to respond. Each general sense differs in the way that receptor protein functions.

- **Touch** is how we experience normal, nondamaging physical light contact to the skin.
- **Pressure** requires a deeper, heavier nondamaging physical stimulus.

- Specialized neurons can detect **vibrations** of the skin.
- **Temperature** is how we perceive different amounts of heat being given off in our surroundings. Changes in temperature are detected by specialized receptors. These receptors are most sensitive to detecting changes in temperature, which is why the

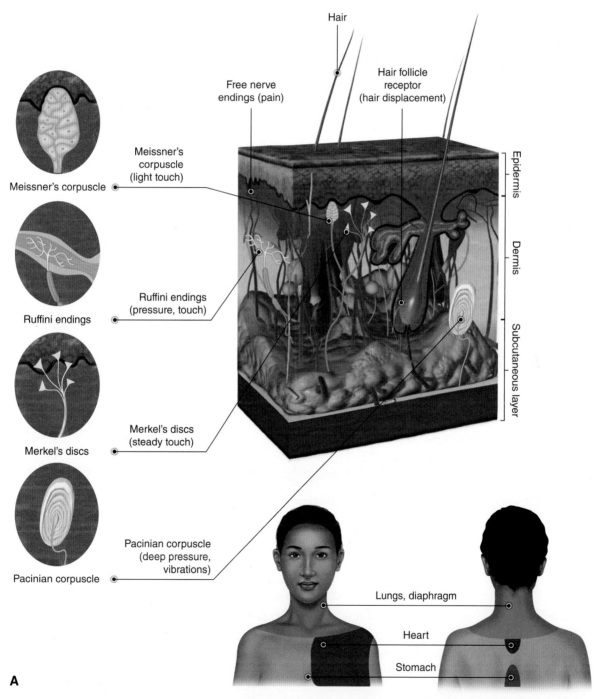

A

FIGURE 6-33AB The general senses do not require specialized organs for detection. (A) The skin contains receptors for touch, pressure, vibration, temperature, and pain.

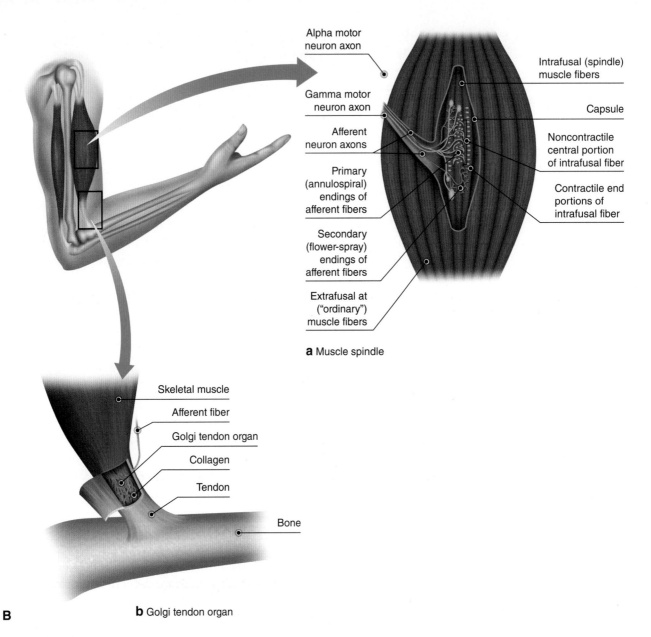

a Muscle spindle

b Golgi tendon organ

B

FIGURE 6-33AB (B) Skeletal muscle contains special sensory structures to detect where the body is in space.

current temperature of your hand will impact how you perceive the temperature of an object.

- When cells become damaged, they release molecules that activate a particular set of neurons that we experience as **pain**.

- The final general sense does not reside in the skin, but the muscles and joints. **Proprioception** is the ability to detect where one's body is in space.

LEARNING OBJECTIVE 6.8.3 **Describe each of the six general senses and the information that each type relays to the brain.**

KEY TERM

thermoreceptors Proteins that detect changes in temperature.

Touch Light touch is detected by neurons located near the skin surface. Receptor proteins in the neuron become activated when the cellular membrane is moved. Anatomical features residing in the upper half of the dermis improve sensitivity.

Pressure Other receptors than the light touch receptors detect heavy pressure. Neurons that encode pressure reside in the deeper layers of the dermis. These neurons have distinct anatomies that allow the receptors in their membrane to respond when deformed. Because of the different location and membrane shape, the neurons that respond to pressure do not respond to light touch.

Temperature The ability to detect changes in temperature is done by **thermoreceptors**. These are proteins that change the amount of their activation over a range of temperatures. Humans are said to have "warm" and "cold" receptors. But these differ only in the ranges in which they are sensitive to temperature changes. So-called warm receptors change their signaling between 25 and 45°C while the so-called cold receptors respond between 10 and 20°C.

Vibration Some neurons in the skin are specialized to respond to rapid oscillations or vibrations. These neurons overlap with the light-touch and deep-pressure neurons. The upper-dwelling light-touch neurons can also detect lower-frequency vibrations, while the lower-dwelling pressure-detecting neurons can also detect higher-frequency vibrations.

Proprioception Proprioception is the ability to detect the body within space. It is because of proprioception that with the eyes closed you can move your hand to touch your nose without opening your eyes. The ability to detect the body is actually derived from the length of your muscles and the position of the joints. Receptors embedded in the muscles and tendons provide stretch information that is used by the central nervous system to provide information about the arrangement of your body parts.

LEARNING OBJECTIVE 6.8.4 **Identify the four special senses.**

LEARNING OBJECTIVE 6.8.5 **Define vision, taste, hearing/balance, and smell.**

Describe each of the four special senses and the information that each relays to the brain.

balance Sense processed by vestibular organs and proprioception that allows us to remain upright.

hearing Ability to detect sound in the world.

smell Ability to detect chemical in the nose.

special senses Senses of the head that use specialized organs or structures to detect stimuli.

taste Ability to detect chemical on the tongue.

vision Ability to detect light and create images.

Special Senses

The **special senses** differ from the general senses because each has specialized organs to perform its role (Figure 6-34). The special senses allow us to detect light (vision), chemicals (taste and smell), sound (hearing), and balance. Each is grouped by the structure that detects them: eyes, ears, nose, and tongue.

Vision The eye is an organ specialized to detect light. Neurons in the eye contain special receptors that respond to light and alter their function. Cells in the eye specialize to detect color, but only in well-lit environments, or detect light in low levels, but only in shades of gray. Our perception of light is perceived as **vision**. Basic visual processing starts in the eye itself before being further processed in the visual centers of the brain.

Taste The tongue is a sensory organ of the mouth. Though mostly a large muscle used while chewing food and critical in speaking, the tongue contains the sensory structures that are perceived as **taste**. Special neurons in the tongue respond to five categories of chemicals (sweet, salty, sour, bitter, and savory). Our full sense of taste requires our sense of smell. This should be evident by the last time you ate your favorite meal with a cold.

Hearing The inner ear contains two distinct special senses encoded by similar types of neurons. One arrangement of these neurons permits for the **hearing** of sound. Pressure waves that are collected by the outer ear structures are amplified in the middle ear and encoded by neurons of the inner ear. Similar to the tuning of the temperature receptors, sound receptors are tuned to respond to particular frequencies of sound.

Balance Another arrangement of the same special neurons that lead to hearing provide our sense of **balance**. Distinct structures of the inner ear provide information about linear and rotational movements of the head in all directions. As a small child, you may have enjoyed spinning in circles to disorient yourself by over-stimulation of these receptors. For many of the same reasons as our hearing deteriorates as we age, you will likely not enjoy or possibly feel ill following spinning in a circle as an adult. The neurons that encode these functions cannot tolerate the same level of stimulation.

Smell Special neurons in the nose detect chemicals in the air that we perceive as **smell**. As opposed to taste which only can detect five classes of chemicals, humans can detect thousands of different odors. This is due to both a greater diversity of receptors that detect odors and a decreased specificity of the

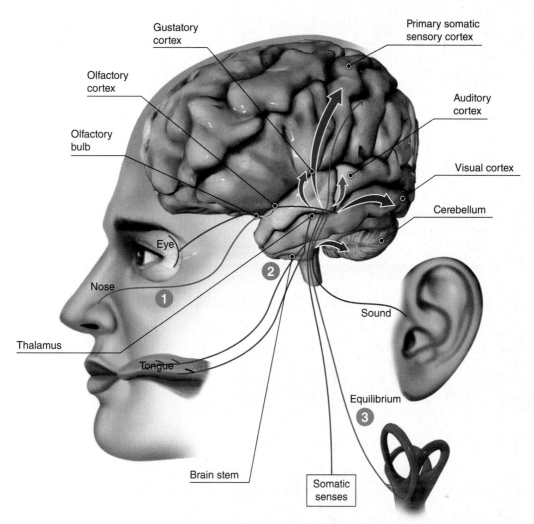

FIGURE 6-34 The special senses are detected by specialized organs in the head. We use our eyes, ears, nose, and mouth to detect vision, hearing, equilibrium, smell, and taste.

receptors for any particular molecule. A perceived odor consists of a mosaic of responses from a collection of neurons each expressing a different odor receptor and being activated to a different extent. Smell is also distinct from all other senses in that it does not travel to the thalamus prior to entering the brain, including a direct connection to the memory center of the brain.

LEARNING OBJECTIVE 6.8.7 Contrast general senses and special senses.

Comparing General Senses and Special Senses

As we discussed, the main difference between the general and special senses is the presence of a specialized organ dedicated to detecting that sense. In both cases, receptor proteins and other cellular specializations help encode the specific stimuli detected by the neuron. But, the general senses are encoded by neurons that extend into the skin, muscles, and tendons. These are structures found throughout the body. The special senses are encoded using specialized sensory structures of the eyes, ears, nose, and tongue. These structures are entirely housed in the head. While the special senses are arguably more complex, both are critical for survival. In fact, losing the ability to detect stimuli from the skin or not receiving information about your body positioning would have a far greater impact on your day-to-day life than losing any of the special senses.

LEARNING OBJECTIVE 6.8.8 Identify the five types of sensory receptors.

LEARNING OBJECTIVE 6.8.9 Describe the functions of each receptor type.

KEY TERMS

chemoreceptors Sensory proteins that detect chemicals in bodily fluids; also related to the perception of smell and taste.

mechanoreceptors Sensory proteins which detect physical deformations of the cellular membrane.

nociceptors Sensory proteins that activate pain neurons.

photoreceptors Sensory proteins in the eye that respond to light.

thermoreceptors Proteins that detect changes in temperature.

TYPES OF SENSORY RECEPTORS

We can categorize the receptors based on the specific type of stimuli that open them. In some cases, these overlap with the general and special senses categorization, but not in all. There are five types of sensory receptors that respond to light (photoreceptors), chemicals (chemoreceptors), physical movements (mechanoreceptors), changes in temperature (thermoreceptors), and damaging or painful stimuli (nociceptors).

Photoreceptors

Photoreceptors are proteins that respond to light. In humans, our photoreceptors are only found in the eye. Changes in light levels cause the neurons that contain the photoreceptors to alter their functioning and permit the detection of light as vision.

Chemoreceptors

Chemoreceptors are broadly defined as proteins that respond to chemicals. In sensory neurons, these chemicals are in the form of smell, taste, and even the pH of the blood (to infer oxygen and carbon dioxide levels). In the nose, chemicals in the air bind to a wide array of chemoreceptors to encode smell. On the tongue, five specific (and distinct from those detecting smell) chemoreceptors bind to chemicals. Our ability to discriminate a wider variety of odors than tastes is due to the difference in the number of chemoreceptors used by these systems. Think about coloring a picture of an ocean. If you are given a single color of blue, you will be limited in how lifelike you can make that drawing. But if you are given several shades of blue and green, you may be able to produce a more vivid image. Having more chemoreceptors allows a greater amount of chemicals to be differentiated and a more vivid "smell picture" to be produced.

Mechanoreceptors

Proteins that allow ions to enter the cell membrane in response to movement of the cell membrane are **mechanoreceptors**. Mechanoreceptors are used to detect a wide range of stimuli. They are the primary type of receptor for detecting light touch, heavy pressure, and vibration. But, as we discuss in unit 6.9, mechanoreceptors are also critical in the ear for detecting sound and maintaining balance.

Thermoreceptors

Thermoreceptors are proteins that can alter their activity in response to a range of changing temperatures. Some thermoreceptors are also activated by certain chemicals. The cool detector, for example, is activated by menthol and the warm detector by capsaicin, the chemical responsible for the heat of chili peppers.

Nociceptors

In our skin and organs, we have specialized neurons, **nociceptors**, for detecting painful or potentially damaging stimuli. Different nociceptors are specialized to process painful temperature, touch, or chemical stimuli. The term *nociceptor* typically refers to the neuron, whereas the terms *photoreceptor, mechanoreceptor,* and *thermoreceptor* could apply to the protein or the neuron that expresses it. For example, nociceptor neurons that respond to physical stimuli must express mechanoreceptor proteins (tuned to ignore nondamaging forms of touch) in order to detect the painful touch.

LEARNING OBJECTIVE 6.8.10 **Explain how receptors stimulate sensory impulses.**

RECEPTORS LINK SENSORY STIMULI AND NEURON FUNCTION

Receptors are the start of all cellular signaling. What signals a cell can respond to are determined by the receptors that they express. Receptors are proteins that can alter their function in the presence of particular stimuli. We have reviewed a variety of different stimuli that can activate sensory receptors leading to our perception of that stimulus. Regardless of what initiates the response, all sensory receptors change the function of the sensory neurons that are expressed in one of two ways (Figure 6-35AB). The receptors can themselves be ion channels. Activation of the receptor allows a particular ion to cross, which makes the cell more or less likely to fire action potentials. Or activation of the receptor leads to an enzyme pathway, which alters neurotransmitter release. Once the stimulus, the sense, is converted to action potentials and neurotransmitter release, the nervous system can process it.

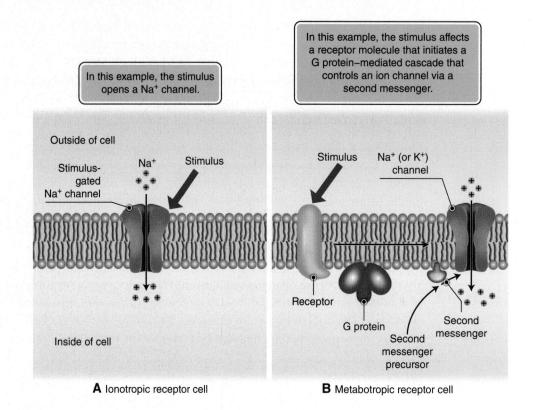

In this example, the stimulus opens a Na⁺ channel.

In this example, the stimulus affects a receptor molecule that initiates a G protein–mediated cascade that controls an ion channel via a second messenger.

Outside of cell

Stimulus-gated Na⁺ channel

Na^+

Stimulus

Stimulus

Na^+ (or K^+) channel

Receptor

G protein

Second messenger precursor

Second messenger

Inside of cell

A Ionotropic receptor cell

B Metabotropic receptor cell

FIGURE 6-35AB Sensory receptors can themselves be ion channels or be linked to enzyme pathways that alter the release of neurotransmitters from the sensory cell.

LEARNING OBJECTIVE 6.8.11 Describe sensation and sensory adaption.

KEY TERMS

sensation Mental experience following stimulation of a sensory structure.

sensory adaptation Changing perception of a continued sensory stimulus.

SENSATION AND SENSORY ADAPTATION

While our receptors determine what stimuli we are capable of detecting, our experience of the world is not a direct representation from those stimuli. Sensation describes the mental experience following stimulation of a sensory structure. For example, if you are walking on a sidewalk in a busy city you may hear numerous sounds. The raw sounds are detected by the ear and sent to the brain. But your experience of these sounds provides meaning to those raw sounds—you can identify the cars driving past, a horn honking, people next to you talking. These experiences would be the sensation of hearing.

Imagine cooking dinner. As you start, the smells are strong and noticeable. But over time the smell is not as strong to you. But, if your friends walked into the room they would strongly smell the delicious meal you were cooking.

Sensory adaptation is a changing perception of a continued stimulus, like the less-noticeable odor of the cooking meal. Many aspects of sensory adaptation are due to properties of the receptors themselves, but some central nervous system processing influences sensory adaption too. However, some stimuli should not be ignored if they persist. Pain is an experience that is indicating damage to the body. If you hold your hand on something hot for a long time, it would be maladaptive to slowly ignore that sensation. Pain does not undergo sensory adaptation. This is because the sensory neurons that encode pain do not alter their activity as the sensory neurons that do undergo adaption will.

LEARNING OBJECTIVE 6.8.12 List the differences between receptors associated with touch, pressure, temperature, and pain.

KEY TERMS

encapsulated Input zones of sensory nerves of the skin which consist of specialized membrane structures used to detect mechanical stimuli.

free nerve endings Input zones of sensory neurons which rely on specialized proteins, rather than membrane specializations, to detect stimuli.

SENSORY NERVE ENDINGS

The cerebral cortex neurons that process, for example, touch and hearing are not structurally or functionally distinct. Each looks similar and will respond to neurotransmitters. What makes them process different information is that the inputs each receives represent different information. Sensory neurons are inherently different from one another. That is because these neurons, by their nature, do not receive input from another neuron. Each sensory neuron is specialized to convert a particular sensory stimulus into an action potential. We can broadly classify them into two groups. **Encapsulated** sensory nerves have membrane specializations, often heavily folded, that are used in detecting the stimulus. Touch and pressure neurons are encapsulated. Other sensory nerves, such as those detecting temperature and pain, have no specialized membrane structures and are referred to as having **free nerve endings**. Proteins in the dendrites of these neurons respond to the sensory stimuli directly.

LEARNING OBJECTIVE 6.8.13 Describe how pain sensations are produced.

KEY TERM

nociception Ability to detect painful stimuli.

PAIN

Pain is the body's response to injury or perceived damage and is referred to as nociception. Specialized neurons encode painful stimuli. We have specialized pain neurons that respond to painful temperature, touch, or chemical stimuli. Many of these neurons respond to more than one type of stimulus. Additionally, pain fibers can be myelinated or unmyelinated. The myelinated fibers process rapid, transient painful stimuli, while activation of the slower unmyelinated fibers encodes dull, persistent pain.

LEARNING OBJECTIVE 6.8.14 Explain the importance of stretch receptors in muscles and tendons.

KEY TERMS

Golgi tendon organ Sensory structure in the tendon that detects stretch in the tendon.

muscle spindle Sensory structure embedded in skeletal muscle that detects changes in the stretch of the muscle.

stretch receptors Specialized sensory structures that detect changes in the size of structures.

STRETCH RECEPTORS

While proprioception is the ability to know where your body is in space, we use this information for far more than finding your finger with your eyes closed. Two main sensory structures provide proprioceptive information. Stretch receptors embedded within the muscles in structures called muscle spindles provide constant information about the length of your muscle. The muscle spindles are critical for your ability to steadily hold an object in front of you with extended arms. Muscle spindles are also responsible for the myotatic stretch reflex, such as the patellar reflex. This common reflex tests for normal spinal function by stretching the quadriceps muscle (via deflecting the patellar tendon). A sensory signal is sent to the spinal cord and makes a connection onto a motor neuron causing the quadriceps muscle to contract an equivalent amount (to compensate for the stretch). This results in a minor kick of the leg.

GOLGI TENDON ORGAN

The other sensory structure providing proprioceptive information is the Golgi tendon organ. Embedded in the tendons attaching muscles to bones, these structures are activated only when the tendon is under a good deal of tension. Their primary purpose is to prevent the muscle from contracting so hard it damages itself. Under large tensions, the Golgi tendon organ prevents the contraction of the muscle it is attached to, thus serving to protect the muscle.

UNIT OBJECTIVE 6.9

Describe the five special senses and their functions.

chemical senses Senses that allow us to detect chemicals in the world around us; smell and taste.

UNIT INTRODUCTION

Many of the senses we perceive require complex organs, not merely specialized cells, to be detected. These special senses are the senses detected in the head by the ear, eye, nose, and tongue, which permit us to sense chemicals, light, and sound in the world around us as well as changes in acceleration and gravity.

CHEMICAL SENSES

Who needs a complicated analytical chemistry lab? You have one in your head already. The chemical senses are how we detect chemicals in the environment around us. We have two forms of chemical senses, the perception of which are interrelated. Both senses require molecules to bind to receptors in the membrane of specialized cells.

LEARNING OBJECTIVE 6.9.1 Describe the sense of taste.

taste Ability to detect chemical on the tongue.

Taste

Taste is the contact-dependent detection of chemicals by receptors on the surface of the tongue. The sense of taste is far less sensitive than smell. This is because the chemoreceptors require contact with the substance, rather than the substantially lower concentration of the chemical being detected that is found in the air. But there are also substantially fewer types of chemoreceptors found on the tongue than in the nose. There are five taste receptors that are completely distinct from the smell chemoreceptors. Embedded inside of pores on the surface of the tongue, the taste chemoreceptors respond to salt, sweet, bitter, sour, or umami (savory) stimuli. Once activated, these cells activate neurons that then travel to the taste center of the insular lobe for further processing. Not all regions of the tongue have the same distribution of taste receptors. For example, the tip is most sensitive to sweet things and the rear is most sensitive to bitter-tasting things. That is not to say the tip cannot taste bitter items, but a larger density of sweet receptors is in this region.

LEARNING
OBJECTIVE **6.9.2** **Describe the sense of smell.**

KEY TERM

smell Ability to detect chemical in the nose.

Smell

Smell is the detection of chemicals in the air by receptors in the back of the nose. As you inhale through the nose, mucus traps some particles in the air. Some of these particles can be detected by the 500–1000 different types of chemoreceptors located in the back of the nose. Once stimulated, the neurons that contain the receptors project their axons through small holes in the skull for furthering processing. The axons of these neurons converge in the olfactory bulb before transmitting the information to a variety of locations throughout the brain, notably the piriform cortex, which contains the amygdala.

LEARNING
OBJECTIVE **6.9.3** **Describe the relationship between smell and taste.**

LEARNING
OBJECTIVE **6.9.4** **Describe how the senses of smell and taste are interpreted.**

The Relationship Between Taste and Smell

At first glance, it might seem redundant to have two chemical sensors in our body. But, they perform distinct roles in distinct manners. The tongue uses only five types of receptors to detect chemicals. These receptors are tucked under folds on the surface of the tongue (Figure 6-36A). The physical location of these receptors requires that the source of the chemical be on the tongue itself. The basic tastes (each with a dedicated receptor) are sweet, sour, salty, bitter, and umami (savory). It is thought that our sense of taste primarily developed to detect poisonous food.

Our sense of smell is much more refined and sensitive than our sense of taste. The nose has several hundred distinct receptors that can bind chemicals in the air (Figure 6-36B). The greater number of receptors, and their ability to bind more broadly to chemicals than most receptors in the body (including taste receptors), provides us with our ability to differentiate thousands of distinct smells. The receptors are in membranes of neurons that have dendrites extending into the nasal cavity. A thin layer of mucus traps chemicals in the air as you breathe. The molecules then bind with the receptors, activating a cascade that leads to smell perception. An interesting aspect of smell processing is the direct connections to the hippocampus, the memory center of the brain. This makes smells have a strong association with memory, which is why you may be reminded of particular events or people as you suddenly smell something associated with them.

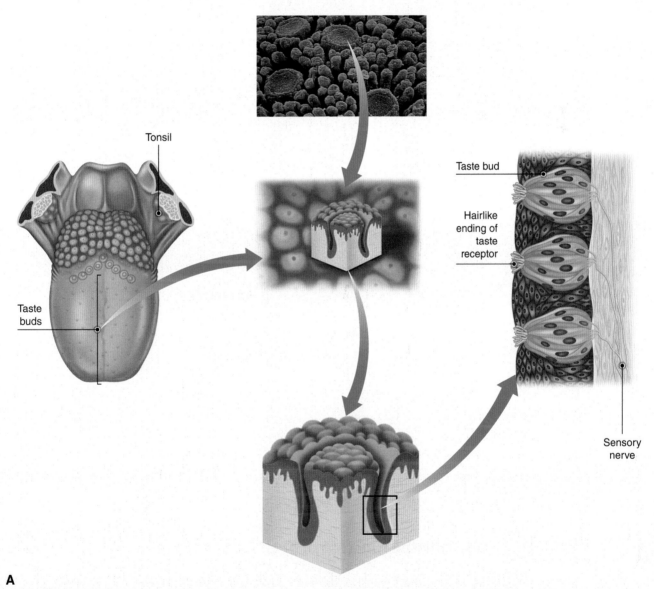

A

FIGURE 6-36AB The chemical senses detect different molecules around us. (A) The tongue has contact-dependent receptors.

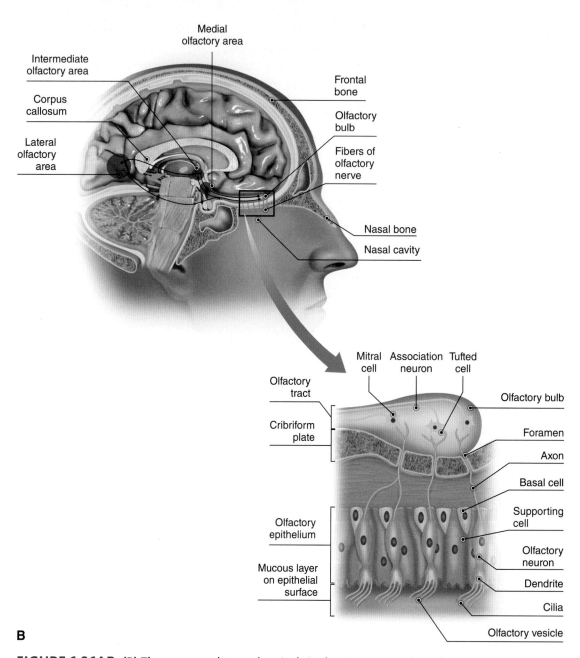

B

FIGURE 6-36AB (B) The nose can detect chemicals in the air. Despite these being separate senses, the perception of them are intermingled.

LEARNING OBJECTIVE 6.9.5 Identify the parts of the ear.

LEARNING OBJECTIVE 6.9.6 Describe the function of each part of the ear.

KEY TERMS

cochlea Sensory structure of the inner ear that detects sound.

eardrum Also known as the tympanic membrane. Boundary membrane between the middle and outer inner that vibrates in response to sound waves.

inner ear Region of the ear that contains the cochlea and vestibular organs.

middle ear Air-filled cavity of the ear that contains the ossicles.

ossicles Small bones found in the middle ear that amplify the sound collected by the outer ear.

outer ear Region of the ear that collects the sound and funnels it toward the sensory structures.

pinnae External portion of the out ear.

vestibular organs Sensory structures in the inner ear that detect equilibrium and balance.

vestibular senses The sensation of body orientation and movement.

ANATOMY OF THE EAR

As you probably know, your ears help you hear. But, did you also know we have cells within our ear that help us with our balance? Your ear is actually a complex sensory organ that detects both hearing and the **vestibular senses**—the sensation of body orientation and movement (Figure 6-37). The ear is separated into three parts: outer, middle, and inner. The **outer ear** consists of the pinnae, the ear canal, and the eardrum. The **middle ear** is an air-filled space that holds the ossicles. The **ossicles** (malleus, incus, and stapes) are the smallest bones of the body; they act to amplify the vibrations of the eardrum and push on the cochlea. The **inner ear** has the sensory structures (cochlea and vestibular organs) that detect the sound waves as well as the vestibular sensory structures. The **cochlea** is a complex, snail shell-shaped organ in the inner ear that has sensory neurons that allow us to hear. The **vestibular organs** are a collection of structures also in the inner ear that allow us to detect gravity as well as linear and angular acceleration.

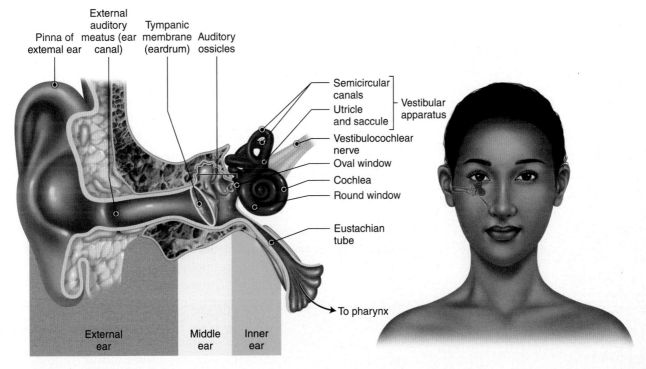

FIGURE 6-37 Anatomy of the ear.

HEARING

The ear is organized both in its anatomy, the relative locations of each structure, and its function (Figure 6-38).

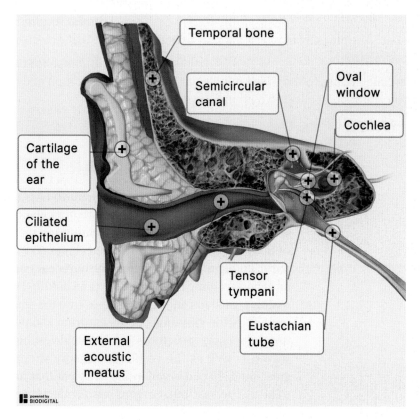

FIGURE 6-38 The ear is made up of three regions, the outer, middle, and inner ear. The outer ear collects the sound; the middle ear amplifies the sound; the inner ear detects the sound.

- Pinnae. The job of the **pinnae** is to collect sound waves and funnel them toward the sensory structures. Human pinnae have folds that allow us to preferentially focus on the frequencies used in speech.
- Tympanic membrane. The eardrum vibrates when sound waves hit it. This is named because it works much like a bongo drum, in reverse. When you play a drum, you physically hit it to cause a sound wave to be emitted. But our eardrum receives the sound wave and transfers that into physical movement.
- Ossicles. The ossicles of the inner ear are three bones connected as levers. Vibrations from the eardrum start a chain of events through the ossicle levers that result in the last bone of the ossicles pushing on a thin membrane on the cochlea. The arrangement of the three ossicles causes an amplification of the force from the eardrum.
- Cochlea. The cochlea is a series of coiled, fluid-filled tubes. As the ossicles push on the cochlear membrane, a wave moves through

the fluid (like in the ocean). The wave vibrates receptors on cells in the cochlea, which change their function to allow us to hear. Due to the structure of the cochlea, different frequencies of sound cause vibrations in discrete areas of the cochlea, and thus only specific sensory neurons are to be activated. The sensory neurons themselves are not tuned to particular frequencies of sounds, but due to their relative location in the cochlea, each is only activated at a specific frequency.

BALANCE

We also use our ears to maintain balance. The vestibular senses only require inner ear structures. Several distinct, but related, structures attached to the cochlea detect changes in gravity and acceleration. This is why you can typically tell when you are upside down even with your eyes closed. Due to the structure of the sensory systems, we can detect linear (forward/backward; up/down) and angular (rotating three-dimensionally) acceleration, but not velocity (or speed). That is why sitting in a chair in your home feels the same as a chair in a train at 60 mph or an airplane at 550 mph. In fact, it is why you can't feel us hurdling through space at a speed of 67,000 mph on Earth's orbit.

The sensory receptors of the vestibular senses are very similar to those used in hearing. The major difference is what causes them to be activated. For hearing, vibrations along the cochlea lead to their activation. For the vestibular senses, the cilia (hairlike cellular extensions) of the sensory neurons are embedded in a gel-like substance. As with the cochlea, the shape of the organs containing the neurons determines what causes their activation. Changes in our body position are separately encoded for all five stimuli detected (two linear and three angular acceleration).

LEARNING OBJECTIVE 6.9.7 Identify the structural components of the eye.

LEARNING OBJECTIVE 6.9.8 Describe each structural component of the eye.

LEARNING OBJECTIVE 6.9.9 Describe the function of each part of the eye.

KEY TERMS

anterior chamber Fluid-filled cavity in the front of the eye.

cornea Thin, transparent membrane covering the eye.

iris Thin membrane between the anterior and posterior chambers of the eye that has the pupil at its center.

lens Gelatinous region of the eye that can change shape to help focus light in the eye.

photoreceptor Sensory proteins in the eye that respond to light.

posterior chamber Fluid-filled cavity between the iris and the lens of the eye.

pupil Opening of the iris that controls the amount of light entering the eye.

retina Rear layer of the eyeball that contains photosensitive neurons.

vitreous chamber Largest of three fluid-filled cavities of the eye between the lens and retina.

THE EYE

Our eye functions very similar to a camera. A camera, like our eye, collects light to make a visual representation of the world. Our eyes are quite complex and sensitive—just get a grain of sand in your eye to realize just how so.

- The outermost component of the eye is the **cornea**. Light travels through the thin, transparent corneal membrane and enters the first of three fluid-filled cavities. The thin cornea is critical to collecting light from a wide area. Its curvature bends light toward the lens.

- The **anterior chamber** is the fluid-filled cavity behind the cornea. It provides nutrients to the surrounding tissues and has immunologically active molecules to protect against foreign particles. In patients with glaucoma, this fluid does not drain well and pressure builds in the area, causing pain and decreased visual ability.

- The **iris** is another thin membrane that lies behind the anterior chambers. The iris is what provides the color of our eyes. A hole at the center of the iris makes the **pupil**. Muscles control the size of the pupil by opening and closing the iris. The larger the hole, the more light enters the eye. Large pupils allow for collecting more light in dark environments. The smaller the hole, the less light that enters the eye. Small pupils prevent the eye from being washed out in bright environments.

- A small fluid-filled cavity behind the iris is known as the **posterior chamber**. Like in the anterior chamber, the fluid here provides nutrients to the surrounding tissues and has immunologically active molecules to protect against foreign particles.

- As light passes through the pupil and posterior chamber, it then crosses the lens. The **lens** contains a gelatinous fluid that can easily change its shape to focus light. The cornea is capable of bending more light than the lens; however, it is not able to be modified. The lens, on the other hand, can change its shape. Small muscles attached to it allow it to flatten and alter the light bending, and thus focus, of the light entering the eye.

- As light continues to travel through the eye, it next enters the large **vitreous chamber**. This final, large fluid-filled cavity makes up the bulk of the eyeball. Its primary role is to maintain the shape of the eyeball and support the lens. The fluid of the vitreous chamber is primarily water and is absent of cells. Two main processes are supported by the vitreous chamber. First is to maintain the shape of the eyeball. The shape of the eye must be predictable. As with our skin, activation of particular sensory receptors indicates a stimulus coming from a particular location. For the skin, that may mean a part of the body. But in the eye, it refers to a portion of the visual world. The bottom portion of the retina, for example, always represents the upper portion of the visual world; and the left portion of the retina always represents the right portion of the visual world. If the sensory neurons in your skin floated around in space, you may confuse a touch on your nose as being on your ear. Likewise, the sensory cells in the back of the retina must maintain their location to accurately encode the location the light is coming from. The vitreous chamber maintains a constant shape of the eyeball so this is possible. The vitreous chamber also helps further bend the light to allow it to spread over a larger amount of the rear of the eyeball.

- Finally, light strikes light-sensitive cells within the **retina**. The retina, which contains the light-sensitive photoreceptors and several other cell layers, forms a layer on the back wall of the vitreous chamber. The **photoreceptor** cells of the retina detect light and make several connections to begin to modify the information before sending it out of the eyeball. Thus, before leaving the retina, the information being detected by the sensory neurons is already processed.

LEARNING OBJECTIVE 6.9.10 Identify the accessory structures of the eye.

LEARNING OBJECTIVE 6.9.11 Identify the functions of the accessory structures of the eye.

KEY TERMS

eye muscles Muscles that attach to the eyelid to cause it to close.

eyebrows Short strip of hair above each eye.

eyelashes Row of hairs that grow on the end of the eyelids.

eyelids Layer of skin that covers the eye to control light, particle, and sweat access to the eyes.

tear ducts Nasal portion of the orbit that excretes a protective fluid.

Accessory Structures of the Eye

Five accessory structures support the eye in sight. The **eyebrows** are a short strip of hair that lie above each eye (Figure 6-39). Their primary role is to prevent sweat or other debris from getting into the eye. We also rely heavily on our eyebrows as a form of nonverbal communication. Similarly, the **eyelashes**, the row of hairs that grow on the end of the eyelids, also prevent small particles from entering the eye. But, bending of the eyelashes serve as a warning that a larger object is too close to the eye in much the same way whiskers function for a cat. The **eyelids** are a layer of skin that covers the eye. By "opening" and "closing," the eyelid controls light, particle, and sweat access to the eye. The eyelids also spread fluid on the surface of the cornea critical to maintain lubrication. The fluid is produced by the **tear ducts** and is released in response to emotions or particles in the eye. The **eye muscles** attach to the eyelid to cause it to close.

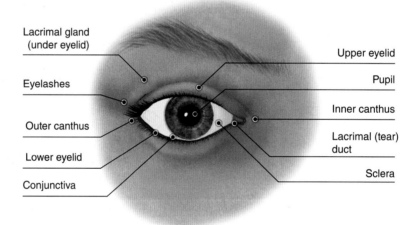

FIGURE 6-39   The accessory structures of the eye protect the eye and help maintain its function.

LEARNING OBJECTIVE 6.9.12   **Identify rods and their visual pigment's function.**

LEARNING OBJECTIVE 6.9.13   **Identify cones and their visual pigment's function.**

LEARNING OBJECTIVE 6.9.14   **Contrast the structure and function of rods and cones.**

KEY TERMS

cones Visual sensory cells specialized to detect color.

rods Visual sensory neurons specialized to detect low light, but only in black and white.

PHOTORECEPTOR CELLS

The retina is a layer on the back of the inner eye (vitreous chamber) that contains many layers of cells involved in visual processing (Figure 6-40). The backmost layer consists of photoreceptors. These are the only light-sensitive cells in our body. We have two types of photoreceptor cells, which differ in their function and location on the retina. We rely on our cones for our best vision.

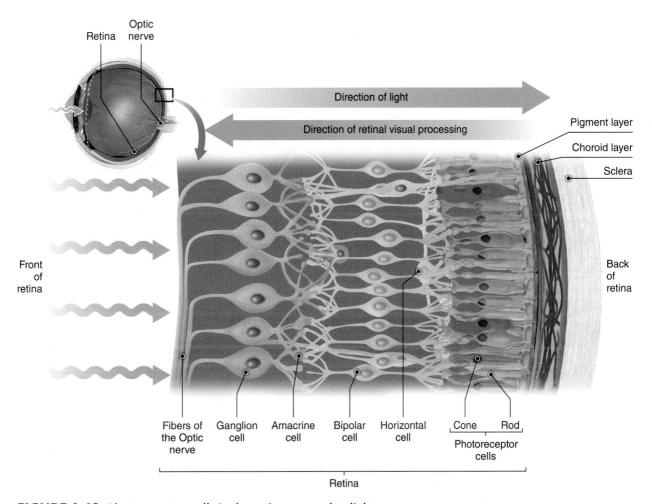

FIGURE 6-40 Photoreceptor cells in the retina respond to light.

The **cones** are light-responsive cells that can detect specific colors. Most people have three types of cones, each most sensitive to a particular color of light. These are named based on the wavelength of light to which they are most sensitive. The S cones detect more short wavelengths of light (420–440 nm; blue), the M cones detect medium wavelengths of light (520–540 nm; green) and the L cones detect longer wavelengths of light (560–580 nm; red). These cones work in pairs to obtain the full color spectrum we perceive. Some individuals lack one or more types of cones, resulting in colorblindness. This does not mean objects of that color are invisible to these individuals. Instead, they have a decreased ability to discriminate between objects of that color. There is a subset of people (mostly female) who are reported to have a fourth type of cone. These individuals can only be detected in the population by using a color discrimination test, and they will perform extremely well. One drawback to cones, however, is they only function in bright conditions. However, the other photoreceptor cell type, **rods**, can detect light under very dim conditions. Rods are unable to differentiate color, resulting in black and white vision. The reason we tend to see in black and white when in dim light (dark room or the evening) is because we primarily rely on rods. The cones are concentrated in one area of the retina, which we rely on for most vision. The rods surround the cones in the periphery of the retina.

Rods and cones have similar structures. Both are long, thin cells, though the rods are slightly longer and thinner. Both photoreceptors are located in the back of the retina with their photosensitive regions facing the rear of the eye. This organization requires light to pass through several layers of cells before striking the rods or cones. In the area of the eye with the best visual ability, the cells are bent in such a way to reduce this. Each photoreceptor cell contains a molecule that can respond to light. When light strikes this molecule, a change inside the cells leads to changes in release of neurotransmitters. There are many versions of these molecules and the specific type determines the wavelengths of light the cell responds to. The rods contain these molecules in a stacked-disc-type structure. The cones, as suggested by their name, have a tapered, cone-like shape with many folds of the cellular membrane in the region that contains the light-sensitive molecules.

LEARNING OBJECTIVE 6.9.15 Explain how the eye refracts light.

KEY TERMS

farsightedness Inability to focus on relatively close objects.

nearsightedness Inability to focus on relatively distant objects.

refraction Bending of light as it passes through different mediums.

REFRACTING LIGHT

Approximately 75% of the back of the eye is covered by the retina. This maximizes the amount of space light that can be detected by the eye. But in order to have light from the world strike the outermost parts of the retina, the light path must be bent. The eye uses **refraction**, or the deflection of light as it passes through different mediums, to bend light as it moves through the eye. This principle is best depicted when a pencil appears disconnected from itself when placed in a glass of water and viewed from the side. Most of the light bending is done by the cornea, mostly due to its curvature. The lens does not bend the light to the same extent, but its ability to change shape allows the amount of refraction to change, ultimately affecting focus. There are muscles attached to the lens that cause it to lengthen when they contract. When the lens is lengthened, the thickness is reduced. Because light travels through less of the lens, the light is less affected and is bent less. Conversely, relaxation of these muscles causes the lens to thicken, resulting in greater bending of the light traveling through. The fluid inside the anterior, posterior, and vitreous chambers also aid in bending the light as it travels to the retina.

Sometimes the refraction provided by the lens, cornea, and fluid-filled chambers does not match the shape of the eyeball. When the eyeball is too long for its focus ability, the light is best focused in front of the retina. This results in nearsightedness, or the inability to focus on objects far away. People who are nearsighted are often able to see close-up objects clearly. On the other hand, some individuals have eyeballs too short for their ability to focus the light. This results in farsightedness, or the inability to focus on near objects. Typically, these individuals can see distant objects clearly.

LEARNING OBJECTIVE 6.9.16 Explain how the brain perceives depth.

LEARNING OBJECTIVE 6.9.17 Explain how the brain perceives distance.

KEY TERMS

depth Ability to see an object three-dimensionally.

distance Ability to determine how far away an object is.

DEPTH AND DISTANCE

Depth is the ability to perceive the world three-dimensionally. This process requires information from both eyes to be processed in the brain. Although each eye is oriented in the same direction (forward) and detect effectively the same visual world, they are slightly offset from one another. You can detect this by closing one eye and placing your thumb to block your view of something in front of your visual field. Then switch eyes and you will notice the object is no longer blocked. But, with both eyes open we do not see two slightly offset images. Our brain combines the images and extracts additional information, which is depth. Subtle differences between the two images are used to provide clues about what object is in front of another object.

However, if you close one eye you will likely still be able to navigate the world reasonably well. This is because our brain uses other things in the image to obtain information about the relative positions of objects in space. Distance refers to the ability to detect the proximity to an object. The great painters of the Renaissance describe this as perspective and the concepts are still used today in movies. From our experience in the world, we know that the same object appears larger when close up than far away. We can also make predictions about the size (and therefore expected distance) based on prior experience, such as seeing a large truck as smaller than a person indicates is further away. The relative movement of an object, such as an airplane flying slowly across the sky, provides information about its distance. You eye also receives feedback from the focal muscles of the lens about whether it is trying to focus on an object that is close or distant.

LEARNING OBJECTIVE 6.9.18 Identify the visual nerve pathways.

KEY TERMS

optic chiasm Location in the brain where visual fibers cross and the optic nerve becomes the optic tract.

optic nerve Cranial nerve II; visualizes sensory information.

optic radiation Axon pathway from the thalamus to the occipital lobe.

optic tract Axon pathway from the optic chiasm to the thalamus.

VISUAL PATHWAYS

As we discussed, information from the left portion of the visual field will be detected by photoreceptor cells in the right side of the retina. Likewise, activity of cells in the left portion of the retina corresponds to the right visual world. This is true in both eyes. However, information is processed in the brain not according to the location of the retina, but the visual world the light is coming from—the right visual world is processed in the left hemisphere and the left visual world is processed in the right hemisphere. Since the left side of both eyes represents the right visual world and vice versa for the right side, neurons representing these signals must come together after leaving the eye.

As we mentioned earlier, the retina contains many layers of cells. In fact, the visual information that is detected by the photoreceptors is altered before ever leaving the retina. There are at least two synapses required for information to leave the retina. Axons from the final layer of cells in the retina make up the optic nerve. The optic nerve leaves the back of the eye toward the brain. As with all sensory information entering the brain, visual information first stops in the thalamus before being transmitted to the occipital lobe in the back of the cerebral cortex. However, before reaching the thalamus the axons need to be reorganized. Information from the left side of the retina of both eyes (representing the right visual world) must travel to the left hemisphere, while information from the right side of the retina of both eyes (representing the left visual world) must travel to the right hemisphere. The optic nerves of both eyes come together at a point termed the optic chiasm. Chiasm means "crossing over." This is the location where the axons representing information from the left part of the right eye switch to the left side of the brain and join with those of the left side of the left eye's retina. Likewise, the axons representing information from the right part of the left eye also cross over to join the axons from the right part of the retina of the right eye. The axons are known as the optic tract. The optic tract are the axons from the optic nerve (there are no synapses in the optic chiasm) reorganized based on the hemisphere they will ultimately terminate. The optic tract then travels to the thalamus. New neurons in the thalamus then project to the occipital lobe in a pathway known as the **optic radiation**. The optical lobe then processes the information with neurons first representing simple visual stimuli (such as orientation of lines) and then representing more complex stimuli (such as simple shapes) and combining as they go to represent complex visual phenomena like buildings (composed of shapes and lines). This hierarchical structure is common for most sensory processing, but is easiest described in terms of vision.

UNIT OBJECTIVE 6.10

Describe pathologies affecting the cells of the nervous system.

UNIT INTRODUCTION

The nervous system is the most complex of the body systems and is very susceptible to damage. There are a variety of disorders caused by or affecting specific cells of the nervous system. Using our knowledge of the role these cells play, we can understand which symptoms are associated with various diseases. In general, a disease can be genetically inherited or acquired through a pathogen or other external stimulus.

LEARNING OBJECTIVE 6.10.1   **Identify common disorders affecting the cells of the nervous system.**

KEY TERMS

Huntington's disease A progressive neurological disorder characterized by uncontrollable movements of the body.

schizophrenia A chronic mental disorder that alters the way a person thinks, feels, acts, and interrupts sensory processing.

COMMON DISORDERS AFFECTING THE CELLS OF THE NERVOUS SYSTEM

Schizophrenia

Schizophrenia is a chronic mental disorder that affects the way a person thinks, feels, acts, and interrupts sensory stimuli. Most individuals with schizophrenia see an onset of symptoms around the age of 18–22. Stress also promotes disease progression, making college students a particularly closely watched group. There is a high genetic link in schizophrenia, with a 50% chance of a monozygotic twin sharing the disease if the other is affected. However, environmental factors likely play a role.

Schizophrenia has two groups of symptoms: positive and negative. Positive symptoms refer to abnormal behaviors that are gained; negative symptoms refer to a loss of a function. Positive symptoms include auditory and/or visual hallucinations, delusions, and excited motor behaviors. Negative symptoms are slowed thought and speech, emotional or social withdrawal, and blunted affect of emotional expression. In the brains of people affected with schizophrenia, we can measure decreased activity in the frontal lobes as well as increased size of the ventricles (due to shrinking of the brain tissue surrounding it).

Treatments for schizophrenia focus on two primary neurotransmitter systems. Typical antipsychotics, which focus on lowering levels of dopamine in the frontal lobe, are effective in decreasing the positive symptoms, especially the movement-related ones. However, some patients do not respond to these drugs and instead use atypical antipsychotics which primarily focus on glutamate signaling. These drugs are effective in treating both the positive and negative symptoms, but may cause weight gain and other motor problems.

Huntington's Disease

Huntington's disease is a progressive neurological disorder caused by a single gene mutation. This disease is characterized by uncontrollable movements of the body but is also associated with cognitive changes including memory impairment, anxiety, depression, and obsessive–compulsive behaviors. Although the normal function of the protein affected by the gene mutation is unknown, a simple blood test provides a diagnosis of Huntington's disease. It is possible to use this test to determine if an individual is afflicted when a family history of Huntington's disease is present prior to symptoms occurring. Genetic counseling is often recommended to individuals with a family history prior to having a child. There is no cure for Huntington's disease. Treatments are ineffective at slowing the progression but can help alleviate symptoms.

LEARNING OBJECTIVE 6.10.2 **Describe the cause, signs, symptoms, and diagnosis of Parkinson's disease.**

KEY TERM

Parkinson's disease A chronic, progressive movement disorder caused by the degradation of the dopamine-producing cells in the area of the brain that initiates movement.

Parkinson's Disease

Parkinson's disease is a chronic, progressive movement disorder in which the dopamine-producing cells in the area of the brain that initiates movements degrade (Figure 6-41). The primary symptoms of Parkinson's disease are tremor, slowness of movement, rigidity, and coordination problems. While it is primarily considered a disease affecting the motor system, there are also cognitive impairments in afflicted individuals. The direct cause of Parkinson's disease is currently unknown, but it is thought to have both genetic and environmental influences.

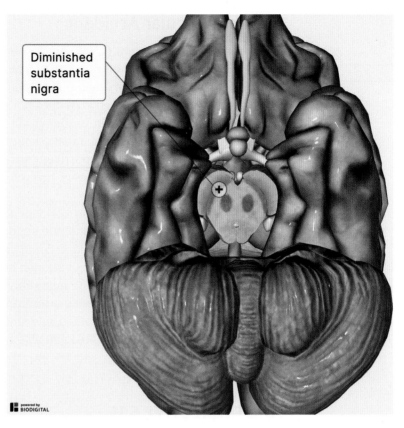

FIGURE 6-41 Parkinson's disease is related to a loss of dopamine-producing neurons in the midbrain.

A confirmed diagnosis of Parkinson's disease is difficult without an autopsy, which specifically measures the loss of the dopamine-containing cells implicated. However, physicians will assess the patient via a medical history and neurological examination. A combination of response to treatment and progression of the disease helps to rule out non-Parkinsonian movement diseases and strengthen the diagnosis. However, there is no cure for Parkinson's disease. Medications for treating Parkinson's are effective in delaying the progression of the disease and primarily focus on various approaches to increase dopamine signaling lost by the dying cells. Deep brain stimulation has become a more common treatment in medication-resistant individuals. This technique implants a neurostimulator that sends impulses to one of many brain areas to help with movement disruptions.

LEARNING OBJECTIVE 6.10.3 Describe the cause, signs, symptoms, and diagnosis of a cerebrovascular accident.

KEY TERM

cerebrovascular accident (CVA) The sudden death of neurons and neuroglia in the brain due to a lack of blood supply to the region. Also known as a stroke.

Cerebrovascular Accident

A **cerebrovascular accident (CVA)**, more commonly known as a stroke, is the sudden death of cells in the brain due to a lack of blood supply to that region. The cells of the brain are very metabolically active and require a constant supply of oxygen. When the disrupted area does not receive blood, the oxygen cannot reach the cells and they begin to die within minutes. Two forms of CVA can occur. An ischemic stroke is the most common and is due to a blockage of the blood vessel by a blood clot. Hemorrhagic strokes occur when the blood vessels feeding an area break. In both cases, an area of the brain does not receive the blood supply it requires.

The exact symptoms of a stroke depend on the area of the brain that is damaged. Common symptoms include sudden weakness of the arm, leg, or face on one side of the body; sudden confusion; sudden vision problems; sudden difficulty with coordination; or sudden headache without a known cause. All symptoms of a stroke come on incredibly rapidly. Diagnosis will include a medical history, particularly paying attention to a history of risk factors such as elevated blood pressure, diabetes, and smoking, as well as a complete neurological exam. A CT scan or MRI can also be used to visualize the damaged areas.

UNIT OBJECTIVE 6.11

Describe pathologies affecting the structural components of a synapse and signal transduction.

UNIT INTRODUCTION

A neuron is a specialized cell for communication both along the axon and between other neurons or other post-synaptic cells, such as muscles, glands, or organs. The synapse is a particularly sensitive area because it relies on signaling outside the cell and many factors can influence function. However, if the axon slows down the action potential propagation, the signals cannot reach the synapse in an efficient manner. In this unit we discuss disorders related to disruptions in neural communication.

LEARNING OBJECTIVE 6.11.1 Identify common disorders affecting the structure and function of a synapse and signal transduction.

KEY TERM

dyskinesia Involuntary, uncontrollable movement of the body typically associated with prolonged treatment for neurological disorders.

COMMON DISORDERS AFFECTING THE STRUCTURE AND FUNCTION OF A SYNAPSE AND SIGNAL TRANSDUCTION

Dyskinesia

Dyskinesia is the involuntary, uncontrollable movement of the body. This can be a standalone disorder, but is often associated with prolonged treatment for drugs that treat Parkinson's disease, antipsychotic medications, or brain injury. The movements range from minor tics of the head or the appearance of fidgeting in the hands to swaying or uncontrollable movements of the body. Diagnosis is difficult and typically relies on behavioral tests as well as blood or imaging to rule out other disorders. Treatments typically involve changing the type or timing of medications causing dyskinesia. Deep brain stimulation can be used when changes in medication are not viable.

LEARNING OBJECTIVE 6.11.2 Describe the cause, signs, symptoms, and diagnosis of organophosphate poisoning.

KEY TERM

organophosphate poisoning A complex response to ingestion of a class of chemicals which prevents the breakdown of acetylcholine in the neuromuscular synapse.

Organophosphate Poisoning

Organophosphates are a class of molecules that inhibit the enzyme that breaks down acetylcholine in the synapse. Organophosphates are commonly used as insecticides, but are also used as medications and even nerve agents. Intentional ingestion or inhalation of organophosphates is a common form of suicide in areas in which the chemicals are common. The molecules can even pass directly through the skin, making chemical-soaked clothing a potential avenue of administration. Regardless of intentional or accidental exposure, organophosphate poisoning results in excessive accumulation of acetylcholine in the synapse. These drugs bind irreversibly with the enzyme, causing long-term blocking. There is an initial hyperstimulation of these receptors followed by a compensation of the post-synaptic cell to reduce activity. Common symptoms include muscle weakness, fatigue, cramps, vomiting, urination, defecation, and excess salivation and tear production. The mnemonic device *SLUDGEM* is often used to remember the symptoms. This corresponds to salivation, lacrimation (tear production), urination, defecation, gastrointestinal distress (cramping), emesis (vomiting), miosis (pupil constriction), and muscle spasm.

Diagnosis of organophosphate poisoning relies on a blood test looking for metabolites of the drugs. Treatments aim to reduce exposure and reverse the chemical effects. Primarily patients should have clothing removed as well as skin cleaned and airways checked for blockages. Two pharmacological treatments can aid in recovery. Pralidoxime displaces the affected enzyme, replacing its activity. Atropine is used to block the receptors that are being overstimulated by the excess acetylcholine.

UNIT OBJECTIVE 6.12

Describe pathologies that affect the basic ways in which the nervous system processes information.

UNIT INTRODUCTION

Neurons, though they come in many shapes and sizes, do not differ greatly in their function. The main determinants of what information a neuron is processing are the inputs. Neurons that receive input from the eyes process vision; those that receive input from the ears process hearing; and those that receive both visual and auditory information are integrating multisensory information. We discuss in this unit how unexpected connections between neurons lead to various disorders.

LEARNING OBJECTIVE 6.12.1 Identify common disorders that affect the way in which the nervous system processes information.

KEY TERM

referred pain Perception of pain in one region of the body when the actual source of the pain is at a distance.

COMMON DISORDERS AFFECTING NERVOUS SYSTEM INFORMATION PROCESSING

Referred Pain

Referred pain is when a person experiences a painful sensation at a location of the body distant from the actual source. It is important to note that this is not imagined pain in any way. There is a real painful stimulus, for example, damage to the heart during a heart attack, but there is an additional painful sensation at other areas, for example, the left arm. There is not a consensus on the exact mechanism, but referred pain is currently thought to be related to pain fibers from the affected area stimulating other neurons in the spinal cord. Nerve damage may also cause referred pain. There is no treatment other than to address the initial painful stimulus.

Describe the condition known as synesthesia.

KEY TERM

synesthesia Abnormal sensory processing in which stimulation of one sensory modality causes a different sensory modality (or cognitive process) to be stimulated.

Synesthesia

Synesthesia is a neurological disorder in which stimulation of one sensory modality causes a different sensory modality (or other cognitive function) to be stimulated. Many forms of synesthesia exist. Some individuals perceive numbers as colors. Many individuals with this form can perform mathematical calculations using colors. Another form is associating sounds with colors. These individuals can literally "see" music. Some individuals associate numbers with locations in space. Interestingly, those with this form of synesthesia are reported to have greater memory than those without it. There are other forms as well. As you can see, people with synesthesia may be considered "improved" over normal-functioning individuals. Many do not recognize their experience as abnormal as they live with it their entire lives, but are more likely to participate in creative activities. The cause for synesthesia is hotly debated. We can say for certain that there is increased crosstalk in the affected domains, but how this occurs has not been determined. There is no treatment and most individuals do not consider the experience negative.

UNIT OBJECTIVE 6.13

Describe pathologies affecting the central nervous system.

UNIT INTRODUCTION

Disorders of the central nervous system help us appreciate all the functions provided by this division of the nervous system. In this section, we discuss various disorders that occur when the central nervous system is damaged or, in some cases, overactive.

Identify common pathologies affecting the central nervous system.

KEY TERMS

Alzheimer's disease A chronic, progressive neurological disorder resulting in dementia, language and mood problems, and other behavioral changes.

concussion Injury to the brain that results in a temporary change in the function of the brain.

meningitis Swelling of the protective layers surrounding the brain and spinal cord.

migraine A painful or throbbing sensation in the head which is often accompanied by nausea, vomiting, or sensitivity to light.

PATHOLOGIES AFFECTING THE CENTRAL NERVOUS SYSTEM

Alzheimer's Disease

Alzheimer's disease is a chronic, progressive neurological disorder that causes brain cells to die, resulting in dementia as well as mood dysregulation, problems with language, loss of motivation, and other behavioral impacts. While some memory loss is a common experience, particularly in older adults, the problems with memory are more substantive and progressive with Alzheimer's disease. Common signs are repeating the same statements, forgetting details of conversations or appointments, getting lost in familiar locations, and even forgetting the names of family members or confusing them with people from their past. The exact cause of Alzheimer's disease is unknown, though both genetic and environmental factors are involved. Definitive diagnosis of Alzheimer's disease requires an autopsy to detect the stereotypical plaques and tangles (buildup of proteins) in the brain (Figure 6-42), but a clinical diagnosis can be performed with a family medical history, neurological exam, family member interviews (to describe the symptoms), and blood tests (primarily to rule out other causes of dementia).

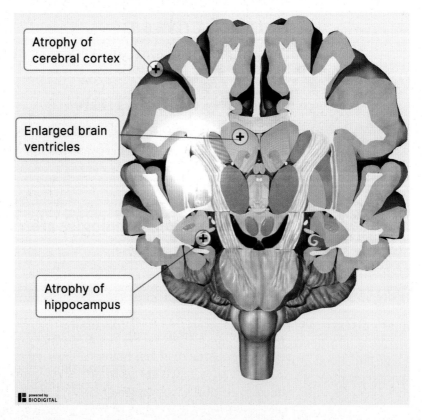

Atrophy of cerebral cortex

Enlarged brain ventricles

Atrophy of hippocampus

FIGURE 6-42 Evidence in the brain of Alzheimer's disease.

There is no cure for Alzheimer's disease and the treatments are focused primarily on relieving the symptoms to elevate the quality of life of the patient.

Concussion

A **concussion** is an injury to the brain that results in a temporary change in function of the brain. Concussions typically are due to a blow to the head or a sudden stopping of the head after moving at a high rate. Often concussions can occur with no external signs of head trauma nor loss of consciousness. People suffering from a concussion will have memory problems, often forgetting the period of time immediately before and after the injury. Depending on the damaged area, a wide array of functions can be affected, including changes in memory, judgment, reflexes, speech, and coordination. Confusion, including an inability to maintain a consistent thought pattern, vomiting, dizziness, and sensitivity to light are tell-tale signs of a concussion. A concussion occurs when the brain is rapidly pushed into the skull. Typically, the cerebrospinal fluid and meninges provide a layer of protection. But, too-rapid acceleration (by hitting the head) or deceleration (by stopping short) makes the brain move with more force than these features can compensate and contact is made. In this way, a concussion can be thought of as a bruised brain. Diagnosis requires neurological testing and may involve brain imaging to look for bleeding or swelling. The best treatment for concussion is preparation and avoidance by wearing protective head gear and avoiding risky activities. Once a concussion occurs, rest is the best approach until symptoms are alleviated. Excessive strain of any kind can prolong the symptoms. A second concussion before the symptoms of the first have been resolved can sometimes result in brain swelling that leads to death.

Meningitis

Meningitis is the swelling of the protective layers (the meninges) surrounding the brain and spinal cord. Meningitis is a result of a pathogenic infection, typically viral. Symptoms include sudden high fever, stiff neck, severe headache (often with nausea), confusion or difficulty concentrating, seizures, and sensitivity to light. The impacts of meningitis depend on the duration of the infection. Brain damage can occur, resulting in hearing loss, memory deficits, and learning disabilities. Seizures, kidney failure, and even death can also occur in extreme cases. While blood culture or neurological imaging may be used for diagnosis, sampling the cerebrospinal fluid via a spinal tap is required for a definitive diagnosis. Depending on the source of the meningitis, treatments may or may not be available. Some vaccines are effective in preventing and antibiotics in treating bacterial meningitis. However, there is no treatment for viral meningitis—time must be taken to allow the virus to run its course.

Migraine

A **migraine** is a painful or throbbing sensation in part or all of the head, often accompanied by nausea, vomiting, and extreme sensitivity to light. In some individuals, the pain can last hours to days, possibly preventing the person from undergoing normal daily activities. Some people with migraines report an aura prior to or during a migraine attack. Some examples of auras include seeing particular shapes or lights, loss of vision, a "pins-and-needles" sensation in the arms and/or legs, and weakness of a body part. A migraine attack may occur several times a week or far less often. Diagnosis of migraine involves medical history and explanation of symptoms. Often brain imaging is used to rule out other causes of severe headaches. A variety of medications are available for treating migraines, with differing effectiveness between individuals. Broadly these medications aim to either prevent the migraine from occurring or treat the pain (or other symptoms) during an attack.

LEARNING OBJECTIVE 6.13.2 Describe the signs, symptoms, and diagnosis of multiple sclerosis.

KEY TERM

multiple sclerosis A presumptive autoimmune disorder resulting in breakdown of the myelin-producing cells of the brain and spinal cord.

Multiple Sclerosis

Multiple sclerosis is thought to be an autoimmune disorder in which the body attacks the myelin-producing oligodendrocytes of the brain and spinal cord. This causes demyelination of the axons, reducing their ability to efficiently send action potentials. Scarring and inflammation of the brain are common indications of multiple sclerosis. The specific cause is currently unknown but is thought to be related to an interaction between genetics and environmental exposure, including viruses. Diagnosis is extremely difficult without an autopsy, but noninvasive imaging techniques may detect the lesions or inflammation. There is no known cure and though some treatments do exist, most have moderate to severe associated adverse effects.

LEARNING OBJECTIVE 6.13.3 Describe the signs, symptoms, and diagnosis of epilepsy.

KEY TERM

epilepsy A group of chronic neurological disorders in which brain activity becomes abnormal, resulting in seizures.

Epilepsy

Epilepsy is a group of chronic neurological disorders in which brain activity becomes abnormal, resulting in seizures. Depending on the area(s) of the brain undergoing the abnormal activity, the symptoms vary widely. A seizure may go completely undetected, may result in a blank stare or confusion, or be more dramatic such as the stereotypical uncontrolled jerking of the arms, legs, and possible rest of body and even loss of consciousness. In some individuals, cognitive symptoms, such as fear or anxiety, can occur due to the seizure.

The exact cause of epilepsy is unknown and can vary by type. Some forms are genetic and inherited within families. Others are caused by head trauma, infection, or developmental disorders. A person with epilepsy may have specific triggers to initiate the seizures (though some are seemingly random). These include lack of sleep, fever, stress, bright or flashing lights, and certain medications or drugs, such as alcohol or nicotine. Though some blood tests can be performed to rule out non-epilepsy seizure-causing disorders, the primary method of diagnosis requires a form of brain recording (typically EEG) while triggering a seizure. Treatments include pharmacological medicines that aim to reduce the seizures, surgery to remove the cells that initiate the seizure, a vagus nerve stimulator that helps reduce seizures, and transition to a ketogenic diet.

UNIT OBJECTIVE 6.14

Describe pathologies affecting the peripheral nervous system.

UNIT INTRODUCTION

The peripheral nervous system, though not as broadly acting as the central nervous system, is still vitally important. Disorders of the peripheral nervous system impact sensory perception, including pain, movement, and control of organs. In this unit we discuss various disorders of the peripheral nervous system. We discuss disorders of the autonomic nervous system, a subdivision of the peripheral nervous system, in the following section.

LEARNING OBJECTIVE 6.14.1 Identify common pathologies affecting the peripheral nervous system.

KEY TERMS

amyotrophic lateral sclerosis (ALS) A chronic, progressive neurological disease that affects the motor neurons of the brain and spinal cord. Also known as Lou Gehrig's disease.

Guillain-Barre syndrome Autoimmune disorder in which the body attacks the peripheral nerve, resulting in pain or muscle weakness.

phantom limb Perceived sensation that an amputated limb is present.

PATHOLOGIES AFFECTING THE PERIPHERAL NERVOUS SYSTEM

Amyotrophic Lateral Sclerosis

Amyotrophic lateral sclerosis (ALS), also known as Lou Gehrig's disease, is a chronic, progressive neurological disease that affects the motor neurons in the brain and spinal cord. ALS is a motor disorder with symptoms of difficulty walking, weakness of the legs and hands, slurred speech, and difficulty maintaining posture. As a progressive disorder, the first symptoms are typically identified in the extremities before spreading to other parts of the body. Some forms of ALS are inherited, but others have no known cause and are likely related to environmental factors or immune malfunctions. Functional test of motor neurons and muscles can be used to diagnose ALS, with many blood or imaging tests used to rule out other potential disorders leading to muscle weakness. While there is no cure for ALS, medications are effective at slowing its progression and medication and a variety of therapies address the symptoms.

Guillain-Barre Syndrome

Guillain-Barre syndrome is a rare autoimmune disorder in which the body attacks the peripheral nerve, resulting in pain or muscle weakness. The first symptoms are typically unexplained sensations, such as tingling in the hands or feet. This is often followed by weakness on both sides of the body. Symptoms of Guillain-Barre syndrome include poor vision, difficulty chewing and swallowing, "pins and needles" in the extremities, pain, and autonomic disruptions including abnormal heart rate, blood pressure, digestive abilities, and bladder control. Guillain-Barre syndrome is now known to be several distinct subtypes, all of which are caused by the immune system attacking an aspect of the peripheral nerve. In some forms the Schwann cells are attacked, causing demyelination. In others the axons themselves are attacked. Because of this, specific diagnosis is difficult. Doctors will take a medical history and possibly examine the cerebrospinal fluid or perform nerve and muscle function tests. The exact cause of Guillain-Barre syndrome is unknown, but infection prior to the symptoms is common. There is no cure. Two treatments aim to speed recovery by either removing the antibodies in the blood attacking the nerves or providing "good" antibodies to counteract the "bad" ones. Even with treatment, full recovery may take 1–3 years.

Phantom Limb

Phantom limb is the perceived sensation that an amputated limb is present. Often, pain is associated as coming from the phantom limb. A classic example of phantom limb pain is described as a missing hand is making a tightly clenched fist without any ability to relax it. Phantom limbs can come following surgical amputation or traumatic injury. It was once thought that phantom limbs were purely psychological, but it is widely accepted that there is a neurological basis. The current belief is the areas of the brain and spinal cord that once represented the amputated limbs become activated by other nearby neurons invading the area left absent from the degeneration of the neurons that once controlled that limb. In this way, phantom limbs are a disease of plasticity. There is no diagnosis as this is a purely subjective disorder. Medications aimed at treating generic pain may be effective in some cases. Other therapies, including viewing the intact limb in a mirror, acupuncture, and spinal cord stimulation, are very successful treatments in many individuals.

LEARNING OBJECTIVE 6.14.2 **Describe the cause, signs, symptoms, and diagnosis of neuropathy.**

KEY TERM

neuropathy Weakness, numbness, or pain resulting from peripheral nerve damage.

Neuropathy

Neuropathy, and in this case specifically peripheral neuropathy, is the weakness, numbness, or pain resulting from peripheral nerve damage. Neuropathy can occur from trauma, infection, metabolic disorders (including diabetes), exposure to chemicals, or even genetic mutations. The symptoms of neuropathy depend on the nerve and extent of the damage. Common symptoms include numbness or tingling in the feet or hands projecting into the limb, sharp or throbbing pain, sensitivity to touch, lack of coordination or muscle weakness, and paralysis. A medical history and neurological exam are used in diagnosis and a variety of blood, imaging, and nerve function tests can be used to determine the specific type (or cause) of neuropathy. Treatments include medications to address the pain or other symptoms as well as therapies, such as electrical stimulation or physical therapy.

LEARNING OBJECTIVE 6.14.3 **Describe the cause, signs, symptoms, and diagnosis of myasthenia gravis.**

KEY TERM

myasthenia gravis Autoimmune neuromuscular disorder characterized by antibodies destroying acetylcholine receptors in muscle tissue.

Myasthenia Gravis

Myasthenia gravis is a chronic autoimmune disease in which the body produces antibodies that attack the acetylcholine receptors in the neuromuscular junction of the synapse between motor neurons and skeletal muscle. This leads to progressive muscle weakness of all skeletal muscles. Typically, the symptoms first occur around the eyes, before spreading to the face, head, and then the arms, legs, and chest. This, unfortunately, may also affect the diaphragm, leading to breathing problems. A hallmark of myasthenia gravis is the symptoms decreasing following periods of rest and becoming worse when active. Blood tests, genetic tests, and muscle recordings are used by a physician to diagnose myasthenia gravis. While there is no cure, the symptoms can be treated through a variety of options, including treating the blood to remove the antibodies, immunotherapy to decrease the body's response to the antibodies, surgery, and medications that alter the activity at the synapse.

UNIT OBJECTIVE 6.15

Describe pathologies affecting the autonomic nervous system.

UNIT INTRODUCTION

The autonomic nervous system regulates organ function and plays a key role in body homeostasis. Disorders that affect the autonomic nervous system cause a wide variety of changes such as heart rate, blood pressure, body temperature, and loss of bowel and bladder control. Some disorders lead to cognitive effects as well. In this unit we discuss disorders of the autonomic nervous system.

LEARNING OBJECTIVE 6.15.1 Identify common pathologies affecting the autonomic nervous system.

KEY TERMS

diabetic autonomic neuropathy Nerve damage of neurons in the autonomic nervous system due to complications of diabetes resulting in autonomic dysregulation.

Shy-Drager syndrome See multiple systems atrophy.

COMMON PATHOLOGIES AFFECTING THE AUTONOMIC NERVOUS SYSTEM

Diabetic Autonomic Neuropathy

Diabetes is a disorder in which glucose is not properly delivered to tissues. Neurons, because of their high metabolic requirements, are particularly susceptible to damage in those with diabetes. Diabetic autonomic neuropathy is nerve damage specifically of neurons of the autonomic nervous system. As the function of these neurons is to regulate organ function, diabetic autonomic neuropathy is particularly dangerous. The specific symptoms depend on which nerves are affected but include dizziness or fainting, problems in urinating, sexual dysfunction, digestive problems, disruptions in normal sweating, slowed pupil response, and exercise intolerance. Diagnosis involves a variety of autonomic functional and blood sugar tests. The primary treatment is to address the underlying diabetes.

Multiple System Atrophy

Multiple system atrophy, also known as Shy-Drager syndrome, is a rare, chronic, progressive neurodegenerative disorder that particularly affects the autonomic nervous system as well as the motor systems. Multiple system atrophy shares many symptoms, and even a cellular marker, with Parkinson's disease. Symptoms include Parkinson's-like motor impairments, such as slowness of movements, tremor, rigidity, poor coordination, and slurred speech, as well as autonomic-specific impairments, including increased likelihood of fainting when getting up rapidly or bladder control problems. The cause of multiple system atrophy is unknown and largely appear seemingly at random. Due to the stated similarity with Parkinson's disease, it is particularly difficult to diagnose. Neurological exams, brain imaging, and autonomic function tests are typically utilized. There is no cure or treatment to slow the progression of multiple systems atrophy. Medications effective in treating Parkinson's disease or treating other symptoms are often used to improve quality of life.

LEARNING OBJECTIVE 6.15.2 Describe the relationship between pheochromocytoma and the autonomic nervous system.

KEY TERM

pheochromocytoma Noncancerous tumor on the adrenal gland that results in excess hormone release causing high blood pressure, headaches, sweating, and other symptoms.

Pheochromocytoma

Pheochromocytoma is a noncancerous tumor on the adrenal gland that results in elevated hormone release from the gland. The hormones produced by the adrenal gland have diverse effects in the body, many of which mimic the effects of the sympathetic nervous system. Keep in mind that the target organ cannot detect the source of a chemical. Even though hormones act over long distances and neurotransmitters are released more locally, the effect on the target organ will not differ. Thus, a wide range of symptoms can occur in pheochromocytoma, including high blood pressure, headaches, sweating, rapid heartbeat, tremors, and shortness of breath. Diagnosis typically involves measuring the amount of epinephrine in the urine over a day, followed by imaging of the adrenal gland to visualize the tumor. The only treatment for pheochromocytoma is surgery to remove the tumor.

UNIT OBJECTIVE 6.16

Describe pathologies affecting sensory functions and the brain interpretation of sensory stimuli.

UNIT INTRODUCTION

We interact with the world around us through our sensory systems. When changes occur in the processing of or interpretation of sensory stimuli, it becomes difficult to accurately understand the world. In this unit we discuss two examples in which changes in stimulus intensity or sensations which do not match reality.

Identify common pathologies affecting sensory functions and the brain's interpretation of sensory stimuli.

sensory processing disorder Condition in which one or more senses are improperly processed by the brain.

COMMON PATHOLOGIES AFFECTING SENSORY FUNCTIONS

Sensory Processing Disorders

Sensory processing disorder is a condition in which one or more senses are improperly processed by the brain. Depending on the individual, this may be hypersensitivity to a particular stimulus or decreased responsiveness to a stimulus. Specific symptoms related to hypersensitivity include extreme responses to sudden or loud sounds, easily distracted, fearful of being touched, or dislike of being in crowds. The symptoms related to decreased sensitivity to stimuli include heightened desire to touch people or objects, lower-than-normal understanding of personal space, uncoordinated movements, high tolerance for pain, difficulty sitting still, and being a "thrill seeker." The causes of sensory processing disorder are not known, though genetic links and changes in brain function have been identified. Both proper diagnosis and treatment utilize behavioral approaches.

Describe how hallucinations are interpreted by the brain.

hallucinations Sensory sensation that appear real but are created without the appropriate sensory input.

Hallucinations

Hallucinations are sensory sensations that appear real but are created without the appropriate sensory input, entirely by the mind. These can occur in any sense, but are often thought about in the visual or auditory domains—seeing an object that is not present or hearing a sound that is not occurring. Hallucinations can be indicative of a psychiatric problem, but also occur in seemingly normal individuals. A common hallucination occurring today is the phantom mobile phone vibration. This is the sensation that a phone in the pocket that it is typically kept in is vibrating. This can occur regardless of the presence of the phone in the pocket and has been reported to occur while the individual is using the phone. The more extreme forms of hallucinations are caused by mental illness, such as schizophrenia or some forms of dementia, drugs, seizures, sensory deprivation, tumors, and other causes. Depending on the cause of the hallucinations (and the extent to which they are affecting the individual), the treatments may range from nothing to antipsychotic medications.

UNIT OBJECTIVE 6.17

Describe pathologies of the four special senses.

UNIT INTRODUCTION

The special senses require specialized organs to interpret sensory stimuli. The intricate nature of these organs provides their ability to function but also make them sensitive to a number of pathologies. In this unit we discuss some disorders of the special senses and how they impact the ability to detect the respective stimulus.

LEARNING OBJECTIVE 6.17.1 **Identify common pathologies of the special senses.**

KEY TERMS

tinnitus Perception of ringing, or other repetitive sounds, in the ears without the sound being present.

vestibular schwannoma Noncancerous tumor on the Schwann cells surrounding the

vestibulocochlear nerve which can result in disruption of auditory or vestibular senses.

COMMON PATHOLOGIES OF THE SPECIAL SENSES

Tinnitus

Tinnitus is the perception of a ringing, or other repetitive sounds, in the ears despite no sound occurring in the world. Tinnitus is a symptom, not a disorder itself, and typically is not indicative of a major problem. Tinnitus can occur with a variety of diseases (especially sinus infections), high blood pressure, brain tumors, or hormonal changes. Some medications and prolonged exposure to loud sounds can also cause tinnitus. The most common form of tinnitus occurs prior to normal hearing loss in older adults. Diagnosis typically relies on the subjective description by the patient, but may involve a hearing test and brain imaging. The best treatment is prevention, as no medications are effective. Hearing aids can help in some cases when the patient also has diminished hearing.

Vestibular Schwannoma

A **vestibular schwannoma** is a noncancerous, typically slow-growing tumor on the Schwann cells surrounding the vestibulocochlear nerve. The size and exact location of the tumor will impact the symptoms experienced, including hearing loss, tinnitus, and balance and coordination problems. An especially large tumor can impinge the facial nerve, leading to weakness or paralysis of the muscles of the face. Only if the tumor presses against the brainstem is there any risk of death. The cause is currently unknown, though an uninherited genetic mutation has been linked to development of a vestibular schwannoma. Diagnosis will involve hearing or coordination tests followed by imaging to visualize the tumor. Treatment may not be necessary and monitoring is the best course of action in that case. Radiation therapy or surgery are the alternate options in more extreme cases.

LEARNING OBJECTIVE 6.17.2 **Describe the signs, symptoms, and diagnosis of sensorineural and conductive hearing loss.**

KEY TERMS

conductive hearing loss Decrease or complete loss of the ability to hear due to something, such as a blockage or infection, preventing sound waves from affecting the inner ear structure.

sensorineural hearing loss Decrease or complete loss of the ability to hear due to damage to the cochlea or vestibulocochlear nerve.

Disorders of Hearing

As we have discussed, the process of hearing involves numerous intricate structures of the inner, middle, and outer ear. Damage to any of these can result in hearing loss. While brain damage can also result in hearing loss, the primary causes are in the ear and can be divided into two main categories, based on the area damaged.

- **Sensorineural hearing loss** is a decrease or complete loss of the ability to hear due to damage to the cochlea or vestibulocochlear nerve. This permanent form of hearing loss is the most common form. This can be due to genetic or developmental factors, head trauma, infection, drug side effects, or even loud noises. A single loud sound, such as a gunshot, or prolonged exposure to loud sounds, such as listening to headphones too loudly for years, can both lead to sensorineural hearing loss. Common locations of damage are the cells in the cochlea that respond to sound or nerve damage. Diagnosis involves obtaining a complete medical history and a variety of specific hearing tests to determine the form of hearing loss. Treatments depend on the severity and location of the damage. Technology surrounding cochlear implants or direct stimulation of the cochlear nerve has made great strides in recent years. It is worth noting that many in the deaf community do not desire treatment nor look at hearing loss as a deficit.

- When the inner ear structures are working properly but something is preventing the sound to reach these structures, it is termed **conductive hearing loss**. Blockages of the ear canal can occur from excess earwax, infection of the outer ear, or abnormal growth causing the ear canal to close. The most common cause in the middle ear is fluid buildup often from infection, which prevents the ossicles from working properly, or a developmental issue with the ossicles. Anything that dampens the sound before reaching the cochlea will result in conductive hearing loss. Conductive forms of hearing loss may be permanent but typically can be corrected. A doctor will obtain a detailed medical history and use various hearing tests to determine the form of hearing loss. Depending on the exact cause of conductive hearing loss will determine the treatment, but may include surgery to remove the blockage, treatment for the underlying condition, or a hearing aid or cochlear implant.

LEARNING OBJECTIVE **6.17.3** **Describe common disorders relating to vision.**

KEY TERMS

cataract Clouding of the lens of the eye leading to a reduction in the sharpness of vision.

glaucoma Group of disease characterized by increased pressure in the eye that can result in vision loss due to damage to the optic nerve.

macular degeneration vision loss due to breakdown of the region of the retina that we most rely on for our most accurate vision.

Disorders of Vision

As humans, we rely heavily on our sense of vision. The eye is an especially complex and sensitive organ. You know this because even the smallest grain of sand in your eye can be extremely painful and may limit vision. Here we focus on some major eye disorders and their causes, symptoms, and treatments.

- **Glaucoma** is a group of diseases that result in optic nerve damage typically due to increased pressure in the eye. A person with glaucoma may first experience peripheral vision loss before extending into central vision. Most forms of glaucoma are not associated with pain, but some forms are painful. The majority of glaucoma is caused by elevated pressure in the anterior chamber of the eye due to poor drainage of the fluid. High pressure in the eye pushes on the optic nerve, causing damage that leads to vision loss. Glaucoma has many correlated genetic factors but can also be caused by external factors such as diabetes or prolonged steroid use. To diagnose glaucoma several eye tests, including visual field and measuring eye pressure, are conducted. There is no cure for glaucoma. Treatments aim at preventing progression of vision loss rather than reversing the effects by lowering eye pressure.

- A **cataract** is the clouding of the lens of the eye causing a reduction in the sharpness of vision. A cataract can also cause vision to obtain a brownish tint due to discoloration in the lens. The symptoms are progressive, including dimmed or clouded vision, sensitivity to light, decreased night vision, rapid prescription changes, and double vision in the affected eye. Cataracts occur during aging as proteins normally found in the lens form abnormal clumps, which cause the cloudy occlusions. Genetics plays a large role in the likelihood of developing cataracts, but other factors such as diabetes, eye trauma, ultraviolet radiation, smoking, and some medications have also been linked. A vision test and visual exam, together with medical history, are used to diagnose cataracts. If the impact of cataracts cannot be addressed with glasses, surgery in which the lens is replaced with an artificial lens is the only treatment.

- **Macular degeneration** is vision loss due to breakdown of the portion of the retina that we primarily rely for our most accurate vision. Macular degeneration is the primary cause of vision loss and typically occurs without pain. Symptoms include visual distortions, reduced vision, requiring brighter light, decreased ability to adapt to low-light situations, and difficulty recognizing faces. Because only a small region of the retina is affected, typically peripheral vision is maintained. The exact cause of macular degeneration is currently unknown, though genetics, age, smoking, high blood pressure, and high cholesterol are linked. An eye doctor will diagnose retina degeneration with a vision test and by examining the back of the retina. There is no cure for macular degeneration and treatments for the common form are mostly ineffective. Some medications can slow the progression of symptoms and new therapies aim at improving the quality of life by helping the patient adapt to the reduced visual abilities.

Chapter 7

The Endocrine System

Chapter Introduction

In this chapter, you learn how the endocrine system is involved in integrating aspects of life, including growth, metabolism, and adaptation, to a constantly changing environment. We also discuss how hormonal imbalances can be recognized, diagnosed, and treated. The endocrine system is the second greatest control system in the body.

UNIT OBJECTIVE 7.1

Explain the role of the endocrine system and hormones in homeostasis.

UNIT INTRODUCTION

When imbalances occur in our body, we have a built-in control system that can easily respond and adjust our internal environment to address the changes. This process is well controlled by the endocrine system.

LEARNING OBJECTIVE 7.1.1 Identify the structure of exocrine glands.

KEY TERMS

exocrine gland Gland that secretes a substance onto the surface of the body using a duct.

exocytosis Process where products are moved from the cytoplasm of the cell to the plasma membrane where they are packaged and ultimately released from the cell.

STRUCTURE OF EXOCRINE GLANDS

The endocrine system is composed of both exocrine and endocrine glands, both of which differ in structure and function. An **exocrine gland** consists of one or more cells that synthesize a product to be secreted onto an epithelial layer when signaled to do so (Figure 7-1AB).

Exocrine glands can either be unicellular or multicellular. Unicellular glands will secrete their products directly onto the surface of epithelial layers or internal body cavities through the process of exocytosis. **Exocytosis** is a process where secretory products are moved from the cytoplasm of the cell to the plasma membrane prepared for secretion, and ultimately released

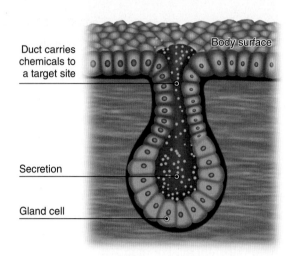

Duct carries
chemicals to
a target site

Body surface

Secretion

Gland cell

A Exocrine gland (has duct)

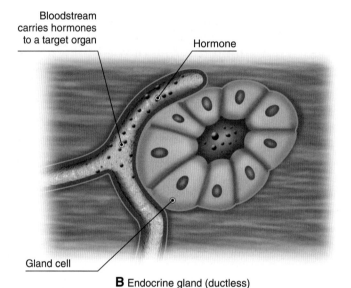

Bloodstream
carries hormones
to a target organ

Hormone

Gland cell

B Endocrine gland (ductless)

FIGURE 7-1AB Exocrine glands excrete their products onto
the body surface (A), while endocrine
glands (B) are ductless and secrete
their hormones into the bloodstream
or surrounding interstitial fluid.

from the cell. Examples of unicellular exocrine glands include mucous and goblet cells that line the internal portions of intestinal and respiratory tracts, both of which secrete mucous to lubricate and protect cellular layers from trauma and pathogenic invasion (Figure 7-2).

Multicellular exocrine glands are structurally more complex and utilize an epithelial duct system that allows for the transfer of the product from where its produced to the epithelial or body cavity surface where it is released. Examples of multicellular glands include gastric, duodenal, sebaceous, mammary, and salivary glands (Figure 7-2).

Exocrine glands

Unicellular
Mucus cells or goblet cells

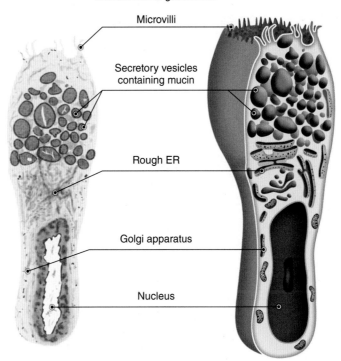

Microvilli

Secretory vesicles
containing mucin

Rough ER

Golgi apparatus

Nucleus

Multicellular
Duct structure

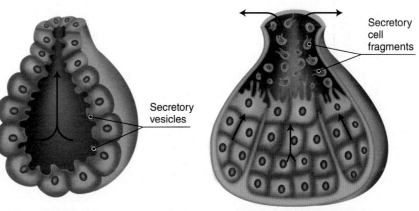

Secretory
cell
fragments

Secretory
vesicles

Merocrine glands secrete
their products by exocytosis

In holocrine glands, the entire
secretory cell ruptures, releasing
secretions and dead cell fragments

FIGURE 7-2 Exocrine glands can be either unicellular or multicellular.
Unicellular glands create their own products and are mostly
represented by mucus or goblet cells.

LEARNING OBJECTIVE **7.1.2** **Describe the function of exocrine glands.**

KEY TERM

comedo A follicle on the skin that becomes clogged with sebum, dead skin cells, and bacteria. Usually occurring in the setting of acne and over-production of androgens that may increase bodily secretions.

FUNCTION OF EXOCRINE GLANDS

Exocrine glands exist to aid in cellular metabolism, tissue lubrication, and protection. Each of these tasks is dependent upon the substance that is made by the cells within the gland. For instance, serous cells aid in intracellular metabolism in the gastrointestinal tract through the exocytosis of proteins and enzymes. The mucous cells that we discussed earlier are more for tissue lubrication of the internal epithelium layers like the mouth, trachea, and esophagus. Along with mucous cells, we have salivary glands located in our mouth that are exocrine glands that secrete enzymes onto the tongue to aid in the beginning of digestion of nutrients.

CLINICAL TIP	Acne, a very common teenage problem, is related to the increase in sebum by sebaceous glands in response to alternating levels of the hormone's testosterone and estrogen. Increased production of sebum can lead to a blockage of the sebaceous duct, causing a comedo. A **comedo** is an obstructed hair follicle that accumulates sebum.

LEARNING OBJECTIVE **7.1.3** **Identify the structure of endocrine glands.**

LEARNING OBJECTIVE **7.1.4** **Describe the function of endocrine glands.**

LEARNING OBJECTIVE **7.1.5** **Contrast the structure and function of exocrine and endocrine glands.**

KEY TERM

extracellular space Fluid surrounding tissue or cells within the body.

STRUCTURE OF ENDOCRINE GLANDS

While exocrine glands are important to the body's overall function, the hormones we discuss later in this chapter are produced by endocrine glands. Therefore, it is important to understand the main difference between structures. Unlike exocrine glands, endocrine glands are considered ductless (Figure 7-1). Made up of thousands of individual cells, these glands can release large amounts of hormones into the surrounding tissue fluid known as the extracellular space. Most of the hormone-producing cells in the endocrine glands are arranged in clusters that maximize their contact between the extracellular space and associated capillaries. This structure allows for the easy passage of secreted hormones into the bloodstream.

FUNCTION OF ENDOCRINE GLANDS

Endocrine glands are responsible for the production and secretion of hormones that regulate growth and a large number of processes involved in everyday homeostasis. In response to stimuli that disrupt our homeostatic balance, specific endocrine glands will begin to secrete their specialized hormones. While exocrine glands like endocrine glands do secrete hormones that aide in maintaining homeostatic imbalances, they also help to regulate body temperature by releasing heat in the form of sweat onto the skin along with regulating the bacterial environment on the surface of the skin. We discuss the major types of hormones and their functions later.

LEARNING OBJECTIVE 7.1.6 List the major function of hormones.

KEY TERMS

hormones Chemical substances, secreted by endocrine glands, that target another tissue in the body.

target cells Cells that can be affected by hormones.

ROLE OF HORMONES

The endocrine system is one of the body's two major regulatory systems. While the nervous system is a rapid response to stimuli, the endocrine system primarily controls processes that require duration and concerted efforts between multiple organs or body systems. To achieve such a continuous process, the endocrine system utilizes hormones, chemical messengers secreted by cells into the extracellular fluid. These messengers travel through the blood and regulate the metabolic function of cells that can be affected by hormones called target cells.

The hormone's entrance into or binding of a cellular receptor on the surface of a target cell initiates a response that can produce three main effects:

- The hormone can cause the cell to uptake more of a product, like glucose.
- The hormone can turn on or turn off the target cell to make new proteins along with additional hormones that can be used for further signaling.

- The hormone can change a cell's shape so it can carry out a specific function.

Depending on the hormone secreted and the target cell to which it binds (which is discussed later in this chapter), there will be a specific response aimed at regulating the overall homeostasis in our body.

For the sake of clarity, we say that hormones have five main roles that contribute to overall homeostasis:

1. Control of growth and development
2. Control of metabolism
3. Maintenance of fluid balances
4. Maintenance of chemical and electrolyte balances
5. Control of various sexual processes

LEARNING OBJECTIVE 7.1.7 Explain how hormones can be classified based on their chemical structure.

KEY TERMS

amines Small modified amino acids.

nonsteroid hormones Hormones created by molecules and chemicals that do not contain a cholesterol compound in the basic structure of the hormone.

steroid hormones Chemical messengers derived from a cholesterol molecule.

CHEMICAL STRUCTURE OF A HORMONE

Hormones vary in their chemical structure, which affects how they interact with a target cell. Generally, there are two types of hormones. Steroid hormones are lipid-based chemical messengers derived from cholesterol. Nonsteroid hormones are composed of three basic building blocks. The first and most simple construct are amines, which are modified amino acids. Next, we have nonsteroidal hormones that are created by peptides. And lastly, we have nonsteroidal hormones created by proteins. Protein-based hormones are far and away from the most abundant type of hormone we have in our body.

LEARNING OBJECTIVE 7.1.8 Identify the structure and function of steroid hormones.

KEY TERM

hydrophobic Nonpolar molecules that repel water.

STEROID HORMONES

Because cholesterol is a chemical compound composed of strictly hydrogen and carbon bonds, it is extremely lipid soluble (Figure 7-3). Lipid-soluble substances can also be described as **hydrophobic**, which are nonpolar molecules that repel water. Interestingly, these hormones pass through the plasma membrane directly into the cell.

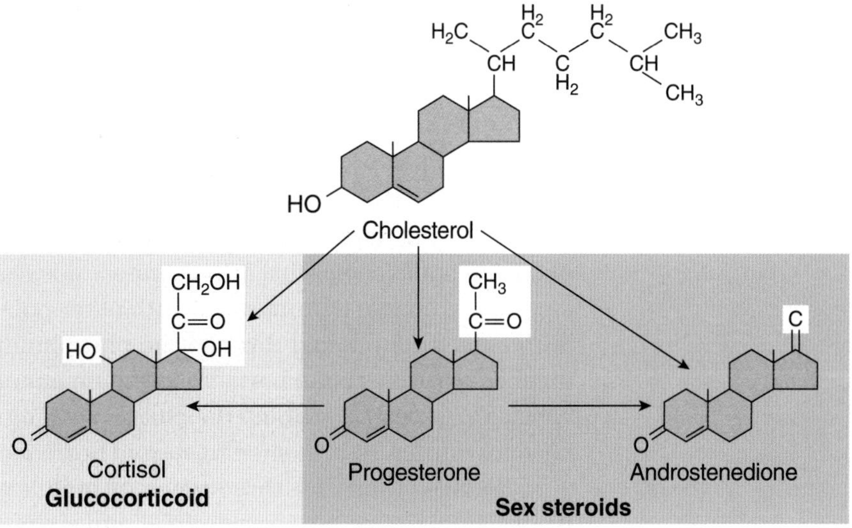

FIGURE 7-3 Cholesterol-based hormones are usually lipid based and contribute to the proper function of steroid hormones.

Gonadal and adrenocortical hormones are examples of hormones derived from cholesterol. Gonadal hormones help us control sexual processes while adrenocortical hormones aid in metabolism, growth and development, fluid balance, and electrolyte balance. Table 7-1 lists examples of each. We discuss their specific functions later in the chapter.

Table 7-1 Classification of Hormones Based on Chemical Structure

CHEMICAL STRUCTURE	SUBTYPE	EXAMPLES
Steroid (cholesterol)	Gonadal	Testosterone, estradiol, progesterone
	Adrenocortical	Aldosterone, cortisol, testosterone, androgens
Nonsteroid	Amino acid	Triiodothyronine, thyroxine, norepinephrine, epinephrine
	Peptide/protein	adrenocorticotropic hormone, antidiuretic hormone, oxytocin, parathyroid hormone, atrial natriuretic peptide, glucagon, insulin, gastrin, leptin

LEARNING OBJECTIVE 7.1.9 Identify the structure and function of nonsteroid hormones.

NONSTEROIDAL HORMONES

The majority of amino acids that create nonsteroidal hormones contain a **hydrophilic** (polar molecules that attract water) side chain. Hydrophilic chains contain a polarized charge that interacts with other polar molecules, prohibiting these hormones from passing through the phospholipid bilayer of the cell. A small number of nonsteroidal hormones contain amino acids with hydrophobic side chains that evenly distribute the charge, making the amino acid nonpolar. This chemical structure is likened to steroid hormones but is very rare.

Because there are three types of building blocks for nonsteroidal hormones, they can be further classified into amines, peptides, and proteins.

Amine Hormones

Amines are modified amino acids that make up melatonin, **catecholamines**, and thyroid hormones (Table 7-1). Generally, these hormones control circadian rhythms, sympathetic nervous system response, and metabolism.

Peptide Hormones

Peptide hormones are formed by short chains of amino acids. Table 7-1 lists examples of each, but generally they are involved in the control of metabolism, fluid, and electrolyte balance.

Protein Hormones

Proteins are composed of longer chains of amino acids, all of which are hydrophilic. Because protein hormones are the most abundant, they are responsible for:

- Reproduction, growth, and development
- Maintenance of electrolyte, water, and nutrient balance
- Cellular metabolism
- Immunologic response

LEARNING OBJECTIVE **7.1.10** Contrast how steroid and nonsteroidal hormones signal their target cells.

KEY TERMS

second messengers Molecules within the cell that respond to a change in environment due to hormonal activation. These signals are responsible for carrying out the specific job of the hormone that attached to the surface of the target cell.

target receptors Molecules inserted into or on the surface of the plasma membrane of a target cell. These compounds allow for hormone activation of the cell.

TARGET CELL ACTIVATION

All major hormones circulate in the bloodstream but only elicit their effects on the tissues that contain their target cells, which express **target receptors**. Target receptors are chemical structures embedded within the plasma membrane, cytoplasm, or nucleus that contain a specific binding site that only the intended hormone can attach to.

It is important to understand that only cells with target receptors for a given hormone will respond to it. For example, many types of cells have receptors for the hormone cortisol. Cortisol is a hormone that we discuss in more detail later on, but because its target receptor can be found on so many different types of tissue, it has widespread effects on the body. Conversely, if a target receptor for a certain hormone is limited to only a certain type of organ, then the hormone will have more of a specialized role.

Regardless of its classification, once a hormone identifies its tissue, target receptors can become activated in one of two ways. The mode of activation depends on the chemical structure of the hormone.

Steroid Hormone Activation

As we discussed, steroid hormones are lipid soluble, allowing them to easily diffuse across the cell membrane of their target cells. Once inside, the hormone binds to its target receptor, allowing it to enter the nucleus and interact with a particular segment of the cell's DNA that causes a secondary response from the cell (Figure 7-4).

Nonsteroidal Hormone Activation

Because nonsteroidal hormones are hydrophilic, they cannot cross the plasma membrane. Therefore, they act on target receptors embedded within the plasma membrane of the target cell. Binding of target receptors on the plasma membrane initiates a hormonal response that will be carried out by **second messengers** inside of the cytoplasm. Second messengers are a group of molecules that relay the signal created by the nonsteroidal hormone and target receptor

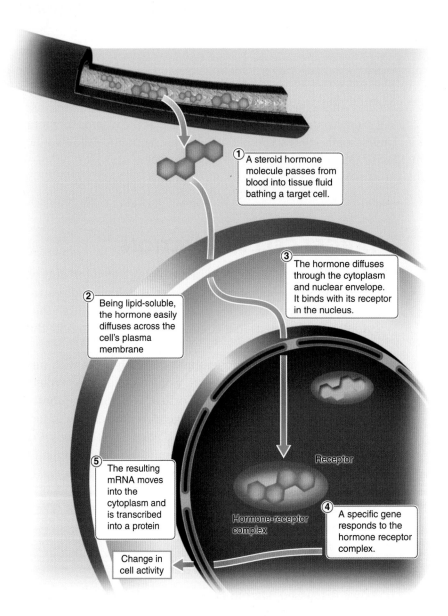

FIGURE 7-4 Because steroid hormones are hydrophobic, they have an ability to cross the plasma membrane without a carrier protein or secondary receptors. This allows the hormone to directly enter the nucleus and alter the DNA complex, creating a specific response by the target cell.

complex. Second messengers will activate other chemicals that participate in cellular secretion, gene activation, or other target cell responses. As a result, nonsteroidal hormones can initiate intracellular changes within the tissue without even crossing the plasma membrane (Figure 7-5).

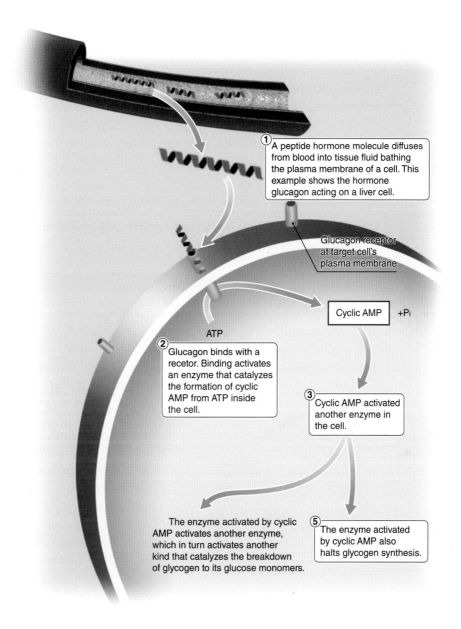

①A peptide hormone molecule diffuses from blood into tissue fluid bathing the plasma membrane of a cell. This example shows the hormone glucagon acting on a liver cell.

Glucagon receptor at target cell's plasma membrane

Cyclic AMP +Pi

ATP

②Glucagon binds with a recetor. Binding activates an enzyme that catalyzes the formation of cyclic AMP from ATP inside the cell.

③Cyclic AMP activated another enzyme in the cell.

The enzyme activated by cyclic AMP activates another enzyme, which in turn activates another kind that catalyzes the breakdown of glycogen to its glucose monomers.

⑤The enzyme activated by cyclic AMP also halts glycogen synthesis.

FIGURE 7-5 Because nonsteroidal hormones are hydrophobic, they cannot pass through the plasma membrane. Therefore, these hormones utilize secondary messengers that begin with a cell surface receptor and internal second messengers that will cause a change in the target cell.

Under normal conditions, insulin, which is a peptide hormone, binds to insulin receptors on cellular membranes of tissues that help to store or utilize glucose. The secondary messengers activated by this hormone-receptor complex creates a glucose transporter, which is protein that is usually stored in the plasma membrane of the target cells, to be placed on the plasma membrane. Placing the glucose transporter on the plasma membrane allows glucose to freely cross into the target cells for storage and utilization.

A patient who continuously consumes a diet high in sugars and carbohydrates causes target cells to be constantly bombarded by insulin. Over time, target cells will develop a tolerance to these high insulin levels and stop responding properly. As a result, less glucose transporters will be embedded within the plasma membrane, leading to an increase in the patient's hyperglycemic state. When this happens, we call these patients *insulin resistant*. Conversely, if there is too much insulin release, then the patient can become dangerously low in blood sugar.

LEARNING OBJECTIVE 7.1.11 Identify common negative feedback mechanisms.

KEY TERM

negative feedback   When a product of the stimulus leads to the decrease or inhibition of the original stimulus that caused the original increase in the product.

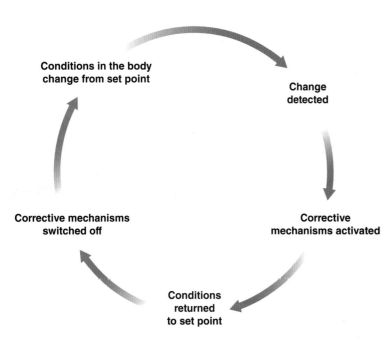

Conditions in the body change from set point

Change detected

Corrective mechanisms switched off

Corrective mechanisms activated

Conditions returned to set point

FIGURE 7-6 Feedback regulation is a cyclical process that begins with an activation of a receptor via a stimulus. This response creates a change that will aim to reduce or feedback upon the original stimulus.

FEEDBACK REGULATION

Because our body is always in a state of dynamic equilibrium, we are constantly adjusting to environmental stimuli. Once we respond to a change in our environment, we have to ensure that we can turn off this response. Therefore, our body has a built-in mechanism known as negative feedback. Negative feedback occurs when the product of a stimulus leads to the decrease or inhibition of the original stimulus that caused it. As a result, the original stimulus in negative feedback loops leads to the creation of its own inhibitor (Figure 7-6).

THERMOREGULATION

Thermoregulation is a classic example of how negative feedback mechanisms work to inhibit the original stimulus.

When body temperature levels rise above 37°C (98.6°F) due to exercise, fever, or hot climates, the hypothalamus becomes activated. Through a series of upregulation of specific hormones (discussed later), the hypothalamic regulatory centers can cause sweat glands to begin to secrete perspiration onto the surface of the skin. This will begin to cool the body and release heat. A reduction in body temperature and return to the normal 37°C benchmark will effectively shut off the hypothalamic regulatory center.

CLINICAL TIP   Think of the body as a giant thermostat in a home heating system. Sensors in the thermostat can detect temperature changes in the home. If the temperature drops below the set point that you have entered into the thermostat, the heating system is activated. Hot air begins to enter the room until the temperature in the room has reached the set point you determined. The heat will then turn off as equilibrium has been reached in the room.

LEARNING OBJECTIVE 7.1.12 Describe how negative feedback mechanisms function.

LEARNING OBJECTIVE 7.1.13 Explain how negative feedback mechanisms control hormone secretions.

KEY TERMS

control center Area in which the input from the receptor is analyzed in the negative feedback loop. Usually the control center is the central nervous system.

effector Area or cells that are responsible for carrying out the response from the control center in the negative feedback pathway.

receptor Type of sensor that monitors the environment and responds to changes in the equilibrium in the negative feedback loop.

stimulus Substance or event invoking a change in a system.

NEGATIVE FEEDBACK LOOP

Almost all hormones act via a negative feedback loop. Therefore, understanding this concept is integral to your overall mastery of the endocrine system.

Regardless of the factor or hormone we are discussing, the negative feedback mechanism is always based on three components. The first component, the **receptor**, is a type of sensor that monitors the environment and responds to changes in the equilibrium. Sensing a change causes the receptor to send input to the control center, the second component. The **control center** analyzes the input it receives from the receptor and determines the appropriate response.

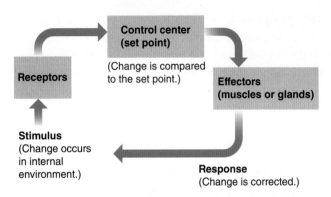

FIGURE 7-7 The feedback mechanism is primarily made up of three steps. The first is the activation of a receptor that then will change the control center. The control center will assess the input information and then create a response that will be carried out by an effector.

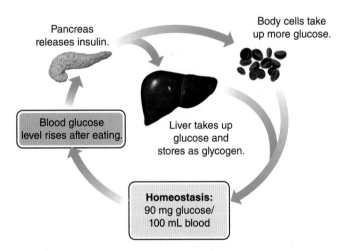

FIGURE 7-8 The insulin feedback mechanism controls hyperglycemia.

Once the control center finalizes the decision on what the set point is, it sends information to the effector. The **effector** provides the means for the control center's response to the original stimulus that initiated the receptor. As a result of the effector generating a response, the original **stimulus** is shut off or reduced to return the situation to homeostatic balance (Figure 7-7).

It is sometimes difficult to grasp these topics unless they are applied to a real-life scenario. So let us now talk about the negative feedback control of blood glucose levels by insulin.

As blood sugar rises, receptors in the islets of Langerhans (specialized cells in the pancreas) become activated. This input is then sent to other specialized cells in the pancreas (the control center). These cells activate beta cells (the effector), causing them to secrete insulin into the bloodstream. This rise in insulin prompts the liver and body tissues to absorb more glucose, removing it from the bloodstream and decreasing the original stimulus that activated this negative feedback loop (Figure 7-8).

In summary, the body's ability to regulate its internal environment is fundamental. Hormones play a massive role in this regulation via negative feedback mechanisms. Some mechanisms are as simple as blood glucose regulation, as others have multiple hormones and hundreds of variables that can disrupt the equilibrium and cause receptors to be activated. Just as there is negative feedback, we also have positive feedback, which is discussed in other chapters as its role is more important in blood clot formation than in hormone function.

LEARNING OBJECTIVE | **7.1.14** | **Discuss how the nervous system plays a role in controlling hormone secretion.**

KEY TERMS

adrenergic receptors Receptor on the surface of cells that cause a sympathetic response.

feed-forward regulation The release of insulin before the rise of blood glucose. This event usually occurs before ingestion of food or continued digestion of food.

hypothalamus Region of the cerebrum that controls body states such as hunger, thirst, and body temperature and regulates hormone release from the pituitary gland.

NEURAL REGULATION

Neural regulation of hormone release is when nervous system input into endocrine cells increases or decreases hormonal secretion. There are three main examples of these processes that we now discuss: innervation of the pancreas, adrenal medulla, and pituitary gland.

Innervation of the Pancreas

As previously discussed, the islets of Langerhans are the control center for insulin release from beta cells. Postganglionic neurons from both the parasympathetic and sympathetic nervous system innervate these cells. When stimulated by the parasympathetic system, beta cells release insulin in a process known as feed-forward regulation. **Feed-forward regulation** is the secretion of insulin in anticipation of the rise of blood glucose from the future ingestion of food or continued digestion of food that contains glucose. Remember, a nickname for parasympathetic nervous system is "rest and digest," so it makes sense that more insulin will be needed to offset the glucose that continues to be absorbed by the gastrointestinal tract.

Conversely, sympathetic innervation of the islets of Langerhans inhibits the release of insulin from the beta cells. We are more sympathetically activated when exercising or assessing a dangerous situation ("fight or flight"), so we need an increase in glucose in our bloodstream so it can be delivered to muscles and our brain to be used as fuel for continued use and thought processing. If we were to increase the rate of insulin release during this time, we would be doing ourselves a disservice, as blood glucose would begin to be stored in tissues and not used for a quick and powerful supply of energy.

Innervation of the Adrenal Medulla

As we discussed, catecholamines are amine hormones that cause a robust sympathetic response (Table 7-1). The two most prominent catecholamines, norepinephrine and epinephrine, are created and stored in the adrenal medulla (more on the details of this process later). When released, these catecholamines bind to **adrenergic receptors**, a type of receptor on the surface of many types of cells that when activated cause a sympathetic response. As a result, it is no surprise that postganglionic nerves associated with the sympathetic nervous system innervate the adrenal medulla and cause their release. An increase in the release of catecholamines serves to potentiate the effects of the fast-acting nervous system so a person stays sympathetically activated for a longer period of time.

Innervation of the Pituitary Gland

The pituitary gland is considered the master regulator of the endocrine system because it releases a significant number of hormones that play an integral part of homeostasis. However, the production and release of these hormones are under neural control. The pituitary is connected to the **hypothalamus**, a part of the brain that is mainly concerned with the regulatory processes necessary for survival. The hypothalamus directly regulates feeding, drinking, sleep, stress, and reproductive responses by stimulating the release of certain hormones from the pituitary gland below it.

In order to regulate the release of hormones, the hypothalamus has nerve fibers that secrete neurotransmitters that directly stimulate cells in the pituitary. Interestingly, the hypothalamus has two ways of doing this. If the hypothalamus wants to create hormones whose cells reside in the posterior pituitary, it simply releases neurotransmitters from the nerve fibers that extend into the posterior pituitary. There are two types of these nerve fibers known as nuclei that we discuss later.

If the hypothalamus wants to stimulate the release of hormones from the *anterior pituitary*, it simply secretes neurotransmitters into the capillary network that connects these two glands. This capillary network is called the hypothalamic hypophyseal portal system (Figure 7-9).

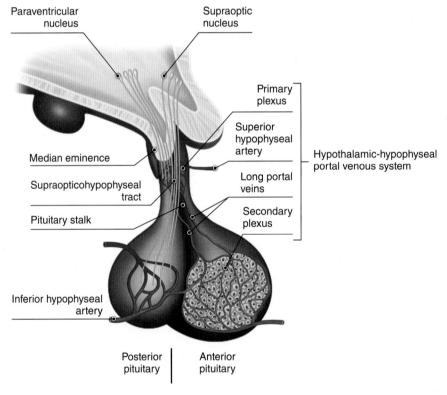

FIGURE 7-9 The hypothalamus is the master regulator of the endocrine system. In order to create changes, this organ is attached to the pituitary gland via blood vessels and nerve tracts. Blood vessels connect the hypothalamus to the anterior pituitary while the posterior is connected via the paraventricular nuclei and supraoptic tracts.

Because of the direct link between the hypothalamus and pituitary glands via innervation and neurotransmitters, the release of subsequent hormones is constantly under regulatory control of the central nervous system. This is how our body ties together the two communication systems and allows us to respond to stimuli both rapidly and for longer periods of time until we can return to equilibrium.

In the next unit, we begin to discuss how all of the glands and specific hormones work together to create a unified response to our ever-changing environment.

UNIT OBJECTIVE 7.2

Describe the major endocrine glands, their location, hormones, and the effects of these hormones.

UNIT INTRODUCTION

Now that we know what hormones do, we can discuss the location of the endocrine organs throughout the body and the types of hormones they secrete.

LEARNING OBJECTIVE 7.2.1 **List the major endocrine glands in the human body.**

ORGANS OF THE ENDOCRINE SYSTEM

Endocrine glands span various areas of our bodies (Figure 7-10). These glands are located within the brain and span the thoracic and abdominopelvic cavities. Endocrine glands exist to react and alter the internal environment of our bodies in response to stimuli.

The endocrine glands are as follows:

Pineal gland
Hypothalamus
Pituitary gland
Thyroid glands
Parathyroid glands
Pancreas
Adrenal glands
Testis
Ovaries

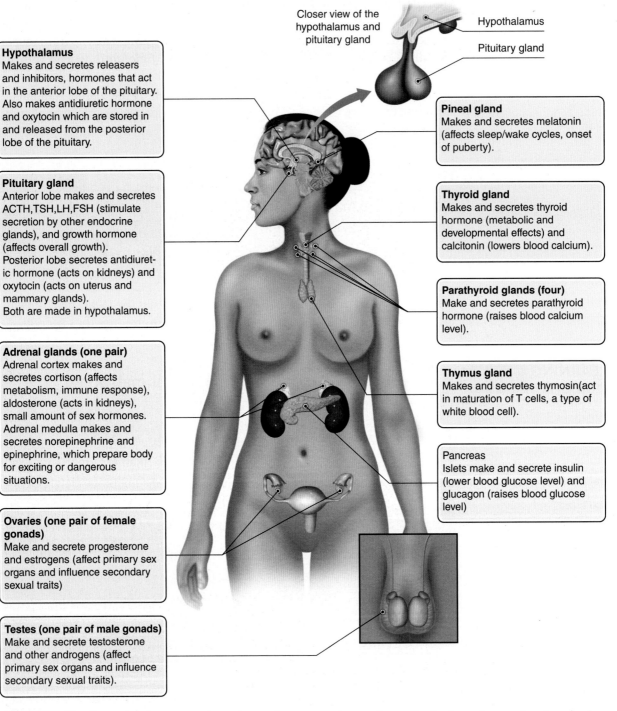

Hypothalamus
Makes and secretes releasers and inhibitors, hormones that act in the anterior lobe of the pituitary. Also makes antidiuretic hormone and oxytocin which are stored in and released from the posterior lobe of the pituitary.

Pituitary gland
Anterior lobe makes and secretes ACTH,TSH,LH,FSH (stimulate secretion by other endocrine glands), and growth hormone (affects overall growth).
Posterior lobe secretes antidiuretic hormone (acts on kidneys) and oxytocin (acts on uterus and mammary glands).
Both are made in hypothalamus.

Adrenal glands (one pair)
Adrenal cortex makes and secretes cortison (affects metabolism, immune response), aldosterone (acts in kidneys), small amount of sex hormones. Adrenal medulla makes and secretes norepinephrine and epinephrine, which prepare body for exciting or dangerous situations.

Ovaries (one pair of female gonads)
Make and secrete progesterone and estrogens (affect primary sex organs and influence secondary sexual traits)

Testes (one pair of male gonads)
Make and secrete testosterone and other androgens (affect primary sex organs and influence secondary sexual traits).

Closer view of the hypothalamus and pituitary gland

Hypothalamus

Pituitary gland

Pineal gland
Makes and secretes melatonin (affects sleep/wake cycles, onset of puberty).

Thyroid gland
Makes and secretes thyroid hormone (metabolic and developmental effects) and calcitonin (lowers blood calcium).

Parathyroid glands (four)
Make and secretes parathyroid hormone (raises blood calcium level).

Thymus gland
Makes and secretes thymosin(act in maturation of T cells, a type of white blood cell).

Pancreas
Islets make and secrete insulin (lower blood glucose level) and glucagon (raises blood glucose level)

FIGURE 7-10 The endocrine system is made up of organs that span the entire body surface and various body cavities.

LEARNING OBJECTIVE 7.2.2 Identify the pineal gland and its anatomical location.

LEARNING OBJECTIVE 7.2.3 Identify the hormone produced by the pineal gland.

LEARNING OBJECTIVE 7.2.4 Describe the action of the hormone produced by the pineal gland.

LOCATION OF THE PINEAL GLAND

The pineal gland is located posteriorly to the third cerebral ventricle lying within the center of the brain and anteriorly to the cerebellum (Figure 7-11).

Melatonin

Melatonin is an amine-based hormone secreted by the pineal gland. It is also considered an indolamine, a type of monoamine hormone that is similar in structure to a catecholamine. It is easy to get melatonin and melanin mixed up,

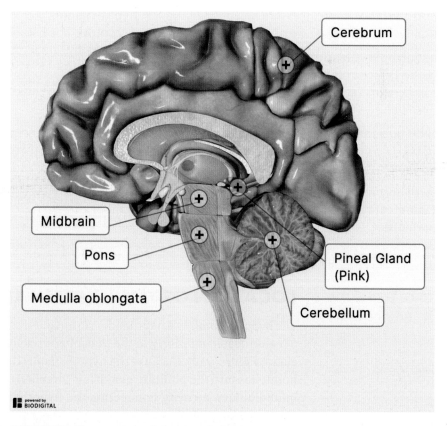

FIGURE 7-11 Location of the pineal gland.

so remember that melanin is the chemical responsible for the hue of our skin and is not associated with the pineal gland.

Recent research suggests that the function of pineal secretion of melatonin is still not well established. Nevertheless, melatonin has been shown to regulate wakefulness and is a hormone that promotes sexual maturation in pubescent women.

LEARNING OBJECTIVE 7.2.5 Identify the hypothalamus and its anatomical location.

LEARNING OBJECTIVE 7.2.6 Identify the hormones produced by the hypothalamus.

LEARNING OBJECTIVE 7.2.7 Describe the actions of the different hormones produced by the hypothalamus.

KEY TERMS

corticotropin-releasing hormone (CRH) Stimulates both the synthesis and the secretion of ACTH.

dopamine Hormone that inhibits prolactin release from the anterior pituitary. This hormone can also affect heart rate, pleasure reception in the brain, and learning.

gonadotropin-releasing hormone (GnRH) Controls the release of gonadotropins, follicle-stimulating hormone, and luteinizing hormone.

growth hormone-releasing hormone (GHRH) Stimulates the secretion of growth hormone.

growth hormone-inhibiting hormone (somatostatin) Inhibits the secretion of growth hormone.

hypothalamic hypophyseal portal system (HHPS) Collection of capillaries that absorbs the hormones from the neuroendocrine cells of the hypothalamus and ensures that they arrive at the anterior pituitary gland.

hypothalamus Region of the cerebrum that controls body states such as hunger, thirst, and body temperature and regulates hormone release from the pituitary gland.

infundibulum End of the fallopian tubes nearest the ovary.

thyrotropin-releasing hormone (TRH) Controls the release of thyroid-stimulating hormone from the pituitary gland that will increase production of thyroid hormones (T3/T4) in the thyroid gland. Usually regulates energy balance, eating patterns, heat production, and prolactin levels.

LOCATION OF THE HYPOTHALAMUS

The hypothalamus is a neuroendocrine gland that contains complex collections of cells located inferiorly to the thalamus while lying superiorly to the pituitary gland (Figure 7-12). Because the hypothalamus directly innervates and secretes hormones into the pituitary gland, it is attached to it through the hypothalamic infundibulum, a cavity connecting the hypothalamus and posterior pituitary gland.

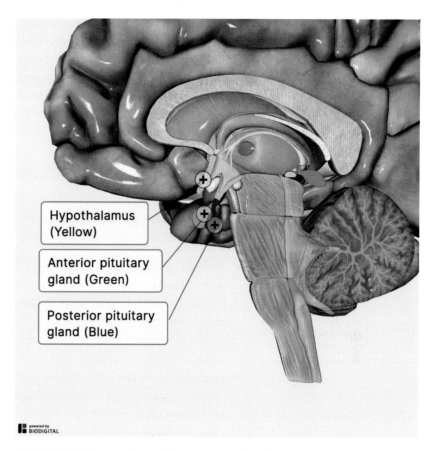

FIGURE 7-12 Location of the pituitary gland and hypothalamus.

HORMONES OF THE HYPOTHALAMUS

The eight hormones of the hypothalamus include:

- Thyrotropin-releasing hormone
- Gonadotropin-releasing hormone
- Corticotropin-releasing hormone
- Growth hormone-releasing hormone
- Growth hormone-inhibiting hormone
- Dopamine
- Oxytocin
- Antidiuretic hormone (ADH)

Because the hypothalamus is directly innervated by the limbic system, its production of hormones is variable on the emotional state or environmental stimuli interacting with the central nervous system. So, depending on the emotional state, the hypothalamus can begin to synthesize specific hormones and release them into the pituitary for storage and subsequent release.

If we dive deeper on this complicated process of neuro and endocrine links between the limbic system, hypothalamus, and pituitary, we see that the hypothalamus utilizes paraventricular and supraoptic nerve tracts to transport hormones to the posterior pituitary. Hormones are delivered to the anterior pituitary via the **hypothalamic hypophyseal portal system (HHPS)**. The HHPS is a collection of capillaries that absorb the hormones from the neuroendocrine cells of the hypothalamus and ensure that they arrive at the anterior pituitary gland.

Hormones that Affect the Anterior Pituitary

Hormones that are released by the hypothalamus, travel through the HHPS, and are delivered to the anterior pituitary have overarching effects on our endocrine system. Below are the six hormones delivered to the pituitary and their function.

- **Thyroid-releasing hormone (TRH).** Controls the release of thyroid-stimulating hormone (TSH) from the pituitary gland, which will increase production of thyroid hormones (T3/T4) in the thyroid gland. TRH also regulates energy balance, eating patterns, heat production, and prolactin levels by increasing our body's overall metabolic rate.
- **Gonadotropin-releasing hormone (GnRH).** Controls the release of gonadotropins, follicle-stimulating hormone (FSH), and luteinizing hormone (LH).
- **Corticotropin-releasing hormone (CRH).** Stimulates both the synthesis and the secretion of ACTH in the corticotropin-producing cells, corticotropes, of the anterior pituitary gland.
- **Growth hormone-releasing hormone (GHRH).** Stimulates the secretion of growth hormone.
- **Growth hormone-inhibiting hormone (somatostatin).** Inhibits the secretion of growth hormone from **somatotropic cells**, the cells that create growth hormone.
- **Dopamine:** Widespread inhibition of prolactin release from the anterior pituitary.

Hormones that Affect the Posterior Pituitary

Oxytocin and ADH are released by the paraventricular and supraoptic nuclei, respectively. Recall that these are the only connections that the hypothalamus has to the posterior pituitary gland where these hormones are stored until their release.

CLINICAL TIP	Begin to think of the hypothalamus as the leader of the endocrine system. Most homeostatic changes can be traced back to this organ. Where the hypothalamus goes, the rest of the endocrine system follows. This is quite evident for the pituitary gland, which is intimately tied to this portion of the brain.

**LEARNING
OBJECTIVE 7.2.8** Identify the anterior pituitary gland and its anatomical
location.

**LEARNING
OBJECTIVE 7.2.9** Identify the hormones produced by the anterior pituitary
gland.

**LEARNING
OBJECTIVE 7.2.10** Describe the actions of the different hormones produced
by the anterior pituitary gland.

KEY TERMS

adrenocorticotropic hormone (ACTH) Promotes release of glucocorticoids and androgens.

chiasmatic groove The upper surface of the sphenoid bone that contains the pituitary gland.

follicle-stimulating hormone (FSH) Stimulates spermatogenesis in males and ovarian follicle maturation in females while also producing estrogen.

growth hormone (GH) Stimulates somatic growth multiple organs while also increasing the levels of insulin growth factors.

hypophyseal fossa Depression within the sella turcica bone indicates where the pituitary gland is located.

insulin growth factors (IGFs) Hormone that plays an important role in growth when stimulated by increased levels of growth hormone.

luteinizing hormone (LH) Promotes testosterone production in males and ovulation in females while also producing estrogen and progesterone.

pituitary gland A pea sized gland that is housed in the sella turcica and is the master regulator of the endocrine system, controlling the activity of numerous hormonesecreting glands.

prolactin (PRL) Hormone within the female reproductive system that stimulates breast tissue to produce breast milk.

sella turcica Depression within the sphenoid bone that allows for the housing of the pituitary gland.

spermatogenesis Production and development of mature sperm.

sphenoid bone Bone of the skull located near the anterior and middle portion of the cranium. This bone houses and protects the pituitary gland along with the hypothalamus.

thyroid-stimulating hormone (TSH) Stimulates the thyroid gland to release triiodothyronine (T3) and thyroxine (T4).

LOCATION OF THE PITUITARY GLAND

The **pituitary gland** is located within the **hypophyseal fossa** of the **sella turcica** within the **sphenoid bone**. Additionally, this gland lies inferior to the hypothalamus and posterior to the **chiasmatic groove** (Figure 7-12).

SUBDIVISIONS OF THE PITUITARY GLAND

As previously mentioned, the pituitary gland is subdivided into the anterior and posterior glands. The anterior pituitary gland is under hypothalamic control via the HHPS and, depending on the levels of certain hormones, can synthesize and secrete six different types of hormones:

- Thyroid-stimulating hormone
- Follicle-stimulating hormone
- Luteinizing hormone (LH)
- Adrenocorticotropic hormone
- Growth hormone (GH)
- Prolactin (PRL)

Conversely, the posterior pituitary is under neuronal control and is responsible for the release of:

- Oxytocin
- Antidiuretic hormone (ADH)

HORMONES OF THE ANTERIOR PITUITARY

After activation by certain hormones produced by the hypothalamus, the anterior can begin to create a specific hormone or more than one of the following hormones (Figure 7-13):

- **Thyroid-stimulating hormone (TSH).** Stimulates the thyroid gland to release triiodothyronine (T3) and thyroxine (T4).
- **Follicle-stimulating hormone (FSH).** Stimulates **spermatogenesis** in males and ovarian follicle maturation in females while also producing estrogen.
- **Luteinizing hormone (LH).** Promotes testosterone production in males, and ovulation in females while also producing estrogen and progesterone.
- **Adrenocorticotropic hormone (ACTH).** Promotes release of glucocorticoids and androgens.
- **Growth hormone (GH).** Stimulates **somatic growth** within liver, muscle, bone, and cartilage while also increasing the levels of **insulin growth factors (IGFs)**.
- **Prolactin (PRL).** Promotes lactation.

CLINICAL TIP

Let's remember that the hypothalamus is the leader of the endocrine system and is directly connected to the pituitary gland. Leaders in any profession usually have more than one way of exerting their leadership qualities. In the case of the hypothalamus, it controls the anterior pituitary gland through blood vessel connections while directing the posterior pituitary gland through neuronal control.

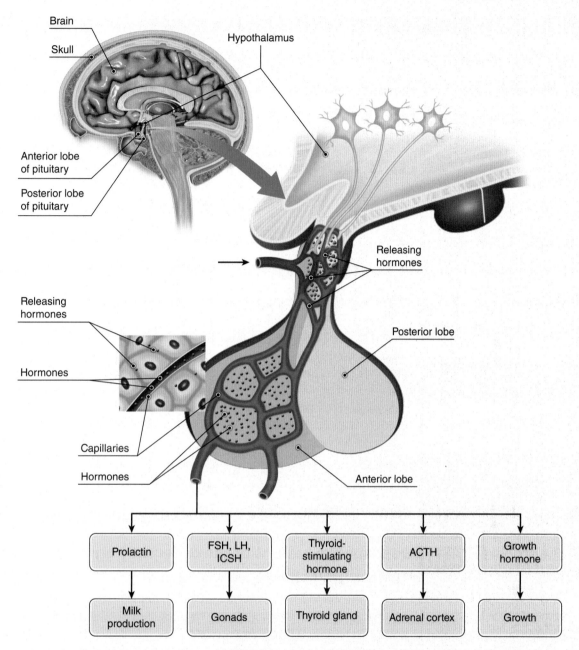

FIGURE 7-13 Interaction between the hypothalamus and pituitary gland along with the secretion of the various hormones controlled by these two organs.

LEARNING OBJECTIVE 7.2.11 Identify the posterior pituitary gland and its anatomical location.

LEARNING OBJECTIVE 7.2.12 Identify the hormones produced by the posterior pituitary gland.

LEARNING OBJECTIVE 7.2.13 Describe the actions of the different hormones produced by the posterior pituitary gland.

KEY TERMS

antidiuretic hormone (ADH) Also known as a vasopressin; hormone secreted by the posterior lobe of the pituitary gland or that increases blood pressure and decreases urine production.

oxytocin Hormone that stimulates uterine contractions and causes the ejection of milk.

LOCATION OF POSTERIOR PITUITARY GLAND

The posterior pituitary gland is located in the anterior portion of the brain at the level of the bridge of the nose. As its name suggests, it is the lobe of the pituitary gland that sits behind the anterior portion of the pituitary.

HORMONES OF THE POSTERIOR PITUITARY

The posterior pituitary is responsible for the release of oxytocin and antidiuretic hormone (ADH). Oxytocin is specifically involved in stimulating uterine contractions during labor while also initiating breast milk ejection and formation of human bonds. ADH is released to stimulate kidney reabsorption of water at the collecting duct. Reabsorption will lead to increased blood volume and widespread vasoconstriction as there is an increase in blood volume requiring an increase in blood pressure.

LEARNING OBJECTIVE 7.2.14 Identify the thyroid gland and its anatomical location.

LEARNING OBJECTIVE 7.2.15 Identify the hormones produced by the thyroid gland.

LEARNING OBJECTIVE 7.2.16 Describe the actions of the different hormones produced by the thyroid gland.

KEY TERMS

basal metabolic rate The smallest amount of energy over a period of time that a person needs to maintain body function.

cholecalciferol Substance produced by the kidneys that helps the body absorb calcium. This compound can be used as a dietary supplement to enhance calcium levels.

direct antagonist Ligand or drug that decreases a biological process by binding to and blocking a receptor.

follicles Small secretory cavity, sac, or gland usually found on the surface of the skin.

isthmus Area between the body of the uterus and the cervix.

thyroglobulin Protein present in the thyroid gland from which thyroid hormones are synthesized.

thyroid gland Gland located superior to the clavicles in the midline of the body responsible for the secretion of hormones involved in metabolism.

LOCATION OF THE THYROID GLAND

The **thyroid gland** is a bilobed gland with multiple **follicles** connected by an **isthmus** that lies anteriorly to the trachea and inferiorly to the thyroid cartilage (Figure 7-14).

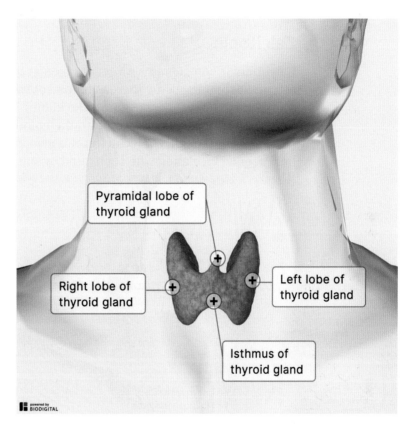

Pyramidal lobe of thyroid gland

Right lobe of thyroid gland

Left lobe of thyroid gland

Isthmus of thyroid gland

powered by BIODIGITAL

FIGURE 7-14 Anatomical location of the thyroid gland.

FOLLICULAR AND PARAFOLLICULAR CELLS OF THE THYROID GLAND

Histologically, thyroid glands are formed by follicular cells, which are responsible for synthesizing **thyroglobulin** and assisting in the production of T3 and T4, the thyroid hormones. T4 is the most abundant form of thyroid hormone and is therefore responsible for most of the hormonal effects. The thyroid gland also contains parafollicular cells that synthesize and secrete calcitonin.

Triiodothyronine and Thyroxine

Triiodothyronine (T3) and thyroxine (T4) arguably have the most diverse effect on our bodies. Primarily, T3 and T4 cause an increase in the **basal metabolic rate**, promote glucose catabolism, enhance nervous system function, promote proper functioning of cardiac myocytes, aid in muscular development, cause the maturation of the skeletal system, ensure proper gastrointestinal motility, regulate female reproduction, and are an integral part of healthy skin.

Because of these widespread effects, T3 or T4 need to be tightly controlled when in the bloodstream. Therefore, these hormones are bound to the plasma protein thyroxin-binding globulin. When bound, T3 or T4 are not active. When finally released from their carrier protein, these thyroid hormones can affect homeostatic levels.

Calcitonin

Calcitonin is considered a **direct antagonist** of PTH and functions to reduce serum calcium levels by increasing osteoblastic activity, increasing excretion of calcium and magnesium at the kidney level, and decreasing **cholecalciferol** synthesis and secretion into the colon to aid in calcium absorption. Interestingly enough, cholecalciferol is also known as vitamin D_3, which can help in bone formation when activated by sunlight on the surface of our skin (Figure 7-15).

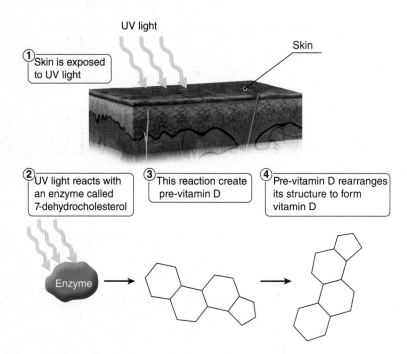

FIGURE 7-15 Cholecalciferol synthesis.

LEARNING OBJECTIVE 7.2.17 Identify the parathyroid glands and their anatomical location.

LEARNING OBJECTIVE 7.2.18 Identify the hormone produced by the parathyroid glands.

LEARNING OBJECTIVE 7.2.19 Describe the action of the hormone produced by the parathyroid glands.

KEY TERMS

calcitriol Synthetic version of vitamin D_3.

distal convoluted tubule Convoluted portion of the nephron between the loop of Henle and the collecting duct. Its function is to concentrate urine prior to its excretion.

hormonal stimuli Relying on the presence of a certain hormone to be activated and create a response within surrounding or distant tissues.

parathyroid glands Small glands located within the thyroid glands that are involved in regulating serum levels of calcium.

LOCATION OF THE PARATHYROID GLANDS

Interestingly, the **parathyroid glands** are four 3–4 mm pea-sized glands located on the posterior aspect of the thyroid gland. Two of the glands are attached to the left and right superior portion and the remaining two are found on the left and right inferior thyroid gland (Figure 7-16).

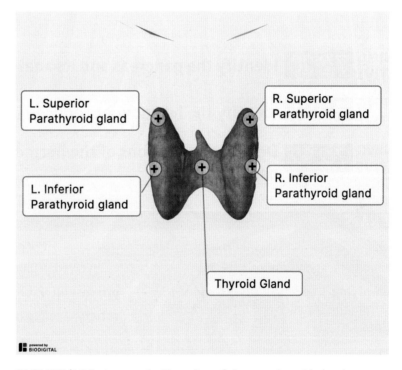

FIGURE 7-16 Anatomical location of the parathyroid gland.

CELLS OF THE PARATHYROID GLANDS

Chief cells are endocrine cells imbedded within the parathyroid tissue that are responsible for the production and secretion of parathyroid hormone (PTH). Surrounding the chief cells are oxyphil cells. Recent research seems to believe that these cells are old or immature forms of chief cells. Most of these cells arise during puberty and really have no bearing on the overall function of the parathyroid gland.

Parathyroid Hormone Release

Unlike many of its counterparts, PTH does not rely on hormonal stimuli, but rather depressed ionized calcium levels in the blood can cause the release of PTH and its targeted effects on bones, the kidneys, and the gastrointestinal tract (GI tract).

Parathyroid Hormone and Bones To increase the amount of free blood calcium, PTH increases osteoclastic activity while simultaneously decreasing osteoblastic activity.

Parathyroid Hormone and Kidneys PTH can also salvage calcium from the kidneys by promoting calcium and magnesium reabsorption in the distal convoluted tubule while increasing potassium excretion. Further changes in the kidney by PTH promote the formation of calcitriol, which will be shuttled to the gastrointestinal tract to increase calcium and vitamin D absorption.

Parathyroid Hormone and the GI Tract Increased calcitriol levels cause an increase in calcium absorption from the ingestion of nutrients and their subsequent digestion in the GI tract.

LEARNING OBJECTIVE 7.2.20 Identify the pancreas and its anatomical location.

LEARNING OBJECTIVE 7.2.21 Identify the hormones produced by the pancreas.

LEARNING OBJECTIVE 7.2.22 Describe the actions of the hormones produced by the pancreas.

KEY TERMS

amylin Peptides that are secreted from beta cells that inhibit glucagon synthesis.

gastric emptying The time it takes for food to empty from the stomach and into the small intestines.

pancreas Gland that regulates multiple hormones involved in glucose control and digestion.

pro-insulin Prohormone precursor to insulin.

satiety Feeling of fullness after eating.

LOCATION OF THE PANCREAS

Located partially posterior to the stomach in the abdomen, the pancreas is about 6 inches in length, with its head attaching to the proximal portion of the duodenum through the pancreatic duct (Figure 7-17). Interestingly, the pancreas is the only endocrine and exocrine gland within the body.

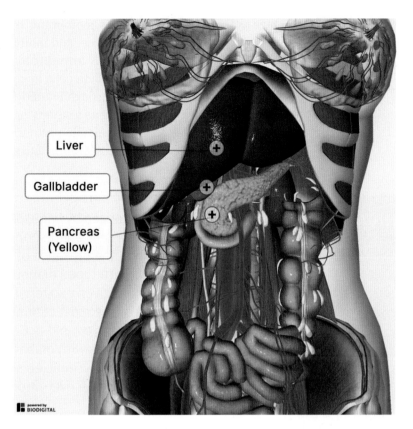

FIGURE 7-17 Anatomical location of the pancreas.

CELLS OF THE PANCREAS

The pancreas is mostly made up of acinar cells, which secrete enzyme-rich fluid into the duodenum during digestion. Within the spaces of acinar cells are the islets of Langerhans cells that contain four types of cells, which secrete different hormones.

Cells of the Islets of Langerhans

The islets contain two major types of cells: alpha cells that secrete glucagon and beta cells that secrete insulin and amylin. Delta cells are responsible for somatostatin release and polypeptide cells are the last but most underresearched portion of the pancreas.

Glucagon A potent peptide hormone, glucagon has significant hyperglycemic effects by breaking down glycogen to glucose, synthesizing glucose from lactic acid and noncarbohydrate materials, and causing the liver to release glucose.

Insulin Insulin is synthesized as a larger part of a peptide hormone called **pro-insulin** and then is broken down just before it is released by the beta cells.

Once active, insulin enhances membrane transport of glucose, inhibits the breakdown of glycogen to glucose, and inhibits the conversion of amino acids from fats and glucose, effectively lowering blood glucose levels.

Amylin   Amylin is released by beta cells in concert with insulin, thus lowering the blood sugar even further through inhibition of glucagon secretion, delaying of gastric emptying, and acting as a satiety agent.

Somatostatin   Like its hypothalamic partner, pancreatic somatostatin inhibits growth hormone and glucagon secretion and slows the rate of gastric emptying.

CLINICAL TIP	Type 1 diabetes is characterized by widespread destruction of beta cells in the pancreas. Beta cells are responsible for the synthesis and secretion of insulin in the presence of elevated blood glucose levels. Because patients with type 1 diabetes have a reduced ability to secrete insulin, they are given exogenous doses of insulin in the form of injections. One of the most common insulin medications is Lantus. Lantus is described as a rapid-acting form of insulin that is administered by most patients with diabetes immediately after eating to alleviate dangerous hyperglycemic episodes. This medication imitates insulin and initiates the ever-important blood glucose negative feedback loop.

LEARNING OBJECTIVE 7.2.23   Identify the adrenal glands and their anatomical locations.

LEARNING OBJECTIVE 7.2.24   Identify the hormones produced by the adrenal glands.

LEARNING OBJECTIVE 7.2.25   Describe the actions of the hormones produced by adrenal glands.

KEY TERMS

adrenal glands   Triangular-shaped glands located superior to the kidneys. These glands are responsible for the production and secretion of hormones involved in cellular metabolism and the regulation of water.

cardio selective   Receptors or hormones that are only located on the myocardium of the heart.

chromaffin cells   Cells located in the adrenal cortex that are responsible for the production and secretion of catecholamines.

zona glomerulosa   Most superficial layer of the adrenal gland responsible for the production of mineralocorticoids.

zona fasciculata   Middle portion of the adrenal gland responsible for the production of glucocorticoids.

zona reticularis   Deepest layer of the adrenal gland responsible for the production of androgens.

LOCATION OF THE ADRENAL GLANDS

The paired adrenal glands are pyramid-shaped organs that lie on the superior portion of the kidneys. These glands are protected slightly by the 12th rib (Figure 7-18).

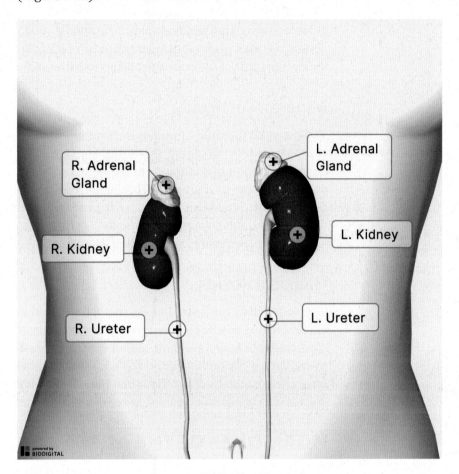

FIGURE 7-18 Anatomical location of the adrenal glands.

Cross-sectional anatomy of the adrenal gland

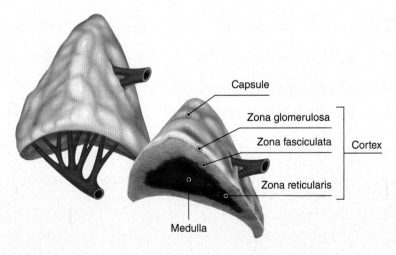

FIGURE 7-19 Functional regions of the adrenal glands.

FUNCTIONAL REGIONS OF THE ADRENAL GLANDS

Each adrenal gland is technically two endocrine glands, one inside of the other. The outer layer, known as the adrenal cortex, can be further subdivided into the zona glomerulosa, zona fasciculata, and zona reticularis. Beneath the cortex is the adrenal medulla, which is a bundle of sympathetic nerves attached to chromaffin cells (Figure 7-19).

HORMONES OF THE ADRENAL CORTEX

The adrenal cortex synthesizes corticosteroids, cholesterol-based hormones that have a variety of effects on the body. Each portion of the cortex houses specific cell types that are specialized to create only one type of corticosteroid.

The most superficial portion of the cortex, the zona glomerulosa, synthesizes mineralocorticoids like aldosterone. The middle and most abundant portion of the cortex, the zona fasciculata, mainly produces glucocorticoids like cortisol, while the deepest part of the cortex produces small amounts of adrenal sex hormones.

Mineralocorticoids

The essential function of mineralocorticoids is to regulate the electrolyte concentrations in extracellular fluids and blood volume. Particularly, aldosterone reduces exertion of sodium from the body by promoting sodium retention and water reabsorption. Furthermore, aldosterone can cause hypokalemia, but only briefly as the long-term effects for hypovolemic episodes must be sustained through continued sympathetic nervous system response, peripheral vasoconstriction, and secondary secretion of ADH from the posterior pituitary.

Glucocorticoids

Glucocorticoids influence energy metabolism and regulate immune responses via fluctuating cortisol levels. Overall, cortisol promotes anti-inflammation and stress reduction along with an increase in blood glucose and insulin levels. Further changes conserve glucose for brain function with protein stores and free fatty acids being used for continued glucose production. Besides metabolism, cortisol can also cause an increase in sympathetic tone.

HORMONES OF THE ADRENAL MEDULLA

Catecholamines are the main hormones produced by the chromaffin cells within the adrenal medulla. Two major types are norepinephrine and epinephrine, with the latter being the most abundant and **cardio selective**.

Androgens

Adrenal-based androgens have little to no effect on the development of secondary sex characteristics but have been shown to have minimal involvement in axillary and pubic hair development along with libido health. Examples include androstadiene and dehydroepiandrosterone (DHEA).

Catecholamines

Catecholamines are the basis for sympathetic response to a stimulus known as the "flight-or-fight" response. When sympathetically activated, the adrenal medulla secretes epinephrine, which quickly increases cardiac output, while norepinephrine causes widespread vasoconstriction. These hormones also attempt bronchodilation to ensure that the maximum amount of air is being perfused to the lungs to supply oxygenated blood that will be needed to fight or run.

Identify the ovaries and their anatomical location.

Identify the hormones produced by the ovaries.

Describe the actions of the hormones produced by the ovaries.

KEY TERMS

estrogen Steroid hormone that promotes the development and maintenance of female characteristics of the body.

ovaries Female reproductive organ located in the pelvic cavity responsible for the secretion of hormones involved in secondary-sex characteristic development and menstruation.

progesterone Steroid hormone that stimulates the uterus to prepare for pregnancy.

LOCATION OF THE OVARIES

The **ovaries** are paired 3.5 cm oval-shaped organs located in the female's abdominopelvic cavity lateral to the uterus (Figure 7-20).

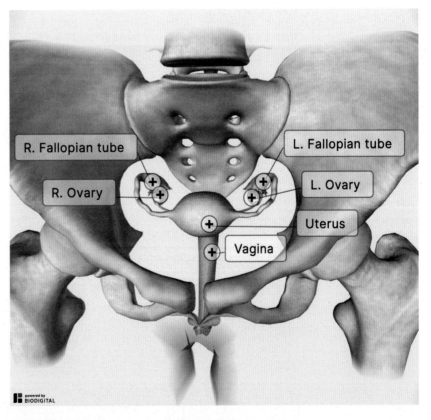

FIGURE 7-20 Anatomical location of the ovaries.

ESTROGEN AND PROGESTERONE

Besides producing ova, or eggs, the ovaries produce several hormones, most importantly, estrogen and progesterone.

- **Estrogen** is responsible for the maturation of the ovaries and other reproductive organs while also contributing to secondary sex characteristics in females, including enlarged breasts and widened hips. Acting with progesterone, estrogen can promote breast development and cyclic changes in uterine mucosa during menstruation.
- **Progesterone** is necessary for implantation of the fertilized egg into the uterus and maintaining a pregnancy. In concert with estrogen, progesterone can aid in breast development and the cyclical changes seen in the endometrial tissue during the menstrual cycle.

LEARNING OBJECTIVE 7.2.29 Identify the testis and its anatomical location.

LEARNING OBJECTIVE 7.2.30 Identify the hormones produced by the testes.

LEARNING OBJECTIVE 7.2.31 Describe the action of the hormones produced by the testes.

KEY TERMS

inhibin A hormone that is produced from the testis and ovary prevents the production of follicle-stimulating hormone (FSH) from the pituitary gland.

Leydig cells Cells responsible in the male for the production of testosterone.

scrotum Pouch of skin containing the testicles.

Sertoli cells Cells responsible in the male for spermatogenesis.

testis Male reproductive organ located in the groin region responsible for the secretion of hormones involved in secondary-sex characteristic development and overall growth.

testosterone Steroid hormone that stimulates the development of male sexual characteristics.

LOCATION OF THE TESTIS

The testis is composed of dense connective tissue and found within the **scrotum** (Figure 7-21), an extra-abdominal skin pouch.

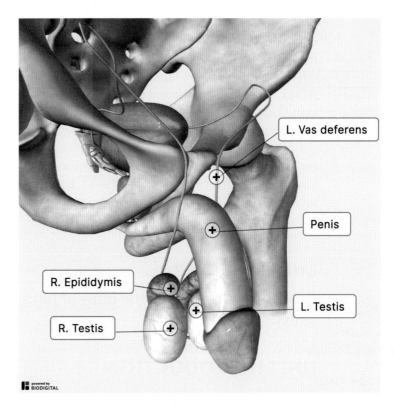

FIGURE 7-21 Anatomical location of the testes.

TESTOSTERONE AND INHIBIN

Both testosterone and inhibin are secreted by the testis, depending on the types of cells that were activated. **Sertoli cells** are under FSH control and can lead to the secretion of the steroid hormones testosterone and inhibin. **Leydig cells** are under LH control and lead to the secretion of testosterone.

In males of prepubescent age, **testosterone** serves as the main catalyst for normal spermatogenesis and the maintenance of proper reproductive health like the continuation of the libido. For males entering or going through puberty, testosterone initiates the maturation of male reproductive organs and the appearance of secondary sex characteristics like axillary hair growth or an appearance of Adam's apple.

As its name suggests, **inhibin** is a hormone secreted by activated Sertoli cells and creates a negative feedback loop, effectively reducing the secretion of FSH from the anterior pituitary.

LEARNING OBJECTIVE 7.2.32 Explain how hormones play a role in homeostasis.

HORMONES' ROLE IN HOMEOSTASIS

The endocrine system plays an important role in homeostasis because hormones regulate the activity of body cells. As you previously learned, hormone release is triggered by a stimulus that will subsequently lead to a response from a certain tissue. In times of homeostatic imbalances, hormones are released to elicit functions that will bring the body back to its fluid equilibrium. Depending on the disruption, the body will secrete specific hormones tasked with reducing or increasing a certain substance or molecule that will bring us back to our steady state. For instance, insulin (as previously discussed) is a hormone that can quickly reverse hyperglycemia and return us to normal blood glucose levels that are within the homeostatic range. Furthermore, we have sex hormones that contribute to menstrual cycles and growth—all important issues that need to be well regulated to remain in homeostasis. There are a multitude of pathways we discuss in of this chapter whose roles become disturbed and lead to major homeostatic imbalances that have significant clinical consequences.

UNIT OBJECTIVE 7.3

Describe the effects on the body of physical and physiological stress.

UNIT INTRODUCTION

Because the endocrine system is designed to respond to changes in our environment, it becomes keenly aware of stress that might disrupt homeostasis. How the body deals with stress has become an important area of interest for endocrinologists, as it can trigger various responses all at once.

LEARNING OBJECTIVE 7.3.1 Describe the characteristics of physical stress on the body.

LEARNING OBJECTIVE 7.3.2 Describe the characteristics of physiological stress on the body.

KEY TERMS

chemical stress Any molecule or substance that can create a stress response in the body. These stressors lead to a disruption in homeostasis.

emotional stress Mental state that can increase a stress response and disruption in homeostatic balance.

stress Feeling of emotion or physical tension.

TYPES OF STRESS

Overall, **stress** refers to any stimulus that can alter our homeostatic balance and cause a physiological response to counteract that stimulus. Our body is subjected to daily stressors that take two major forms: physical and physiological.

Physical Stress

The most common type of physical stress is an acute injury that causes cellular damage and localized inflammation. Injuries happen every moment in our body as blood vessels rupture, cells are being destroyed, or pathogens are trying to invade our tissues. These microscopic injuries promote a vigorous stress response that we will discuss, but it's important to remember that physical stress is not just what you can see happen to a person's body such as weightlifting or a black eye from a fight, it can also be smaller everyday wear-and-tear that we cannot see. Despite the size of the stress, there is still a response.

Physiological Stress

Unlike direct injury to a tissue or organ system, physiological stress can be undetected or unseen. There are two types of physiological stressors, emotional and chemical, that can affect the endocrine system and cause a widespread range of symptoms.

     Emotional stress can be an uncomfortable state of mind brought on by a patient's response to trauma or underlying mental condition. This mental state will elicit transformations in a patient's baseline hormone levels such as cortisol, which we discuss later.

     Chemical stress relates to an alteration of the internal homeostatic environment by reducing or increasing certain chemicals in our bloodstream such as hormones, toxins, or electrolytes. Because these molecules contain a molecular component that has the ability to modify cells that they encounter, chemical stress can easily lead to the breakdown of cells and tissue.

LEARNING OBJECTIVE 7.3.3 Contrast the characteristics of physical and physiological stress on the body.

LEARNING OBJECTIVE 7.3.4 Identify the characteristics of the general stress response.

LEARNING OBJECTIVE 7.3.5 Describe the general stress response.

LEARNING OBJECTIVE 7.3.6 Identify the signs of long-term stress on the body.

LEARNING OBJECTIVE 7.3.7 Explain how long-term stress affects the body and homeostasis in a negative manner.

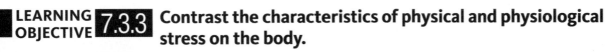

KEY TERM

cytokines Proteins that play a regulatory function in the immune system.

CHARACTERISTIC RESPONSES OF PHYSICAL AND PHYSIOLOGICAL STRESS

Because physical stress can cause localized cell death, there is an initiation of a pro-inflammatory response that will target the damaged area. Local cellular response causes a release of inflammatory **cytokines**. These cytokines include histamine, bradykinins, prostaglandins, and leukotrienes. Elevated levels of these immunomodulators will cause a local vasodilation of the tissue, leading to the infiltration of leukocytes. White blood cells will begin to clear the local infection and prevent further infection. Once edema, cellular debris, and infections are cleared, there will be the arrival of fibrous tissue. This fibrous tissue creates the scars that we may see on a patient's body after surgery or a deep laceration. These events are examples of physical stress that begin to manifest into physiological stress responses.

Physiological stress causes a more systemic reaction where changes in emotional states and chemical imbalances can be an acute or chronic response (Figure 7-22).

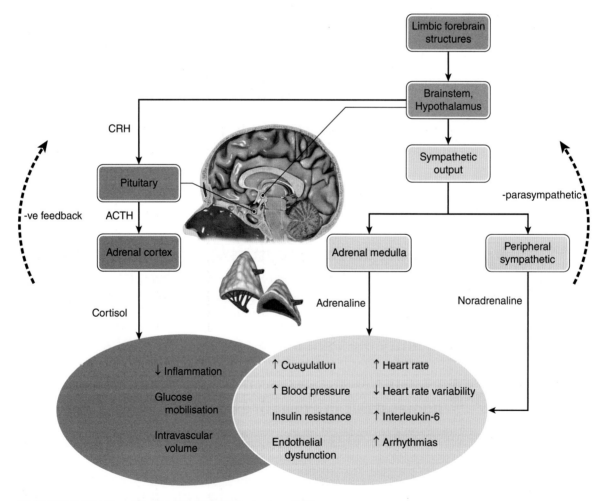

FIGURE 7-22 The effects of stress on the human body.

Acute Physiological Stress

Acute physiological changes cause an increased heart rate, blood pressure, and metabolism along with bronchodilation, alterations in blood flow to areas of the body that need to be perfused to accomplish a certain task, and a reduction in both gastric and urinary function. We in the medical field refer to this physiological response as a "flight-or-fight" reaction where our body becomes primed to decide whether to retreat or defend itself in the face of external stimuli.

Chronic Physiological Stress

Prolonged exposure to physiological stress will begin to change the underlying physiology in an individual's body. There will be an increase in water retention leading to an increase in blood pressure. There is also a significant reduction in immune function not only leading to increased susceptibility for illness but also an opportunity for physical stress reactions to fester and become infected.

GENERAL STRESS RESPONSE

When a short-term stressor activates the body to fight-or-flight status, the sympathetic nervous system responds to hypothalamic nerve signals. These stimuli travel down the efferent nervous system and into the adrenal medulla where norepinephrine and epinephrine are released. With few exceptions, these hormones exert the same effects as described in the acute physiological stress reaction. However, catecholamines last a few seconds or minutes, underlying the need to quickly assess a situation and respond to it.

Conversely, when a long-term stressor activates the body, the hypothalamus activates the adrenal cortex. Here, we can again see the difference between the nervous and endocrine system: one is fast-acting and the other is a more progressive change in response to a chronic stimulus. Activation of the adrenal cortex is accomplished through the increase in CRH and ACTH. Both mineralocorticoids and glucocorticoids are released and contribute to the chronic characteristics described above. Notably, aldosterone contributes to the blood volume issues while cortisol, the hormone most clinicians consider the "stress hormone," alters brain function, cellular metabolism, and immune response.

As a result, patients reporting consistent levels of chronic stress should be evaluated for neurochemical and behavioral changes, extensive weight loss or gain, or recent illnesses.

UNIT OBJECTIVE 7.4

Describe common pathologies affecting endocrine glands, their hormones, and their functions.

UNIT INTRODUCTION

One of the most important issues that health care professionals deal with is the loss of proper endocrinological function. Experiencing an increase in or lack of a certain hormone can have devastating effects on our overall health and requires medical management to handle the issue.

KEY TERMS

circadian rhythm Internal body clock that regulates the sleep–wake pattern.

insomnia Inability to sleep.

somnolence Sleepy, drowsy.

THE CIRCADIAN RHYTHM

The circadian rhythm is defined as a 24-hour cycle that includes periods of wakefulness and sleep. Mostly influenced by retinal receptors that sense light that leads to the pineal gland secretion of melatonin, the circadian rhythm is both sensory and hormonal based. With increase in melatonin, there is an increase in wakefulness and a decrease in levels that leads to somnolence and fatigue (Figure 7-23).

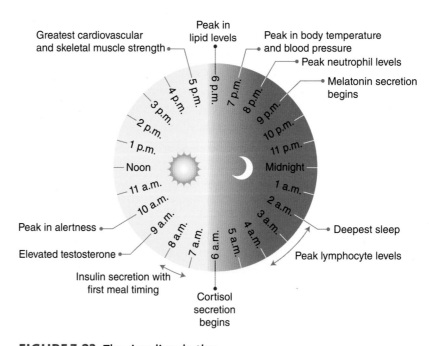

FIGURE 7-23 The circadian rhythm.

PINEAL GLAND DYSFUNCTION

With an over secretion of melatonin due to enhanced light reception or an adenomatous growth within this region of the brain, we would expect patients to be hyperactive or possess insomnia-based traits as they attempt to fall asleep. Conversely, patients with a hyposecretion of the hormone will lead to daytime somnolence.

Other secondary functions of the pineal gland include the timing of sexual maturation and appetite. Everchanging levels of melatonin could also disrupt the rhythmic patterns of these physiological responses.

LEARNING OBJECTIVE 7.4.2 Identify common disorders affecting the hypothalamus.

HYPOTHALAMIC DISORDERS

Recall that the hypothalamus is the leader of the endocrine system, so any disorder is going to have widespread and possibly detrimental effects. Disorders of the hypothalamus include:

- Birth defects where neural tracts are improperly formed, which halts the proper formation of neuroendocrine signals needed for communication between the hypothalamus and pituitary.
- Prader-Willi syndrome, which causes a reduction in gestational growth hormone and subsequent hypothalamic development that will ultimately delay growth in a developing child, leading to milestone delays and cognitive issues.
- Eating disorders and other malnourished states, which deplete the hypothalamus of vital minerals and vitamins needed for proper hormone production.
- Tumors that can begin to infiltrate properly functioning hypothalamic tissue and cause dysregulation.
- Head trauma, which can alter the neural wiring so crucial to the hypothalamus and pituitary relationship.
- Autoimmune diseases targeting neuroendocrine cells that will begin to destroy endocrine cells in the hypothalamus and decrease their function.

LEARNING OBJECTIVE 7.4.3 Identify common disorders affecting the pituitary gland.

KEY TERMS

hemochromatosis Disorder where the body holds onto too much iron. These iron molecules are stored in the liver and skin causing liver damage, diabetes mellitus, and bronze discoloration of the skin.

sarcoidosis Chronic disease of unknown cause that results in the enlargement of lymph nodes in many parts of the body and the widespread deposition of immune complexes. This abnormal tissue can cause scar tissue formation and destruction of normal tissue within the pulmonary and cardiovascular system leading to respiratory or cardiac failure.

PITUITARY DISORDERS

Like hypothalamic disorders, pituitary dysregulation can have wide-ranging effects and clinical presentations. There are two main types of pituitary disorders.

- Nontumor pituitary diseases. Nonpituitary diseases include sarcoidosis, hemochromatosis, and infection of the pituitary gland. Sarcoidosis is an autoimmune disease that causes widespread inflammation in our body and causes fibrous scar tissue to form, particularly in our lungs and lymph nodes. Hemochromatosis is a disease where the body stores too much iron and usually affects the liver.

- Tumor-based pituitary diseases. Though rare, pituitary adenomas are the most common cause of pituitary dysfunction and should be kept on the list of differential diagnoses with patients with vision changes and vague symptoms that might indicate systemic homeostatic imbalances.

LEARNING OBJECTIVE 7.4.4 Describe the signs, symptoms, diagnosis, and treatment of diabetes insipidus.

KEY TERMS

desmopressin Synthetic version of ADH. Usually used to replace ADH or to clinically determine ADH levels.

hydrochlorothiazide Loop diuretic that can help in removing water via the kidneys.

tubular necrosis Breakdown and damage to the nephron tubule of the kidney.

vascular collapse Failure of circulation most likely due to volume issues.

DIABETES INSIPIDUS

At its core, diabetes insipidus (DI) is either a deficiency of ADH or an insensitivity to ADH. Deficiencies of ADH indicate that the issues are centrally located where the posterior pituitary lacks adequate levels of ADH. This is the most common reason for DI and results from autoimmune destruction of the posterior pituitary and head trauma that causes neural delays between the hypothalamus and pituitary. This is known as neurogenic diabetes insipidus or central DI (Figure 7-24).

An insensitivity to ADH indicates that the kidneys do not respond to ADH levels. These disruptions result from kidney destruction due to certain prescription drug use or tubular necrosis. This is known as nephrogenic diabetes insipidus. There are also patients who may experience congenital insensitivities to ADH where from birth, the receptors within their nephrons do not respond adequately to ADH secretion.

Clinically, patients suspected of having either central or nephrogenic DI will have polydipsia, polyuria, and nocturia. Many times, these patients will also be hypernatremic as water is being constantly excreted rather than reabsorbed. Secondary to these electrolyte imbalances, patients will develop dehydration and vascular collapse.

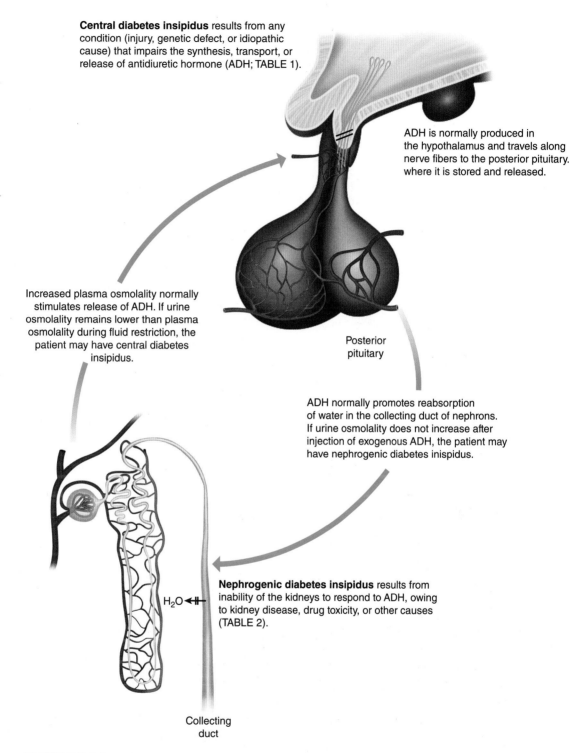

Central diabetes insipidus results from any condition (injury, genetic defect, or idiopathic cause) that impairs the synthesis, transport, or release of antidiuretic hormone (ADH; TABLE 1).

ADH is normally produced in the hypothalamus and travels along nerve fibers to the posterior pituitary, where it is stored and released.

Increased plasma osmolality normally stimulates release of ADH. If urine osmolality remains lower than plasma osmolality during fluid restriction, the patient may have central diabetes insipidus.

Posterior pituitary

ADH normally promotes reabsorption of water in the collecting duct of nephrons. If urine osmolality does not increase after injection of exogenous ADH, the patient may have nephrogenic diabetes inisipidus.

H_2O

Nephrogenic diabetes insipidus results from inability of the kidneys to respond to ADH, owing to kidney disease, drug toxicity, or other causes (TABLE 2).

Collecting duct

FIGURE 7-24 Diabetes insipidus pathophysiology.

Diagnosis

DI can be qualified as central or nephrogenic by performing a fluid deprivation test. Here, water is withheld from the patient and it is suspected that patients will begin to create highly concentrated urine in order to hold onto all of the water that they have. In DI patients, withholding water will not change their urine concentration as ADH continues to be absent. Furthermore, a **desmopressin** test can be performed and if the patient responds to this test by producing correctly concentrated urine, then the issue is of central DI origin. Continued production of diluted urine indicates that there is a nephrogenic DI present.

Treatment

Central DI can be treated with administration of synthetic ADH to replace the inadequate amounts, whereas nephrogenic DI can be treated with a low-sodium diet, fluid restriction, and **hydrochlorothiazide**. If a patient is in a severe hypovolemic state, we can fluid-resuscitate them with one-half normal saline (0.45% saline solution).

LEARNING OBJECTIVE 7.4.5 Describe the signs, symptoms, diagnosis, and treatment of pituitary dwarfism.

KEY TERMS

exogenous External source or administration of a substance.

hyposecretory Decreased secretory capacity.

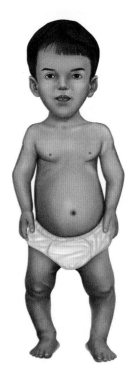

FIGURE 7-25 This toddler with pituitary dwarfism has a significant short stature along with shortened extremities due to the lack of GH secretion.

PITUITARY DWARFISM

Pituitary dwarfism is directly related to a reduced ability of the anterior pituitary to secrete normal amounts of growth hormone. Therefore, the anterior pituitary is in a **hyposecretory** state.

Clinically, the hyposecretory state leads to reduction in stature along with growth throughout infancy and childhood (Figure 7-25). Adults who experience pituitary dwarfism will experience increased blood pressure, hyperlipidemia, decreased cardiac output, and decreased bone mass.

Diagnosis

Specific blood levels of growth hormone are obtained when there is a suspicion of pituitary dwarfism. Clinical findings such as short stature, developmental delays, and chronic ear infections in children are sometimes definite manifestations of this disease.

Treatment

Because the pituitary is in a hyposecretory state, **exogenous** growth hormone must be administered to increase blood levels. Over time, replacement will lead to an increase in growth during the childhood years along with an improvement in overall health in adults.

LEARNING
OBJECTIVE 7.4.6 **Describe the signs, symptoms, diagnosis, and treatment of gigantism.**

KEY TERMS

neoplastic A collection of cells that have developed due to abnormal cell or tissue growth.

somatotropinoma Mass that has developed in the pituitary gland that is oversecreting growth hormone.

GIGANTISM

If the anterior pituitary can exist in a hyposecretory state, then it can also exist in a hypersecretory state. Gigantism is a result of an over secretion of growth hormone most commonly caused by a somatotropinoma.

Diagnosis

Gigantism can be elucidated by measuring the levels of GH in the blood. Patients with gigantism present with glucose intolerance due to a chronically elevated hyperglycemic state. There is also diffuse enlargement of the hands, feet, and skull. Space will begin to develop within a patient's teeth and coarse facial features will develop. A deepened voice may be heard accompanied by diffuse weight gain.

Treatment

Neoplastic tissue that is causing the gigantism must be surgically removed to abate the symptoms. Therefore, ear, nose, and throat neurosurgeons will perform transsphenoidal resection surgery to remove the somatotropinoma.

LEARNING
OBJECTIVE 7.4.7 **Describe the signs, symptoms, diagnosis, and treatment of acromegaly.**

LEARNING
OBJECTIVE 7.4.8 **Compare gigantism and acromegaly.**

KEY TERM

hypertrophic Increasing in size.

ACROMEGALY

Like gigantism, acromegaly is a result of an over secretion of growth hormone. The only discernable difference between acromegaly and gigantism is that gigantism is a childhood disorder usually characterized by macro features developing before the closure of the growth plates. Once growth has stopped, any increased release of growth hormone that causes features to become **hypertrophic** is classified as acromegaly.

Diagnosis

Along with elevated GH levels, patients with acromegaly will also display increased levels of IGF-1. Imaging studies like magnetic resonance imaging of the brain could display an increase in pituitary size that might indicate an overproduction of GH.

Treatment

Like gigantism, surgical resection of the neoplastic tissue is considered goldstandard treatment, but effects can also be regulated by pharmacologic interventions in the adult population. For instance, bromocriptine, a dopamine agonist, will cause the widespread inhibition of growth hormone released from the anterior pituitary.

LEARNING OBJECTIVE 7.4.9 Identify common disorders affecting the thyroid gland.

KEY TERM

thyroiditis Mass that has developed in the pituitary gland that is oversecreting growth hormone.

THYROID DISORDERS

Diseases of the thyroid gland are some of the most common disorders that health care professionals encounter. Health care professionals must commit most of these disorders to memory because of their widespread prevalence. Diseases of the thyroid can be further broken down into hypothyroid or hyperthyroid states.

Hypothyroid Diseases

Hypothyroid diseases are classified as a decrease in thyroid function and include Hashimoto's thyroiditis, lymphocytic thyroiditis, postpartum thyroiditis, de Quervian's thyroiditis, and medication-induced thyroiditis. All these disease states seem to have an autoimmune component where the destruction of the thyroid tissue leads to a downregulation of thyroid hormone release. These diseases can also be caused by thyroid nodule carcinomas, the most common being papillary carcinoma.

Hyperthyroid Diseases

Hyperthyroid diseases are classified as an increase in thyroid function and include Graves' disease, toxic multinodular goiter (TMG), toxic adenoma, and TSH secreting adenoma. Except for the TSH-secreting adenoma, which is pituitary based, there seems to be a hypertrophic growth of follicular cells within the thyroid that cause the additional release of T3 and T4. This state can also be caused by thyroid nodule carcinomas.

CLINICAL TIP

Lab Results Rules

For all endocrine disorders, there can be an issue within the hypothalamus, pituitary gland, or the target organ. Depending on the where the issue lies, the diagnosis can range from a tertiary, secondary, or primary problem. Tertiary endocrine disorders arise from hypothalamic dysregulation while secondary disorders are due to pituitary problems. Issues directly within the target tissue are deemed primary disorders. To determine where the issue is, health care professionals use blood tests to measure the hormone levels to see where the problem is located.

So, with this knowledge let us apply it to the thyroid gland: If a patient has an elevated level of TSH that has caused a hyperthyroid state with elevated T3 and T4 levels, the problem is most likely located in the pituitary gland. Here, we see an elevation of both TSH and T3 and T4 levels.

To simplify things even further: If laboratory levels are going in the *same* (either both increased or decreased) direction, it is a secondary or tertiary endocrine disorder. So, if TSH is high and T3/T4 is high, then we have a secondary or tertiary hyperthyroidism (to further investigate whether this is an issue with the pituitary or hypothalamus would require specialized testing from an endocrinologist).

If laboratory values are *opposite* (one value increased and one value decreased), it is a primary endocrine disorder because the target organ is secreting an abundance of hormone that is negatively feeding back on its stimulus. So, low TSH and high T3/T4 indicates a primary hyperthyroid disorder.

LEARNING OBJECTIVE 7.4.10 Describe the signs, symptoms, diagnosis, and treatment of hypothyroidism.

KEY TERMS

Hashimoto's thyroiditis Autoimmune disorder that leads to the destruction of the thyroid gland causing a hypothyroid state.

hypothyroidism Disease state where the thyroid gland produces decreased amounts of thyroid hormones.

HYPOTHYROIDISM

Hypothyroidism is defined by the widespread decrease of blood T3 and T4 levels. Regardless of whether this is a primary, secondary, or tertiary problem, the follicular cells within the thyroid gland are failing to secrete adequate levels of T3 and T4. Patients with hypothyroidism will present with a multitude of symptoms that sometimes do not immediately correlate with one hormonal issue. What is important to remember is that T3 and T4 have some of the most far-reaching effects when it comes to hormones, so health care professionals must always be vigilant of symptoms that arise around the same time and point to a decrease in thyroid hormone levels.

Clinically, the patient with hypothyroidism will report cold intolerance, weight gain, dry and thickened skin, lateral eyebrow thinning, fatigue, constipation, bradycardia, and hypoglycemic symptoms.

Diagnosis

Hypothyroidism is commonly diagnosed using the blood concentrations of TSH and free T4 (FT4). TSH levels will give a depiction of pituitary involvement while FT4 will quantify the level of actively available thyroid hormone. Elevated TSH levels with normal and low FT4 are diagnosed as primary and subclinical hypothyroid disorders, respectively. Low TSH and Low FT4 levels are diagnosed as secondary or tertiary hypothyroidism.

Treatment

Health care professionals must be well educated on the treatment of hypothyroid disease. Mainstay treatment has been exogenous hormone replacement using levothyroxine. This drug is synthetic T4 and will correct the hypothyroid state. Notably, TSH levels should be checked every 6 weeks to see if the dose of levothyroxine is appropriate.

CLINICAL TIP	In the United States, Hashimoto's thyroiditis is the most common cause of hypothyroidism. **Hashimoto's thyroiditis** is an autoimmune disorder that causes the widespread reduction of thyroid tissue. Worldwide, the most common cause of hypothyroidism is iodine deficiency due to inadequate nutrition.

LEARNING OBJECTIVE 7.4.11 **Describe the signs, symptoms, diagnosis, and treatment of hyperthyroidism.**

KEY TERMS

gynecomastia Enlargement of breast tissue usually related to hormone imbalance or hormone therapy.

hyperthyroidism A disease state where the thyroid gland produces increased amounts of thyroid hormones.

HYPERTHYROIDISM

Hyperthyroidism is defined by the widespread increase of blood T3 and T4 levels. Regardless of whether this is a tertiary, primary, or secondary problem, the follicular cells within the thyroid gland are overproducing T3 and T4.

Patients with hyperthyroidism will present with complaints of heat intolerance, weight loss, moist and soft skin, presence of a mass near their thyroid, anxiety, palpitations, tremors, weakness, diarrhea, tachycardia, **gynecomastia**, and hyperglycemia.

Diagnosis

Hyperthyroidism is classically diagnosed by TSH and FT4. Elevated TSH levels with high levels of FT4 are diagnosed as secondary or tertiary hyperthyroidism. Low TSH and normal to low FT4 levels are diagnosed as subclinical or primary hyperthyroidism, usually due to a toxic goiter that is causing the inappropriate release of T3 and T4.

Treatment

Treatment of hyperthyroidism is based on managing the inappropriate secretion of hormone while addressing the life-threatening issues such as tachycardia and subsequent hypertension. Radioactive iodine therapy can be used to destroy the thyroid gland as the injection will cause the uptake of iodine by the thyroid gland, but its radioactive properties will lead to cell death. Long-term levothyroxine therapy must then be started in these patients. Surgical resection of the overactive tissue may also lower T3 and T4 levels. Therefore, patients may undergo subtotal or total thyroidectomies depending on the severity of their condition. Reducing secondary symptoms, such as tachycardia, can be done by prescribing beta blockers or other heart rate-controlling medications.

CLINICAL TIP   Hyperthyroidism can be accompanied by life-threatening periods of thyrotoxicosis where a patient may experience dangerously elevated blood pressures or heart failure due to sustained cardiac output. To stop these situations, methimazole or Propylthiouracil (PTU) can be used.

LEARNING OBJECTIVE 7.4.12   **Describe the signs, symptoms, diagnosis, and treatment of Graves' disease.**

KEY TERMS

exophthalmos Abnormal protrusion of the eyeballs.

pretibial myxedema Localized lesions of the skin around the tibia as a result of increase in fat deposits due to Graves' disease.

GRAVES' DISEASE

Graves' disease is the most common form of hyperthyroidism in women ages 20–40 years old. This is an autoimmune disorder where TSH autoantibodies are created, causing a significant decrease in TSH levels. The decrease in TSH levels is so significant that the thyroid gland has an unregulated hyperthyroid response.

Patients with Graves' disease present with hyperthyroid complaints along with exophthalmos, a specific finding in patients with this disease (Figure 7-26). **Exophthalmos** is due to the increased fat pad size behind the orbit that forces the eye to sit more anteriorly. Patients can also display **pretibial myxedema**, which are swollen and reddish pitting plaques on their shins.

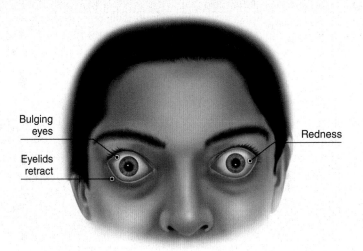

Bulging eyes

Eyelids retract

Redness

FIGURE 7-26 Patient with exophthalmos.

Diagnosis

As previously mentioned, a depressed TSH level and elevated FT4 will signal a primary hyperthyroid condition like Graves' disease. However, antibody tests can confirm the diagnosis as a positive result of thyroid-stimulating immunoglobulins can almost confirm this disease.

Treatment

First-line treatment for Graves' disease is radioactive iodine therapy followed by a thyroidectomy or medication in times of thyrotoxicosis. With correct management and titration of the levothyroxine to optimal levels after destruction of the gland, this hyperthyroid state is well managed.

LEARNING OBJECTIVE 7.4.13 **Identify common disorders affecting the parathyroid glands.**

PARATHYROID DISORDERS

The parathyroid gland can have disorders that cause hyper- and hypoparathyroid states.

Hyperparathyroid Disorders

The most common parathyroid gland disorder is a parathyroid adenoma followed closely by inappropriate parathyroid hyperplasia. Due to the interplay between the parathyroid glands and kidneys, chronic renal failure or recent renal transplant can be causes of hyperparathyroid gland disorder. Because the damage to the kidney is so severe in chronic renal failure, it can no longer reabsorb calcium, effectively decreasing blood calcium levels and leading to an overproduction of PTH by the parathyroid glands.

Hypoparathyroid Disorders

Hypoparathyroid disorders result from tissue trauma during a thyroidectomy or complete removal during a parathyroidectomy. Additionally, autoimmune disorders that attack chief cells within the parathyroid glands can lead to the overall depression of PTH and cause a chronic hypoparathyroid state.

LEARNING OBJECTIVE 7.4.14 **Identify common disorders affecting the pancreas.**

PANCREATIC DISORDERS

Pancreatic disorders can lead to an abundance of issues, many of which can be debilitating and life-threatening. In later chapters we discuss the diseases of pancreatic carcinomas and acute and chronic pancreatitis, but in this chapter, it is important to understand that disorders like diabetes type 1 and type 2 endocrine diseases of the pancreas can cause lifelong changes and require pharmaceutical intervention. Medical treatments are usually aimed at regulating the process of glucose production and release.

LEARNING OBJECTIVE 7.4.15 Describe the signs, symptoms, diagnosis, and treatment of type 1 diabetes mellitus.

TYPE 1 DIABETES MELLITUS

Type 1 diabetes mellitus is considered an autoimmune disorder where antibodies are created against pancreatic beta cells located within the islets of Langerhans. Destruction of these cells causes an insulin deficiency that most commonly presents in children or young adults.

Patients with type 1 diabetes are usually asymptomatic until their blood glucose levels become so unregulated that the kidneys begin to excrete excess sugar in the urine. In order to get rid of the excess sugar, patients experience polyuria, polydipsia, and polyphagia, along with significant weight loss. Patients with chronically uncontrolled diabetes may develop neuropathy, retinopathy, nephropathy, and vascular complications like coronary disease, peripheral vascular disease, and possible stroke. Hypoglycemic episodes can also affect some of these patients as their glucose becomes so unregulated that the body overcompensates when trying to rid itself of excess sugar. Patients will develop tremors, palpitations, nervousness, and tachycardia along with headache, confusion, and slurred speech.

Diagnosis

Once a patient presents to the clinic with the symptoms of glucose intolerance, it is imperative to begin testing glucose levels. Normal fasting blood glucose levels fluctuate between 70 and 100 mg/dl, and in order to assess how far a patient deviates from the norm, there are three types of tests that can be carried out:

- Fasting plasma glucose: Patient must fast for at least eight hours and the glucose level should be above 126 mg/dl on two separate occasions.
- Two-hour glucose tolerance test: Two hours after eating, the glucose level is checked and should be above >200 mg/dl.
- Hemoglobin A1C: Indicates average blood glucose level for the past four months. Any level above 6.5% is considered a diagnostic criterion for diabetes.

Treatment

The overarching treatment plans for patients with type 1 diabetes is to modify diet, exercise, and lifestyle changes accompanied by pharmacological management. Most patients with type 1 diabetes will need exogenous insulin to increase the storage capability of their cells and, depending on the severity of their disease or adherence to a healthy lifestyle, they may need different types of insulin. Currently, there are four types of insulin on the market, ranging from rapid-acting to long-acting. Rapid-acting insulin medications are encouraged for the postprandial spike while long-acting insulin can last up to 24 hours and can offer overnight coverage.

LEARNING OBJECTIVE 7.4.16 Describe the signs, symptoms, diagnosis, and treatment of type 2 diabetes mellitus.

KEY TERMS

diabetic ketoacidosis (DKA) Complication of diabetes that occurs when the body produces high levels of acidic ketones due to the increased breakdown of fats for energy use.

type 2 diabetes mellitus Most common type of diabetes where an individual's body no longer responds to insulin due to an overall increase in glucose levels.

TYPE 2 DIABETES MELLITUS

Ninety percent of all diabetics in the United States are diagnosed with type 2 diabetes. Unlike type 1 diabetes, type 2 diabetes mellitus is based on insulin resistance or relative insulin secretion by the pancreatic beta cells. Patients more susceptible to type 2 diabetes carry comorbidities such as a positive family history, hypertension, hyperlipidemia, and obesity.

Many times, patients with type 1 and type 2 diabetes are unaware of their symptoms until increased urine output or other chronicities like neuropathy occur. There are also situations where patients can experience diabetic keto-acidosis (DKA). DKA is a condition where patients experience nausea, vomiting, and abdominal pain because of dangerously elevated glucose levels. DKA is a medical emergency and requires aggressive treatment.

Diagnosis

Like patients diagnosed with type 1 diabetes, type 2 diabetics must undergo the same diagnostic tests as those suspected of having type 1 diabetes. Notably, patients should be assessed in a timely manner because there is no telling how long the type 2 diabetes has been present or within an uncontrolled state.

Treatment

Patients with type 2 diabetes should strive for dietary and lifestyle modifications with the addition of medication if the hemoglobin A1C test is above 7.0% even after attempted changes. Currently, there is only one agreed-upon medication regimen and that is that every patient regardless of their test results should be started on metformin (Glucophage). Second and third-line medications along with insulin injections can later be added by the health care professional depending on the side effects, personal preference, and insurance coverage. To date, there are eight classes of hyperglycemic agents all with debatable strength and efficacy.

LEARNING OBJECTIVE 7.4.17 Describe the signs, symptoms, diagnosis, and treatment of gestational diabetes mellitus.

GESTATIONAL DIABETES

During pregnancy, a women's body is more prone to uncontrollable glucose levels. The stress of gestation can lead to hyperglycemic and hypoglycemic episodes that become further unregulated as the woman progresses through her pregnancy. Risk factors for gestational diabetes are similar to type 2 diabetes and interestingly enough, 50% of mothers diagnosed with **gestational diabetes** will develop full type 2 diabetes at some point.

Clinically, these patients present the same as patients with type 1 and type 2 diabetes. There may be an increased reporting of polyuria or neuropathy secondary to either the pregnancy or the onset of gestational diabetes.

Diagnosis

Gestational diabetes usually presents after the 24th week of gestation and should be screened for in the third trimester. Again, the screening tools used are the same as for patients with type 1 and type 2 diabetes. Specifically, the 3-hour oral glucose tolerance test is the gold standard for gestational diabetes. A glucose level above 200 mg/dl after this time point will indicate gestational diabetes.

Treatment

Because of the added factor that the unborn fetus is going to be affected by the mother's increasing blood glucose levels, there is a need to adequately adjust these levels. The mother should be encouraged to eat a well-balanced meal that avoids complex sugars or carbohydrates. Physical activity should be impressed on patients and injectable insulin can be used for maintenance until the birth of the child.

LEARNING OBJECTIVE 7.4.18 **Contrast the three forms of diabetes mellitus.**

DIFFERENCES BETWEEN FORMS OF DIABETES MELLITUS

When assessing patients with similar clusters of symptoms that are highly suspicious for diabetes mellitus, it is important to know the differences in how each disease presents. This will guide your questions and the treatment plan that you and the health care team will adhere to.

As previously discussed, diabetes mellitus can be classified as type 1, type 2, or gestational. Of the three, type 1 diabetes has the strongest genetic link and its age of onset is usually young and sudden. This differs from type 2 diabetes, which is usually an acquired disorder over a long period of time and diagnosed most often in adults. As its name suggests, gestational diabetes is only seen in women who may develop insulin resistance during their pregnancy. Most of these women will develop lifelong diabetes even after they give birth.

Patients with type 1 diabetes usually present with low levels of insulin due to the fact that they lack genes needed for its proper synthesis. Patients with type 2 diabetes can present with normal to increased levels of insulin as their body attempts to self-regulate the larger amounts of sugar that it is seeing from a patient's dietary intake.

LEARNING OBJECTIVE 7.4.19 **Contrast diabetes insipidus and diabetes mellitus.**

DIABETES INSIPIDUS AND DIABETES MELLITUS

Yes, it may be confusing to walk into the office and see that a patient's chief complaint is polydipsia and polyuria, but you can easily discern between the two by remembering what hormone is responsible for each disease. ADH is more often associated with DI while insulin dysregulation is related to DM. Furthermore, strong history-taking skills and evaluation of a patient's lifestyle will assist you in reaching a correct diagnosis.

LEARNING OBJECTIVE 7.4.20 **Identify common disorders affecting the adrenal glands.**

KEY TERM

Addison's disease A disorder that occurs when your body produces too little of cortisol.

ADRENAL DISORDERS

Recall that the adrenal gland is composed of two differing portions. The adrenal cortex is more responsible for corticosteroid release and is therefore more susceptible to adenomatous disorders that cause neoplastic changes. However, many adrenal cortex disorders are a direct result of physician practices. We talk about this later in the chapter.

Lying deeper within the gland, we have the adrenal medulla, which is extremely susceptible to neoplastic changes that will cause unregulated catecholamine release. The most common disorder within this tissue layer is a pheochromocytoma.

CLINICAL TIP	Pheochromocytomas are an extremely rare type of tumor. The classic triad of a pheochromocytoma is called PHE: palpitations, headaches, and excessive sweating. Diagnosis includes the quantification of epinephrine and norepinephrine metabolic waste products within a 24-hour urine sample. Remember, the only treatment is surgical resection of the tissue, and therefore you must always consider this condition if you cannot find a true diagnosis.

LEARNING OBJECTIVE 7.4.21 Describe the signs, symptoms, diagnosis, and treatment of Addison's disease.

ADDISON'S DISEASE

Addison's disease causes widespread destruction of the zona glomerulosa and fasciculata within the adrenal gland. Due to the destruction, aldosterone and cortisol are no longer properly secreted. Mostly caused by autoimmune diseases, Addison's disease can be further complicated by infections, vascular accidents, or metastatic diseases that affect the kidney. What we just read was a description of primary Addison's disease because we were talking about the destruction of the target organ. Secondary and tertiary Addison's disorders do exist, with secondary Addison's disease being an interesting concept.

Secondary Addison's disease is usually caused by medications. In secondary Addison's disease, we have a reduction in ACTH, leading to a depression in cortisol levels because the patient has been on prescription steroid use. Exogenous glucocorticoid use for inflammatory or autoimmune diseases can effectively shut off the normal cortisol system, leading to a widespread depression of cortisol levels.

Clinically, all of these patients present with symptoms indicative of low to no cortisol. Patients will complain of weakness, fatigue, myalgia, abdominal pain, syncope, hyponatremia, hyperkalemia, anorexia, hypo- or hyperglycemia, and skin hyper- or hypopigmentation dependent upon the type of Addison's disease they have as melatonin skin changes are dependent upon ACTH levels (Figure 7-27ABC).

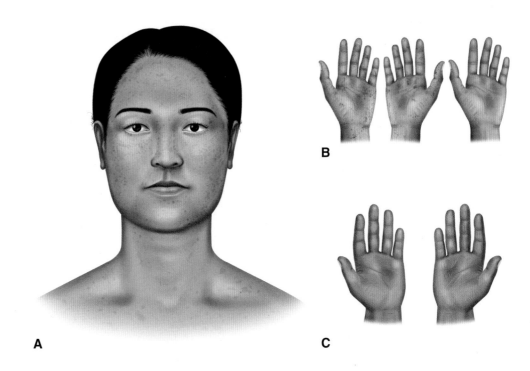

FIGURE 7-27ABC A patient's clinical manifestations can vary depending on the type of Addison's disease they have, but many patients will typically present with an increased skin pigmentation.

Diagnosis

Patients should be tested with high-dose ACTH stimulation tests to see if any changes will occur while also being subjected to CRH stimulation tests that will determine if the issue is within the pituitary or adrenal glands.

Addison's disease also effects aldosterone secretion because ACTH also controls this hormone's release. Therefore, aldosterone will be significantly reduced in the patient's blood. This is significant because aldosterone is intricately involved in reabsorbing or excreting molecules from the kidney based on the body's needs for fluid and electrolytes. As a result, less aldosterone will lead to a patient becoming hypokalemic and hypernatremic. You will learn more about where this hormone acts and its particular function in a separate chapter.

Treatment

Because both mineralocorticoids and glucocorticoids are significantly inhibited, hormone replacement therapy is the mainstay of treatment. Hydrocortisone along with fludrocortisone are the pharmacological interventions, but continuous monitoring is warranted. At any time, additional cortisol may be needed to respond to a stressful situation.

LEARNING
OBJECTIVE 7.4.22 **Identify common disorders affecting the ovaries.**

KEY TERM

dermoid cystic teratomas Tumor made up of several different types of tissues.

OVARIAN DISORDERS

The most common ovarian disorders are usually benign but can mimic those of neoplastic disease, usually requiring considerable care and elucidation of the true cause. Disorders can range from ovarian cysts, ovarian cancer, dermoid cystic teratomas, and polycystic ovarian syndrome. Not surprisingly, all these disorders are connected one way or another to FSH and LH.

LEARNING
OBJECTIVE 7.4.23 **Describe the signs, symptoms, diagnosis, and treatment of polycystic ovarian syndrome.**

KEY TERMS

hirsutism Condition of male-pattern hair growth in the female population. Usually occurring on the face.

polycystic ovarian syndrome (PCOS) Condition in women where higher than normal levels

of male hormones are produced leading to hirsutism, diabetes, and possible infertility.

POLYCYSTIC OVARIAN SYNDROME

Polycystic ovarian syndrome (PCOS) is an endocrine syndrome caused by an overactivation within the hypothalamus–pituitary–ovarian axis. As previously learned, female reproductive organs are under the control of LH and FSH, which will lead to alterations in the levels of estrogen and progesterone in the body. In patients with PCOS, this balance becomes disrupted, leading to an increased level of LH with no negative feedback mechanisms to reduce its release.

Diagnosis

As a result of the above, ovarian androgens like estrogen and its precursor molecule, testosterone, begin to increase; however, there is no change in progesterone. As we have learned, progesterone is responsible for the release of the ovum and the beginning of menstruation, but women with PCOS have depressed levels because of the increased levels of estrogen and testosterone. Therefore, PCOS patients will begin to complain of amenorrhea and hirsutism, unwanted male pattern hair growth due to increased levels of testosterone.

Interestingly enough, this axis also has some secondary control over insulin release, which makes matters worse. Patients begin to become insulin resistant, which only increases the severity of their clinical picture because now they begin to develop diabetes and obesity.

Treatment

Because PCOS is a diagnosis of exclusion and cannot be treated until other options are addressed, treatment usually includes oral contraceptives that are used to reduce androgens and stabilize the menstrual cycle. Spironolactone, an androgen inhibitor, has been shown to have great control over the hormonal imbalances seen in PCOS. And, as always, there are diet and lifestyle changes that can be done as PCOS has shown to have a direct correlation to obesity and type 2 diabetes.

LEARNING OBJECTIVE 7.4.24 Identify common disorders affecting the testis.

KEY TERMS

hydroceles Swelling in the scrotum that occurs when fluid collects in the tissue surrounding the testicle.

testicular torsion Twisting of the spermatic cord that inhibits blood supply to a testicle, which is a medical emergency.

varicoceles Swelling or an increase in size of the veins that supply the scrotum and testicles.

DISORDERS OF THE TESTIS

Like the ovaries, the testis is subject to benign and neoplastic growths like testicular cancers. Further complications can arise in the form of varicoceles which is an enlargement of the veins around the testicle, hydroceles which is a medical condition in which fluid becomes trapped around the testicle, and testicular torsion which is an acute medical emergency. Specific to the endocrine system, hypogonadism can be a direct consequence of decreased blood testosterone levels indirectly related to either GnRH or FSH and LH release. Smaller than normal testicles should always be investigated, especially if there has been a noticeable change in size.

UNIT OBJECTIVE 7.5

Describe common pathologies related to physical and physiological stress on the body.

UNIT INTRODUCTION

Chronic stress not only is annoying for our psyche, but its constant presence can begin to alter normal physiologic conditions that can be life-threatening.

LEARNING OBJECTIVE 7.5.1 **Describe the effects of physical and physiological stress on blood pressure.**

STRESS AND BLOOD PRESSURE

Stressful situations produce a surge of hormones when we are in a stressful situation. Controlled by sympathetic tone and catecholamine release, there is widespread vasoconstriction and increased cardiac output. Together, these physiological changes raise blood pressure where chronic stress can continue to perpetuate these issues. Physically, vasoconstriction and cardiac output could make your skin sweaty, your pupils dilate to intake information, and a focus only found through stimulant release.

LEARNING OBJECTIVE 7.5.2 **Describe the effects of physical and physiological stress on normal sleep patterns.**

STRESS AND SLEEP

Stress can physiologically inhibit melatonin release by upregulating excitatory hormones and neurotransmitters within the CNS. Further melatonin depression will only continue to deepen already altered sleep patterns and behaviors. Physically, patients may feel more agitated, lethargic, on edge, or delirious.

LEARNING OBJECTIVE 7.5.3 **Describe the effects of physical and physiological stress on body weight.**

STRESS AND BODY WEIGHT

An ever-present sympathetic stimulatory tone leads to tachycardia and an increased metabolic state which will relate to widespread weight loss. Furthermore, cortisol released during stressful situations will only increase metabolic rate and basal body temperatures. Physically, joints and bones may feel better while cardiac and pulmonology function will increase, barring any development of an eating disorder, which can accompany stressful situations and anxiety.

Chapter 8

The Blood

Chapter Introduction

Blood is the connection between everything in our body. This liquid tissue is the river through which all biological products and processes flow. Modern medicine still views blood as an important snapshot of what is happening within a patient. Health care professionals examine this tissue more often than any other when trying to determine the cause of a disease. In this chapter we describe the functions of blood, its components, and the many diseases that can arise from this life-sustaining fluid.

UNIT OBJECTIVE 8.1

Describe the characteristics of blood and blood cells.

UNIT INTRODUCTION

Blood is the transporting fluid. It has the ability to carry nutrients from the digestive tract to cells along with oxygen and other metabolic wastes while fighting pathogens. In this unit, we learn about the different parts of blood and how they contribute to carrying out a variety of functions.

LEARNING OBJECTIVE 8.1.1 Describe the overall function of blood and its role in homeostasis.

KEY TERM

formed elements Living cellular components of the blood.

BLOOD'S OVERALL FUNCTION

Blood performs numerous types of functions, with the most prominent job being the movement of substances from one area of the body to the next. Transportation allows for blood to be oxygenated by the lungs, metabolic wastes to be cleared, and hormones to be delivered to target organs. Blood is also a master regulator of our body's internal environment. Such tasks as temperature control, pH monitoring, and assessment of fluid volume are all essential roles to which blood contributes. These types of regulatory mechanisms are described in other chapters.

Blood further maintains homeostasis by contributing to the immune system and stopping blood loss. The factors controlling these functions are known as formed elements and are the living cellular components of our blood.

LEARNING OBJECTIVE 8.1.2 Identify the formed elements in blood.

LEARNING OBJECTIVE 8.1.3 Describe the formed elements in blood.

KEY TERMS

agranulocytes White blood cells that do not contain packets of chemicals that can activate the immune system. Examples include leukocytes and monocytes.

erythrocytes Red blood cells found in blood that contain hemoglobin and carry oxygen throughout the body.

erythropoiesis Process of creating red blood cells.

granulocytes White blood cells that contain immunologic chemicals packaged in small granules. Examples include neutrophils, eosinophils, and basophils.

hemoglobin Protein containing a red pigment that can bind and transport oxygen.

leukocytes White blood cell; circulates throughout the body and plays an important part in the body's immune response and reaction to foreign bodies and disease.

leukopoiesis Process of creating new white blood cells within the bone marrow.

megakaryocytes Large bone marrow cell that acts as the precursor to platelets.

platelets Formed elements that help to form blood clots.

plasma Liquid portion of blood that contains proteins and clotting factors.

COMPOSITION OF BLOOD

At its core, blood is classified as a type of connective tissue with a liquid extracellular matrix. Blood is considered a connective tissue because it consists of cells (formed elements) surrounded by an extracellular matrix, which in the case of blood is the liquid blood plasma (Figure 8-1).

Unlike typical connective tissue, blood lacks collagen and elastic fibers. We discuss why blood is still considered a connective tissue later but for now let us talk about the specific formed elements and plasma.

There are three types of formed elements, the most abundant being erythrocytes. Outside of the health care community, erythrocytes are known as red blood cells (RBCs). Erythrocytes normally comprise 45% of the volume of a blood sample, with just one microliter (uL) containing 4.7–6 million RBCs! To clarify this even further, one eye drop is equivalent to 50 uL, meaning we are talking about microscopic levels of liquid that still contain that

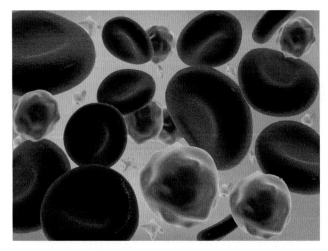

FIGURE 8-1 Under microscopy, RBCs are reddened circles that will deliver oxygen throughout the blood. Surrounding these formed elements is plasma, which is depicted by the white spaces. Other formed elements include WBCs, which usually are stained purple in microscope smears. Here we see a certain type of WBC in the bottom left corner.

many RBCs. Therefore, it makes sense that RBCs are only about 7.5 um in diameter. These cells are shaped like biconcave discs and appear red and light in color under a microscope. Erythrocytes are formed through a process known as erythropoiesis, which is discussed later. Once erythropoiesis is complete, mature RBCs lack a nucleus (known as anucleate) and most organelles. Without a nucleus, RBCs lack the ability to divide and multiply or repair cellular damage. This inability to repair any damage that occurs to the cell accounts for their relatively short 120-day lifespan. Lacking a nucleus and organelles makes RBCs a highly specialized type of cell whose main job is to transport oxygen and carbon dioxide throughout the body. This process is carried out by hemoglobin, a protein that makes up RBCs and easily binds to oxygen.

The second type of formed element is leukocytes, or white blood cells (WBCs). WBCs account for only 1% of formed elements, with 4000–11,000 WBCs for each microliter of blood. Despite their low numbers, WBCs are an integral part of the immune system and our defense against disease. As a result, WBCs use the bloodstream as a mode of transportation to areas of damage or infection.

Unlike RBCs, WBCs possess nuclei and organelles. These organelles are essential for the continued immune response that leukocytes will initiate when they reach a local area of damage or infection. Leukocytes are created through a process known as leukopoiesis, a process that is explained in greater detail shortly.

Leukopoiesis will yield the five main types of leukocytes. These leukocytes can further be separated into granulocytes and agranulocytes. Granulocytes are leukocytes that contain secretory packets within their cytoplasm-containing compounds that will activate other parts of the immune system, destroying pathogens or creating a global immune response. The three granulocytes are neutrophils, eosinophils, and basophils. Agranulocytes, as their name suggests, are leukocytes without secretory packets in their cytoplasm. There are two types of agranulocytes, monocytes and lymphocytes. Specifics on these cell types are discussed later.

The final type of formed element is platelets, even though they are not technically cells. Platelets are fragments of megakaryocytes, a cell that is produced during leukopoiesis. Megakaryocytes are large cells that get trapped within the bone marrow as they try to exit the small capillaries that lead to the systemic circulatory system. As a result, platelets are actually fragmenting the megakaryocyte, which break off and exit the capillaries in the bone marrow.

LEARNING OBJECTIVE 8.1.4 Identify the components of the liquid portion of blood.

LEARNING OBJECTIVE 8.1.5 Describe the physical properties of plasma.

LEARNING OBJECTIVE 8.1.6 Describe the functions of the various plasma components.

KEY TERM

albumin Plasma protein found in the blood that creates and maintains blood's colloid osmotic pressure.

COMPOSITION OF PLASMA

Blood plasma is a straw-colored, sticky fluid comprising 55% of the whole blood volume. Plasma is 90% water, with the other 10% composed of numerous different dissolved solutes. These dissolved molecules include nutrients, gases, hormones, wastes, and products of cell activity, proteins, and electrolytes. Table 8-1 summarizes the major plasma components.

Table 8-1 Composition and Description of Various Plasma Components

TYPE	DESCRIPTION	
WATER	Dissolves solutes and absorbs heat for redistribution	
	SUBTYPE	**DESCRIPTION**
SOLUTES	**Electrolytes**	Includes Na^+, K^+, Ca^{2+}, Mg^{2+}, Cl^-, PO_{3-}, SO_{2-}, HCO_{3-}, H^+
	Plasma proteins	Albumin
		Gamma globulins
		Fibrinogen
	Nonprotein nitrogenous substances	Urea, uric acid, creatinine, and ammonium salts
	Gases	Oxygen and carbon dioxide
	Hormones	Steroid and nonsteroid hormones

Electrolytes vastly outnumber the other substances and play an integral role in maintaining osmotic pressure, normal blood pH, and cell function. Plasma proteins are the other important part of plasma as they serve a variety of functions. There are three main types of plasma proteins. The first and most abundant is **albumin**. Synthesized by the liver, albumin acts as a carrier to shuttle certain molecules through circulation while also contributing to normal blood pH and plasma osmotic pressure. Additional proteins like gamma globulins are antibodies released during an immune response. Finally, fibrinogen, a plasma protein created by the liver, is an important part of the clotting cascade.

Smaller components of plasma include molecules that are by-products of cellular metabolism. Most of these substances will be excreted by the kidneys. Other cellular metabolites are dissolved within the plasma, like carbon dioxide that can be replaced by oxygen within the capillaries. Furthermore, hormones that target distant endocrine organs will either be dissolved in the blood or bind to plasma proteins.

Because the body is constantly trying to maintain a fluid balance between electrolytes, proteins, and cellular metabolites, the composition of plasma varies continuously. Small changes can easily disrupt the homeostatic balance of plasma composition as an increase in cellular activity can lead to a buildup of nitrogenous wastes or lactic acid.

CLINICAL TIP

Plasma holds the formed elements within suspension but is less dense than the cellular components of blood. Therefore, plasma can be easily separated from RBCs, WBCs, and platelets via centrifugation (Figure 8-2). Spinning a blood sample can separate the main components of the blood so the plasma or formed elements can be measured.

For instance, patients with a suspected electrolyte imbalance can be further worked up by obtaining a blood sample that is then subjected to centrifugation. Plasma is then isolated, and electrolyte levels can be measured with greater accuracy.

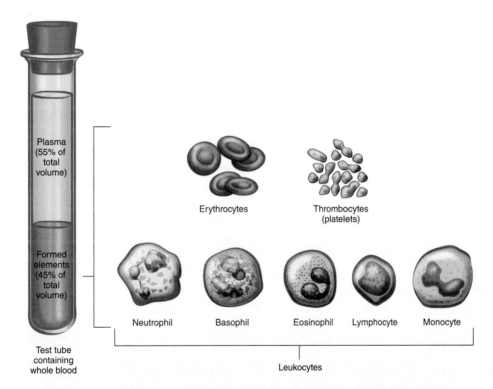

Plasma (55% of total volume)

Formed elements (45% of total volume)

Test tube containing whole blood

Erythrocytes

Thrombocytes (platelets)

Neutrophil   Basophil   Eosinophil   Lymphocyte   Monocyte

Leukocytes

FIGURE 8-2 Traveling at hundreds of RPMs a minute, plasma and formed elements begin to separate based on their density. RBCs sink to the bottom while plasma stays at the top of the test tube due to the amount of weight and contents the cell holds.

LEARNING OBJECTIVE 8.1.7 Identify hematopoietic stem cells.

LEARNING OBJECTIVE 8.1.8 Describe the process of hematopoiesis.

HEMATOPOIETIC STEM CELLS

Formed elements of blood all arise from undifferentiated precursor cells known hematopoietic stem cells (HSCs). HSCs will begin to transform into RBCs, WBCs, or platelets depending on the body's current need and chemical messengers (known as hematopoietic factors).

Depending on the hormones and growth factors present, there are two cell types that begin to form the formed elements. The first cell type is known as a myeloid progenitor cell. Myeloid progenitor cells are the precursors for RBCs, megakaryocytes, eosinophils, basophils, neutrophils, monocytes (that can turn into macrophages), and dendritic cells. The second cell type is lymphoid progenitor cells, which will eventually lead to the creation of natural killer cells, T cells, and B cells. Figure 8-3 shows the pathway of erythrocyte and leukocyte differentiation.

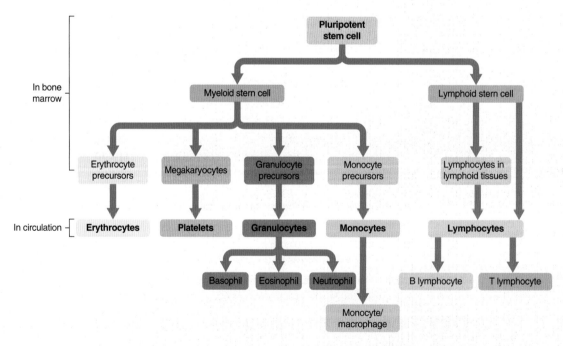

FIGURE 8-3 Once the bone marrow is activated by hematopoietic factors, the hematopoietic stem cells begin to differentiate into these specific pathways. As maturation continues, cells become more specialized and eventually end up manifesting into fully functional portions of the immune and circulatory systems.

HEMATOPOIESIS

The process of blood cell differentiation is called **hematopoiesis**. The hematopoietic stem cells are located within the red marrow of the pectoral and pelvic girdles, humerus, and femur. Hematopoiesis can be further broken up into two specific types of cell differentiation: erythropoiesis and leukopoiesis. Erythropoiesis is the process of forming new RBCs by initiating myeloid progenitor cell production and subsequent erythrocyte production. Erythropoiesis can be increased for a variety of reasons that will be covered later in this chapter. Overall, any reduction in the number of RBCs, reduced hemoglobin, or decreased oxygen levels in the blood will cause the increase in levels of erythropoietin. **Erythropoietin** is a hormone that binds to HSCs in the red marrow and begins the process of erythropoiesis (Figure 8-4).

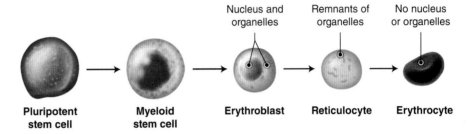

FIGURE 8-4 Erythropoiesis is a highly specialized mechanism that ultimately results in an increase of functional RBCs that can be used for increased oxygen delivery. Initiation of hematopoietic stem cells into myeloid progenitor cells begins this process and continues to specialize into reticulocytes and finally erythrocytes. These mature RBCs exit the bone marrow and enter into the systemic circulatory system.

CLINICAL TIP

Reticulocytes account for about 2% of all circulating blood in healthy people. Therefore, complete blood counts (CBC) usually contain reticulocyte counts, a quantification of what percentage of the RBCs are reticulocytes. Reticulocyte counts above or below the normal range indicate abnormal rates of RBC production and are a result of a multitude of disorders that can include anemias, thalassemias, cancers, internal bleeds, or pneumonia.

If erythropoiesis is responsible for RBC production, then leukopoiesis is the process of WBC production. Because certain immune cells arise from differing progenitor cells, myeloid or lymphoid, the signal is specific to the cell needed to fight the present pathogen. When our body is infected, the pathogen can be of various types. Usually the pathogen is a bacteria or virus, but sometimes it's a fungus. Certain WBCs have a propensity to fight certain pathogens creating a difference in stimuli that might increase myeloid progenitor cells over lymphoid progenitors.

Therefore, most of leukopoiesis is driven by interleukins and colony-stimulating factors. **Interleukins** are specialized glycoproteins released by WBCs to recruit more of that certain type of WBC. These interleukins will stimulate specific **colony-stimulating factors (CSFs)** embedded within the bone marrow that will begin to differentiate the HSC into the needed WBC type.

For example, cancer patients undergoing chemotherapy that suppresses bone marrow are given intravenous CSFs. These CSFs stimulate the production of WBCs in an attempt to promote an intact immune system. The process of leukopoiesis is summarized in Figure 8-5.

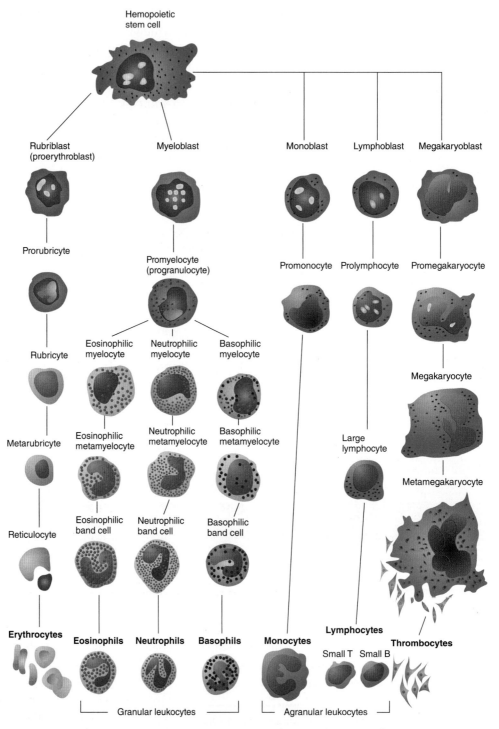

FIGURE 8-5 CSFs and interleukins are the main driving forces behind the development of new WBCs. Despite the type of WBC being created, its lineage can be traced back to an increase in a certain type of CSF or interleukin level. As CSF and interleukins enter the bone marrow, they act upon the hematopoietic stem cells and begin to differentiate them into the desired cell.

LEARNING OBJECTIVE 8.1.9 Identify red blood cells and their structural characteristics.

KEY TERMS

anucleate Cells that are without a nucleus.

hemoglobin Protein containing a red pigment that can bind and transport oxygen.

micro-thrombosis Small thrombosis usually affecting small capillaries that can lead to infarctions.

sickle cell anemia Inherited form of anemia in which there aren't enough healthy red blood cells to carry adequate oxygen throughout the body.

thalassemia Blood disorder that decreases the proper formation of hemoglobin within the red blood cell structure.

RED BLOOD CELLS

As we have discussed, RBCs are created by a process known as erythropoiesis, which can be controlled by the amount of erythropoietin, hemoglobin, and oxygen in the body. Changes in any of these levels will specifically affect the number of mature RBCs that are created.

Interestingly, mature erythrocytes are anucleate, meaning that they do not contain a nucleus. RBCs also lack most organelles, preventing these cells from actively dividing after being released into the bloodstream.

Oxygen binds to erythrocytes via hemoglobin, a protein that makes RBCs red and binds easily and reversibly to oxygen. Hemoglobin (Hb) is made up of a heme group that is comprised of an iron atom and a protein globin of four polypeptide chains, two alpha (α) and two beta (β) chains (Figure 8-6). Each hemoglobin molecule can carry four oxygen molecules, and one RBC has over 250 million hemoglobin molecules. This means that if we do the math, one RBC allows for the transport of one billion molecules of oxygen!

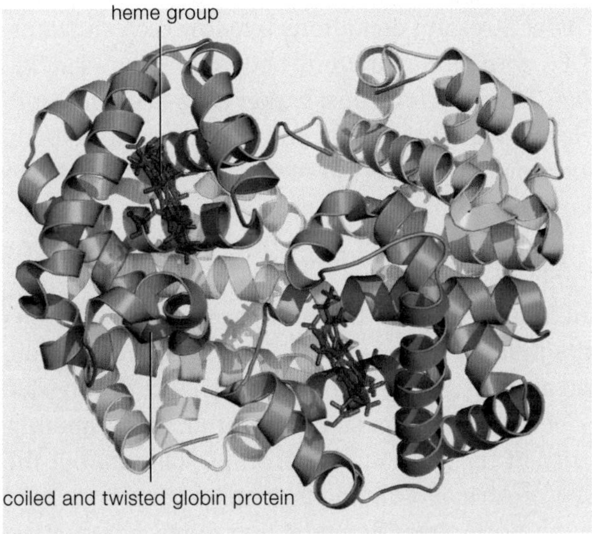

heme group

coiled and twisted globin protein

FIGURE 8-6 RBCs develop a biconcave shape and are anucleate. RBCs are formed by a heme molecule and iron molecule. These molecules bind oxygen and allow for its transport throughout the circulatory system.

ABNORMAL HEMOGLOBIN

Production of abnormal hemoglobin is a genetic variant that can cause debilitating effects for patients. All hemoglobinopathies (abnormal hemoglobin disorders) can be classified into two types: thalassemias or abnormal hemoglobin structures. Thalassemias are a result of underproduction of normal globin subunits. This loss of normal hemoglobin subunits leads to a decrease in the oxygen-binding ability of the RBC. These red blood cells are also dysmorphic, meaning that they lose their normal biconcave doughnut shape, which can cause them to become lodged in capillary beds. The inappropriate structure also increases the fragility of the RBC, leading to shorter lifespans and destruction as they begin to occlude the blood vessels they are lodged in. For instance, a nice round biconcave RBC will easily travel through

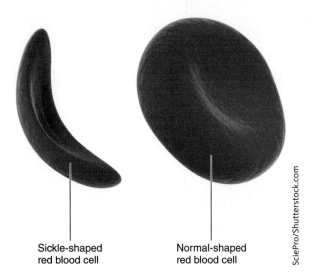

Sickle-shaped
red blood cell

Normal-shaped
red blood cell

SciePro/Shutterstock.com

FIGURE 8-7 Due to the improper coding of genes that create RBCs, those with a sickle cell shape develop an elongated and noncircular appearance under a microscope. This change in shape also makes it more difficult to transfer oxygen and easily move through small capillaries.

a small circular blood vessel, whereas a polygonal, noncircular RBC that are usually the by-products of thalassemias might get stuck in the blood vessel and cause complications that could lead to death.

Structural abnormalities in the globin proteins are different from thalassemias because they are a qualitative, not quantitative, problem. These genetic diseases result in the abnormal structure of one of the globin chains, either α or β. Genetic alterations lead to different amino acids being coded for the formation of the chain, impairing its ability to properly fold and bind to oxygen (Figure 8-7).

Sickle Cell Trait and Disease

The most common structural abnormality disease is sickle cell trait, which is an autosomal recessive disease. Autosomal recessive diseases are quite rare as both parents have to have the abnormal gene and then pass it onto their child. For sickle cell trait, this abnormal gene affects the formation of the hemoglobin β chain. We denote this change in the hemoglobin structure by indicating the position in the peptide chain that was improperly coded along with the new amino acid that was inserted. As a result, people with sickle cell trait are denoted as HbS.

Interestingly enough, carrying the HbS trait confers some protection against malaria and has thus survived in the gene pool of sub-Saharan African descendants and, to a lesser extent, eastern Mediterranean and Middle Eastern ethnic groups. However, under stressful conditions like low oxygen states, sickness, and dehydration, RBCs with HbS mutations become rigid and sickle shaped due to improper folding. These grossly misshapen cells occlude capillary beds that can eventually lead to an obstruction and infarction if the body remains in a stressful state for a prolonged period of time. It is important to remember that hemoglobin molecule formation is not dependent on one gene but on many genes. Therefore, just because an individual has inherited one abnormal gene from their parents does not mean that every hemoglobin molecule will be improperly formed in their body. But, if a person of the various ethnicities listed above inherits multiple copies of the HbS genetic mutation, they may progress to **sickle cell disease**. Sickle cell disease is more severe due to a higher percentage of sickled RBCs than in sickle cell trait. Consequently, sickle cell trait is found in 8–10% of the African American population, but the *disease* is found in about 0.002% of African Americans.

Sickle cell trait and disease both alter the usual and correct formation of hemoglobin and RBC structure. This mutation causes RBCs to look sickled under a microscope. With less surface area and decreased oxygen-binding capacity, patients with sickle cell trait and disease can easily become fatigued in times of high stress. Complications, while rare, can manifest themselves as infarctions and intense pain as the RBCs begin to occlude smaller vessels and capillaries.

Recent illnesses can stress the body, creating a hypoxic state, and under lower oxygen conditions, this sickle-shaped RBC becomes more pronounced as the β chains stick together. This increased stiffening of the RBC reduces the surface area needed to bind oxygen. Eventually, the stiffness of the RBC will cause it to rupture or build up in smaller vessels that cannot accommodate the change from a circular smooth RBC to a hardened crescent-shaped molecule. We call this phenomenon **micro-thrombosis**. Often patients with sickle cell disease will have splenic infarcts frequently, resulting in a small nonfunctional spleen that may end up being surgically removed (Figure 8-8).

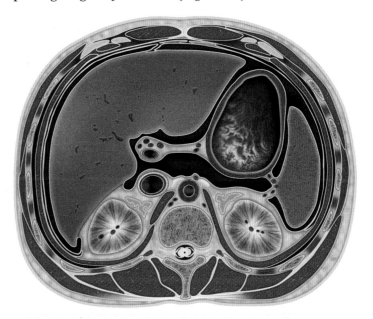

FIGURE 8-8 Abdominal CT scan of a patient admitted to the emergency department in a sickle cell crisis. On the left side the spleen has some changes in its color due to the ischemia of that area of the spleen. This part of the spleen may quickly become necrotic and could lead to surgical removal.

LEARNING OBJECTIVE 8.1.10 **Describe the function of red blood cells.**

KEY TERM

hemoglobin buffer system Chemical process that hemoglobin undergoes in order to balance blood pH.

RED BLOOD CELL FUNCTIONS

Overall, RBCs have two main functions in the body. The most commonly known function of the RBC is to transport oxygen from the lungs and deliver it to the tissues of the body. In the lungs oxygen molecules received from inspired air will be bound to the hemoglobin molecules within the RBC. Once the RBC reaches the capillary bed of a target organ, the oxygen molecules uncouple from the hemoglobin structures and exit the capillaries via fenestrations into the interstitial space and into the cell. At this point carbon dioxide (CO_2), a by-product of cellular metabolism, diffuses into the capillaries and binds to the free hemoglobin. As a result, RBCs transport CO_2 back to the lungs where it will exit the body during exhalation (Figure 8-9AB).

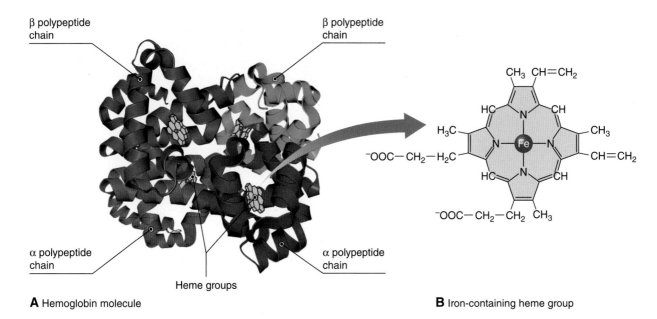

A Hemoglobin molecule

B Iron-containing heme group

FIGURE 8-9AB Hemoglobin is responsible for the binding of oxygen and subsequently carbon dioxide when it is transported back to the lungs. This bond is essential to the function of RBCs in the body.

Even though most CO_2 is expired, some remains within the RBCs because this molecule can be used to manage any sudden changes in systemic acidity or alkalinity via the **hemoglobin buffer system**. This idea of blood being a buffering system is covered more completely in Chapter 16.

LEARNING OBJECTIVE 8.1.11 Identify the normal lab values for number of red blood cells, hemoglobin, and hematocrit.

KEY TERM

hematocrit (Hct) Blood test that measures the volume percentage of red blood cells in blood.

NORMAL RBC VALUES

Complete blood count results will always offer a snapshot of the number of total RBCs within the bloodstream. Normal RBC numbers for males range from 4.7 to 6.1 million cells per microliter of blood, while females have a range between 4.2 and 5.4 million cells per microliter (recall our eyedrop example from earlier). Because the average body contains about 5–6 liters of blood, we can do simple math and reveal that there are roughly 25 trillion RBCs in our body at any given time! Fluctuating levels of RBCs vary depending on certain disease processes. Increases in number usually signal a genetic disorder. What is more concerning are decreases in RBC production, as they signal an underlying issue with nutrients available for cell production, blatant RBC destruction, or outright loss of RBCs via hemorrhage.

NORMAL HEMOGLOBIN VALUES

As we have learned, hemoglobin is specifically integrated into red blood cells during their formation. Hemoglobin will give us a quick snapshot of our oxygen-carrying capacity. Normally, males have 13.5–17.5 grams of hemoglobin per deciliter of blood, while females have 12.0–15.5 grams per deciliter.

Deciliters are vastly different than microliters. While microliters measure microscopic drops of blood, deciliters are one-tenth of a liter, or 100 mL. This is a volume we can see with our own eyes. It would be like pouring 10% of a liter of soda into a glass to have with our slice of pizza.

Again, like RBCs, fluctuating levels of hemoglobin have various pathologies but illustrate an overall increase in whole blood when compared to plasma. Decreased levels of hemoglobin are usually a result of hemorrhaging or a reduced ability to create this protein properly.

NORMAL HEMATOCRIT VALUES

Hematocrit (Hct) measures the proportion of RBCs in a percentage of blood (Figure 8-10). The number directly reflects the volume that the RBCs occupy in that sample of blood we mentioned earlier (see Clinical Tip). Therefore, a hematocrit can be expressed as the ratio of RBCs to every other blood product that we have discussed thus far. Males should have a hematocrit of 45–52% and females typically have a Hct of 37–48%. Increased hematocrits have various pathologies but illustrate an overall increase in production of RBCs or their increased contribution to the overall spun-down sample. Decreased levels of hemoglobin usually stem from hemorrhage or a reduced ability to create RBCs properly.

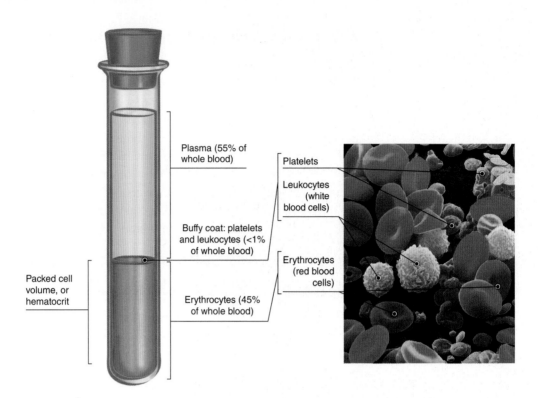

Plasma (55% of whole blood)

Platelets

Leukocytes (white blood cells)

Buffy coat: platelets and leukocytes (<1% of whole blood)

Erythrocytes (red blood cells)

Packed cell volume, or hematocrit

Erythrocytes (45% of whole blood)

FIGURE 8-10 Centrifugation of blood will easily quantify the percentage of RBCs in a sample of blood. The hematocrit can be affected by multiple factors that can either increase or decrease in value in the sample of blood.

LEARNING OBJECTIVE 8.1.12 Explain why red blood cell counts are important.

KEY TERM

hypercoagulable state Increased predisposition to form clots.

IMPORTANCE OF RBC LEVELS

Because RBCs comprise most of our blood compartment, any alteration in their number could have significant impacts on our overall physiology. Remember that RBCs are the main cell that transports oxygen and is responsible for removal of CO_2 and any significant decrease will lead to poor oxygenation of tissues along with a reduced ability to remove potent toxins from the interstitial spaces. Conversely, increases in RBCs can also be detrimental. Any increase in RBC, Hgb, and Hct is also important to document as an improper overproduction presents issues with adequate normal RBC, WBC, platelet, and protein function. Increases in any levels above normal ranges can also lead to an increase in the viscosity of blood, causing a **hypercoagulable state**, a condition in which there is an increased tendency toward blood clotting.

LEARNING OBJECTIVE 8.1.13 **Explain how the number of red blood cells present in a sample of blood can be used to diagnose disease.**

Decreased RBC, Hemoglobin, and Hematocrit Levels

Decreased levels of RBCs or the tests that express its overall contribution to whole blood can indicate several diseases that affect the overall quantity of RBCs and their proper function. Diseases or states accompanied by a decrease in RBC levels include anemias, which is the complete loss of blood, destruction of RBCs via hemolytic disorders, or underproduction because of nutritional deficiencies. Renal failure can also potentiate decreases in these values because we lose the ability to secrete EPO, a topic we discuss later in this chapter. Cancers along with a growing fetus during pregnancy can utilize iron and B_{12}, a vitamin needed for the correct synthesis of RBCs. Additionally, certain medication classes like antibiotics and nonsteroidal anti-inflammatory drugs (NSAIDs) can decrease these levels as they interfere with proper absorption of nutrients needed to create RBCs within the bone marrow.

Increased RBC, Hemoglobin, and Hematocrit Levels

Increased levels of RBCs or the tests that show an overview of its contribution to whole blood, can indicate several diseases that are affecting the overall quantity of RBCs or their proper function. Diseases or states that can be inferred by an increase in RBC levels include polycythemias which are a class of genetic disorders that elevate the Hct count. Other diseases that create a hypoxic environment like chronic obstructive pulmonary disease, chronic bronchitis, smoking, or cancer will also lead to elevated values as our body attempts to make more RBCs that can capture more oxygen.

CLINICAL TIP	Dehydration can falsely lead one to believe that there is an increase in Hct, Hgb, and RBCs because they are occupying more space in the blood sample since there is less water to create the plasma layer.

LEARNING OBJECTIVE 8.1.14 **Describe the life cycle of a red blood cell.**

KEY TERMS

bile Yellow or greenish alkaline fluid secreted by the liver and passed into the duodenum where it aids in the absorption of fat.

bilirubin Pigment formed by the breakdown of hemoglobin and excreted in the bile.

biliverdin By-product of heme synthesis.

ferritin Blood cell protein that contains iron.

hemosiderin A deposit or collection of iron after it has been broken down from RBCs.

RED BLOOD CELL LIFE CYCLE

The usual lifespan of an RBC is 100–120 days because their anucleate state prohibits them from synthesizing new proteins, growing, or dividing. After a mature RBC enters the systemic circulation system from the bone marrow, its hemoglobin begins to degrade, reducing the cell's ability to carry oxygen. Because mature RBCs are anucleate, they lack the ability to repair cellular damage sustained from traveling through arteries and veins. Damaged RBCs are eventually destroyed by macrophages found in the spleen, liver, and bone marrow (Figure 8-11).

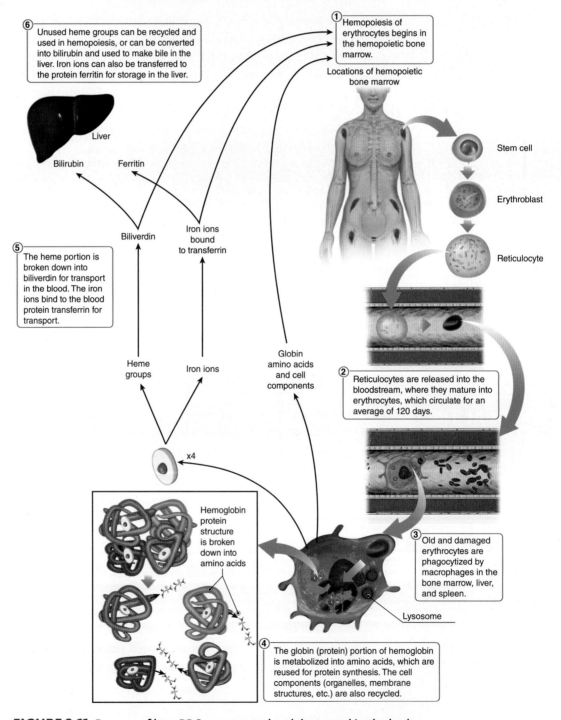

6. Unused heme groups can be recycled and used in hemopoiesis, or can be converted into bilirubin and used to make bile in the liver. Iron ions can also be transferred to the protein ferritin for storage in the liver.

1. Hemopoiesis of erythrocytes begins in the hemopoietic bone marrow.

Locations of hemopoietic bone marrow

Liver

Bilirubin   Ferritin

Stem cell

Erythroblast

Reticulocyte

Biliverdin   Iron ions bound to transferrin

5. The heme portion is broken down into biliverdin for transport in the blood. The iron ions bind to the blood protein transferrin for transport.

Heme groups   Iron ions

Globin amino acids and cell components

2. Reticulocytes are released into the bloodstream, where they mature into erythrocytes, which circulate for an average of 120 days.

x4

Hemoglobin protein structure is broken down into amino acids

3. Old and damaged erythrocytes are phagocytized by macrophages in the bone marrow, liver, and spleen.

Lysosome

4. The globin (protein) portion of hemoglobin is metabolized into amino acids, which are reused for protein synthesis. The cell components (organelles, membrane structures, etc.) are also recycled.

FIGURE 8-11 Process of how RBCs are created and destroyed in the body.

During destruction, the heme structure and globin protein begin to dissociate. The globin portion of hemoglobin is further metabolized into its specific amino acids, which are also recycled for future hemoglobin production.

The liver has a unique ability to salvage the iron group of the heme molecule and bind it to ferritin or hemosiderin, two proteins that assist in iron storing. Iron is reused again for new hemoglobin formation; the remaining portion of heme is broken down into biliverdin and further into bilirubin, a yellow pigment that is secreted into the GI system and renal tubules. Bilirubin is also responsible for the pigmentation of bile, a solution secreted by the gallbladder to aid in the breakdown of fats.

LEARNING OBJECTIVE 8.1.15 Define erythropoietin.

LEARNING OBJECTIVE 8.1.16 Explain the role erythropoietin plays in red blood cell production.

KEY TERMS

chemoreceptors Sensory proteins that detect chemicals in bodily fluids; also related to the perception of smell and taste.

erythropoietin (EPO) Hormone that increases red blood cell production.

ERYTHROPOIETIN

Erythropoietin (EPO) is a glycoprotein that will directly stimulate erythropoiesis within the red marrow. The overall signal that causes a release of EPO is the drop in normal blood oxygen levels (Figure 8-9). Specialized oxygen receptors, known as chemoreceptors most commonly found in the kidney, will measure the concentration of oxygen within the blood. If a drop of oxygen concentration is sensed, chemoreceptors will signal the release of factors that are sensitive to low concentrations of oxygen that will subsequently accelerate EPO release. Additionally, males tend to have higher levels of erythropoietin when compared to women due to the direct stimulation of EPO production via testosterone. This is why males have higher levels of RBCs, Hgb, and Hct.

There are three specific conditions that will increase EPO levels:

- Reduced numbers of RBCs due to hemorrhage or inappropriate destruction due to inherited hemolytic diseases or improper blood transfusions (discussed later)
- Insufficient RBC production because of nutritional deficits like folate or vitamin B_{12}
- Reduced availability of oxygen that calls for more RBCs and hemoglobin to capture all the available inhaled oxygen molecules

LEARNING OBJECTIVE 8.1.17 **Explain why erythropoietin is used illicitly by professional athletes.**

EPO DOPING

Athletes that engage in highly aerobic activities like professional cyclers or marathon runners have been known to inject themselves with a synthetic EPO that elicits the same effects as the endogenous hormone. By injecting EPO, athletes can increase their stamina and performance by increasing RBC numbers, effectively expanding their oxygen-carrying capacity. Having more RBCs than the average athlete will allow the body to effectively shunt more blood and energy to the athlete's already taxed muscles during competition. One downside that many of these athletes overlook is that as they are exercising, they become dehydrated, further concentrating their already thick blood. The increasing viscosity of the blood can get stuck to the endothelial tissues of arteries and veins, causing a formation of a thrombus and putting these individuals at risk for clotting, strokes, and myocardial infarction.

LEARNING OBJECTIVE 8.1.18 **Identify the five types of white blood cells.**

LEARNING OBJECTIVE 8.1.19 **Classify the five types of white blood cells as either granulocytes or agranulocytes.**

LEARNING OBJECTIVE 8.1.20 **Describe the function of each of the five white blood cell types.**

KEY TERMS

defensins Peptides that kill foreign cells by poking holes in cell membranes and cell walls.

leukocytosis Increased white blood cell counts usually due to an immune response or neoplastic syndrome.

WHITE BLOOD CELLS

Accounting for less than 1% of the total blood volume, white blood cells are far less numerous than red blood cells. However, WBCs are critical to our defense against disease, and through the process of leukocytosis, can increase rapidly in number. By mounting an immune response to pathogens and recruiting additional immune cells, these cells are integral in the maintenance of our overall health.

White blood cells can be grouped into two major categories based on structural and chemical characteristics. Granulocytes contain obvious membrane-bound cytoplasmic granules that will be used to destroy pathogens or enhance an immune response. Agranulocytes lack obvious granules but still have important functions in immune surveillance.

Granulocytes

Granulocytes characteristically have a lobed nucleus and are much larger and short lived when compared to RBCs. These types of cells also contain cytoplasmic granules packed with chemicals that can prompt immune response or the breakdown of pathogens. For instance, some granulocytes contain digestive enzymes that metabolize the bacteria's cell wall causing it to lyse, while other cells have antimicrobial proteins known as **defensins**. Depending on the type of infection, there is a specialized response from one of the three granulocytes (Figure 8-12).

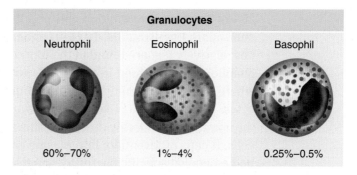

FIGURE 8-12 Granulocytes contain neutrophils, eosinophils, and basophils in varying concentrations among all blood products.

Neutrophils Neutrophils are the most abundant type of WBC and granulocyte. The neutrophil cytoplasm contains very fine granules. One type contains hydrolytic enzymes that are classified as a type of lysosome while the second type contains defensins. Neutrophils are our body's first line of defense against bacterial infections. Their numbers can rapidly expand during acute infections, attracted to sites of inflammation. Once the neutrophil engulfs the bacteria, it begins to degrade the bacteria using the two specific types of granules within their cytoplasm. Some neutrophils are partial to fungi, especially *Candida*, the fungus involved in yeast infections and thrush.

Eosinophils The second type of granulocytes is eosinophils. They contain large coarse granules that have unique digestive enzymes. Unlike neutrophils, eosinophils do not specifically digest bacteria, but rather mount the first attack against parasitic worms such as tapeworms and pinworms. These worms are usually ingested via undercooked food and typically insert themselves into the respiratory or digestive mucosa. Eosinophils also play a complex role in asthma and allergies that is beginning to be better illustrated through research. Briefly, it is hypothesized that eosinophils contribute to tissue damage that occurs in the immune process that only worsens inflammation and bronchoconstriction seen in asthma and allergic reactions.

Basophils Lastly, basophils are the rarest white blood cell and type of granulocyte. Their cytoplasm contains large, coarse granules containing histamine, an inflammatory chemical that acts as a vasodilator and attracts other white blood cells to the inflamed site. Histamine release usually accompanies inflammatory processes along with asthma and allergies. Inflammation can manifest itself in many ways, but is usually accompanied by mucus accumulation, possible disruption of the tissue layers, and a feeling of warmth or signs of infection.

Interestingly, the other granule inside of the basophils is heparin, an anticoagulant molecule that prevents the blood from clotting and has little to do with immunity. We discuss blood coagulation in greater detail later in this chapter.

Agranulocytes

Agranulocytes (Figure 8-13) include lymphocytes and monocytes, which lack granules and act functionally different than granulocytes. They too are larger than RBCs but have spherical-shaped nuclei. Lymphocytes account for about 25% of the total white blood cell population and are the second-most abundant behind neutrophils. Large numbers of lymphocytes exist in the body, but relatively few are found in the bloodstream. As their name suggests, most lymphocytes are found in the lymph nodes and lymphoid tissues and organs where they play a crucial role in immunity. There are two types of lymphocytes: T lymphocytes (T cells) and B lymphocytes (B cells). T cells function in the immune response by directly acting against virus-infected cells and tumor cells. B cells differentiate into plasma cells, which will eventually create antibodies against specific bacteria. Functions of T-cells and B-cells are described further in Chapter 12.

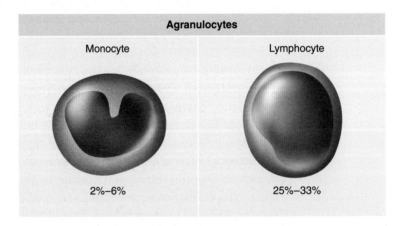

FIGURE 8-13 Agranulocytes include lymphocytes and monocytes in varying concentrations among all blood products.

Monocytes are the largest white blood cell when it comes to cell size. When circulating monocytes leave the bloodstream and enter tissues, they differentiate into highly mobile macrophages that become active phagocytes. These macrophages can engulf viruses, certain intracellular bacterial parasites, cellular debris from broken-down tissue or pathogens, and chronic infections such as tuberculosis.

Macrophages are also important in activating lymphocytes to mount a further immune response. This is explained more in Chapter 12.

LEARNING OBJECTIVE **8.1.21** Identify blood platelets.

LEARNING OBJECTIVE **8.1.22** Describe the origin of platelets and how that relates to their structure.

LEARNING OBJECTIVE **8.1.23** Explain the function of platelets.

KEY TERMS

platelets Formed elements that help to form blood clots.

thrombocytopenia Condition of low blood platelet count.

thrombocytosis Increase in clot formation.

thrombophilia Abnormality of blood coagulation that increases the risk of thrombosis by having too many platelets produced.

thrombopoietin Hormone that controls platelet production.

PLATELETS

Platelets, also called thrombocytes, are fragments of cells and are about one-fourth the size of a lymphocyte. They are classified as a formed element in the blood along with RBCs and WBCs. Platelets are used in the clotting process to form a plug when a tear or injury occurs to the lining of a blood vessel. By sticking to the endothelial cells of the blood vessels, platelets begin to initiate a fast and localized response to a vessel injury. We discuss this process in more detail shortly.

Megakaryocyte Development

After HSCs are activated by the hormone **thrombopoietin**, they begin to differentiate into a megakaryoblast. This cell undergoes continuous maturation until a megakaryocyte is formed (Figure 8-14). Because of the sheer size of the megakaryocyte, it becomes trapped in the capillaries where it begins to release cytoplasmic extensions without organelles or portions of the nuclei into the blood. The plasma membrane quickly regenerates around the cytoplasmic fragments, creating what we know as platelets.

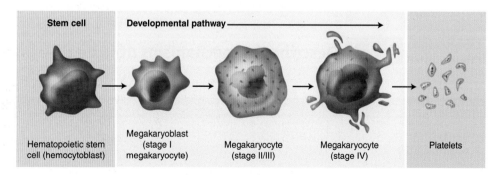

FIGURE 8-14 Megakaryocytes develop into platelets after undergoing multiple differentiation steps. Once activated by certain cell receptors, a megakaryoblast will quickly become a megakaryocyte that will manifest platelets once it becomes lodged in the capillaries around the bone marrow.

Platelet Counts

It is estimated that each microliter of blood contains 150,000–400,000 platelets. Because they have no way to reproduce or repair themselves, platelets only last about 10 days. Platelet counts over 400,000 are considered **thrombocytosis** and actually can have a detrimental effect on a patient's health because now they are more at risk of clotting. Patients who have depressed levels of platelets, known as **thrombocytopenia**, can have issues with bleeding as any small damage to vessels could be life-threatening without enough platelets to plug up the damage in the epithelium. Collectively, any type of platelet disorder when increased or decreased is considered a **thrombophilia**.

CLINICAL TIP	For reasons unknown or known by a health care professional, a patient's platelet count could dip below 20,000. At this point, this patient is extremely vulnerable to cerebral hemorrhaging and imminent death. It is of utmost importance to quickly address this number and devise a treatment plan with the medical care team in order to increase this patient's platelet levels as soon as possible.

UNIT OBJECTIVE 8.2

Explain the process of hemostasis.

UNIT INTRODUCTION

As blood flows through our circulatory system, it is expecting all of the vessels to be intact. But we know that most vessels can undergo trauma and even become damaged to a point where blood cells can leak out and cause bleeding. In order to correct this potentially life-threatening situation, the body undergoes a process known as hemostasis.

LEARNING OBJECTIVE 8.2.1 Define hemostasis.

LEARNING OBJECTIVE 8.2.2 Identify the three steps in hemostasis.

LEARNING OBJECTIVE 8.2.3 Describe the mechanisms utilized to achieve hemostasis.

KEY TERMS

coagulation The process by which the blood thickens to form blood clots.

fibrin A protein that is activated the clotting cascade that binds to platelets, forming a plug around the area of blood vessel damage.

hemostasis Stoppage of bleeding and the first step in wound healing.

prostacyclin Platelet aggregation inhibitor.

vascular spasm A quick tightening of a blood vessel that happens immediately after vessel damage in attempts to prevent significant blood loss.

HEMOSTASIS

Normally, blood flows freely past an intact blood vessel, but when the vessel is broken, blood will end up leaking out of that hole. Therefore, it is the job of the platelets to plug that hole and achieve **hemostasis**, or halting the bleeding.

The three steps to hemostasis are (Figure 8-15) vascular spasm, platelet plug formation, and coagulation.

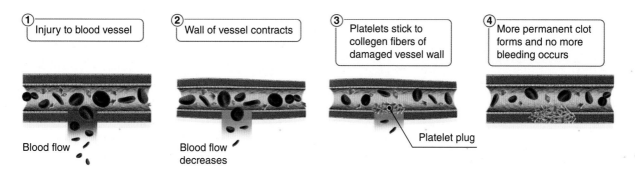

| ① Injury to blood vessel | ② Wall of vessel contracts | ③ Platelets stick to collegen fibers of damaged vessel wall | ④ More permanent clot forms and no more bleeding occurs |

Blood flow

Blood flow decreases

Platelet plug

FIGURE 8-15 Hemostasis is quickly achieved by platelet plug formation after a vessel is retracted from the site of injury. Soon after, blood clotting begins and further repairs the endothelial damage that just occurred.

Vascular Spasm

During hemostasis, three steps occur rapidly in order to achieve proper clotting. In the first step, vasoconstriction around the area of injury creates what is known as a **vascular spasm**. The vasoconstriction is controlled by local pain receptors that relay the message to the central nervous system and cause the muscle surrounding the area of trauma to contract around the vessel, constricting it in order to stop large amounts of blood from exiting the damaged area. Chemical messengers can cause a vascular spasm and vasoconstriction that will impede blood flow to this area for as long as 30 minutes after the injury occurs.

Platelet Plug Formation

In the second step of hemostasis, platelets begin to aggregate (collect) at the break within the vessel wall. Interestingly, platelets do not adhere to the surface of cells that create vessels, but to the collagen fibers under the damaged cellular layer. Normally, intact cells will release nitric oxide and **prostacyclin**, a prostaglandin that causes vasodilation-inhibiting platelet aggregation.

Coagulation

The last step of hemostasis is **coagulation**, a process that forms a blood clot via platelets and the protein threads of fibrin. Recall that **fibrin** is a threadlike protein that is dissolved within the blood that, when activated, can help achieve hemostasis (Table 8-1). When bound to the platelets, the fibrin threads will create a meshlike structure over the tear in the vessel wall (Figure 8-16). How fibrin is activated and used to repair breaks is a multistep process that is complex.

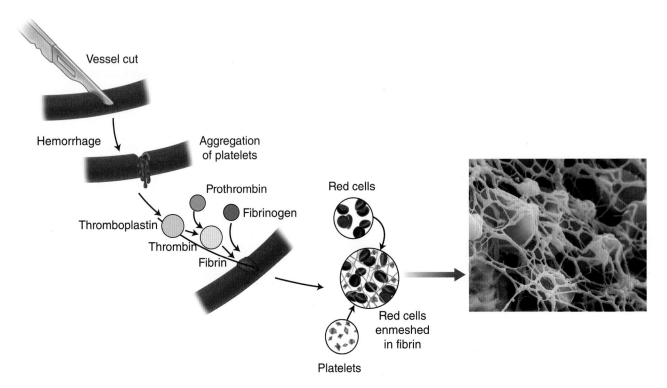

FIGURE 8-16 Clot formation is the final step of hemostasis and ensures that the vessel is nearing the final stage of repair. Fibrin is integral in this process as it acts as a glue between platelets and other blood products. We can see fibrin under electron microscopy, illustrated by the white strands.

LEARNING OBJECTIVE **8.2.4** Identify the coagulation cascade's extrinsic pathway, intrinsic pathway, and common pathway.

LEARNING OBJECTIVE **8.2.5** Explain how the coagulation cascade is initiated for both the intrinsic and extrinsic pathways.

KEY TERMS

clotting factors Substances in blood plasma that are involved in the clotting process.

clotting factor III Surface glycoprotein that can initiate the clotting cascade when activated.

CLOTTING FACTORS

To transform fibrin threads to a sticky protein complex that binds to platelets is a process controlled by clotting factors. **Clotting factors** are plasma proteins synthesized by the liver (except clotting factor III, the tissue factor) and circulate in the bloodstream until they are activated. (Some health care professionals will refer to these proteins as procoagulants because they promote coagulation.) Activation of the clotting factors will turn them into enzymes, which will activate the next clotting factor in the sequence (Figure 8-17), ultimately ending in a properly formed fibrin protein ready to be bound to a platelet.

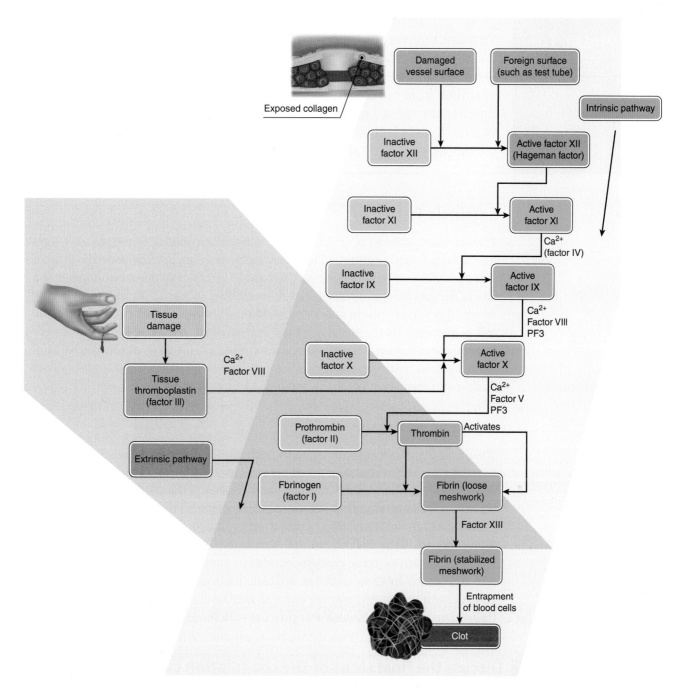

FIGURE 8-17 The coagulation pathway is dependent upon 13 different types of clotting factors that control the next step of clot formation. Activation of both the intrinsic and extrinsic pathways allow for the common pathway to be turned on. Here we have the transformation of prothrombin to thrombin, which directly causes fibrin, a part of the plasma, to become a solid and form a clot near the area of injury.

There are 13 different types of clotting factors numbered I to XIII involved in this cascade. They remain inactive until mobilized by the clotting factor that controls their behavior or an event like vessel injury. These clotting factors can initiate either the intrinsic, extrinsic, or both pathways.

Vitamins that we absorb from our diet are essential for numerous life functions, especially coagulation. Vitamin K is directly involved in the synthesis of clotting factors II, VII, IX, X. Failure to acquire vitamin K from our diet (malabsorption), or liver disease (hepatitis) will significantly reduce production of these clotting factors. Therefore, vitamin K–deficient patients may be more susceptible to increased blood loss, especially after an injury.

Extrinsic Pathway

The extrinsic pathway is activated from substances outside of the blood. Therefore, this pathway is controlled by the actual vessel damage that occurred instead of the platelet response to the injury. Damaged vessel cells release chemicals and one of them is known as tissue factor, or clotting factor III. At its core, clotting factor III is a glycoprotein imbedded within the plasma membrane, and when the cell is damaged its plasma membrane is destroyed, releasing the glycoprotein into the bloodstream and activating the extrinsic pathway. As a result, activation of the extrinsic pathway is a very quick response to severe tissue trauma and will lead to clot formation within 15 seconds of suspected tissue damage.

Intrinsic Pathway

The intrinsic pathway accompanies the extrinsic pathway in the clotting cascade; however, this pathway is dependent upon factors within the bloodstream, not tissue damage. This makes the intrinsic pathway slower than the extrinsic pathway because it relies on negatively charged surfaces. Recall that intact cells and most proteins within our body are negatively charged and, as we have learned, vessel injury will reveal the internal surface of collagen fibers, a highly negative surface.

Accompanying these changes, activated platelets are also negatively charged and will control intrinsic pathway activation. Consequently, clotting factors that control the intrinsic pathway are not activated until platelets arrive at the area of tissue damage, making it a slower process with more intermediate steps.

LEARNING OBJECTIVE 8.2.6 **Discuss the final steps of the coagulation cascade that result in a stable fibrin clot.**

KEY TERMS

factor X Clotting factor involved in the common pathway that is responsible for initiating the common pathway.

factor XIII (fibrin-stabilizing factor) Molecule that increases the stability of the fibrin clot.

prothrombin activator Complex of a dozen blood coagulation factors usually occurring as a result of blood loss or trauma.

thrombin Principal enzyme in hemostasis that continues that activation of the coagulation pathway and formation of stable fibrin complex.

Common Pathway

Even though the activation and steps of the intrinsic and extrinsic pathways differ, they both reach a common goal of activating clotting factor X (Factor X). **Factor X** is the common enzyme within the clotting cascade that when activated will complex with a Ca2+ ion and clotting factor V to form prothrombin activator. As a result, **prothrombin activator**, an enzyme, will directly catalyze a protein known as prothrombin (clotting factor II) into its active form of thrombin.

Thrombin is another enzyme that will transition the soluble fibrin into the protein gel that can bind to platelets. Here, we can see that we have reached the end of the clotting cascade. We have achieved our end goal of activating thrombin that will allow fibrin to glue to platelets and form a structural meshwork of a blood clot.

Blood Clot Stabilization

To ensure that the solid fibrin we just intricately created is not damaged, we stabilize the core of this protein with **factor XIII (fibrin-stabilizing factor)**, an enzyme activated by thrombin, and bind newly created fibrin strands together. Cross linking further stabilizes the clot, effectively sealing the hole until the blood vessel can be permanently repaired.

LEARNING OBJECTIVE 8.2.7 Explain how the process of hemostasis is stopped once initiated.

KEY TERM

anticoagulants Molecules that decrease clotting.

ANTICOAGULANTS

Under normal circumstances, the blood is a delicate balance between clotting factors and **anticoagulants**, factors that inhibit clotting. But once a vessel is damaged, activated clotting factors overcome the number of anticoagulants to create a hypercoagulable state. However, once a ruptured vessel is stabilized, cellular factors that initiated the extrinsic pathway are decreased, and platelets halt recruitment, inhibiting the intrinsic pathway. The intact cells once again begin to secrete antithrombotic substances like nitric oxide and prostacyclin. Numbers of platelets decrease, and anticoagulant factors begin to once again control the internal blood vessel environment (Figure 8-18).

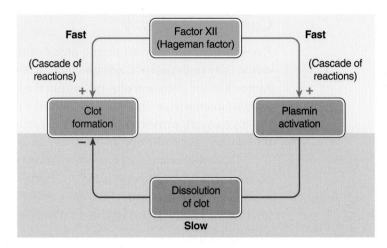

FIGURE 8-18 To destroy the clot just formed by the clotting cascade, there are other proteins that degrade this fibrin after the vessel injury is repaired.

Identify reasons why blood coagulation would need to be prevented.

KEY TERMS

atrial fibrillation Abnormal heart rhythm characterized by chaotic contractions of the atria.

thromboembolic disorders Formation of blood clots in blood vessels. Usually caused by a hypercoagulable state.

thrombocytosis Increase in clot formation.

Indications for the Use of Anticoagulants

Numerous chronic health conditions are considered **thromboembolic disorders**, or conditions that cause undesirable clot formation. Despite the body's many regulatory systems, undesirable intravascular clotting can occur with diseases that cause or include:

- Atherosclerosis
- Inflammation
- Irregular cardiac arrhythmias
- Increased platelet counts, or **thrombocytosis**
- Increased periods of blood stasis (blood not moving)

Thrombi and Emboli

The conditions above place the body in a hypercoagulable state, leading to the formation of a **thrombus**, a clot that develops and persists in an unbroken vessel. Conditions that roughen the vascular epithelium are usually the precursor for the development of thrombus, as we have learned that any conditional changes in the vessel wall can initiate the clotting cascade. Therefore, atherosclerosis, inflammation, and blood stasis due to bedridden conditions can all alter the internal environment of the blood vessel and lead to death of those tissues. For instance, atherosclerosis coronary arteries can lead to myocardial infarction (heart attack).

Other medical conditions like **atrial fibrillation** (cardiac arrhythmia), an irregular rhythm of atrium contractions in the heart, can create thrombi that transition to embolus, a clot that breaks away or is transported to another area of the body. These thrombi are a result of blood staying in the atrium due to the irregularity of the heart rate, and when an embolism enters a blood vessel that is too small for it to pass through, it will cause a blockage of blood to the organ proceeding the clot. As a result, many clots end up in the pulmonary capillaries and cause a pulmonary embolus, or even worse travel to cerebral arteries and cause a stroke. Because of these dangerous consequences, patients with atrial fibrillation are routinely anticoagulated.

LEARNING OBJECTIVE 8.2.9 **Explain how blood coagulation can be prevented physiologically.**

KEY TERMS

antithrombin III Molecule that inhibits the coagulation pathway by decreasing the number of co-factors that are needed to stimulate clotting.

heparin Anticoagulant that is used to decrease the clotting ability of the blood.

protein C Blood coagulation factor involved in creating a hypercoagulable state.

MECHANISMS OF ANTICOAGULATION

Normally, three homeostatic mechanisms exist to prevent blood coagulation. The first revolves around a negative feedback mechanism that inactivates active clotting factors after the clotting process has begun. This swift removal will prevent the improper coagulation of blood over time. Clotting factors will only work if their concentrations rise over certain thresholds, so actively depressing their numbers prevents coagulation.

Second, rapid and continuous blood flow through arteries keeps its composition less viscous and likely to stick to the vessel wall and create minor damage. Also, clots do not usually form in moving blood because activated clotting factors are washed away and transported to other areas of normal vessel content that will effectively inactivate their function.

The third mechanism involves blocking the fibrinogen from inappropriately turning into fibrin. These chemicals include **antithrombin III**, a protein present that quickly inactivates any thrombin protein not bound to fibrin. **Protein C**, a protein produced by the liver that is vitamin K dependent, will depress the intrinsic pathway when active clotting is not needed. And lastly, **heparin**, a naturally occurring anticoagulant stored within basophils, will be secreted and enhance the activity of antithrombin III.

KEY TERMS

aspirin Pain reliever and blood thinner used for minor aches and its anticoagulation properties via the inhibition of COX 1 and 2 receptors.

Factor 10(a) Clotting factor involved in the common pathway that is responsible for initiating the common pathway.

warfarin (Coumadin) Anticoagulant that is used to decrease the clotting ability of the blood by inhibiting the metabolism of vitamin K and its production of clotting factors.

ANTICOAGULANT DRUGS

Recent developments in pharmacology have provided a wealth of options providers can use to prevent inappropriate blood coagulation in their patients (Figure 8-19). Despite newer drugs, there is still a heavy reliance on aspirin, heparin, and warfarin.

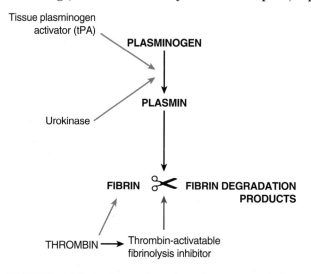

FIGURE 8-19 Anticoagulant drugs have expanded exponentially in the past few decades. Here we see the mechanisms of action of most of the medications that practitioners use on a daily basis for anticoagulation.

Aspirin is a prostaglandin-based drug that inhibits thromboxane, a potent activator of platelets. Some new drugs like clopidogrel (Plavix), ticagrelor (Brillinta), prasugrel (Effient), dipyridamole/aspirin (Aggrenox), and Ticlodipine (Ticlid) are also antiplatelet medications.

Heparin is used to increase the already potent effects of endogenously made heparin. Administered as an injectable, heparin is most commonly used in a hospital setting for blood transfusions. Other individuals who have conditions like atrial fibrillation are prescribed warfarin (coumadin), a medication that inactivates the production of clotting factors from vitamin K.

Interestingly, warfarin has been replaced by more novel anticoagulants that depress the actions of Factor 10 and Factor 10(a), the metabolically active portion of Factor X that helps to create the prothrombin activator mechanism. These drugs include but are not limited to:

- apixaban (Eliquis)
- dabigatran (Pradaxa)
- rivaroxaban (Xarelto)

LEARNING OBJECTIVE 8.2.11 Explain the process of clot resolution.

KEY TERMS

fibrinolysis Breakdown of fibrin in blood clots leading to thinning of the blood.

plasmin Enzyme that degrades blood plasma proteins.

plasminogen Precursor to plasmin.

platelet-derived growth factor (PDGF) Growth factors that regulate cell growth and division of platelets.

tissue plasminogen activator (tPA) Treatment for the destruction of emboli within the body. Mostly used for the breakdown of emboli in the setting of strokes.

BLOOD CLOT DESTRUCTION

Even as the environment returns to normal, the clot just formed is not an appropriate long-term solution to the damage. Therefore, as platelets begin to plug the hole, they secrete **platelet-derived growth factor (PDGF)**, a chemical messenger that will stimulate the growth of new blood vessel walls. Further healing will promote **fibrinolysis**, a process that destroys the clot and removes it from the vessel wall.

Furthermore, **plasmin**, a derivative of the plasma protein **plasminogen**, is also activated by intact vessel cells that release of **tissue plasminogen activator (tPA)**. Plasminogen is also activated by Factor 12 and thrombin to create a negative feedback and decrease the formation of new clots (refer back to Figure 8-18 for more of an illustrative look at this process). In total, fibrinolysis begins within two days and continues slowly over several days until the clot finally dissolves.

UNIT OBJECTIVE 8.3

Describe the importance of blood groups and their role in blood transfusions.

UNIT INTRODUCTION

Because blood plays such a primary role in a variety of metabolic processes, it is necessary to maintain both the quantity and quality of it in our body. As a result, if we were to lose blood it would be essential to replace it with the correct type of blood from a donor or from some of our own frozen material that we might have donated before a large surgery. If the blood is not properly transfused, there are significant consequences that can be potentially life-threatening.

LEARNING OBJECTIVE 8.3.1 Define antigen, antibody, and agglutination.

KEY TERMS

agglutination Clumping of blood particles that are of differing types. Usually a result of a mismatched transfusion.

antibody Immune system proteins produced in response to a specific antigen that non-self cells for destruction.

antigen Surface protein that creates a certain label on the cell. Usually used to distinguish differing blood types.

ANTIGEN

The surface of RBCs, and other cells in our body for that matter, contain a glycoprotein and glycolipid group known as an **antigen**. The presence or absence of this surface marker delineates the type of blood a patient may have (Figure 8-20).

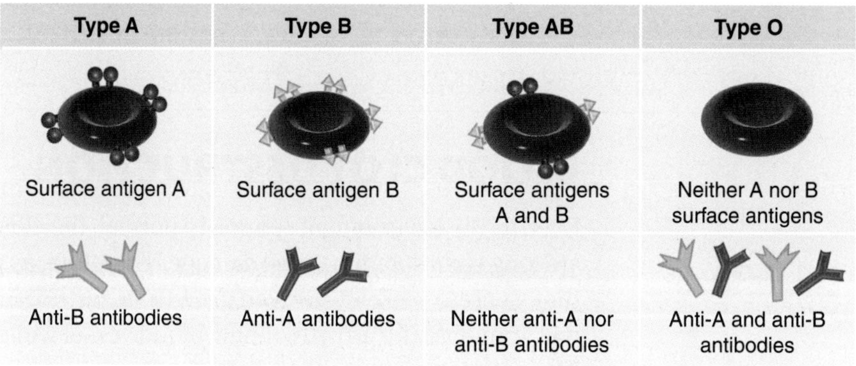

Type A	Type B	Type AB	Type O
Surface antigen A	Surface antigen B	Surface antigens A and B	Neither A nor B surface antigens
Anti-B antibodies	Anti-A antibodies	Neither anti-A nor anti-B antibodies	Anti-A and anti-B antibodies

FIGURE 8-20 Blood types will contain biological markers that determine the type of blood patients have. These antigens dictate what type of blood transfusions a patient can safely get. Antibodies produced by the body are the *opposite* of what the antigen is.

ANTIBODY

Circulating in the bloodstream are antibodies against antigens that are not present on the body's RBCs. **Antibodies** are proteins produced to counteract a specific antigen. As a result, when we receive a blood transfusion from a donor with antigens on their RBCs that the recipient blood has antibodies to in their plasma, the patient may undergo a significant and life-threatening reaction due to the antibody attack of the donor's blood. This process is known as a transfusion reaction, which we discuss later.

AGGLUTINATION

If a patient is exposed to donor blood that has antigens on the surface of their RBCs that the patient has antibodies for, then a defense mechanism known as agglutination will be triggered. **Agglutination** occurs when the mixing of incompatible blood causes antibodies and antigens to bind to one another, leading them to clump together. These clumps can clog small blood vessels, severely damaging tissues (Figure 8-21).

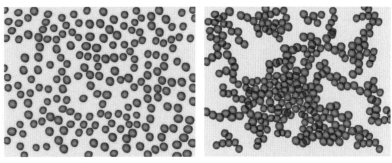

Compatible blood cells   Incompatible blood cells

FIGURE 8-21 Microscopic representation of the agglutination process. Incompatible blood types will cause the destruction of the blood shown on the second slide. Here, Type B blood was treated with Type A blood, which caused its immediate destruction due to the antibody interactions.

LEARNING OBJECTIVE 8.3.2 Identify the antigens, antibodies, and blood types of the ABO system of blood typing.

ABO BLOOD TYPES

As previously discussed, antigens act as indicators of the type of cells that we have. In humans, there are two types of RBC antigens that are genetically inherited, coded, formed, and inserted on the surface of newly forming RBCs. These antigens are A and B antigens. Individuals with A antigens on the surface of their RBCs are known as "Type A" and those with B antigens are "Type B." Some people inherit genes from their parents that code for A and B antigens, making them "Type AB." Conversely, patients that do not inherit these genes have neither A or B antigens on the surface of their RBCs. These patients are labeled as "Type O" (Figure 8-20).

Because we learned that antibodies bind to antigens and can cause agglutination, it would be deadly if "Type A" patients were to make A antibodies. Therefore, the antibodies that these individuals make is the opposite of the antigen present on their surface. What's more, "Type AB" individuals do not have any circulating antibodies because they have both A and B antigens on their RBCs, while "Type O" patients have both A and B antibodies in their serum (Figure 8-20).

LEARNING OBJECTIVE 8.3.3 Identify the antigens, antibodies, and blood types of the Rh system of blood typing.

KEY TERMS

hemolysis Breakdown of red blood cells.

Rh factor Protein found on the surface of red blood cells.

RH BLOOD GROUPS

Worldwide, there are 52 types of Rh antigens that can be present or absent from the surface of RBCs. These antigens are referred to as **Rh factors**, and about 85% of the United States population is Rh factor positive (Rh+), meaning that their RBCs express a specific Rh antigen (for convenience, many blood type and screen tests will report both the ABO blood group along with the Rh status; e.g., A+).

Interestingly, Rh factors have no standing on a person's production of Rh antibodies. Therefore, a person who is Rh– does not make anti-Rh factor antibodies unless exposed to a blood transfusion that is from a Rh+ individual. Then, the immune system becomes sensitized and subsequent exposure to Rh+ blood will create a major agglutination reaction, leading to **hemolysis** or the destruction of RBCs.

LEARNING OBJECTIVE 8.3.4 Explain the process of blood typing.

KEY TERM

blood typing Testing of a sample of blood to determine an individual's blood group.

BLOOD TYPING

Blood typing is a laboratory test (Figure 8-21) used to determine a person's blood type before the initiation of a blood transfusion. This information will allow for the correct type of blood to be infused and avoid significant transfusion reactions to occur.

Blood typing begins by obtaining a blood sample from the recipient and placing a drop on a microscope slide. Serum with anti-A or anti-B antibodies is added to the blood sample in order to see if the sample will begin agglutination and hemolysis. Agglutination is shown by the significant changes in the RBC sample or cellular fragments appearing. Interpreting this information will allow for the correct transfusion, as agglutination would signal that the recipient's blood contains antigens that will be destroyed by that specific blood type. Furthermore, type AB will show agglutination changes when both serums are added, while Type O will reveal no changes in blood sample characteristics due to the lack of surface antigens.

Because it is so critical that blood groups be compatible, cross matching is also done where the donor's blood is added to the recipient's blood in the same process as above. Extensive cross matching should also be done in reverse where the donor's blood is added to the recipients to ensure proper blood transfusion. Notably, Rh factor testing is done in the same way.

LEARNING OBJECTIVE 8.3.5 Define universal donor and universal recipient.

Universal Donor

Individuals who are Type O are known as universal donors due to the absence of antigens on the surface of their blood. This characteristic allows these donors to give blood to any other type without the concern of an attack from antibodies of the recipient.

Universal Recipient

Individuals who are Type AB+ are known as universal recipients due to the absence of antibodies in their blood. This characteristic allows recipients to get blood from any other blood type without the concern that the donor's blood will be degraded by antibodies.

LEARNING OBJECTIVE 8.3.6 Describe the results of transfusing mismatched blood types on the red blood cells.

KEY TERMS

infarctions The reduction or loss of blood supply to a specific organ.

transfusion reactions Inappropriate blood destruction due to the mismatch of surface antigens and antibodies between the donor and the host.

TRANSFUSION REACTIONS

When mismatched blood is given to a donor, a transfusion reaction occurs in which the recipient's plasma antibodies attack the donor's RBCs. Almost immediately, agglutination occurs where the complexes begin to block small blood vessels and they begin to rupture. Rupture releases hemoglobin and activates macrophages and the subsequent death of other injured RBCs.

These events quickly lead to three major problems. The first, and most concerning, is that the transfused blood cannot transport oxygen due to the major loss of hemoglobin. Second, this free hemoglobin begins to travel to the kidney and injure the nephrons, leading to kidney failure. The last issue is that the clumped and dying RBCs in the small vessels are creating infarctions, an obstruction of blood supply to an area of tissue beyond the clot. Prolonged ischemia will lead to cell death in the areas starved for oxygen (Figure 8-22).

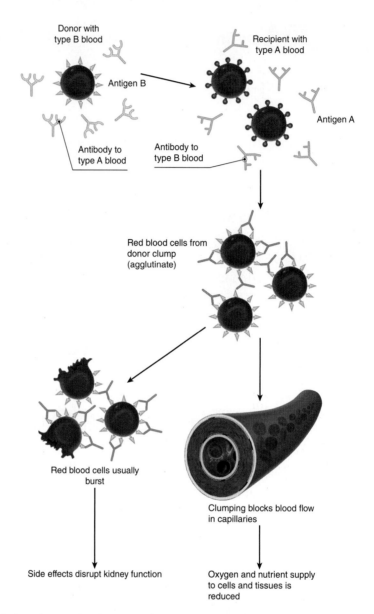

FIGURE 8-22 An example of an agglutination reaction that will ultimately lead to a significant transfusion reaction if not corrected quickly.

LEARNING OBJECTIVE 8.3.7 Describe the physical signs and symptoms of a mismatched blood transfusion.

CLINICAL MANIFESTATIONS OF MISMATCHED BLOOD TRANSFUSIONS

Patients experiencing a transfusion reaction are most likely to present with hypotension and tachycardia because of the significant ischemia from the widespread clumping and clogging of small arteries feeding major organs.

Further complications arise as the patient begins to develop abdominal pain along with nausea and vomiting. If not corrected quickly, these patients can quickly become septic and die.

UNIT OBJECTIVE 8.4

Describe pathologies affecting blood cells and the functions of blood.

UNIT INTRODUCTION

Like any other type of tissue, blood can become distorted, damaged, and diseased. Because of its overarching effects on the body, any type of imbalance can cause a variety of issues. In this unit, we will uncover why these diseases happen and learn how they present.

LEARNING OBJECTIVE 8.4.1 **Identify the cause, symptoms, and treatment for the most common types of anemia.**

KEY TERMS

extrinsic anemias Acquired forms of anemia not related to genetic components.

intrinsic anemias Inherited disorders that can lead to anemia. The most common inherited anemias are sickle cell anemia and thalassemia.

intrinsic factor Substance secreted by the stomach that enables the body to absorb vitamin B_{12}.

melena Blood-tinged feces usually containing a dark red or brown hue.

pica Eating disorder that involves ingesting items that are not typically thought of as food, such as paint or clay.

sickle cell anemia Inherited form of anemia in which there aren't enough healthy red blood cells to carry adequate oxygen throughout the body.

tenesmus Painful defecation.

thalassemia Blood disorder that decreases the proper formation of hemoglobin within the red blood cell structure.

ANEMIA

The word *anemia* can give providers nightmares because it can signal a variety of diseases from straightforward to more complex. At their core, anemias are caused by

1. increased blood loss,
2. increased RBC destruction, or
3. decreased RBC production.

The diseases that underly these three main causes are much more complicated to tease out and treat, but most assessments begin with an interpretation of a CBC.

CBC values like RBC count, Hgb, or Hct can elucidate the true amount of RBC within the system. But other values can be explored as well. Take the reticulocyte count, for example. An elevated reticulocyte count will show that the body is trying to produce more RBCs over a shorter amount of time. The why behind that mechanism is not so easily determined. Is it because the patient is bleeding and the body is responding to blood loss or is it that RBCs are being destroyed by a transfusion reaction or another hemolytic event? Or is it none of the above and the body is inappropriately putting out new RBCs due to a cancerous reaction? Here we try to understand some of the most common reasons why anemias occur.

Blood Loss

Hemorrhagic anemias are caused by blood loss either acutely or chronically. Acute blood loss focuses more on traumatic events such as a stab wound or motor vehicle accident. Patients presenting with acute blood loss will be pale to gray in color, hypotensive, tachycardic, and in various stages of consciousness as they begin to lose enough blood volume needed to perfuse their brain. Acute blood loss is a medical emergency commonly seen in emergency rooms and requires rapid evaluation and treatment with

1. IV fluids to expand the blood volume for perfusion purposes,
2. blood transfusions to ensure proper oxygenation of tissues, and
3. an investigation into and closure of the wound or tear that is causing the bleed.

Chronic blood loss is a slight yet persistent loss of RBCs. Patients usually present with generalized pallor, fatigue, muscle weakness, and malaise. If the chronic blood loss is due to a slow internal bleed from gastric ulcers, hemorrhoids, or other areas of the GI tract, the patient may complain of blood-tinged stools (**melena**), pain in their epigastric region, **tenesmus** (painful defecation), or frank blood in their vomit. Treatment is usually investigating the cause of the bleed and then medications or surgical intervention to address the specific issue.

RBC Destruction

The class of anemias that destroy RBCs are known as hemolytic anemias. These diseases cause an increase in RBC destruction with little to no replacement of dead RBCs. Hemolytic anemias can be classified into two types: intrinsic and extrinsic.

Intrinsic Anemias These anemias are inherited disorders with a genetic component. The most common two within this type are sickle cell anemia and thalassemia. We have previously discussed these two diseases as being hemoglobinopathies, but they can be further classified as hemolytic in nature.

Briefly, **sickle cell anemia** presents as quite asymptomatic unless the patient is in a hypoxic state. Many people are only diagnosed with sickle cell if there are indications for genetic testing during the early stages of birth, and individuals may never experience a sickle cell crisis. Treatment of sickle cell disease includes a variety of approaches that focus on pain management and

IV hydration for an active crisis, to a broader treatment plan that attempts to increase RBC production with folic acid supplementation (a precursor to erythrocyte production) and regular transfusions.

Thalassemia can range from being harmless to life-threatening depending on how many globin chains are affected by the improper folding or protein sequencing. Patients with significant thalassemia (major deformities in the α or β chains) will present as pale and fatigued and have bone pain, hepatosplenomegaly, iron overload, and reticulocytosis (increased reticulocytes on CBC). Treatment regimens are aimed at the severity of the disease, but all try to overcome the oxygen deficit the patient is experiencing. Therefore, management is focused on blood transfusions, iron chelation therapy to remove the improper depositing of iron in areas outside of heme groups, and splenectomies in rare cases to ensure that RBCs are not being destroyed and have a chance to bind to oxygen regardless of their shape. Genetic counseling and conservative management is usually offered to patients with minor thalassemia that do not experience any adverse effects.

Extrinsic Anemias These anemias are acquired disorders with a possible autoimmune component or overreaction to certain physiological states. The most common type of extrinsic hemolytic anemia is disseminated intravascular coagulation, which is discussed shortly.

Decreased RBC Production

A number of problems can decrease erythrocyte production from the lack of raw materials needed to induce erythropoiesis to the complete failure of the marrow itself. It is also possible that EPO levels are severely depressed leading to an over decrease in RBC production (see earlier explanation of EPO). Notably, iron-deficiency anemia is a lack of iron consumption in the diet or a secondary result of hemorrhagic anemias that we discussed above. Iron-deficiency anemia is one of the most common type of anemias and usually affects females more than males. Patients afflicted with this type of anemia may present with pallor, fatigue, muscle weakness, and general malaise. Specifically, patients with this anemia develop **pica**, a condition of ingesting nonedible materials like clay or chalk. Reasons as to why this happens remain unknown, but it should always be in the back of your mind when evaluating a patient for anemia. The mainstay treatment of this type of anemia is iron supplementation with ferrous sulfate and vitamin C replacement.

Pernicious Anemia Pernicious anemia is another common type of anemia that arises from a decrease in the building blocks of RBCs. Pernicious anemia is specific to a lack of B_{12} absorption of the GI tract due to an autoimmune destruction of the cells responsible releasing **intrinsic factor**, a factor essential for vitamin B_{12} uptake (Figure 8-23). Therefore, RBC production within the red marrow subsides and histological stains of RBCs are created that are giant (macrocyte) and immature and lack hemoglobin. Therefore, these patients present with anemic-like symptoms, gait abnormalities, memory loss, dementia, anorexia, and diarrhea. Treatment for pernicious anemia includes B_{12} injections until symptoms subside. Additionally, absence of folate (vitamin B_9) has the same effects on RBCs, while hypothyroidism, ETOH abuse, and liver disease can all contribute to this clinical presentation of anemia.

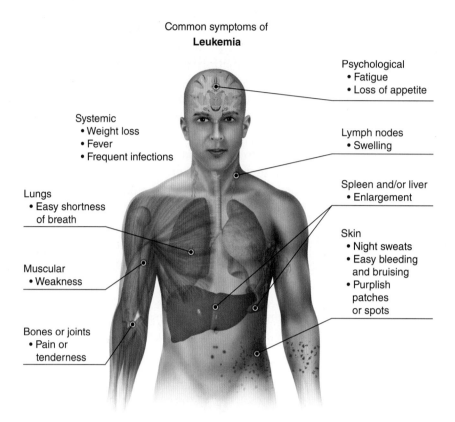

Common symptoms of
Leukemia

Psychological
• Fatigue
• Loss of appetite

Systemic
• Weight loss
• Fever
• Frequent infections

Lymph nodes
• Swelling

Spleen and/or liver
• Enlargement

Lungs
• Easy shortness
  of breath

Skin
• Night sweats
• Easy bleeding
  and bruising
• Purplish
  patches
  or spots

Muscular
• Weakness

Bones or joints
• Pain or
  tenderness

FIGURE 8-23 Bone marrow biopsy shows total replacement of normal hematopoietic cells with lymphoblasts with convoluted or folded nuclei. Also shown are the clinical manifestations that accompany leukemia.

Aplastic Anemia Aplastic anemia is the last reason why RBC production may be decreased. This type of anemia refers to the direct destruction of red marrow due to drugs, viruses, or radiation. Anemic-like symptoms along with immune suppression and clotting abnormalities also plague these patients as HSCs have been destroyed. Treatment of aplastic anemias includes blood transfusions, with long-term management being a bone marrow transplant to reset the damaged and improper red marrow.

LEARNING OBJECTIVE 8.4.2 Identify common causes of increased white blood cell counts.

INCREASED WBCs

Overproduction of leukocytes usually signals one of two events going on behind the scenes. The first is an acute or chronic immune reaction. The increases in WBC are a proper response to a pathogen and will likely rid the disease from the body and return to normal levels depending on the pathogenic progression. The other reasons that WBCs increase in number are due to various types of blood-based or solid cancers. In this case, there is an improper increase in WBC production that will cause immature cells to develop, leading to further immune suppression and cancer metastasis. Many times, elevated WBC counts on a CBC are the only clue to an underlying cancer.

LEARNING OBJECTIVE 8.4.3 Describe the general signs, symptoms, and treatment of leukemia.

LEUKEMIAS

The term leukemia literally translates to "white blood." This term refers to the group of cancerous conditions involving the overproduction of abnormal WBCs. Because WBCs come in all shapes and sizes with differing progenitor cells, leukemias are named based on the type of cell they are overproducing. For instance, myelogenous leukemia indicates that there is an overproduction of myeloid progenitor cells (NEUTROPHILS, EOSINOPHILS, BASOPHILS, OR MONOCYTES). The most severe type of leukemia is acute lymphoblastic leukemia, which can also cause an increase in platelets and RBCs. This disease normally affects children and is luckily a highly curable disease.

Signs and Symptoms

The main problem with leukemia is the creation of one single type of predominantly immature blood cells that begin to crowd out the properly functioning cells in the blood (Figure 8-23). Furthermore, the massive replication of stem cells crowds out the normal stem cells leading to a greatly decreased production of certain cell types and a greatly increased production of the other cell type. Therefore, patients with suggested leukemia present with fever, malaise, weight loss, muscle weakness, anemia, clotting issues, and heat and cold intolerances.

Treatment

Because the underlying issue with leukemias is that there is an overproduction of malfunctioning cells, sometimes the best treatment is a hard reset of the signals that control this overgrowth. In medicine, the hard reset is known as radiation treatment, which functions to knock out all of or the majority of the bone marrow stem cells that are contributing to this disease. After radiation a patient usually undergoes a bone marrow transplant from a correctly matched donor and newly and properly functioning stem cells from the donor begin to rebuild the necessary blood cells. As you can imagine, this treatment comes with many complications as it is effectively knocking out the immune system by destroying WBCs, leaving patients immunocompromised and open to opportune infections that might cause secondary problems and even death.

Recently, there have been advances in leukemia treatments where antileukemic drugs can specifically target the improperly functioning cells and destroy them. This approach is more like utilizing a small, sharp scalpel to make an incision compared to the radiation treatment, which is like a machete (it will get the job done but cause a much larger and complicated incision).

UNIT OBJECTIVE 8.5

Describe pathologies affecting the process of hemostasis.

UNIT INTRODUCTION

If we recall, hemostasis means to "stop the bleed," but there exist some diseases that make this process quite difficult to achieve. Here, we learn about the underlying pathologies of hemophilia.

LEARNING OBJECTIVE 8.5.1 **Describe the signs, symptoms, diagnosis, and treatment of hemophilia.**

KEY TERMS

cryoprecipitate Type of prepared plasma that contains fibrinogen, von Willebrand factor, Factor 8, Factor 9, and fibronectin. Usually used to substitute significant blood loss or a decrease in clotting factors.

fresh frozen plasma Blood product made from the plasma portion of the blood that can be unfrozen in the hospital during an emergency situation and provided to a patient that may be deficient of clotting factors.

hemophilia Rare disorder in which the blood doesn't clot normally.

petechiae Tiny, circular, nonraised patches that appear on the skin or in a mucous or serous membrane. Usually is a sign of bleeding under the skin.

PTT Test Measurement that calculates the time it takes for a blood clot to form.

INR A measurement on how much time it takes for a patient's blood to clot. An elevated INR means that the patient's blood is too thin while a decreased level means that the blood is too prone to clotting.

purpura Tiny raised patches that can appear on the skin. Usually a result of bleeding under the skin.

HEMOPHILIA

Hemophilia refers to the collection of rare disorders that decreases the clotting ability of the blood. Depending on the type of hemophilia a patient possesses, they have a deficiency in a clotting factor that negatively affects the clotting cascade, creating an uncoagulable state. Hemophilia almost exclusively affects males as they have X-linked recessive traits.

Signs and Symptoms

Hemophilia patients usually do not present with petechiae or purpura, two dermatological findings of ruptured blood vessels and excessive bleeding. This is because hemophilia is not a platelet disorder, but rather a clotting cascade issue. Therefore, clinical manifestations include bleeding in weight-bearing joints due to the excessive trauma and mechanical stress along with excessive hemorrhaging after sustaining a trauma, surgery, or lacerations.

Diagnosis

Establishing the presence of a hemophilia disorder is quite straightforward. Physicians will routinely order a PTT test, or partial thromboplastin time, which measures how quickly your blood clots. Normal clotting times range from 11 to 13.5 seconds from initiation of the clotting test to formation of the blood clot. Many physicians will use the international normalized ratio (INR) to assess the time needed for a blood sample to clot. Normal values fall within 0.8–1.1. Because hemophilia patients express less clotting factor, their PTT test results and INR levels will be above the standard times. In review, If your INR is higher than the range above, that means your blood clots more slowly than desired. A lower INR means your blood clots more quickly than desired.

Treatment

Depending on the type of hemophilia a patient has, there are varying treatment options. One fact does remain the same: The overall goal is to replace the patient's supply of missing clotting factors. Recombinant and synthetic clotting factors are routinely injected into these patients in order to ensure proper clotting in the event of vessel damage. In emergency situations, fresh frozen plasma and cryoprecipitate are routinely used. Fresh frozen plasma is a blood product made from the plasma portion of the blood and can be unfrozen in the hospital during an emergency situation. Because it is composed of plasma, this product has all of the essential clotting factors needed to reverse the bleed. Cryoprecipitate is a more specific concentration of prepared plasma that contains fibrinogen, von Willebrand factor, Factor 8, Factor 9, and fibronectin.

LEARNING OBJECTIVE 8.5.2 Describe the signs, symptoms, diagnosis, and treatment of a deep vein thrombosis.

KEY TERMS

D-dimer test Test used to measure the by-products of clot destruction. Usually carried out when there is a suspicion for a hypercoagulable; estate in the blood.

deep vein thrombosis (DVT) Blood clot that forms in a vein deep in the body.

DEEP VEIN THROMBOSIS

Deep vein thrombosis (DVT) occurs when a blood clot forms in one of the deep veins of the body (Figure 8-24). The most common areas for DVTs to develop are within in the calves and near the popliteal artery on the posterior aspect of the knee. As we have been discussing, any state that makes our body more prone to blood clots can be a risk factor for the development of a thrombus.

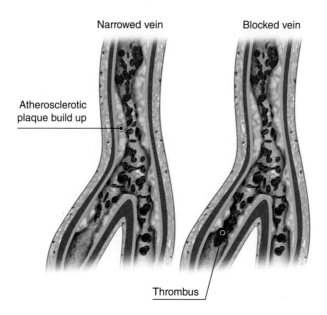

Narrowed vein   Blocked vein

Atherosclerotic
plaque build up

Thrombus

FIGURE 8-24 Pathology of a deep vein thrombosis.

CLINICAL TIP

The three most distinguishing features that you will get from a patient's history that should prompt you to think about a DVT or thrombus are known as Virchow's Triad. They consist of:

- Venous stasis (prolonged sitting or no movement of blood)
- Endothelial damage (vessel damage due to atherosclerosis or surgery)
- Hypercoagulability

Signs and Symptoms

Patients with DVTs usually have significant physical findings that can lead you to a correct diagnosis. Many times, they will have unilateral swelling of a lower extremity, warm skin, and a palpable cordlike structure that represents the obstructed vein. The patient may also complain of calf pain or tenderness along with some bruising. Other signs of a massive DVT would be pale and cold skin below the thrombus area as a result of an infarction and reduced blood flow.

Diagnosis

Because DVTs can become life-threatening if the thrombus turns into an embolus or leads to significant obstruction of an artery, there must a quick assessment of the person's lower extremities. The mainstay diagnostic tool is a venous duplex ultrasound that looks for compression of the vein due to the presence of a blood clot. Further imaging like a venous arthrogram is warranted if the ultrasound does not detect the issue. Further lab tests like a **D-dimer test** will detect degraded fibrin products that might indicate the presence of a clot (this test is not that useful considering that fibrin is constantly being broken down and recycled in the body even if we do not have a DVT).

Treatment

Once a DVT has been confirmed, the patient must be given anticoagulation therapy. As discussed above, there is a multitude of options in the arsenal for accomplishing this task, but mainstay treatment for DVTs is heparin or warfarin. Other Factor 10 and 10a inhibitors are sometimes used, but because heparin and warfarin have the ability to decrease a multitude of clotting factors, they can be more effective in patients with recurring or chronic DVTs.

LEARNING OBJECTIVE 8.5.3 Describe the signs, symptoms, and treatment of disseminated intravascular coagulopathy.

KEY TERMS

disseminated intravascular coagulopathy (DIC) Widespread hemorrhaging after clots are destroyed or used up. Usually a condition that is preceded by massive trauma where the body needs to quickly use clotting factors in attempts to stop blood loss.

thrombocytopenia Condition of low blood platelet count.

DISSEMINATED INTRAVASCULAR COAGULOPATHY

Disseminated intravascular coagulopathy (DIC) refers to a pathological activation of the coagulation system due to infections, malignancies, obstetrical complications, or massive tissue injuries. DIC is considered a life-threatening condition because of how quickly it can create a dangerously low hypercoagulable state due to the rapid consumption of clotting factors, platelets, and coagulation proteins. Without proper replacement, the patient will begin to hemorrhage profusely.

Signs and Symptoms

Patients with DIC usually present with widespread hemorrhaging at the mouth, nose, and skin and in the GI tract. Simultaneously, large clots that formed out of the immediate increase in coagulation become trapped in the kidney, liver, and respiratory system. As a result, the thrombi can reduce circulation and cause respiratory distress, abnormal liver function, and gangrene if tissues are not properly perfused.

Diagnosis

The excessive consumption of clotting factors will reveal an elevated PT and INR time along with severe **thrombocytopenia**, a massive reduction in the number of platelets if the blood sample is subjected to histology or CBC. Furthermore, fibrinogen levels will be decreased as it is being converted to fibrin with the rising levels of thrombin. Other findings significant with DIC is an increase in fibrinolysis over time as the clots begin to dissolve along with elevated D-dimer results.

Treatment

The goal of DIC treatment is to assess and treat the underlying cause while also infusing fresh frozen plasma, which will give stable amounts of new clotting factors and platelets that can be used to halt the hemorrhaging. Platelet transfusions will also provide the necessary numbers of these cells to ensure that the patient does not bleed to death while we assess the condition.

UNIT OBJECTIVE 8.6

Describe pathologies related to blood typing and transfusions.

UNIT INTRODUCTION

During pregnancy, there are various conditions that health care providers are responsible for assessing and adequately treating. Many times, the routine obstetrics visits serve to screen for issues that will arise during labor or shortly after. One of the most life-threatening conditions is erythroblastosis fetalis.

LEARNING OBJECTIVE 8.6.1 Describe the cause, signs, symptoms, diagnosis, and prophylaxis of erythroblastosis fetalis.

KEY TERMS

bilirubin Pigment formed by the breakdown of hemoglobin and excreted in the bile.

erythroblastosis fetalis Abnormal presence of erythroblasts in the blood usually found in newborns or mothers with nonmatching Rh surface proteins.

RhoGAM Medication used to prevent Rh antibody development in an Rh negative mother after childbirth.

ERYTHROBLASTOSIS FETALIS

An important issue related to the Rh factor occurs in pregnant Rh− women who are carrying Rh+ babies. The first pregnancy usually results in the delivery of a healthy baby, but once bleeding occurs, the Rh+ blood of the baby can enter the mother's systemic circulatory system. Immunologic awareness of the Rh+ factor will prompt the immune system to create anti-Rh antibodies.

These anti-Rh antibodies will become an issue in the mother's second pregnancy if her baby is Rh+ as the anti-Rh antibodies will pass through the placental blood supply and cause hemolytic destruction of the baby's RBCs, a condition known as erythroblastosis fetalis.

Signs and Symptoms

Rh+ babies born to mothers with anti-Rh antibodies will experience severe hemolytic anemia, jaundice, kernicterus (brain damage due to jaundice), and a condition known as fetal hydrops where fluid accumulates in the pleural spaces, especially the pericardium, which causes congestive heart failure. As you can see, anti-Rh antibodies can be extremely detrimental to a newborn, warranting quick diagnosis and treatment.

Diagnosis

Throughout gestation, the baby is subjected to the mother's blood supply so there is a prolonged period where the child can be exposed to these anti-Rh antibodies. If erythroblastosis fetalis is suspected, the mother should be typed and screened for their presence and fetal monitoring should begin in the second trimester. Monitoring techniques include amniotic fluid analysis and percutaneous umbilical blood sampling that will look for increased bilirubin, a by-product of RBC destruction, or decreased Hct. Either one of these results warrants further workup in order to protect the baby.

Prophylaxis and Treatment

Because the pathophysiology behind erythroblastosis fetalis is understood, there are ways to completely prevent its occurrence. Every mother at her first prenatal visit is typed and screened for Rh factor. If she is determined to be Rh–, her child will be typed and screened during the second trimester to evaluate if prophylaxis treatment needs to be given during her pregnancy or childbirth.

If a Rh+ baby is being born to a Rh– mother, these individuals will receive 300 mcg of a drug known as RhoGAM. RhoGAM is an immunoglobulin that contains anti-RH antibodies. When given to a mother at 28 weeks and then again within 72 hours of delivery, these antibodies will be present in the mother's system and agglutinate with any Rh+ blood that may come from the baby during pregnancy and childbirth. Through agglutination, RhoGAM can inhibit the mother's immunologic response to the Rh+ blood, preventing her from creating her own antibodies that would be harmful to her next Rh+ child. As a result, the mother never becomes sensitized and the agglutinated anti-Rh antibodies and RH+ blood is quickly destroyed by macrophages inside the circulatory system.

Despite our best efforts, some mothers will fail to be prophylaxed with RhoGAM, leaving their next children at risk for erythroblastosis fetalis. If this is the case and it is confirmed by diagnosis, health care providers should aggressively treat the child in utero with RBCs via umbilical vein delivery in order to replace the rapidly dying blood cells. If the child has already been delivered, providers should perform exchange perfusions where the newborn's blood is removed and replaced with Rh− blood (Figure 8-25).

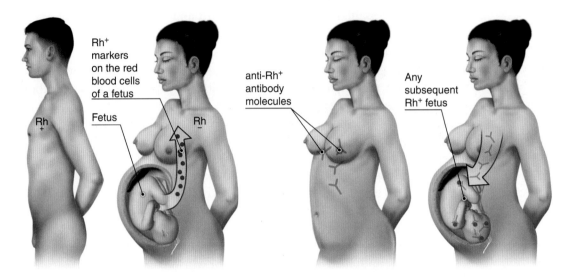

FIGURE 8-25 Theory for administration for RhoGAM.

Chapter 9

The Cardiovascular System

Chapter Introduction

The cells and tissues of the body need oxygen in order to survive, and the cardiovascular system works hard to deliver life-sustaining oxygenated blood through thousands of miles of blood vessels to trillions of cells. The cardiovascular system is driven by the powerful heart, which pumps over 100,000 times each day and billions of times in a lifetime to transport blood through a system of blood vessels that regulate blood pressure and blood flow in addition to transporting oxygen and carbon dioxide.

UNIT OBJECTIVE 9.1

Describe the components of the cardiovascular system.

UNIT INTRODUCTION

In order to transport blood throughout the body, the cardiovascular system must contain a pump and a series of pathways connecting the heart with the lungs, organs, and tissues. The heart serves as the pump that pushes blood through a complex series of blood vessels. These blood vessels begin with the large-diameter and muscular arteries, which branch to smaller arterioles and then to tiny capillary networks. Substances move between the capillaries and tissues. For example, oxygen moves out of capillaries and carbon dioxide moves in. The remaining deoxygenated blood moves back to the heart by way of smaller venules and veins. The heart then transports this blood to the lungs for oxygenation and the journey begins again.

LEARNING OBJECTIVE 9.1.1 Identify the structures of the cardiovascular system.

KEY TERMS

arteries Thick tubular structures that carry blood away from the heart.

arterioles Smaller vessels branching from arteries.

capillaries Smallest blood vessels consisting of one layer of simple squamous epithelium.

veins Tubular structures carrying blood toward the heart.

venules Vascular structures of the venous system that are smaller than veins and connect veins with capillaries.

STRUCTURES OF THE CARDIOVASCULAR SYSTEM

The primary structures of the cardiovascular system include the heart and thousands of miles of blood vessels. The blood vessels can be further broken down into arteries, arterioles, capillaries, venules, and veins. Arteries are typically the largest blood vessels, with a thick muscular layer. The arteries branch to form smaller arterioles, which help to distribute blood to small, complex capillary networks. The tiny capillaries are very thin and allow for exchange of substances between the blood and tissues. Oxygenated blood that is full of nutrients enters the capillaries at the arterial end, allowing for the oxygen and nutrients to be transported into the tissues by diffusion. Carbon dioxide and waste products diffuse back into the capillaries, allowing for deoxygenated blood to exit at the venous end. The deoxygenated blood moves back to the heart through a series of vessels containing one-way valves called venules and veins.

LEARNING OBJECTIVE 9.1.2 Identify the location of the heart in the body.

KEY TERMS

apex Apex of the heart is the inferior point of the heart.

base Chemical compound that ionizes when placed in a liquid and has the ability to bind to free hydrogen ions. The solution could also be called alkaline and has a pH greater than 7 (7.45 when used in reference to the human body).

esophagus Smooth muscle structure located between the pharynx and stomach that is part of the alimentary canal that carries substances from the mouth to the stomach.

fibrous connective tissue Tough connective tissue containing collagen fibers.

loose connective tissue

mediastinum Area in the thoracic cavity between the lungs.

pericardium Fibrous tissue structure that contains the heart.

sternum Bone located in the anterior portion of the thorax that has three divisions (manubrium, body, xiphoid process) and connects to the ribs and clavicles.

thoracic cavity Hollow area of the body located in the chest or thoracic area.

trachea Respiratory air passage containing C-shaped hyaline cartilage rings beginning at the inferior border of the larynx and extending to the primary bronchi.

LOCATION OF THE HEART IN THE BODY

The heart is located in the thoracic cavity deep to the sternum and medial to the lungs in an area between the lungs known as the mediastinum (see Figure 9-1). The mediastinum contains the heart, esophagus, trachea, blood vessels, nerves, and membranes surrounding the heart. A fibrous connective tissue membrane known as the **pericardium** must be dissected away in order to view the heart.

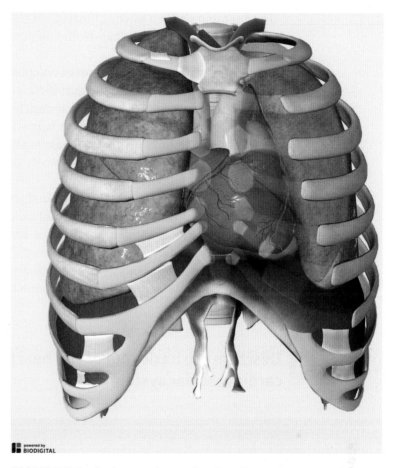

FIGURE 9-1 The heart is located within the mediastinum of the thoracic cavity. It is medial to the lungs, superior to the diaphragm, and anterior to the spinal column.

The heart is shaped like a blunt cone and is about the size of an adult fist. The inferior point of the cone points downward and to the left and is called the **apex** and the superior portion is called the **base**. More of the heart resides left of the midline of the **thoracic cavity** than on the right. The apex is located at the level of the fifth or sixth rib. The great vessels of the heart connect to structures in the base, which is located at about the second rib.

LEARNING OBJECTIVE 9.1.3 Describe the general function of the heart.

FUNCTION OF THE HEART

The primary cardiovascular system function of the heart is to pump blood through the blood vessels which are organized into three **circulatory circuits.** The heart contains hollow chambers for receiving and pumping blood.

These chambers are lined with cardiac muscle which is stimulated by specialized tissue that generates electrical impulses. Cardiac muscle responds to these impulses by contracting and generating pressure inside of the hollow chambers which pushes blood first from the receiving chambers to the pumping chambers and then from the pumping chambers out to the lungs and body.

Although the heart can contract completely on its own, the nervous system works to regulate heart rate through the autonomic nervous system. The heart receives feedback from the nervous system by way of sensory receptors in blood vessels. Input from the sympathetic nervous system promotes an increase in heart rate, while input from the parasympathetic nervous system promotes a decrease in heart rate. Both systems work to maintain a constant flow of blood through the circulatory circuits.

The three circulatory circuits include the **pulmonary**, **systemic**, and **coronary circulatory pathways**. The pulmonary circuit is a pathway for blood to flow from the body to the lungs for oxygenation. Once blood becomes oxygenated by the lungs, it flows through the much larger systemic circuit to the tissues of the body. The heart tissue also needs a constant supply of oxygenated blood in order to function and this blood is supplied by the coronary circuit.

LEARNING OBJECTIVE 9.1.4 **Describe the basic role of the heart within the cardiovascular system.**

KEY TERMS

deoxygenated blood Blood containing low oxygen levels after passing through tissue capillaries.

oxygenated blood Blood containing high oxygen levels after passing though capillaries in the lungs.

oxygenation Process of increasing oxygen levels in the blood.

THE ROLE OF THE HEART WITHIN THE CARDIOVASCULAR SYSTEM

The primary function of the heart is to pump **deoxygenated blood** to the lungs for **oxygenation** and then to deliver **oxygenated blood** to the body. In addition to oxygen and carbon dioxide, the blood carries nutrients and waste products. The heart contributes to regulation of blood volume and pressure by hormonal secretions and input from the autonomic nervous system works to control heart rate and blood pressure.

LEARNING OBJECTIVE 9.1.5 Identify arteries, veins, and capillaries based on their structure.

KEY TERMS

capillaries Smallest blood vessels consisting of one layer of simple squamous epithelium.

tunica externa Outer layer of an artery or vein.

tunica intima Inner layer of an artery or vein.

tunica media Middle muscular layer of an artery or vein.

vasoconstriction Narrowing of blood vessels.

vasodilation Process of dilating or widening a blood vessel through relaxation of smooth muscle.

STRUCTURE OF ARTERIES, VEINS, AND CAPILLARIES

Arteries, veins, and capillaries are hollow, tubular vessels that transport blood to the heart, lungs, and body. These hollow vessels serve as pathways for blood flow from the heart to the tissues of the body. Arteries are typically the largest and thickest vessels and carry blood from the heart to smaller, branching vessels called arterioles. Arterioles branch to form the smallest vessels called capillaries. Capillaries allow for exchange of substances between the blood and tissues. After substance exchange occurs, capillaries transport blood to venules, which feed into larger veins that transport blood back to the heart. Despite their similar function, each type of vessel has a different structure.

Arteries

Arteries are composed of three layers (see Figure 9-2). The outer layer, or **tunica externa**, consists of elastic and collagen fibers. The larger vessels have walls so thick that they contain tiny blood vessels that carry nutrients to the tissue in the vessel wall. Nerve fibers also innervate arteries. The middle layer, or **tunica media**, is thicker in arteries than in veins. It primarily consists of smooth muscle with some elastic fibers. The smooth muscle in the tunica media allows for constriction (**vasoconstriction**) and dilation (**vasodilation**) of the arteries. The nervous system has some control over the diameter of arteries in order to control blood pressure. Also, blood vessels are able to constrict when damaged to reduce the loss of blood. The inner layer, or **tunica interna**, consists of an inner thin layer of simple squamous epithelium called the endothelium anchored to another layer by a basement membrane. The basement membrane anchors the endothelium to a layer called the internal elastic lamina consisting of elastic fibers.

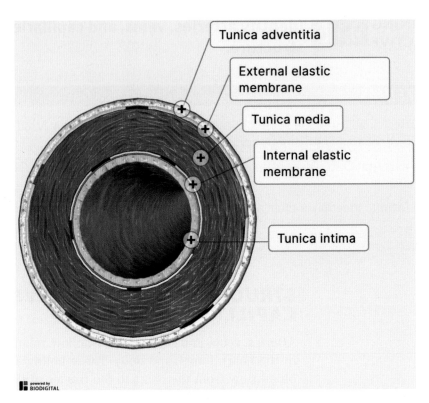

FIGURE 9-2 The wall of an artery has three layers, with the thickest being the tunica media.

Veins

Veins, like arteries, contain three layers (see Figure 9-3). However, the middle layer, or tunica media, is not as thick as in arteries. Veins have larger lumens than arteries, and many veins contain one-way valves that only allow blood to flow to the heart. Valves in veins help to transport blood to the heart and are assisted by muscular contraction. For example, during exercise more blood flow is needed to supply oxygenated blood to the tissues. Muscle contraction works to constrict veins by increasing the pressure inside. The increased pressure pushes blood toward the heart by way of the one-way valves, only allowing blood to flow toward the heart.

Large veins can vasoconstrict and do so in situations of blood loss in order to help to conserve blood. When significant blood is lost, the sympathetic nervous system stimulates veins to constrict in an effort to return blood to the heart. Although the constriction in veins is limited, the system allows for nearly normal blood flow when up to 25% of blood is lost.

Capillaries

Capillaries are the smallest blood vessels in the body. They carry blood to the venous system and allow for the exchange of substances between the blood and the tissues. Capillaries form complex networks and it is estimated there

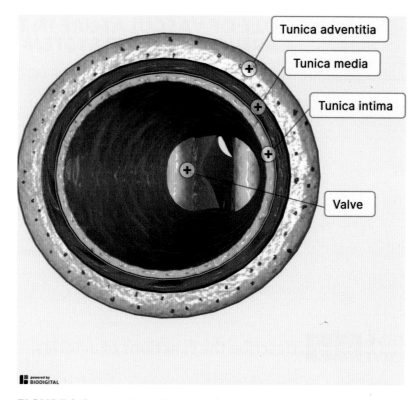

FIGURE 9-3 Veins have the same three layers as an artery, but their tunica media is very thin and they have valves to prevent the backflow of blood.

are about one billion capillaries in the human body. Blood flow to capillaries is controlled by small smooth muscles called precapillary sphincters where the capillary branches form an arteriole.

Capillaries are extensions of the endothelium of arteries. They consist of simple squamous epithelium and a **basement membrane** that allows a good degree of permeability for substance exchange. Capillaries are more numerous in areas with high metabolic activity, such as muscle and nerve tissue. Permeability also varies according to metabolic demand. For example, capillaries in the liver and spleen are more permeable than those in smooth or skeletal muscle. Most substances are exchanged by diffusion, but other transport mechanisms involved include filtration and osmosis.

LEARNING OBJECTIVE 9.1.6 **Describe the overall role of the vasculature in the cardiovascular system.**

ROLE OF VASCULATURE IN THE CARDIOVASCULAR SYSTEM

Blood vessels (vascular system) play an important role in the cardiovascular system. In addition to transporting blood, the vascular system helps to regulate blood flow and blood pressure by constricting (vasoconstriction) and dilating (vasodilation).

Adjusting the pressure inside of blood vessels helps to maintain a continuous flow of blood through the vascular system. For example, arteries can respond to a decrease in blood pressure by constricting. The thick muscular layer (tunica media) in arteries receives input from the sympathetic nervous system, which causes the smooth muscle to contract resulting in an increase in pressure. Some veins can constrict as well to help maintain a constant flow of blood to the heart. Likewise, relaxing the smooth muscle layer in both arteries and veins promotes vasodilation. Vasodilation decreases pressure inside of vessels and decreases blood flow.

LEARNING OBJECTIVE 9.1.7 Describe the functions of arteries.

KEY TERMS

pulmonary artery Arteries branching off the pulmonary trunk that carry deoxygenated blood to the lungs.

shunt Act of moving blood to other parts of the body.

vasoconstricting Process of constricting or narrowing a blood vessel.

vasodilating Dilating or widening of a blood vessel from relaxation of smooth muscle.

FUNCTION OF ARTERIES

Arteries carry blood away from the heart. With the exception of the **pulmonary artery**, the blood is oxygenated and transported to the tissues of the body. The arteries can also help to regulate blood flow and blood pressure by **vasoconstricting** and **vasodilating**. For example, when body temperature drops, arteries can **shunt** blood away from the extremities and to the core of the body in order to conserve heat. Also, when blood pressure drops, arteries can vasoconstrict in order to increase blood pressure.

Arteries branch to form smaller vessels called arterioles. Arterioles, like arteries, contain three layers, including a thick middle layer (tunica media). Arterioles work to adjust blood pressure entering the capillaries. They do this by contracting and relaxing the smooth muscle in the tunica media, causing vasoconstriction and vasodilation. Blood pressure must remain low in the fragile capillaries or they would burst. The arterioles work to eliminate forceful bursts of blood and promote a steady, continuous stream of blood to the capillaries.

LEARNING OBJECTIVE 9.1.8 Describe the basic function of veins.

one-way valves Valves in the venous system that only allow blood flow toward the heart.

FUNCTION OF VEINS

Veins carry blood toward the heart. With the exception of the pulmonary veins, the blood is deoxygenated and transported to the heart so that it can be pumped to the lungs for oxygenation. Since blood pressure is lower in veins, pressure to move blood back to the heart is, in part, generated external to veins by muscular contraction. The blood moves through veins toward the heart through a series of one-way valves.

Venules carry deoxygenated blood from capillaries to the larger veins. Like veins, venules have three layers. The inner endothelial layer consists of stratified squamous epithelium. The middle layer is thinner than arterioles and contains smooth muscle and elastic fibers and the outer layer consists of fibrous connective tissue. The thin layers of venules make them porous, allowing substances to move from the blood to the tissue.

LEARNING OBJECTIVE 9.1.9 Identify the arteries and veins that compose the pulmonary circuit.

KEY TERMS

pulmonary circuit System of blood vessels that bring deoxygenated blood from the heart to the lungs for oxygenation and then transport oxygenated blood back to the heart.

pulmonary trunk Great vessel of the heart exiting the right ventricle.

right and left pulmonary arteries Arteries carrying deoxygenated blood from the pulmonary trunk to the lungs.

right and left pulmonary veins Veins extending from the lungs to the left atrium carrying oxygenated blood.

THE PULMONARY CIRCUIT

Blood is carried from the heart to the lungs and then back to the heart by way of the pulmonary circuit (see Figures 9-4, 9-5, and 9-6).

The arteries and veins of the pulmonary circuit include:

- Pulmonary trunk
- Right and left pulmonary arteries
- Right and left pulmonary veins

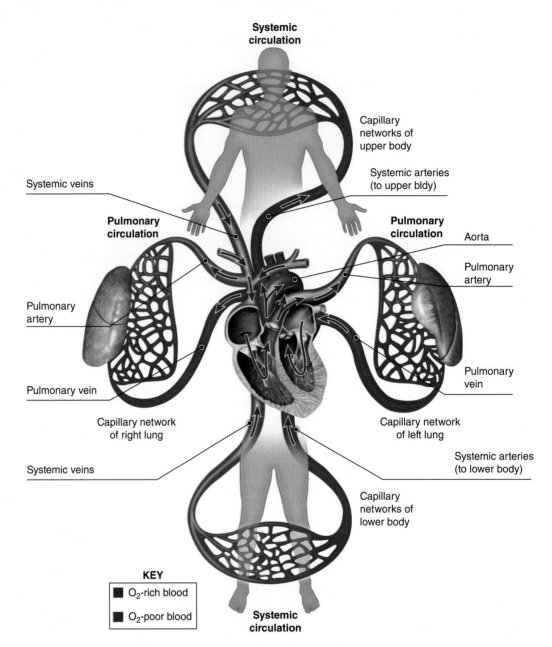

FIGURE 9-4 The pulmonary and systemic circuits of the cardiovascular system. The pulmonary circuit is represented by the lung images on the right and left of the figure, while the system circuit is represented by the upper portion of the body at the top and the lower portion of the body at the bottom.

The pulmonary circuit begins with the pathway of deoxygenated blood from the heart to the lungs. Deoxygenated blood flows from the right ventricle to the **pulmonary trunk**, which branches into the **right and left pulmonary arteries**. The deoxygenated blood enters the lungs and becomes oxygenated. The oxygenated blood then flows through the **right and left pulmonary veins** to the left atrium of the heart. Blood will then move from the heart to the body by way of the **systemic circuit**.

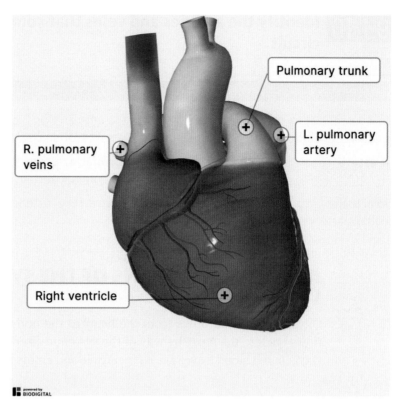

FIGURE 9-5 Anterior view of the coronary circuit.

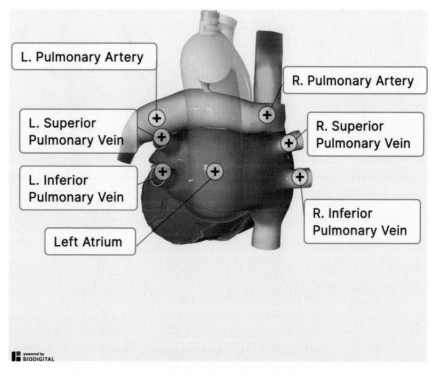

FIGURE 9-6 Posterior view of the pulmonary circuit.

LEARNING OBJECTIVE 9.1.10 Identify the arteries and veins that compose the systemic circuit.

KEY TERMS

aorta Large blood vessel exiting the left ventricle, known as a great vessel of the heart.

brachiocephalic artery Artery branching off the aorta.

common carotid arteries Arteries branching from the brachiocephalic artery on the right and aorta

on the left carrying blood to the internal and external carotid arteries.

common iliac arteries Paired inferior branches off the abdominal aorta.

subclavian artery Arteries located below the clavicle.

ARTERIES AND VEINS OF THE SYSTEMIC CIRCUIT

Oxygenated blood flows from the heart to the body and deoxygenated blood flows back to the heart by way of the systemic circuit (see Figure 9-7 and 9-8). Oxygenated blood leaves the left ventricle and enters the aorta. The aorta arches

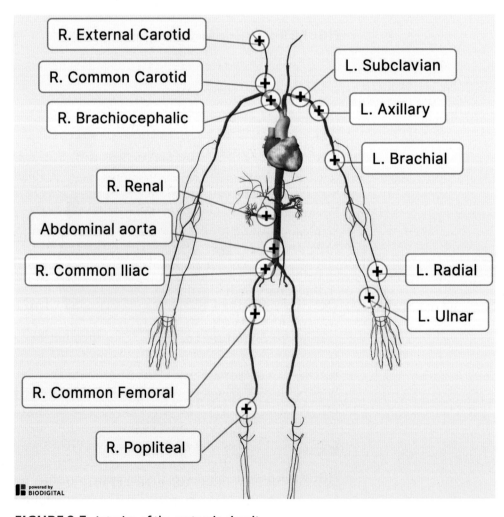

FIGURE 9-7 Arteries of the systemic circuit.

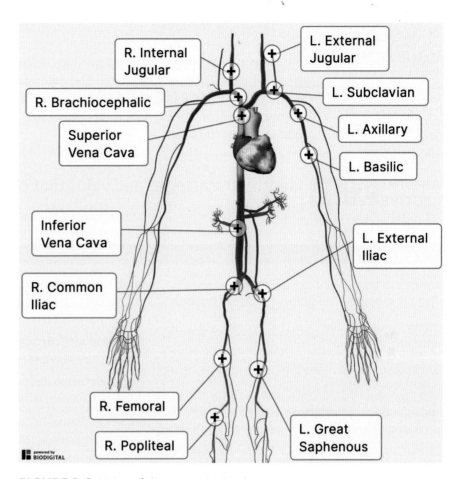

FIGURE 9-8 Veins of the systemic circuit.

and extends inferior to become the thoracic aorta before passing through the diaphragm to become the abdominal aorta. Branches of the abdominal aorta supply the organs of the abdomen. The abdominal aorta then divides to become the right and left **common iliac arteries**. The common iliac arteries divide into internal and external iliac arteries, with the external iliac arteries exiting the abdominal cavity to supply the lower extremities.

There are three major branches of the aorta that supply the head, neck, and upper extremities. These include the **brachiocephalic**, left common carotid, and left subclavian arteries. The brachiocephalic divides into right common carotid and **subclavian arteries**. The **common carotid arteries** supply the head and subclavian arteries supply the upper extremities.

Veins return blood from the tissues to the heart. There are deep veins and superficial veins. Deep veins carry deoxygenated blood from the tissues of the upper extremity by way of the radial and ulnar veins, which merge into the brachial vein. The brachial vein carries blood to the axillary vein, which becomes the subclavian vein. The subclavian vein becomes the brachiocephalic vein, which merges with the superior vena cava. Superficial veins of the upper extremity include the cephalic (lateral), basilic (medial), and median cubital vein in the elbow region. The head and neck regions are drained by the internal and external jugular veins along with the vertebral vein. These veins connect with the subclavian vein.

Tissues of the lower extremities are drained by the deep veins, which include the anterior and posterior tibial veins and fibular veins, which drain into the popliteal veins. The popliteal veins drain into the femoral veins, which merge with the external iliac veins. The external iliac veins enter the abdominopelvic cavity and merges with the common iliac veins, which drain into the inferior vena cava. The inferior vena cava brings the deoxygenated blood to the right atrium of the heart.

LEARNING OBJECTIVE 9.1.11 Identify the arteries and veins that compose the coronary circuit.

KEY TERMS

circumflex artery Branch of the left coronary artery that wraps around the left side of the heart.

coronary sinus Cardiac vein that empties into the right atrium.

great cardiac vein Large vein located on the heart that connects with the coronary sinus.

left anterior descending artery Branch of the left coronary artery located in the interventricular sulcus.

marginal artery Refers to a branch of the right coronary artery.

middle and posterior cardiac veins Veins of the coronary circuit that drain the area supplied by the marginal and circumflex arteries.

right and left coronary arteries Part of the coronary circuit or circulatory pathway.

right posterior descending artery Artery that is a branch of the right coronary artery.

small cardiac vein Refers to a portion of the coronary circulatory circuit that drains blood into the great cardiac vein.

ARTERIES AND VEINS OF THE CORONARY CIRCUIT

Cardiac muscle in the heart requires a constant supply of oxygenated blood, since oxygen is needed to produce ATP needed for the heart to contract. Some people wrongly assume that the heart is able to obtain the oxygen and nutrients it requires from the blood traveling through its chambers. Instead, a group of blood vessels known as the coronary circuit supply the heart with oxygenated blood and return deoxygenated blood to the venous system (see Figures 9-9 and 9-10).

Arteries of the coronary circuit branch from the aorta. There are two main arteries, which include the right and left coronary arteries. The right coronary artery divides into two smaller arteries that supply both ventricles, the right atrium, and the posterior one-third of the interventricular septum. These include the right posterior descending and marginal arteries. The left coronary artery supplies both ventricles, the left atrium, and the anterior two-thirds of the interventricular septum. The left coronary artery divides into the left anterior descending and circumflex arteries.

Veins of the coronary circuit include the coronary sinus, great cardiac vein, and anterior, middle, and posterior cardiac veins. All of these veins drain deoxygenated blood from the myocardium. The coronary sinus empties into the right atrium. The great cardiac vein connects to the coronary sinus and receives blood from smaller branches including the posterior, middle, and small cardiac veins.

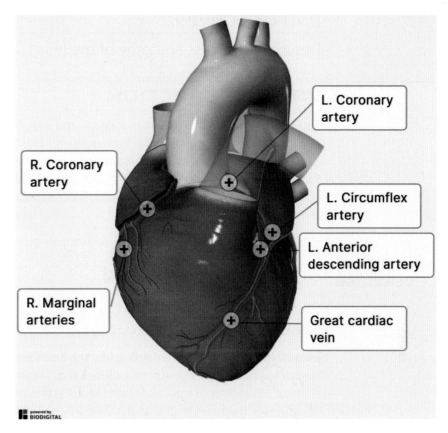

FIGURE 9-9 Anterior view of the coronary circuit.

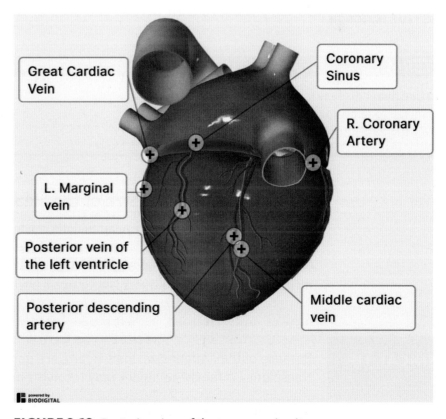

FIGURE 9-10 Posterior view of the coronary circuit.

UNIT OBJECTIVE 9.2

Describe the gross anatomy of the heart.

UNIT INTRODUCTION

The basic design of the heart is elegant and simple and allows it to perform its vital function of keeping the human body alive. The heart contains hollow chambers with strong muscular walls and a system of valves for directing blood flow to the great vessels that enter and exit carrying blood to the lungs and body. This section examines the heart's basic structure by presenting the gross anatomy of the heart.

LEARNING OBJECTIVE 9.2.1 Describe the size of the heart.

SIZE OF THE HEART

Despite its large role in maintaining life, the heart is a relatively small organ. The human heart is about the size of a closed fist. The width of the heart at its base is about 3.5 inches (8 cm) wide, and its length is about 5 inches (12 cm). The thickness of the heart wall is about 2.5 inches (6 cm).

LEARNING OBJECTIVE 9.2.2 Identify factors that affect the size of the heart.

KEY TERM

congestive heart disease Disease characterized by damage to heart muscle and enlargement of the ventricles of the heart.

Factors Affecting the Size of the Heart

Factors affecting the size of the heart include gender, age, body size, and pathology. Male hearts are generally larger than female hearts. Adults hearts are larger than children's hearts and body size is correlated with heart size. Pathologies such as congestive heart disease can cause an enlarged heart.

CLINICAL TIP | Because of their larger size, male hearts are generally used in heart transplants. A female recipient may receive a male heart.

LEARNING OBJECTIVE 9.2.3 Describe the heart's position within the thoracic cavity.

mediastinum Area in the thoracic cavity between the lungs.

POSITION OF THE HEART

The heart is positioned in the middle of the chest (thoracic cavity), just deep to the sternum and in the area between the lungs known as the mediastinum. The posterior portion of the heart is anterior to the thoracic vertebrae at about the level of T5 to T8. More of the heart resides left of the midline of the thoracic cavity, with the apex of the heart pointing to the left.

LEARNING OBJECTIVE 9.2.4 Identify the great vessels of the heart.

KEY TERMS

aorta Large blood vessel exiting the left ventricle, known as a great vessel of the heart.

great vessels Large vessels entering and exiting the heart.

inferior vena cava Large vein carrying blood to the right atrium.

left atrium Hollow chamber of the heart that receives oxygenated blood from the lungs carried by the pulmonary veins.

left ventricle Hollow chamber in the heart that contracts and pushes blood out of the heart.

pulmonary arteries Arteries branching off the pulmonary trunk that carry deoxygenated blood to the lungs.

pulmonary trunk Great vessel of the heart exiting the right ventricle.

pulmonary veins Blood vessels carrying oxygenated blood from the lungs to the left atrium.

right atrium Hollow chamber on the right side of the heart that receives blood from the superior and inferior vena cavae.

right ventricle Hollow chamber in the right side of the heart that pushes blood to the pulmonary trunk.

GREAT VESSELS OF THE HEART

The blood vessels entering and exiting the heart are known as the great vessels (see Figures 9-11 and 9-12). These include the superior and inferior vena cava, which bring deoxygenated blood to the right atrium; the pulmonary trunk, which sends deoxygenated blood from the right ventricle to the pulmonary arteries and lungs; the pulmonary veins, which bring oxygenated blood to the left atrium; and the aorta, which sends oxygenated blood from the left ventricle to the body.

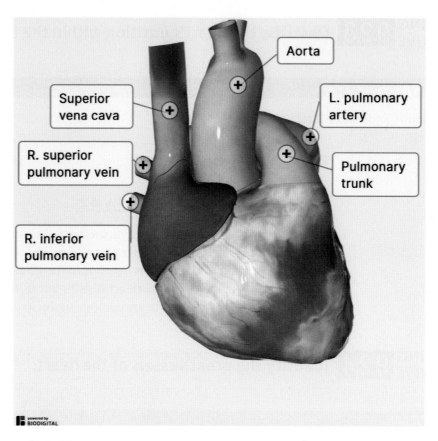

FIGURE 9-11 Anterior view of the great vessels of the heart.

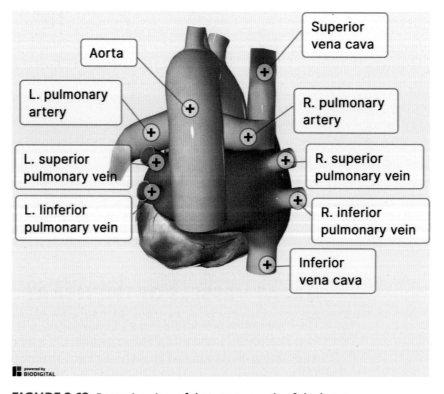

FIGURE 9-12 Posterior view of the great vessels of the heart.

LEARNING OBJECTIVE 9.2.5 **Identify the four chambers of the heart.**

KEY TERMS

atria Hollow chamber of the heart that acts as a receiving chamber for blood entering the heart.

ventricle Hollow structure in the heart that pushes blood out.

CHAMBERS OF THE HEART

The inner portion of the heart consists of hollow chambers. There are two receiving chambers called **atria**, and two pumping chambers called ventricles (see Figure 9-13). There are two chambers on each side of the heart, including the right atrium and right **ventricle** and left atrium and left ventricle.

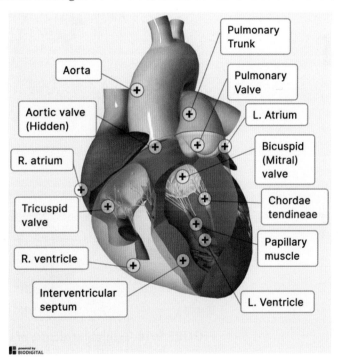

FIGURE 9-13 Internal structures of the heart.

LEARNING OBJECTIVE 9.2.6 **Identify the four chambers of the heart using the heart's external anatomical features.**

KEY TERMS

auricle Irregularly shaped structure overlying the atria.

left atrium Hollow chamber of the heart that receives oxygenated blood from the lungs carried by the pulmonary veins.

left ventricle Hollow chamber in the heart that contracts and pushes blood out of the heart.

right atrium Hollow chamber on the right side of the heart that receives blood from the superior and inferior vena cavae.

right ventricle Hollow chamber in the right side of the heart that pushes blood to the pulmonary trunk.

EXTERNAL ANATOMY OF THE HEART

The anterior surface of the heart primarily consists of the **right ventricle**. The **right atrium** is visible superior to the right ventricle just deep to an irregularly shaped structure called the **auricle**. The inferior surface primarily consists of the **left ventricle** with a small portion of the right ventricle. The right border of the heart consists of the right atrium and the left border consists of the left ventricle. The **left atrium** is just above the left ventricle and, like the right atrium, is covered by an auricle (See Figure 9-14).

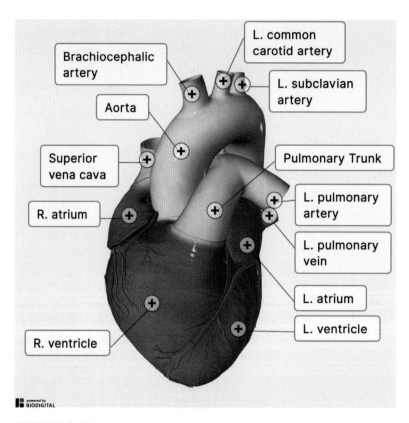

FIGURE 9-14 External structure of the heart.

LEARNING OBJECTIVE 9.2.7 Identify the layers of the pericardium.

THE PERICARDIUM

The heart is surrounded by a membrane known as the **pericardium**. The pericardium includes the outer fibrous pericardium and inner serous pericardium. The serous pericardium consists of two layers, which include the parietal and visceral pericardium (see Figure 9-15).

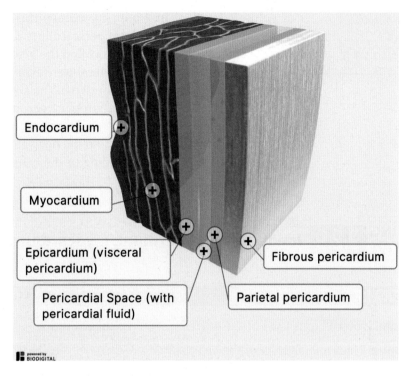

FIGURE 9-15 Layers of the pericardium and wall of the heart.

LEARNING OBJECTIVE 9.2.8 **Describe the structure and function of each layer of the pericardium.**

KEY TERMS

dense connective tissue Type of fibrous connective tissue found in ligaments and tendons.

epicardium Outer fibrous layer of the heart.

fibrous pericardium Outer portion of the heart containing fibrous connective tissue.

parietal pericardium Outer layer of the fibrous structure that contains the heart known as the pericardium.

pericardium Fibrous tissue structure that contains the heart.

serous pericardium Portion of the pericardium that contains the visceral and parietal pericardium.

visceral pericardium Portion of the pericardium located on the surface of the heart.

Structure and Function of the Pericardium

The outer portion of the pericardium consists of **dense connective tissue** and is called the **fibrous pericardium**. It attaches to the diaphragm, sternum, and outer layer of the great vessels. The inner portion of the pericardium is called the **serous pericardium** and consists of two layers, each consisting of epithelial cells. The outer layer lines the inside of the **fibrous pericardium** and is called the **parietal pericardium**. The inner layer connects to the outer surface of the heart and is called the **visceral pericardium**. The visceral pericardium is also known as the outer layer of the heart or **epicardium**. A thin pericardial cavity exists between the parietal and visceral pericardia filled with pericardial fluid, a slippery serous fluid that prevents friction and irritation.

The pericardium helps to hold the heart in the mediastinum and provides a barrier to help prevent overfilling of the heart and protect the heart against infection.

LEARNING OBJECTIVE 9.2.9 Identify the epicardium, myocardium, and endocardium.

KEY TERMS

epicardium Outer fibrous layer of the heart.

myocardium Thick middle layer of the heart wall consisting of cardiac muscle.

endocardium Inner layer of the heart.

LAYERS OF THE HEART

The heart contains three layers, which include the outer epicardium, middle myocardium, and inner endocardium. The outer layer, or **epicardium**, is also known as the visceral pericardium. The epicardium is a thin superficial layer consisting of epithelial cells and adipose tissue. The **myocardium** is a thick layer consisting of cardiac muscle. The inner **endocardium** is a thin layer consisting of epithelium and connective tissue that lines the inner portion of the heart and is consistent with the inner linings of the blood vessels.

LEARNING OBJECTIVE 9.2.10 Describe the function of the epicardium, myocardium, and endocardium.

Function of the Heart Layers

The epicardium is considered a serous membrane that helps to reduce friction while the heart is contracting and relaxing. The myocardium performs the contractions of the heart, which move blood through the circulatory pathways. The myocardium also contains specialized cardiac muscle tissue that conducts electrical impulses through the muscular wall. The endocardium lines the inner surface of the heart and valves and provides a smooth surface for blood flow.

CLINICAL TIP	An infection of the endocardium is known as endocarditis. Endocarditis is a serious and potentially fatal condition caused by bacteria or fungi.

LEARNING OBJECTIVE 9.2.11 Explain why the myocardium thickness differs between the left and right ventricle.

Differences in Myocardium Structure

The myocardium is consistent throughout the heart; however, there are some differences in myocardium thickness in each of the ventricles. The differences directly relate to the function of each side of the heart. The myocardium of the left ventricle is thicker due to the action of pumping blood to the entire body, which requires more force than the right side's job of pumping blood from the heart to the lungs.

LEARNING OBJECTIVE 9.2.12 Identify the four valves in the heart.

KEY TERMS

aortic valve Semilunar valve located near the junction of the aorta and left ventricle.

atrioventricular valves Heart valves located between the atria and ventricles.

bicuspid valve Also known as the mitral valve, located between the left atrium and ventricle and containing two cusps.

mitral valve Also known as the bicuspid valve, a valve containing two cusps located between the left atrium and ventricle.

pulmonary trunk Great vessel of the heart exiting the right ventricle.

pulmonary valve Semilunar valve located in the pulmonary trunk near its connection to the right ventricle.

semilunar valves Valves located in the pulmonary trunk and aorta containing three cusps.

tricuspid valve Atrioventricular valve containing three cusps and located between the right atrium and ventricle.

HEART VALVES

The heart contains four valves (see Figure 9-16ABCD). The two **atrioventricular valves** are located between each atrium and ventricle. The right atrioventricular valve has three cusps and is called the **tricuspid valve**. The left atrioventricular valve has two cusps and is called the **bicuspid** or **mitral valve**. There are two valves located in each of the great vessels exiting the heart and are known as **semilunar valves**. The **pulmonary valve** is located at the junction of the **pulmonary trunk** and right ventricle. The aortic valve is located at the junction of the aorta and left ventricle. The semilunar valves contain three cusps, each in the shape of a half moon.

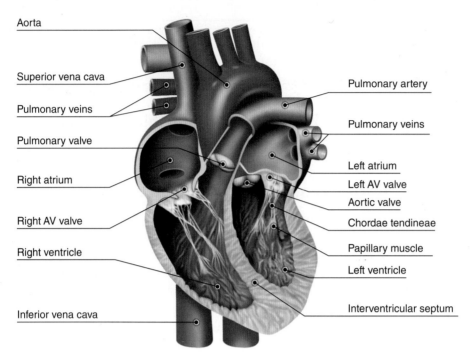

A Location of the heart valves in a longitudinal section of the heart

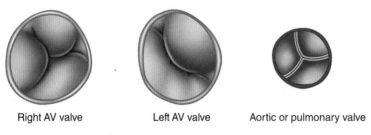

Right AV valve   Left AV valve   Aortic or pulmonary valve

B Heart valves in closed position, viewed from above

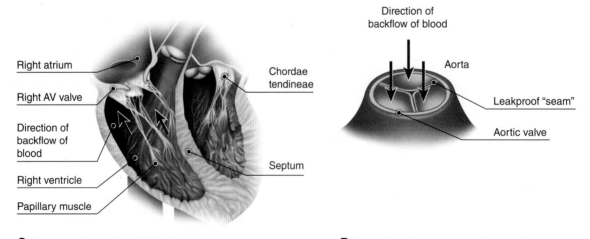

C Prevention of eversion of AV valves

D Prevention of eversion of semilunar valves

FIGURE 9-16ABCD A) A longitudinal section of the heart that contains the four heart valves. B) The tricuspid, mitral, and semilunar valves as seen from above. C) The function of the valves is to prevent the backflow of blood, so their structure is one that supports this function. D) The pressure within the aorta becomes higher than that in the left ventricle when the ventricle relaxes, causing aback pressure that forces the aortic valve shut.

LEARNING OBJECTIVE 9.2.13 Describe the function of heart valves.

Function of the Heart Valves

The atrioventricular valves prevent the backflow of blood into each atrium during contraction (systole) of the ventricles. Each cusp of an atrioventricular valve is attached to small, string-like structures made of collagen called chordae tendineae. The chordae tendineae attach to papillary muscles on the walls of the ventricles. These valves are controlled by pressure. When the ventricular pressure increases during contraction, the valves close, keeping blood from leaking into the atria. During ventricular systole, the papillary muscles contract to maintain a tight seal between the atria and ventricles by preventing prolapse of the atrioventricular valves.

The semilunar valves are one-way valves that open during ventricular contraction, allowing blood to flow into the pulmonary trunk and aorta. Like the atrioventricular valves, these valves are controlled by pressure and prevent backflow of blood into the ventricles during relaxation (diastole).

LEARNING OBJECTIVE 9.2.14 Contrast the location and structure of the four heart valves.

Structure of the Heart Valves

The one-way valves of the heart have similar functions; however, some differences exist in their structure. The atrioventricular valves consist of cusps anchored to the walls of the ventricles by chordae tendineae. The tricuspid valve located between the right atrium and ventricle contains three cusps, while the bicuspid located between the left atrium and ventricle contains two. The semilunar valves contain a similar structure, with each valve consisting of three cusps. The structure of the semilunar valves helps to maintain a tight seal between the ventricles, pulmonary trunk, and aorta. This is in contrast to the structure of the atrioventricular valves, which require chordae tendineae and papillary muscles to prevent leakage of blood into the atria during ventricular systole.

LEARNING OBJECTIVE 9.2.15 Explain the importance of heart valves in cardiac physiology.

KEY TERMS

compliant Referring to the elastic component of a structure.

prolapse Bulging or collapsing of a heart valve.

regurgitation Abnormality of heart valves characterized by leaking.

stenosis Narrowing, usually refers to narrowing of a vessel or heart valve.

Heart Valves and Cardiac Physiology

The heart valves help to direct the blood flow through the heart. Problems in heart valve function include stenosis and prolapse. In stenosis, the valve narrows due to calcification or scar tissue and becomes less compliant, resulting in a greater workload for the heart and subsequent weakening of the ventricular myocardium. Prolapsed valves do not close properly with one or more cusps bulging upward during ventricular contraction, sometimes causing blood to leak into the atrium (regurgitation).

CLINICAL TIP Mitral valve prolapse typically presents with an abnormal clicking sound (murmur). Symptoms include a rapid heart rate, dizziness, shortness of breath, fatigue, and chest pain. Treatments include medications and, in severe cases, the mitral valve may be replaced.

UNIT OBJECTIVE 9.3

Describe the structure and function of the cardiac electrical conduction system.

UNIT INTRODUCTION

Contractions of the heart are controlled by a specialized electrical system embedded in the muscular walls of the heart. This system works to provide a consistent rhythm of contractions that are timed to allow the heart to pump blood efficiently. Although regulated by the nervous system, the heart can beat entirely on its own since its electrical system can generate its own action potentials. This unit examines the cardiac electrical conduction system.

LEARNING OBJECTIVE 9.3.1 Identify the components of the electrical conduction system of the heart.

atrioventricular bundle Section of nodal tissue located inferior to the atrioventricular node and at the superior junction of the ventricles capable of generating action potentials at 20–40 beats per minute.

atrioventricular (AV) node Section of nodal tissue located at the inferior portion of the right atrium at the junction of the right atrium and ventricles capable of generating action potentials at 40–60 bpm.

gap junctions Hollow, water-filled cylinders that allow things like nutrients and ions to pass between neighboring cells; most commonly found in cardiac cells and embryonic cells.

intercalated discs Specialized cell junctions found in cardiac muscle.

internodal pathways Specialized pathways in cardiac muscle that carry electrical impulses between nodes.

nodal cells Specialized cardiac muscle cells that can generate action potentials.

Purkinje fibers Specialized muscle fibers containing cells that conduct electricity located in the walls of the ventricles.

sinoatrial (SA) node Area of specialized cardiac muscle that can generate action potentials; sets the heart's rhythm.

ELECTRICAL CONDUCTION SYSTEM OF THE HEART

The heart contains cells that generate action potentials called **nodal cells**. Electrical impulses generated by nodal cells travel to cardiac muscle by way of **intercalated discs** and **gap junctions** along specific pathways called **internodal pathways** (see Figure 9-17). These pathways begin at an area in the posterior–superior region of the right atrium known as the **sinoatrial (SA) node**. The SA node, also known as the primary pacemaker, generates the electrical impulses that will regulate the rhythm of the heart and has the quickest rate of depolarization. Impulses from the SA node travel to the **atrioventricular (AV) node** located at the inferior portion of the right atrium near the interatrial septum. The AV node delays the impulse to allow the atria to fully contract and push blood into the ventricles, prior to allowing the signal to pass into the ventricles. The impulse then moves to the **atrioventricular bundle** (bundle of His) located at the junction of the ventricles in the superior portion of the interventricular septum.

Impulses from the atrioventricular bundle move along two branches called the right and left bundle branches that move though the interventricular septum toward the apex of the heart. Fast-conducting **Purkinje fibers** located in the myocardium of the ventricles carry impulses through the myocardium. The Purkinje fibers allow for ventricular contraction to begin at the apex and end toward the base of the heart. Contraction of the apex before the base helps to push blood to the pulmonary trunk and aorta.

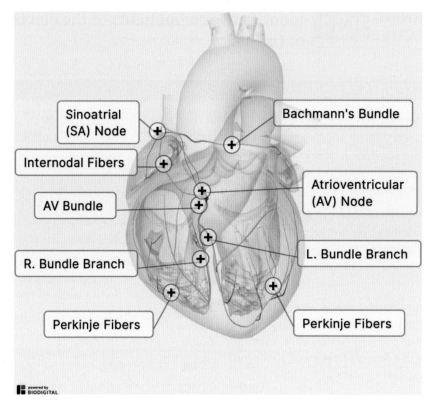

FIGURE 9-17 The cardiac conduction system.

LEARNING OBJECTIVE 9.3.2 List the parts of the electrical conduction system by the order in which they are stimulated.

KEY TERMS

atrioventricular bundle Section of nodal tissue located inferior to the atrioventricular node and at the superior junction of the ventricles capable of generating action potentials at 20–40 beats per minute.

atrioventricular node Section of nodal tissue located at the inferior portion of the right atrium at the junction of the right atrium and ventricles capable of generating action potentials at 40–60 bpm.

internodal pathways Specialized pathways in cardiac muscle that carry electrical impulses between nodes.

Purkinje fibers Specialized muscle fibers containing cells that conduct electricity located in the walls of the ventricles.

sinoatrial node Area of specialized cardiac muscle that can generate action potentials; sets the heart's rhythm.

Flow of Electrical Impulses Across the Heart

Electrical impulses flow across the heart by following specific routes called internodal pathways. The impulses begin at the sinoatrial node and flow through the heart in the following order:

1. Sinoatrial node
2. Internodal pathways

3. Atrioventricular node
4. Atrioventricular bundle
5. Right and left bundle branches
6. Purkinje fibers

Electrical impulses are generated by the sinoatrial node. These impulses promote contraction of the right atrium. The impulses then travel to the left atrium and the atrioventricular node. Impulses from the sinoatrial node reach the left atrium by way of an internodal pathway called Bachmann's bundle in order to promote contraction of the left atrium. Impulses reaching the atrioventricular bundle travel to the atrioventricular bundle, which relays these impulses to the right and left bundle branches, and fast-conducting Purkinje fibers, which promote contraction of the ventricles.

LEARNING OBJECTIVE 9.3.3 Identify the following aspects of an electrocardiogram: P-wave, QRS complex, T-wave, isoelectric line, PR interval, ST segment.

LEARNING OBJECTIVE 9.3.4 Explain how the waves and complexes of an ECG relate to the flow of electricity through the electrical conduction system.

KEY TERMS

cardiac cycle Sequence of mechanical and electrical events allowing the heart to contract and move blood.

isoelectric line Reference line in the ECG representing the baseline or zero voltage.

PR interval The section on an ECG between the beginning of the P-wave and beginning of the R-wave.

PR segment The section on an ECG between the end of the P-wave and beginning of the R-wave.

P-wave ECG waveform that represents ventricular repolarization.

QRS complex ECG waveform that represents ventricular depolarization and atrial repolarization.

ST segment ECG measurement that begins at the end of the QRS complex and ends at the beginning of the T-wave.

T-wave Portion of an ECG just after the QRS complex that represents ventricular repolarization.

THE ELECTROCARDIOGRAM

The electrocardiogram (ECG) is a test that measures the electrical activity of the heart and represents events in the cardiac cycle. The ECG presents a display plotting electrical voltage against time. A standard ECG consists of three primary waveforms that rise and fall on a baseline or reference line called the isoelectric line. ECGs are read from left to right, beginning with a waveform forming a small upward and downward curve called the P-wave. The P-wave is followed by a complex wave consisting of a small, sharp downward spike (Q-wave), large upward spike (R-wave), and small downward spike (S-wave), collectively called the **QRS complex**. Another small upward and downward curved line called the **T-wave** follows the QRS complex.

The ECG represents the electrical events of the cardiac cycle. These events include depolarization and repolarization occurring in areas of cardiac muscle. The P-wave represents depolarization of the atria, which occurs just prior to contraction (systole). The QRS complex represents the combined electrical activity from both ventricular depolarization, which occurs just before systole, and atrial repolarization, which occurs when the atria are beginning to relax (diastole). However, the magnitude of the ventricular depolarization, essentially overrides the small signal produced by atrial repolarization. The T-wave represents ventricular repolarization, which occurs as the ventricles are going into diastole.

As we discuss the different portions of the ECG, please refer to Figure 9-18. The distance between the beginning of the P-wave and beginning of the QRS

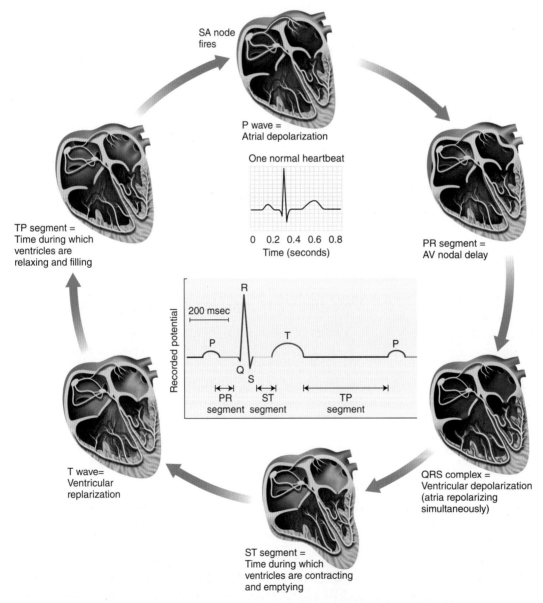

FIGURE 9-18 The electrocardiogram (ECG) represents the electrical activity in the heart associated with contraction and relaxation of the hearts chambers.

complex is known as the PR interval. The PR interval is used to assess the conduction of electrical impulses from the atria to the ventricles. Between the end of the P-wave and beginning of the QRS interval is a flat line called the PR segment. The PR segment represents the true isoelectric line. The ST segment is measured between the end of the QRS interval and beginning of the T-wave. The ST segment represents the isoelectric line between ventricular depolarization and repolarization.

CLINICAL TIP	Abnormalities of the PR interval are often associated with conduction blocks in which impulses are delayed or blocked between the atria and ventricles.

The distance from the end of the QRS complex to the end of the T-wave is called the ST segment. The end of the QRS complex represents the J point, which indicates the start of the ST segment. The ST segment is abnormal in a number of cardiac pathologies.

CLINICAL TIP	The ST segment is often elevated in myocardial ischemia (MI; heart attack).

LEARNING OBJECTIVE 9.3.5 Describe what the ECG of a healthy adult should look like.

KEY TERMS

P-wave ECG waveform that represents ventricular repolarization.

QRS complex ECG waveform that represents ventricular depolarization and atrial repolarization.

ST segment ECG measurement that begins at the end of the QRS complex and ends at the beginning of the T-wave.

T-wave Portion of an ECG just after the QRS complex that represents ventricular repolarization.

The Normal ECG

The ECG of a healthy adult should contain all of the waves (P-wave, QRS complex, T-wave) with the appropriate shapes and distances between them. Each group of waves (P, QRS, T) should occur with a distance between them representing the normal heart rate of 60–100 beats per minute (bpm). The duration of the P-wave should be between 0.08 and 0.10 seconds. The QRS complex should range between 0.08 and 0.12 seconds and the T-wave should range between 0.10 and 0.25 seconds. A normal PR interval will range from 0.12 to 0.20 seconds and the ST segment should have the appropriate shape.

UNIT OBJECTIVE 9.4

Describe the actions of the cardiac cycle.

UNIT INTRODUCTION

All of the events that work in concert in the heart to allow it to pump blood are collectively called the cardiac cycle. The cardiac cycle consists of electrical, mechanical, and physiological processes that work together in a precise manner. This unit examines the actions of the cardiac cycle.

LEARNING OBJECTIVE 9.4.1 Identify the path of blood through the heart.

KEY TERMS

deoxygenated blood Blood containing low oxygen levels after passing through tissue capillaries.

oxygenated blood Blood containing high oxygen levels after passing though capillaries in the lungs.

BLOOD FLOW THROUGH THE HEART

Blood follows a specific pathway through the heart. The right atrium of the heart receives deoxygenated blood from the superior and inferior vena cava as well as the coronary sinus. Blood flows from the right atrium through the tricuspid valve to the right ventricle where it is pushed through the pulmonary valve to the pulmonary trunk. The pulmonary trunk divides into right and left pulmonary arteries, which carry blood to the lungs.

The lungs provide a constant supply of oxygen to the blood and provide a pathway for release of carbon dioxide. Once blood is oxygenated by the lungs, it flows through the right and left pulmonary veins to the left atrium of the heart. Blood flows from the left atrium through the bicuspid (mitral) valve to the left ventricle, where it is pushed through the aortic valve to the aorta. The aorta then carries the oxygenated blood to the tissues of the body.

LEARNING OBJECTIVE 9.4.2 Describe atrial systole, atrial diastole, ventricular systole, and ventricular diastole.

LEARNING OBJECTIVE 9.4.3 Explain the relationship between atrial systole and ventricular diastole.

THE CARDIAC CYCLE

During a single heartbeat, the heart must deliver deoxygenated blood to the lungs and oxygenated blood to the body. The series of events that accomplishes this task is called the cardiac cycle.

LEARNING OBJECTIVE 9.4.4 **Explain the relationship between atrial diastole and ventricular systole.**

Ventricular Filling

During the first phase of the cardiac cycle, the atria and ventricles are in a relaxed state referred to as diastole. During this phase, pressure is greater in the vena cavae and pulmonary veins than in the atria, promoting blood flow from the vessels into the atria. Deoxygenated blood flows from the superior and inferior vena cavae to the right atrium, while oxygenated blood flows from the four pulmonary veins into the left atrium. Electrical impulses generated by the sinoatrial node travel to the atrioventricular node, Bachmann's bundle, and atrioventricular bundle, causing depolarization of the atria as represented by the P-wave of the ECG.

Pressure changes control the opening and closing of the heart valves. Blood flow into the atria produces a greater pressure than in the ventricles, promoting opening of the one-way atrioventricular valves, allowing blood to flow into the ventricles. This passive flow of blood accounts for approximately 70% of ventricular filling. The relaxed ventricles also produce a lower pressure than in the pulmonary trunk and aorta, causing the one-way semilunar valves to close.

Atrial Systole

Atrial systole (contraction) occurs next in the cycle. Blood flows past the open atrioventricular valves and into the ventricles. The remaining 30% of ventricular filling occurs during this phase. The total volume of blood in the ventricles at the end of this phase is about 130 ml and is known as end diastolic volume. Ventricular pressure remains low enough to keep the semilunar valves closed. Electrical impulses travel from the atrioventricular bundle to the right and left bundle branches and Purkinje fibers, causing depolarization of the ventricles and represented by the QRS complex in the ECG.

Ventricular Systole

The next phase of the cycle is marked by contraction of the ventricles (systole) while the atria relax (diastole). Pressure increases in the ventricles, allowing blood to flow back toward the atria. This backflow of blood, along with the increased ventricular pressure, promotes closing of the atrioventricular valves and opening of the semilunar valves. Just prior to the opening of the semilunar valves, the closed but contracting ventricles undergo a period of isovolumetric contraction during which there is no movement of blood. The movement of blood out of the ventricles marks the ventricular ejection phase. Blood flows from the right ventricle to the pulmonary trunk and from the left ventricle to the aorta. The ventricles begin to repolarize as represented by the T-wave in the ECG.

The amount of blood exiting the ventricles during systole is about 70–80 ml and is known as stroke volume. The amount of blood remaining in the ventricles at the end of systole would then be the end diastolic volume (130 ml) minus the stroke volume (70–80 ml), which is about 50–60 ml. This value is known as end systolic volume. Upon completion of this phase, the cycle repeats.

LEARNING OBJECTIVE 9.4.5 **Locate the four anatomical points used to auscultate heart sounds.**

KEY TERMS

auscultation Examination of the sounds of the heart.

Erb's point Auscultation point heard at the third left intercostal space at the left border of the sternum.

intercostal space The space between two ribs.

mid-clavicular line Imaginary anatomical line extending inferior along the thorax from the middle of the clavicle.

LISTENING TO THE HEART: AUSCULTATION POINTS

As part of a cardiovascular assessment, a practitioner may listen to the heart by using a stethoscope. Listening to heart sounds is known as auscultation and can reveal abnormalities of cardiac function. The heart sounds are produced by various cardiac events such as closing of the valves and the movement of blood through the heart (see Figure 9-19).

The heart valves can be heard at several anatomical points. The aortic valve can be heard at the second right intercostal space at the right border of the sternum. The pulmonary valve can be heard at the second left intercostal space at the left border of the sternum. Closing of both atrioventricular valves can be heard at the third left intercostal space at the left border of the sternum, which is known as Erb's point. The tricuspid valve is heard at the fourth left intercostal space at the left border of the sternum and the bicuspid (mitral) valve is heard at the fifth intercostal space at the mid-clavicular line.

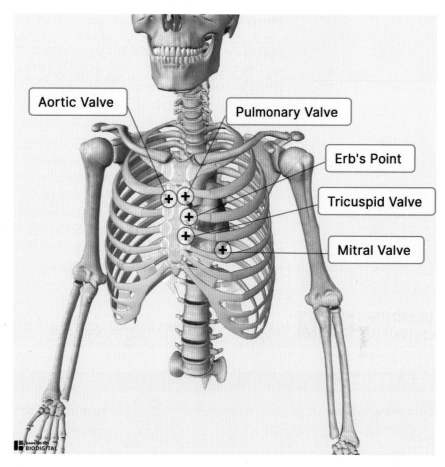

FIGURE 9-19 The anatomical landmarks for listening to the heart valves are as follows: Tricuspid valve- 4th left intercostal space, Mitral valve- 5th left intercostal space at the mid-clavicular line, Pulmonary valve- 2nd left intercostal space, Aortic valve- 2nd right intercostal space. Erb's point is located at the 3rd left intercostal space.

LEARNING OBJECTIVE **9.4.6** Describe the normal S1 and S2 heart sounds and how they are created.

KEY TERM

ventricular filling Portion of cardiac cycle characterized by filling of the ventricles with blood.

Heart Sounds

During auscultation, a practitioner will hear the familiar "lub-dub" sound of the cardiac cycle. The first heart sound (S1), or "lub" sound, is produced by closing of the atrioventricular valves, which occurs at the beginning of ventricular systole. The second heart sound (S2), or "dub" sound, is produced by the closing of the semilunar valves, which occurs at the end of ventricular systole and the beginning of ventricular diastole. The period between S1 and S2 represents ventricular systole. Likewise, the period between S2 and S1 represents ventricular diastole.

A third sound (S3) can sometimes be heard between S2 and S1. This sound results from **ventricular filling** and can be heard in children and athletes. It also arises in congestive heart failure. The fourth sound (S4) occurs just before S1 and is not often heard. It is considered abnormal in adults. This sound is produced by contraction of the atria forcefully pushing blood against a stiff ventricle, which can result from heart failure.

LEARNING OBJECTIVE 9.4.7 Identify common causes of heart murmurs.

KEY TERMS

diastolic murmurs Abnormal heart sounds occurring during diastole.

ejection Referring to ejection fraction which is a measure of the blood exiting the left ventricle with each contraction.

patent ductus arteriosus Hollow tubular structure between the aorta and pulmonary trunk that should close after birth but remains open.

regurgitation Abnormality of heart valves characterized by leaking.

stenosis Narrowing, usually refers to narrowing of a vessel or heart valve.

systolic murmurs Abnormal heart sounds occurring during contraction, or systole, of the ventricles of the heart.

Heart Murmurs

Abnormal heart sounds are known as murmurs and can result from a variety of problems. Murmurs typically indicate problems with heart valves.

Murmurs occurring during the interval between S1 and S2 are called **systolic murmurs**. Systolic murmurs can be divided into murmurs caused by **regurgitation** and **ejection**. Murmurs occurring during the interval between S2 and S1 are known as **diastolic murmurs**. Diastolic murmurs are caused by **stenosis** (narrowing) of the bicuspid or tricuspid valves, or **regurgitation** of the aortic or pulmonary valves.

There are also continuous murmurs that are heard throughout the cardiac cycle. These are caused by blood flow from a higher pressure structure to a lower pressure structure. For example, a condition known as **patent ductus arteriosus** can produce a continuous murmur. The ductus arteriosus is a vessel that carries blood between the pulmonary trunk and aorta in the fetus and should close at birth. A patent ductus arteriosus remains open after birth, allowing some blood flow that can be heard by auscultation.

KEY TERMS

crescendo–decrescendo murmurs Abnormal heart sounds characterized by an increase followed by a decrease in loudness.

crescendo murmurs Abnormal heart sounds characterized by an increase in loudness.

Auscultation of Heart Murmurs

Heart valve defects causing heart murmurs produce abnormal sounds during auscultation. The sounds are caused by abnormal blood flow through structures of the heart such as valves. The abnormal blood flow produces noise that can vary by pitch or intensity. Practitioners will note the timing in relation to S1 and S2, location, quality, pitch, and intensity of a murmur. For example, some murmurs increase in intensity over time (**crescendo murmurs**) whereas others first increase, then decrease in intensity (**crescendo–decrescendo murmurs**).

CLINICAL TIP Prolapse of the mitral valve usually produces a murmur with a mid-systolic click, which results from the left ventricle contracting and pushing the valve closed. Bulging cusps of a valve produce clicking sounds upon closing.

KEY TERM

autonomic nervous system Division of the peripheral nervous system that regulates organ function; composed of the sympathetic and parasympathetic nervous systems.

THE AUTONOMIC NERVOUS SYSTEM AND THE CARDIAC CYCLE

The heart rate must adjust in order to meet the varying demands of the body. Heart rate is controlled by the nervous and endocrine systems. For example, the **autonomic nervous system** continuously adjusts the heart rate and force of contraction of myocardium to maintain blood pressure and blood flow to the tissues.

LEARNING OBJECTIVE 9.4.11 **Describe the effects of the parasympathetic nervous system on heart rate.**

KEY TERMS

cardiac accelerator nerves Group of sympathetic nervous system nerves arising from thoracic spinal nerve roots that travel to the sinoatrial node.

cardiac plexus Group of nerves that connect the autonomic nervous system to the heart.

vagus nerve Cranial nerve X; sensory and motor nerves extending to the visceral organs.

The Cardiac Plexus

The **cardiac plexus** connects the autonomic nervous system to the heart. The cardiac plexus sends sympathetic neurons to the SA and AV nodes. These neurons are called **cardiac accelerator nerves**. The parasympathetic nervous system also sends neurons to the SA and AV nodes via the **vagus nerve** (cranial nerve X).

The autonomic nervous system impulses originate in the cardiac control centers in the medulla oblongata. The sympathetic nervous system works to increase the heart rate and force of contraction; the parasympathetic nervous system has the opposite effect.

LEARNING OBJECTIVE 9.4.12 **Describe the effects of the parasympathetic nervous system on the cardiac cycle.**

KEY TERMS

autonomic nervous system Division of the peripheral nervous system that regulates organ function; composed of the sympathetic and parasympathetic nervous systems.

baroreceptor Sensory receptor that senses pressure.

cardiac accelerator nerves Group of sympathetic nervous system nerves arising from thoracic spinal nerve roots that travel to the sinoatrial node.

cardiac plexus Group of nerves that connect the autonomic nervous system to the heart.

chemoreceptors Sensory proteins that detect chemicals in bodily fluids; also related to the perception of smell and taste.

glossopharyngeal nerve Cranial nerve IX; sensory and motor information of the throat and neck.

vagus nerve Cranial nerve X; sensory and motor nerves extending to the visceral organs.

Sensory Receptors

Sensory information about the cardiovascular system originates in **baroreceptors** and **chemoreceptors**. These receptors are innervated by the **glossopharyngeal nerve** (cranial nerve IX). The baroreceptors monitor changes in pressure whereas chemoreceptors monitor changes in blood levels of oxygen, carbon dioxide, and pH (see Figure 9-20).

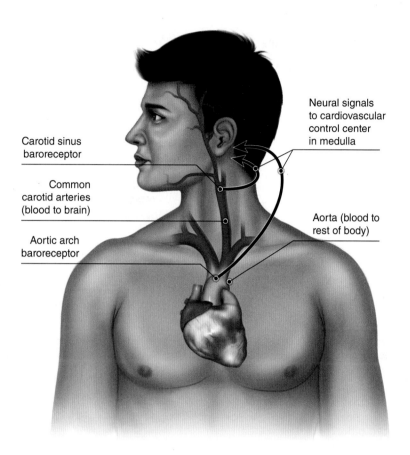

Carotid sinus baroreceptor

Common carotid arteries (blood to brain)

Aortic arch baroreceptor

Neural signals to cardiovascular control center in medulla

Aorta (blood to rest of body)

FIGURE 9-20 Baroreceptors monitor blood pressure and feed this information to the cardiac control center in the brain. Based on this information, the brain can stimulate the heart to increase blood pressure, reduce stimulation to decrease blood pressure, or do nothing to keep blood pressure the same.

For example, when a person rises from a supine to a sitting position, there is a temporary drop in blood pressure in the head. This is sensed by baroreceptors in the carotid sinus. The sensory information travels via the glossopharyngeal nerve to the cardiac control centers to produce a subsequent increase in heart rate via the sympathetic pathway.

The sympathetic neurotransmitter is norepinephrine (NE), which works to speed up the heart.

The Bainbridge reflex (atrial reflex) occurs with an increase in stretch of the atrial walls. The atrial walls stretch in response to an increase in venous pressure, causing more blood to flow into the atria. The reflex results in an increase in sympathetic activity and decrease in parasympathetic activity, which speeds up the heart to help move the increased volume of blood into the ventricles. The increased movement of blood into the ventricles results in a decrease in venous pressure. The Bainbridge reflex then helps to compensate for increases in venous pressure.

Norepinephrine and acetylcholine have both neurotransmitter and hormonal action. NE and epinephrine are both secreted by the adrenal medulla. Epinephrine, which is also called adrenaline, is similar in chemical structure to norepinephrine and likewise has a similar effect on the heart. These hormones are secreted in response to stress and exercise. Thyroid hormone also has a similar action to NE and increases heart rate.

UNIT OBJECTIVE 9.5

Describe the structure and functions of the body's vasculature.

UNIT INTRODUCTION

Blood is pumped through nearly 100,000 miles of blood vessels as it completes its journey through the body, bringing oxygenated blood to the tissues and then back to the heart so it can be pumped to the lungs for more oxygen. This complex system of blood vessels can be organized into vascular circuits or pathways, each completing a specific function. This unit examines the body's vasculature and major vascular circuits.

LEARNING OBJECTIVE 9.5.1 Identify the major vascular circuits.

KEY TERMS

pulmonary circuit System of blood vessels that bring deoxygenated blood from the heart to the lungs for oxygenation and then transport oxygenated blood back to the heart.

systemic circuit System of blood vessels carrying blood from the heart to the body.

vascular circuits Systems of blood vessels that work together to carry blood to specific parts of the body.

MAJOR VASCULAR CIRCUITS

Blood flows through the body by way of major vascular circuits. Oxygenated blood flows from the heart to the body and deoxygenated blood flows back to the heart by way of the systemic circuit. Deoxygenated blood flows to the lungs from the heart and oxygenated blood flows from the lungs to the heart through the pulmonary circuit. Blood is delivered to heart muscle tissue by way of the coronary circuit.

LEARNING OBJECTIVE 9.5.2 Describe the path of blood through the systemic circuit.

KEY TERMS

abdominal aorta Portion of the aorta just after it passes below the diaphragm and before it divides into the common iliac arteries.

accessory hemiazygos vein Vein located on the left side of the vertebral column.

anterior and posterior tibial arteries Arteries extending below and continuing from the popliteal artery.

aorta Large blood vessel exiting the left ventricle, known as a great vessel of the heart.

aortic bodies Series of chemoreceptors located in the aortic arch.

aortic sinus Widening of the aorta just above the aortic valve that serves as a location for baroreceptors.

ascending aorta Portion of the aorta between the left ventricle and aortic arch.

ascending lumbar veins Veins located in the thoracic cavity that contribute to the azygos vein.

axillary artery Lateral continuation of the subclavian artery.

axillary vein Lateral continuation of the subclavian vein.

azygos vein Vein that runs along the right side of the thoracic vertebrae. It empties into the superior vena cava.

basilar artery Artery formed by the union of the vertebral arteries.

basilic vein Medial superficial vein of the upper extremity.

brachial vein Continuation of the axillary vein.

brachiocephalic trunk Artery branching off the aorta on the right side and dividing into the right subclavian and right common carotid arteries.

bronchial artery Referring to the lungs. For example, the bronchial arteries supply the lungs with oxygenated blood.

cavernous sinuses Cavities that serve the venous system by draining the ophthalmic veins.

celiac trunk artery Branch of the abdominal aorta.

cephalic vein Lateral superficial vein of the upper extremity.

Circle of Willis (cerebral arterial circle) System of arteries that provides blood to the brain.

common carotid artery Arteries branching from the brachiocephalic artery on the right and aorta on the left carrying blood to the internal and external carotid arteries.

common hepatic artery Arteries in the abdominal cavity that supply the stomach and liver.

common iliac vein Inferior branch of the inferior vena cava.

cystic veins Veins in the abdominal cavity that drain the gallbladder.

deep femoral artery Continuation of the external iliac arteries located in the thighs.

deep palmar arch Arteries located in the palms of the hands.

descending genicular artery Branch of the femoral artery supplying the area around the knee.

dorsal and plantar arches Arteries supplying the inferior portion (plantar) and superior portion (dorsal) of the foot.

dorsalis pedis artery Branch of the tibial artery located in the ankle.

dorsalis pedis vein Vein in the ankle that becomes the anterior tibial vein.

dural sinuses Hollow areas in the meninges that carry venous blood.

esophageal artery Arteries supplying the esophagus.

external iliac vein Vein in the pelvis that connects the femoral and common iliac veins.

falx cerebri Section of dura mater located in the longitudinal fissure that separates the right and left hemispheres of the brain.

femoral arteries Continuation of the external iliac arteries located in the thighs.

femoral circumflex artery Branch of the femoral artery located in the upper thigh.

femoral vein Continuation of the external iliac vein located in the thigh.

fibular artery (peroneal artery) Inferior and lateral branch of the popliteal artery.

gonadal artery Arteries located in the abdominal and pelvic cavities.

gonadal veins Veins located in the pelvis that drain the testes and ovaries.

great saphenous vein Superficial medial vein in the upper portion of the lower extremity.

hemiazygos vein Vein located on the left side of the vertebral column that originates from the posterior intercostal and left ascending lumbar veins.

hepatic portal system System of veins carrying digestive substances from the digestive system to the liver.

hepatic veins Vein located in the abdominal cavity that drains blood from the liver.

humeral circumflex artery Branch of the brachial artery.

inferior phrenic artery Small artery branching from the aorta that supplies the diaphragm.

inferior phrenic veins Veins in the abdominal cavity that drain the diaphragm.

inferior sagittal sinus Hollow area that is part of the venous system located between the hemispheres of the brain.

internal and external carotid arteries Branches of the common carotid arteries.

internal and external iliac arteries Inferior branches of the common iliac arteries.

internal and external jugular veins Veins located in the neck draining structures of the head and neck and connecting to the subclavian veins.

internal iliac vein Branch of the common iliac vein.

left gastric artery Arteries in the abdominal cavity that supply the stomach and liver.

lumbar artery Parietal branches of the abdominal aorta.

medial and lateral plantar arteries Arteries in the foot.

medial and lateral plantar veins Veins in the foot.

median cubital vein Vein located in the anterior portion of the elbow.

median sacral artery Parietal branches of the abdominal aorta.

mediastinal artery Branch of the thoracic aorta.

middle cerebral artery One of three major paired arteries that supply the cerebrum.

middle sacral artery Small artery that branches from the posterior portion of the abdominal aorta and extends along the lower lumbar vertebrae and sacrum.

ophthalmic veins Veins in the skull draining the eye.

ophthalmic artery Artery supplying the eye.

pericardial artery Referring to the pericardium.

popliteal artery Artery located behind the knee.

popliteal vein Vein located behind the knee.

posterior communicating arteries Arteries that are part of the Circle of Willis that supply blood to the brain.

posterior intercostal artery Veins located in the posterior thorax.

posterior tibial vein Vein located in the lower leg.

radial artery Arteries in the forearm that originate from the brachial arteries.

radial vein Veins in the forearm that transport blood to the brachial vein.

renal artery Arteries located in the abdominal cavity that supply the kidneys.

renal veins Veins carrying blood from the kidneys located in the abdominal cavity.

right and left common iliac arteries Arteries branching inferior from the abdominal aorta.

right and left coronary arteries Part of the coronary circuit or circulatory pathway.

right and left suprarenal arteries Arteries carrying blood to the adrenal glands.

sigmoid sinuses Hollow areas in the skull that carry venous blood from the posterior venous sinus.

small saphenous vein Vein located in the lower leg.

splenic artery Branch of the abdominal aorta that brings blood to the spleen.

straight sinus Hollow vascular area that drains the inferior sagittal sinus.

subclavian arteries Arteries located below the clavicle.

subclavian vein Vein located below the clavicle.

subcostal artery Referring to below the ribs.

superficial arch Arteries located in the palms of the hands.

superficial dorsal venous arch System of veins in the foot that drain into the Great Saphenous vein.

superior and inferior mesenteric arteries Arteries in the abdominal cavity supplying the mesentery with blood.

superior and inferior vena cava Large veins carrying deoxygenated blood to the right atrium.

superior phrenic artery Arteries located in the thoracic cavity that branch from the thoracic aorta.

systemic circuit System of blood vessels carrying blood from the heart to the body.

thoracic aorta Portion of the aorta below the arch extending into the thoracic cavity.

transverse sinuses Hollow venous area on the outside of the brain.

ulnar artery Arteries in the forearm that originate from the brachial arteries.

ulnar collateral arteries Small arteries branching off the ulnar arteries.

ulnar vein Veins in the forearm that transport blood to the brachial vein.

vertebral arteries Arteries located in the transverse foramen of vertebrae.

vertebral veins Veins located in the transverse foramen of vertebrae.

BLOOD FLOW THROUGH THE SYSTEMIC CIRCUIT

Once oxygenated by the lungs, blood flows from the heart to the rest of the body by way of the **systemic circuit**. The systemic circuit begins with the aorta and ends with the superior and inferior vena cava, which supply blood to the right atrium (see Figure 9-21).

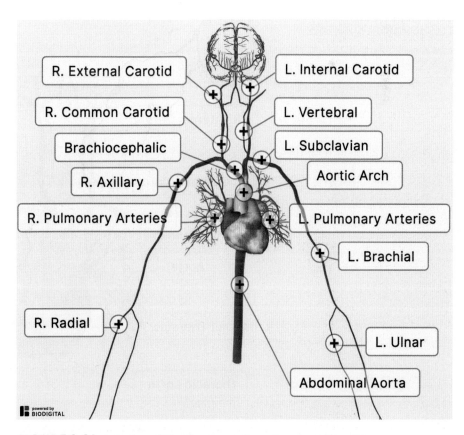

FIGURE 9-21 Arteries of the thorax, neck, and upper extremities.

Aorta

The **aorta** exits the left ventricle and becomes the **ascending aorta**. At the junction of the aorta and left ventricle is an enlargement known as the **aortic sinus**. The aortic sinus contains the **aortic bodies**, which are chemoreceptors that sense changes in chemical concentration and send this information back to the nervous system. The ascending aorta curves, forming the arch of the aorta, and extends inferior to become the **thoracic aorta**. It then passes through the diaphragm to become the **abdominal aorta**.

The **right and left coronary arteries** arise from the aorta shortly after it emerges from the aortic valve. Along the arch of the aorta are three branches. From left to right, these include the brachiocephalic trunk, left common carotid, and left **subclavian arteries**. The **brachiocephalic trunk** divides into the right common carotid and right subclavian arteries.

The thoracic aorta contains both visceral branches to organs and parietal branches to structures of the body wall. The visceral branches include the **pericardial, bronchial, esophageal,** and **mediastinal arteries**. The parietal branches include the **posterior intercostal, subcostal,** and **superior phrenic arteries** (see Figure 9-22).

Abdominal Arteries

The thoracic aorta pierces the diaphragm and becomes the abdominal aorta. The abdominal aorta terminates with a bifurcation producing the **right and left common iliac** and **middle sacral arteries**. The visceral branches of the abdominal

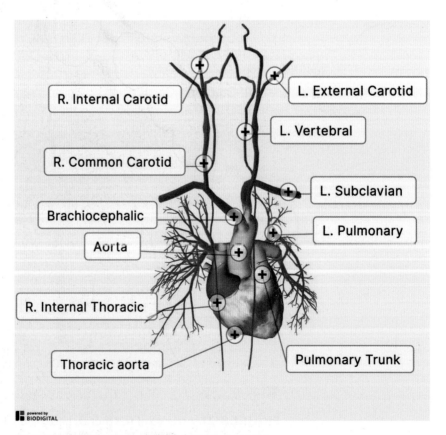

FIGURE 9-22 Arteries of the thorax and neck.

aorta include the **celiac trunk**; **right and left suprarenal**, **renal**, and **gonadal arteries**; and the **superior and inferior mesenteric arteries**. The parietal branches include the **inferior phrenic**, **lumbar**, and **median sacral arteries**.

The celiac trunk divides into the **splenic**, **left gastric**, and **common hepatic arteries**. The splenic artery supplies the spleen and some of the arteries to the stomach. The left gastric artery supplies the stomach and part of the esophagus. The common hepatic artery supplies arteries for the liver, stomach, gallbladder, and small intestine.

The right and left common iliac arteries divide and become the **internal and external iliac arteries** at the level of the lumbosacral junction. The internal iliac arteries supply the urinary bladder, genitalia, walls of the pelvis, and medial thigh. The external iliac arteries continue to the lower extremities (see Figure 9-23).

Arteries of the Lower Extremities

The external iliac arteries emerge from under the inguinal ligament as the **femoral arteries**. The **deep femoral artery** branches from the femoral artery and gives rise to the **femoral circumflex artery**. The femoral artery continues distally and gives rise to a branch known as the **descending genicular artery** that supplies

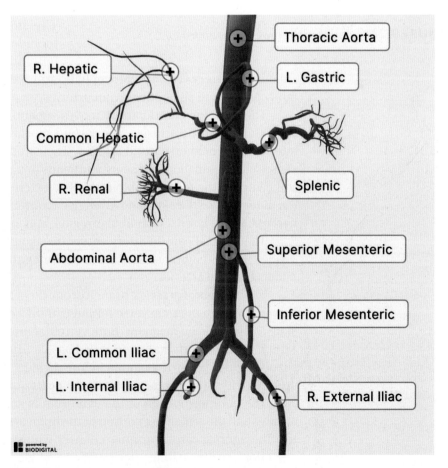

FIGURE 9-23 Arteries of the abdomen.

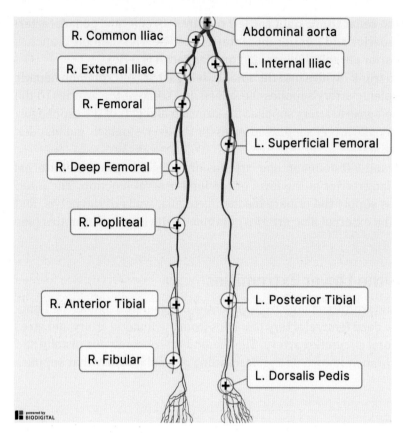

FIGURE 9-24 Arteries of the lower extremities.

the area around the knee. The femoral artery pierces the adductor longus muscle and emerges as the **popliteal artery**, which branches to become **anterior and posterior tibial arteries**. The **fibular artery (peroneal artery)** branches from the posterior tibial artery.

The anterior tibial artery becomes the **dorsalis pedis artery** at the ankle, which branches and supplies the foot. The posterior tibial divides into the **medial and lateral plantar arteries**. These arteries supply the plantar area of the foot. The smaller divisions of the plantar arteries connect with the dorsalis pedis artery to form the **dorsal and plantar arches** of the foot (see Figure 9-24).

Arteries of the Head and Upper Extremity

The initial branches of the aorta include the brachiocephalic trunk, left common carotid artery, and left subclavian artery. The brachiocephalic trunk divides to form the right common carotid and right subclavian arteries.

The common carotid artery moves superior and divides into the **internal and external carotid arteries**. The carotid sinus is located at the junction of the internal and common carotid arteries. The carotid sinus is a baroreceptor that senses changes in blood pressure and sends this information to the cardiac control center in the medulla oblongata. The external carotid artery continues on the outer part of the skull and gives rise to arteries that supply the esophagus, neck, pharynx, larynx, mandibular region, and face.

The internal carotid artery enters the skull through the carotid canal and divides into three branches. These are the **ophthalmic**, anterior cerebral, and **middle cerebral arteries**.

The **vertebral arteries** branch from the subclavian arteries and extend upward through the transverse foramen of the cervical vertebrae and enter the skull at the foramen magnum. Both vertebral arteries merge to form the **basilar artery**. Both the vertebral arteries and basilar arteries give rise to branches that supply various parts of the brain before dividing to form the posterior cerebral arteries, which then branch to form the **posterior communicating arteries**.

The anterior portion of the cerebrum is supplied by the internal carotid arteries and the remaining portion of the brain is supplied by the vertebral arteries. The internal carotid arteries connect with the basilar artery by way of two posterior communicating arteries. The resulting vascular structure forms a ring called the circle of Willis (cerebral arterial circle) (see Figure 9-25). This structure allows for some redundancy in supply to the brain as it can receive blood from either the vertebral arteries or internal carotid arteries.

The subclavian artery continues under the clavicle and gives rise to the internal thoracic artery, vertebral artery, and thyrocervical trunk. The subclavian artery emerges from under the clavicle to form the **axillary artery**, which branches to form the **humeral circumflex artery**. The axillary artery continues along the arm to become the brachial artery, which gives rise to the deep brachial artery and the **ulnar collateral arteries**. At the elbow, the brachial artery divides to form the **radial** and **ulnar arteries**. At the wrist the radial and ulnar arteries reconnect to form the **superficial** and **deep palmar arches**, which, in turn, supply the digital arteries of the fingers.

Veins of the Systemic Circuit

The veins of the systemic circuit drain into the **superior and inferior vena cava** that connect with the right atrium of the heart. The superior vena cava is formed by the union of the right and left brachiocephalic veins. Each brachiocephalic vein is formed by two branches, including the subclavian and jugular veins. The **subclavian veins** drain the veins of the head and neck. The subclavian drains the shoulder and upper extremity.

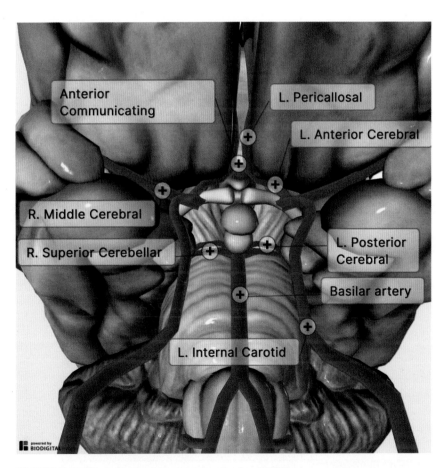

FIGURE 9-25 Arteries forming the Circle of Willis.

Veins of the Upper Extremity

Two superficial veins and one deep vein from the upper extremity connect with the lateral portion of the subclavian vein. The superficial veins include the cephalic vein (lateral) and the basilic vein (medial). Both of these veins extend to the distal upper extremity. The deep vein is the axillary vein, which is a continuation of the subclavian vein as it emerges from the inferior aspect of the clavicle. The axillary vein extends into the arm and becomes the brachial vein, which divides into the radial and ulnar veins. Like the arteries of the upper extremities, the radial and ulnar veins also connect at the deep palmar arch. The median cubital vein resides in the anterior portion of the elbow and connects with the cephalic and basilic veins. The cephalic and basilic veins both connect at the superficial palmar arch. The median antebrachial vein is located in the forearm area and connects the radial and ulnar veins (see Figure 9-26).

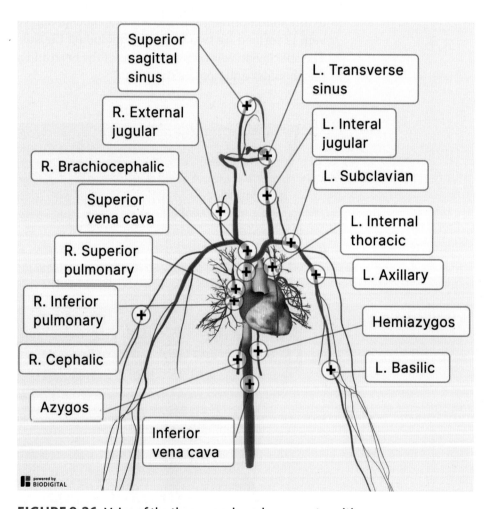

FIGURE 9-26 Veins of the thorax, neck, and upper extremities.

| CLINICAL TIP | The superficial veins of the arm are commonly used for blood draws and IVs. These include the medial cubital, cephalic, and basilic veins. |

Veins of the Head and Neck

The head and neck are drained by the **internal and external jugular veins** and the **vertebral veins** (see Figure 9-27). The drainage begins with the **dural sinuses**. The dural sinuses are located in the meninges between the periosteal and meningeal layers in the dura mater of the brain. The superior and inferior dural sinuses are located in the **falx cerebri**. The **inferior sagittal sinus** located deep between the two hemispheres drains into the **straight sinus**. The superior sagittal and straight sinuses in turn drain into the **transverse sinuses**. These drain into the **sigmoid sinuses**, which are continuous with the internal jugular vein. The **cavernous sinuses** drain the **ophthalmic veins** and also connect with the internal jugular vein.

The internal jugular veins exit the brain at the jugular foramen. As they proceed inferior to the subclavian, they receive blood from the superficial temporal and facial veins.

The external jugular veins are superficial veins of the head that drain the superficial structures of the face and head. They drain into the subclavian veins. The vertebral veins drain the area around the cervical vertebrae.

Veins of the Thorax

The **azygos vein** originates from the right **ascending lumbar veins** and right posterior intercostal veins. The azygos vein is not a paired vein and runs along the right side of the thoracic vertebrae. It empties into the superior vena cava. The

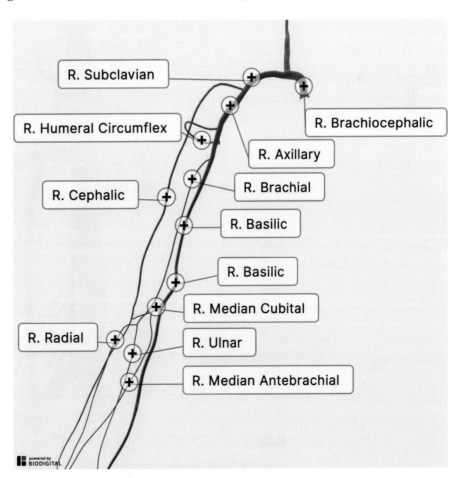

FIGURE 9-27 Veins of the upper extremities.

azygos vein connects the superior and inferior vena cavae and functions as an alternative route for blood flow to the right atrium if the superior or inferior vena cava is blocked (see Figure 9-28).

The **hemiazygos vein** lies on the left side of the vertebral column and originates from the posterior intercostals and left ascending lumbar veins. A continuation of the hemiazygos vein is the **accessory hemiazygos vein**, which extends superior.

Veins of the Abdomen and Lower Extremity

The veins of the abdomen and lower extremity drain into the inferior vena cava.

Deoxygenated blood carrying nutrients from the digestive system empties into the **hepatic portal system**. This blood flows to the liver, which extracts the nutrients for use in metabolism. The veins that drain into the hepatic portal vein have the same names as the arteries in the digestive system. These include the superior mesenteric, inferior mesenteric, and splenic veins (see Figure 9-28).

A series of lumbar veins are located in the posterior abdominal wall and drain into the inferior vena cava and the **ascending lumbar veins**. The **gonadal**

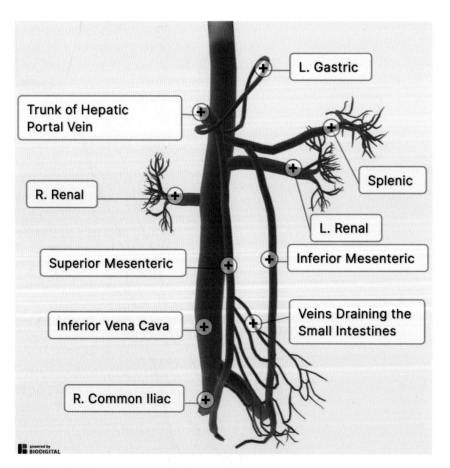

FIGURE 9-28 Veins of the thorax and abdomen.

veins drain the testes and ovaries. The right gonadal vein drains into the inferior vena cava while the left gonadal vein empties into the left renal vein. The **renal veins** drain the kidneys.

The **hepatic veins** drain blood from the liver to the inferior vena cava. The **cystic veins** drain the gallbladder and connect with the hepatic veins and the **inferior phrenic veins** drain the diaphragm.

Veins of the Lower Extremity

A number of veins of the lower extremity originate from the **medial and lateral plantar veins**, which drain into the **posterior tibial vein**. The fibular or peroneal vein drains into the posterior tibial vein. The **dorsalis pedis vein** at the ankle becomes the anterior tibial vein, which becomes the popliteal vein at the posterior knee (see Figure 9-29).

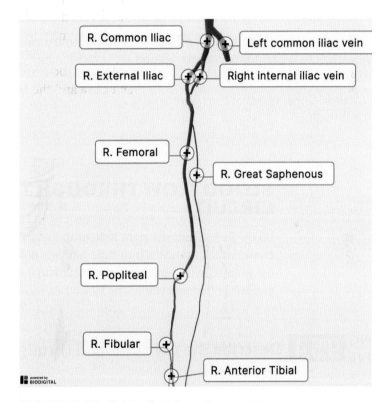

FIGURE 9-29 Veins of the lower extremities.

The **popliteal vein** ascends into the thigh region and becomes the **femoral vein**. The femoral vein becomes the **external iliac vein** and combines with the **internal iliac vein** to become the **common iliac vein** that unites with the inferior vena cava.

The **superficial dorsal venous arch** of the foot becomes the **great saphenous vein**, which is a long superficial vein located on the medial side of the leg that connects with the external iliac vein. The **small saphenous vein** also originates from the dorsal venous arch and courses more laterally before connecting with the great saphenous vein.

> **CLINICAL TIP**   Due to its connection with the left renal vein, the left gonadal vein can cause swelling of the scrotum with cancer of the kidney.

There are also clinical consequences related to the left vein of the testicle and its connection to the left renal vein; kidney infections and even cancer of the kidney can spread to the left testicular vein. This causes the blood to gather, leading to dilated (expanded) veins in the scrotum.

LEARNING OBJECTIVE 9.5.3 Describe the path of blood through the pulmonary circuit.

KEY TERMS

pulmonary arteries Arteries branching off the pulmonary trunk that carry deoxygenated blood to the lungs.

pulmonary trunk Great vessel of the heart exiting the right ventricle.

pulmonary veins Blood vessels carrying oxygenated blood from the lungs to the left atrium.

BLOOD FLOW THROUGH THE PULMONARY CIRCUIT

Blood flows from the right side of the heart to the lungs through the **pulmonary trunk**, which branches into right and left **pulmonary arteries**. The blood becomes oxygenated in the lungs and travels back to the left side of the heart through the right and left **pulmonary veins**. The heart then moves the blood to the rest of the body.

LEARNING OBJECTIVE 9.5.4 Describe the path of blood through the coronary circuit.

KEY TERMS

circumflex arteries Branch of the left coronary artery that wraps around the left side of the heart.

coronary arteries Branches off the aorta that carry blood to heart muscle.

coronary sinus Cardiac vein that empties into the right atrium.

great cardiac vein Large vein located on the heart that connects with the coronary sinus.

interventricular septum Heart muscle located between the ventricles.

interventricular sulcus Indentation or groove between the ventricles on the anterior portion of the heart.

left anterior descending artery Branch of the left coronary artery that extends along the interventricular sulcus.

left coronary artery Artery originating from the aorta to supply the left side of the heart.

marginal artery Refers to a branch of the right coronary artery.

middle cardiac vein Vein extending from the apex of the heart along the posterior interventricular sulcus that drains into the cardiac sinus.

posterior cardiac vein Vein extending along the posterior wall of the left ventricle and draining into the cardiac sinus.

posterior interventricular artery Coronary artery located in the posterior interventricular sulcus connecting with the left anterior descending artery.

right posterior descending artery Artery branching off the right coronary artery.

small cardiac vein Vein draining blood from the right side of the heart to the coronary sinus.

BLOOD FLOW THROUGH THE CORONARY CIRCUIT

The two primary arteries of the coronary circuit include the right and left **coronary** arteries (see Figure 9-30). The right coronary artery divides into the **right posterior descending** and **marginal arteries**. The right posterior descending artery supplies the posterior walls of both ventricles. The right posterior descending artery merges with the anterior interventricular artery. The right

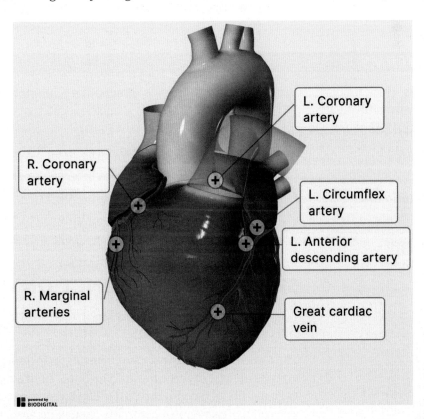

FIGURE 9-30 Coronary arteries and veins.

marginal artery supplies the lateral right side of the heart. The **left coronary artery** divides into the **left anterior descending artery** located in the **interventricular sulcus** and **circumflex artery**. The left anterior descending artery supplies the **interventricular septum** and anterior walls of both ventricles. The circumflex artery supplies the left atrium and posterior wall of the left ventricle.

There is some anatomical variation in the arrangement of coronary arteries. In 85% of the population, the left coronary artery gives rise to the left anterior descending artery, but in the remaining 15%, the left coronary artery gives rise to both right and left descending arteries. In 4% of the population, there is only one coronary artery that supplies the entire heart. The coronary circulation can include many anastomoses (connections) between arteries along with additional routes for blood flow to the heart. These additional (collateral) routes serve as supportive networks to help provide oxygen and nutrition but may not be enough to sustain heart muscle if one of the coronary arteries is blocked.

The **great cardiac vein** can be seen on the anterior side of the heart in the interventricular sulcus and on the posterior side of the heart connecting with the coronary sinus. The great cardiac vein receives blood from smaller branches, including the posterior, middle, and small cardiac veins. The **posterior cardiac vein** drains the areas supplied by the marginal and circumflex arteries. The **middle cardiac vein** drains the areas supplied by the **posterior interventricular artery** and the **small cardiac vein** drains the area around the posterior right atrium and ventricle. The anterior cardiac veins drain the area around the right ventricle and connect to the right atrium. The coronary sinus is a large vein that drains deoxygenated blood from the myocardium of the heart and empties into the right atrium.

LEARNING OBJECTIVE `9.5.5` **Describe the structure and function of arteries and arterioles.**

KEY TERMS

arteries Thick tubular structures that carry blood away from the heart.

arterioles Smaller vessels branching from arteries.

capillaries Smallest blood vessels consisting of one layer of simple squamous epithelium.

metarteriole Area between arteriole and capillary containing a precapillary sphincter muscle.

precapillary sphincter Circular smooth muscle located between an arteriole and capillary.

tunica externa Outer layer of an artery or vein.

tunica interna Inner layer of an artery or vein.

tunica media Middle muscular layer of an artery or vein.

STRUCTURE AND FUNCTION OF ARTERIES AND ARTERIOLES

Structure of Arteries

The arterial system consists of **arteries**, **arterioles**, and **capillaries**. The largest arteries consist of three layers. The outer **tunica externa** consists of elastic and collagen fibers (see Figure 9-31). The larger vessels also contain minute blood vessels that carry nutrients to the tissue and are innervated by nerve fibers.

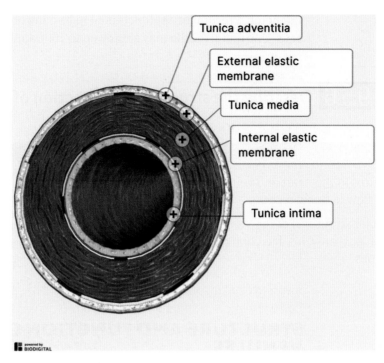

FIGURE 9-31 Cross-section of an artery.

The middle layer (**tunica media**) is thicker in arteries than in veins and consists of smooth muscle with some elastic fibers. The smooth muscle in the tunica media allows for constriction (vasoconstriction) and dilation (vasodilation). The nervous system helps to control blood pressure by adjusting the diameter of arteries. Arteries can also constrict when damaged to reduce the loss of blood.

The inner layer (**tunica interna**) consists of an inner thin layer of simple squamous epithelium called the endothelium anchored to another layer by a basement membrane. The basement membrane anchors the endothelium to a layer called the internal elastic lamina consisting of elastic fibers.

Function of Arteries

Some arteries contain more elastic connective tissue and serve to mediate blood pressure near the heart. These arteries will expand and contract in order to provide a continuous flow of blood to other blood vessels. For example, without this dampening effect there would be abrupt changes in pressure in blood vessels, which can eventually lead to damage.

The elastic arteries near the heart give rise to arteries with a thick tunica media known as muscular arteries. These arteries function to maintain blood pressure and subsequent blood flow throughout the body by vasoconstricting.

Structure and Function of Arterioles

Arteries branch to form smaller structures called arterioles. Arterioles help to control blood flow to various parts of the body by way of vasoconstriction and vasodilation. The end of the arteriole that connects with capillaries narrows and becomes a metarteriole containing a round smooth muscle called a **precapillary** sphincter. Precapillary sphincters help to control the flow of blood to capillary beds. One **metarteriole** may supply up to 100 capillaries, forming a capillary bed.

LEARNING OBJECTIVE 9.5.6 Describe the structure and function of veins and venules.

KEY TERMS

valves Structures in the heart and veins that only allow blood flow in one direction.

venules Vascular structures of the venous system that are smaller than veins and connect veins with capillaries.

STRUCTURE AND FUNCTION OF VEINS AND VENULES

The venous system begins at the venous end of capillaries. Oxygen and carbon dioxide exchange occurs in capillaries and deoxygenated blood is carried by the venous vessels.

Venules

Venules begin at the ends of capillaries and carry blood to the veins. Venules are very small and similar in structure to capillaries. They allow for substance exchange and merge to form larger-diameter veins.

Veins

Veins, like arteries, contain three layers. However, the middle layer or tunic media is not as thick as in arteries. Veins have larger lumens than arteries and many veins contain **valves** that only allow blood to flow toward the heart. Veins can vasoconstrict and do so during blood loss in order to conserve blood. When significant blood is lost, the sympathetic nervous system stimulates veins to constrict in an effort to return blood to the heart. This allows for nearly normal blood flow when up to 25% of blood is lost.

Blood Flow in Veins

Pressure in the arterial system is greatest at the left ventricle and decreases throughout the system. For example, blood pressure is greater in the aorta than in arterioles and even less in capillaries. In order to create pressure to move blood back to the heart, veins rely on a system of one-way valves. Many veins are located next to muscles. Muscle contraction produces an external pumping force on veins that helps to move blood to the heart. The movement of the diaphragm also contributes to venous flow along with the subsequent changes in pressure in the thoracic cavity (see Figure 9-32AB).

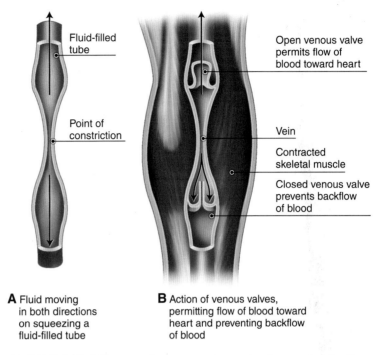

A Fluid moving in both directions on squeezing a fluid-filled tube

B Action of venous valves, permitting flow of blood toward heart and preventing backflow of blood

FIGURE 9-32AB Muscular contraction and valves assist the flow of blood in veins on its path back to the heart.

LEARNING OBJECTIVE 9.5.7 Describe the structure and function of capillaries.

KEY TERMS

basement membrane Material secreted by both the epithelial cells above it and the connective tissue cells below it; forms the basal surface and anchors epithelium in place.

endothelium Simple squamous epithelium found lining blood vessels, lymphatic vessels, and the heart.

precapillary sphincters Circular smooth muscle located between an arteriole and capillary.

simple squamous epithelium Epithelial tissue consisting of one layer of flat squamous cells.

STRUCTURE AND FUNCTION OF CAPILLARIES

Capillaries are the smallest blood vessels in the body. They carry blood to the venous system and allow for the exchange of substances between the blood and the tissues. Capillaries form complex networks and it is estimated that there are about one billion capillaries in the human body. Blood flow to capillaries is controlled by small smooth muscles called precapillary sphincters.

Capillaries are extensions of the endothelium of arteries. They consist of simple squamous epithelium and a basement membrane that allows a good degree of permeability for substance exchange. Capillaries are more numerous in areas with high metabolic activity such as muscle and nerve tissue. Permeability also varies according to metabolic demand. For example, capillaries in the liver and spleen are more permeable than those in smooth or skeletal muscle. Most substances are exchanged by diffusion, but other transport mechanisms include filtration and osmosis (see Figure 9-33).

Feature	Arteries	Arterioles	Capillaries	Veins
Number	Several hundred*	Half a million	10 billion	Several hundred*
Special features	Thick, highly elastic, walls; large radii*	Highly muscular, well-innervated walls; small radii	Very thin walled; large total cross-sectional area	Thin walled compared to arteries; highly distensible: large radii*
Functions	Passageway from the heart to organs; pressure reservoir	Primary resistance vessels; determine distribution of cardiac output	Site of exchange; determine distribution of extracellular fluid between plasma and interstitial fluid	Passageway to the heart from organs; blood reservoir

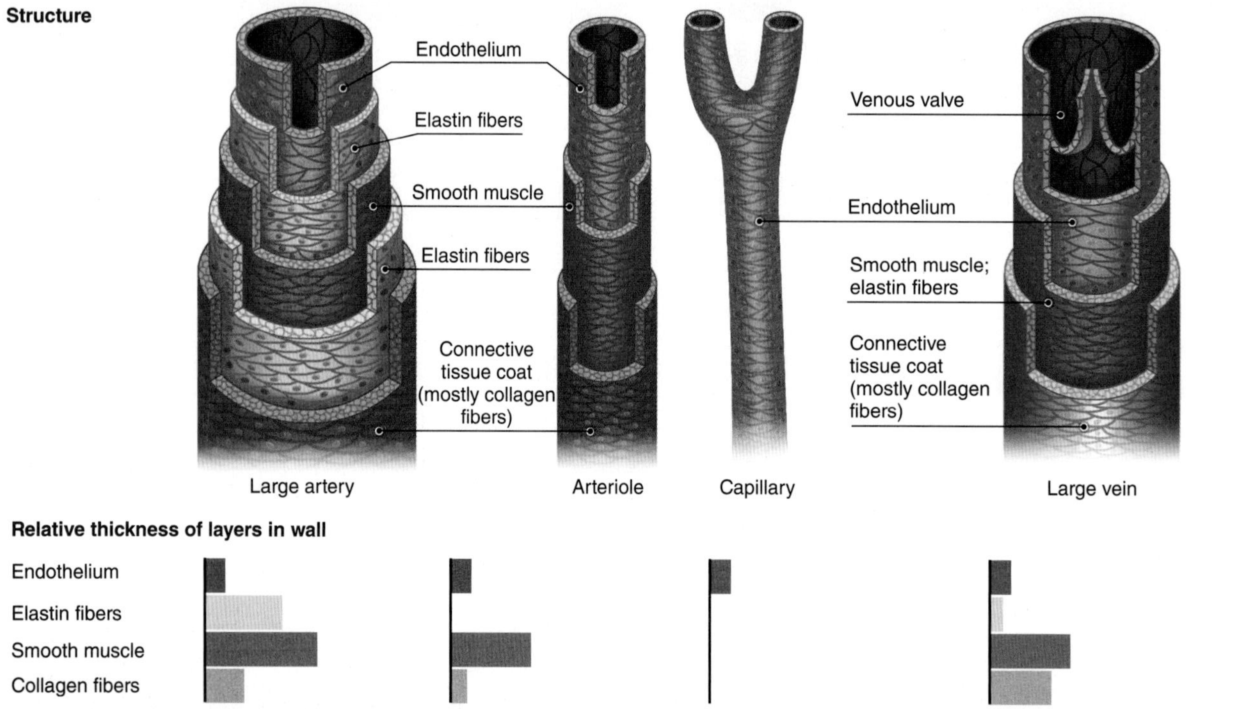

Structure

*These numbers and special features refer to the large arteries and veins, not to the smaller arterial branches or venules

FIGURE 9-33 Structure of arteries, veins, and capillaries.

UNIT OBJECTIVE 9.6

Describe the signs, symptoms, and diagnosis of common pathologies that affect the gross anatomy of the heart.

UNIT INTRODUCTION

As with many organs of the body, the heart can be affected by disorders and diseases. These range from genetic abnormalities to chronic disease processes that eventually affect the heart. This unit examines the signs, symptoms, and diagnosis of common pathologies that affect the heart.

LEARNING OBJECTIVE 9.6.1 **Identify common disorders affecting the gross anatomy of the heart.**

atrial septal defect Perforation of the atrial septum allowing blood to flow between atria.

coarctation of the aorta Narrowing of the aorta.

d-transposition of the great arteries Condition characterized by reversal of the aorta and pulmonary trunk.

ductus arteriosus Fetal circulatory pathway between the aorta and pulmonary trunk.

fossa ovalis Indentation located in the interatrial septum that is a remnant of fetal circulation.

ligamentum arteriosum Remnant of fetal circulation, a ligament that forms from the ductus arteriosum.

Tetralogy of Fallot Genetic heart defect characterized by four abnormalities: ventricular septal defect (hole between the ventricles), stenosis of the pulmonary valve, enlargement of the right ventricle (right-ventricular hypertrophy), and an aorta that is positioned to receive blood from both ventricles (overriding aorta).

ventricular septal defect Birth defect characterized by perforations in the ventricles.

ANATOMICAL HEART DISORDERS

Patent Ductus Arteriosus

The **ductus arteriosus** is a vessel that allows fetal blood to travel from the pulmonary trunk to the aorta. After birth, this vessel closes and eventually becomes the **ligamentum arteriosum** (see Figure 9-34). In some cases, the ductus arteriosus remains open after birth. A patent ductus arteriosus causes additional blood to move from the aorta into the pulmonary arteries, resulting in lung congestion.

Coarctation of the Aorta

Coarctation of the aorta is a narrowing of the aorta (see Figure 9-34). This condition causes increased pressure in the left ventricle because the heart must contract more forcefully to push blood through the constriction. The increased left-ventricular pressure can result in enlargement of the left ventricle (hypertrophy) and eventually, left-ventricular heart failure.

Atrial Septal Defect

Before birth, blood passes from the right to left atria through a hole called the foramen ovale. This passageway closes at birth and eventually fuses to become the fossa ovalis. In some cases, the foramen ovale does not close (patent foramen ovale). In other cases, the tissue between the atria (atrial septum) contains perforations or is nonexistent, called **atrial septal defect** (see Figure 9-34A-E). All of these result in movement of blood between the atria.

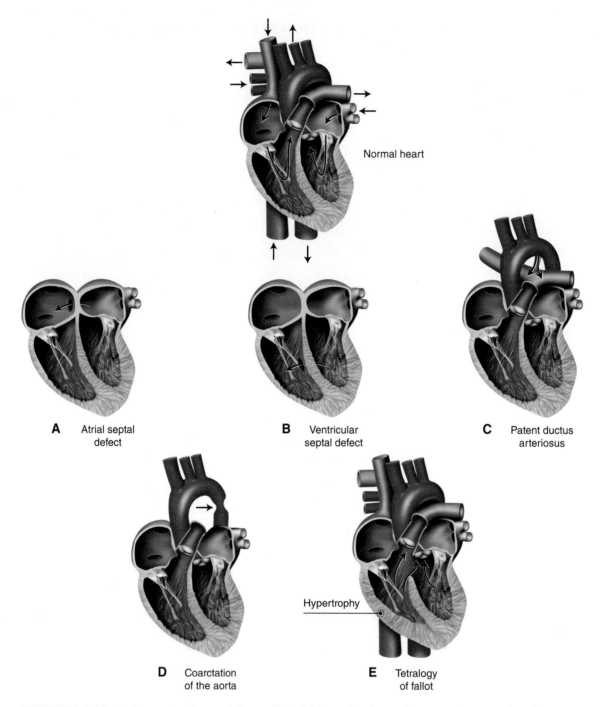

FIGURE 9-34A-E Congenital heart defects. A) Atrial Septal Defect. B) Ventricular Septal Defect. C) Patent ductus arteriosus. D) Coarctation of the Aorta. E) Tetralogy of Fallot.

A patent foramen ovale causes the movement of oxygenated blood from the left side of the heart to the right side where it mixes with deoxygenated blood. This can result in lower oxygen levels in blood traveling to the body.

d-Transposition of the Great Arteries

d-Transposition of the great arteries is a condition characterized by a reversal of the main vessels exiting the heart. In this case, the aorta and pulmonary trunk are reversed. The pulmonary trunk connects to the arch of the aorta and the aorta connects to the pulmonary arteries. This results in deoxygenated blood bypassing the lungs and flowing to the body (see Figure 9-35).

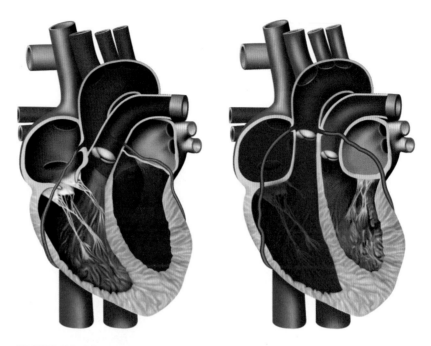

FIGURE 9-35 Transposition of the great arteries. Notice the reversal of the aorta and pulmonary trunk.

This condition is treated by surgery by one of two procedures. In an arterial switch procedure, the pulmonary artery and aorta are moved to their normal locations. In an atrial switch procedure, a passageway is created between both atria. This allows deoxygenated blood to flow to the left ventricle and pulmonary trunk and oxygenated blood to flow to the right ventricle and aorta. The atrial switch procedure requires the right side of the heart to pump blood to the body and can result in long-term complications such as irregular heartbeat and heart failure.

Tetralogy of Fallot

Tetralogy of Fallot is a congenital disorder that includes four abnormalities: a ventricular septal defect (hole between the ventricles), stenosis of the pulmonary valve, enlargement of the right ventricle (right-ventricular hypertrophy), and an aorta that is positioned to receive blood from both ventricles (overriding aorta) (see Figure 9-34).

Ventricular Septal Defect

The ventricular septum develops during fetal development. If the septum does not fully develop, or contains perforations, blood will flow between the ventricles. A ventricular septal defect will cause the heart to work harder and can result in lung congestion (see Figure 9-34).

Truncus Arteriosus

In normal hearts, two large vessels exit the ventricles (pulmonary trunk and aorta). Truncus arteriosus is a congenital disorder in which both vessels develop as one. This vessel is positioned so that it carries blood from both ventricles (see Figure 9-36).

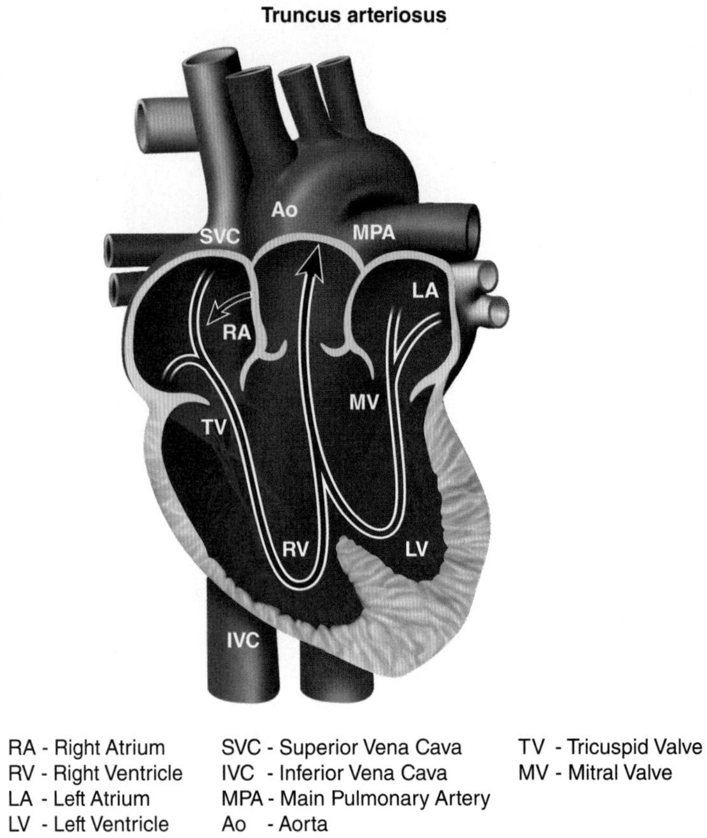
Truncus arteriosus
Ao
SVC
MPA
LA
RA
MV
TV
RV
LV
IVC
RA - Right Atrium
RV - Right Ventricle
LA - Left Atrium
LV - Left Ventricle
SVC - Superior Vena Cava
IVC - Inferior Vena Cava
MPA - Main Pulmonary Artery
Ao - Aorta
TV - Tricuspid Valve
MV - Mitral Valve

FIGURE 9-36 Truncus arteriosus. Notice how there is one large artery leaving the heart that splits to become the aorta and pulmonary trunk.

LEARNING OBJECTIVE 9.6.2 **Describe the signs, symptoms, and diagnosis of a pericardial tamponade.**

KEY TERMS

pericardial tamponade Condition arising from fluid buildup in the pericardium that inhibits ventricular contraction.

pericarditis Inflammation of the pericardium.

Pericardial Tamponade

Pericardial tamponade is a condition in which fluid builds up in the pericardium. This condition can result from trauma, cancer, inflammation (**pericarditis**), kidney failure, radiation treatments, or surgery. The additional fluid puts pressure on the heart, causing a decrease in the amount of blood the heart can pump (decrease in cardiac output) (see Figure 9-37).

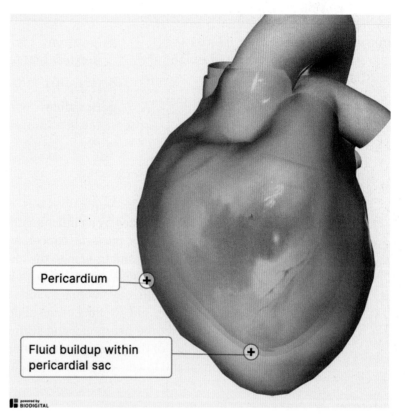

Pericardium

Fluid buildup within pericardial sac

FIGURE 9-37 This image is a of a pericardial effusion, which can result in a pericardial tamponade.

Signs and symptoms of cardiac tamponade include low blood pressure (hypotension); chest pain with radiation to the neck, shoulders, or back; rapid breathing; weak pulse; anxiety; dizziness; fainting; and loss of consciousness.

A practitioner will look for the presence of Beck's triad, which includes hypotension, distended neck veins, rapid heart rate (tachycardia) with decreased heart sounds. Tests including ultrasound, chest x-ray, electrocardiogram, computed tomography (CT), and magnetic resonance imaging (MRI) scans of the heart will help in identifying this condition.

Treatment for pericardial tamponade can include:

- Pericardiectomy: Surgery to remove a portion of the pericardium to relieve pressure on the heart.
- Pericardiocentesis: Insertion of a needle into the pericardium to remove fluid.
- Thoracotomy: Surgery to drain blood from around the heart.

Less invasive treatment such as pericardiocentesis is recommended first before performing more invasive surgical treatments. Once the patient is stabilized, supportive treatment can include medications for lowering blood pressure, oxygen, and intravenous fluids for maintaining normal fluid volume.

LEARNING OBJECTIVE 9.6.3 Describe the signs, symptoms, and diagnosis of pericarditis.

KEY TERMS

blood urea nitrogen Blood test that measures urea nitrogen, a waste product, in the blood and can help to indicate organ disease.

C-reactive protein Protein blood marker that is used to indicate inflammation.

palpitations Heartbeats that are fast, strong, or irregular that can be felt.

pericarditis Inflammation of the pericardium.

pericardium Fibrous tissue structure that contains the heart.

Pericarditis

Pericarditis is characterized by an inflammation of the pericardium. Pericarditis can be caused by viruses, bacteria, cancer, autoimmune disorders, myocardial infarction, medications, and trauma to the chest.

Pericarditis can cause severe, sharp chest pain that radiates to the left shoulder and neck. Other symptoms include shortness of breath, palpitations, fever, cough, fatigue, and swelling of the abdomen and lower extremities. Pericarditis can restrict the heart, causing stiffness of the ventricular walls. This reduces the ability of the heart to pump blood resulting in congestion of blood in the abdomen and lower extremities, which leads to edema (see Figure 9-38).

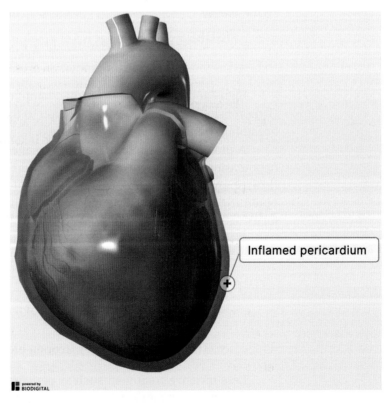

Inflamed pericardium

powered by
BIODIGITAL

FIGURE 9-38 Pericarditis.

A practitioner will conduct a variety of tests including auscultation (pericarditis produces a characteristic pericardial rub sound), an ECG, blood tests to look for increased creatine, **blood urea nitrogen** (BUN), and **C-reactive protein**. Imaging studies such as ultrasound, MRI, CT, and x-ray may be performed.

LEARNING OBJECTIVE 9.6.4 Describe the signs, symptoms, and diagnosis of hypertrophic cardiomyopathy.

KEY TERMS

hypertrophic cardiomyopathy Type of heart disease characterized by thickening of the muscular walls of the heart.

obstructive cardiomyopathy Enlargement of a heart ventricle that obstructs blood flow out of the ventricle.

Hypertrophic Cardiomyopathy

Hypertrophic cardiomyopathy is a genetic disorder causing thickening of the ventricles (usually the left ventricle). The thickened left ventricle can affect the function of the bicuspid (mitral) valve, causing blood to leak into the left atrium when the valve is closed. Sometimes, the ventricular septum enlarges and obstructs blood flowing out of the ventricle (**obstructive cardiomyopathy**). This occurs because the inner portion of the ventricle enlarges due to the stiffness of the external portion. Volume decreases inside of the ventricle causing reduced function that can lead to serious consequences including death. Hypertrophic cardiomyopathy can cause sudden cardiac arrest in young people and athletes.

Hypertrophic cardiomyopathy is difficult to identify due to the lack of symptoms. In some cases, the condition presents with shortness of breath, chest pain, arrhythmias, palpitations, and fainting after exertion.

To diagnose hypertrophic cardiomyopathy, a practitioner will perform a variety of tests including an ECG, echocardiogram to examine the thickness of the ventricles, stress ECG, as well as imaging studies including cardiac MRI.

UNIT OBJECTIVE 9.7

Describe common pathologies that affect the electrical conduction system of the heart.

UNIT INTRODUCTION

Some heart disorders result from problems with the electrical system of the heart. These can range from mild disturbances of heart rhythm to potentially lethal heart rhythms. This unit examines common pathologies that affect the electrical conduction system of the heart.

Identify the following abnormal ECGs: sinus bradycardia, sinus tachycardia, and asystole.

KEY TERMS

asystole ECG reading indicating no contraction of the heart.

sinus bradycardia Heart rate lower than the normal 60–100 beats per minute.

sinus tachycardia Regular heart rhythm greater than 100 beats per minute.

syncope Commonly known as fainting and characterized by a loss of consciousness from decreased blood flow to the brain.

vasovagal Parasympathetic stimulus carried by the vagus nerve: cranial nerve X.

vasovagal and syncope A loss of consciousness from decreased blood flow to the brain caused by an emotional stimulus.

SINUS BRADYCARDIA, SINUS TACHYCARDIA, AND ASYSTOLE

The normal heart rate is between 60 and 100 beats per minute. **Sinus bradycardia** is a heart rate below 60 beats per minute, and **sinus tachycardia** is a heart rate above 100 beats per minute. The absence of electrical activity in the heart (flat line on an ECG) is known as **asystole**.

Sinus Bradycardia

Bradycardia can be seen in athletes and is a normal response to cardiovascular fitness. However, an abnormally slow heart rate can occur when the vagus nerve (cranial nerve X) sends impulses to the heart. This is known as the **vasovagal** response and can cause fainting (vasovagal **syncope**).

Other causes of bradycardia include heart muscle damage from a myocardial infarction or heart disease, infection, electrolyte imbalances, inflammation of heart tissues (myocarditis), sleep apnea, and medications used to slow down the heart.

Sinus Tachycardia

In sinus tachycardia the sinoatrial node stimulates the heart to beat at a faster rate (greater than 100 beats per minute). There are many causes of sinus tachycardia, which include emotional stress, medications, thyroid disorders, heart muscle damage, and anemia. Many people experience an isolated incident of sinus tachycardia, which does not require treatment. In more frequent cases, the underlying cause of sinus tachycardia must be treated.

Asystole

Asystole results from cardiac arrest and presents with no electrical signal on an ECG. There are many causes of cardiac arrest including myocardial infarction, shock, severe electrolyte imbalances, trauma, and infection. Asystole must be treated immediately or death will occur within a few minutes. Treatment usually consists of administering an electric shock to the heart (defibrillation).

LEARNING OBJECTIVE 9.7.2 Identify the following abnormal ECGs: atrial fibrillation, supraventricular tachycardia, ventricular tachycardia, and ventricular fibrillation.

LEARNING OBJECTIVE 9.7.3 Describe the relationship between sudden cardiac arrest and the following arrhythmias: ventricular tachycardia, ventricular fibrillation, and asystole.

KEY TERMS

atrial fibrillation Abnormal heart rhythm characterized by chaotic contractions of the atria.

paroxysmal supraventricular tachycardia Rapid heart rate that originates from tissue located above the ventricles.

supraventricular tachycardia Fast but regular heartbeat caused by nodal tissue located above the ventricles.

ventricular fibrillation Chaotic abnormal heart rhythm in which the ventricles do not contract.

ventricular tachycardia Regular heart rhythm greater than 100 beats per minute.

ATRIAL FIBRILLATION, VENTRICULAR FIBRILLATION, SUPRAVENTRICULAR TACHYCARDIA, AND VENTRICULAR TACHYCARDIA

Atrial Fibrillation

Atrial fibrillation is characterized by an absence of P-waves on an ECG. Action potentials in the atria are produced at a rapid, chaotic rate and the ECG will display low-level irregular waveforms between QRS complexes. QRS complexes are abnormal patterns known as an "irregularly irregular" rate due to groups of action potentials reaching the atrioventricular node.

Atrial fibrillation is one of the most common arrhythmias and increases in incidence over the age of 65. Signs of atrial fibrillation include palpitations, fatigue, dizziness, shortness of breath, and chest pain. Some people are not aware they have atrial fibrillation. This condition increases the risk of stroke by four to five times. Treatment includes medications to help control and maintain a normal heart rhythm and anticoagulant medications to inhibit the formation of blood clots.

NORMAL RATE AND RHYTHM

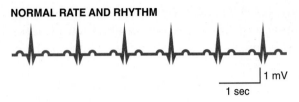

1 mV

1 sec

ABNORMALITIES IN RATE

Tachycardia

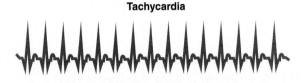

ABNORMALITIES IN RHYTHM

Premature ventricular contraction

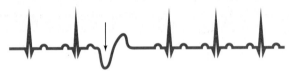

Ventricular fibrillation

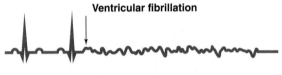

Complete heart block

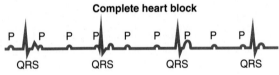

P P P P P P P P P

QRS QRS QRS QRS

CARDIAC MYOPATHIES

Myocardial infarction (heart attack)

FIGURE 9-39 Common cardiac arrhythmias are a result of abnormalities in rate, rhythm, or myopathies.

Ventricular Fibrillation

Ventricular fibrillation is characterized by the ventricles contracting in a rapid, chaotic fashion. The ventricles quiver and cannot pump blood during ventricular fibrillation. Since there is no organized contraction of the ventricles, the ECG presents with a low-level chaotic waveform (see Figure 9-39).

Ventricular fibrillation is a very serious problem and is a medical emergency because it can lead to cardiac arrest. The primary symptom of ventricular fibrillation is loss of consciousness with concurrent unresponsiveness of the patient. Ventricular fibrillation can be caused by damage to heart muscle from a myocardial infarction or abnormal electrical impulses originating in the ventricles. This condition must be treated immediately with defibrillation.

Supraventricular Tachycardia

Supraventricular tachycardia (paroxysmal supraventricular tachycardia) is characterized by a rapid, regular rhythm usually between 150 and 250 beats per minute on an ECG. In supraventricular tachycardia, the QRS complexes appear normal and close together. Due to the rapid rate, the T-waves of the previous beats will cover the P-waves of the next beat.

Supraventricular tachycardia (SVT) is caused by electrical impulses originating in areas of the heart above the ventricles or in the atria or atrioventricular node. Many people experience episodes of SVT without needing treatment. People with SVT may experience palpitations, shortness of breath, dizziness, fainting, or sweating. There are many causes of SVT including consumption of stimulants such as caffeine or alcohol, smoking, heart disease, thyroid disorders, and asthma medications. SVT is not life-threatening and is usually treated with lifestyle modifications.

Ventricular Tachycardia

Ventricular tachycardia is characterized by a rapid contraction of the ventricles at a rate greater than 100 beats per minute. The ECG presents with QRS complexes in close proximity to one another. Sustained ventricular tachycardia lasts longer than 30 seconds. Nonsustained ventricular tachycardia lasts less than 30 seconds (see Figure 9-38).

Ventricular tachycardia is caused by abnormal electrical impulses originating from the ventricles. It can progress to more severe arrhythmias such as ventricular fibrillation and asystole if left untreated. Symptoms range from mild to severe and include palpitations, dizziness, shortness of breath, chest pain, loss of consciousness, and sudden cardiac arrest. Ventricular tachycardia can be treated with medications, cardioversion (electrical shock), defibrillation, or surgery.

UNIT OBJECTIVE 9.8

Describe common pathologies that affect the cardiac cycle.

UNIT INTRODUCTION

A complex series of events must occur in order to move blood through the heart. These include the generation and transport of timed electrical impulses through the heart, contraction of the atria and ventricles, and the opening and closing of the heart valves. Collectively, these events are known as the cardiac cycle. Many of the problems that affect the heart also affect the cardiac cycle. This unit examines those pathologies that have an effect on the cardiac cycle.

LEARNING OBJECTIVE 9.8.1 Identify common disorders affecting the cardiac cycle.

CARDIAC CYCLE DISORDERS

Disorders affecting the cardiac cycle include electrical problems (arrhythmias), genetic and anatomical deformities, infection, inflammation, and heart failure.

Patent Ductus Arteriosus

A patent ductus arteriosus is a passageway for blood to flow from the pulmonary trunk to the aorta. The function of the ductus arteriosus is to provide a route for blood to bypass the fetal lungs, which are filled with amniotic fluid. The ductus arteriosus should close at birth. However, if it remains open, blood can flow from the aorta back to the pulmonary trunk and into the lungs due to the higher pressure in the aorta.

    A patent ductus arteriosus affects the cardiac cycle. The increased blood in the lungs can lead to increased pressure in the pulmonary arteries (pulmonary hypertension), which puts additional stress on the heart. This can lead to heart failure.

Coarctation of the Aorta

Coarctation of the aorta is characterized by a narrowing of the aorta. This condition affects the cardiac cycle by way of increasing pressure in the left ventricle, causing the heart to work harder to pump blood to the body and eventually causing heart failure.

Describe the signs, symptoms, and diagnosis of heart failure.

KEY TERMS

angiography Imaging of blood vessels using contrast media and x-rays.

congestive heart failure Type of heart disease characterized by damage to heart muscle resulting in the inability of the heart to pump blood.

diastolic failure Type of heart failure that affects ventricular filling.

echocardiogram Imaging test using high-frequency sound waves (ultrasound).

myocardial biopsy Test of cardiac muscle performed by inserting a device in a blood vessel that collects a small amount of heart muscle tissue.

natriuretic peptide Hormone secreted by the atria that promotes reduction of sodium reabsorption in the kidneys with a net effect of water loss.

systolic failure Type of heart failure that affects contraction of the ventricles.

Congestive Heart Failure

Congestive heart failure (CHF) occurs when damage to the heart results in the inability of the ventricles to adequately pump blood. This leads to buildup of fluid in the abdomen and lower extremities. The heart attempts to adapt to heart failure by causing the ventricles to enlarge and increasing the heart rate as the heart struggles to maintain cardiac output. Heart failure can affect the right ventricle (right-sided heart failure) or left ventricle (left-sided heart failure). Heart failure can also affect the pumping ability of the ventricles (**systolic failure**) or the ability of the ventricles to fill (**diastolic failure**).

CHF can be caused by hypertension, heart muscle damage from a myocardial infarction, infection, cardiomyopathy, arrhythmias, or valvular problems. Due to the left ventricle's decreased function, blood pressure increases in the pulmonary circulation, causing pulmonary edema. Fluid builds up in the lungs and interferes with the exchange of oxygen and carbon dioxide, causing hypoxia (low blood oxygen levels), breathing difficulties, and shortness of breath (see Figure 9-40).

Heart failure signs and symptoms include:

- Shortness of breath on exertion
- Swelling in the abdomen (ascites) and/or extremities
- Fatigue
- Inability to perform activities
- Coughing with pink, bloody sputum from pulmonary edema
- Fluid retention
- Increased urination
- Chest pain

Heart failure is diagnosed with a variety of tests, including:

- Chest x-ray to determine if the heart is enlarged.
- ECG to determine the presence of arrhythmias.

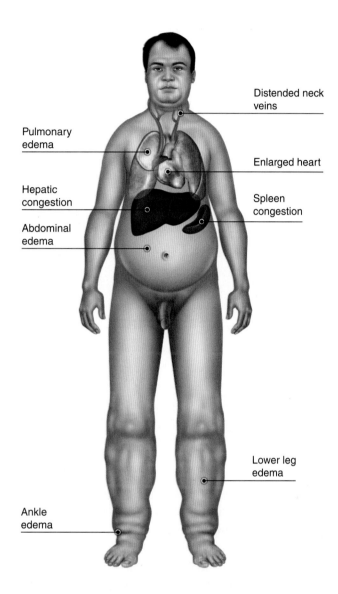

Distended neck veins

Pulmonary edema

Enlarged heart

Hepatic congestion

Spleen congestion

Abdominal edema

Lower leg edema

Ankle edema

FIGURE 9-40 Signs and symptoms of congestive heart failure include: pulmonary edema, edema of the lower extremities, edema of the abdomen, enlarged heart, congestion of the spleen and liver, and distended neck veins.

- **Echocardiogram** to determine the size and thickness of the heart walls along with assessing the movement of blood through the heart.
- Blood tests to assess the levels of **natriuretic peptide**, a hormone that helps to control fluid volume.
- Stress test to assess how the heart functions during periods of exertion.
- Imaging studies such as CT and MRI to assess the size of the heart and ventricles.

- **Angiography** to assess the coronary arteries that supply the heart muscle with oxygenated blood.
- **Myocardial biopsy** in which small samples of heart muscle are taken from an instrument inserted through a vein in the neck or groin.

LEARNING OBJECTIVE 9.8.3 Describe the effects of heart failure on the cardiac cycle.

KEY TERM

ventricular systole Contraction of the ventricles.

Heart Failure and the Cardiac Cycle

Heart failure has the following effects on the cardiac cycle:

Increased heart rate due to sympathetic activity. The sympathetic nervous system increases the heart rate in an attempt to maintain blood flow through the heart (cardiac output). The increased heart rate can also increase blood pressure.

During the first phase of the cardiac cycle, the atria and ventricles are in a relaxed state, referred to as diastole. Blood flows into the atria and ventricles, with about 70% of the total blood entering the ventricles. Heart failure can cause a decreased amount of blood to fill the ventricles. Stiffness of the ventricular walls inhibit the ability of the ventricles to stretch and result in decreased filling.

During the **ventricular systole** phase of the cardiac cycle, heart failure can result in decreased blood flow out of the ventricles (decreased cardiac output).

LEARNING OBJECTIVE 9.8.4 Contrast right-sided heart failure and left-sided heart failure.

KEY TERMS

diastolic heart failure Type of heart failure that affects ventricular filling.

systolic heart failure Type of heart failure that affects contraction of the ventricles.

Right-Sided Versus Left-Sided Heart Failure

Heart failure can affect the right and/or left side of the heart. Left-sided heart failure can affect the filling of the ventricles (**diastolic heart failure**) and the pumping of the ventricles (**systolic heart failure**). In diastolic heart failure, stiffness of the ventricular wall interferes with its ability to relax and stretch. This results in problems with the amount of blood entering the ventricle. In systolic heart failure, the ventricular wall is damaged, resulting in the inability to pump blood out of the ventricle (decreased ejection fraction). The ventricle enlarges in an attempt to compensate for the reduced ability to pump blood.

Pressure in the pulmonary vasculature increases with left-sided heart failure. This causes fluid to build up in the tiny structures (alveoli) that exchange oxygen and carbon dioxide between the lungs and the blood, resulting in pulmonary edema.

In right-sided heart failure, the right ventricle becomes damaged in response to left-sided heart failure. Left-sided heart failure causes an increase in pressure in the right side of the heart. This increase in blood pressure can damage the right side of the heart, causing blood to back up in the abdomen and extremities (edema).

UNIT OBJECTIVE 9.9

Describe common pathologies affecting the body's vasculature.

UNIT INTRODUCTION

The body's blood vessels can be affected by disease processes that range from structural abnormalities to progressive chronic disease. This unit examines common pathologies affecting the body's blood vessels.

LEARNING OBJECTIVE 9.9.1 Identify common disorders affecting the body's vasculature.

KEY TERMS

carotid artery stenosis Narrowing of the carotid artery.

coronary artery disease (CAD) Narrowing of the inner lumen of coronary arteries usually from atherosclerotic plaquing.

COMMON VASCULAR DISORDERS
Carotid Artery Stenosis

Carotid artery stenosis is the narrowing of the carotid arteries in the neck. These arteries supply the arteries to the brain and face. Carotid artery stenosis is caused by the formation of plaques on the inner lining of the arteries from atherosclerosis.

The decreased blood flow to the brain resulting from narrowing of the carotid arteries can cause dizziness, fainting, and small strokes called transient ischemic attacks (TIA) that come from small blood clots forming in the carotid arteries. TIAs present with the symptoms of stroke, which include numbness, paralysis on one side of the body, blurred vision, difficulty speaking, and headaches. However, symptoms of TIAs last for a short time period but are often warning signs of an upcoming stroke (see Figure 9-42).

Carotid artery stenosis is diagnosed with imaging studies including ultrasound, MRI, CT, and cerebral angiography. This condition can be treated with a procedure in which a small tube or stent is placed in the carotid artery called carotid angioplasty (see Figure 9-43). It can also be treated surgically by a procedure in which the endothelium is removed, called endarterectomy.

Coronary Artery Disease

Coronary artery disease (CAD) is the narrowing or blockage of the coronary arteries, which supply the heart with blood. CAD is caused by the formation of plaque on the inner lining of the arteries from atherosclerosis (see Figures 9-41 and 9-44).

Coronary artery disease can lead to a myocardial infarction (MI) whereby reduced blood flow causes damage to heart muscle. Pieces of plaque can break off and cause clotting and blockage of the artery. Signs of an MI include chest pain in the area of the sternum with radiation to the left arm, jaw, or back; indigestion; nausea; sweating; shortness of breath; and dizziness (see Figure 9-45).

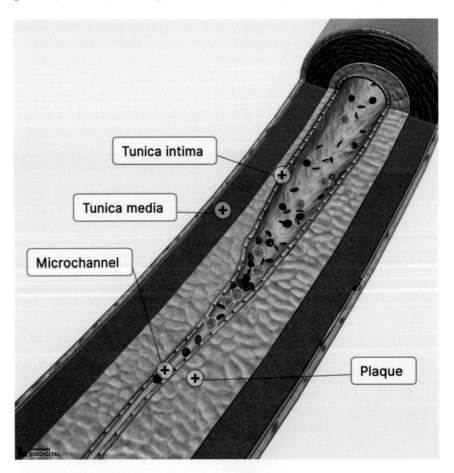

FIGURE 9-41 Complete obstruction of the blood vessel due to atherosclerosis.

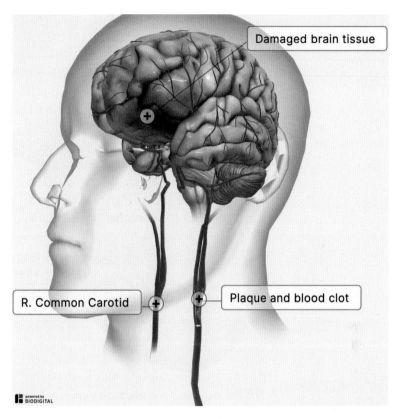

FIGURE 9-42 Ischemic stroke caused by an obstruction of the internal carotid artery.

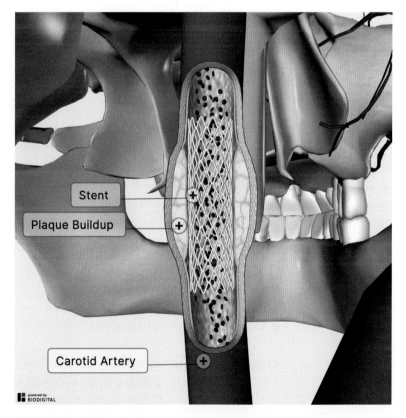

FIGURE 9-43 A stent located in the right carotid artery.

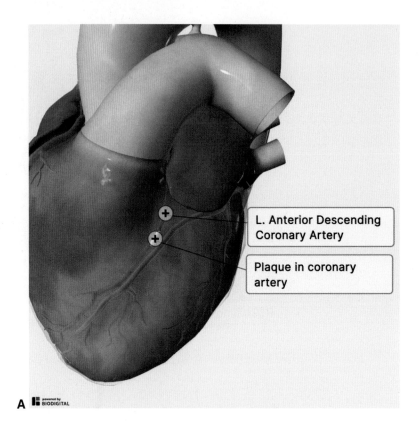

A

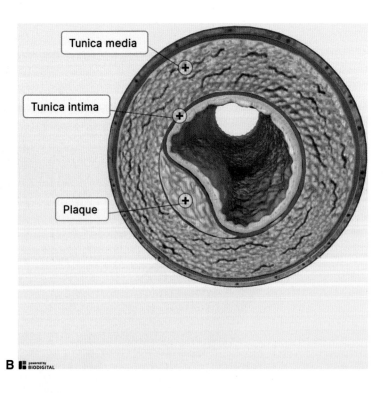

B

FIGURE 9-44ABC A) Plaque in coronary artery partially obstructing the flow of blood. B) Moderate atherosclerosis of a coronary artery. C) Severe atherosclerosis of a coronary artery. (*Continued*)

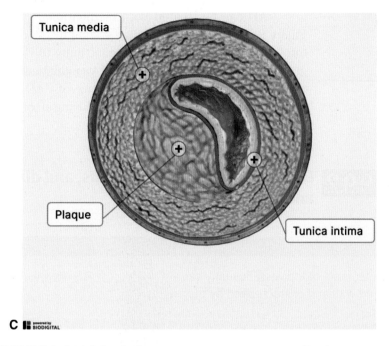

C

FIGURE 9-44ABC A) Plaque in coronary artery partially obstructing the flow of blood. B) Moderate atherosclerosis of a coronary artery. C) Severe atherosclerosis of a coronary artery.

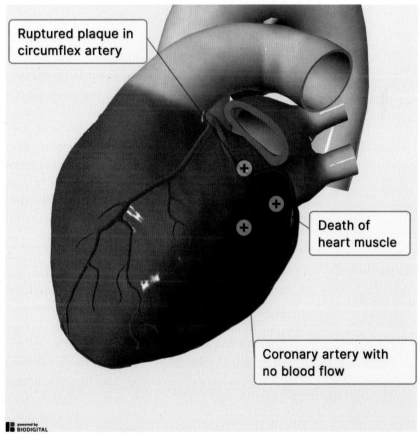

FIGURE 9-45 Obstruction of the left circumflex coronary artery. This obstruction of the coronary artery has resulted in necrosis (tissue death) of the myocardium supplied by the coronary artery.

CAD can be treated with medications, catheterization or surgery (see Figure 9-44). Medications called statins work to lower blood levels of cholesterol, which has been shown to contribute to CAD. Other medications may be given to lower blood pressure or to vasodilate arteries. Prevention is an important factor in decreasing the incidence of CAD and includes positive lifestyle changes such as quitting smoking, reducing alcohol intake, consuming a healthy diet, and exercising.

LEARNING OBJECTIVE 9.9.2 Describe the signs, symptoms, and diagnosis of an aneurysm.

KEY TERM

aneurysms Defect in a blood vessel usually caused by a weakened wall and characterized by bulging of the vessel.

ANEURYSMS

Aneurysms result from the weakening of an artery's walls. Aneurysms can have no symptoms until they rupture. In some cases, aneurysms can produce blood clots due to the turbulent blood flow through the vessel. Ruptured aneurysms can cause sudden pain, dizziness, rapid heart rate, nausea and vomiting, low blood pressure, and shock. Aneurisms occur more frequently in males. Risk factors for aneurysms include high blood pressure (hypertension), smoking, obesity, and atherosclerosis.

Types of aneurysms include cerebral, aortic, and those involving peripheral vessels (Figure 9-46). The most common of these is the abdominal aortic aneurysm (AAA). Abdominal aortic aneurysms have two common morphologies, sacular (Figure 9-48) and fusiform (Figure 9-49). Sacular aneurysms are often found midway between the end of the thoracic aorta and where the aorta splits into the left and right common iliac arteries. Fusiform aneurysms, on the other hand, typically develop right before the aorta splits into the left and right common iliac arteries. A ruptured aneurysm is a medical emergency and, in some cases, there is a low survival rate. Unruptured aneurysms can be treated with stents or grafts to help provide strength to the arterial walls. These can be inserted surgically or with a catheter.

In a dissecting aortic aneurysm, blood tears through the inner endothelial lining of the aorta, causing the other layers to rupture and producing severe, sharp chest pain. This aneurysm has a relatively low survival rate with about 20% of patients dying before reaching the hospital (see Figure 9-47).

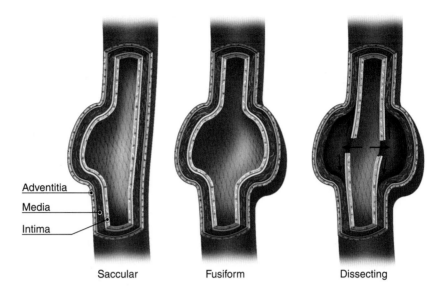

Adventitia
Media
Intima

Saccular   Fusiform   Dissecting

FIGURE 9-46 The three common types of aneurysms. The first image is of a saccular aneurysm, the second is a fusiform aneurysm, and the third is a dissecting aneurysm. Notice in the dissecting aneurysm that blood can flow between the tunica intima and tunica media.

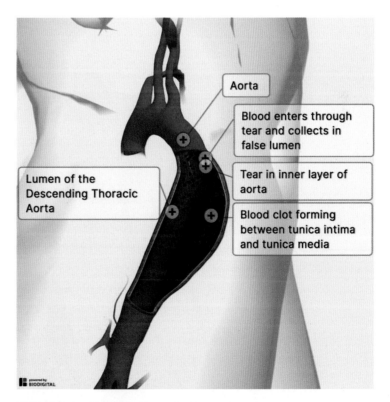

Aorta

Blood enters through tear and collects in false lumen

Lumen of the Descending Thoracic Aorta

Tear in inner layer of aorta

Blood clot forming between tunica intima and tunica media

FIGURE 9-47 Dissection of a thoracic aorta aneurysm.

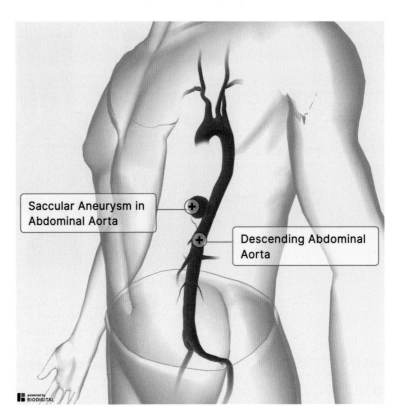

FIGURE 9-48 A saccular aneurysm of the abdominal aorta.

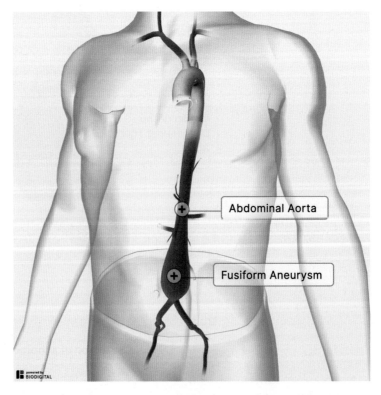

FIGURE 9-49 A fusiform aneurysm of the abdominal aorta.

LEARNING OBJECTIVE 9.9.3 Describe the signs, symptoms, and diagnosis of a dissecting abdominal aortic aneurysm.

abdominal aorta Portion of the aorta just after it passes below the diaphragm and before it divides into the common iliac arteries.

abdominal ultrasound Imaging test of the abdominal region using high-frequency sound waves.

dissecting abdominal aortic aneurysm Weakening of the wall of the abdominal aorta causing bulging and eventual tearing of the artery.

Abdominal Aortic Aneurysm (AAA)

The lower portion of the aorta located below the diaphragm is called the **abdominal aorta**. An abdominal aortic aneurysm is a bulging of the artery that can slowly grow over a period of years. If the aneurysm ruptures, it is called a **dissecting abdominal aortic aneurysm**. The dissection process occurs from blood pushing through the inner endothelial lining of the abdominal aorta, causing the other layers to rupture. Rapid blood loss can then occur as blood moves into the abdominal cavity. These aneurysms occur more frequently in males over the age of 60. Risk factors include high blood pressure, atherosclerosis, smoking, trauma, infection, diabetes, inflammation, vascular disease, and genetics.

Symptoms of an AAA include a pulsating mass in the abdominal region and deep pain in the abdomen. This condition can also cause low back pain. AAAs are diagnosed with a complete examination followed by various imaging tests that can include CT scans, MRI, and **abdominal ultrasound**. They can also be discovered on routine physical examinations whereby a practitioner will discover a pulsating mass in the abdomen. Occasionally, calcification of the abdominal aorta will occur allowing the aneurysm to be seen on x-ray. The rupture of a AAA is a medical emergency, with about half of patients dying before reaching the hospital.

LEARNING OBJECTIVE 9.9.4 Describe the signs, symptoms, and diagnosis of Raynaud's phenomenon.

autoimmune syndrome Syndrome in which the body's antibodies destroy tissue.

nailfold capillaroscopy Test performed with special optical equipment on fingernails or toenails to investigate the circulatory function of the small capillaries.

paresthesia Abnormal sensation in a part of the body, sometimes referred to as numbness or tingling.

Raynaud's phenomenon Circulatory disorder characterized by reduced circulation to the hands or feet.

rheumatoid arthritis Autoimmune disorder causing destruction of the joints of the body.

systemic lupus erythematosus Autoimmune disorder, commonly referred to as lupus, characterized by inflammation of body tissues.

RAYNAUD'S PHENOMENON

Raynaud's phenomenon occurs when arteries in the hands and feet vasoconstrict in response to cold temperatures or stress. The hands and feet can change color and turn white, red, or blue. In addition to feelings of cold, patients can also experience **paresthesia** (numbness and tingling) in the hands or feet. The phenomenon lasts for about 15 minutes, until the extremities can heat up. In primary Raynaud's, the phenomenon occurs without any illness and usually affects women under 30 years of age. Secondary Raynaud's occurs as a complication of another illness, usually an **autoimmune syndrome** such as **systemic lupus erythematosus** or **rheumatoid arthritis**.

Raynaud's is usually not serious, but in some cases can cause problems related to loss of blood flow such as sores and gangrene. Raynaud's is diagnosed by evaluation of history and physical examination. In addition, tests such as a **nailfold capillaroscopy** can be performed to evaluate blood vessels at the tips of the fingers.

Chapter 10

The Respiratory System

Chapter Introduction

Oxygen is an essential requirement for the cells of our bodies, and our respiratory system ensures a constant supply of this vital element. We cannot survive without oxygen for even a few minutes before cell death begins to occur. In addition to supplying oxygen, the respiratory system removes carbon dioxide and helps to regulate blood pH, secretes enzymes, houses immune system cells, and allows us to speak.

UNIT OBJECTIVE 10.1

Describe the structure and general functions of the respiratory system.

UNIT INTRODUCTION

The respiratory system is vital to our survival and performs a variety of functions. It includes two main sections. The upper respiratory system acts as a passageway that warms and cleans the air entering our bodies. The lower respiratory system performs the exchange of oxygen and carbon dioxide with the blood. In addition to moving air containing oxygen and carbon dioxide into our bodies, the respiratory system performs functions related to blood pH regulation, enzyme secretion, and immunity.

LEARNING OBJECTIVE 10.1.1 Identify the general functions of the respiratory system.

LEARNING OBJECTIVE 10.1.2 Describe the general functions of the respiratory system.

KEY TERMS

acidic Pertaining to an acid; a value lower than 7 on the pH scale.

alkaline Chemical compound that ionizes when placed in a liquid and has the ability to bind to free hydrogen ions. The solution could also be called a base and has a pH greater than 7 (7.45 when used in reference to the human body).

alveoli Smallest functional units of the lung; structures in which the exchanges of gases occur.

intrathoracic Area inside of the thoracic cavity.

larynx Portion of respiratory system located between the pharynx and trachea that contains the vocal cords.

true vocal chords Thick portions of the vocal cords (vocal folds) that vibrate and produce sound.

RESPIRATORY SYSTEM FUNCTIONS

The respiratory system has a variety of functions. In addition to moving air inside and outside of the body in order to provide a source of oxygen and to remove carbon dioxide, the respiratory system helps to regulate the pH of the blood, assists the immune system in protecting the body from pathogens, and allows us to speak.

The general functions of the respiratory system include ventilation, external and internal respiration, regulation of blood pH, production of sound by the vocal chords, and immunity.

Ventilation. Air entering and exiting the lungs is known as ventilation. Air moves from higher to lower pressure and expansion of the lungs during inhalation lowers intrathoracic pressure, allowing air to move in. Likewise, contraction of the lungs increases the pressure, pushing air out of the lungs.

External Respiration. Once inside of the lungs, oxygen can move into the blood by diffusion by way of small capillaries surrounding the smallest structures of the lungs (alveoli). Likewise, carbon dioxide diffuses out of the blood and into the alveoli to be expelled during exhalation. The movement of oxygen and carbon dioxide between the lungs and blood is known as external respiration.

Internal Respiration. The movement of oxygen and carbon dioxide in and out of cells is internal respiration.

Regulation of Blood pH. Carbon dioxide is stored in the blood and has a direct effect on hydrogen ion concentration. A faster respiratory rate decreases carbon dioxide and hydrogen ion concentration in the blood. This has the effect of making the blood more alkaline. Likewise, a slower breathing rate will increase carbon dioxide and hydrogen ion concentration, making the blood more acidic. The respiratory system can adjust the breathing rate to help to regulate blood pH.

Production of Sound. Our voice is produced by air causing the vocal cords in the larynx to vibrate. The respiratory system projects air into the larynx and past the membranous folds known as the true vocal chords. Muscles in the larynx help to control the vibration of the vocal cords to change the pitch of the sound of our voice.

Immunity. Portions of the respiratory system are lined with pseudostratified columnar epithelium, which works to trap pathogens in mucous and transport them to the digestive tract where hydrochloric acid in the stomach destroys them. The respiratory system cells also secrete antimicrobial peptides, which help to protect the lungs from pathogens.

LEARNING OBJECTIVE 10.1.3 Identify external, internal, and cellular respiration.

LEARNING OBJECTIVE 10.1.4 Describe external, internal, and cellular respiration.

KEY TERMS

cellular respiration Series of reactions occurring in the cell that converts glucose to ATP.

diffusion Passive movement of substances from an area of high concentration to lower concentration until reaching equilibrium.

external respiration Process by which gas exchange occurs between the alveoli and the blood.

internal respiration Movement of oxygen and carbon dioxide into and out of cells by way of diffusion.

reaction pathways Systems of chemical reactions.

EXTERNAL, INTERNAL, AND CELLULAR RESPIRATION

Oxygen moves by diffusion from the smallest functional units of the lungs called alveoli through the capillary walls to the blood. Carbon dioxide moves from the blood by diffusion through the capillary walls to the alveoli. This process is called external respiration (Figure 10-1).

After oxygen is transported to the tissues, it diffuses across capillary walls to the cells of the tissues. Oxygen can now enter the cells. Likewise, carbon dioxide produced by the cells moves out of the cells so that it can be transported by the blood to the lungs for removal during exhalation. The movement of oxygen and carbon dioxide into and out of the cells is known as internal respiration (Figure 10-1).

Oxygen and substances derived from food (carbohydrates, lipids, proteins) are needed by cells to produce ATP. Cells contain a series of catabolic reaction pathways that convert these digested substances to energy (ATP). These reactions require a constant supply of oxygen. The use of oxygen by cells to make ATP is known as cellular respiration.

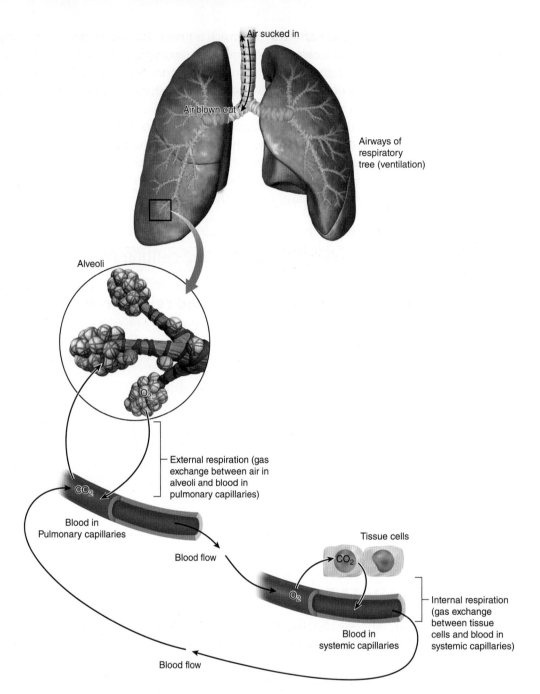

FIGURE 10-1 External respiration involves the exchange of oxygen and carbon dioxide between the lungs and blood while oxygen and carbon dioxide are exchanged between the blood and tissues in internal respiration.

External Respiration

External respiration includes the movement of oxygen and carbon dioxide between the lungs and the blood. This movement occurs by diffusion and is driven by differences in pressure. Oxygen enters the lungs at a higher pressure than blood in the pulmonary arteries entering the lungs. The difference in pressure in the alveoli versus the pulmonary arteries promotes the movement of oxygen from the alveoli to the deoxygenated blood in the pulmonary arteries. Since oxygen is lipid soluble, it can move through the phospholipid bilayers of alveoli and capillaries.

The pulmonary arteries also carry carbon dioxide at a higher pressure than in the alveoli. Since carbon dioxide is also lipid soluble, it can diffuse across the phospholipid bilayers of the capillaries and alveolar membrane and follow its pressure gradient into the lungs.

Internal Respiration

The blood carries oxygen to the tissues so that it can move into the tissues and provide a constant supply of oxygen for producing energy. Likewise, carbon dioxide in the tissues must be transported by the blood to the lungs so that it can be removed from the body. The process of moving oxygen and carbon dioxide between the blood and tissues is known as internal respiration. Blood in capillaries surrounding tissue carries oxygen at a higher pressure than the tissues. Oxygen follows its pressure gradient and diffuses from the blood to the tissues and into cells. Cells use the oxygen for producing ATP by way of a series of reaction pathways.

Cellular Respiration

Once oxygen reaches the tissues, the cells of the tissues use oxygen to produce energy in the form of ATP. There are two types of cellular reaction pathways that produce ATP. Aerobic pathways use oxygen, whereas anaerobic pathways do not. The majority of ATP in the body is produced by the aerobic pathways.

LEARNING OBJECTIVE 10.1.5 **Explain why respiration is so vital to human survival on a cellular level.**

RESPIRATION AND HUMAN SURVIVAL

Many of the body's physiological processes are powered by ATP. For example, sodium and potassium gradients power neurons, muscle cells (skeletal, smooth, and cardiac), urine formation, and many other processes. These gradients are produced and maintained by active transport proteins such as the sodium-potassium pump that use ATP. Since oxygen plays a vital role in cellular respiration, the constant supply of oxygen by the respiratory system is required for producing ATP and keeping the body alive.

LEARNING OBJECTIVE 10.1.6 **Identify the organs that compose the respiratory system.**

KEY TERMS

bronchi Air passages extending from the trachea and entering the lungs.

bronchioles Smaller branches from tertiary bronchi that attach to alveoli.

larynx Portion of respiratory system located between the pharynx and trachea that contains the vocal cords.

nasal cavity Air passageway located behind the maxillary bones and above the hard palate.

pharynx Partially shared passageway for the respiratory and digestive systems beginning at the posterior nasal cavity and extending to the trachea.

sinuses Hollow chambers within the bones of the skull.

trachea Respiratory air passage containing C-shaped hyaline cartilage rings beginning at the inferior border of the larynx and extending to the primary bronchi.

vomer Bone located in the nasal cavity that, along with the perpendicular plate of the ethmoid bone, forms the nasal septum.

THE RESPIRATORY SYSTEM

The respiratory system (Figure 10-2) consists of air passageways and the lungs. The respiratory system can be divided into the upper and lower respiratory systems. The upper respiratory system consists of the nose and nasal cavity, the sinuses, the pharynx, and the portion of the larynx above the vocal cords. The lower respiratory system consists of the portion of the larynx including the vocal cords and below, the trachea, the bronchi, the bronchioles, and the lungs and alveoli.

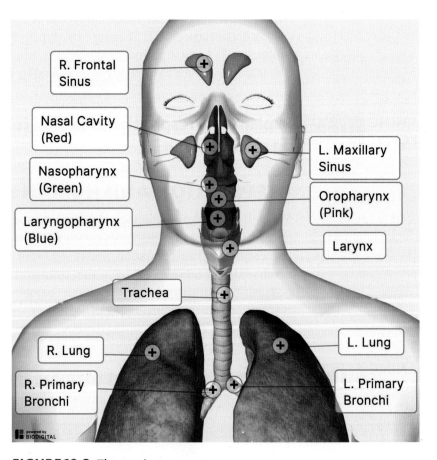

FIGURE 10-2 The respiratory system.

Describe the structure of the organs that compose the respiratory system.

Describe the functions of each organ that composes the respiratory system.

KEY TERMS

arytenoid Small paired cartilage on the posterior portion of the larynx.

cardiac notch Indentation in the area where the heart contacts the left lung; also known as a cardiac impression.

ciliated pseudostratified columnar epithelium Type of epithelium characterized by one row of columnar cells that contain cilia.

conchae Protrusions located on the inner surface of the nasal cavity that help to create turbulent air flow.

corniculate Small paired cartilage on the posterior portion of the larynx.

cricoid cartilage Cartilage located on the anterior portion of the larynx just below the thyroid cartilage.

cuneiform Small paired cartilage on the posterior portion of the larynx.

epiglottis Cartilaginous structure in the larynx that closes it off when swallowing to prevent the movement of substances into the trachea.

ethmoid Deep bone in the skull that contributes to the nasal septum and orbit.

Eustachian tubes Small passageways between the middle ear and nasal cavity.

glottis Triangular space formed in the larynx when the vocal cords are relaxed.

lamina propria Thin layer of loose connective tissue located beneath epithelial cells.

laryngopharynx Lowermost portion of the pharynx.

nasopharynx Portion of the pharynx that extends from the posterior portion of the nasal cavity to the soft palate.

oropharynx Portion of the pharynx extending from the soft palate to the epiglottis.

palatine bones Bones of the skull contributing to the posterior portion of the hard palate.

parietal pleural membrane Membrane of the lungs that attaches to the inside of the thoracic cavity.

pharyngeal tonsils Masses of lymphoid tissue located in the pharynx.

pleural fluid Fluid secreted by the parietal pleural membrane.

simple squamous epithelium Epithelial tissue consisting of one layer of flat squamous cells.

surfactant Substance secreted by type II alveolar cells that decreases surface tension in the alveoli.

thyroid cartilage Large cartilage wrapping around the larynx.

trachealis muscle Smooth muscle located in the trachea that helps to regulate air flow into the lungs by constricting or dilating the trachea.

Type I pneumocytes Mucous-producing cells located in alveoli that form part of the respiratory membrane through which gas exchange occurs between the alveoli and capillaries.

Type II pneumocytes Surfactant-secreting cells located in the alveoli.

visceral pleural membrane Portion of the pleural membrane attached to the surface of the lungs.

ORGANS OF THE RESPIRATORY SYSTEM
Nose and Nasal Cavity

Air moves into the upper respiratory system through the nose at the nostrils (external nares) and enters the nasal cavity (see Fig. 10-3). The nasal cavity (nasal vestibule) is lined with **ciliated pseudostratified columnar epithelium** with goblet cells. Beneath the epithelium is a highly vascular area known as the **lamina propria**. Vessels in the lamina propria help to heat and humidify the air. The nasal cavity also contains bony protuberances called nasal **conchae**. There are superior, middle, and inferior conchae. The purpose of the conchae is to create a turbulent flow of air that works to warm the air and provide more contact with the nasal mucosa so that particles can be picked up by the mucosa. The turbulent air can also reach the upper nasal cavity containing sensory receptors for smell.

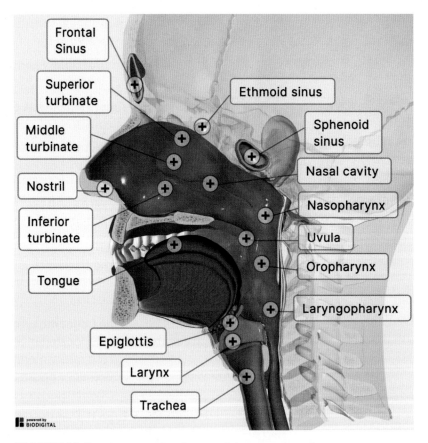

FIGURE 10-3 Nose, mouth, pharynx, larynx, and trachea.

The nasal septum divides the nasal cavity into right and left sections. The nasal septum is formed by two bones. The superior portion consists of the perpendicular plate of the **ethmoid** bone, and the inferior portion consists of the **vomer** bone. The anterior portion of the nasal septum consists of cartilage.

Located between the conchae are the superior, middle, and inferior meatuses, which are small grooves allowing air flow between the nasal cavity, paranasal sinuses, and nasolacrimal ducts.

The floor of the nasal cavity consists of the hard palate. The anterior portion of the hard palate is formed by the maxilla and the posterior portion is formed by the palatine bones. The hard palate separates the nasal and oral cavities. Just posterior to the hard palate is the soft palate and uvula.

The Pharynx

Air passing through the internal nares enters the upper portion of the pharynx known as the nasopharynx. The nasopharynx begins posterior to the conchae and extends inferiorly to the soft palate. The soft palate raises to close off the nasopharynx during swallowing to prevent substances from moving into it. The nasopharynx is lined with ciliated pseudostratified columnar epithelium with mucous-secreting goblet cells. Mucous traps bacteria and debris and the cilia move these through the nasopharynx so they can be swallowed. The nasopharynx also contains connections from the Eustachian tubes. The pharyngeal tonsils (adenoids) are also located in the nasopharynx.

Inferior to the nasopharynx is the oropharynx, which extends from the soft palate to the epiglottis. The oropharynx is a shared passageway for the movement of air to the trachea and digestive substances on their way to the esophagus. The palatine and lingual tonsils are located in the oropharynx. The oropharynx is lined with stratified squamous epithelium.

The most inferior portion of the pharynx is the laryngopharynx, which extends from the tip of the epiglottis to the larynx. The laryngopharynx is also a shared pathway with the digestive tract and is lined with stratified squamous epithelium.

The Larynx

The larynx (Figure 10-4) begins at the base of the tongue and extends to the trachea. The larynx consists of nine cartilages that are interconnected with muscles and ligaments. Three of these cartilages are unpaired and include the thyroid and cricoid cartilages and the epiglottis. The largest of the cartilages is the thyroid cartilage (Adam's apple). Inferior to the thyroid cartilage is the cricoid cartilage. The epiglottis is an elastic cartilage flap that closes during swallowing to keep substances from moving into the trachea and air passages. Smaller, paired cartilages include the arytenoid, corniculate, and cuneiform cartilages.

The larynx contains the vocal cords, which consist of two sets of paired ligaments that extend from the arytenoid to the thyroid cartilages (Figure 10-5). One set of ligaments (superior set) are called the false vocal cords. The inferior set is called the true vocal cords. When the vocal cords are relaxed, they form a triangular space for air passing through to the lungs called the glottis. The larynx is lined with pseudostratified columnar epithelium. The vocal cords are covered by a mucous membrane.

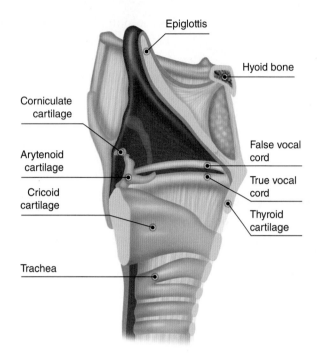

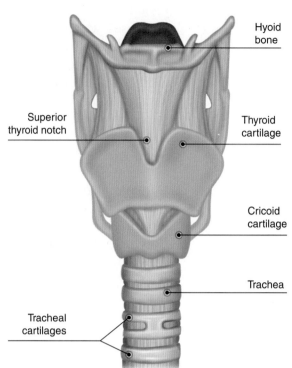

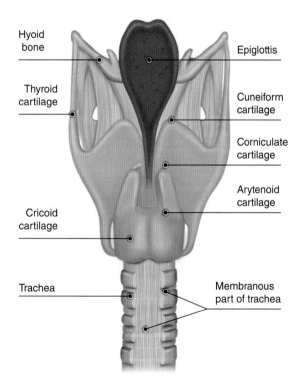

FIGURE 10-4 The larynx.

Different pitches in the voice are produced by vibrations of the vocal cords. Vibration of smaller areas of the vocal cords results in higher pitches. Males typically have longer vocal cords than females, which results in lower pitches.

The Trachea

Air travels from the larynx to the trachea. The trachea is a tubular structure consisting of dense connective tissue and C-shaped rings of hyaline cartilage (Figure 10-6A). The trachea is lined with ciliated pseudostratified columnar epithelium with goblet cells, just like the nasal cavity. The cilia move substances upward toward the larynx and esophagus for swallowing. The 20 C-shaped cartilage rings do not completely encircle the trachea but are open at the posterior side. The posterior section of the trachea also contains a ligament and smooth muscle known as the **trachealis muscle**. The trachealis muscle can contract and constrict the trachea so that air can move through the trachea with more force for coughing or sneezing. The trachea usually ends at about the level of the fifth thoracic segment.

The inferior end of the trachea divides into right and left bronchi at an area known as the carina. The carina is the last tracheal cartilage and forms a cartilage division between the two bronchi.

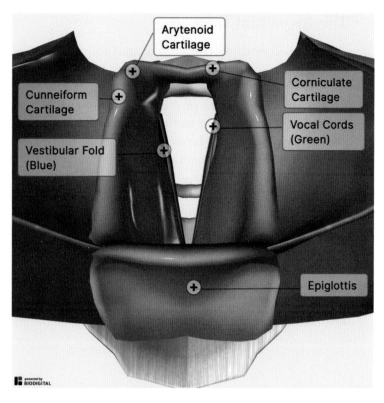

FIGURE 10-5 The vocal cords.

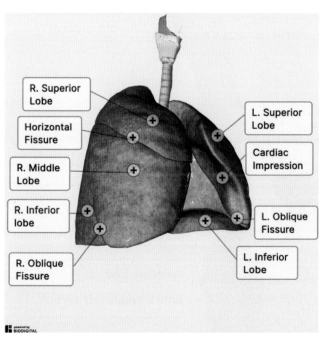

FIGURE 10-6A Lobes and fissures of the lungs.

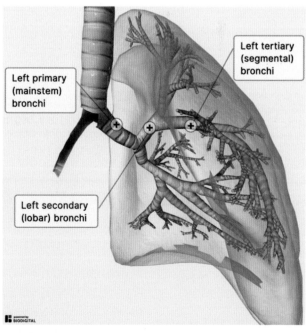

FIGURE 10-6B Primary, secondary, and tertiary divisions of the bronchial tree.

The Bronchial Tree

The trachea ends at the carina and divides into two tubular structures called the right and left primary bronchi. The bronchi then divide into smaller branches called secondary or lobar bronchi and then even smaller branches called tertiary or segmental bronchi (Figure 10-6B). The structure of the bronchi is similar to the trachea with incomplete cartilage rings and smooth muscle. As the bronchi get smaller, there is less cartilage and more smooth muscle until reaching the tertiary bronchi that consists entirely of smooth muscle and epithelium (Figure 10-7). The smooth muscle can constrict and dilate the bronchi to help control the amount of air flowing into the lungs. Constriction and dilation of the bronchi are controlled by the autonomic nervous system. Sympathetic stimulation promotes dilation while parasympathetic stimulation promotes constriction.

The bronchi continue to branch and form small bronchioles that divide to form terminal bronchioles, which mark the end of the air conduction pathway. Smooth muscle begins to disappear as the terminal bronchioles give rise to the respiratory bronchioles. Gas exchange begins at the respiratory bronchioles,

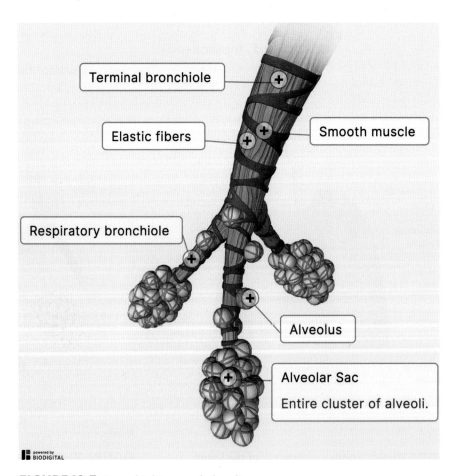

Terminal bronchiole

Elastic fibers

Smooth muscle

Respiratory bronchiole

Alveolus

Alveolar Sac
Entire cluster of alveoli.

powered by
BIODIGITAL

FIGURE 10-7 Bronchial tree and alveoli.

which connect with the alveolar ducts. The alveolar ducts give rise to alveoli. Alveoli are considered the functional unit of the lung and consist of small hollow areas for gas exchange. The alveolar ducts and alveoli are lined with **simple squamous epithelium** that allows for gas exchange. These simple squamous epithelial cells are known as **Type I pneumocytes**. The alveoli also contain other cells known as **Type II pneumocytes**. These cells secrete a substance known as **surfactant** that helps to decrease the surface tension in the alveoli, allowing them to remain open for gas exchange. The lungs contain about 300 million alveoli.

The Lungs

The lungs are two cone-shaped structures residing in the thoracic cavity that are soft, pliable, and spongelike in nature. The inferior portion of each lung reaches to the diaphragm. The superior portion extends about one inch above each clavicle. The right lung contains three lobes (superior, middle, and inferior) and is larger than the left lung, which contains two lobes (superior and inferior). The lobes are separated by fissures. The right lung includes a horizontal and oblique fissure while the left lung only contains an oblique fissure. The medial surface of each lung contains an area known as the hilum where blood vessels, lymphatics, nerves, and bronchi enter and exit. The left lung also contains the **cardiac notch**, which is an indentation for the heart.

The lungs are surrounded by two serous pleural membranes (Figure 10-8). The surface of each lung contains a **visceral pleural membrane** that closely

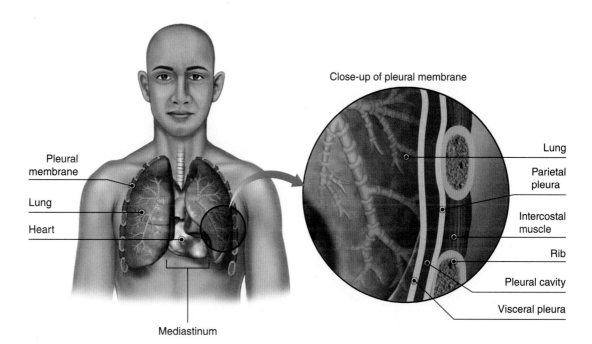

Close-up of pleural membrane

Pleural membrane

Lung

Heart

Mediastinum

Lung

Parietal pleura

Intercostal muscle

Rib

Pleural cavity

Visceral pleura

FIGURE 10-8 Pleural membranes.

adheres to the lung's surface. Lining the interior of the thoracic wall is the **parietal pleural membrane**. The pleural membranes form a space between them that is filled with **pleural fluid**, which helps to reduce friction and holds the membranes together. The pleural membranes form a connection that helps to keep the lungs inflated. Loss of this connection, such as in the case of air entering the pleural space, can cause the lungs to collapse.

CLINICAL TIP	Respiratory sounds can be heard by holding a stethoscope over different parts of the thorax. This is called an auscultation examination.

CLINICAL TIP	The lower lobes of both lungs are more posterior than the other lobes. Auscultation of the lower lobes is performed on the posterior thorax.

UNIT OBJECTIVE 10.2

Describe the mechanism and control of breathing.

UNIT INTRODUCTION

From the moment we take our first breath, and throughout our lives until we take our last, our respiratory systems function to bring oxygen-containing air into our bodies and move carbon dioxide containing air out. This unit examines the mechanism and control of breathing.

LEARNING OBJECTIVE 10.2.1 Define inspiration (inhalation) and expiration (exhalation).

INHALATION AND EXHALATION

When we breath, air enters the lungs during inhalation and exits during exhalation. Air moves into and out of the lungs according to changes in pressure. Air will follow a pressure gradient and move from an area of higher pressure to an area of lower pressure. Inhalation is the movement of air into the lungs by way of creating a lower intrathoracic pressure than atmospheric pressure. Exhalation is the movement of air out of the lungs resulting from a higher intrathoracic pressure than atmospheric pressure.

LEARNING OBJECTIVE 10.2.2 Identify the process of inhalation.

LEARNING OBJECTIVE 10.2.3 Describe the process of inhalation.

KEY TERMS

Boyle's Law Law stating that the pressure of a gas is inversely proportional to its volume.

pectoralis minor Deep muscle in the anterior thorax connecting to the rib cage and scapula.

pleural cavity Space between the visceral and parietal pleural membranes surrounding the lungs.

pulmonary ventilation Movement of air into and out of the lungs.

respiratory cycle Cycle consisting of inhalation and exhalation.

scalene group Group of muscles in the neck.

serratus anterior Muscle located on the lateral rib cage and extending to the anterior portion of the scapula.

sternocleidomastoid Muscle located in the lateral cervical region extending from the mastoid process to the clavicle and sternum.

Process of Inhalation

Inhalation and exhalation depend on changes in lung volume and air pressure. One cycle of inspiration and expiration is called a **respiratory cycle**. The movement of air in and out of the lungs is known as **pulmonary ventilation**. Air moves into the lungs and to the alveoli where oxygen and carbon dioxide diffuse between the alveoli and blood. It is important to maintain good air flow to the alveoli (alveolar ventilation) at all times.

Air is a gas and gases move according to changes in pressure. Gas will move from areas of higher pressure to areas of lower pressure. Pressure in the lungs must be lower than atmospheric pressure for air to move into the lungs.

Expansion of the thoracic cavity causes the lungs to expand because of the **pleural cavity**. The pleural membranes secrete a fluid that forms a bond between the membranes. The force of this bond results in a pressure that is about 4 mm Hg below atmospheric pressure. This intrapleural pressure results from the elastic force of the lungs contracting along with surface tension in the alveoli working to compress the alveoli opposing the force created by expanding the thoracic cavity. If the fluid bond did not exist, the lungs would collapse to about 5% of their normal size.

During inhalation (Figure 10-9), the diaphragm contracts and pulls downward, increasing the volume of the thoracic cavity. The external intercostal muscles also contract and expand the ribcage. The increased volume decreases the pressure inside of the lungs and air flows from higher pressure outside the lungs to lower pressure inside the lungs. Other muscles besides the diaphragm and external intercostals are involved in respiration when greater amounts of air need to be moved into the lungs. Muscles assisting in inhalation include the **sternocleidomastoid**, **serratus anterior**, **pectoralis minor**, and **scalene group**.

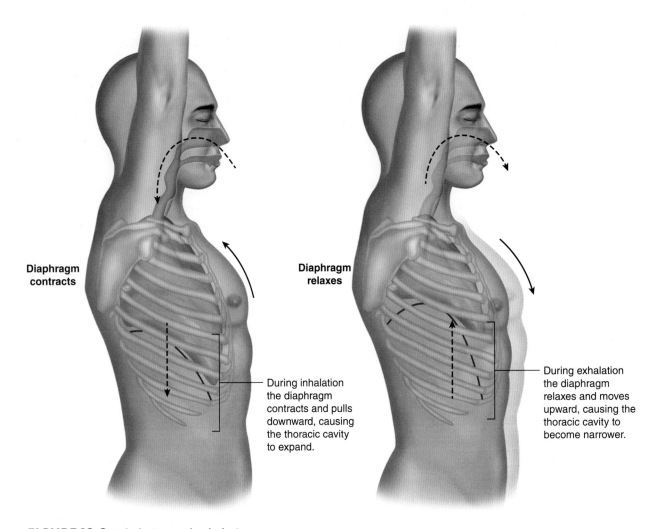

Diaphragm contracts

During inhalation the diaphragm contracts and pulls downward, causing the thoracic cavity to expand.

Diaphragm relaxes

During exhalation the diaphragm relaxes and moves upward, causing the thoracic cavity to become narrower.

FIGURE 10-9 Inhalation and exhalation.

Boyle's Law **Boyle's Law** relates pressure and volume. It can be represented by:

P = 1/V
P = pressure
V = volume

Molecules of a gas will move at random within an enclosed space, producing pressure on the walls of the space. The same amount of gas in a smaller space will exert a greater pressure than when in a larger space. So, increasing the volume will lower the pressure for a given temperature and vice versa. According to Boyle's Law (Figure 10-10), pressure and volume are inversely related. For example, when the lungs expand, the pressure inside of the lungs decreases.

Container A   Container B   Container C

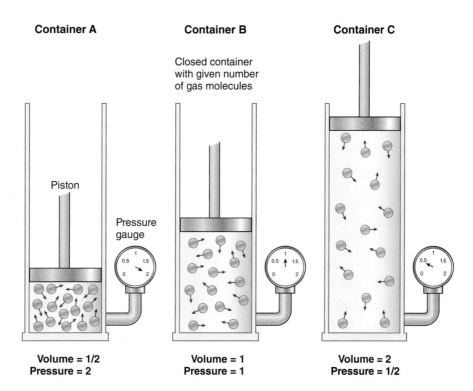

Closed container
with given number
of gas molecules

Piston

Pressure
gauge

Volume = 1/2   Volume = 1   Volume = 2
Pressure = 2   Pressure = 1   Pressure = 1/2

FIGURE 10-10 Each container has the same number of gas molecules. Since the volume of container A is the smallest, we know that the pressure would be the highest. If the gas was transferred to container B, the volume increases so the pressure would drop. The same would be true if we moved the gas to container C, as the volume is even greater than that of A or B. This illustrates the principle in Boyle's law, that pressure and volume are always inversely related; as one increases the other will always decrease.

CLINICAL TIP   Some cases of chronic obstructive pulmonary disease can cause the accessory muscles of inhalation to hypertrophy, causing patients to develop a thick neck and barrel chest.

LEARNING OBJECTIVE 10.2.4 Identify the process of exhalation.

LEARNING OBJECTIVE 10.2.5 Describe the process of exhalation.

KEY TERMS

abdominals Referring to the abdominal musculature.

compliance Pertaining to the elastic property of the lungs; ability of lung tissue to stretch and relax.

emphysema Lung disease characterized by damage to the alveoli resulting in large air pockets.

internal intercostals Deep muscles locate between the ribs that function to pull the ribs together.

surfactant Substance secreted by type II alveolar cells that decreases surface tension in the alveoli.

transverse thoracic Thin muscle located on the inner surface of the anterior thoracic wall.

Process of Exhalation

Compliance represents the lung's ability to expand. The more compliant the lung, the easier it will expand. As the lungs become less compliant, they require more force to expand. The tissue structure of the lungs, flexibility of the thoracic cage, and production of **surfactant** all affect compliance. For example, people with **emphysema** have increased compliance due to the breakdown of lung tissue.

During exhalation (see Figure 10-9), the diaphragm relaxes, decreasing the volume of the thoracic cavity. The elastic fibers of the lungs work to move the lungs back to their original shape and the pressure increases, moving air out of the lungs. Resting exhalation is considered a passive process. Muscles assisting in exhalation include the **internal intercostals**, **transverse thoracic**, and **abdominals**.

LEARNING OBJECTIVE 10.2.6 Define tidal volume, inspiratory reserve volume, expiratory reserve volume, residual volume, vital capacity, and total lung capacity.

KEY TERMS

expiratory reserve volume Lung volume representing the amount of air leaving the lungs during a maximal exhalation in addition to tidal volume.

inspiratory reserve volume Amount of air that enters the lungs during a maximal inhalation in addition to tidal volume.

residual volume Amount of air remaining in the lungs after a maximal exhalation.

spirometer Device used to measure volumes of air entering and exiting the lungs.

tidal volume Amount of air entering or exiting the lungs during resting breathing.

total lung capacity Amount of air residing in the lungs including residual volume.

vital capacity Amount of air entering and exiting the lungs during a maximal inhalation and exhalation; sum of tidal volume, inspiratory reserve volume, and expiratory reserve volume.

RESPIRATORY RATES AND VOLUMES

The normal adult respiratory rate is about 12–18 breaths per minute. For children, the rate is about 18–20 breaths per minute. Respiratory volumes can be measured with a device called a **spirometer**. The spirometer can measure the amount of air entering or exiting the lungs during resting or forceful breathing (Figure 10-11AB).

The volume of air moved into or out of the lungs in a resting inhalation or exhalation is known as **tidal volume** and is about 500 ml.

Inspiratory reserve volume (IRV) is the maximum amount of air that can be inhaled in addition to tidal volume. IRV is usually about 3300 ml in males and 1900 ml in females.

Expiratory reserve volume (ERV) is the maximum amount of air that can be exhaled in addition to tidal volume. ERV is about 1000 ml.

Residual volume (RV) is the amount of air remaining in the lungs after a maximal exhalation. RV is about 1200 ml in males and 1100 ml in females.

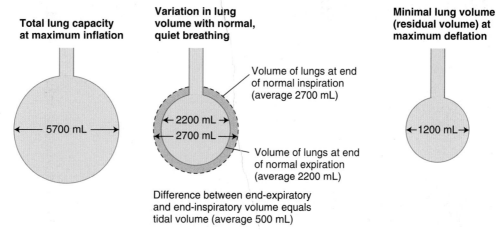

Total lung capacity at maximum inflation

5700 mL

Variation in lung volume with normal, quiet breathing

Volume of lungs at end of normal inspiration (average 2700 mL)

2200 mL
2700 mL

Volume of lungs at end of normal expiration (average 2200 mL)

Difference between end-expiratory and end-inspiratory volume equals tidal volume (average 500 mL)

Minimal lung volume (residual volume) at maximum deflation

1200 mL

(a) Normal range and extremes of lung volume in a healthy young adult male

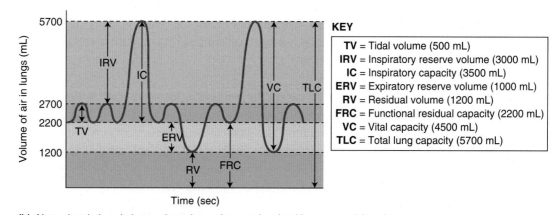

KEY

TV = Tidal volume (500 mL)
IRV = Inspiratory reserve volume (3000 mL)
IC = Inspiratory capacity (3500 mL)
ERV = Expiratory reserve volume (1000 mL)
RV = Residual volume (1200 mL)
FRC = Functional residual capacity (2200 mL)
VC = Vital capacity (4500 mL)
TLC = Total lung capacity (5700 mL)

(b) Normal variations in lung volume in a spirogram in a healthy young adult male

FIGURE 10-11AB Spirometry measures the volume of air entering and exiting the lungs.

Combining respiratory volumes gives us respiratory capacities. These include vital capacity, inspiratory capacity, functional residual capacity, and total lung capacity.

Vital capacity is the maximal amount of air that can move in and out of the lungs in a single breath. It is the sum of tidal volume, inspiratory reserve volume, and expiratory reserve volume. It is about 4800 ml in males and 3400 ml in females.

Total lung capacity is the total volume of air in the lungs. It is the sum of vital capacity and residual volume. It is about 6000 ml in males and 4500 ml in females.

LEARNING OBJECTIVE 10.2.7 Define inspiratory capacity, expiratory capacity, functional residual volume, and dead space.

LEARNING OBJECTIVE 10.2.8 Describe the four respiratory air volumes and the four respiratory air capacities.

RESPIRATORY CAPACITIES

Inspiratory capacity is the amount of air that can move into the lungs after resting inhalation and exhalation. Inspiratory capacity is the sum of tidal volume and inspiratory reserve volume.

Functional residual capacity is the air remaining in the lungs after a resting inhalation and exhalation. Functional residual capacity is the sum of expiratory reserve volume and residual volume. Functional residual capacity helps to keep the lungs inflated after exhalation and acts as a reserve of air available for gas exchange.

Some air enters the lungs but does not contribute to gas exchange. Areas of the respiratory system including the trachea, bronchi, and respiratory bronchioles do not have the gas exchange structures present in the alveoli such as a thin epithelial membrane surrounded by capillaries. The air in these structures is known as anatomical dead space. A very small volume of air does not participate in gas exchange in the alveoli. This tiny volume of air constitutes physiological dead space.

LEARNING OBJECTIVE 10.2.9 Define minute volume and alveolar minute volume.

LEARNING OBJECTIVE 10.2.10 Explain minute volume and alveolar minute volume.

MINUTE VOLUME AND ALVEOLAR MINUTE VOLUME

The amount of air entering or exiting the respiratory tract in one minute is known as the minute volume. The minute volume is a gross measurement of gas volume and does not represent the amount of air reaching the alveoli for gas exchange. This is due to respiratory structures that do not possess a respiratory membrane that allows the movement of oxygen and carbon dioxide. These structures constitute what is known as anatomic dead space. The anatomic dead space must be subtracted from the minute volume in order to determine the **alveolar minute volume**, which is the amount of air reaching the alveoli in one minute.

LEARNING OBJECTIVE 10.2.11 **Explain how minute volume and alveolar minute volume are calculated.**

Calculating Minute Volume and Alveolar Minute Volume

The respiratory minute volume (minute volume) is the amount of air inhaled or exhaled in one minute. We can calculate the minute volume by multiplying the tidal volume by the number of breaths per minute. For example, in a resting adult:

RMV = Breaths/min $\times$ Tidal volume

If breaths/min = 15 and tidal volume = 500 ml

Respiratory minute volume (RMV) = 7500 ml or 7.5 liters

The minute volume indicates how much air has entered the respiratory system. However, not all of the air inhaled reaches the alveoli. This is because of the air in the respiratory passages known as anatomic dead space. To calculate the amount of air reaching the alveoli (alveolar minute volume):

Alveolar minute volume = Breaths per minute $\times$ (Tidal volume $-$ Anatomic dead space)

Anatomic dead space is usually 150 ml.
Example 1: Normal resting breathing

AMV = 12 $\times$ (500 $-$ 150)

AMV = 4200 ml or 4.2L

Example 2: Rapid shallow breathing

AMV = 20 $\times$ (200 $-$ 150)

AMV = 1000 ml or 1.0 L

Can you see that less air reaches the alveoli with rapid shallow breathing than in normal resting breathing?

LEARNING OBJECTIVE 10.2.12 **Define nonrespiratory air movements.**

LEARNING OBJECTIVE 10.2.13 **Identify common nonrespiratory air movements.**

NONRESPIRATORY AIR MOVEMENTS

Besides supplying oxygen and removing carbon dioxide, the respiratory system produces air movements that do not contribute to gas exchange. These are known as nonrespiratory air movements. These air movements are produced by changes in pressure that are caused by contractions of the diaphragm and accessory muscles and closing of the epiglottis.

Nonrespiratory air movements occur every day. For example, speech is produced by forcing air through the larynx, causing the vocal cords to vibrate. We also laugh at things we interpret as funny, and cough and sneeze when we are ill. Other nonrespiratory air movements include singing, whistling, and burping.

LEARNING OBJECTIVE 10.2.14 **Identify the locations of respiratory control in the brain.**

KEY TERMS

limbic system Deep brain region often called the emotional brain that processes emotion, memory, and reward.

medulla oblongata Region of the brainstem that controls respiratory and cardiovascular functions.

neural control centers Groups of neurons located in the pons and medulla oblongata of the brainstem that work to regulate respiration.

phrenic nerve Paired nerves consisting of cervical nerve roots (C3, C4, C5) that innervate the diaphragm.

pons Region of the brainstem regulating breathing, heart rate, blood pressure, hearing, equilibrium, and other functions.

RESPIRATORY CONTROL CENTERS

Breathing is controlled by groups of neurons located in the brainstem that send information to the phrenic nerve, which controls the diaphragm muscle at the base of the thoracic cavity (Figure 10-12). These neural centers monitor substances in the blood including oxygen and carbon dioxide, along with blood pH. Changes in these substances stimulate the neural control centers to increase or decrease the breathing rate based on the metabolic demands of the body.

The pons contains the pontine respiratory group and the pneumotaxic center. The medulla oblongata contains paired groups of neurons in the ventral and dorsal portions. These are called the dorsal and ventral respiratory groups and are collectively known as the medullary respiratory center. Other areas of the brain that influence breathing include the cerebral cortex and limbic system.

LEARNING OBJECTIVE 10.2.15 **Describe the function of the respiratory control centers.**

Function of Respiratory Control Centers

Control of respiration occurs in the brainstem at the respiratory control centers (Figure 10-12). These centers monitor substances in the blood and adjust the respiratory rate to ensure a constant supply of oxygen to the tissues and a blood pH within the normal range of 7.35 to 7.45. The respiratory control centers sense changes in blood P_{O_2}, P_{CO_2}, and hydrogen ion concentration, which directly relate to pH.

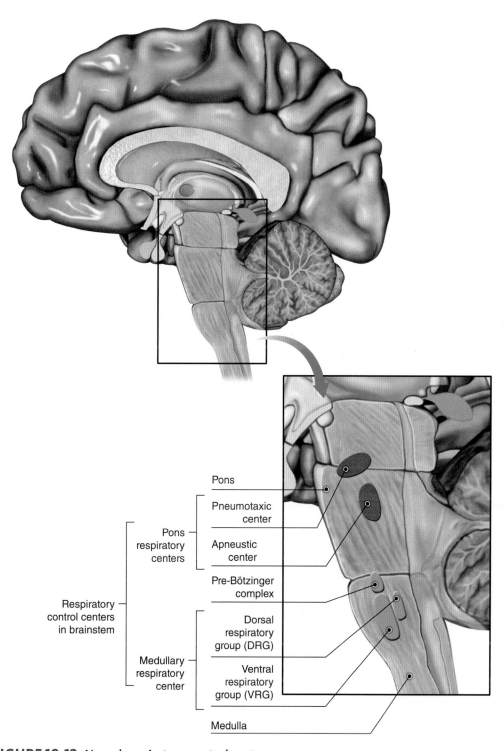

FIGURE 10-12 Neural respiratory control centers.

LEARNING OBJECTIVE 10.2.16 Explain the control mechanisms of normal breathing.

KEY TERMS

aortic body Series of chemoreceptors located in the aortic arch.

apneustic center Respiratory center in the pons portion of the brainstem.

carotid bodies Chemoreceptors located in the carotid arteries near the bifurcation where the common carotid becomes the internal and external carotid arteries.

chemoreceptors Sensory proteins that detect chemicals in bodily fluids; also related to the perception of smell and taste.

dorsal respiratory group Paired group of neurons located in the posterior portion of the medulla oblongata that work to regulate breathing rate and rhythm.

Hering-Breuer reflex Protective reflex in the lungs preventing overinflation by inhibiting neural respiratory centers.

hypercapnia Condition characterized by abnormally high carbon dioxide levels in the blood.

hypocapnia Condition characterized by lower than normal carbon dioxide levels in the blood.

hypoxia Condition characterized by low oxygen levels in the blood.

medullary respiratory center Area in the medulla oblongata that contains the ventral and dorsal groups of neurons that contribute to respiratory control.

pneumotaxic center Neural control center located in the pons that works to inhibit inhalation.

pontine respiratory group Group of respiratory control neuron; also known as the pneumotaxic center.

ventral respiratory group Group of neurons located in the anterior portion of the medulla oblongata that work to control forceful breathing.

MECHANISMS OF NORMAL BREATHING
Neural Control of Breathing

Neural control of respiration begins in the brainstem in the pons and medulla oblongata. The medulla oblongata contains the **medullary respiratory center**. The medullary respiratory center consists of two groups of neurons called the dorsal and ventral respiratory groups (Figure 10-12).

The **dorsal respiratory group** consists of two groups of neurons located in the posterior area of the medulla oblongata. This group is primarily responsible for contraction of the diaphragm for regulation of the breathing rate. The neurons receive input from other parts of the brain and receptors that sense changes in concentrations of gases and pH.

The **ventral respiratory group** stimulates the external and internal intercostals and abdominal muscles. This group is active in forceful breathing.

The pons contains the **pontine respiratory group**. This center works with the centers in the medulla and helps to fine-tune breathing rate and rhythm. The **pneumotaxic center** also receives input from other centers in the brain.

The **apneustic center** also resides in the pons. The pneumotaxic center inhibits the apneustic center to help control exhalation. However, if damage to the brainstem occurs, a patient can exhibit apneustic breathing. This consists of a very slow respiration rate with a deep inhalation held for 10–20 seconds, followed by shallow and brief exhalations that provide little pulmonary ventilation.

All of the above respiratory centers innervate the phrenic and intercostal nerves. The phrenic nerve innervates the diaphragm.

Neural Events of Breathing

For normal resting breathing, the following neural events occur. The dorsal respiratory group becomes active sending a message along the phrenic nerves to contract the diaphragm and external intercostal muscles, causing air to move into the lungs. This is followed by inhibition of the dorsal respiratory group, causing relaxation of the respiratory muscles and passive exhalation.

For forceful breathing, both dorsal and ventral respiratory groups are active, causing the respiratory muscles and accessory muscles to contract. Part of the ventral respiratory group that innervates the muscles of expiration is inhibited, promoting air movement into the lungs. This is followed by inhibition of the dorsal respiratory group while the ventral respiratory group is activated. The muscles of inspiration relax while the muscles of expiration contract, expelling air from the lungs.

Breathing is not entirely unconscious. We can decide to breathe deeply or stop breathing by holding our breath. The cerebral cortex provides connections to the brainstem centers for breathing. The limbic system also affects breathing. For example, strong emotions can speed up breathing.

Sensory Feedback for Breathing

Chemoreceptors sensing changes in concentration of oxygen and pH are involved in controlling respiration. Central chemoreceptors are located in the brain and medulla oblongata. Peripheral chemoreceptors are located in the carotid arteries and aortic arch. The carotid bodies are located in the internal carotid arteries near the bifurcation of the common carotid arteries. The aortic body is located in the arch of the aorta. The carotid bodies connect to the medulla via the glossopharyngeal nerve (CN IX). The aortic body connects to the medulla oblongata via the vagus nerve (CN X).

Peripheral chemoreceptors detect changes in blood oxygen levels. If oxygen levels drop, the peripheral chemoreceptors first become more sensitive to P_{CO_2} and have little effect on respiration. However, if O_2 continues to decrease (below 60 mm Hg), the peripheral chemoreceptors stimulate the neural respiratory centers to increase the breathing rate.

Central chemoreceptors are more sensitive to blood carbon dioxide levels. As P_{CO_2} levels increase, central chemoreceptors stimulate the neural respiratory centers to increase the breathing rate in an attempt to decrease carbon dioxide in the blood.

The medulla oblongata senses changes in pH by way of carbon dioxide diffusion. CO_2 moves across the blood-brain barrier and into the cerebrospinal fluid (CSF). Bicarbonate (HCO_3^-) remains in the blood. This results in an inverse relationship between arterial P_{CO_2} and the pH of CSF. For example, as P_{CO_2} decreases, the pH of CSF increases, which causes the neural respiratory centers to decrease the breathing rate. If P_{CO_2} remains abnormally low for longer periods (a few days), special choroid plexus cells promote the movement of HCO_3^- into CSF. The system essentially resets for different levels of P_{CO2}.

Overall, increased blood levels of carbon dioxide result in an increased rate and depth of breathing. The respiratory centers are very sensitive to changes in P_{CO2}. Small increases in P_{CO2} can cause large increases in respiratory rate. A greater than normal P_{CO2} is called **hypercapnia**, while a lower than normal P_{CO2} is called **hypocapnia**.

Neural respiratory centers are also sensitive to changes in P_{O2}, but changes in P_{CO2} account for the majority of respiratory regulation. If P_{O2} levels decrease while P_{CO2} levels remain normal, there will be a subsequent increase in respiration rate. A lower than normal P_{O2} is called **hypoxia**. Small changes in P_{O2} do not cause an appreciable stimulation of the respiratory centers.

Hering-Breuer Reflex

Another neural control mechanism is the **Hering-Breuer reflex**. This reflex is a protective mechanism and prevents over-inflation of the lungs. Stretch receptors on the walls of the bronchi and bronchioles send impulses to the vagus nerve and to the medulla oblongata during forceful breathing. The impulses inhibit the respiratory centers and produce exhalation.

CLINICAL TIP Spinal cord injuries can affect patients' ability to breathe on their own. Injuries above the C4 or C5 levels can affect the function of the diaphragm and require a ventilator for breathing. Some injuries to thoracic and lumbar spinal levels will affect the function of the accessory muscles of breathing whereby patients will have trouble with coughing and sneezing.

LEARNING OBJECTIVE 10.2.17 **Describe the various factors that influence the rate, depth, and rhythm of breathing.**

KEY TERMS

amygdala Region of the limbic system involved in processing emotion.

chemoreceptors Sensory proteins that detect chemicals in bodily fluids; also related to the perception of smell and taste.

hippocampus Region of the limbic system involved in memory storage.

hyperventilation Increase in breathing rate greater than the normal rate of 12–25 breaths per minute.

hypothalamus Region of the cerebrum that controls body states such as hunger, thirst,

and body temperature and regulates hormone release from the pituitary gland.

hypoventilation Abnormally low breathing rate less than the normal rate of 12–25 breaths per minute.

limbic system Deep brain region often called the emotional brain that processes emotion, memory, and reward.

precentral gyri Gyrus in the frontal lobe just anterior to the central sulcus that processes motor information.

FACTORS THAT INFLUENCE BREATHING RATE, DEPTH, AND RHYTHM

Brainstem

Primary control of breathing occurs in the respiratory centers in the brainstem. These centers rely on feedback from central sensory receptors (**chemoreceptors**) in the brain and brainstem and peripheral chemoreceptors in the aortic body and carotid sinuses. These chemoreceptors monitor blood concentrations of carbon dioxide, oxygen, and hydrogen ions, which directly relate to pH. The respiratory centers respond to feedback by increasing or decreasing the breathing rate by sending impulses to the diaphragm and accessory muscles by way of the phrenic nerve.

Carbon Dioxide and pH Carbon dioxide plays an important role in regulating breathing rate. Carbon dioxide is lipid soluble and capable of moving across the blood-brain barrier by diffusion. Central chemoreceptors are sensitive to changes in carbon dioxide levels in the blood. Increased levels of blood carbon dioxide promote the formation of carbonic acid, which dissociates into bicarbonate and hydrogen ions. Increased hydrogen ion concentration lowers blood pH. The respiratory centers respond to the decrease in pH by increasing breathing rate in an attempt to release carbon dioxide through exhalation and subsequently decrease blood concentration of carbon dioxide.

Oxygen Peripheral chemoreceptors are sensitive to changes in blood oxygen concentration. Most of the oxygen carried is transported in the blood by hemoglobin, but a small amount is dissolved in plasma. The peripheral chemoreceptors are sensitive to the dissolved oxygen, so a large change in oxygen levels is required to initiate a response by the chemoreceptors. If the blood oxygen concentration drops below about 60 mm Hg, the chemoreceptors stimulate the respiratory centers to increase breathing rate.

Cerebral Cortex

The cerebral cortex allows for voluntary control of breathing by overriding the brainstem centers. Humans can consciously increase (**hyperventilation**) or decrease (**hypoventilation**) breathing rate. The voluntary motor cortex located in the **precentral gyri** of the frontal lobes is responsible for conscious control of breathing.

Emotions

The **limbic system** includes the **amygdala**, **hippocampus**, and **hypothalamus** and is important in producing emotional experiences and memory. The limbic system can also affect breathing. For example, emotional states of fear, anxiety, or excitement can increase breathing rate while states of calmness and relaxation can decrease breathing rates.

UNIT OBJECTIVE 10.3

Explain the process of gas exchange and transport.

UNIT INTRODUCTION

Once oxygen-containing air enters our bodies, oxygen needs to get to the tissues so that life-sustaining energy can be produced by the cells. Carbon dioxide, the by-product of energy production, must then be removed by way of the blood and exhaled by the lungs. This unit examines the process of gas exchange and transport.

LEARNING OBJECTIVE 10.3.1 Identify the structure of the respiratory membrane.

LEARNING OBJECTIVE 10.3.2 Describe the structure of the respiratory membrane.

KEY TERMS

alveolar epithelium Tissue lining the inside of the alveolus (simple squamous epithelium).

capillary epithelium Thin tissue lining capillaries consisting of simple squamous epithelium.

respiratory membrane Membrane consisting of the alveolar and capillary membrane in which gas exchange occurs.

THE RESPIRATORY MEMBRANE

The exchange of oxygen and carbon dioxide occurs across the **respiratory membrane**. Air enters the respiratory system and is transported from the upper respiratory system to the trachea, bronchi, bronchioles, and alveoli. Gas is exchanged between the alveoli and surrounding capillaries. The respiratory membrane consists of the alveolar and capillary walls.

The respiratory membrane consists of three layers, including the **alveolar epithelium**, **capillary epithelium**, and the combined basement membranes of both epithelial layers. Simple squamous epithelium lines the alveoli and capillaries. The respiratory membrane is very thin and surrounds each of the 300 million alveoli in the lungs to produce a very large surface area for gas exchange.

LEARNING OBJECTIVE 10.3.3 Identify the function of the respiratory membrane.

LEARNING OBJECTIVE 10.3.4 Explain the function of the respiratory membrane.

diffusion Passive movement of substances from an area of high concentration to lower concentration until reaching equilibrium.

partial pressures Pressure exerted by a single gas in a mixture of gases.

Function of the Respiratory Membrane

Gas exchange occurs at the respiratory membrane. Oxygen and carbon dioxide can readily diffuse across the extremely thin membrane with a large combined surface area. **Diffusion** across the membrane occurs from differences in **partial pressures** of oxygen and carbon dioxide in the alveoli and blood. Oxygen will diffuse from the alveoli to the blood in alveolar capillaries and carbon dioxide diffuses from the blood to the alveoli.

Cells of the alveoli include Type I alveolar cells, Type II alveolar cells, and macrophages. Type I alveolar cells produce the simple squamous epithelium lining the alveoli. Type II alveolar cells are cuboidal epithelial cells that secrete surfactant. Surfactant works to decrease surface tension in the alveoli. Without surfactant, the force created by surface tension would cause the alveoli to collapse. Macrophages work to remove debris from the inner surface of the alveoli.

Alveoli contain tiny pores that allow air to move between alveoli. This helps to equalize pressure throughout the lungs and provides an alternative pathway for air to move into alveoli if bronchioles collapse.

LEARNING OBJECTIVE 10.3.5 Define partial pressure.

LEARNING OBJECTIVE 10.3.6 Describe partial pressure.

Henry's Law Law stating the amount of gas in a liquid is proportional to its partial pressure.

partial pressure gradient Difference in partial pressure on both sides of a membrane.

P_{CO2} Partial pressure of carbon dioxide.

P_{O2} Partial pressure of oxygen.

PARTIAL PRESSURE

Many gases contain more than one individual gas and are considered mixtures of various gases. The mixture of gases exerts a pressure known as the total pressure of the gas. Each gas in the mixture also exerts a pressure known as the partial pressure. The partial pressure then is the pressure an individual gas exerts in a mixture of gases occupying the same volume (Figure 10-13).

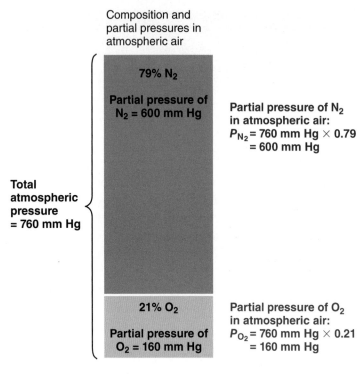

Composition and partial pressures in atmospheric air

79% N₂

Partial pressure of N₂ = 600 mm Hg

Partial pressure of N₂ in atmospheric air:
P_{N_2} = 760 mm Hg × 0.79 = 600 mm Hg

Total atmospheric pressure = 760 mm Hg

21% O₂

Partial pressure of O₂ = 160 mm Hg

Partial pressure of O₂ in atmospheric air:
P_{O_2} = 760 mm Hg × 0.21 = 160 mm Hg

FIGURE 10-13 Partial pressure is the pressure exerted by a gas in a mixture of gases.

The pressure each gas produces in the mixture of gases is known as the partial pressure of the gas. We can represent the partial and total pressure of a gas such as air as follows:

$$P(\text{nitrogen}) + P(\text{oxygen}) + P(\text{water vapor}) + P(\text{carbon dioxide}) = P(\text{air}) = 760 \text{ mm Hg}$$

For example, if oxygen produces 20.9% of the total pressure of air, then 20.9% of 760 mm Hg is about 159 mm Hg. The partial pressure of oxygen is 159 mm Hg. We can denote partial pressure with a capital P preceding the chemical symbol an element such as P_{O_2} or P_{CO_2}.

Partial pressure can be thought to be analogous to concentration. **Henry's Law** states that at a given temperature the amount of gas in a solution is directly proportional to the partial pressure of the gas. Gas, like other substances, follows a gradient, so we can say that gas follows a **partial pressure gradient**. For example, oxygen will move from a P_{O_2} of 100 mm Hg to a P_{O_2} of 80 mm Hg.

LEARNING OBJECTIVE 10.3.7 Explain the role partial pressure plays in the diffusion of gases.

KEY TERMS

emphysema Lung disease characterized by damage to the alveoli resulting in large air pockets.

interstitial space Fluid compartment surrounding cells.

solubility Ability of a substance to dissolve in water.

solubility coefficient Volume of a substance that can be dissolved by a unit volume of solvent at a specified pressure and temperature.

Partial Pressure and Gas Exchange

Air enters the respiratory tract and is warmed and humidified. It eventually reaches the alveoli and mixes with the air resident there. Alveolar air differs from atmospheric air. For example, alveolar air contains more carbon dioxide than atmospheric air.

After reaching the alveoli, gases diffuse across the respiratory membrane and into the surrounding capillaries. The P_{O_2} of alveolar air is about 104 mm Hg and the P_{CO_2} is about 40 mm Hg. The P_{O_2} of deoxygenated blood is about 40 mm Hg and the P_{CO_2} is about 45 mm Hg (Figure 10-14). Oxygen and carbon dioxide both diffuse in opposite directions across the respiratory membrane. Oxygen diffuses from the alveolus to the blood (P_{O_2} of 104 mm Hg to P_{O_2} of 40 mm Hg) and carbon dioxide diffuses from the blood (P_{CO_2} of 45 mm Hg) to the alveolus (P_{CO_2} of 40 mm Hg) (Figure 10-14).

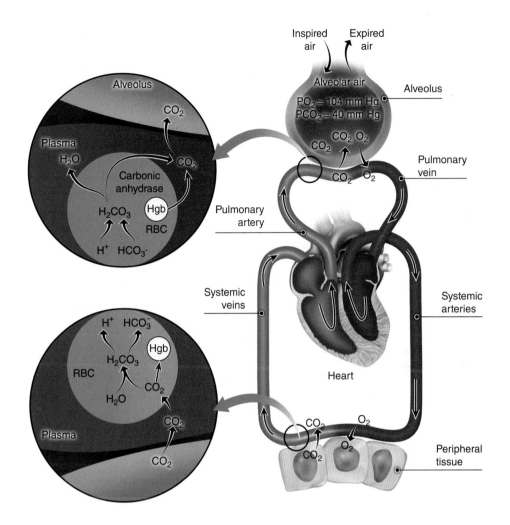

FIGURE 10-14 Movement of oxygen and carbon dioxide between the lungs, blood, and tissues.

Other factors affecting the diffusion of gases include the **solubility**, the size of the concentration gradient, and the surface area and thickness of the respiratory membrane.

The solubility of a gas in liquid is represented by the **solubility coefficient**, which is the amount of gas that can be dissolved in a given amount of solvent under a standard pressure of 1 atmosphere. Substances with higher solubility coefficients will dissolve more readily than those with lower solubility coefficients. For example, the solubility coefficient for oxygen is 0.024 and for carbon dioxide is 0.57. Carbon dioxide is much more soluble (or able to dissolve) in water than oxygen. Both oxygen and carbon dioxide can easily move across the respiratory membrane. Damage to the respiratory membrane affects the diffusion of oxygen before affecting carbon dioxide due to the increased solubility of carbon dioxide. Damage to the respiratory membrane can cause internal oxygen levels to decrease to dangerous levels. Giving supplemental oxygen helps to increase the concentration of oxygen and aid diffusion.

The respiratory membrane's total area is about 70 square meters. Some diseases can adversely affect the respiratory membrane. These include emphysema and lung cancer. **Emphysema** creates large chambers within the lung that decrease the surface area of the respiratory membrane. Lung cancer produces tumors that decrease surface area as well.

Partial pressure and the subsequent pressure gradient can change by increasing or decreasing alveolar ventilation. Breathing slowly and deeply lowers alveolar P_{CO2} as more C_{O2} exits the lungs with each breath.

Oxygenated blood leaves the pulmonary circulation and enters the systemic circulation for distribution to the tissues. The P_{O2} of oxygenated blood is 104 mm Hg and the P_{CO2} is 40 mm Hg in the pulmonary circulation. The oxygenated blood mixes with blood from the bronchial veins, causing the P_{O2} to decrease to 95 mm Hg. Blood leaving the pulmonary circulation and entering the systemic circulation has a P_{O2} of 95 mm Hg.

Oxygenated blood eventually reaches the tissues. The P_{O2} in the **interstitial space** is about 40 mm Hg and decreases to about 20 mm Hg in the cells. Oxygen diffuses down its partial pressure gradient and enters the interstitial space and cells. The blood is now deoxygenated with a P_{O2} of 40 mm Hg.

Carbon dioxide is produced in the cells as a by-product of metabolism. Tissue P_{CO2} is about 46 mm Hg in the cells and about 45 mm Hg in the interstitial space. The P_{CO2} of oxygenated blood is about 40 mm Hg. Carbon dioxide diffuses from the interstitial space to the blood. The resulting P_{CO2} of deoxygenated blood leaving the tissues is then 45 mm Hg.

Deoxygenated blood returns to the lungs where the alveolar P_{CO2} is about 40 mm Hg. Carbon dioxide then diffuses to the alveoli and is expelled with each exhaled breath.

LEARNING OBJECTIVE 10.3.8 **Identify the ways oxygen is transported in the blood.**

LEARNING OBJECTIVE 10.3.9 **Explain how oxygen is transported in the blood.**

KEY TERMS

deoxyhemoglobin Hemoglobin molecule that forms when oxygen is released by hemoglobin.

hemoglobin Protein containing a red pigment that can bind and transport oxygen.

oxyhemoglobin Molecule that forms when oxygen combines with hemoglobin.

OXYGEN TRANSPORT IN THE BLOOD

One of the primary functions of blood is to transport oxygen to the tissues. Red blood cells transport most of the oxygen in blood because they contain hemoglobin, which gives blood its red color. Hemoglobin is a protein molecule consisting of four chains, with each chain containing a heme compound. Oxygen can attach to the heme portion of **hemoglobin**, forming **oxyhemoglobin** and giving blood a bright red color. Under normal circumstances, a small amount of oxygen is dissolved in plasma. However, if P_{O2} were to increase such as in breathing 100% oxygen, or in a hyperbaric chamber, the amount of oxygen dissolved in plasma increases. Henry's Law states that the amount of oxygen dissolved in plasma is proportional to P_{O2}. Each hemoglobin molecule can bind with four oxygen molecules. Hemoglobin releases oxygen to form **deoxyhemoglobin**, giving blood a dull red, sometimes deep purple color. There are almost 300 million hemoglobin molecules in one red blood cell. Hemoglobin can respond to changes in P_{O2}, pH, and temperature.

LEARNING OBJECTIVE 10.3.10 Identify the ways carbon dioxide is transported in the blood.

LEARNING OBJECTIVE 10.3.11 Explain how carbon dioxide is transported in the blood.

KEY TERMS

bicarbonate ion Ionic form of bicarbonate (HCO_3^-).

carbaminohemoglobin Hemoglobin molecule formed by the attachment of carbon dioxide.

carbonic anhydrase Enzyme in red blood cells that promotes the formation of carbonic acid from carbon dioxide and water.

chloride shift Movement of chloride ions into red blood cells as bicarbonate ions exit.

respiratory acidosis Blood pH lower than 7.35 caused by a decrease in breathing rate or inability of the lungs to expel carbon dioxide.

CARBON DIOXIDE TRANSPORT IN THE BLOOD

Carbon dioxide must be carried by the blood from the tissues to the lungs, so it can be expelled from the body during exhalation. Carbon dioxide is transported in the blood by three mechanisms. These include carbon dioxide dissolved in plasma, carbon dioxide combining with hemoglobin, and storage of carbon dioxide by the bicarbonate ion.

About 7% of the total carbon dioxide in blood is dissolved in plasma. Carbon dioxide also combines with hemoglobin to form a compound known as carbaminohemoglobin. About 23% of carbon dioxide is transported as carbaminohemoglobin. The majority of carbon dioxide (about 70%) is transported in the form of bicarbonate ion (Figure 10-15).

$$H_2O + CO_2 \leftrightarrow H_2CO_3 \leftrightarrow H^+ + HCO_3^-$$

Carbon dioxide in the blood combines with water to form carbonic acid. Carbonic acid is a weak acid that dissociates into hydrogen ions and bicarbonate ions. The above reaction also occurs in red blood cells with the addition of the carbonic anhydrase enzyme. Carbon dioxide diffuses into red blood cells and encounters the enzyme carbonic anhydrase to form carbonic acid. Bicarbonate ions diffuse out of the red blood cells into the plasma. In order to maintain ionic stability, chloride ions move into the red blood cell. The movement of chloride ions in exchange for bicarbonate is called the chloride shift.

Chloride ions are transported by facilitated diffusion through membrane transport proteins. If chloride ions were to remain inside the red blood cell, the buildup of negative charges would change the electrical potential of the red blood cell. Hydrogen ions in the red blood cells will bind to hemoglobin.

Both reactions in blood plasma and the red blood cells are reversible with either the storage or release of carbon dioxide. For example, in areas of low P_{CO2} such as in the alveoli, the reaction will work in the direction to release C_{O2} for removal by the lungs. In other words, carbon dioxide is converted from its storage form for release by the lungs. In areas of high P_{CO2} such as in the tissues, the reaction will work in the direction to produce the bicarbonate ion. In other words, carbon dioxide will be stored in the blood for transport to the lungs.

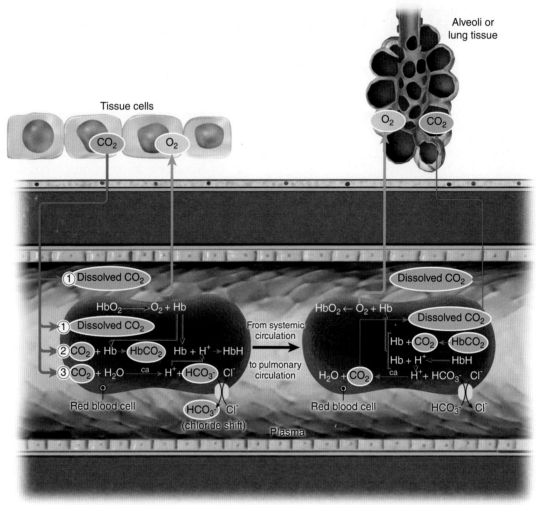

ca = carbonic anhydrase

FIGURE 10-15 Carbon dioxide transport in the blood. Carbon dioxide picked up at the tissue level is transported in the blood to the lungs in three ways: (1) physically dissolved, (2) bound to hemoglobin (Hb), and (3) as bicarbonate ion (HCO_3).

Respiratory Acidosis

Because most of the carbon dioxide is transported by the bicarbonate ion with subsequent release of hydrogen ions, a buildup of carbon dioxide in the blood will produce a lower pH. Carbon dioxide and water combine to form carbonic acid in the blood. Carbonic acid dissociates into bicarbonate and hydrogen ions. If the respiratory system cannot release enough carbon dioxide, the subsequent production of hydrogen ions makes the blood acidic. This is known as **respiratory acidosis** and can result from obstructive diseases such as emphysema or chronic bronchitis. For example, holding your breath can produce an increase in carbon dioxide in the blood. The cells continue to produce carbon dioxide, but the lungs are not removing it through exhalation. Carbon dioxide builds up in the blood producing the hydrogen ion by-product and the blood begins to become more acidic.

Likewise, carbon dioxide in the blood will decrease with hyperventilation. In this case, too much carbon dioxide is removed by the lungs and the hydrogen ion concentration subsequently decreases.

CLINICAL TIP	Respiratory acidosis primarily occurs from a lung disease such as asthma, emphysema, or COPD in which the lungs are not able to expel enough carbon dioxide. Symptoms of respiratory acidosis range from headache and confusion to coma and death.

CLINICAL TIP	Respiratory alkalosis can occur from disorders that increase the breathing rate such as panic disorder, and pulmonary embolism. Symptoms of respiratory alkalosis include anxiety, lightheadedness, and tremors. Respiratory alkalosis can also mimic symptoms of pneumonia.

LEARNING OBJECTIVE 10.3.12 Describe gas exchange in both the pulmonary and systemic circuits.

KEY TERMS

pulmonary circuit System of blood vessels that bring deoxygenated blood from the heart to the lungs for oxygenation and then transport oxygenated blood back to the heart.

systemic circuit System of blood vessels carrying blood from the heart to the body.

GAS EXCHANGE IN THE PULMONARY AND SYSTEMIC CIRCUITS

Oxygen and carbon dioxide move between the blood and tissues in the pulmonary and systemic circuits. The **systemic circuit** brings oxygenated blood to the tissues and returns deoxygenated blood to the heart. The arteries in the systemic circuit contain blood with a higher partial pressure of oxygen (P_{O_2}) than the tissues. When this blood reaches the capillaries in the tissues, oxygen follows its partial pressure gradient and diffuses into the tissues. The tissues also contain a higher P_{CO_2} than the blood, so carbon dioxide follows its partial pressure gradient and diffuses from the tissues to the capillaries. The resulting deoxygenated blood is carried by the venous system to the heart (see Figure 10-14).

The **pulmonary circuit** transports blood from the heart to the lungs for oxygenation and then back to the heart for transport to the body. Oxygen in deoxygenated blood in the pulmonary capillaries in the lungs has a lower partial pressure than inhaled air in the alveoli. This allows for diffusion of oxygen across the respiratory membrane and into the capillaries. Likewise, the partial pressure of carbon dioxide is higher in the capillaries than in the alveoli, allowing for diffusion of carbon dioxide from the blood to the alveoli. The lungs expel carbon dioxide during exhalation.

LEARNING OBJECTIVE 10.3.13 Explain the oxygen-hemoglobin dissociation curve.

KEY TERMS

Bohr effect Changes in hemoglobin's affinity for oxygen binding from changes in pH.

Haldane effect changes in hemoglobin's affinity for carbon dioxide binding from changes in pH.

metabolic demand Referring to the action of cell metabolism.

oxygen-hemoglobin saturation (dissociation) curve Mathematical curve representing the percent saturation of hemoglobin on the vertical axis and the partial pressure of oxygen on the horizontal axis.

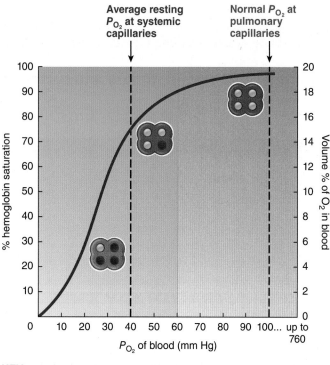

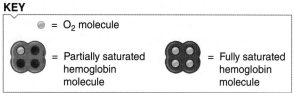

KEY

= O_2 molecule

= Partially saturated hemoglobin molecule

= Fully saturated hemoglobin molecule

FIGURE 10-16 Oxygen-hemoglobin dissociation curve. Hemoglobin increases oxygen binding in areas of higher P_{O_2} and decreases oxygen binding in areas of lower P_{O_2}.

OXYGEN-HEMOGLOBIN DISSOCIATION CURVE

Oxygen Binding to Hemoglobin

The degree of oxygen binding to hemoglobin can be represented by what is known as an **oxygen-hemoglobin saturation (dissociation) curve** (Figure 10-16). If all of the hemoglobin is fully bound with oxygen molecules, then the saturation is 100%.

By examining the saturation curve, we see that in areas of lower P_{O_2}, hemoglobin tends to release oxygen. Hemoglobin decreases its affinity for oxygen binding. Low areas of PO_2 (tissues) require a constant supply of oxygen to the cells. For example, at a P_{O_2} of about 40 mm Hg, hemoglobin is about 75% saturated. This means that about 23% of the oxygen bound to hemoglobin was released. The remaining 75% of oxygen acts like a reserve in case P_{O_2} becomes lower. In the tissues, small changes in P_{O_2} can have a large effect on the release of oxygen. This helps to ensure the tissues receive enough oxygen so they can function properly.

In areas of higher P_{O_2}, we see that hemoglobin is almost completely saturated (about 98%). This means that hemoglobin increases its affinity for oxygen binding. For example, at the alveolar P_{O_2} of 104 mm Hg, we can see that hemoglobin is 98% saturated. Even if P_{O_2} drops to 80 mm Hg we see that hemoglobin is still 95.8% saturated.

Factors Affecting Oxygen and Carbon Dioxide Binding to Hemoglobin

Effects of pH on Hemoglobin Saturation The functional characteristics of hemoglobin can change. Hemoglobin saturation is affected by changes in pH, temperature, and P_{CO_2}.

As pH decreases, more free hydrogen ions bind to hemoglobin and change its function by causing it to release oxygen more readily. We can say that in areas of lower pH, hemoglobin decreases its affinity for oxygen binding. Likewise, in areas of increased pH, hemoglobin will increase its affinity for oxygen binding. This change in binding affinity for oxygen is a result of the **Bohr effect**.

Hemoglobin also changes with respect to carbon dioxide binding at the same time it changes for oxygen binding. As pH decreases, hemoglobin increases its affinity for carbon dioxide binding. Likewise, in areas of increased pH, hemoglobin will decrease its affinity for carbon dioxide binding. These changes in hemoglobin function for carbon dioxide are a result of the **Haldane effect**.

Effects of P_{CO_2} on Hemoglobin Saturation An increase in P_{CO_2} has the same effect as a decrease in pH. Hemoglobin again decreases its affinity for oxygen binding. Release of hydrogen ions and bound carbon dioxide work to produce this effect.

Effects of Temperature on Hemoglobin Saturation Increased temperatures also decrease hemoglobin's affinity for oxygen binding. Hemoglobin works to release oxygen into the tissues during times of increased metabolism such as with exercise or fever.

The changes in hemoglobin's function with decreases in pH, increases in P_{CO_2}, and temperature can be represented by a right shift in the saturation curve. Likewise, in areas of higher pH, lower P_{CO_2}, and decreased temperature, hemoglobin resumes its normal function. We can say the saturation curve shifts to the left of its normal position.

Effects of Exercise on Hemoglobin Saturation For example, exercise will cause an increased **metabolic demand** in the tissues and subsequent need for oxygen supply and removal of carbon dioxide. P_{CO_2} increases in skeletal muscle tissue with a subsequent increase in hydrogen ion concentration resulting in a lower pH. By-products of anaerobic metabolism such as lactic acid also work to decrease pH.

The decrease in pH causes a right shift in the hemoglobin saturation curve. Hemoglobin works to release oxygen in the tissues and pick up carbon dioxide more readily. At the lungs, pH is in the normal range. Hemoglobin then works to release carbon dioxide and bind with oxygen for transport to the tissues. The saturation curve then shifts to the right in skeletal muscle and then back to the left in the lungs.

UNIT OBJECTIVE 10.4

Describe common pathologies affecting the structure and function of the respiratory system.

UNIT INTRODUCTION

A variety of diseases can affect the structure and function of the respiratory system These range from genetic disorder to chronic diseases. This unit examines diseases that affect the respiratory system's structure, which subsequently affects its function.

KEY TERMS

adenocarcinoma Type of lung cancer that forms in glands.

aspiration Inhalation of nonair substances into the trachea.

asthma Disease characterized by constriction of the bronchial air passages resulting in a decrease in airflow into and out of the lungs.

chronic bronchitis Chronic inflammation of the bronchial air passages characterized by a productive cough lasting greater than three months.

cleft palate Genetic condition that results in incomplete closure of the hard or soft palate.

large cell carcinoma A type of lung cancer that accounts for a small portion of lung cancers and originates from epithelial tissue.

laryngitis Condition characterized by inflammation of the larynx.

lung carcinoid Cancerous lung tumor made of cells from the neuroendocrine system.

mononucleosis Contagious disease typically caused by the Epstein-Barr virus that causes swollen lymph nodes and swollen liver or spleen.

nasal polyps Small, noncancerous growths on the inside of the nasal cavity.

nasal septum Bony structure consisting of the perpendicular plate of the ethmoid bone and vomer bone.

neuroendocrine Pertaining to the nervous and endocrine systems.

non-small cell lung cancer Most common type of lung cancer consisting of subtypes including squamous cell carcinoma, adenocarcinoma, and large cell carcinoma.

perpendicular process of the ethmoid bone Bony process of the ethmoid bone extending inferior.

pharyngitis Inflammation of the pharynx.

pleural effusion Fluid buildup in the pleural cavity.

pneumoconiosis Lung disease caused by inhaling toxic substances such as coal dust resulting in lung fibrosis.

pneumonia Lung infection caused by viruses or bacteria characterized by fluid buildup in the lungs.

pulmonary fibrosis Formation of scar tissue in the lungs.

sinusitis Inflammation of the sinuses of the skull.

small cell lung cancer Type of lung cancer originating from neuroendocrine cells that can spread rapidly.

squamous cell carcinoma Type of skin cancer that appears as scaly, red, painful areas that bleed and do not heal and that grow slowly and rarely spread.

COMMON RESPIRATORY SYSTEM PATHOLOGIES AFFECTING STRUCTURE AND FUNCTION

Pathologies of the respiratory system can affect the upper or lower respiratory tracts. Pathologies include infection, inflammation, cancer, and structural deformities. Examples of infectious pathologies include sinusitis, laryngitis, and pharyngitis. Structural deformities include deviated nasal septum, nasal polyps, and cleft palate.

Sinusitis

Sinusitis is an inflammation and swelling of the nasal mucosa (Figure 10-17). Sinusitis can be acute or chronic if it lasts greater than 12 weeks. It can be caused by bacterial or viral infections (common cold), small benign growths in the nasal cavity (nasal polyps) that block drainage of nasal secretions, or deviation of the nasal septum (formed by cartilage and the ethmoid and vomer bones).

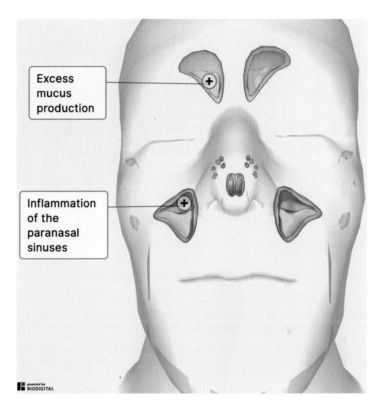

Excess mucus production

Inflammation of the paranasal sinuses

FIGURE 10-17 Sinusitis is an inflammation of the sinuses.

Nasal Polyps

Nasal polyps are small, noncancerous (benign) growths in the nasal cavity (Figure 10-18). These soft structures tend to hang downward in a teardrop configuration and can inhibit air flow and nasal secretions. Nasal polyps are caused by chronic inflammation of the nasal mucosal membrane.

Deviated Nasal Septum

The nasal septum is formed by the **perpendicular process of the ethmoid bone**, vomer bone, and cartilage. It divides the nasal cavity into equal right and left sections. A misaligned or deviated nasal septum is not centered and creates unequal right and left chambers of the nasal cavity (Figure 10-19). This can interfere with air flow through the nasal cavity and can promote infection. A deviated nasal septum can also cause sleep apnea.

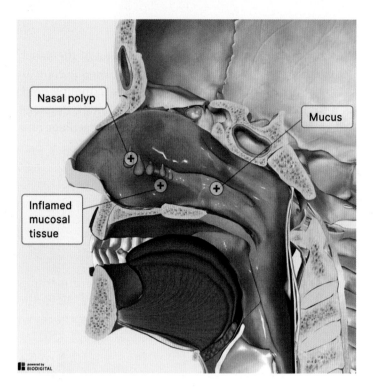

FIGURE 10-18 Nasal polyps.

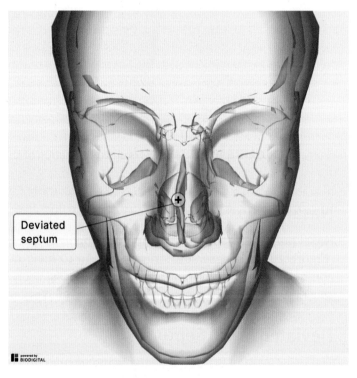

FIGURE 10-19 Deviated nasal septum.

Asthma

Asthma is a disease characterized by chronic inflammation of the air passages. The smooth muscle in the bronchi and bronchioles respond to inflammation by constricting and reducing air flow. Symptoms of asthma include wheezing, coughing, and shortness of breath. The severity of the symptoms can vary from mild to severe and, in some cases, be triggered by exercise. The exact cause of asthma is unknown but is thought to be a combination of genetic and environmental factors, and potentially hygiene. The hygiene hypothesis suggests that asthma results from a decreased exposure to pathogens during childhood. Exposure to pathogens during childhood results in a milder response than in adulthood by triggering the immune system, which develops more resistance to asthma as an adult.

Lung Cancer

Lung cancer is a disease in which the cells of the lung become abnormal and divide frequently to produce a tumor. Lung cancer cells also metastasize or spread to other parts of the body. Most lung cancers fall into two categories: **non-small cell lung cancer** and **small cell lung cancer**. **Lung carcinoid** tumors are a third type of lung cancer. Non-small cell lung cancer is the most common type and consists of subtypes including **squamous cell carcinoma**, **adenocarcinoma**, and **large cell carcinoma**. Adenocarcinomas begin in mucous-secreting cells in the outer margins of the lungs.

Squamous cell carcinoma begins in the squamous epithelial cells lining the inner air passages of the lungs. Large cell carcinoma is a fast-growing cancer that can occur in any part of the lung. Small cell cancer (oat cell cancer) is a fast-growing cancer that is **neuroendocrine** in origin, meaning it begins in nerve and hormone-secreting cells in the lungs. Small cell cancer can also metastasize most often to the brain, bones, and liver. Lung carcinoid tumors are also neuroendocrine tumors that grow in the air passages in the lungs. Lung cancer tumors can multiply and grow, resulting in inhibition of gas exchange.

The number one risk factor for lung cancer is smoking. Smoking includes cigarettes, cigars, pipes, and any tobacco products. Even smoking occasionally or just a few cigarettes a day can increase the risk of lung cancer. Not only does cigarette smoking increase the risk for lung cancer, but it also increases the risk for many other cancers including stomach, colon, liver, pancreatic, laryngeal, renal, urinary bladder, and leukemia. Tobacco smoke contains thousands of toxic chemicals, many of which are directly linked to cancer. Quitting smoking can decrease the risk for cancer, but those who have smoked continue to have a higher risk than those who have not smoked. Secondhand smoke also increases the risk for lung cancer and has been linked to increased respiratory infections, asthma, ear infections, heart disease, and sudden infant death syndrome.

Pneumonia

In **pneumonia**, the lungs become inflamed usually from exposure to a bacterial or viral infection. Pneumonia can also occur from other diseases such as COPD, congestive heart failure, cystic fibrosis, and diabetes and exposure to various fungi and parasites. In some cases, pneumonia results from **aspiration** (inhalation) of a substance such as food, drink, or saliva. In pneumonia, the alveoli can fill with mucous or pus, decreasing the lungs' ability to perform gas exchange. Symptoms of pneumonia can range from mild to life-threatening with the severity depending on the cause and health of the subject.

CLINICAL TIP	Part of a lung examination includes tapping on the thorax, known as percussion. Air-filled spaces will produce a resonant sound while fluid-filled spaces such as in pneumonia produce a dull sound.

Pleural Effusion

Pleural effusion is characterized by fluid buildup in the pleural space (between the visceral and parietal pleura) (Figure 10-20). The excess fluid can occur from congestive heart failure, kidney or liver disease, cancer, and infections. Symptoms vary depending on the severity of the disease and can range from slight chest discomfort to dyspnea (shortness of breath) and pleuritic chest pain, which is a sharp pain that increases during inhalation.

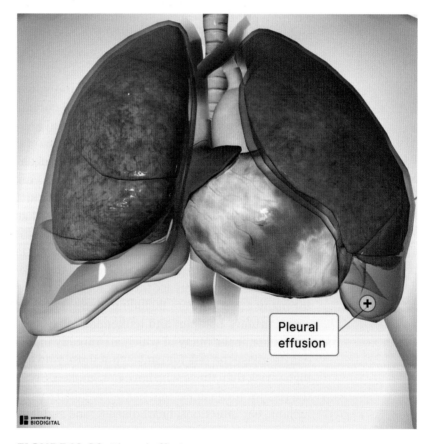

FIGURE 10-20 Pleural effusion.

Pharyngitis

Pharyngitis or sore throat is an inflammation of the pharynx from a bacterial (group A streptococcus) or viral infection. Symptoms include a painful, itchy throat along with fever, headache, nasal congestion, swollen lymph nodes, and fatigue. Pharyngitis from viral causes usually resolves in a few days to a week. However, pharyngitis from mononucleosis can continue for a much longer period. Bacterial pharyngitis can require antibiotic treatment.

Laryngitis

Laryngitis is an inflammation of the larynx, which produces the voice. Laryngitis can be caused by bacterial or viral infections, trauma to the vocal cords, allergies, autoimmune disorders, and gastric reflux. Since the larynx produces the voice, laryngitis can alter the pitch of the voice. Severe laryngitis can be very dangerous due to swelling that can block the airway by obstructing the glottis (opening to the trachea).

Pneumoconiosis

Pneumoconiosis is a term used to describe lung diseases caused by inhaled substances including silicon, asbestos, and coal dust. Pneumoconiosis usually occurs from occupational exposure to these substances. The substances remain in the lungs for long periods of time, resulting in inflammation and scar formation (fibrosis). The extent of the disease depends on the particle size, with smaller particles moving further into the lungs. The severity of pneumoconiosis can vary from no symptoms to life-threatening.

Pulmonary Fibrosis

Pulmonary fibrosis (interstitial lung disease) is characterized by scarring (fibrosis) of lung tissue. Pulmonary fibrosis is caused by exposure to substances such as asbestos, autoimmune disease such as rheumatoid arthritis, and can be idiopathic (no known cause). In pulmonary fibrosis, the healing ability of the lungs is impaired, resulting in formation of fibrotic tissue that decreases lung function. There is no cure for pulmonary fibrosis, but some medications can slow the progress of the disease.

Laryngeal Cancer

Cancer of the larynx most commonly originates in the epithelial tissues (squamous cells). Symptoms include a lump in the throat, hoarseness of the voice, sore throat, wheezing, and difficulty swallowing. The treatment depends on the location and severity of the disease and can include radiation, chemotherapy, and surgery.

LEARNING OBJECTIVE **10.4.2** Describe the cause, signs, symptoms, and diagnosis of a pneumothorax.

KEY TERM

pneumothorax Lung condition whereby air becomes trapped between the pleural membranes of the lungs.

PNEUMOTHORAX

A **pneumothorax** is characterized by the presence of air between the visceral and parietal pleura (pleural space) (Figure 10-21). Pneumothorax can be idiopathic (without apparent cause) or can occur from a traumatic injury or underlying diseases such as asthma, COPD, pneumonia, or tuberculosis. In some cases, a small blister of air called a bleb can rupture and release air into the pleural space, causing a pneumothorax. Air in the pleural space causes loss of the negative pressure that helps to keep the lungs inflated, so collapse of the lung can occur. In a condition known as tension pneumothorax, the air causes an increase in intrathoracic pressure. This buildup of pressure can cause lung collapse that leads to cyanosis and puts pressure on the heart and blood vessels, which can decrease cardiac output. Tension pneumothorax is a life-threatening disorder and requires immediate decompression through insertion of a chest tube.

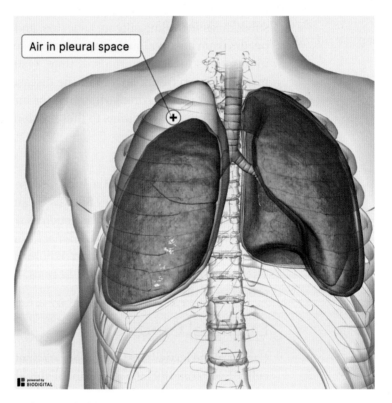

FIGURE 10-21 Pneumothorax.

Signs and Symptoms

Symptoms will depend on the severity of the pneumothorax. These can range from a mild shortness of breath (dyspnea) to severe shortness of breath accompanied by sudden, severe, sharp chest pain. Other symptoms include cyanosis from decreased blood oxygenation, rapid breathing, rapid heart rate (tachycardia), and coughing. Lungs sounds will be absent on the side of the collapsed lung. A tension pneumothorax can cause complete lung collapse and change the position of the heart and major vessels, resulting in a life-threatening situation.

Diagnosis

Diagnosis is based on evaluating the pleural space. A physician will evaluate lung sounds with a stethoscope. Other physical examination signs include a rapid pulse, low blood pressure, and low blood oxygen levels. Imaging studies such as a chest x-ray, CT scan, or ultrasound help to visualize the air and evaluate lung collapse.

LEARNING OBJECTIVE 10.4.3 Describe the cause, signs, symptoms, and diagnosis of pulmonary tuberculosis.

KEY TERM

pulmonary tuberculosis Disease caused by a bacterium (*Mycobacterium tuberculosis*) that produces an infection with a chronic cough containing bloody sputum.

PULMONARY TUBERCULOSIS

Pulmonary tuberculosis (TB) is a disease caused by the bacterium *Mycobacterium tuberculosis*. TB primarily attacks the lungs and can also spread to other parts of the body such as the brain, kidneys, and spine. Exposure to the bacterium can occur from water droplets expelled from an infected person by coughing or sneezing. The bacterium can remain dormant in latent tuberculosis. Latent tuberculosis is not contagious but can eventually develop into an active form. Active tuberculosis causes symptoms and is contagious.

In many cases, patients experience an initial exposure to tuberculosis (primary tuberculosis) followed by a dormant period in which the virus is encapsulated by immune system cells forming granulomas. The bacterium in a granuloma can survive for years and cause an active (post-primary) infection. A depressed or compromised immune system can often lead to active tuberculosis infection. Examples of diseases and conditions that can lead to a depressed or compromised immune system are HIV/AIDS, organ and/or tissue transplants, and other chronic infections.

Signs and Symptoms

Tuberculosis can cause the following symptoms:

Persistent sputum-producing cough that lasts several weeks
Hemoptysis
Fatigue, fever, and weight loss
Pain with breathing
Excessive night sweats

Diagnosis

Diagnosing tuberculosis centers on evaluating the lungs and identifying the *Mycobacterium tuberculosis* bacterium. Presence of the bacterium can be determined by using a skin test in which a small amount of purified protein derivative tuberculin is injected intradermally. Formation of a red, raised bump indicates a positive test and the presence of the bacterium. The test is not 100% reliable and false positives can occur when a patient has been vaccinated using the bacillus Calmette-Guerin vaccine. This vaccine is used in countries with a high tuberculosis infection rate. Physicians may also perform a chest x-ray to look for granulomas and damaged lung tissue. Sputum cultures testing for acid-fast bacilli may also be used to help diagnose the disease.

UNIT OBJECTIVE 10.5

Describe common pathologies affecting the mechanism and control of breathing.

UNIT INTRODUCTION

Some diseases affect the structures that control respiratory function, such as the parts of the nervous system that control breathing. This unit examines common pathologies that affect the mechanism and control of breathing.

LEARNING OBJECTIVE 10.5.1 Identify common pathologies affecting the mechanism and control of breathing.

KEY TERMS

cerebrovascular accident The sudden death of neurons and neuroglia in the brain due to a lack of blood supply to the region. Also known as a stroke.

embolism Condition resulting from material (e.g., clot, lipid, gas) lodged in a blood vessel.

multiple sclerosis A presumptive autoimmune disorder resulting in breakdown of the myelinproducing cells of the brain and spinal cord.

myelin Wrapping of glial cell membrane around an axon that acts to speed up conduction of action potentials.

COMMON PATHOLOGIES AFFECTING THE MECHANISM AND CONTROL OF BREATHING

Some common pathologies affecting the control of breathing include spinal cord injury, multiple sclerosis, and cerebrovascular accident.

Spinal Cord Injury

Damage to the spinal cord from trauma, tumors, or multiple sclerosis can affect breathing. Spinal cord trauma to the cervical spine in the area of the C3, C4, and C5 spinal segments can result in the inability of the nervous system to send impulses to the diaphragm and breathing muscles, causing a loss of breathing function.

Multiple Sclerosis

Multiple sclerosis is an immune disease that results in damage to myelin in the nervous system cells. Myelin helps to conduct nervous system impulses between the nervous system and muscles, organs, or glands. Damage to myelin can impede the signals from the nervous system to respiratory muscles, resulting in weakness that can cause respiratory problems such as lung infections, aspiration, and respiratory failure.

Cerebrovascular Accident

A cerebrovascular accident (CVA) affecting the brainstem occurs when a blockage such as an embolism or ruptured blood vessels hemorrhages in the pons and medulla. The pons and medulla contain the respiratory control centers, which can be affected by a CVA. The severity of symptoms depends on the areas of the brainstem involved and the extent of cell damage and can range from mild temporary symptoms to coma and death.

LEARNING OBJECTIVE 10.5.2 Explain how head trauma can affect the rate, depth, and rhythm of breathing.

KEY TERMS

carbon monoxide poisoning Condition that occurs when carbon monoxide builds up in the blood from inhalation of carbon monoxide.

Cheyne-Stokes breathing Abnormal breathing pattern characterized by cycles of deep and shallow breathing.

hyponatremia Condition characterized by abnormally low sodium levels in the blood (lower than 136 meq/L).

tachypnea Rapid breathing greater than 20 breaths per minute.

traumatic brain injury Injury to nervous tissues of the brain resulting from head trauma.

TRAUMATIC BRAIN INJURY AND THE RESPIRATORY SYSTEM

A force to the head (blow, jolt, bump) can cause an injury to the brain and brainstem known as a traumatic brain injury (TBI). TBI can affect the respiratory centers in the brainstem and cause alterations in breathing rate, depth, and rhythm.

TBI can result in abnormal breathing patterns including irregular breathing, periodic breathing, and tachypnea (increased breathing rate). A TBI affecting the pons and medulla oblongata is associated with irregular breathing. An abnormal breathing pattern, known a Cheyne-Stokes breathing, can occur from increased intracranial pressure resulting from TBI.

Cheyne-Stokes breathing is characterized by a repeating cyclical pattern of fast and deep breathing that becomes shallow and stops producing periods of apnea. The pattern lasts from 30 seconds to 2 minutes and repeats continuously. Cheyne-Stokes breathing can also occur in patients experiencing congestive heart failure, hyponatremia (low blood sodium), and carbon monoxide poisoning.

KEY TERMS

apnea Stopped breathing.

hypertension High blood pressure as indicated by a systolic pressure greater than 130/80 mm Hg.

impotence Inability of a male to achieve an erection.

insomnia Inability to sleep.

polysomnogram Sleep study in which physiological processes such as blood oxygen levels, brain waves, pulse, and breathing are monitored during sleep.

SLEEP APNEA

Sleep apnea is a disorder characterized by periods of **apnea** (stopped breathing) during sleep. Sleep apnea can be caused by obstructions in the upper air passages of the respiratory system, most commonly the tissues in the back of the throat. Sleep apnea can also be caused by disorders affecting the central nervous system and respiratory centers that result in the inability to send impulses to the diaphragm to control breathing. Patients suffering from sleep apnea can stop breathing hundreds of times per night, with each period lasting up to a minute or longer. Sleep apnea is more prevalent in males than in females. It can eventually cause **hypertension**, cardiovascular disease, weight gain, **impotence**, and problems with memory.

There are three primary types of sleep apnea: obstructive, central, and complex. In obstructive sleep apnea, the muscles of the throat relax and obstruct the airway. In central sleep apnea, the respiratory control center fails to communicate with the breathing muscles. Complex sleep apnea is a combination of obstructive and central sleep apneas. Sleep apnea can be caused by structural problems such as large tonsils, large tongue, small jaw, large neck, and large overbite. It can also be caused by smoking, obesity, and age.

Signs and Symptoms

Conditions associated with sleep apnea include obesity, daytime sleepiness, waking with a sore throat or dry mouth, and morning headaches.

Other signs and symptoms of sleep apnea include loud snoring and **insomnia**.

Diagnosis

Physicians may perform a sleep study test known as a **polysomnogram**. These tests can be performed in a sleep center or at home. Patients are connected to equipment to monitor physiology during sleep by technicians. The equipment monitors heart and breathing rates, movements, and blood oxygen levels. Patients may also be given a home test that includes a small monitor that measures breathing, heart rate, and blood oxygen levels.

During a polysomnogram, the total sleep time, sleep efficiency, sleep latency, sleep stages, arousals, and awakenings are recorded. Sleep efficiency is the total sleep time divided by the total recording time. Patients with sleep apnea awaken repeatedly throughout the night and have poor sleep efficiency. Sleep latency is the amount of time it takes to fall asleep. In normal individuals this is about 15 minutes but in sleep-deprived individuals, it can be shorter. The sleep stages are determined by examining brain wave activity and range from light to deep sleep. Arousals and awakenings are periods in which sleep is interrupted and are followed by lighter stages of sleep. The test also measures how many times a patient will stop breathing (apnea) during the test.

UNIT OBJECTIVE 10.6

Describe common pathologies affecting gas exchange and transport.

UNIT INTRODUCTION

Once air enters the respiratory system, oxygen and carbon dioxide must be transported by the blood to the tissues and back. Some diseases interfere with this process. This unit examines common pathologies affecting gas exchange and transport.

LEARNING OBJECTIVE 10.6.1 Identify common disorders that affect the process of gas exchange and transport.

KEY TERM

granulomas Small mass of inflamed tissue that is granular in appearance.

COMMON DISORDERS AFFECTING GAS EXCHANGE AND TRANSPORT

Disorders affecting gas exchange include chronic obstructive pulmonary disease, pulmonary fibrosis, lung cancer, pneumonia, asthma, pneumoconiosis, and pulmonary tuberculosis.

Chronic obstructive pulmonary disease can result in decreased gas exchange due to decreased ventilation and a decrease in the alveolar surface area available for gas exchange, which results from emphysema. Pulmonary tuberculosis and fibrosis also produce space-occupying lesions or exudate that reduce the capability for gas exchange across the respiratory membrane.

Tuberculosis is a disease in which a bacterium produces tumorous structures called **granulomas** in the lungs. TB can also cause the formation of scar tissue in the lungs. The granulomas can open, releasing the bacteria that causes scar tissue formation and inflammation. The alveoli can break apart, resulting in a decrease in surface area for gas exchange.

LEARNING OBJECTIVE **10.6.2** **Describe the cause, signs, symptoms, and diagnosis of chronic obstructive pulmonary disease.**

KEY TERMS

asbestos Silicate substance that acts as a carcinogen in lung tissue.

barrel chest Thoracic deformity produced in chronic obstructive pulmonary disease from the hypertrophy of respiratory muscles.

chronic bronchitis Chronic inflammation of the bronchial air passages characterized by a productive cough lasting greater than three months.

chronic obstructive pulmonary disease (COPD) Chronic lung disease that includes chronic bronchitis and emphysema.

cor pulmonale Enlargement of the right side of the heart occurring from lung disease.

emphysema Lung disease characterized by damage to the alveoli resulting in large air pockets.

forced expiratory volume Test performed with a spirometer in which a subject performs a maximal exhalation directly after a maximal inhalation as quickly as possible.

forced vital capacity Amount of air measured by a forced expiratory volume test.

silica dust Dust occurring from working with materials containing silica such as quartz.

CHRONIC OBSTRUCTIVE PULMONARY DISEASE

Chronic obstructive pulmonary disease (COPD) is a combination of diseases including chronic bronchitis and emphysema. In chronic bronchitis, the bronchi and bronchioles become inflamed, causing increased mucous production and bronchoconstriction that can impede ventilation. Emphysema is characterized by damage to the alveoli, which break apart and form large spaces. This creates a smaller surface area for gas exchange. COPD is a progressive disease and is usually caused by long-term exposure to substances that irritate lung tissue such as cigarette smoke or occupational substances such as asbestos and silica dust.

Diagnostic tests used to confirm COPD include spirometry, chest x-ray, CT, and blood tests. Spirometry measures volumes of air entering or exiting the lungs. Measurements used to diagnose COPD include forced expiratory volume in one second (FEV1) and forced vital capacity (FVC). Forced expiratory volume is the volume of air that exits the lungs during one second of maximal exhalation. Forced vital capacity is the amount of air entering and exiting the lungs during a maximal inhalation and exhalation. FEV1 and FVC are decreased in obstructive diseases due to the decrease in air flow. The FEV1/FVC ratio can be used to help diagnose COPD. In normal individuals, the FEV1/FVC ratio is between 70 and 85%, depending on age. Patients with COPD exhibit ratios lower than the lower normal limit.

A chest x-ray and CT can visualize signs of COPD, and blood testing can indicate low oxygen content in arterial blood.

| **CLINICAL TIP** | Patients with COPD will often assume a position of leaning forward with their hands on their knees (tripod position) when sitting and breathe through pursed lips. |

Chronic Bronchitis

Chronic bronchitis is characterized by long-term inflammation of the bronchial tree that results in increased mucous production. Patients with chronic bronchitis have a productive cough. Chronic bronchitis can result in thickening of the mucous membrane and dilation of the bronchi (bronchiectasis). Progression of the disease results in obstruction of the bronchi and bronchioles, which decreases air flow into the lungs. Along with the chronic cough, patients may experience difficulty breathing (dyspnea), low blood oxygen levels (hypoxia), and high blood carbon dioxide levels (hypercapnia). As the disease progresses, the damaged lungs can cause edema and right-sided heart failure (**cor pulmonale**), which can eventually be fatal.

Emphysema

Emphysema is characterized by increased mucous production in the alveoli. The mucous causes air to become trapped, resulting in inflation and eventual destruction of the alveoli. As the alveolar membrane breaks apart, the alveoli fuse with adjacent alveoli, creating large spaces that can trap more air. The area for gas exchange decreases, which decreases oxygenation of the blood. Patients with emphysema can get air into the lungs, but due to the trapped air in the alveoli, they struggle to exhale. As patients struggle to exhale, the increased activity of the respiratory muscles can lead to hypertrophy and formation of a **"barrel chest"** (Figure 10-22). Weight loss can occur from the amount of energy expended in order to breathe. Symptoms of emphysema include coughing, wheezing, dyspnea, and hypoxia due to the decreased gas exchange. As the disease advances, it can cause increased resistance to blood flow in the lungs. This causes increased blood pressure in the pulmonary arteries and can lead to right-sided heart failure (cor pulmonale).

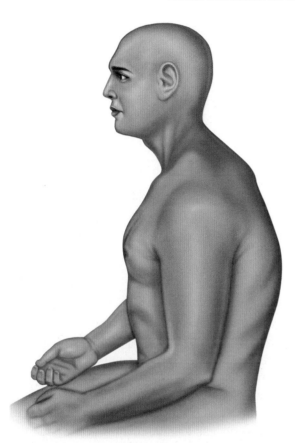

FIGURE 10-22 Patients with emphysema can exhibit a barrel chest and breathe through pursed lips.

CLINICAL TIP	Patients with chronic bronchitis are often referred to a "blue bloaters" due to cyanosis and edema while patients with emphysema are referred to as "pink puffers" due to minimal cyanosis and breathing with pursed lips.

LEARNING OBJECTIVE **10.6.3** **Describe the cause, signs, symptoms, and diagnosis of cystic fibrosis.**

CYSTIC FIBROSIS

Cystic fibrosis (CF) is a disease of genetic origin. CF is an **autosomal recessive** condition caused by mutations of the **cystic fibrosis transmembrane conductance regulator** gene. The defective gene affects chloride transport in cells that create thick mucus secretions that block ducts and air passages in the lungs.

Signs and Symptoms

Signs and symptoms of CF result from the thick mucus causing infections and blocking passageways in organs. Patients with CF have very salty skin due to excess chloride excretion from sweat glands and exhibit difficulty breathing, productive cough, shortness of breath, and frequent sinus and lung infections. CF is sometimes identified by parents discovering that their baby's skin has a salty taste after kissing the child. Besides lung impairment, the disease causes the blockage of **pancreatic ducts**, which can inhibit secretion of digestive substances and cause damage to the pancreas. This can lead to inflammation of the pancreas (**pancreatitis**), or **malabsorption** from a lack of pancreatic enzymes needed for digestion. In a majority of cases, males with CF are also infertile due to a genetic absence of the vas deferens, which carries sperm from the epididymis to the ejaculatory duct. Patients with CF can also exhibit clubbing or enlargement of the fingers and toes, which occurs in a number of respiratory disorders.

Diagnosis

Diagnosis of CF centers on identifying the defective gene, mucous analysis, and levels of a pancreatic substance (**immunoreactive trypsinogen**). Identification of the defective genes can be done by prenatal genetic testing. After birth, infants can be tested with a **sweat chloride test** that measures the amount of chloride in the baby's sweat. The test is performed by wiping a small amount of medication on the baby's skin to stimulate the sweat glands followed by collection of the sweat. The sweat is then analyzed for a high chloride level. Newborns can also be screened through a blood test that examines levels of an immunoreactive trypsinogen, which tends to be high in CF.

Chapter 11

The Lymphatic System

Chapter Introduction

The lymphatic system could be mistaken for a subdivision of the cardiovascular system, as it plays a very important role in returning fluids to the cardiovascular system. Aside from helping fluids and small solutes return to the cardiovascular system, the lymphatic system transports lipids from the site of absorption in the GI system back to the bloodstream and assists the immune system in the defense of our body against disease.

UNIT OBJECTIVE 11.1

Identify the structural components and functions of the lymphatic system.

UNIT INTRODUCTION

As we progress through this unit, we explore the structure of the lymphatic system, how this structure impacts the physiological actions of the system, and how it interacts with other organ systems. Lymphatic vessels are structurally very similar to veins, as they have thin walls, contain valves, and carry fluid under low pressure. As they carry this fluid back toward the heart, they have a similar function to veins. However, you will discover as we move through this unit that the lymphatic system has other important functions as well. The vessels and organs comprising the lymphatic system are seen in Figure 11-1.

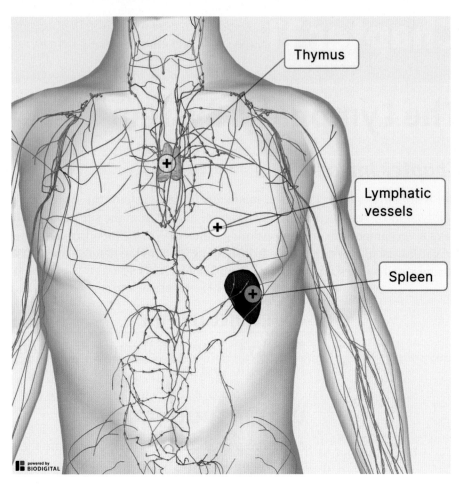

FIGURE 11-1 Vessels and organs of the lymphatic system.

LEARNING OBJECTIVE 11.1.1 Identify the functions of the lymphatic system.

LEARNING OBJECTIVE 11.1.2 Explain the role of the lymphatic system in transporting excess interstitial fluid back to the circulatory system.

KEY TERMS

colloid Substance that is dispersed evenly throughout another substance.

edema Localized area of excess fluid.

immunity Body's ability to defend itself.

interstitial fluid Fluid found in interstitial spaces (space between cells).

osmotic Liquid that has the tendency to absorb through a semipermeable structure or membrane.

FUNCTIONS OF THE LYMPHATIC SYSTEM

The lymphatic system is a collection of cells and biochemicals that travel through lymphatic vessels and the organs and glands that produce them. The lymphatic network, which assists in circulating body fluids, is closely associated with the cardiovascular system. The lymphatic system performs three vital functions in the body: return of excess interstitial fluid to the bloodstream, absorption of fats from the gastrointestinal tract, and defending against disease. Without the lymphatic system returning excess interstitial fluid back to the cardiovascular system, tissues throughout the body would become edematous and systemic blood pressure would fall. The lymphatic system is also the primary means of transporting lipids from where they are absorbed in the intestinal tract to where they are processed. The immune system is also closely linked with the lymphatic system, as many of the cells and structures that are part of the lymphatic system also provide both defense against disease and immunity against future infection.

Return of Excess Interstitial Fluid to the Cardiovascular System

The hydrostatic pressure in a blood capillary filters water and small molecules from the plasma into the interstitial space. This plasma-like fluid, known as interstitial fluid, contains nutrients, gases, small proteins, and hormones, but does not include plasma proteins as they are too large to pass through the openings in the capillary walls. The plasma proteins remaining within the blood vessel create an osmotic effect, known as the plasma colloid osmotic pressure. The osmotic pressure of these proteins helps to draw some of the fluid that was filtered back into the blood capillaries. Even though the pressure gradient of the plasma proteins in the capillaries favors water reabsorption, roughly 25% of the filtered fluid remains in the interstitial spaces. Lymphatic capillaries absorb this excess fluid in the interstitial spaces and transport it back to the bloodstream. If the lymphatic system did not exist, the excess fluid that could not be reabsorbed by blood capillaries would cause localized tissue swelling, which is known as edema. This resulting edema can be seen in Figure 11-2.

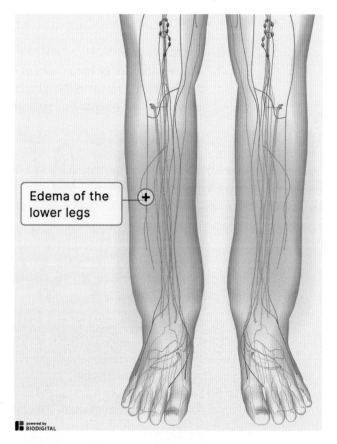

Edema of the lower legs

FIGURE 11-2 Peripheral edema of the legs.

LEARNING OBJECTIVE **11.1.3** Explain the role of the lymphatic system in transporting lipids absorbed from the GI tract.

KEY TERMS

chylomicrons Protein and fat globules found in lymph and blood.

cisterna chyli Enlarged sac in the abdomen that eventually leads to the thoracic duct.

endoplasmic reticula Network of tubes within the cytoplasm of the cell with a role in synthesizing proteins and lipids.

fatty acid molecules Fat molecules that are digested in the small intestines.

lacteals Vessels in the small intestine that are part of the lymphatic system.

lipoprotein Molecules that contain lipids and proteins.

villi Projections or small, finger-like structures located on the plicae circulares of the small intestine to promote the absorption of digested food; a villus is composed of numerous microvilli which are used for increasing the surface area of the wall of the intestine.

Transportation of Lipids

Enzymes from the pancreas and intestinal mucosa help to digest fat molecules in the small intestine. The resulting fatty acid molecules that remain after digestion are absorbed through the wall of the small intestines and into the specialized lymphatic capillaries through the following steps:

1. The **fatty acid molecules** dissolve in the epithelial cell membranes of the intestinal **villi** and diffuse through the villi.
2. The **endoplasmic reticula** of the cells use the fatty acids and synthesize them into fat molecules, very similar to those previously digested.
3. These fats gather into clusters that become encased by protein.
4. The resulting large molecules of **lipoprotein** are called **chylomicrons**, and they make their way to the lymphatic **lacteals** (Figure 11-3). These lacteals are specialized lymphatic capillaries found in the villi of the small intestine.

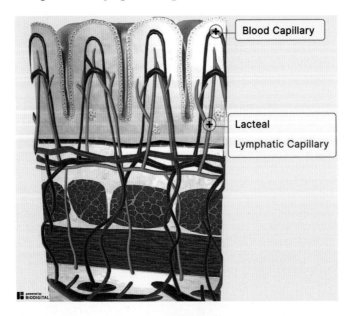

FIGURE 11-3 Lacteal (lymphatic capillary) of the gastrointestinal system.

5. Smooth muscle contractions in the villi help to empty the lacteals into the **cisterna chyli**, which is an enlargement of the thoracic duct. The lymph then carries the chylomicrons to the bloodstream, where the fats are transported to muscle and adipose cells.

LEARNING OBJECTIVE 11.1.4 **List the structures lymph fluid flows through from capillaries to venous circulation.**

KEY TERM

lymphatic trunks Vessels that lead to larger lymphatic structures.

PATH OF LYMPHATIC FLOW THROUGH THE BODY

The lymphatic system is a network of vessels that transport excess interstitial fluid and lipids to the subclavian veins of the thorax. Lymphatic capillaries are blind-ended and join together and form lymphatic vessels. The vessels lead to larger lymphatic structures, called **lymphatic trunks**, which have ducts that join the veins in the thorax (Figure 11-4). Interspersed along these vessels are lymph nodes, whose structure and function we discuss shortly.

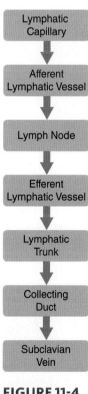

FIGURE 11-4
Path of lymph fluid flow through the lymphatic system.

LEARNING OBJECTIVE 11.1.5 Identify the structure of a lymphatic vessel.

LEARNING OBJECTIVE 11.1.6 Describe the structure of a lymphatic vessel.

KEY TERMS

anchoring filaments Structure in skin containing elastic fibers that have a role in fluid movement throughout the body.

viscera Organs in cavities of the body.

STRUCTURE OF LYMPHATIC VESSELS

Lymphatic vessels are very much like those of veins, but have thinner walls and contain lymph nodes at intervals along their length. Lymphatic vessels of the skin travel in loose subcutaneous tissue and generally follow veins. Lymphatic vessels of the **viscera** usually follow arteries, forming units around them. Each lymphatic vessel has three layers: an endothelial lining, a middle layer of smooth muscle and elastic fibers, and an outer layer of connective tissue (Figure 11-5). The epithelial surfaces of the lymphatic walls are attached to surrounding connective tissue by thin protein filaments called **anchoring filaments**. When edema has occurred in the tissues, the swelling pulls on the anchoring filaments that make the openings between the cells even larger so that more fluid can flow into the lymph capillaries to try to compensate for the edema. Because lymph is transported at low pressure, lymphatic vessels have semilunar valves similar to those of veins to prevent the backflow of lymph. The larger lymphatic vessels lead to lymph nodes, which are specialized organs. The vessels merge into larger lymphatic trunks after leaving the lymph nodes and eventually deliver their lymph into two main channels, the thoracic duct and the right lymphatic duct.

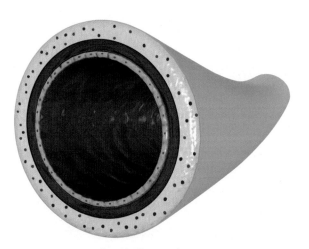

Lymphatic vessel

FIGURE 11-5 Structure of a lymphatic vessel.

Lymphatic Capillaries

Lymphatic capillaries are microscopic, closed-ended tubes (Figure 11-3). These capillaries extend into the interstitial spaces, forming a network that parallels the blood capillaries in the body. Just as the walls of blood capillaries are a single layer of squamous epithelial cells, so are the lymphatic vessels. This single layer of cells is called endothelium. These thin walls allow tissue fluid (interstitial fluid) from the interstitial space to enter the lymphatic capillaries. Once the interstitial fluid has entered the lymphatic capillaries, it is called lymph. The lymphatic capillaries join together to form lymph vessels.

Normally, more fluid leaves the blood capillaries than returns to them due to a difference in hydrostatic and osmotic pressure. The closed-ended lymphatic capillaries collect the excess fluid and return it to the venous circulation through lymphatic vessels. Lymph capillaries are structured to specifically return small proteins to the cardiovascular system that have leaked out of blood capillaries. The epithelial cells that form the walls of lymphatic capillaries overlap but are not attached to each other. This allows flaps to be created that function like one-way valves. These minute openings between endothelial cells that make up the lymph capillary wall allow fluids to flow easily into the lymph capillary but prevent the flow of fluid out of the capillary.

Lymphatic Trunks and Collecting Ducts

The lymphatic trunks drain lymph from particular areas of the body and are named for those areas. For example, the lumbar lymphatic trunk drains lymph from the lower limbs, lower abdominal wall, and pelvic organs; the intestinal trunk drains the abdominal organs; the intercostal and broncho-mediastinal trunks drain lymph from parts of the thorax; the subclavian trunk drains the upper limbs; and the jugular trunks drain portions of the neck and head. The lymphatic trunks then join one of two collecting ducts: the thoracic duct or the right lymphatic duct.

LEARNING OBJECTIVE 11.1.7 Identify the structure of a lymph node.

LEARNING OBJECTIVE 11.1.8 Describe the structure of a lymph node.

KEY TERMS

afferent vessels Lymphatic vessels leading to a lymph node.

efferent vessels Lymph vessels that leave the lymph nodes.

germinal centers Central areas of lymph nodes where a small number of B lymphocytes are produced.

lymphadenitis Inflammation of lymph nodes.

lymphangitis Bacteria and debris that accumulate in the sinuses of a lymph node, resulting in inflammation of the superficial lymph nodes.

medullary chords Inner region of a lymph node where lymphocytes are arranged in strands.

parenchyma Tissue of an organ that enables the organ to function.

trabeculae Tissue that provides structural support to spongy bone.

STRUCTURE OF A LYMPH NODE

Lymph nodes are oval, bean-shaped structures, with a slight indentation on one side, located along the length of lymphatic vessels (Figure 11-6). This indentation is called a hilus, or hilum. The lymphatic vessels leading to a lymph node (**afferent vessels**) enter at various points on the node's convex surface, but the

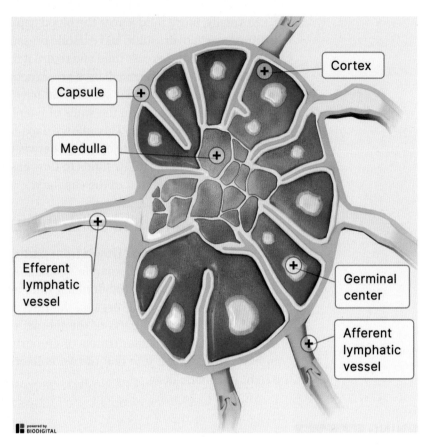

FIGURE 11-6 Internal structures of the lymph node.

lymph vessels leaving the lymph node (**efferent vessels**) exit from the hilum. Blood vessels also leave at the hilum. Each node is covered by a capsule of thick, dense connective tissue that extends into the node. These extensions into the node are called **trabeculae**. Inside the capsule is a network of reticular fibers and cells, which make up the framework of lymph nodes. The **parenchyma** of a lymph node is specialized into two regions: the cortex and the medulla. The outer cortex contains densely packed B lymphocytes and macrophages arranged in masses called lymphatic nodules, or lymphatic follicles. These lymphatic nodules contain central areas known as the **germinal centers** where a small number of B lymphocytes are produced (the majority of lymphocytes are produced in the bone marrow). The inner region of a lymph node is called the medulla where lymphocytes are arranged in strands, called **medullary chords**. These chords also contain macrophages and plasma B cells.

The spaces in a lymph node are known as lymphatic sinuses. The lymphatic sinuses are a complex network of chambers and channels where lymph circulates. Lymph enters a lymph node through afferent lymphatic vessels, moving slowly through the lymph sinuses, and leaves through efferent lymphatic vessels. Bacteria and debris can accumulate in the sinuses of a lymph node, resulting in inflammation of the superficial lymph nodes (**lymphangitis**) that appear as red streaks under the skin. Inflammation of the lymph node itself often follows, called **lymphadenitis**, with an enlarged lymph node that can be painful.

11.1.9 Identify the thoracic duct and right lymphatic duct.

11.1.10 Identify the portion of the body drained by the thoracic duct and the portion drained by the right lymphatic duct.

KEY TERMS

right lymphatic duct Short vessel that begins just inferior to the clavicle on the right side of body.

thoracic duct Large lymph duct of the lymphatic system; begins as the cisterna chyli.

THORACIC DUCT AND RIGHT LYMPHATIC DUCT

The **thoracic duct** and **right lymphatic duct** are relatively small vessels (Figure 11-7). Their primary purpose is to return lymph to venous circulation at the venous angle between the internal jugular vein and the subclavian vein on either side of the body.

Thoracic Duct

The thoracic duct (Figure 11-7) begins in the abdomen as a swollen lymphatic vessel called the cisterna chyli. The cisterna chyli is located near the L1 and L2 vertebrae. The thoracic duct ascends along the vertebral bodies of the inferior

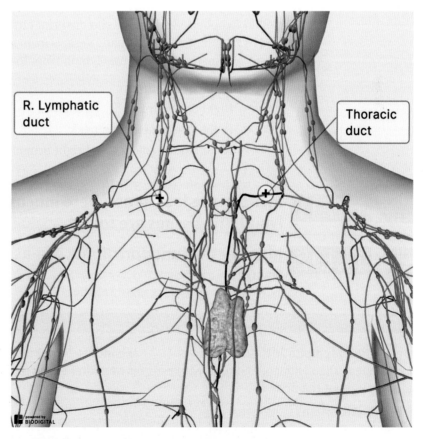

FIGURE 11-7 Right lymphatic duct and thoracic duct, both highlighted in purple.

thoracic vertebrae and passes through the aortic hiatus of the diaphragm into the thoracic cavity. In the thorax, it travels superiorly on the midline alongside the aorta before crossing to the left side of the vertebral column between the T4 and T6 vertebral levels. The thoracic duct then empties into the venous system at the angle between the left subclavian vein and the left internal jugular vein. The many valves within the thoracic duct make this vessel appear beaded; however, in a living person the duct may be small and colorless, making it vulnerable during surgery. The thoracic duct drains the following portions of the body:

- Drains directly into thoracic duct:
  ° Left side of thorax
  ° Left upper limb
  ° Left side of head and neck
  ° Left side of trachea and left bronchi
- Drains into cisterna chyli:
  ° Abdomen
  ° Pelvis
  ° Both lower limbs

Right Lymphatic Duct

This is a short vessel that begins just inferior to the clavicle on the right side of body (see Figure 11-7). It empties into the venous system at the angle between the right subclavian vein and the internal jugular vein. Rather than forming from a swollen lymphatic vessel like the cisterna chyli, the right lymphatic duct is formed by the merging of lymphatic vessels from the upper limb, head, and neck. The right lymphatic duct receives lymph from the following:

- Right side of thorax
- Right upper limb
- Right side of head and neck
- Right side of trachea and right bronchi

LEARNING OBJECTIVE 11.1.11 Identify the locations where mucosa-associated lymphatic tissues are found.

LEARNING OBJECTIVE 11.1.12 Identify the function of mucosa-associated lymphatic tissue.

KEY TERMS

mucosa-associated lymphatic tissues Groups of lymphocytes called lymphoid nodules within mucosa throughout the body.

primary lymphatic organs Sites where new lymphatic cells are formed and matured.

secondary lymphatic organs Organs that monitor and filter extracellular fluids.

LYMPHATIC ORGANS

The organs of the lymphatic system are described as either primary lymphatic organs or secondary lymphatic organs.

- Primary lymphatic organs are sites where new lymphatic cells are formed and matured. These include red bone marrow and the thymus.
- Secondary lymphatic organs monitor and filter extracellular fluids. Lymph nodes, tonsils, mucosa-associated lymphatic tissue, and the spleen are all considered secondary lymphatic organs.

Mucosa-Associated Lymphatic Tissues

Mucosa-associated lymphatic tissues (MALT) are unencapsulated lymphoid tissues that contain lymphocytes within mucosa throughout the body. Some areas where MALT can be found are in the lining of the gastrointestinal, urinary, genital, and respiratory tracts. MALT is often subdivided based on its location in the body. For example:

- Gastrointestinal-associated lymphatic tissue (GALT): This refers to groups of diffuse lymphoid nodules in the mucosa of the gastrointestinal tract.
- Bronchus-associated lymphatic tissue (BALT): This tissue refers to groups of diffuse lymphoid nodules in the mucosa of bronchi and the lungs.
- Vulvo-vaginal-associated lymphatic tissue (VALT): This describes groups of diffuse lymphoid nodules in the skin of the vulva and mucosa of the vagina.

No matter where in the body it is found, MALT plays an important role in protecting the body against infection in tissues that open to the external environment.

LEARNING OBJECTIVE 11.1.13 Identify the function of lymph nodes.

KEY TERMS

lymph nodes Encapsulated ovoid structures found along lymph vessels.

ovoid Oval shaped.

Lymph Nodes

Lymphocytes exist in small groupings throughout the body, for example in MALT, or they may be found grouped together inside of lymph nodes (Figure 11-8AB). Lymph nodes are encapsulated ovoid structures found along lymph vessels.

Their primary purpose is to filter lymph before it returns to venous circulation. The cells of the lymph nodes seek out foreign invaders, such as viruses and bacteria, as well as potentially tumorigenic cells. To facilitate this function, lymphatic vessels must both go into and out of lymph nodes. As discussed previously, vessels entering the lymph nodes are called afferent lymphatic vessels, and vessels exiting the lymph nodes are called efferent lymphatic vessels.

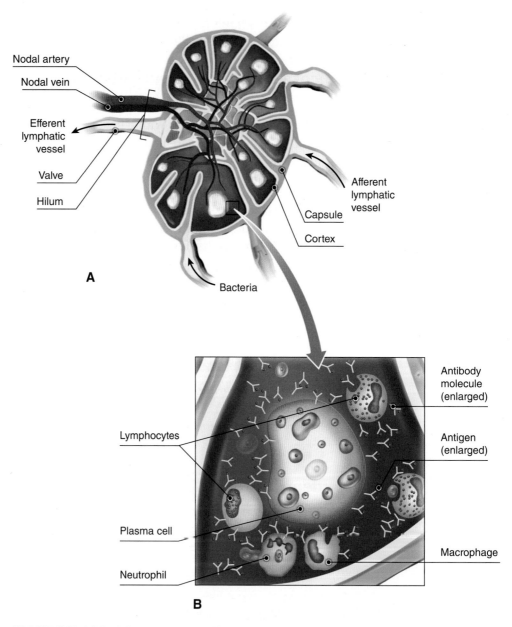

FIGURE 11-8AB (A) Cross section of a lymph node. The arrows indicate the flow of lymph. (B) Microscopic section of lymph node showing how bacteria are destroyed within lymph nodes.

LEARNING
OBJECTIVE **11.1.14** **Describe the function of mucosa-associated lymphatic tissue and lymph nodes.**

KEY TERMS

antigen-presenting cell Phagocytic cells that have engulfed foreign invaders and placed the foreign invaders' antigens on their own cell surface to present it to other cells in the immune system.

antigens Chemical groups, such as proteins and polysaccharides, on the surface of a cell that can stimulate an immune response.

lymphocytes Agranulocytic white blood cells which primarily function in the adaptive immune system; T cells and B cells.

macrophages Type of white blood cell found in areolar connective tissue; functions as part of the body's immune system and engulfs and breaks down cells and cellular debris.

Mucosa-Associated Lymphatic Tissue Function

MALT primarily helps prevent infection of tissues that open to the external environment. This refers to areas of the body such as the gastrointestinal, urinary, genital, and respiratory tracts, as these are all directly exposed to components of the external environment. This makes them particularly susceptible to infection. Prevention of infection primarily relies on **lymphocytes**, which are found within MALT. Lymphocytes are a type of immune system cells that have the ability to identify and destroy foreign invaders of the body. More details on the immune system and the many functions of lymphocytes are discussed in Chapter 12.

Lymph Node Function

Lymph nodes (Figure 11-9) contain lymphocytes, along with other types of immune system cells. These cells include **macrophages** (Figure 11-8) and **antigen-presenting cells**. These cells are discussed in greater detail in Chapter 12, but it is important to note that these cells have two important roles in fighting infection and foreign invaders:

- Macrophages and lymphocytes (Figure 11-8) have the ability to destroy foreign invaders.
- Antigen-presenting cells display foreign invaders (**antigens**) to B cells and T cells so that those lymphocytes can mount a unique and focused response against that particular invader.

As lymph enters afferent vessels and flows to lymphatic nodules within lymph nodes, macrophages, lymphocytes, and antigen-presenting cells perform the above functions on any foreign invaders that are detected. Some foreign invaders are destroyed here, but those that are not destroyed exit through efferent vessels with appropriate antigens. These antigens are recognized by the immune system, which will mount a unique response to destroy the foreign cells or viruses.

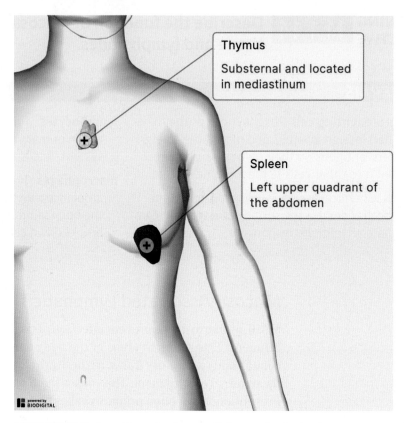

Thymus

Substernal and located in mediastinum

Spleen

Left upper quadrant of the abdomen

powered by
BIODIGITAL

FIGURE 11-9 Location of spleen and thymus in the body.

LEARNING OBJECTIVE 11.1.15 Identify the structure of the spleen.

LEARNING OBJECTIVE 11.1.16 Describe the structure of the spleen.

KEY TERMS

concave Curve inward.

convex Curve outward.

splenic artery Branch of the abdominal aorta that brings blood to the spleen.

splenic vein Vein that takes deoxygenated blood away from the spleen.

Spleen Structure

The spleen is an oval-shaped organ found in the abdomen (Figure 11-9). It is located in the left upper quadrant of the abdomen, just inferior to the diaphragm. It is oriented parallel to the long axis of the body and has a **concave** side and **convex** side (Figure 11-10). The concave side faces medially and the convex side faces laterally. The concave side features openings for the **splenic artery** and **splenic vein**. The splenic artery brings oxygenated blood to the spleen and the splenic vein takes deoxygenated blood away from the spleen. It has two main tissue types, referred to as red pulp and white pulp.

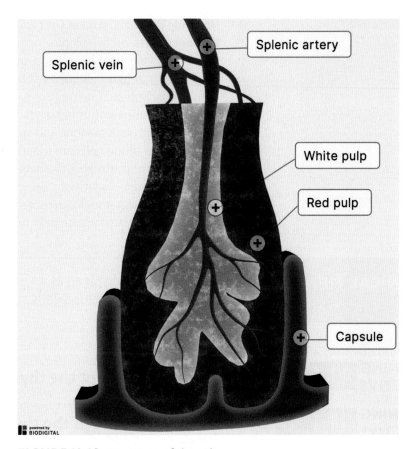

powered by
BIODIGITAL

FIGURE 11-10 Structure of the spleen.

LEARNING OBJECTIVE 11.1.17 Identify the function of the spleen.

LEARNING OBJECTIVE 11.1.18 Describe the function of the spleen.

KEY TERM

sinuses Hollow chambers within the bones of the skull.

Spleen Function

The red pulp and white pulp of the spleen serve two main functions: to remove old and damaged red blood cells and to protect the body from foreign invaders.

- White pulp is comprised of secondary lymphoid tissue. While it monitors extracellular fluid, the B cells within this tissue produce antibodies that help the immune system mount specific and unique responses to foreign invaders.

- Red pulp contains **sinuses** (or cavities), where blood cells collect, that are separated by splenic cords. Splenic cords are strands of connective tissue that consist of a loose network of reticular fibers and reticular cells. The splenic cords contain white and red blood cells. Splenic macrophages, one of the white blood cells found in splenic cords, phagocytize old red blood cells. In this way blood sent through cavities and splenic cords is filtered and old or damaged red blood cells are identified and destroyed. As the red blood cells are destroyed, the hemoglobin inside of them begins to leak into the bloodstream. Specific macrophages in the spleen break down the hemoglobin molecules so that the iron and amino acids can be used to create new red blood cells in the bone marrow.

CLINICAL TIP	Think of the red pulp of the spleen as an obstacle course of red blood cells. Only the healthiest red blood cells survive the obstacle course.

LEARNING OBJECTIVE 11.1.19 Identify the structure of the thymus.

LEARNING OBJECTIVE 11.1.20 Describe the structure of the thymus.

KEY TERMS

cortex Outer layer of an organ.   **medulla** Inner layer of an organ.

Thymus

Another lymphatic organ comprised of lymphatic tissue is the thymus (Figure 11-11). The thymus, which contains two irregularly shaped lobes, spans the inferior region of the neck and the anterior region of the superior thoracic cavity.

The bulk of the thymus is located between the heart and sternum. Its lobes are further separated into thymic lobules, which feature an outer **cortex** and inner **medulla**. The cortex of the thymic lobule contains developing T lymphocytes. The medulla of the thymic lobule contains large, loosely arranged lymphocytes. The defining characteristic of the medulla is the presence of thymic corpuscles (Hassall's corpuscles). Thymic corpuscles are large aggregates of epithelial cells unique to the thymus that secrete cytokines to regulate the activity of dendritic cells.

Unlike most other organs, the structure of the thymus changes dramatically over time. The thymus is fully functional at birth. It is a relatively large organ in infancy and childhood. Beginning in puberty and following adolescence, the thymus begins to deteriorate. The thymus is replaced by fat in adulthood as T-cell formation and differentiation are reduced. It can begin fully functioning again in an adult if the body requires rapid formation of new T cells; however, this does not happen immediately due to previous deterioration of the thymus.

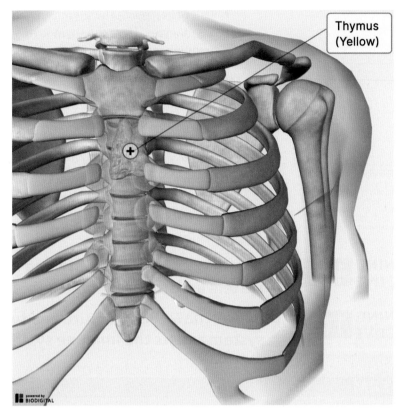

FIGURE 11-11 Location of the thymus in the body.

LEARNING
OBJECTIVE   11.1.21   **Identify the function of the thymus.**

LEARNING
OBJECTIVE   11.1.22   **Describe the function of the thymus.**

LEARNING
OBJECTIVE   11.1.21   **Identify the function of the thymus.**

LEARNING
OBJECTIVE   11.1.22   **Describe the function of the thymus.**

KEY TERMS

immunocompetent Immune system that functions normally.

pluripotential Undifferentiated stem cell.

T cells Specialized immune cells created in the thymus.

Thymus Function

The main function of the thymus is to create specialized cells called **T cells**. T cells play an important role in the body's immune response. T cells are created through a multitude of steps involving bones and the thymus:

- The precursor cells to T cells are formed in the bone marrow during fetal development. These **pluripotential** cells are called lymphoid stem cells. Lymphoid stem cells differentiate into lymphocytes in the bone marrow. The lymphocytes then travel from the bones to the thymus through the bloodstream.

- Once they reach the thymus, lymphocytes are renamed thymocytes. Here the thymocytes mature and become **immunocompetent** (that is, they are capable of undergoing an immune response). To become immunocompetent, thymocytes must learn to recognize foreign invaders and healthy cells belonging to the body. In this process, accessory proteins CD4, CD8, and TCR are added to the surface of the thymocytes. The creation of T cells is highly regulated by a hormone called thymosin that is created within the thymus gland.
- Once matured and immunocompetent, T cells leave the thymus to participate in the immune system. For more details on their role in the immune response, see Chapter 12.

LEARNING OBJECTIVE 11.1.23 Identify how the structure and function of the lymphatic system assists the immune system.

LEARNING OBJECTIVE 11.1.24 Explain how the structure and function of the lymphatic system assists the immune system.

KEY TERM

antibodies Immune system proteins produced in response to a specific antigen that non-self cells for destruction.

LYMPHATIC SYSTEM AND IMMUNE SYSTEM

As we've discussed throughout this chapter, the lymphatic system plays key roles in assisting the immune system. This is achieved not only through the structure of the lymphatic system, but also the functions of the lymphatic system.

One of the more prominent ways the lymphatic system assists the immune system is through filtration. Lymph that is filtered through lymph nodes is filled with **antibodies** added by plasma cells within the lymph node (Figure 11-6). These antibodies help the immune system recognize foreign cells as invaders and allow them to mount specific, unique responses to invaders. Another important way that the lymphatic system assists the immune system is by developing and maintaining cells that are integral to the immune response:

- T cells, which are originally created in bone, migrate to the thymus where they mature.
- B cells, which are created and matured in bone or lymph nodes, can be found in the spleen and other lymphatic tissue.

Finally, the lymphatic system helps carry out immune functions by assisting in the identification of foreign invaders and in helping the body mount an immune response to those invaders.

- When the cels maintained by the lymphatic system locate a cell with a particular antigen, macrophages arrive and begin to phagocytize the invader.

- The fragments of antigens created by macrophages, called antigen-presenting cells, alert T cells to the presence of infection in the body.
- T cells begin an immune response (discussed in greater detail in Chapter 12).

UNIT OBJECTIVE 11.2

Describe common pathologies affecting the lymphatic system.

UNIT INTRODUCTION

When it is functioning normally, the lymphatic system plays an important role in maintaining and protecting the body. Not only does it work closely with the immune system to protect, identify, and eliminate foreign invaders, it also plays a role in filtering out old and damaged cells from blood. However, there are several pathologies that may affect how the lymphatic system functions. Common disorders of the lymphatic system may cause a variety of symptoms, as well as alter normal functioning of the human body. There are two different classifications of disorders related to the lymphatic system: those pathologies that directly alter the lymphatic system and those pathologies that either use the lymphatic system to access other regions of the body or are affected by lymphatic system functions.

LEARNING OBJECTIVE 11.2.1 Identify common disorders of the lymphatic system.

KEY TERMS

edema Localized area of excess fluid.

lymphoma Also called lymphatic cancer; condition in which lymphocytes begin to mutate and duplicate rapidly and out of control.

COMMON LYMPHATIC DISORDERS

Lymphatic disorders are classified as those pathologies that directly influence the lymphatic system's functions and structures. There are two common disorders that directly influence how the lymphatic system functions: lymphoma and edema.

Lymphoma

One lymphatic disorder is lymphoma, which may also be called lymphatic cancer. In this condition, lymphocytes begin to mutate and duplicate rapidly, causing out-of-control growth of both healthy and damaged lymphocytes. This causes lymph nodes to become filled with cancerous cells. It may also lead to damaged lymphocytes spreading to other areas of the body. This overgrowth of unhealthy cells alters the lymphatic system's ability to assist in immune functions and to carry out other functions in the body. There are many different types of lymphoma, but the two most common types are non-Hodgkin's lymphoma and Hodgkin's lymphoma. The difference between these two relates to the types of cells present in the tumor. Both lymphomas arise from B cells; however, Hodgkin's lymphoma will also contain special, giant cells called Reed-Sternberg cells. The cause of lymphoma is unclear.

Edema

Edema is another condition that directly influences the structure and functions of the lymphatic system. It is classified as swelling that is caused by an accumulation interstitial fluid. This may occur when lymphatic vessels or lymph nodes are damaged. If lymph is blocked by cancer cells or inflamed vessels, interstitial fluid will be unable to drain into lymphatic capillaries. Ultimately the blocked fluid will accumulate distal to the damaged vessel or lymph node. Edema is discussed in greater detail shortly.

LEARNING OBJECTIVE 11.2.2 Identify the diseases and disorders that use the lymphatic system to access other regions of the body.

KEY TERMS

lymphangitis Bacteria and debris that accumulate in the sinuses of a lymph node, resulting in inflammation of the superficial lymph nodes.

metastasis When cancer cells from tumors near lymphatic vessels enter lymph and spread to and infect other locations in the body.

DISEASES THAT TRAVEL IN THE LYMPHATIC SYSTEM

In addition to diseases directly altering the structure and function of the lymphatic system, there are also conditions that use the lymphatic system to spread throughout the body. Most commonly, these diseases are different forms of cancer and infection.

- Cancer: **Metastasis**, or the spread of cancer cells, occurs in advanced stages of most cancers. Cancer cells move through the body using a variety of methods depending on where they arise; for example, cancer in the intestines can easily travel to the liver through the abdominal veins. As we have seen, the lymphatic system is a diffuse structure with widespread vessels and nodes. Cancer cells can enter the lymphatic system via any nearby lymph vessels or nodes to spread the disease to other areas of the body (Figure 11-12).

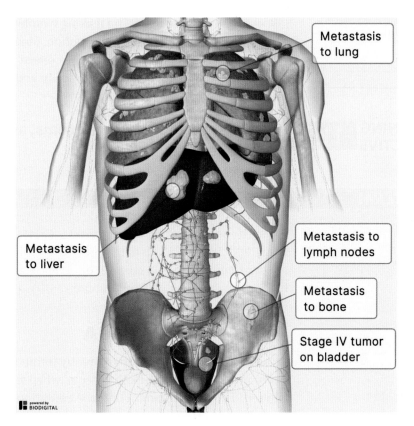

FIGURE 11-12 How cancer may use the lymphatic system to travel throughout the body.

- Infection: Noncancerous foreign invaders can also use the lymphatic system to spread an infection throughout the body. This might occur when an infectious invader enters a damaged lymph node. Since the lymph node is not functioning normally, the infectious cell may pass through the lymph node without being detected. This allows it to travel to other regions of the body. It may also lead to a condition in which the tissue of the lymphatic system becomes infected by a foreign invader. This infection of lymphatic tissue is called **lymphangitis**. Lymphangitis may occur in a variety of ways, but may most commonly occur after foreign invaders enter the body and the lymphatic system through a wound.

- Venom: Certain types of venom use the lymphatic system to enter the bloodstream. This is determined by the size of the biologically active proteins within the venom. Venom from spiders or scorpions contains relatively small proteins that can pass directly through the fenestrations in blood capillaries, but venom from snakes contains proteins that are too large to enter the blood capillaries. Instead, proteins in snake venom are absorbed into lymphatic vessels that have larger openings than the blood capillaries. The venom then travels through the lymphatic system and enters the bloodstream via the thoracic or right lymphatic ducts. Once within the lymphatic system, some proteins in venom are capable of damaging the walls of lymphatic vessels, causing lymph to leak. The leaking lymph results in edema, which is discussed in the next section. Medical treatments to combat the effects of venom typically consist of intravenous injections of antibodies for the biologically active peptides in the venom.

11.2.3 **Describe the signs, symptoms, and diagnosis of peripheral edema.**

KEY TERM

peripheral edema Swelling that occurs when lymphatic vessels are unable to drain excess interstitial fluid.

PERIPHERAL EDEMA

In addition to pathologies that directly influence and use the lymphatic system, there are also pathologies that occur when the lymphatic system's function is altered. The most common of these conditions is peripheral edema.

Peripheral edema is defined as tissue swelling that occurs when lymphatic vessels are unable to drain excess interstitial fluid. This inability to drain interstitial fluid may be caused by a variety of things, including:

- Damage to lymph nodes that occurs during surgery
- Cancer cells blocking lymphatic vessels
- Cancer treatments that damage lymph nodes
- Infection of lymph nodes

Most commonly, peripheral edema presents in the arm or leg and may make the affected limb feel heavy. The affected limb will also appear to be swollen. Other signs and symptoms of peripheral edema include the following:

- Restricted range of motion
- Recurring infections
- Discomfort and aching
- Skin feels tight and may thicken

Peripheral edema is diagnosed using a variety of methods. A thorough physical examination and medical history are important and will help the health care provider begin to determine the cause of edema. Magnetic resonance imaging (MRI) and computer tomography (CT) scans can reveal areas of damage to the lymphatic system. Depending on the patient's symptoms and history, an ultrasound may also be ordered, as it can detect obstructions in lymphatic tissues. Radioactive dye may be used in conjunction with diagnostic imaging, as it can allow health care providers to visualize the flow of lymph through lymphatic vessels and nodes.

Although there is no cure for peripheral edema, there are several treatments that may help manage the symptoms of the condition. This may include compression, massage, and specialized exercises. If edema is caused by underlying infection, treating the infection to reduce inflammation may also help as well. Additionally, peripheral edema may be treated with medications, such as diuretics, which encourage the patient's body to expel excess fluid. For example, furosemide, a medication that acts on the kidneys to promote water loss through urine, is frequently used in the treatment of edema.

LEARNING OBJECTIVE 11.2.4 Explain how a radical mastectomy often leads to edema of the upper limb on the affected side.

MASTECTOMY AND EDEMA

Edema of the upper limb may commonly occur in patients who have undergone a radical mastectomy. This occurs because mastectomy may include removal of several axillary lymph nodes in order to be sure that all cancerous tissue is removed and to reduce the likelihood that surrounding lymph nodes will spread cancerous cells throughout the body (Figure 11-13). However, removal of these lymph nodes not only changes how the lymphatic system works but may also cause damage to remaining lymph vessels and axillary lymph nodes.

In a normal-functioning lymphatic system, lymph from the upper limb typically travels through lymphatic vessels in the arm to the subclavian lymphatic vessels and enters axillary lymph nodes along its journey. However, lymphatic vessels and axillary lymph nodes damaged by a mastectomy may be unable to bring lymph from the arm to subclavian lymphatic vessels. This causes lymph to become trapped in the arm, which leads to edema of the affected side.

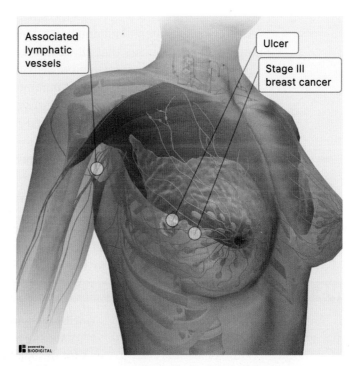

FIGURE 11-13 Patient with breast cancer that has metastasized to a nearby lymph node.

Chapter 12

The Immune System

Chapter Introduction

The immune system consists of many organs, cells (white blood cells), and chemicals that work together to protect the body from foreign invaders. The components of the immune system are somewhat unique because they are not all physically connected to one another like components of other body systems (like the skeletal system). Even though they are not physically connected, the components of the immune system function together to maintain health. If something foreign enters the body (such as bacteria, viruses, other parasites, or even cells from another human), the immune system will detect these foreign entities and remove or destroy them. It operates as a sort of defense system to prevent or diminish attacks by these potentially harmful entities. In addition to fighting foreign cells, the immune system also works to eliminate cancerous cells of the body. Finally, the immune system cooperates with other body systems to heal any damaged tissues and restore the body to a state of homeostasis.

UNIT OBJECTIVE 12.1

Describe the immune system's components, functions, and role in homeostasis.

UNIT INTRODUCTION

As previously stated, the immune system is comprised of many different structures and components that all work together to protect the body from foreign invaders. The immune system consists of two separate parts called the innate immune system and the adaptive immune system. The two parts of the immune system are interconnected with some overlapping functions, although they each have different components. The primary role of both categories of the immune system is to prevent infection by pathogens and destroy foreign invaders that enter the body. In addition, the immune system works to destroy cancer cells in the body.

LEARNING OBJECTIVE 12.1.1 Identify the functions of the immune system.

KEY TERMS

alloantigens Antigens on the cell surface of other humans; antigens from the same species.

antibodies Immune system proteins produced in response to a specific antigen that non-self cells for destruction.

antigens Chemical groups, such as proteins and polysaccharides, on the surface of a cell that can stimulate an immune response.

autoantigens "Self" antigens; antigens on our own body cells.

heteroantigens Antigens on the cell surface of a microorganism; antigens from another species.

immune system Diverse system of the body that protects it from foreign invaders; includes white blood cells and lymphoid organs.

immunocompetent Immune system that functions normally.

immunocompromised Immune system that isn't functioning properly.

infection Condition arising from having a microorganism living in and reproducing in the body.

infectious disease Condition arising from an infection that is damaging the body.

lysis Popping or bursting of a cell.

opportunistic infections Infection that occurs in immunocompromised individuals due to opportunistic pathogens.

pathogen Microorganism that can cause disease.

phagocytosis Process by which white blood cells engulf, digest, and excrete foreign cells.

THE IMMUNE SYSTEM

There are several purposes of the immune system. The overall function of the immune system is to protect the health of the human body by preventing attack from certain microorganisms, known as pathogens, and the chemicals and toxins that they release. A **pathogen** is any organism that can cause disease in an **immunocompetent** host. This may include bacteria (as seen in Figure 12-1), protozoa, fungi, and helminths (worms) (Figure 12-2). While viruses are not technically considered living organisms, we do consider them pathogens because they can cause disease. Pathogens that only cause disease in **immunocompromised** individuals are known as opportunistic pathogens. These cause **opportunistic infections**. This distinction is discussed in greater detail in the section "Immunodeficiency Disorders."

Many body systems work together to preserve health and prevent infection. For example, consider the life cycle of white blood cells, which are a key component in many immune system functions:

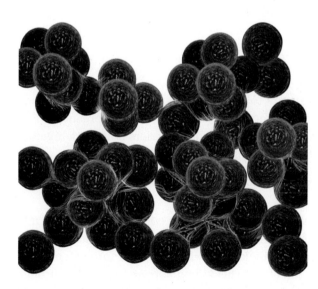

FIGURE 12-1 *Staphylococcus*. There are many types of *Staphylococcus* bacteria that live on the skin and mucous membranes. Some are essentially harmless while others can make us sick.

- White blood cells circulate through the bloodstream and lymphatic vessels so that they will be able to come into contact with pathogens in numerous parts of the body.

- Organs that you learned about in previous chapters, such as the bone marrow and thymus, serve as places of production and maturation for the white blood cells.

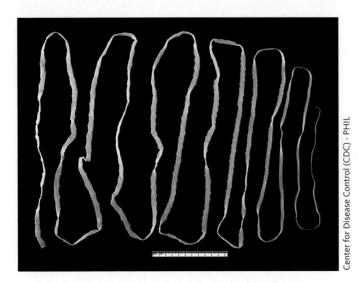

Center for Disease Control (CDC) - PHIL

FIGURE 12-2 *Taenia saginata. Taenia* is a type of tapeworm that can infect humans who eat raw or undercooked beef.

- Other lymphoid organs, such as the spleen and lymph nodes, house some of these white blood cells and provide optimal environments for the white blood cells to attack and kill foreign materials.

All parts of the immune system are necessary and important for optimal health. If any part is not functioning appropriately, infection and disease may occur. It is important for us to understand how each part functions and how the system functions as a whole in order to fully understand conditions that influence the immune system's ability to function at its full capacity, such as the condition in this chapter's clinical scenario.

Protection against pathogens and other foreign substances is achieved through three main immune system functions.

Defense from Attack

The immune system defends other organs and tissues of the body from attack by attempting to prevent entry, infection, and infectious disease by pathogens. The terms *infection* and *infectious disease* are sometimes used interchangeably but are not really the same thing.

- **Infection** means an organism is living in the body and actively reproducing. The organism may or may not be damaging the body.
- If the organism is harming the cells and tissues of the body in any way, the result is **infectious disease**.

The immune system attempts to defend the body against infection and infectious disease by providing barriers to prevent entry of these organisms into the body. The body has both physical and chemical barriers that work together to prevent entry and replication of pathogens in the body.

Killing Pathogens

If pathogens enter the body, various immune system components will begin to kill them to try to prevent infectious disease. White blood cells and chemicals in the innate immune system can quickly and efficiently kill foreign cells and prevent the establishment of infection. This killing happens primarily through a process called phagocytosis as well as through cell lysis by the complement system. In addition, some chemicals prevent the pathogen from replicating.

- **Phagocytosis**: Action of certain white blood cells (Figure 12-3AB) in which they engulf and break down a foreign cell or particle to kill it.
- Complement system: Group of proteins that work together to directly lyse foreign cells. **Lysis** means the popping or bursting of a cell.

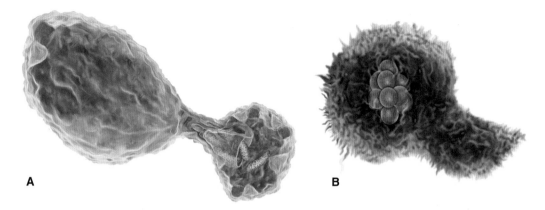

A   B

FIGURE 12-3AB White blood cells known as phagocytes have the ability to perform phagocytosis, which is when the phagocyte engulfs and kills pathogens. Phagocyte engulfing (A) bacteria and (B) fungus.

The **immune system** also includes very specific mechanisms to remove infection and protect the body in case of future attack. These specific mechanisms involve cells and proteins that are part of the adaptive immune system. Its components recognize a cell's **antigens**, which are unique chemical groups attached to each cell that can trigger an immune response. Antigens may be chemicals on the surface of a foreign cell or a free-floating chemical or toxin. Once the adaptive immune system recognizes a foreign antigen, it develops very specific fighting mechanisms to remove these antigens. Part of this specific response is the production of antibodies. **Antibodies** (Figure 12-4) are proteins produced by the immune system to bind to and fight the antigen. With each exposure, the adaptive immune system "remembers" how to fight the antigen, learns to fight it a little bit better, and can ultimately result in immunity against the antigen.

Recognition of Self Versus Non-Self

In order for the immune system to function appropriately, it must be able to distinguish the difference between your own cells and the cells of foreign invaders. This task is achieved by detecting the type of antigen that the white blood cell has come in contact with. Your white blood cells can recognize the difference between antigens on your own body cells and antigens on foreign cells. Antigens on your own body cells are called **autoantigens**, and your immune system does not attack them. Attacking your own cells would result in cell damage and disease. Antigens that are on foreign cells from another human, such as those that would enter your body during a blood

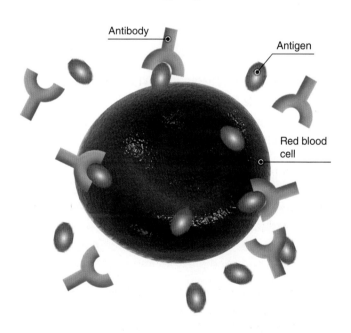

Antibody

Antigen

Red blood cell

FIGURE 12-4 Cells of the adaptive immune system produce antibodies that can bind to foreign antigens. Antibodies bind to the alloantigens on a red blood cell. This type of reaction could occur if a patient received a blood transfusion from the wrong blood type that would contain alloantigens that are foreign to the patient.

transfusion, are called **alloantigens**. If alloantigens are very different than your own antigens, your body may attack them. Antigens that are on microorganisms are called **heteroantigens**. Your body must recognize that heteroantigens are foreign and fight them quickly to maintain health and homeostasis.

It can be helpful to think of the parts of the immune system as groups of soldiers always working to prevent attack, but who are prepared to fight attackers as necessary. The white blood cells are the soldiers who are constantly patrolling the area they protect (your body) by traveling the roads around the area (blood and lymphatic vessels) looking for foreign invaders (antigens). When the soldiers detect the foreign invader, they will stop and fight to make sure the invader does not enter the area further. Think of the innate immune system as the guards, fencing, and weapons designed to keep the attackers out. If attackers get in, the adaptive immune system soldiers will go to their hideouts (lymphatic organs) and will use their "weapons" (antibodies) to remove the invaders and neutralize the attack.

LEARNING OBJECTIVE 12.1.2 Identify the components of the innate immune system.

LEARNING OBJECTIVE 12.1.3 Identify the functions of the innate immune system.

LEARNING OBJECTIVE 12.1.4 Describe the functions of the innate immune system.

KEY TERMS

agranulocytes White blood cells that do not contain packets of chemicals that can activate the immune system. Examples include leukocytes and monocytes.

basophils Granulocytic white blood cells which function in allergic responses and inflammation.

cytokines Proteins that play a regulatory function in the immune system.

defensins Peptides that kill foreign cells by poking holes in cell membranes and cell walls.

diapedesis Process of white blood cells squeezing through blood vessel walls to enter the tissues.

eosinophils Granulocytic white blood cells which function in the destruction of helminths and participate in allergic responses.

granulocytes White blood cells that contain immunologic chemicals packaged in small granules. Examples include neutrophils, eosinophils, and basophils.

heparin Anticoagulant that is used to decrease the clotting ability of the blood.

histamine Chemical released during inflammation that causes smooth muscle contraction and blood vessel dilation.

innate Natural and inborn such as innate immunity.

interferons Innate immune system chemicals which inhibit viral replication.

leukocyte White blood cell; circulates throughout the body and plays an important part in the body's immune response and reaction to foreign bodies and disease.

lymphocytes Agranulocytic white blood cells which primarily function in the adaptive immune system; T cells and B cells.

monocytes Agranulocytic white blood cells which perform phagocytosis.

neutrophils Agranulocytic white blood cells with segmented nuclei which perform phagocytosis.

ubiquitous State of being in many places in the earth.

THE INNATE IMMUNE SYSTEM

As briefly mentioned, the immune system is often discussed in terms of two subcategories: the innate immune system and the adaptive immune system. The innate immune system includes the first and second lines of defense. The general function of these two lines of defense is to prevent pathogens and other foreign cells and substances from entering the body. When something foreign is able to gain access to the body, the functions of the innate immune system attempt to immediately rid the body of the foreign structure.

Physical and chemical barriers that help prevent pathogens from entering the body are considered the first line of defense. The first line of defense is not truly an immune response since it does not involve the fighting of organisms; however, it is an important defense mechanism in the protection of the body since it works to prevent the establishment of infections.

The innate immune system also includes the second line of defense. The second line of defense consists of a group of white blood cells and chemicals in the innate immune system that quickly and efficiently kill foreign cells and prevent the establishment of infection. The second line of defense kills pathogens primarily through phagocytosis and cell lysis by the complement system. In addition, some chemicals prevent the pathogen from replicating. In this way, if an organism has made its way past our first line of defense, the second line of defense can remove the organism from the body.

Innate can be defined as natural and inborn. Therefore, the innate immune system is something that all healthy people are born with. It is ready to work immediately to protect the body against pathogens through naturally present body functions. Characteristics of the innate immune system include the following:

- It is something that all healthy people possess from birth.
- It is nonspecific, reacting essentially the same way to every foreign substance.
- It is ready to work immediately when exposed to a pathogen. It does not require prior exposure to learn how to work.
- Its response does not change with subsequent exposures. For example, it doesn't matter if you've been exposed to the same pathogen 50 times, the innate immune system will react the same way during the 50th exposure as it did during the first exposure.

The innate immune system has two main components: white blood cells and antimicrobial chemicals.

WHITE BLOOD CELLS

The scientific name for a white blood cell is a **leukocyte**. As discussed in Chapter 8, leukocytes are an integral part of innate immunity. As you learned in the section on the cardiovascular system, leukocytes are produced in the bone marrow from a specialized type of stem cell. Once the leukocytes are produced, they must go through a process of maturation. This process either occurs in bone marrow or the thymus. When they are mature, they circulate through the bloodstream and lymphatic vessels looking for pathogens to fight.

As a review, there are five main types of leukocytes as well as an associated type of cell called dendritic cells that work together in the immune system (Figure 12-5). These cells can be divided into two categories, called granulocytes and agranulocytes.

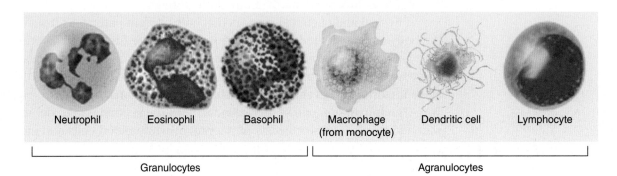

| Neutrophil | Eosinophil | Basophil | Macrophage (from monocyte) | Dendritic cell | Lymphocyte |

Granulocytes   Agranulocytes

FIGURE 12-5 Five main types of leukocytes and a dendritic cell. Notice how the eosinophil and basophil have large obvious granules. Neutrophils also have visible granules, but they are much smaller and are not visible here.

Granulocytes

Granulocytes are the first main category of leukocytes. These cells are called **granulocytes** because they contain visible granules that can be seen when looking through a microscope. You'll notice these granules clearly in Figure 12-5. Three types of granulocytes are neutrophils, eosinophils, and basophils.

- **Neutrophils** are the most common white blood cell found in your body (Figure 12-5). Approximately 50–75% of all white blood cells are neutrophils. Neutrophils are one of the main phagocytic cells in the body. Their primary job is to find pathogenic bacteria, engulf it, and remove it from the body. Neutrophils also clean up and destroy your own cells when they are damaged. They circulate through the blood and then move into the tissues when necessary by squeezing through the blood vessel walls. This process is called **diapedesis**.

- **Eosinophils** are present in the body in much smaller amounts than neutrophils. Only 1–3% of your white blood cells are eosinophils. Eosinophils fight against parasites like helminths and participate in allergic reactions (which are discussed in more detail later in this chapter).

- **Basophils** make up only 0–2% of your circulating white blood cells. Basophils have histamine and heparin in their granules. **Histamine** is a chemical that causes smooth muscle contraction and blood vessel dilation. **Heparin** is an anticoagulant that prevents blood from clotting. These two chemicals play an important role in the process of inflammation and allergic reactions, which are discussed in greater detail later in this chapter.

As mentioned in Chapter 8, a CBC (complete blood count) is a blood test that gives the number of red blood cells, white blood cells, and platelets in a sample of the patient's blood. It can be used to identify certain diseases related to blood, such as leukemia, which is a disorder involving the overproduction of certain white blood cells. A CBC may also include a differential, which counts the numbers of the five main types of white blood cells. On a differential lab report, neutrophils may be referred to using different names, such as neutrophils, segmented neutrophils, segs, or even PMNs, which stands for polymorphonuclear neutrophils.

Agranulocytes

The second category of leukocytes is called agranulocytes (see Figure 12-5) because usually no granules can be seen when looking at them in a microscope. The two types of **agranulocytes** are monocytes (also called macrophages) and lymphocytes.

- **Monocytes**: 2-10% percentage of circulating white blood cells are monocytes. These cells are called monocytes when they are circulating through the bloodstream. They have the ability to leave the blood and go into the tissues looking for pathogens. Once inside the tissues, they are known as macrophages (Figure 12-6). Along with neutrophils, monocytes and macrophages are very efficient phagocytic cells. They move throughout the body looking for pathogens and dead or damaged body cells, which they engulf and destroy.

- Dendritic cells are thought to be related to macrophages. They live in the tissues and are often found in places like the skin. Dendritic cells have long projections coming off of their cell bodies that allow them to make quick contact with antigens. Like macrophages, when they find antigens, they will phagocytize them. Dendritic cells and macrophages are important links between the innate immune system and the adaptive immune system. This link is discussed in later sections of this chapter.

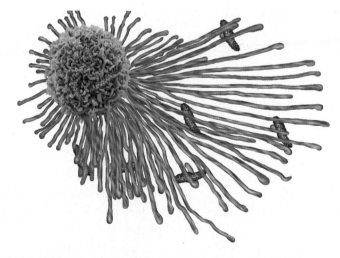

FIGURE 12-6 Macrophage (blue) makes contact with foreign antigens on bacterial cells (purple), preparing to kill the bacteria.

- **Lymphocytes** make up the remaining 20–40% of white blood cells. There are two main types of lymphocytes: B cells and T cells. B cells and T cells are a key component of the adaptive immune system and are discussed in detail later in this chapter.

CLINICAL TIP	When you see the letter *a* at the beginning of a word in medical terminology, it means "not" or "without." For example, the word *agranulocyte* is a cell without granules.

ANTIMICROBIAL CHEMICALS

A variety of proteins produced by the innate immune system can also kill pathogens (Table 12-1).

Table 12-1 Innate Immune System Components

INNATE IMMUNE SYSTEM COMPONENT	GENERAL FUNCTION
Leukocytes	Phagocytosis
Defensins	Poking holes in microbial cell membranes and cell walls
Cytokines	Regulate the growth and function of leukocytes and other types of cells
Interferon	Inhibit viral replication

- **Defensins** are peptides that are produced by a variety of cells and tissues. They kill foreign cells by poking holes in the cell membrane or cell wall of the pathogen.
- **Cytokines** are small proteins that help regulate both the innate and adaptive immune systems. There are many different types of cytokines in the body. In general, they help to regulate the growth and function of many cells, including leukocytes.
- One important group of cytokines that function in the innate immune system are interferons. **Interferons** inhibit the replication of viruses, which are a type of foreign invader in the body. Viruses are not living things. They must infect your body by entering your cells and directing your cells to replicate them (Figure 12-7). Once they have replicated, they will burst from the cell and the newly replicated viruses will each infect other cells. A virally infected cell can produce interferons. When viruses burst from a cell, the cell releases interferons. The interferons then bind to receptors on nearby cells to prevent the virus from entering and replicating within them. Some interferons may also interfere with the growth of cancer cells.

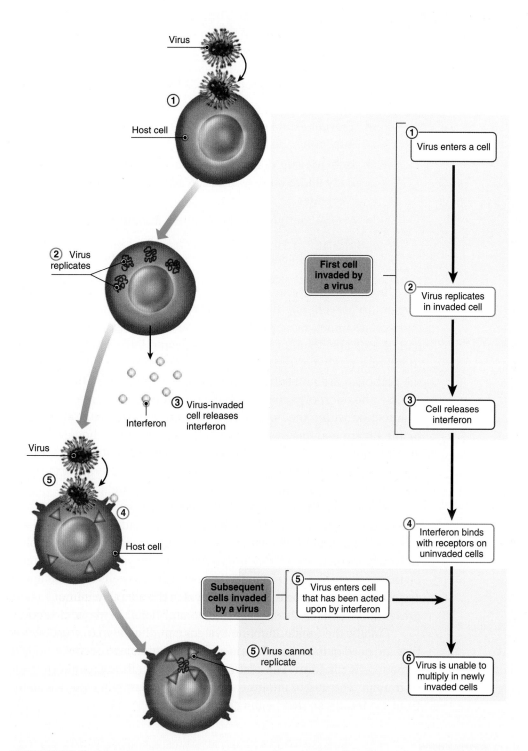

FIGURE 12-7 What happens when a virus invades a body cell and interferon is produced to block the replication of the virus in nearby cells.

FUNCTIONS OF THE INNATE IMMUNE SYSTEM

Microorganisms are ubiquitous. The term **ubiquitous** means that microorganisms are everywhere. They are found in or on virtually every surface of the earth, including in and on the human body. Many of these organisms are not harmful, but some are pathogens. If we come into contact with these pathogens every day of our lives, multiple times a day, why are we not always sick?

Part of the answer lies in the functions of the innate immune system. The innate immune system functions to:

- Prevent entry of foreign cells by providing barriers to those cells
- Recognize pathogens and defend against non-self
- Prevent establishment of organisms in the body, which prevents infection
- Help prevent disease by keeping pathogens that have entered the body under control until the adaptive immune system can begin working
- Present antigens to the adaptive immune system to begin adaptive responses
- Clear damaged human cells from the body

Remember that the first line of defense provides physical and chemical barriers to prevent anything foreign from entering the body. As long as these barriers are intact, most pathogens never make their way inside the body. If a pathogen is able to enter the body, the second line of defense will begin trying to kill and remove the pathogen. Leukocytes recognize that the antigens on the pathogen are non-self and will begin to attack. If pathogens can be killed quickly, the microorganism may never be able to replicate enough to establish an infection within the body. Even if infection does occur, killing of pathogens by the innate immune system can help keep those pathogens from producing large numbers and spreading through the body. Since the innate immune system goes to work immediately, it will try to keep these pathogens in check until the much slower adaptive immune system is ready to fight.

In addition, the innate immune system serves as an important link to the adaptive immune system through antigen presentation. As we discuss in the next section about phagocytosis, not all leukocytes can perform phagocytosis. However, the leukocytes that do perform phagocytosis put antigenic fragments on their cell surface to "present" these antigens to cells of the adaptive immune system. This antigen presentation activates the adaptive immune response. This presentation process is discussed in greater detail in the next section.

Finally, the innate immune system can phagocytize your own cells when they are dead or damaged. This is a natural response to clear the body of old cells so new cells can form. This also occurs if your cells are damaged from infection or trauma. The innate immune system leukocytes will clear the damaged cells from the tissues so that healing may occur.

LEARNING OBJECTIVE 12.1.5 List the seven types of innate defense mechanisms.

LEARNING OBJECTIVE 12.1.6 Describe the function of the seven types of innate defense mechanisms.

KEY TERMS

antigen presentation Process in which MHC molecules along with antigen attach to the cell surface of the phagocyte to allow immune cells to distinguish between self-cells and other cells.

cilia Hair-like projections that move in a wavelike manner that support movement.

complement cascade Set of reactions that occur after the complement system is activated in which protein triggers the activation of the next protein.

inflammation Generalized, localized response to cellular injury in order to prevent the spread of infection.

lysozyme Enzyme in tears and saliva that can poke holes in bacterial cell walls.

membrane attack complex (MAC) Group of proteins that form to drill holes and small pores in the membranes of foreign cells to cause lysis of foreign cells.

MHC molecule Unique molecules that help the immune system to recognize self versus non-self.

opsonins Groups of proteins that coat foreign cells during opsonization.

opsonization Coating of foreign cells with proteins to help with phagocytosis.

perforins Chemicals released by NK cells that kill foreign cells.

permeability Quality of a membrane that allows molecules to pass through it.

phagolysosome Phagosome that has joined together with a lysosome to digest a foreign cell.

phagosome Endocytic vesicle within a phagocytic cell containing an engulfed foreign cell.

pseudopods Extensions of a cell's membranes to make "false feet."

pyrogens Chemicals that raise the temperature set point of the hypothalamus.

natural killer (NK) cell Specialized type of lymphocyte that functions in the second line of defense.

vasoconstriction Narrowing of blood vessels.

vasodilation Process of dilating or widening a blood vessel through relaxation of smooth muscle.

INNATE DEFENSE MECHANISMS

Seven main defense mechanisms protect the body as part of the innate immune system. These mechanisms function as part of the first and second lines of defense. The innate defense mechanisms include:

- Physical barriers
- Chemical defenses
- Species resistance
- Natural killer (NK) cell
- Inflammation
- Fever
- Phagocytosis

The first line of defense is comprised of physical barriers, species resistance, and some of the chemical defenses. The second line of defense includes the actions of NK cells, inflammation, fever, and phagocytosis. The complement system, a type of chemical defense, is also a second line of defense.

Physical Barriers

The primary function of physical barriers in the innate immune system is to prevent entry of microorganisms and other foreign substances into the body. Physical barriers include the skin, mucous membranes, cleansing actions, and excretory and expelling actions.

- Skin. Skin makes an excellent barrier to prevent invasion by foreign molecules. Epithelial cells in the outer layer of the skin (the stratum corneum) are packed together and are interwoven with keratin. The result is a thick, strong, waterproof layer that most pathogens cannot break through. As long as the skin is intact with no scrapes, breaks, or cuts, the majority of the body is protected against foreign invaders.

- Mucous membranes. Mucous membranes line surfaces of the respiratory, digestive, and urogenital systems and help to prevent the entry of foreign invaders through these areas. The presence of mucous on these membranes creates a surface that is difficult for bacteria to stick to. This prevents bacteria from attaching to surfaces and inhibits their entrance to the body. In addition, epithelial cells in the respiratory system have **cilia** that sweep foreign pathogens up and out of the bronchi, toward the pharynx. From the pharynx, the pathogens will be swallowed where many will be killed due to the strongly acidic pH.

- Cleansing actions. The cleansing action of the tears, saliva, and urine are mechanical barriers that also help prevent attachment and entry of pathogens. Tearing of the eyes helps to wash away microbes that could enter through the eyes. The saliva continually flushes microbes out of the mouth and into the stomach. The urinary tract also washes away microbes by moving urine through the ureters, through the bladder, and out of the body through the urethra.

- Expelling and excretory actions. Sneezing (Figure 12-8), coughing, vomiting, and defecation all act as mechanical barriers designed to remove microbes that have entered the respiratory and digestive systems.

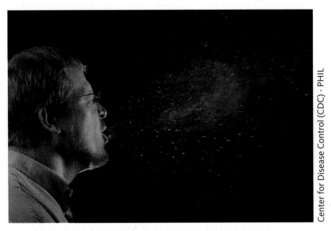

Center for Disease Control (CDC) - PHIL

FIGURE 12-8 A man in the process of sneezing. Sneezing is one method that the immune system uses to rid the body of pathogens and other foreign molecules.

CLINICAL TIP   Microbes spread easily between people through sneezing. It is important to cover a sneeze with a tissue.

Chemical Barriers

There are several chemical defenses that are part of the first line of defense as well. Chemical defenses create conditions that make survival of microbes difficult. Chemical defenses in the first line of defense include lysozyme, defensins, and acidity:

- Lysozyme in tears and saliva. **Lysozyme** is an enzyme that pokes holes in bacterial cell walls.

- Defensins. As mentioned previously (Table 12-1), defensins are peptides made by numerous cells and tissues of the body that destroy microbial cell membranes.

- Acidity. Most microorganisms cannot survive and reproduce in an acidic pH. The stomach contains hydrochloric acid, which is a very strong acid. Most microbes cannot survive the strongly acidic pH of the stomach. The vagina is also acidic due to the presence of an acid called lactic acid, which helps prevent the growth of many microorganisms. Even the skin has an acidic pH that can inhibit the growth of some microbes.

The Complement System The complement system is a chemical defense that is part of the second line of defense. The complement system consists of a large number of plasma proteins that work together to enhance the actions of the immune system and to help clear foreign cells from the body. The complement system is a complex system consisting of over 30 proteins. The proteins circulate through your bloodstream in an inactive form. They can be activated directly by substances on a microbial cell wall or by recognizing an antibody combined with an antigen. Once the system is activated, each protein triggers the activation of the next protein in a set of reactions known as the **complement cascade**.

There are two main functions of the complement cascade: opsonization and cell lysis.

- **Opsonization** is the coating of a foreign cell with proteins, known as **opsonins**. Opsonization enhances the process of phagocytosis. When a foreign cell has been coated with opsonins, such as complement proteins, phagocytic cells have an easier time recognizing that it is foreign and are able to make physical contact with the cell to start phagocytosis.

- Cell lysis, discussed previously, refers to the direct killing and bursting of a foreign cell. Several complement proteins can join together to form a complex known as the **membrane attack complex (MAC)**. The MAC acts as a sort of drill. It drills through the foreign cell membrane to form holes or small pores (Figure 12-9). The foreign cell will then burst (lyse) in the process.

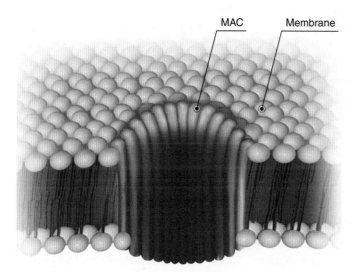

MAC   Membrane

FIGURE 12-9 MAC (blue) embedded in a microbial cell membrane (pink). The MAC pokes holes or pores into the cell membrane to kill the microbe.

Species Resistance

Species resistance refers to the genetic makeup of an individual that makes them naturally resistant to certain pathogens that cause disease in other species. For example, there are certain diseases that affect cats and dogs but do not affect humans. Likewise, there are diseases that affect humans that do not affect cats and dogs.

One explanation for species resistance is that certain pathogens must attach to receptors on the host cell in order to invade the cell. Organisms of different species have different receptors on their cells. A virus that can attach to a receptor on a dog's cell may not be able to infect human cells because humans are missing that particular receptor. Another explanation for species resistance is the difference in temperature between different organisms. Most microbes have a narrow temperature range that is optimal for their growth. They may grow really well in one type of species, but another species could be slightly too warm or too cold for optimal growth of the microbe.

Natural Killer Cell

A **natural killer (NK) cell** is a specialized type of lymphocyte that functions in the second line of defense. The function of NK cells is to seek out and kill foreign cells and microorganisms that have managed to enter into the body. They play a key role in killing virally infected cells and cancer cells. NK cells release chemicals called **perforins**. Perforins can damage the cell membranes of foreign cells, leading to cell lysis. NK cells also release cytokines, which, as discussed previously, enhance the response of other immune cells. NK cells are very unique because other types of lymphocytes, such as T cells and B cells, function as part of the adaptive immune system. In addition, the other lymphocytes react very specifically to their foreign targets, while NK cells function in a more nonspecific way as part of the innate immune system.

Inflammation

Imagine that you are walking across your lawn barefoot when you step on a rusty nail. The nail punctures your skin (creating a break in the first line of defense) which damages the cells and tissues in your foot. The second line of defense must now kick in to clean up the cellular damage in your foot and to prevent the entry and spread of microorganisms through the open wound.

When a part of the body has been damaged due to injury, trauma, or infection, the secondary defense mechanism known as inflammation will begin. **Inflammation** is the innate immune system's general, localized response to cellular injury. Its main function is to prevent spread of microorganisms.

When an injury occurs, the first actions the body takes to protect itself are vasoconstriction and the formation of a blood clot. **Vasoconstriction** refers to the narrowing (constricting) of blood vessels in the damaged area. Constricting blood vessels reduces blood flow in the damaged area. This is important because it prevents blood loss from the injury that you have sustained until a blood clot can form. When the risk of blood loss has stopped, the process of inflammation can occur.

Inflammation can be summarized in the following three main steps and in Figure 12-10.

1. **Vasodilation.** This refers to the widening (dilation) of localized blood vessels in the area of the injury or disease. Injured cells release the chemical histamine. Histamine triggers vasodilation (Figure 12-10, parts 2 and 3).

The result of vasodilation is that more blood flows to the affected area. The flow of blood into the damaged area brings in white blood cells to fight any invading pathogens (Figure 12-10, part 1). The blood also carries chemical components to the injured area that help fight an infection if it occurs (Figure 12-10, part 1).

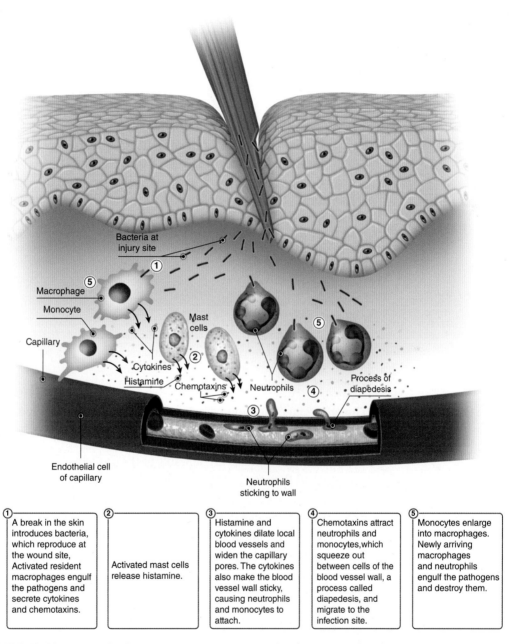

① A break in the skin introduces bacteria, which reproduce at the wound site, Activated resident macrophages engulf the pathogens and secrete cytokines and chemotaxins.	② Activated mast cells release histamine.	③ Histamine and cytokines dilate local blood vessels and widen the capillary pores. The cytokines also make the blood vessel wall sticky, causing neutrophils and monocytes to attach.	④ Chemotaxins attract neutrophils and monocytes,which squeeze out between cells of the blood vessel wall, a process called diapedesis, and migrate to the infection site.	⑤ Monocytes enlarge into macrophages. Newly arriving macrophages and neutrophils engulf the pathogens and destroy them.

FIGURE 12-10 Steps of inflammation using an example of a puncture in the skin due to a situation such as stepping on a rusty nail, allowing bacteria to enter through the wound.

2. **Permeability** of capillaries increases. The endothelial layer of the capillaries will separate slightly, allowing for increased permeability. Some of the blood plasma as well as various antimicrobial chemicals can leak out of the bloodstream and into the tissues to help prevent infection of the tissues. This permeability also allows the phagocytic white blood cells to leave the blood vessel and travel into the tissue through the process of diapedesis, as described earlier (Figure 12-10, part 4).

3. Phagocytosis occurs. Phagocytic cells, such as neutrophils and macrophages, will perform phagocytosis on any bacteria or other foreign particles that have entered (Figure 12-10, part 5). In addition to performing phagocytosis, the white blood cells secrete cytokines, which act to bring additional white blood cells to the area to fight foreign invaders. The phagocytic cells clean up the area by killing microorganisms that have entered and by digesting the damaged cells from the injured person's body. Another type of white blood cell, a mast cell, may secrete histamine in response to the foreign invader. The white blood cells themselves may die when they have completed the cleanup. The combination of the dead tissue cells, dead white blood cells, and dead microorganisms can lead to the appearance of pus in the area. When all damage is cleared, tissues will begin to heal.

There are five cardinal signs that can be seen in a patient with inflammation. They are:

1. Redness
2. Heat
3. Swelling
4. Pain
5. Loss of function

The three mechanisms of inflammation described above lead to these cardinal signs:

- Heat and redness are a result of the vasodilation and increased blood flow to the affected area.
- Increased capillary permeability leads to swelling as fluid leaks into the tissues.
- As fluid builds in the tissues, pressure is put on nearby nerve endings, leading to pain.
- All of these things together lead to loss of function.

Fever

A fever is any rise of body temperature above the normal set point for the body. A normal body temperature is near 98.6°F (37°C), although it can vary slightly from person to person. Normal body temperature is regulated by a region of the brain called the hypothalamus. Normal maintenance of body temperature may be disrupted when the body is exposed to pyrogens. **Pyrogens** are substances that raise the temperature set point in the hypothalamus above normal. Pyrogens may be released directly from a microorganism. For example, some bacteria release toxins that act as pyrogens. Our own phagocytic white blood cells can also release pyrogens during the process of phagocytosis.

Fever is a part of the innate immune response because it prevents the replication of some microbes. Many microbes grow and replicate best around normal human body temperature. If that body temperature rises, their growth and replication will slow down and possibly even stop. In addition, fever actually enhances your immune response. It speeds up the process of phagocytosis. It also enhances the action of interferon to prevent replication of viruses in body cells.

Phagocytosis

Phagocytosis is one of the most important defense mechanisms in the innate immune system. It is part of the immune system's second line of defense to kill pathogens when they do make their way into the body. The term *phagocytosis* comes from a Greek word meaning "to eat." Phagocytosis is the action of certain white blood cells called phagocytes. Phagocytes engulf, destroy, and digest microorganisms and other foreign cells. Phagocytes can also degrade your own cells when they become old or diseased. This allows nonfunctioning cells to be removed from the body so that new cells can take their place. The most active phagocytes in the human body are neutrophils and monocytes/macrophages.

Phagocytosis has four steps (Figure 12-11):

1. Physical contact: The first step in phagocytosis is that the phagocyte must make direct physical contact with the microbe. At this stage, receptors on the surface of the phagocyte recognize that the microbe is foreign and that it needs to be removed from the body.

2. Formation of the phagosome: The phagocyte will then extend its cell membrane into projections called **pseudopods**. The pseudopods will surround and engulf the microbe, bringing the microbe inside of the phagocyte. The microbe will end up inside of an endocytic vesicle in the white blood cell. The vesicle is called a **phagosome**.

3. Formation of the phagolysosome: The phagosome will join together with a cellular organelle called a lysosome. Lysosomes are full of digestive enzymes that can degrade microorganisms. When the phagosome and the lysosome join together, they make a new structure called the **phagolysosome**.

4. Digestion and excretion: Digestive enzymes will be released into the phagolysosome, killing the microorganism. The microorganism will be destroyed. Its remaining waste products and antigen fragments will be excreted from the phagocyte. These antigen fragments will attach to MHC molecules inside the cell. **MHC molecules** are molecules that help the immune system recognize the difference between self and non-self. MHC genes code for MHC molecules. They are unique to each individual person.

   Antigenic fragments combined with MHC molecules will attach to the cell surface of the phagocyte in a process called **antigen presentation**. This allows immune cells to recognize self (MHC) and non-self (antigen). The phagocyte that contains the attached foreign antigens is now known as an antigen-presenting cell. Antigen-presenting cells help stimulate the adaptive immune system.

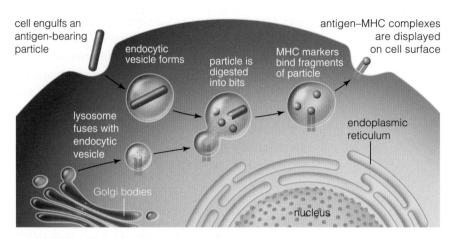

cell engulfs an
antigen-bearing
particle

endocytic
vesicle forms

particle is
digested
into bits

MHC markers
bind fragments
of particle

antigen–MHC complexes
are displayed
on cell surface

lysosome
fuses with
endocytic
vesicle

endoplasmic
reticulum

Golgi bodies

nucleus

FIGURE 12-11 Phagocytic white blood cell performing phagocytosis on an antigen-bearing particle, such as a bacterial cell.

LEARNING OBJECTIVE 12.1.7 Identify the components of the adaptive immune system.

LEARNING OBJECTIVE 12.1.8 Identify the function of adaptive immunity.

LEARNING OBJECTIVE 12.1.9 Describe the functions of adaptive immunity.

LEARNING OBJECTIVE 12.1.10 Identify the two types of lymphocytes.

KEY TERMS

cell-mediated immunity Action of the adaptive immune system mediated by T cells.

humoral immunity Action of the adaptive immune system mediated by antibodies.

plasma cell Activated B cell that secretes antibodies.

THE ADAPTIVE IMMUNE SYSTEM

The adaptive immune system includes the third line of defense. If a pathogen has made its way into the body and past the first and second lines of defense, the adaptive immune system will begin fighting the pathogen to kill it, remove it from the body, and preserve the health of the body. The third line of defense is very specific and involves the actions of lymphocytes and antibodies to target and remove specific antigens.

The word *adaptive* refers to the ability of this part of the immune system to change, adjust, and improve with time. While people are born with some components of the adaptive immune system, this part of the immune system takes time and exposure to antigens in order to fully develop and be able to protect the body.

Like the innate immune system, the main components of the adaptive immune system are white blood cells. The white blood cells that are active in adaptive immunity are the lymphocytes, specifically the lymphocytes called T cells and B cells.

There are two divisions of the adaptive immune system:

1. **Cell-mediated immunity.** This is the action of T cells. There are two main types of T cells (cytotoxic T cells and helper T cells). Their actions are detailed in the next sections of this chapter.

2. **Humoral immunity.** The term *humoral immunity* originates from the term *humor*, which means "in the serum." Humoral immunity refers to the actions of antibodies that move through the serum and the way those antibodies respond to antigens. Antibodies are produced by a specific type of B cell called a **plasma cell.**

FUNCTIONS OF THE ADAPTIVE IMMUNE SYSTEM

The adaptive immune system has the same basic function of the innate immune system, which is to destroy any foreign invaders or toxins that they produce. As covered in the next section, certain white blood cells (lymphocytes) that are a part of the adaptive immune system destroy pathogens to maintain health and rid the body of infection. These lymphocytes mount a very specific attack against particular antigens to destroy the organism and remove the antigen.

The adaptive immune system has a much more important function, however, because it functions to induce immune memory or immunity. When lymphocytes learn to fight a particular foreign entity, it results in immunologic memory, which means the cells "remember" how to best fight and kill that invader. If you are exposed to the same pathogen again, this immune memory will allow you to mount the adaptive immune response much faster and much more effectively than it did the first time you were exposed. This is discussed in detail in the next section.

LEARNING OBJECTIVE 12.1.11 Identify the functions of T lymphocytes and B lymphocytes.

LEARNING OBJECTIVE 12.1.12 Describe the functions of T lymphocytes and B lymphocytes.

LEARNING OBJECTIVE 12.1.13 Describe the activation mechanism of T lymphocytes and B lymphocytes.

KEY TERMS

antigen-presenting cells Phagocytic cells that have engulfed foreign invaders and placed the foreign invaders' antigens on their own cell surface to present it to other cells in the immune system.

cytotoxic T cells T cells that kill virally infected cells and cancer cells.

differentiate Specialization of cells.

helper T cells T cells that help activate B cells by secreting cytokines.

immunity Body's ability to defend itself.

memory T cells T cells that remember how to fight a particular antigen.

proliferation Cloning and increase in number of cells.

T Lymphocytes

Like all other white blood cells, lymphocytes arise from stem cells in the bone marrow. As mentioned previously, there are two main types of lymphocytes: the T cells and the B cells. T cells are formed in the bone marrow, but they are in an immature state while there. They are not prepared to fight. Before they are ready to fight pathogens, they must become mature (Figure 12-12). The T cells will leave the bone marrow and travel to the thymus, where they will mature.

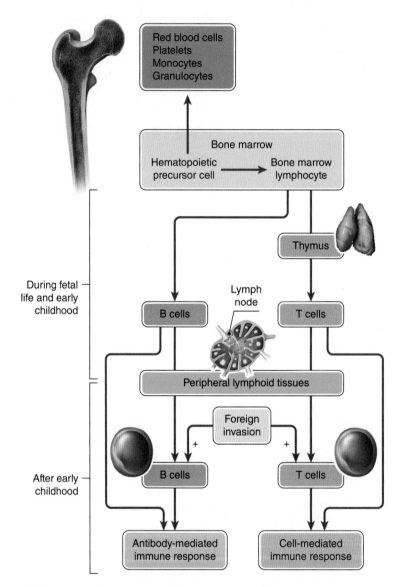

FIGURE 12-12 Summary of the development, maturation, and immune response of B and T cells.

| CLINICAL TIP | Both thymus and T cells start with the letter *T*, so you can remember that T cells mature in the thymus. |

Once T cells are mature, they will leave the thymus and begin to circulate through the blood, "looking" for foreign cells to fight (Figure 12-12). Some T cells will stay in various lymphatic organs such as the lymph nodes or spleen in order to fight foreign invaders that may circulate through these organs.

There are three different types of T cells at work in the process of adaptive immunity:

- **Cytotoxic T cells.** Cytotoxic T cells (also called killer T cells) have the ability to directly kill our own cells that are infected with viruses, foreign cells, and even cancerous tumor cells (Figure 12-13AB). They secrete perforins that destroy the cell by poking holes in its cell membrane. Cytotoxic T cells are also called CD8+ cells, referring to a specific cell marker found on the surface of the cell.

- **Helper T cells.** As the name implies, the job of helper T cells is to help other immune system cells. Specifically, helper T cells help activate B cells by secreting cytokines. Helper T cells are called CD4+ cells.

- **Memory T cells.** Memory T cells have the ability to "remember" the pathogen that they have come into contact with. This memory allows the cells to fight that pathogen much faster if they come into contact with it in the future.

Activation of T Cells Even though T cells are mature when they leave the thymus, they are still not in fighting mode. They are circulating throughout the body in an inactive form. Before they are ready to fight, they must be activated. Activation of T cells requires interaction with the innate immune system.

Remember that white blood cells of the innate immune system will perform phagocytosis on a foreign cell. The phagocytic white blood cell will engulf the foreign cell, kill and digest it, and place the destroyed cell's fragments (antigens) on the surface of the white blood cell. This allows it to "present" the antigens to the rest of the immune system, which is referred to as **antigen-presenting cells** (Figure 12-14). Antigen-presenting cells, such as macrophages, neutrophils, and dendritic cells, present the antigens to T cells in order to activate the T cell.

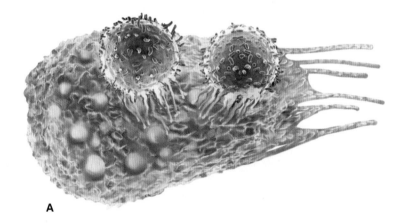

A

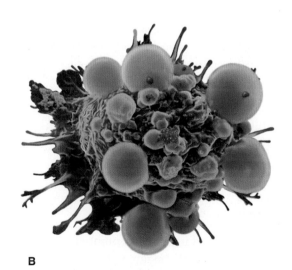

B

FIGURE 12-13AB (A) Cytotoxic T cells killing a cancerous cell. (B) Dying cancer cell.

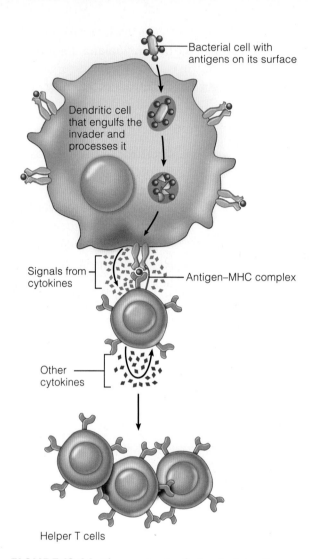

FIGURE 12-14 Phagocytosis of a bacterial cell by a dendritic cell. Following phagocytosis, the antigen is presented along with MHC on the cell surface to activate a helper T cell.

The steps of T cell activation (Figure 12-15) are as follows:

1. An antigen-presenting cell will present an antigen on its cell surface. The antigen will be combined with an MHC molecule. T-cell activation requires antigen be combined with MHC.
2. Receptors on the T cell will make physical contact with the antigen/MHC complex.
3. The T cell will become activated and will proliferate. **Proliferation** means that the cell will be cloned and increase in numbers. When T cells proliferate, they will also **differentiate**, meaning they will specialize so that each type of T cell will have a separate job. Some of the clones will be cytotoxic T cells, some will be helper T cells, and some will be memory T cells.

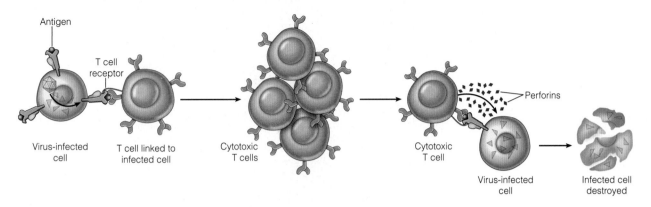

FIGURE 12-15 Cytotoxic T cell being activated to fight a virally infected cell.

After activation, cytotoxic T cells will be ready to destroy their target cells by secreting perforins. Memory T cells will be able to be quickly activated in the case of future exposures to the pathogen. Helper T cells will be ready to help activate B cells by secreting cytokines.

B Lymphocytes

Like T cells, B lymphocytes develop from stem cells in the bone marrow. They go through many stages of development, but they do not need to leave the bone marrow in order to mature. Once mature, they will leave the bone marrow to circulate through the blood and travel through the lymphatic organs looking for foreign cells to fight.

CLINICAL TIP Both bone marrow and B cells start with the letter *B*, so you can remember that B cells mature in the bone marrow.

Activation of B Cells B cell activation requires two things:

1. An antigen must fit the shape of the B cell receptor and
2. Helper T cells must secrete cytokines to assist with B cell activation.

B cells have small, Y-shaped receptors on their cell surfaces (Figure 12-16). These receptors have ends that can fit together with antigens. Each type of B cell only has receptors that can fit together with one type of antigen. For example, if a B cell has receptors that can bind to an antigen on the bacteria *Streptococcus*, that same B cell will not be able to bind to antigens from the bacteria *E. coli*. This accounts for the specificity of the adaptive immune system. There are many different B cells moving throughout the body, each one primed to fight a different type of antigen.

CLINICAL TIP Think of the fit between B cell receptors and antigens like puzzle pieces that must fit perfectly together.

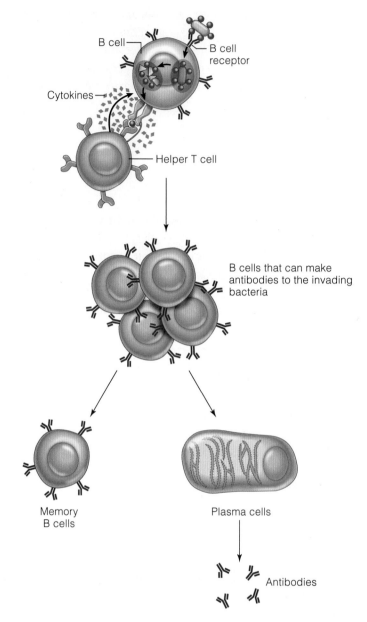

FIGURE 12-16 B cell with a bacterial antigen that has bound to its receptor. With the assistance of the helper T cell, the B cell is activated and will proliferate and differentiate, forming memory B cells and plasma cells. The plasma cells will secrete antibodies to help fight more of the antigens.

If a B cell encounters an antigen that fits the shape of its receptor, it can become activated. Activated helper T cells will secrete cytokines, which will assist in this process (Figure 12-16). When the B cell activates, it will proliferate and differentiate into plasma cells and memory B cells. Plasma cells will produce and secrete antibodies that can float throughout the serum.

Antibodies are actually the receptors that were originally attached to the B cell (Figure 12-17). The antibodies are very specific to that particular antigen. Antibodies do not destroy foreign cells—their role in immune response is to enhance the actions of other parts of the immune system. For example, antibodies can act as opsonins, enhancing the process of phagocytosis. Antibodies can also agglutinate bacteria and some foreign cells, making them stick together so that it is easier for phagocytes to kill them. Antibodies can also neutralize viruses and toxins. Finally, certain types of antibodies can activate the complement system, leading to destruction of the foreign cells.

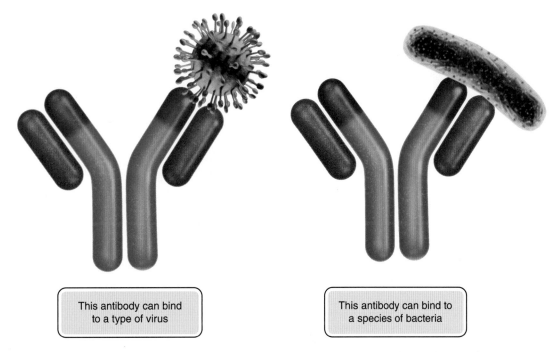

This antibody can bind to a type of virus

This antibody can bind to a species of bacteria

FIGURE 12-17 Two different antibodies: one that can bind to a virus and one that can bind to a bacterium.

Memory B cells retain the "memory" of how to create antibodies to that particular antigen. If the antigen is encountered again in the future, memory B cells can mount a quick response, potentially leading to immunity. **Immunity** refers to the ability of the body to become resistant to pathogens.

LEARNING OBJECTIVE 12.1.14 Contrast the defensive functions of the innate and adaptive immune systems.

COMPARING INNATE AND ADAPTIVE IMMUNITY

Both the innate and adaptive immune systems work together to maintain the health of the body. However, as we've discussed, their defensive functions are significantly different from one another (Figure 12-18).

Timeframe for response (Table 12-2): While the innate immune system is ready to go to work immediately, the adaptive immune system takes time to develop to its full potential. The adaptive immune system doesn't begin working to destroy a pathogen until several days after exposure to the pathogen.

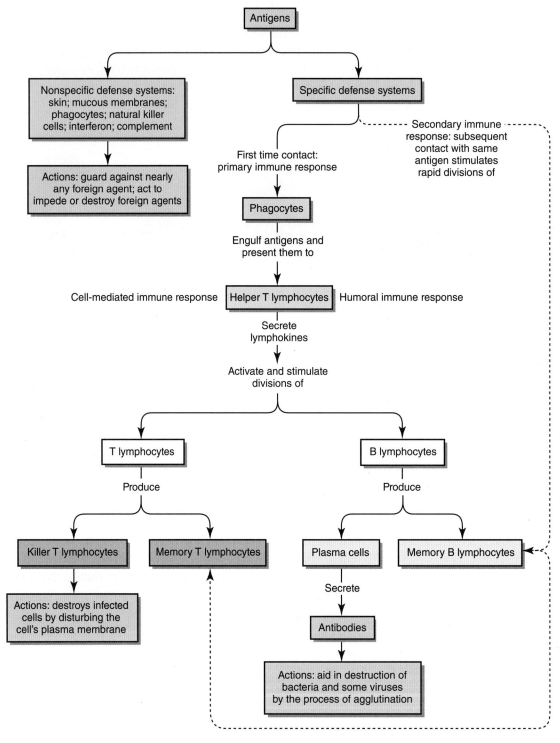

FIGURE 12-18 Actions of the innate and adaptive immune systems.

- Specificity: The innate immune system is very nonspecific. This means it will react to every foreign entity essentially the same way. The adaptive immune system, however, is extremely specific and is based on fighting each antigen with a very specific antibody. The response varies for each pathogen and each antigen. This results in more efficient destruction of the pathogen.

Table 12-2 Innate and Adaptive Immune Systems

BRANCH OF THE IMMUNE SYSTEM	TIMEFRAME FOR RESPONSE	SPECIFICITY	RESULTS IN IMMUNITY?	LINES OF DEFENSE	EXAMPLES
Innate	Immediate	Nonspecific	No	First and second lines of defense	Skin, mucous membranes, phagocytic WBCs, complement system
Adaptive	Many days	Very specific	Yes	Third line of defense	B and T lymphocytes, antibodies

- Response over time (Table 12-2): The innate immune system has the same response with every encounter to the pathogen. In the adaptive immune system, the response improves with each exposure. Memory cells remember how to fight a pathogen and can mount a quicker and stronger immune response with each subsequent exposure. This results in immune memory, leading to immunity.

LEARNING OBJECTIVE 12.1.15 Identify the parts of an immunoglobulin molecule.

KEY TERMS

fragment antigen binding (Fab) Part of the immunoglobulin molecule that binds to antigens.

fragment constant (Fc) Bottom portion of the immunoglobulin that attaches to the B cells to form receptors.

immunoglobulin Immune system protein; another name for an antibody.

ANTIBODY STRUCTURE

Antibodies are also called immunoglobulins. "Immuno" refers to the immune system and "globulin" means protein, so an immunoglobulin, or antibody, is an immune system protein. They are also sometimes called gamma globulins since they circulate in the gamma portion of the blood. Immunoglobulins are made of four protein chains hooked together by disulfide bonds. The four protein chains hook together in a "Y" formation (Figure 12-19). The long parts of the Y are called the heavy chains of the immunoglobulin. The shorter parts are called the light chains.

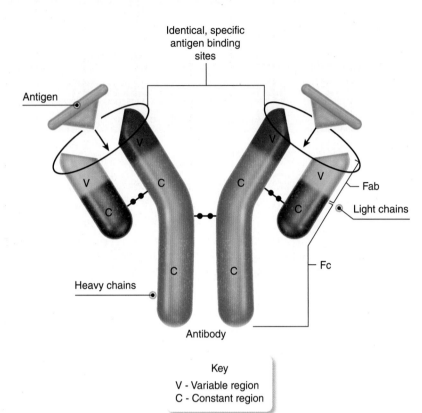

Key

V - Variable region
C - Constant region

FIGURE 12-19 Y-shaped immunoglobulin molecule. The Fab region binds antigens. Only one certain antigen can fit together with the immunoglobulin.

The bottom portion of the immunoglobulin molecule is called the constant region of the molecule or the **fragment constant (Fc)**. The Fc region attaches to the B cells to form the B-cell receptors. The other ends of the molecule are called the variable regions or the **fragment antigen binding (Fab)**. As the name implies, this is the part of the molecule that binds to antigens. Remember that each antibody can only bind to one specific antigen. These ends are variable, meaning that the variable region of one antibody is different than the variable region of another antibody so that they can bind different antigens.

LEARNING OBJECTIVE 12.1.16 Identify the five types of immunoglobulins.

LEARNING OBJECTIVE 12.1.17 Describe the five types of immunoglobulins.

LEARNING OBJECTIVE 12.1.18 Describe the function of each type of immunoglobulin.

KEY TERMS

IgG Smallest immunoglobulin; most predominant antibody secreted into serum; secondary response antibody.

IgA Immunoglobin present on mucous membranes and body secretions, such as tears, saliva, and breast milk; prevents bacterial cells from attaching to mucous membranes.

IgE Antibody found on certain white blood cells; plays a role in allergic reactions and inflammation.

IgD Antibody found in low numbers throughout the body. Most commonly found on surface of B cells.

IgM Largest antibody; primary response antibody and is the first released when exposure to pathogen occurs.

CLASSES OF IMMUNOGLOBULINS

There are five different types, or classes, of immunoglobulins (Figure 12-20). The structure of the constant region on the heavy chain is what determines the class that the immunoglobulin belongs to. Each has a slightly different structure and function. They are named IgG, IgA, IgE, IgD, and IgM (Ig stands for immunoglobulin).

Secreted antibodies

IgG Main antibody in blood; activates complement, neutralizes toxins; protects fetus and is secreted in early milk.

IgA Abundant in exocrine gland secretions (e.g., tears, saliva, milk, mucus), where it occurs in the form *shown here*. Interferes with binding of pathogens to body cells.

Membrane-bound antibodies

IgE Anchored to surface of basophils, mast cells, eosinophils, and some dendritic cells. IgE binding to antigen induces anchoring cell to release histamines and cytokines. Factor in allergies and asthma.

IgD   B cell receptor.

IgM   B cell receptor, as a monomer. Also is secreted as pentamer (group of five), as shown here.

FIGURE 12-20 Shape and functions of each of the five subclasses of immunoglobulins (also called antibodies).

- **IgG**. IgG is the predominant antibody secreted into the serum. It is the smallest antibody and is in a monomer form (one Y). Because it is so small, it can easily cross the placenta in pregnant women (passive immunity is discussed in greater detail in the section "Active Versus Passive Immunity."). This provides some passive immunity to the newborn. IgG antibodies can also activate the complement system. IgG is considered the secondary immune response antibody (primary and secondary responses are discussed in more detail in the next section). IgG antibodies take a while to develop when you are exposed to a pathogen, but they are considered protective. IgG is also secreted from memory cells. If you have a high number of IgG antibodies to a particular pathogen, you are considered immune to that pathogen.

- **IgA**. IgA is present on mucous membranes and body secretions such as tears, saliva, and breast milk. The passage of IgA in breast milk can give some passive immunity to breast-fed infants. IgA prevents bacterial cells from attaching to mucous membranes. It also helps to neutralize toxins. IgA may either be in a monomer form or a dimer (two Y's attached together by their Fc regions).

- **IgE**. IgE is found bound to white blood cells that play a role in allergies and inflammation, such as eosinophils and basophils. When IgE binds to these cells, it can trigger the release of histamine from these cells, leading to allergy symptoms.

- **IgD**. IgD is found in very low numbers in the body. Most of it is found on the surface of B cells, where it serves as a B cell receptor.

- **IgM**. IgM is the largest antibody. When it is secreted, it is in the form of a pentamer (five Y's attached together). IgM is called the primary response antibody. It is the first one released when you first come into contact with a foreign cell. IgM is not secreted from memory cells, so it does not confer permanent immunity. IgM is good at activating the complement system to help destroy foreign cells. It is too large to cross the placenta, so it does not provide passive immunity to the newborn, but it is the first antibody that infants will make when exposed to pathogens.

LEARNING OBJECTIVE 12.1.19 Identify primary and secondary immunity.

LEARNING OBJECTIVE 12.1.20 Describe primary and secondary immunity.

LEARNING OBJECTIVE 12.1.21 Contrast the primary and secondary immune responses.

KEY TERMS

primary immune response Immune responses that occur the first time the immune system comes in contact with a pathogen.

secondary immune response Immune response that occurs with secondary and subsequent

exposures to pathogen; response begins almost immediately and includes a higher amount of antibodies than primary immune response.

titer Laboratory test to check the number of a particular antibody in the blood.

PRIMARY AND SECONDARY IMMUNITY

The very first time in a person's life that they are exposed to a foreign antigen, their immune system will begin to produce antibodies. This is called the **primary immune response**.

Remember the long process of activation that has to occur for B and T cells to become activated before antibodies can be produced. Because of this, the primary immune response can take several weeks to reach full strength. The first antibody that will be made during this response is IgM, and it will be made in fairly low levels. Much later in the response, low levels of IgG will also be made.

If the person is exposed to the same antigen again, later in life, they have already produced memory cells that remember how to fight that pathogen. Activation and secretion of antibodies occurs much quicker and the response is much stronger. As you can see in Figure 12-21AB, the response begins almost immediately, and higher amounts of antibodies are produced than with the primary response. This is referred to as a **secondary immune response**. Small amounts of IgM will be produced in the secondary response, but extremely high levels of IgG will be produced very quickly and work to help remove the foreign entity. Since the immune response happens so quickly, the patient may not feel sick and may not even know that the antigen has entered their body before it is dealt with by the immune system.

Vaccines

Vaccines (also called immunizations) work based on these ideas of primary and secondary immune responses. When someone is given a vaccine, they are given a weakened or killed version of the organism that their health care provider wants to protect them against. This first exposure to the organism triggers the

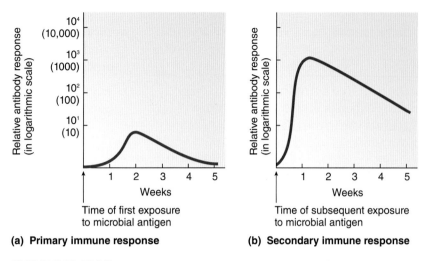

(a) **Primary immune response**   (b) **Secondary immune response**

FIGURE 12-21AB Primary immune response occurs the first time a person is exposed to an antigen; secondary immune response occurs with subsequent exposures.

primary immune response. Since the organism is weakened or killed, the patient will not get sick from the organism. Their immune system will respond, however, and memory cells will be made. Then, if the person gets exposed to the actual organism during the course of life, their memory cells already remember how to fight that pathogen. The secondary immune response will kick in to remove the pathogen before the person even knows that they have come into contact with it.

Occasionally, a health care provider may order a titer for a patient. A **titer** is a laboratory test in which a patient's IgG levels are tested to see if a person is immune to a particular disease. For example, if a health care provider orders a measles titer, the patient's blood will be tested for high levels of IgG specific for the measles virus. If the antibodies are found in high enough levels, the person is considered immune to measles.

LEARNING OBJECTIVE 12.1.22 Identify active and passive immunity.

LEARNING OBJECTIVE 12.1.23 Describe active and passive immunity.

LEARNING OBJECTIVE 12.1.24 Contrast active and passive immunity.

KEY TERMS

active immunity Immune condition where a person produces antibodies.

artificially acquired active immunity Immune condition where a person is introduced to a microorganism through medical means and develop their own antibodies to the microorganism.

artificially acquired passive immunity Immune condition where a person is given someone else's antibodies through a medical procedure.

naturally acquired active immunity Immune condition where a person is exposed to a microorganism in the course of daily life and make antibodies to the microorganism.

naturally acquired passive immunity Immune condition where a person is given someone else's antibodies through the course of natural life.

passive immunity Immune condition where a person is given someone else's antibodies.

COMPARING ACTIVE AND PASSIVE IMMUNITY

There are many different ways in which a person might be protected against a particular pathogen. The person's own immune system can fight a pathogen in a process known as active immunity, or the person can get assistance from someone else's immune system in a process known as passive immunity (Table 12-3).

Table 12-3 Types of Immunity

	NATURAL IMMUNITY	ARTIFICIAL IMMUNITY
Active	A person gets a disease and recovers.	Vaccination causes the body to create antibodies that will defend against disease.
Passive	Mother provides antibodies and immunity across the placenta (IgG) or via breast milk (IgA).	Serum, immunoglobulins, or antitoxins provided by another person or animal.

Active Immunity

Active immunity (Table 12-3) means that the person's immune system is producing antibodies to fight the pathogen. Active immunity is a result of the T- and B-cell activation processes previously described. Upon exposure to an antigen, the person's adaptive immune system will be activated, and they will produce antibodies to help fight the pathogen. Active immunity takes time to develop, but when it does it can result in long-lasting immunity. There are two subcategories of active immunity:

- **Naturally acquired active immunity.** This is the type of immunity developed when a person is exposed to an antigen as part of their normal lives and produces antibodies to fight it. For example, a child is exposed to the measles virus. The child produces memory cells and antibodies to neutralize the virus. Since the child's own immune system is producing the antibodies and the virus was contracted through normal life activities, this is termed *naturally acquired active immunity.*

- **Artificially acquired active immunity.** This is the type of immunity developed when a person is exposed to an antigen in the form of a vaccine and then they produce antibodies to fight it. For example, a parent takes their child to the pediatrician to receive the measles vaccine. The child is given a weakened version of the measles virus that cannot give the child the measles disease. The child will develop memory cells and antibodies to neutralize the weakened virus. The memory cells will remember how to fight the virus if the child is exposed to the actual measles virus later in life. Since the child's own immune system is still producing the antibodies, this is still active immunity; however, it is artificially acquired since the exposure came through a vaccine rather than normal daily activities.

Passive Immunity

The second process for protection against a pathogen is passive immunity. In **passive immunity** (Table 12-3), the person is receiving antibodies that were made in a different person. The person's own immune system is not making the antibodies. Passive immunity can be very beneficial to babies since they have never been exposed to antigens before. Passive immunity can also help people who are immunocompromised due to disease, chemotherapy, or medications that have suppressed their immune system. Immunocompromised individuals may not be able to produce their own antibodies due to a weakened immune system. Passive immunity gives only short-term protection since the person is not activating their own lymphocytes or creating their own memory cells. There are also two subcategories of passive immunity:

- **Naturally acquired passive immunity.** This is a response that occurs when a person is given someone else's antibodies through normal life experiences. Naturally acquired passive immunity occurs through either breastfeeding or when the mother's IgG antibodies can cross the placenta. As mentioned previously, this type of immunity is only temporary because the baby's own immune system is not being activated; however, it is a beneficial, short-term protection for the baby against certain pathogens.
- **Artificially acquired passive immunity.** This is when a person is given someone else's antibodies through medical means. These antibodies are typically given through an IV to help protect immunocompromised patients. IgG may also be given as a treatment post-exposure to bloodborne infections such as HIV, hepatitis B, and hepatitis C. Artificially acquired passive immunity also includes instances when a patient is given antibodies that come from animals, for example, when antivenom is given to counteract a snake bite.

Identify the four types of hypersensitivity.

Describe the four types of hypersensitivity.

KEY TERMS

allergens Antigens that stimulate allergic reactions.

anaphylaxis Systemic, rapid reaction to an allergen that causes life-threatening respiratory and circulatory dysfunction.

autoimmune Immune condition that results from making antibodies that attack self-antigens.

degranulation Cellular process that causes release of histamine, which enables immune response.

hypersensitivity Increased sensitivity of the immune system leading to an elevated immune response.

sensitization First exposure to an allergen.

HYPERSENSITIVITY REACTIONS

Sometimes the immune system has an increased, exaggerated response to certain antigens. "Hyper" means increased or a lot of something, so these types of reactions are called hypersensitivity reactions. **Hypersensitivity** is an increased sensitivity of the immune system leading to an elevated immune response. There are four categories of hypersensitivity reactions, discussed next.

Type I Hypersensitivity Reactions

Type I hypersensitivity is more commonly known as an allergy (Table 12-4). These are immediate, exaggerated immune responses to certain antigens known as **allergens**. Allergies are thought to have a genetic link and seem to run in families. The specific allergy isn't inherited; however, genetics may make someone more inclined to develop a particular allergy. For example, one family member may have an allergy to pollen, while another has an allergy to mold.

Table 12-4 Types of Hypersensitivity

HYPERSENSITIVITY	CAUSE	EXAMPLES
Type I	IgE antibodies	Seasonal allergies; allergies to mold, peanuts, bee venom
Type II	IgM or IgG antibodies	Transfusion reactions, autoimmune hemolytic anemia
Type III	IgM or IgG antibodies	Systemic lupus erythematosus, rheumatoid arthritis
Type IV	T cells	Poison ivy, PPD test for tuberculosis

Allergic reactions occur in two stages (Figure 12-22), similar to the primary and secondary immune response.

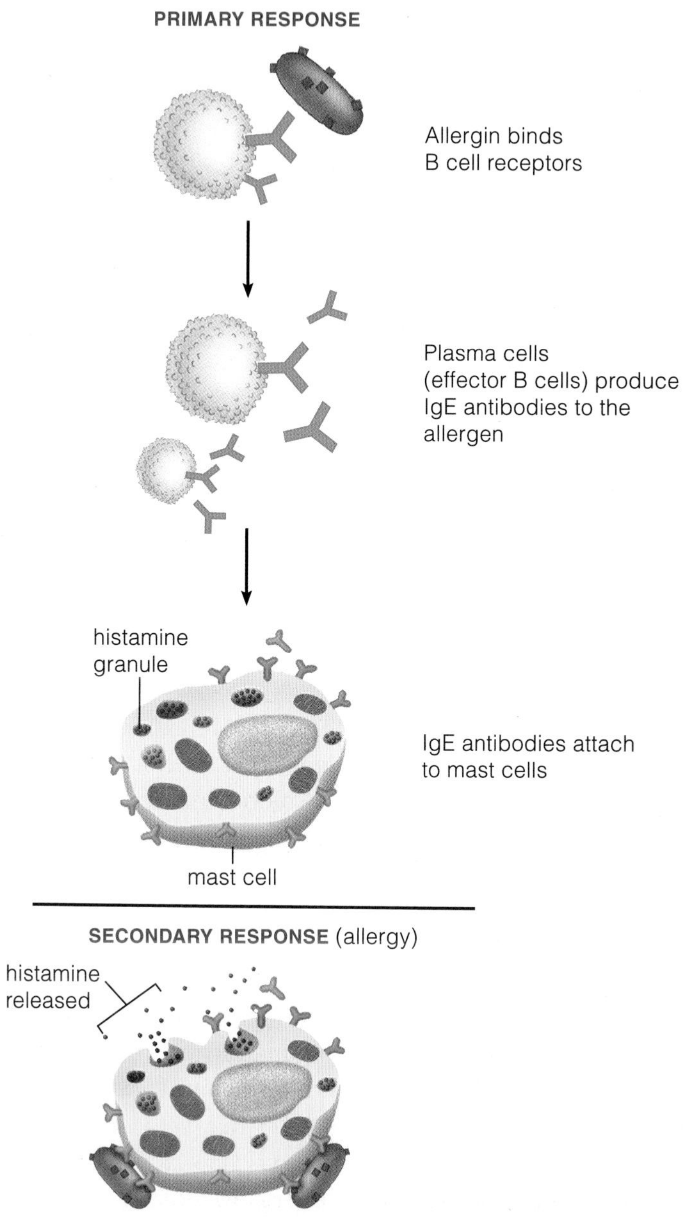

PRIMARY RESPONSE

Allergin binds
B cell receptors

Plasma cells
(effector B cells) produce
IgE antibodies to the
allergen

histamine
granule

IgE antibodies attach
to mast cells

mast cell

SECONDARY RESPONSE (allergy)

histamine
released

FIGURE 12-22 How allergic responses develop within the body.

- **Sensitization.** The first stage of an allergic reaction is called sensitization. Sensitization is the first exposure to the allergen. When the person is exposed to the antigen, B cells will be activated. The resulting plasma cells will produce IgE antibodies. These IgE antibodies will bind to white blood cells, such as eosinophils, basophils, and mast cells. Memory cells are also formed that remember how to respond to the allergen.

- **Degranulation.** In second and subsequent exposure to allergens, degranulation of white blood cells occurs. The white blood cells bound to antigens can remain in the person's body for years, ready to "fight" the allergen when exposed. If the allergen makes its way into the person's body a second time, the reaction will be immediate. The allergen will bind to two adjacent IgE antibodies on the surface of the white blood cells. The binding of the allergen triggers the degranulation of the white blood cell, resulting in the release of histamine and other chemicals from the cells. The histamine and other chemicals cause what we think of as allergy symptoms, including (but not limited to) the following:

  ° Rhinitis (runny nose)
  ° Itchy eyes and nose
  ° Sneezing
  ° Rashes, hives, and swelling
  ° Diarrhea
  ° Asthma and trouble breathing

Anaphylaxis is a systemic, rapid reaction to an allergen that causes respiratory and circulatory dysfunction. It is a serious condition that may be fatal. Anaphylaxis can cause a sudden drop in blood pressure, swelling of the respiratory passages that inhibit breathing, and can even make the heart stop beating. Certain allergies—such as allergies to peanuts, latex, and bee stings—are known for causing anaphylaxis.

Type II Hypersensitivity Reactions

Type II hypersensitivity reactions are very different from type I. Unlike type I, type II reactions are generally mediated by IgG or IgM antibodies rather than IgE (Table 12-4). These antibodies are triggered by antigens on the surface of cells that come from another person or even rarely by a lack of tolerance to our own self-antigens. The reaction of antibodies to our own antigens is called an **autoimmune** response. Type II hypersensitivity reactions result in destruction of the foreign cell or self-cell. When the antibody binds to the antigen on the cell, the complement system will be activated, resulting in lysis of the cell.

A common type of type II hypersensitivity reaction is a transfusion reaction. If a person receives blood from someone with a different blood type (e.g., a person with Type A blood receives blood from a donor with Type B blood), antibodies will bind to the foreign antigens on the foreign blood cells. Binding of the antibody will activate the complement system, and the complement system will destroy the foreign blood cells.

Type II hypersensitivity also occurs in the autoimmune disease called autoimmune hemolytic anemia. In this condition, the person's own antibodies start to attack the person's own red blood cell antigens. This results in activation of the complement system and lysis of the person's own red blood cells, leading to anemia.

Type III Hypersensitivity Reactions

Type III hypersensitivity reactions are the result of immune complexes that form between soluble antibody and antigen (Table 12-4). Type III reactions also involve IgG or IgM antibodies. These antibodies bind to antigens that are not attached to a cell, but rather are soluble and floating around in the bloodstream. The antigen and antibody can join together, forming a complex that can lodge itself in various tissues of the body. When stuck in the tissues, this complex can cause tissue destruction due to phagocytosis or activation of the complement system.

Systemic lupus erythematosus (SLE) and rheumatoid arthritis are examples of autoimmune diseases caused by type III hypersensitivities. In SLE, antibodies are directed against DNA. Immune complexes are formed that can deposit in many different organs, damaging those organs. In rheumatoid arthritis, immune complexes deposit in the joints, causing damage. Autoimmune diseases are discussed in the next section.

Type IV Hypersensitivity Reactions

Type IV reactions are not caused by antibodies at all (Table 12-4) but by the actions of T cells. After exposure to certain antigens, T cells will be sensitized to the antigen. After repeated exposure, the T cells will accumulate in the skin and will attract other white blood cells that can cause inflammation of the skin. Type IV reactions are called delayed-type hypersensitivity reactions because they can take up to several days to be noticeable.

Contact dermatitis is a common example of a type IV hypersensitivity. This type often occurs due to exposure to antigens in poison ivy. The allergen can travel through the top layers of the skin, where it will come into contact with T cells. Subsequent exposure causes the T cells to accumulate and recruit other white blood cells that can damage the skin, resulting in the itchy rash associated with poison ivy.

Type IV hypersensitivity reactions are also used in a common test to see if a person has been exposed to tuberculosis. This test is called the PPD test, which stands for purified protein derivative. A person is infected with a derivative from the bacterium *Mycobacterium tuberculosis*, which is the bacterium that causes tuberculosis. If the person has been exposed to tuberculosis before, a type IV hypersensitivity reaction will cause a red, hardened raised area around the site of injection. Forty-eight to 72 hours after the injection, the patient will return to the physician to have the area measured to determine if they have been previously exposed to tuberculosis.

UNIT OBJECTIVE 12.2

Describe common pathologies of the immune system.

UNIT INTRODUCTION

As we have discussed, the immune system is a very important system for maintaining health of the human body. When functioning properly, the immune system can protect us from diseases caused by bacteria, viruses, and other pathogens. Unfortunately, there are a number of pathological conditions that can arise that alter the immune system's ability to function properly.

LEARNING OBJECTIVE 12.2.1 Identify common pathologies of the immune system.

KEY TERMS

acquired Something a person develops.

agammaglobulinemia No detectable antibodies in the blood.

congenital Something a person is born with.

hypogammaglobulinemia Low levels of antibodies in the blood.

immunodeficiency Decrease in immune function leading to low levels of immune cells or chemicals.

opportunistic pathogens Microorganisms that do not usually cause disease but can in immunocompromised patients.

true pathogens Microorganisms that can cause disease in healthy patients with fully functioning immune systems.

IMMUNODEFICIENCY DISORDERS

An **immunodeficiency** is a deficiency in one or more of the immune system's cells or molecules. Immunodeficiency disorders can have a serious negative impact on the health and lifespan of the individual that is suffering from the disease. Without all immune system cells and molecules working like they are supposed to, a patient suffering from this condition is more likely to get sick and even die from common microorganisms that we are all exposed to every day. These patients not only get sick from **true pathogens** (pathogens that can cause disease in a healthy host), but also from **opportunistic pathogens** (organisms that don't usually cause disease unless an individual is immunocompromised). Immunodeficiency disorders can be congenital (something the person is born with) or acquired (something they develop later in life). The disorder can result from a lack of B cells and antibodies, T cells, or a combination of many different factors.

Congenital Immunodeficiencies

Congenital immunodeficiencies are usually inherited diseases that an individual is born with. A lack of B cells, T cells, or a combination of many factors can result in the individual having a poorly functioning immune system.

- B cell disorders: B cell immunodeficiencies result in a decreased amount of antibody production, leading to either hypogammaglobulinemia or agammaglobulinemia. Remember that antibodies may sometimes be called gamma globulins. "Hypo" means decreased and "a" means without. So, hypogammaglobulinemia means that a person has a decreased quantity of antibodies being produced. Agammaglobulinemia means that the person has no antibodies being produced. Sometimes, only one particular class of antibody is missing; IgA deficiencies are the most common. In other cases, multiple classes of antibodies are not being produced.

  For most people with one of these conditions, the main cause of illness is frequent, recurrent bacterial infections. These infections may result in death if serious enough. Treatments, such as IV IgG, may extend the lifespan of the individual by providing artificially acquired passive immunity.

- T cell disorders: T cell disorders can cause many different issues for the patient since T cells play a role in both cell-mediated and humoral immunity. A defect in cytotoxic T-cell production or maturation would result in problems with direct killing of foreign cells. A defect in helper T-cell production or maturation could result in problems stimulating B cells to produce antibodies.

- Severe combined immunodeficiency (SCID): SCID is a group of diseases that affects both B- and T-cell function. The disease may result in the presence of B and T cells that are not functional, or even in a complete absence of all types of lymphocytes. There are many different genetic causes of the various types of SCID. Regardless of the cause, the result is an individual who is severely immunocompromised. Without a functioning immune system, the individual is susceptible to many microorganisms, even those that are not generally considered to be pathogenic. People with SCID often have a drastically reduced lifespan, possibly not living past the age of 2 years old. Bone marrow transplants are effective in some patients by providing new stem cells that can produce new B and T cells. Bone marrow transplants are currently the best option for increasing the lifespan of individuals with SCID.

Acquired Immunodeficiencies

Acquired immunodeficiencies are something that can develop throughout the course of a person's life, instead of something they are born with. Some acquired immunodeficiencies are the result of treatment of another condition. For example, patients with cancer often undergo chemotherapy. Chemotherapy will kill the cancerous cells in the patient's body, but it can also kill normal, healthy cells, like those of the immune system. This would result in an acquired immunodeficiency in which the patient's immune system would not be able to effectively kill and remove pathogens in the body.

Acquired Immunodeficiency Syndrome Other acquired immunodeficiencies are due to an infectious disease. AIDS is an acquired immunodeficiency caused by an infectious disease. In fact, AIDS stands for acquired immunodeficiency syndrome. It is caused by a virus called the human immunodeficiency virus (HIV). HIV is transmitted through contact with contaminated blood and body fluids. This most commonly occurs through sexual contact, mother-to-baby transmission, or being stuck with a needle that came in contact with a patient who has HIV. Once in the body, the HIV invades the immune system cells, primarily the helper T (CD4+) cells. It replicates within these cells, destroying them. The immune system has a difficult time fighting the virus, due to the fact that it primarily infects the immune system cells themselves.

If the patient's helper T-cell count gets low enough, the patient becomes more susceptible to both true pathogens and opportunistic pathogens. Initial HIV infections may have little to no symptoms, but AIDS is diagnosed once the helper T cells drop below 200 cells/mm^3. Once the patient has full-blown AIDS, opportunistic infections become common. These opportunistic pathogens may eventually kill the AIDS patient. In addition to being susceptible to more microbial diseases, patients are also more susceptible to certain cancers (remember that one role of the immune system is to kill cancer cells). One of these common cancers in AIDS patients is called Kaposi sarcoma (Figure 12-23). Kaposi sarcoma is a rare disease that causes reddish-purple lesions on the skin.

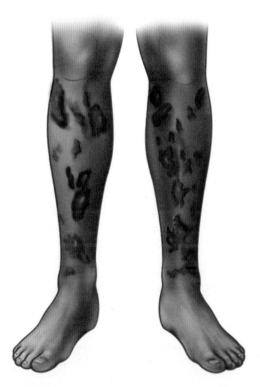

FIGURE 12-23 AIDS patient with Kaposi sarcoma.

LEARNING OBJECTIVE 12.2.2 Explain the role the immune system plays in transplanted tissue rejection reactions and graft-versus-host reactions.

TRANSPLANTED TISSUE REJECTION REACTIONS

Organ transplants are important lifesaving procedures. When a patient has an organ that is not functioning, they may receive an organ transplant from another person. Many different types of organs can be transplanted, including kidneys, corneas, pieces of skin, portions of the liver, and many others. Remember that human cells have MHC molecules that help our immune system to recognize self and non-self. Each person's MHC molecules are slightly different. Because of this, when a person receives an organ transplant from another source, the immune system is able to recognize that those body cells have slightly different MHC molecules and may begin to attack them, which damages the donated organ.

When the patient's immune system detects the donated organ is foreign, it will initiate an attack that can cause tissue rejection. Cytotoxic T cells play a major role in the tissue rejection reaction and will begin to kill cells on the transplanted tissue. Antibodies against the tissue may also be developed. The transplanted organ may ultimately die. The more foreign the organ is, the more extreme the rejection reaction will be. For this reason, transplants from an identical twin's organs would work best and transplanted organs from a family member would be the next best option.

Immunosuppressant medications may be given to the transplant recipient to help minimize the chances of a rejection reaction. These medications can also cause additional problems, however, because they essentially leave the recipient immunocompromised and susceptible to pathogens.

GRAFT-VERSUS-HOST REACTIONS

In some cases, not only can the recipient reject the donor tissue, but the donor tissue (the graft) can reject the host (the recipient). This phenomenon is known as graft-versus-host disease. Graft-versus-host disease is most common in stem-cell transplants. Sometimes these transplants result in mature donor T cells being transplanted. These donor T cells will detect the recipient's cells as foreign and begin to attack them, often by releasing cytokines that can damage the recipient's cells. Immunosuppressive drugs or the removal of T cells from the transplant can help minimize this risk.

LEARNING OBJECTIVE **12.2.3** **Identify common autoimmune diseases and the body systems they affect.**

KEY TERMS

autoantibodies Antibodies directed against self-antigens.

hyperthyroidism A disease state where the thyroid gland produces increased amounts of thyroid hormones.

hypothyroidism Disease state where the thyroid gland produces decreased amounts of thyroid hormones.

molecular mimicry Body is exposed to, and makes antibodies against, an antigen that is similar in structure to a self-antigen, which can result in cross-reactivity of the antibody.

AUTOIMMUNE DISEASES

As we have discussed, in order for the immune system to function properly, it must be able to distinguish between self and non-self. It should recognize when a cell is foreign and attack it and remove it from the body. It should also recognize when cells belong to us and exhibit tolerance to them. In other words, the immune system should not attack self-antigens.

Sometimes the immune system loses this self-tolerance. The result is an autoimmune disease. An autoimmune disease results when the patient's own immune system begins to attack the patient's own cells. Antibodies that are formed, which can attack the patient's own antigens, are called **autoantibodies**.

The exact cause of autoimmunity is not known, but there are many different potential causes. Most types of autoimmunity have a genetic link, although there isn't one particular gene that has been identified to cause these diseases. It's possible that during development, a patient's T cells may not "learn" how to properly distinguish between self and non-self, resulting in autoimmunity. Another hypothesis is that of molecular mimicry. **Molecular mimicry** is the idea that the body gets exposed to a pathogen that has an antigen that is very similar to the person's own antigens. When antibodies are made against the pathogenic antigen, those same antibodies can cross-react with the patient's own antigens.

There are many different types of autoimmune diseases, each with different types of autoantibodies. Clinical manifestations of the disease depend on what type of antibody is formed and which body tissues it will attack.

Autoimmune Thyroid Diseases

Autoimmune thyroid diseases are very common. These diseases result in autoantibodies that attack the cells of the thyroid gland. The thyroid gland is a small gland in the neck that produces the thyroid hormones thyroxine (T4) and triiodothyronine (T3). Thyroid hormones are necessary for the proper functioning and metabolism of many body cells. If autoantibodies attack the thyroid gland, they can damage the thyroid gland and prevent it from functioning properly, affecting the levels of these hormones.

Hashimoto's Disease Hashimoto's disease, also called Hashimoto's thyroiditis, is an autoimmune disease resulting in hypothyroidism. **Hypothyroidism** means that the thyroid gland is producing decreased amounts of the thyroid hormones T3 and T4. Without adequate levels of circulating T3 and T4, many of the patient's body cells will be affected. Some common symptoms of hypothyroidism include the following:

- Goiter (an enlarged thyroid; Figure 12-24)
- Fatigue
- Depression
- Weight gain
- Sensitivity to cold
- Dry and brittle hair and skin
- Joint and muscle pain

Graves' Disease Graves' disease, although caused by a similar mechanism as Hashimoto's disease, results in hyperthyroidism. In **hyperthyroidism**, increased levels of the thyroid hormones are produced. Symptoms

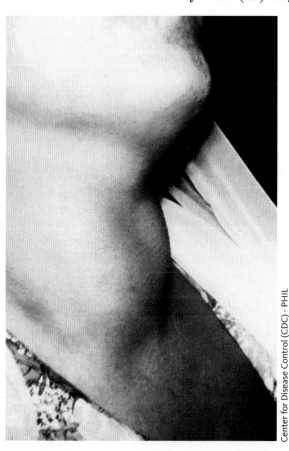

Center for Disease Control (CDC) - PHIL

FIGURE 12-24 Goiter (an enlarged thyroid gland).

are essentially the opposite of what you would see with Hashimoto's disease. Common symptoms of Graves' disease include weight loss, anxiety and nervousness, heat intolerance, rapid heart rate, and protruding eyes.

Multiple Sclerosis

Multiple sclerosis (MS) is an example of an autoimmune disease that can affect an entire system. In the case of MS, the central nervous system is affected. Autoantibodies bind to the myelin sheath in the nervous system, stimulating an additional immune response by T cells and macrophages. This immune response causes the formation of lesions in the brain and spinal cord called plaques. Symptoms can vary depending on the parts of the nervous system affected. Examples of symptoms may include weakness or paralysis in limbs, problems with eyesight, numbness and tingling, dizziness, and fatigue.

Chapter 13

The Gastrointestinal System

Chapter Introduction

While sitting down to enjoy a tasty meal is often considered a relaxing experience, it requires the gastrointestinal system to kick into high gear. Food that is consumed must be broken down into a form that is usable by the body to promote health and growth and prevent disease. In this chapter, we learn how the GI system breaks down and digests the food we consume into absorbable nutrients and expels waste.

UNIT OBJECTIVE 13.1

Describe the general structure and functions of the digestive system.

UNIT INTRODUCTION

Digestion is essential to life; at its most basic, it breaks down food into smaller parts until they can be absorbed by the human body, providing fuel to power the body's activities. As the body digests food, it breaks it down into the nutrients that can be used, absorbs these nutrients into the bloodstream, and then rids the body of any wastes.

LEARNING OBJECTIVE 13.1.1 Identify the general functions of the digestive system.

LEARNING OBJECTIVE 13.1.2 Describe the general functions of the digestive system.

KEY TERMS

absorption Passage of digested food materials from the digestive tract of an individual into the cardiovascular and lymphatic systems for distribution to the body's cells.

alimentary canal The long muscular tube of the digestive system that transports ingested materials from the mouth to anus; site of mechanical and chemical digestion.

chemical digestion Molecular breakdown of food by bile and enzymes secreted throughout the digestive system.

digestion Breakdown of the large food materials into smaller particles by mechanical and chemical digestion.

excretion Discharge of waste from the body.

mechanical digestion Physical breakdown of food.

peristalsis Process of smooth muscle contraction along the GI tract that forces material to move further along the tract.

secretion Discharge of enzymes to aid in the breakdown of bolus materials.

FUNCTIONS OF THE DIGESTIVE SYSTEM

The functions of the digestive system include transportation, secretion, digestion, absorption of nutrients, and excretion of waste. Food is propelled forward and transported through the digestive system by peristalsis, or muscular contractions of the mouth, pharynx, esophagus, and small and large intestine (collectively, these organs make up the alimentary canal). Digestion is the breakdown of consumed food into a form that is absorbable by the body. This occurs as a result of both physical breakdown and the secretion of chemicals that deconstruct food into small particles. It is estimated that the body secretes about 9 liters of digestive juices to aid with digestion in a single day! Absorption occurs once food is broken down into a form that the body is able to process. Absorption does not begin until consumed food enters the stomach, and the majority of nutrient absorption occurs in the intestines.

Mechanical digestion is just as it sounds: the physical breakdown of food. This occurs by chewing and the churning or mixing of food as it moves through the digestive system. Chemical digestion is the molecular breakdown of food by bile and enzymes secreted throughout the GI system. These chemical compounds break fats, proteins, and carbohydrates down into small absorbable structures. While chemical digestion of carbohydrates and starches is initiated upon food entering the mouth, chemical digestion continues in the stomach, and the majority of chemical digestion occurs much further down in the small intestine.

Waste excretion occurs through defecation. This is the physical passing of indigestible substances from the body. Regular defecation is necessary to prevent accumulation of waste products within the digestive system.

LEARNING OBJECTIVE 13.1.3 Identify the alimentary canal.

LEARNING OBJECTIVE 13.1.4 Describe the general anatomical characteristics of the alimentary canal.

THE ALIMENTARY CANAL

The alimentary canal is a portion of the digestive system. It consists of a one-way tube compromised of a network of hollow GI system organs with multiple segments that are separated by sphincters. The alimentary canal begins at the mouth, where food enters the body, and ends at the anus, where solid waste exits the body. Additional alimentary canal organs between these two openings include the pharynx, esophagus, stomach, small intestine, large intestine, and rectum (Figure 13-1). The alimentary canal is long and measures up to 30 feet (approximately 9 meters) in length. This is comparable in size to a three-story building! Because the mouth and anus open to the outside environment, the lumen or inner lining of the alimentary canal is considered an external body surface.

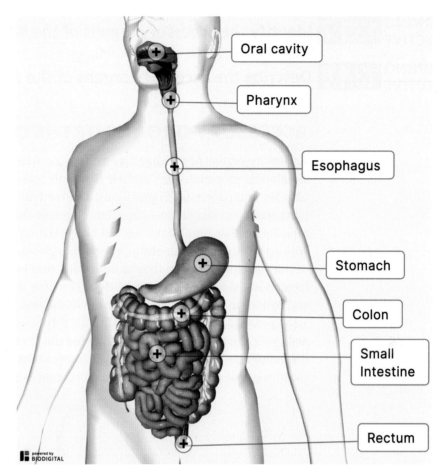

FIGURE 13-1 The organs of the alimentary canal are the pharynx, esophagus, stomach, small intestine, large intestine, and rectum.

LEARNING OBJECTIVE 13.1.5 Identify the general function of the alimentary canal.

LEARNING OBJECTIVE 13.1.6 Describe the general function of the alimentary canal.

Function of the Alimentary Canal

The alimentary canal functions as a pathway to move food through the body. The organs of the alimentary canal work with accessory organs of the digestive system to digest food as it moves through the canal. Mechanical and chemical digestion converts food into a form that can be absorbed by the blood and lymphatic vessels for use by the body. Protein and carbohydrate nutrients are absorbed by mucosal cells and transported across the wall of the alimentary canal by blood vessels. Lipids or fatty acids are transported across the wall of the alimentary canal by lymphatic vessels or lacteals. Materials unable to be absorbed are expelled as solid waste.

LEARNING OBJECTIVE **13.1.7** Identify the accessory organs of the digestive system.

LEARNING OBJECTIVE **13.1.8** Describe the accessory organs of the digestive system.

ACCESSORY ORGANS OF THE DIGESTIVE SYSTEM

Accessory organs of the digestive system aid with digestion but are not part of the alimentary canal. They include the teeth, tongue, salivary glands, liver, gallbladder, and pancreas (Figure 13-2). The teeth and tongue initiate digestion by participating in mechanical digestion. Together they work to prepare consumed food for further breakdown by the body. The salivary glands are also located within the mouth and function as secretory glands to initiate chemical digestion of polysaccharides. The liver, gallbladder, and pancreas are secretory organs located in the abdomen (Figure 13-3). The liver is the largest gland in the body and resides in the upper right quadrant of the abdomen. Immediately below this is the pear-shaped gallbladder containing three ducts: the hepatic, common bile, and cystic ducts. The pancreas lies behind the stomach and in close proximity to the duodenum of the small intestine. Chemicals excreted by the organs continue the process of chemical digestion as food moves through the body.

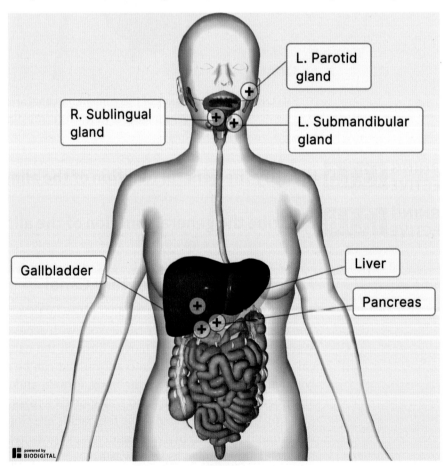

FIGURE 13-2 The teeth, tongue, salivary glands, liver, gallbladder, and pancreas are accessory organs of the digestive system.

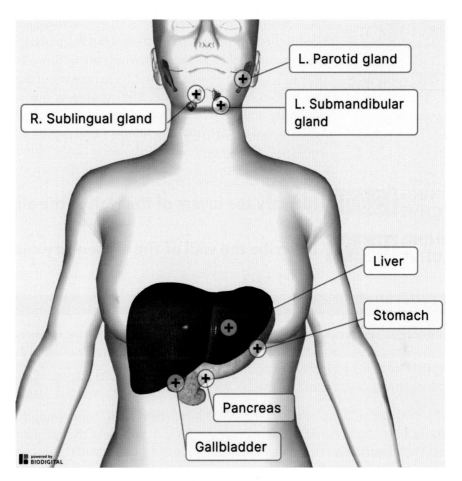

FIGURE 13-3 The liver, gallbladder, and pancreas are secretory organs located within the abdomen. Also shown are the salivary glands found in the mouth and head.

LEARNING OBJECTIVE 13.1.9 Describe the general functions of the accessory organs of the digestive system.

KEY TERMS

bile Yellow or greenish alkaline fluid secreted by the liver and passed into the duodenum where it aids in the absorption of fat.

chyme Digested, viscous, semifluid contents of the intestine.

Functions of Accessory Organs of the Digestive System

The teeth and tongue contribute to mechanical digestion as they tear, compress, and move food within the mouth. Salivary glands in the mouth excrete saliva to moisten and lubricate food as it moves through the alimentary canal. The digestive enzyme amylase is present in saliva and initiates chemical digestion by breaking polysaccharides (i.e., carbohydrates and starches) down into simple sugars that are more easily digested later in the digestive process. The molecular breakdown of food continues as it moves through the digestive system and encounters digestive enzymes secreted from glands located in the pancreas, liver, and gallbladder. These enzymes break down fats, proteins, and carbohydrates. While the stomach is not an accessory organ, it also secretes enzymes that further break down food. **Bile** consists of bile salts, cholesterol, bilirubin, and water and is excreted from glands in the liver and stored in the gallbladder. When mixed with **chyme**, a combination of gastric secretions and food that has been partially digested, it contributes to further breakdown fat.

LEARNING OBJECTIVE 13.1.10 Identify the layers of the wall of the alimentary canal.

LEARNING OBJECTIVE 13.1.11 Describe the wall of the alimentary canal.

KEY TERMS

enteric nervous system One of the main part of the autonomic nervous system, consisting of a meshlike system of neurons that govern the functions of the gastrointestinal tract.

mucosa Innermost layer of the alimentary canal.

muscalaris Part of the alimentary canal that covers the submucosa, consisting of a double layer of smooth muscle that promotes contractions and the movement of chyme.

serosa Outermost layer or external covering of the wall of the alimentary canal.

submucosa Layer of connective tissue located below a mucous membrane.

tenia coli Three smooth muscle strips on the outside of the ascending, transverse, descending, and sigmoid colon; contract lengthwise to produce the bulges in the colon.

LAYERS OF THE ALIMENTARY CANAL WALL

The alimentary canal wall is composed of four layers. From the innermost layer to outermost layer this includes the **mucosa, submucosa, muscalaris,** and **serosa.** Each layer consists of a different tissue type that is directly related to a specific role in the digestion of food (Figure 13-4).

Mucosa

The mucosa is the innermost layer of the alimentary canal. It is a mucous membrane that extends the entire distance of the alimentary canal and is in direct contact with food and chyme. The mucosa contains three layers and is comprised of both epithelium cells and connective tissue. Digestion, secretion and absorption occur via the epithelium or innermost layer. Mucus produced in the epithelium can promote the movement of food through the alimentary canal and protect organs from potential damage due to contact with digestive enzymes. The mucosa is surrounded by a middle layer or lamina propria. This is a connective tissue that includes lymphatic vessels and blood vessels. These absorb and transport valuable nutrients. The lamina propria is covered by the muscularis mucosa or a thin layer of smooth muscle. The structure of mucosae

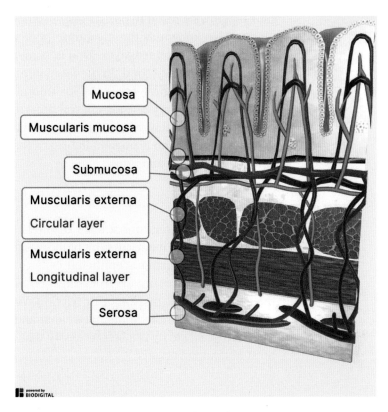

FIGURE 13-4 The four layers of the alimentary canal are the mucosa, submucosa, muscalaris, and serosa.

of alimentary canal organs varies in response to the organ's environment and function. For example, folds in the small intestine increase absorption by providing an increase in surface area and columnar pits are present in the stomach to aid in secretion.

Submucosa

Directly below the mucosa and connecting it to the muscularis is the submucosa consisting of connective tissue. This allows the organ to regain its shape following distention due to the passage or storage of food. Embedded within this are secretory glands, large blood and lymph vessels, and nerves. The submucosal plexus is also found here. This is a nerve fiber network that makes up part of the **enteric nervous system**, which sends signals from the gut to the central nervous system, which then sends signals back to adjust intestinal function.

Muscularis

The muscularis covers the submucosa and consists of a double layer of smooth muscle that promotes contractions and the movement of chyme. Rhythmic contraction of thick circular muscle layers enveloped by an outer muscle layer that runs lengthwise result in peristalsis. A layer of nerves referred to as Auerbach's plexus, also known as the myenteric plexus, regulates peristalsis. An oblique muscle provides a third layer. This is present only within the stomach to promote the churning of food. In the large intestine, the outer longitudinal muscle is separated into three **tenia coli**, or thin muscle strips, to create texture and pouches. Involuntary muscle contractions are regulated by nerves of the autonomic nervous system. Skeletal muscle provides the body with voluntary control over movements and is present in organs that are not automatically controlled, such as the tongue and anus.

Serosa

The serosa is the outermost layer of the alimentary canal. It consists of loose connective tissue, innervated by blood vessels and nerves, and is covered by a single layer of squamous epithelial cells to form an organ border. The serosa functions to protect organs from the abdominal cavity. Serous fluid secreted by the cells decreases resistance or friction. Visceral peritoneum is present in the abdominal area of the alimentary canal and on the surface of the muscularis. The peritoneal cavity is a serous cavity that encompasses the area surrounding most abdominal organs.

LEARNING OBJECTIVE 13.1.12 Identify gastrointestinal mixing movements.

LEARNING OBJECTIVE 13.1.13 Explain how contents of the gastrointestinal system are mixed and moved.

KEY TERM

segmentation Mixing movement that combines chyme with gastric solutions.

MOVEMENT AND MIXING OF GI CONTENTS

Distention triggers peristalsis or the forward movement of chyme. Contraction of a muscle ring behind a stimulating mass of chyme propels it forward. Contractions occur intermittently and continue repeatedly in order to move the mass toward the anus. Hormone regulation controls the rate of peristalsis, allowing adequate time for digestion and absorption to occur. Rapid peristalsis does not allow adequate time for digestion or nutrient absorption and results in diarrhea. Slow peristalsis prevents chyme from moving forward at an adequate rate and can result in constipation. Mixing movements combine chyme with digestive secretions to promote digestion. Mixing occurs mainly with constrictive mixing movements and to a much lesser extent through the movement that occurs during peristalsis. During forward propulsion, the mass spins. While minimal, this helps to accommodate the mixing of digestive substances and promotes absorption. Propulsion into an area that meets resistance of a closed sphincter results in a mixing as the chyme churns without forward movement. This can mimic cutting or kneading of contents.

Segmentation is a mixing movement. Instead of moving chyme forward, repeat constrictive contractions within the alimentary canal organs prevent forward momentum. This causes the breakdown and then reconstitution of chyme with gastric secretions. This is followed by eventual relaxation of the small intestine resulting in forward propulsion.

LEARNING OBJECTIVE 13.1.14 Identify the effects of the sympathetic nervous system on the alimentary canal.

LEARNING OBJECTIVE 13.1.15 Describe the effects of the sympathetic nervous system on the alimentary canal.

KEY TERM

sympathetic nervous system Region of the autonomic nervous system that activates the fight-or-flight response.

SYMPATHETIC NERVOUS SYSTEM

Your environment and stress level impacts the functions of organs along your alimentary canal. The sympathetic nervous system is one portion of the autonomic nervous system. It controls your body's fight-or-flight response by telling it when to prepare for action, both physical and mental. The sympathetic nervous system is activated at a time of stress, fear, or danger. When activated, it triggers your body to conserve energy for survival. Blood is moved to vital organs, such as the heart and lungs, to provide energy to pump blood and oxygen to the brain, and away from the organs of the alimentary canal such as the stomach and intestines. This, combined with a lack of nerve stimulation, slows the digestive process. GI system movement slows as digestion and defecation are not considered lifesaving necessities. The breakdown, absorption, and excretion of solid waste are slowed. The urethral and anal sphincters are constricted, which inhibit voiding. Abdominal bloating and constipation can result.

LEARNING OBJECTIVE 13.1.16 Identify the effects of the parasympathetic nervous system on the alimentary canal.

LEARNING OBJECTIVE 13.1.17 Describe the effects of the parasympathetic nervous system on the alimentary canal.

KEY TERM

parasympathetic nervous system Portion of the autonomic nervous system (ANS) that promotes digestive and excretory processes.

PARASYMPATHETIC NERVOUS SYSTEM

The **parasympathetic nervous system** is the second portion of the autonomic nervous system. While the sympathetic nervous system protects you from danger and, as a result, slows digestion, the parasympathetic nervous system is all about rest and relaxation. As a result, it promotes digestion. During an identified state of relaxation and homeostasis, blood pressure and heart rate are regulated at low, normal levels. There is increased nerve stimulation to the alimentary canal, which encourages secretion of digestive enzymes, such as saliva and gastric acid, and peristalsis. This results in increased gastrointestinal activity. Increased blood flow stimulates gastric movement, resulting in promotion of nutrient absorption and waste excretion through the movement of chyme.

LEARNING OBJECTIVE 13.1.18 Contrast the effects of the sympathetic and parasympathetic nervous systems on the alimentary canal.

COMPARING SYMPATHETIC AND PARASYMPATHETIC NERVOUS SYSTEM EFFECTS ON THE ALIMENTARY CANAL

The sympathetic and parasympathetic nervous system have differing effects on digestive functions within the alimentary canal. Generally, in situations when one division predominates over the other, opposite effects occur. For example, when activities of the sympathetic nervous system take over, blood will shift away from the alimentary canal and there will be a decrease in digestive enzyme secretion, peristalsis, and digestion of food. When activities of the parasympathetic nervous system dominate, there is increased enzyme secretion and peristalsis, resulting in active digestion of food and regular bowel movements (Table 13-1).

Table 13-1 Sympathetic and Parasympathetic Effects of Alimentary Canal Responses

ALIMENTARY CANAL RESPONSE	SYMPATHETIC (FIGHT OR FLIGHT)	PARASYMPATHETIC (RELAXATION AND BALANCE)
Blood flow	Shifting of blood away from organs of alimentary canal results in decreased nutrient absorption	No effect
Digestive enzyme secretion	Decreased	Increased
Peristalsis	Decreased	Increased
Digestion of food	Slowing of the digestive process can result in bloating, diarrhea, and constipation	Activation of the digestive process can result in a regular bowel movement routine and stools of normal consistency

UNIT OBJECTIVE 13.2

Describe the structures and functions of the mouth, pharynx, and esophagus.

UNIT INTRODUCTION

The mouth, pharynx, and esophagus make up part of the upper gastrointestinal tract. Digestion begins in the mouth. The pharynx and esophagus move the bolus from the mouth to the stomach, where digestion continues.

LEARNING OBJECTIVE	**13.2.1**	**Identify the important anatomical structures within the mouth.**
LEARNING OBJECTIVE	**13.2.2**	**Describe the important anatomical structures within the mouth.**
LEARNING OBJECTIVE	**13.2.3**	**Describe the functions of the important anatomical structures found within the mouth.**

KEY TERM

mastication Chewing.

STRUCTURES WITHIN THE MOUTH

Food enters the alimentary canal through the mouth. The teeth and tongue are located within the oral cavity. The salivary glands are an accessory organ present in the oral cavity that play a vital role in digestion (Figure 13-5).

Teeth

Deciduous teeth (commonly referred to as "baby teeth") begin to erupt at around 6 months old and continue until around 2 years old. At this point, the mouth will contain 20 deciduous teeth. The adult mouth contains 32 teeth (16 in each jaw), including four wisdom teeth that are frequently extracted in late adolescence (Figure 13-6). Tooth function is determined by the shape of the tooth (Table 13-2).

Tongue

The tongue is a combination of muscles that are attached to the floor of the mouth. It is often thought of in regard to the taste buds that coat it. This is understandable as taste and texture often determine our response to foods placed within the mouth. Aside from taste, the tongue works with the teeth to assist with chewing and swallowing, playing an important role in mechanical digestion.

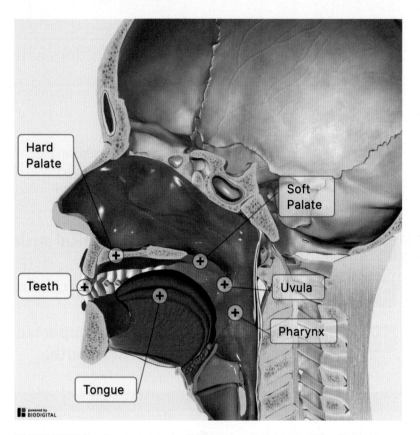

FIGURE 13-5 The structures within the mouth that aid in digestion are the teeth, tongue, and salivatory glands (sublingual gland, parotid glands, and submandibular gland).

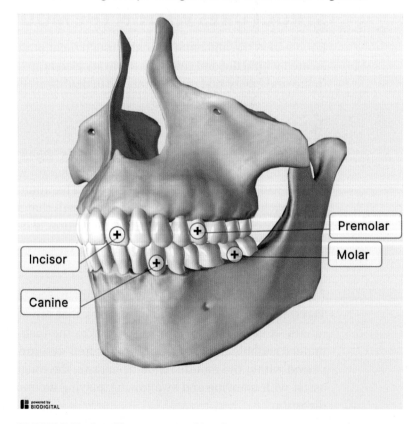

FIGURE 13-6 Different types of teeth.

Table 13-2 Functions and Shapes of Different Teeth

TYPE OF TOOTH	SHAPE	FUNCTION
Molar	Wide with flat crown	Crush, grind
Premolar or bicuspid	Wide with flat crown	Crush
Canine	Pointed	Tear, pierce
Incisor	Chisel	Bite, cut

Functions of Teeth and Tongue

Mastication is the breakdown of food by the teeth. Chewing and grinding mechanically alters the physical state of food, increasing the surface area of the food so that it can be broken down efficiently by enzymes during digestion. When we chew, the tongue moves food within the mouth, against the cheek, and between teeth. Movement of a food bolus in the mouth by the tongue encourages contact with various types of teeth to promote thorough mechanical digestion and shapes the food into a small bolus for swallowing.

Function of Salivary Glands

Sensory response to the presence and taste or smell of food stimulates the salivary glands to produce saliva; it is the enzyme salivary amylase that initiates chemical digestion. Various compositions and consistency of saliva moisten the mouth, lubricate food, and initiate carbohydrate breakdown.

LEARNING OBJECTIVE **13.2.4** **Describe the parts of a tooth.**

KEY TERMS

cementum Substance that encloses the dentin of the root of a tooth.

crown Portion of the tooth that is found over the gum line.

dentin Bonelike substances found in teeth.

Enamel Hard, calcareous substance that is used for the formation of a thin layer capping the teeth to protect the teeth from wear and acids.

gingiva tissue Area around the root of the tooth that helps keep the tooth in place.

periodontal ligament Group of specialized connective fibers that attach a tooth to the alveolar bone.

pulp Center of the tooth that contains blood and nerves.

ANATOMY OF A TOOTH

A tooth consists of the crown or portion visible above the gum line and a root that is below the gum line and contained in the bone of the jaw by the periodontal ligament. This is covered by a thin mucosal tissue referred to as gingiva tissue. While the crown is responsible for mechanical breakdown of food, the root anchors the tooth in place and connects it to the blood and nerves of the body. Both are covered by a mineral surface. **Enamel**, a very hard mineral substance, covers the crown and a slightly less firm and thinner mineral called **cementum** covers the root. **Dentin** is a hard but porous tissue that lies below the mineral surface. Nutrients are able to pass through this permeable layer. Blood and nerves are contained in the center of the tooth or **pulp** cavity and root canal (Figure 13-7).

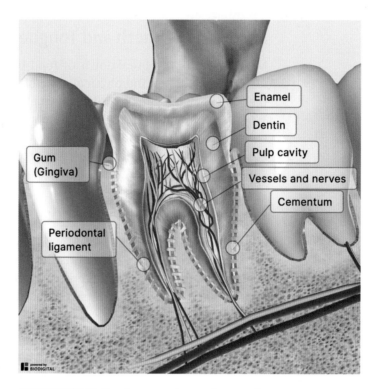

FIGURE 13-7 Teeth are made up of enamel, cementum, dentin, and the pulp, which contains blood and nerves.

LEARNING OBJECTIVE 13.2.5 Describe how different types of teeth are meant for different types of food.

TOOTH FUNCTION BASED ON TOOTH SHAPE

We have learned that various teeth of various shapes perform different functions. Based on this, certain teeth are better suited for various types of food based on the action needed to break the food down. For example, meat must be bitten into and torn while leafy vegetables must be ground. Incisors have sharp edges and are used to bite into a piece of meat, canines are pointed and used to tear the meat into a proper-sized piece, and molars have ridges that are used to crush and grind leafy vegetables.

LEARNING OBJECTIVE 13.2.6 Identify the major parts of the pharynx and esophagus.

KEY TERMS

esophagus Smooth muscle structure located between the pharynx and stomach that is part of the alimentary canal that carries substances from the mouth to the stomach.

pharynx Partially shared passageway for the respiratory and digestive systems beginning at the posterior nasal cavity and extending to the trachea.

THE PHARYNX AND ESOPHAGUS

The pharynx or throat is comprised of skeletal muscle with an interior mucous membrane coating. This connects to the esophagus, which leads to the stomach. The esophagus is a collapsible tube comprised of muscle and lined with mucosa that is positioned behind the trachea or windpipe.

LEARNING OBJECTIVE 13.2.7 Describe the major parts of the pharynx and esophagus.

KEY TERMS

esophageal hiatus An opening in the diaphragm, the esophagus passes through the esophageal hiatus and joins the stomach.

laryngopharynx Lowermost portion of the pharynx.

nasopharynx Portion of the pharynx that extends from the posterior portion of the nasal cavity to the soft palate.

oropharynx Portion of the pharynx extending from the soft palate to the epiglottis.

The pharynx is divided into three sections: the nasopharynx, oropharynx, and laryngopharynx. The nasopharynx lies behind the nasal cavity, the oropharynx behind the oral cavity, and the laryngopharynx behind the larynx. Both the nasopharynx and oropharynx open to the lungs and play a role in respiratory system function. The laryngopharynx leads to the esophagus. Contractions of circular muscles provide peristalsis to move food forward, providing a direct passage for food along the alimentary canal.

The esophagus connects the pharynx to the stomach. Just prior to the stomach opening, the esophagus passes through the diaphragm via an opening called the esophageal hiatus. Sphincter muscles, specifically the upper esophageal sphincter, are located at the top of the esophagus and contract to prevent food and digestive secretions from entering the airway. This occurs with vomiting, eating, and breathing. A second sphincter muscle, the lower esophageal sphincter, lies just prior to the stomach opening. This contracts to prevent stomach contents from traveling backward and entering the esophagus. The upper esophageal sphincter can be voluntarily controlled while the lower esophageal sphincter is involuntary.

LEARNING
OBJECTIVE **13.2.8** Identify the actions involved in the swallowing mechanism.

KEY TERMS

deglutition Process of swallowing.

epiglottis Cartilaginous structure in the larynx
that closes it off when swallowing to prevent the
movement of substances into the trachea.

ACTIONS IN THE SWALLOWING MECHANISM

Deglutition, or swallowing, is a complicated process that requires closure of
the airway, as well as peristalsis and mucosal lubrication to move food forward.
When you swallow, the tongue moves the food bolus from the mouth to the
pharynx and then to the esophagus, while shutting the epiglottis. The swallowing process occurs in three phases: the voluntary phase, pharyngeal phase, and
esophageal phase.

LEARNING
OBJECTIVE **13.2.9** Explain the mechanism involved in swallowing.

KEY TERM

esophageal sphincter Sphincters that close the
esophagus when food is not being swallowed;
the upper esophageal sphincter surrounds the
upper part of the esophagus, and the lower
esophageal sphincter surrounds the lower part
of the esophagus at the junction between the
esophagus and stomach.

Voluntary Phase

The first phase of swallowing is voluntary. Upon completion of chewing, the
swallowing mechanism is activated. This begins with muscles securing the
mouth shut as a bolus of food is pushed back into the oropharynx by an up-and-
backward movement of the tongue.

Pharyngeal Phase

The second phase of swallowing is involuntary and controlled by the medulla
oblongata. The pharyngeal muscles repeatedly contract and relax to move the
food bolus through the pharynx. Neurological receptors activate and send
impulses to structures in the mouth, specifically the uvula and soft palate, to

prevent aspiration by closing the nasopharynx; to the muscles of the trachea to constrict; and cause the epiglottis to shut off the larynx and the trachea. The food bolus enters the esophagus following relaxation of the upper esophageal sphincter.

Esophageal Phase

The esophageal phase is also involuntary and controlled by the medulla oblongata. Peristalsis continues to propel the food bolus to the stomach. In the esophagus, various muscles work together. Circular muscles of the muscularis pinch the tube closed as longitudinal muscles contract to decrease tube length. Movement is aided by lubrication from esophageal gland secretion of mucous. The lower **esophageal sphincter** is activated by distention and opens to allow passage of the food bolus into the stomach (Figure 13-8ABC).

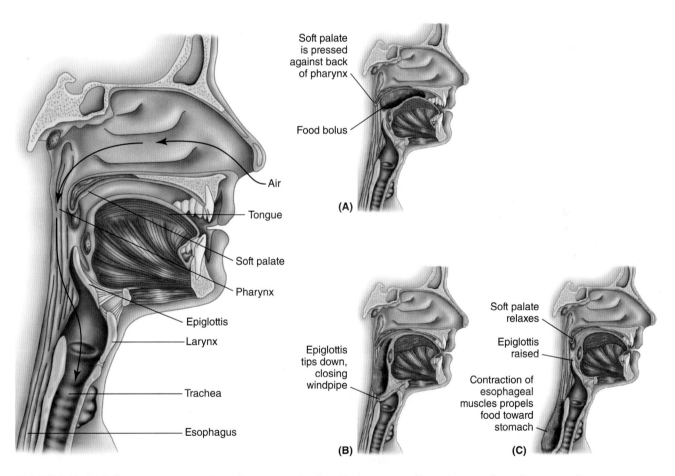

FIGURE 13-8ABC Three phases of swallowing as the food bolus moves from the mouth to the stomach.

UNIT OBJECTIVE 13.3

Describe the structure and functions of the stomach.

UNIT INTRODUCTION

The stomach muscle continues mechanical digestion. Its functions include the collection and storage of food, digestion, and movement of partially digested food.

LEARNING OBJECTIVE 13.3.1 Identify the stomach.

LEARNING OBJECTIVE 13.3.2 Describe the anatomical characteristics of the stomach.

KEY TERMS

body Central and the largest portion of the stomach.

cardia Part of the stomach that encloses the gastroesophageal sphincter.

gastric fundus Round portion of the stomach located above and to the left of the cardia.

greater curvature Boundary of the stomach that forms a long, convex curve on the left from the opening for the esophagus to the opening of the duodenum.

lesser curvature Part of the stomach that extends between the cardiac and pyloric orifices, forming the right border.

pyloric sphincter Connection or link between the stomach and the starting point of the duodenum that controls the emptying of the stomach contents into the small intestine.

pylorus Narrow inferior part of the stomach; also known as the antrum.

rugae Large mucosal folds of the stomach.

THE STOMACH

The stomach is a J-shaped organ. It is hollow and pouchlike. The stomach lies in the upper left portion of the abdomen immediately between the esophagus and the small intestine of the alimentary canal.

The stomach is secured in the abdomen by peritoneal tissue. The **lesser curvature** or medial portion of the stomach curve is attached to the liver while the **greater curvature** or lateral and larger portion of the stomach curve is attached to a portion of the abdominal wall. There are four regions of the stomach organ. The stomach and esophagus meet below the diaphragm at the **cardia**. The dome-shaped upper portion of the stomach pouch is the **gastric fundus**, which opens to the center and largest portion of the stomach referred to as the **body**. The stomach narrows and connects to the duodenum of the small intestine at the **pylorus**. The **pyloric sphincter** is a sphincter muscle that contracts and relaxes to control the emptying of stomach contents into the small intestine. When the stomach is without food it collapses inward upon itself, forming **rugae** or folds (Figure 13-9).

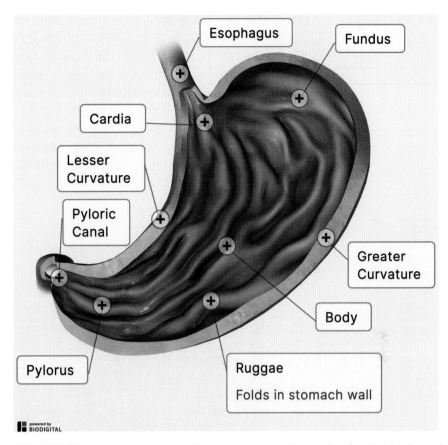

FIGURE 13-9 The main parts of the stomach are the cardia, fundus, body, and pylorus.

LEARNING OBJECTIVE 13.3.3 Describe the physiological characteristics of the stomach.

KEY TERM

gastric pit Indentations in the stomach that denote entrances to the gastric glands.

Physiological Characteristics of the Stomach

In addition to the four layers present in each alimentary canal organ, an inner oblique muscle layer is present in the muscularis of the stomach. This aids stomach churning and mechanical digestion.

Multiple glands secrete gastric fluids or gastric juice in the stomach to aid with chemical digestion. Gland openings consist of small dots, referred to as **gastric pits**, that line the epithelium. These gastric pits are connected to tube-shaped gastric glands that produce the gastric juice, including a variety of digestive enzymes (which are discussed in greater detail later in the chapter). The larger portion of the stomach, namely the fundus and body, are home to larger glands. The parietal cells located in the gastric glands found in the fundus and cardia produce intrinsic factor. Without intrinsic factor, vitamin B_{12} will not be absorbed by the body later on in the digestive process.

A mucosal barrier protects the stomach from damage and self-digestion. This is comprised of a neutralizing mucous coating, tight epithelial cells, and stem cells located at junctions of gastric glands and gastric pits. The mucous coating provides both a barrier and neutralizes acid. Tightly packed epithelial cells prevent the seepage of gastric juice to inferior tissue layers while stem cells quickly repair and replace damaged epithelial tissue. Bacteria introduced to the stomach are eradicated by the secretion of stomach acid (Figure 13-10).

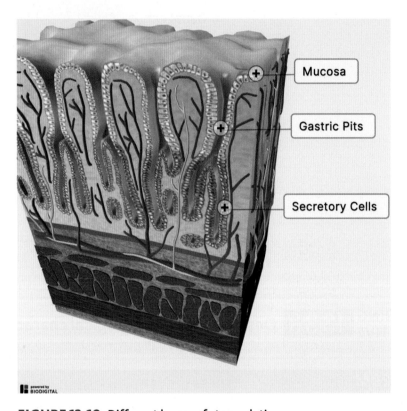

Mucosa

Gastric Pits

Secretory Cells

FIGURE 13-10 Different layers of stomach tissue.

LEARNING OBJECTIVE 13.3.4 Describe the major functions of the stomach.

Functions of the Stomach

The stomach has multiple functions in the digestive process including collection and storage of food, digestion, and movement of partially digested food.

Food is collected in the stomach and can be stored in the fundus before it is mixed with chyme. Chyme can also be stored for limited periods of time in the stomach. This will occur if chyme is present in the duodenum. In this instance, gastric emptying will be temporarily delayed until the duodenum is prepared to handle it.

Gastric juice secretion and physical churning occurring in the stomach breaks down food both chemically and mechanically. The composition of food impacts the length of the digestive process and time to movement to the duodenum, with foods high in carbohydrates moving along faster than those high in protein. The churning of the stomach contents can vary from gentle to strong. The intensity of mixing waves strengthen as food moves downward through the stomach toward the pylorus. The combination of gastric secretions and physical churning prepares food for further processing in the intestines. Not much is absorbed by the stomach; however, water, alcohol, and aspirin can pass easily through the stomach mucosa into the blood.

UNIT OBJECTIVE 13.4

Describe the structure and functions of the small intestine.

UNIT INTRODUCTION

The small intestine is actually quite long; the "small" in its name comes from the small size of its diameter. It is the organ responsible for digestion and almost all absorption of nutrients that occur during the digestive process.

LEARNING OBJECTIVE 13.4.1   **Identify the general functions of the small intestine.**

LEARNING OBJECTIVE 13.4.2   **Describe the general functions of the small intestine.**

KEY TERM

ileocecal sphincter   Valve that separates the small intestine from the large intestine.

THE SMALL INTESTINE

The small intestine is the organ of the alimentary canal responsible for digestion and almost all of the absorption of nutrients that occurs during the digestive process. It is the largest part of the alimentary canal, typically 3–5 meters in length in a living person. The small intestine starts at the pyloric sphincter and ends at the **ileocecal sphincter**, where the large intestine begins (Figure 13-11).

Almost all chemical digestion takes place in the small intestine. The food breakdown process continues in the small intestine by mixing chyme from the stomach with pancreas enzymes and liver and gallbladder bile salts. This prepares various nutrients, such as carbohydrates, protein, and fat, for absorption. During the chyme's 3- to 6-hour journey, almost all of the nutrients and water will be absorbed into the bloodstream.

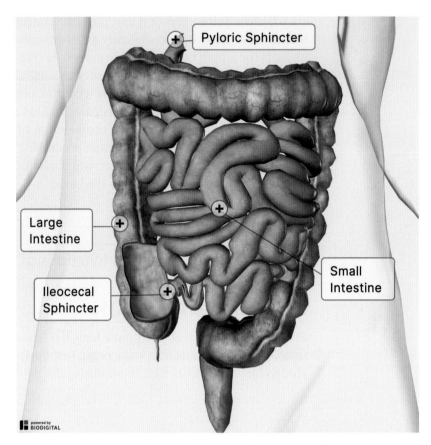

Pyloric Sphincter

Large Intestine

Small Intestine

Ileocecal Sphincter

powered by BIODIGITAL

FIGURE 13-11 The small intestine begins at the pyloric sphincter and ends at the ileocecal sphincter.

LEARNING OBJECTIVE 13.4.3 Identify the duodenum, jejunum, and ileum.

KEY TERM

duodenorenal flexure Border between the duodenum and the jejunum.

THE DUODENUM, JEJUNUM, AND ILEUM

The term *small intestine* is a bit of a misnomer as the small intestine is the longest organ of the alimentary canal. What the word *small* refers to is the narrow diameter of the organ (generally from 2.5 to 4 cm). The small intestine contains three parts: the duodenum, jejunum, and ileum. The duodenum is the part closest to the stomach; it cups the pancreas head and extends to the connection of the duodenum and jejunum or duodenorenal flexure. At this point the jejunum, which is the midsection of the small intestine, continues to the ileum, which constitutes the longest and final portion of the small intestine (Figure 13-12).

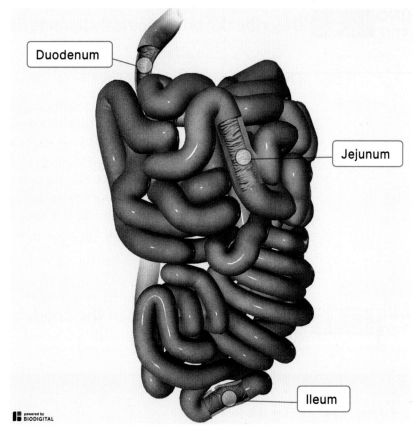

FIGURE 13-12 The small intestine is made up of the duodenum, jejunum, and ileum.

LEARNING OBJECTIVE 13.4.4 Describe the anatomical characteristics of the duodenum.

KEY TERMS

major duodenal papilla Rounded projection at the opening of the common bile duct and pancreatic duct that is the primary mechanism for the secretion of bile and other digestive enzymes.

sphincter of Oddi Muscular valve that controls the flow of digestive juices through the hepatopancreatic duct into the second part of the duodenum.

Duodenum Anatomy

The duodenum extends from the base of the stomach at the pyloric sphincter in a C-shape as it wraps around the pancreas head. Small openings, including the **major duodenal papilla**, are present along the duodenum to allow enzymes from the pancreas and gallbladder to enter the small intestine. Hormone regulation of the **sphincter of Oddi**, which is part of the major duodenal papilla, controls the flow of bile and pancreatic enzymes.

LEARNING OBJECTIVE **13.4.5** **Describe the physiological characteristics of the duodenum.**

Duodenum Physiology

The duodenum is divided into four parts: the superior part (SD), the descending part (DD), the horizontal part (HD), and the ascending part (AD). It is important to note that these parts of the duodenum are not physically distinct from one another. In addition to the names previously stated, the parts of the duodenum are also commonly referred to as the first part, second part, third part, and fourth part. The superior part of the duodenum is the only part that is not attached to the posterior abdominal wall; as such, it is the only part of the duodenum that is movable. Pancreatic juices and bile are emptied into the descending part of the duodenum.

LEARNING OBJECTIVE **13.4.6** **Describe the functions of the duodenum in relation to digestion.**

KEY TERM

ampulla of Vater Cavity where the common bile duct and the pancreatic duct open into the major duodenal papilla.

Duodenum Function

The duodenum regulates the emptying of the stomach into the small intestine. It is where chyme is processed so that the body can easily absorb nutrients as it passes through the intestines. Chyme enters the duodenum through the pyloric sphincter after it has been mixed with hydrochloric acid in the stomach. An alkaline mixture is then secreted from the Brunner's glands in the mucosa of the duodenum to neutralize the hydrochloric acid present in the chyme. This protects the duodenum and also helps the chyme arrive at a pH level that is conducive to chemical digestion. Once the chyme reaches the ampulla of Vater, it is mixed with pancreatic juices and bile from the liver and gallbladder.

Contractions in the duodenum support the mixing of chyme with bile and pancreatic enzymes. This mixing further breaks down the lipids, proteins, and carbohydrates, completing the process of chemical digestion. Slow peristalsis contributes to digestion and of absorption of nutrients while pushing chyme toward the jejunum. Small contractions of the intestinal wall, or segmentation, also helps to mix the chyme with the secretions and aid the rate of digestion.

LEARNING OBJECTIVE **13.4.7** **Describe the anatomical characteristics of the jejunum.**

Jejunum Anatomy

The jejunum begins at the duodenojejunal flexure. This is a sharp bend in the small intestine where the duodenum meets the jejunum. The jejunum is a continuation of the hollow small intestine that lies between the duodenum and ileum without any differentiation from either. It is bordered on three sides by the large intestine and secured to the abdominal cavity by abdominal mesentery. Mucus is produced by goblet cells in the mucosa to lubricate chyme.

LEARNING OBJECTIVE 13.4.8 Describe the physiological characteristics of the jejunum.

KEY TERMS

microvilli Cellular membrane profusions that increase the absorptive area of the cell for diffusion.

villi Projections or small, finger-like structures located on the plicae circulares of the small intestine to promote the absorption of digested food; a villus is composed of numerous microvilli which are used for increasing the surface area of the wall of the intestine.

Jejunum Physiology

Folds in the wall of the jejunum increase the surface area available for absorption of nutrients from chyme. The surface area of the jejunum is covered in finger-like projections of mucosa called villi. The villi increase the surface area available to absorb the nutrients from chyme. Each epithelial cell on the surface of the jejunum contains microvilli to assist in the transport of nutrients—including sugar fructose, amino acids, small peptides, vitamins, and glucose—through the jejunum and ileum.

LEARNING OBJECTIVE 13.4.9 Describe the functions of the jejunum in relation to digestion.

Jejunum Function

The jejunum functions to absorb nutrients from chyme. The majority of nutrients absorbed as food passes through the alimentary canal occurs in the jejunum.

LEARNING OBJECTIVE 13.4.10 Describe the anatomical characteristics of the ileum.

Ileum Anatomy

The ileum continues from the junction with the jejunum and connects to the large intestine at the ileocecal sphincter. Similar to the jejunum, it is bordered on three sides by the large intestine and secured to the abdominal cavity by abdominal mesentery. The movement of chyme from the small intestine to the large intestine is controlled by the ileocecal sphincter.

Describe the physiological characteristics of the ileum.

Describe the functions of the ileum in relation to digestion.

KEY TERM

Peyer's patches Aggregated lymphatic follicles found at the region of the small intestine.

Ileum Physiology

The ileum is the longest portion of the small intestine and is more muscular, with an increased vascular and lymphatic network than is found in the other portions of the small intestine. Lymphatic tissue masses located in the ileum are referred to as **Peyer's patches**.

Ileum Function

Remaining nutrients, including vitamin B_{12} and bile salts, are absorbed through the ilium before digested food moves into the large intestine. The hormones gastrin, secretin, and cholecystokinin are secreted by the cells of the ileum into the blood. Cells in the lining of the ileum secrete the enzymes protease and carbohydrase to accomplish the final digestion of proteins and carbohydrates in the lumen of the intestine.

Describe the functions of Peyer's patches.

PEYER'S PATCHES

Lymphatic Peyer's patches work with the immune system to identify toxins and infectious agents in the intestines. Microfold cells form the outer layer of lymph node clusters. These are specialized cells that can identify and obliterate pathogens in isolation without activation of the full immune system. They are concentrated in the ileum because this region contains a large number of bacteria that need to be prevented from entering the bloodstream.

Describe how the products of digestion are absorbed.

KEY TERM

motilin Hormones secreted in the small intestine that control interdigestive contractions.

ABSORPTION OF DIGESTIVE PRODUCTS

Repeated forcing of chyme against the mucosa of the small intestine by segmentation promotes absorption. The small intestine boasts a large surface area for absorption due to folds in the lining. Specialized cells within the small intestine mucosa absorb the products of digestion into the blood and lymph while other various cells secrete mucous and enzymes to protect the intestinal lining from the digestion process. After the majority of the chyme is absorbed, decreased distention of the small intestine triggers the secretion of motilin, a hormone that results in a change from segmentation contractions to motility movements. Each contraction slowly moves food down the small intestine toward the large intestine.

UNIT OBJECTIVE 13.5

Describe the structure and function of the large intestine.

UNIT INTRODUCTION

The large intestine is the last part of the gastrointestinal tract. Water is absorbed here; the remaining waste materials are stored here as feces before defecation occurs.

LEARNING OBJECTIVE 13.5.1 Identify the general functions of the large intestine.

LEARNING OBJECTIVE 13.5.2 Describe the general functions of the large intestine.

KEY TERM

feces Semisolid mass of indigestible food materials in the large intestine.

THE LARGE INTESTINE

The large intestine is shorter than the small intestine; it is because of the size of its diameter (approximately 7 cm) that it is referred to as large. The cecum, colon, rectum, and anus are the four regions that comprise the large intestine. It is responsible for absorption and fecal elimination. It surrounds the small intestine on three sides.

Function of the Large Intestine

The large intestine absorbs water and any remaining nutrients from chyme residue. The colon also absorbs any vitamins, such as vitamin K, thiamine, and riboflavin, that are created by colonic bacteria. What remains results in the formation of feces, or stool, to be expelled as solid waste. Stool is made up of undigested food, bacteria, water, epithelial cells from mucosa of the alimentary tract, and inorganic salts.

LEARNING OBJECTIVE 13.5.3 Identify the cecum and appendix.

LEARNING OBJECTIVE 13.5.4 Describe the anatomical characteristics of the cecum and appendix.

LEARNING OBJECTIVE 13.5.5 Describe the physiologic characteristics of the cecum and appendix.

LEARNING OBJECTIVE 13.5.6 Describe the functions of the cecum and appendix.

THE CECUM AND APPENDIX

The cecum is the first portion of the large intestine. The appendix is attached to the cecum.

The cecum is the short, pouchlike region of the large intestine that is below the ileocecal valve at the junction of the small and large intestine. It is a blind pouch, with one end closed. The appendix is attached to the closed end in the form of a tube-like structure with a winding shape. The open end of the cecum attaches to the ascending colon. It is considered to be the beginning of the large intestine and is generally on the right side of the body. Contents of the ileum are deposited into the cecum's pouchlike structure. In herbivores, the cecum stores food material for bacteria to break down; however, because this no longer occurs in the human cecum, it is just a pouch. The main function of the cecum is to absorb salt and water. It also lubricates the matter that remains with mucous from its internal wall.

The appendix is a blind-ended tube that is connected to the cecum. It averages 9 cm in length and 6 mm in diameter. The appendix is located in the lower right quadrant of the abdomen and is about 2 cm beneath the ileocecal valve. The appendix doesn't have a digestive function. It is made up of lymph tissue and it may attack parasites or bacteria present in food. The function of the appendix remains unclear. However, it is a reservoir for the accumulation of bacteria; it is not considered a required organ but may play a role in immune response.

LEARNING OBJECTIVE 13.5.7 Identify the ascending, transverse, descending, and sigmoid colon.

LEARNING OBJECTIVE 13.5.8 Describe the anatomical characteristics of the ascending, transverse, descending, and sigmoid colon.

KEY TERM

haustra Pouches in the colon.

THE COLON

The colon is shaped like a box. The first vertical portion directly off the cecum is the ascending colon; this portion of the large intestine makes a right-angle turn toward the liver at the hepatic flexure and is followed by the horizontal transverse colon. The spleen bends at the left splenic flexure, creating the vertical descending colon. The descending colon makes a midline medial turn. This portion has an S shape and is referred to as the sigmoid colon (Figure 13-13).

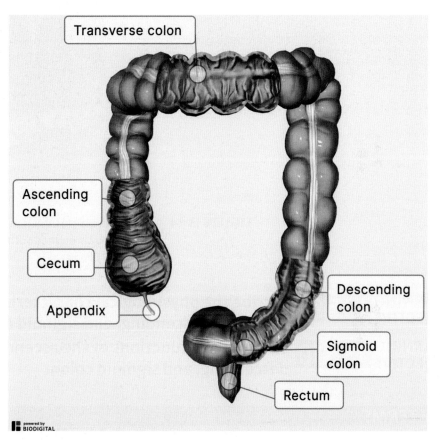

FIGURE 13-13 Four parts of the large intestine are the cecum, colon, rectum, and anus.

Colon Anatomy

The large intestine or colon contains the same layers of tissue found throughout the organs of the alimentary canal with a circular and longitudinal layer of muscularis (Figure 13-14). It contains three bands of smooth muscle, referred to as tenia coli. **Haustra** are the small pouches of the colon that give the colon its segmented appearance. The haustra are formed because the tenia coli, which runs the length of the colon, are shorter than the colon; the saclike appearance that results are the haustra.

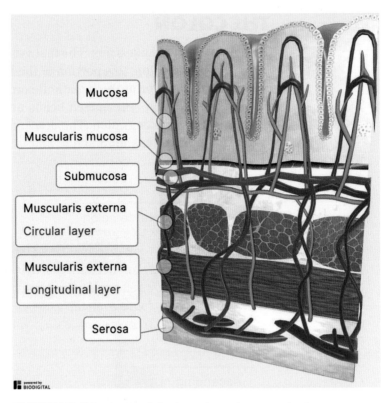

Mucosa

Muscularis mucosa

Submucosa

Muscularis externa
Circular layer

Muscularis externa
Longitudinal layer

Serosa

powered by
BIODIGITAL

FIGURE 13-14 Layers of the large intestine contain the same tissue found throughout other organs of the alimentary canal.

LEARNING OBJECTIVE 13.5.9 Describe the physiological characteristics of the ascending, transverse, descending, and sigmoid colon.

LEARNING OBJECTIVE 13.5.10 Describe the functions of the ascending, transverse, descending, and sigmoid colon.

KEY TERMS

flatus Gas generated in the stomach or bowels.

saccharolytic fermentation Breakdown of carbohydrates by bacteria.

Colon Physiology

Muscular contractions move food through the large intestine and aid in absorption. The mucosa is primarily comprised of cells for absorption. Goblet cells secrete mucus for lubrication and protect the organ wall, but few enzyme-secreting cells are present and there are no digestive secretions.

Colon Function

Slow contractions of the large intestine are triggered by passage of chyme from the ileum into the large intestine. This combined with slow peristalsis promotes absorption of water. Mass movement contractions are strong with the intention of quickly propelling stool to the rectum for defecation. In the ascending colon, the process of extracting water and other nutrients from waste materials for recycling begins. The remaining unwanted waste material moves upward toward the transverse colon by peristalsis. Solid waste is stored in the descending colon. The sigmoid colon expels solid waste and gases from the digestive tract. Its curve allows gas to be expelled from the body without simultaneously releasing feces.

Digestive enzymes are not secreted in the large intestine. Despite this, chemical digestion still occurs due to the bacterial flora found in the colon. **Flatus** or gas consists of methane gas, hydrogen, and carbon. This is produced as a by-product of **saccharolytic fermentation** or the breakdown of carbohydrates by bacteria. Foods containing complex carbohydrates and sugars that are unable to be digested produce increased amounts of flatus. Mucus is secreted for lubrication.

LEARNING OBJECTIVE 13.5.11 Identify the rectum and anus.

LEARNING OBJECTIVE 13.5.12 Describe the anatomical characteristics of the rectum and anus.

LEARNING OBJECTIVE 13.5.13 Describe the physiological characteristics of the rectum and anus.

LEARNING OBJECTIVE 13.5.14 Describe the functions of the rectum and anus.

KEY TERMS

rectal ampulla Place in the rectum where feces is stored before their release via the anal canal.

rectal valves Crescent-like folds located in the rectal ampulla caused by infoldings of the circular muscle and submucosa.

THE RECTUM AND ANUS

The rectum is the distal end of the large intestine. It connects the sigmoid colon to the anus, the opening where stool is excreted from the body.

The rectum has three bends in its structure, which create **rectal valves**. The rectum ends with the **rectal ampulla**, which is where feces is stored until it is released. While the rectum does not contain teniae coli or haustra, it does have strong smooth muscle layers that are used to expel feces from the body.

Three bends in the structure of the rectum create rectal valves. These are not sphincter valves. They support the weight of stool to prevent rapid dumping into the anus and an urgent need to defecate. The rectum stores feces temporarily until defecation.

The anus contains two sphincter muscles. Smooth muscle makes up the internal anal sphincter. Control of this is involuntary. The external anal sphincter is voluntary and is comprised of skeletal muscle. The anus contains two sphincter muscles. Pressure receptors in the anus work with the brain to relax sphincters when defecation is appropriate. The anus controls the discharge of feces from the body.

LEARNING OBJECTIVE 13.5.15 **Explain the mechanism of defecation.**

KEY TERM

Valsalva maneuver Action that involves closure of the glottis while contracting abdominal and diaphragm muscles to induce defecation.

DEFECATION

Feces pass through the sigmoid colon into the rectum. Rectal wall stretching activates the parasympathetic nervous system, specifically a defecation reflex. Voluntary control is maintained over the external anal sphincter. When it is deemed an appropriate time for defecation, rectal muscle contraction pushes stool out of the body. Use of a Valsalva maneuver can assist with the passage of stool. This is a voluntary action that involves closure of the glottis while contracting abdominal and diaphragm muscles.

UNIT OBJECTIVE 13.6

Discuss the structure and functions of the gastrointestinal system's accessory structures.

UNIT INTRODUCTION

Accessory structures of the gastrointestinal system contribute to digestion but are not part of the digestive tract. They release hormones, enzymes, and other secretions that aid in the digestive process. These accessory structures are important because, without them, the digestive organs would not be able to function properly.

LEARNING OBJECTIVE 13.6.1 **Identify each gland and accessory organ of the digestive system.**

ACCESSORY ORGANS AND GLANDS OF THE GASTROINTESTINAL SYSTEM

Accessory organs and glands of the digestive system include the teeth, tongue, salivary glands, gastric or stomach glands, liver, gallbladder, and pancreas.

LEARNING OBJECTIVE 13.6.2 Describe the structure of the salivary glands.

Salivary Glands

In humans, there are three salivary glands, which consist of various lobes and are located in the mouth (Table 13-3). These glands secrete via a network of ducts located in various locations within the oral cavity (Figure 13-15).

Table 13-3 Salivary Glands

GLAND	LOCATION	LOBES PRESENT	DUCT LOCATION
Parotid gland	Anterior to the ears	Two	Second molar on the upper palate
Submandibular glands	Inferior to the jaw	Two	Below the tongue
Sublingual glands	Bilateral sides of the tongue and inferior to the mouth floor	One	Bilaterally near the incisors

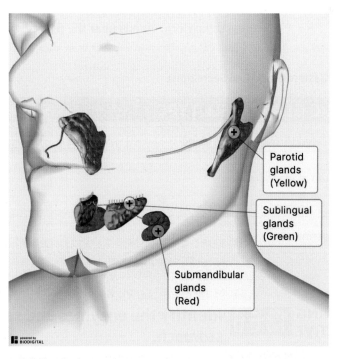

FIGURE 13-15 The salivary glands shown in relation to the jaw.

LEARNING OBJECTIVE 13.6.3 Identify the enzymes and secretions produced by the salivary glands.

LEARNING OBJECTIVE 13.6.4 Describe the enzymes and secretions of the salivary glands and their role in digestion.

Saliva Saliva is produced and secreted by the salivary glands. The parotid glands are the largest of the salivary glands; they produce about 20% of the saliva secreted in the mouth. While smaller, the submandibular glands produce approximately 70% of the saliva secreted in the mouth and the sublingual glands produce approximately 10%. Saliva is a combination of mucus, water containing electrolytes, bicarbonate, antibacterial compounds, and amylase enzyme. The parotid and submandibular glands produce mostly serous cells, while the sublingual glands produce mostly mucus.

Saliva lubricates the food bolus for swallowing and maintains moisture of the oral mucosa. Bicarbonate maintains an alkaline environment while antibacterial compounds prevent bacterial overgrowth. The amylase enzyme initiates chemical digestion by breaking down starch into simple sugars.

LEARNING OBJECTIVE 13.6.5 Describe the structure of the stomach's glands.

Stomach Glands

The stomach contains multiple types of gastric glands (Table 13-4). Each varies by location in the stomach and enzyme secreted. Cardiac gastric glands are at the top of the stomach, followed by gastric glands in the center of the stomach and by pyloric glands near the pyloric sphincter.

Table 13-4 Gastric Gland Cell Secretions

GASTRIC GLAND CELL TYPE	SECRETION
Parietal, located throughout the gland	Intrinsic factor Hydrochloric acid
Chief, located at gland base	Pepsin Renin
Mucous neck, located in the neck of gastric pits	Mucus
Enteroendocrine	Gastrin Other hormones that impact digestion

LEARNING OBJECTIVE 13.6.6 Identify the enzymes and secretions produced by the stomach.

LEARNING OBJECTIVE 13.6.7 Describe the enzymes and secretions of the stomach and their role in digestion.

Enzymes and Secretions

Cardiac and pyloric glands secrete mucus while the gastric glands secrete enzymex containing digestive juices. The enzyme secreted is related to the cell composition of the gland. Enzymes, especially those that digest protein, are produced and secreted in an inactive form. This is to protect the body's own cells; they are activated when exposed to stomach acid and other enzymes.

Role of Enzymes and Secretions Intrinsic factor is required for absorption of vitamin B_{12} in the intestine. This is vital for red blood cell production. Hydrochloric acid is responsible for protein digestion and bacterial eradication. The enzyme pepsin breaks down protein while renin separates milk products. Mucus is a protective secretion. It dilutes acid strength and coats the stomach to prevent damage from exposure to digestive juices. Gastric acid release is stimulated by gastrin.

LEARNING OBJECTIVE 13.6.8 Identify the hormones controlling the release of secretions and enzymes from the stomach.

Release of Secretions and Enzymes Gastric secretion occurs in three phases that can occur separately or simultaneously. The cephalic phase occurs in anticipation of food entering the alimentary canal. Thoughts, sights, and smells of food can activate the cerebral cortex and trigger this prior to food entering the alimentary canal. The parasympathetic nervous system becomes activated and stimulates the gastric glands to release gastric juice. Additional gastric juice is secreted in response to partially digested food.

The gastric phase requires food to move into the stomach to be activated. Amino acids and peptides of partially digested food stimulate gastric functions. Stomach distention and increases in pH stimulates hydrochloric acid release. Acetylcholine secreted by parasympathetic nerve fibers, as well as histamine and gastrin secreted from enteroendocrine G cells, further stimulate gastric secretions.

The intestinal phase and release of intestinal gastrin occurs with the movement of chyme into the duodenum. This stimulates enteroendocrine cells in the intestine, resulting in stimulation and release of pancreas and gallbladder secretions as well as communication to the stomach to slow the movement of chyme.

LEARNING OBJECTIVE 13.6.9 Describe the structure of the liver.

THE LIVER

The liver is located in the upper right abdominal quadrant, almost entirely enclosed by the rib cage. When viewed from the top, it is comprised of two lobes: a large right lobe and a smaller left lobe (Figure 13-16). When viewed from below, two additional lobes are visible: the caudate and quadrate lobes (Figure 13-17). The liver is primarily composed of numerous structural units called liver lobules. These lobules are roughly hexagonal in shape and composed of hepatocytes (liver cells); they are stacked like bricks in a wall. These are congregated around hepatic sinusoids due to their blood storage and porous tissue. Blood enters the liver through the hepatic portal vein. From there, it enters the hepatic veins and empties through the vena cava. Between hepatocyte cells are bile canaliculus ducts that store bile.

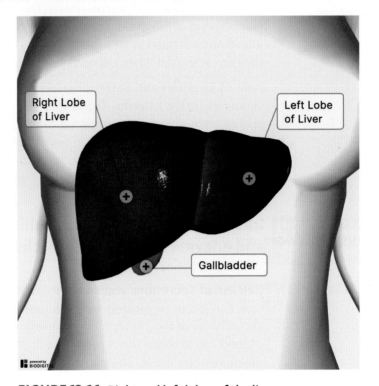

FIGURE 13-16 Right and left lobes of the liver.

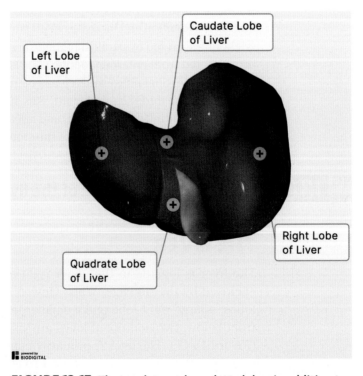

FIGURE 13-17 The caudate and quadrate lobes in addition to the right and left lobes.

LEARNING OBJECTIVE 13.6.10 Describe the functions of the liver.

Function of the Liver

The main job of the liver is to filter the blood from the digestive tract before it goes to the rest of the body; it processes nutrients after they are absorbed from the small intestine. The liver is also able to break down and convert ammonia that is produced during digestion into urea. The hepatocytes in the liver are responsible for producing proteins that the body uses for blood clotting and to maintain fluid in the circulatory system. The liver also manufactures cholesterol, triglycerides, and carbohydrates and it turns glucose into glycogen. It also produces and secretes bile into the duodenum. Bile is produced by the liver, stored in the gallbladder, and used for fat digestion in the duodenum. Finally, the liver acts as a storage unit for the body, storing vitamins B_{12}, A, D, and K, as well as folic acid and iron.

LEARNING OBJECTIVE 13.6.11 Describe the secretions produced by the liver and their role in digestion.

LEARNING OBJECTIVE 13.6.12 Identify the hormones controlling the release of secretions and enzymes from the liver.

Liver Secretions

Bile is a dark green or yellowish-brown fluid that functions to break fat into smaller components, making digestion easier. Bile salts are a component of bile; their purpose in bile is to aid in the absorption of fats and fat-soluble vitamins, such as vitamins B_{12}, A, D, and K. Bile salts also aid in the elimination of cholesterol from the body and in the reduction of bacteria from the digestive system. Without bile salts, cholesterol would crystalize and form gallstones. Bilirubin is the chief bile pigment produced as a waste product during the breakdown of red blood cells. Bilirubin is absorbed from the blood by the liver cells, excreted into bile, and metabolized by bacteria in the small intestine. One of the by-products of the breakdown of bilirubin is what gives feces its brown color.

Hormones of Liver Secretion

Bile is formed in the liver but stored in the gallbladder. Release of the hormone cholecystokinin from the duodenum stimulates bile release from the gallbladder. Bile travels from the gallbladder to the duodenum via the bile duct.

LEARNING OBJECTIVE 13.6.13 Describe the structure of the gallbladder.

KEY TERMS

biliary tree Bile ducts and gallbladder.

Hartmann's pouch Mucosal fold at the junction of the neck of the gallbladder and the cystic duct.

gallstones A small, hard, mass formed in the gallbladder from bile components such as cholesterol, bile salts, and bilirubin.

THE GALLBLADDER

The gallbladder is a saclike organ that is pear shaped and resides between the right and left liver lobes. It is surrounded by peritoneum. It is comprised of a fundus, body, and neck. The fundus is the upper round portion that lies just below the liver. The body is the largest portion of the organ. It lies against the liver and above the duodenum. The neck narrows into the cystic duct that extends to the biliary tree, which is a network of ducts. The cystic duct extends from the gallbladder while the hepatic duct extends from the liver. Both meet to form the common bile duct that leads to the duodenum. It is at this meeting place of the gallbladder and the cystic duct that a mucosal fold known as Hartmann's pouch is formed. Cholelithiasis can result from lodgment of gallstones in this location (Figure 13-18). Gallstones are formed in the gallbladder from bile components such as cholesterol, bile salts, and bilirubin. Gallstones form when there is an inconsistency in the makeup of bile, resulting in hard stones that may block the bile duct, causing cramping in the upper right part of the abdomen.

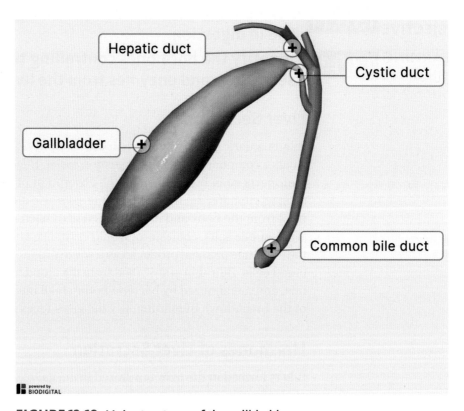

FIGURE 13-18 Main structures of the gallbladder.

LEARNING OBJECTIVE 13.6.14 Describe the function of the gallbladder and its role in bile storage and secretion.

LEARNING OBJECTIVE 13.6.15 Identify the hormones controlling the release of secretions and enzymes from the gallbladder.

Function of the Gallbladder

The gallbladder stores and concentrates bile after it is formed in the liver. It releases bile into the duodenum for digestion of fats.

Hormones of Gallbladder Secretion

The release of the hormone cholecystokinin is caused by fatty acids and amino acids in chyme as it enters the duodenum. This activates the release of bile from the gallbladder. Cholecystokinin is transported to the gallbladder via the blood. It stimulates contraction of the muscularis layer of the gallbladder, pushing bile into the cystic duct and further into the common bile duct and into the duodenum.

LEARNING OBJECTIVE 13.6.16 Describe the structure of the pancreas.

KEY TERM

hepatopancreatic ampulla Cavity where the common bile duct and the pancreatic duct open into the major duodenal papilla; also known as the ampulla of Vater.

THE PANCREAS

The pancreas is located on the left of the abdomen. This organ is comprised of glandular tissue and appears bumpy. It extends from its widest part at the duodenum to a narrower portion at the spleen. The pancreatic duct unites with the bile duct from the liver in the wall of the duodenum, forming the **hepatopancreatic ampulla** (Figure 13-19). This opens into the duodenum and a valve controls the release of bile and pancreatic juice.

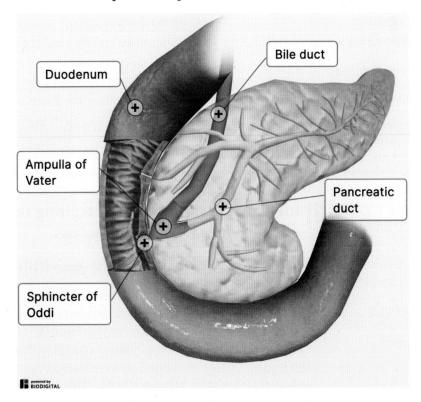

FIGURE 13-19 The pancreas in relation to other digestive organs.

The pancreas contains both exocrine and endocrine parts. In its role as an exocrine gland, the pancreas secretes enzymes that break down proteins, lipids, carbohydrates, and nucleic acid during digestion. These enzymes are released into small ducts that get larger and eventually form the main pancreatic duct. This duct drains into the duodenum. In its role as an endocrine gland, the pancreas houses mini-endocrine glands called the islets of Langerhans. These glands release hormones, such as insulin and glucagon, directly into the bloodstream to regulate blood sugar levels.

LEARNING OBJECTIVE 13.6.17 Identify the enzymes and secretions produced by the pancreas.

LEARNING OBJECTIVE 13.6.18 Describe enzymes and secretions of the pancreas and their role in digestion.

Enzymes and Secretions of the Pancreas and Their Role in Digestion

Pancreatic juice is secreted from the pancreas. This consists of multiple digestive enzymes, water, salts, and bicarbonate. Pancreatic enzymes secreted include proteases, pancreatic amylase, pancreatic lipase, ribonuclease, and deoxyribonuclease as well as trypsin, chymotrypsin, and carboxypeptidase. The various pancreatic enzymes function on various constituents of chyme (Table 13-5).

Table 13-5 Pancreatic Enzyme's Effect on Chyme

PANCREATIC ENZYME	DIGESTIVE FUNCTION ON CHYME
Protease	Breaks down proteins
Pancreatic amylase	Breaks down glycogen and starches
Pancreatic lipase	Breaks down large fat molecules, triglycerides, into smaller fatty acids and monoglycerides
Ribonuclease (RNA)	Breaks RNA into sugar ribose, and nitrogen bases
Deoxyribonuclease (DNA)	Breaks DNA into sugar deoxyribose and nitrogenous bases
Trypsin, chymotrypsin, and carboxypeptidase	Break proteins into amino acids

LEARNING OBJECTIVE 13.6.19 Identify the hormones controlling the release of secretions and enzymes from the pancreas.

Pancreas Secretion and Enzyme Release

Pancreas secretion and enzyme release is controlled by the hormone secretin and cholecystokinin. Secretin is made and released by the duodenum in response to movement of acidic chyme from the stomach to the small intestine. This activates the release of pancreatic juice that is able to buffer the stomach acidity. Cholecystokinin is also released from the duodenum in response to chyme that is high in protein and fat. This stimulates the release of pancreatic juice containing enzymes to break down protein and fat.

UNIT OBJECTIVE 13.7

Describe common pathologies affecting the overall structure and function of the gastrointestinal system.

UNIT INTRODUCTION

Many disorders of the gastrointestinal system are common. These disorders occur when organs within the digestive system don't function as intended and cause problems with digesting food or discomfort or pain. Different types of cancers affect the gastrointestinal system as well. While some of these are quite common, others are less frequent.

LEARNING OBJECTIVE 13.7.1 Identify common disorders affecting the overall structure and function of the gastrointestinal system.

KEY TERMS

constipation Infrequent bowel movement or difficulty emptying bowels.

diarrhea Increased frequency of defecation, usually with liquid stools.

dysphagia Inability to swallow normally.

gastroesophageal reflux disease (GERD) Backflow of stomach acid or gastric juice, or fluids and food into the esophagus from the stomach.

gallstones An abnormal, small, hard mass that is formed in the gallbladder from bile components.

hemorrhoids The inflammation and enlargement of rectal veins.

irritable bowel syndrome Chronic condition of a group of symptoms, such as cramping. bloating, abdominal pain, constipation and diarrhea, that affect the large intestine.

pancreatitis Disorder characterized by inflammation of the pancreas.

GASTROINTESTINAL SYSTEM DISORDERS

Many common disorders can impact the structure and function of the GI system. These can include:

- Tooth loss: Because the salivary glands are activated by chewing, tooth loss can result in reduced saliva production. Other results of tooth loss are inhibited enzyme production, which affects the breakdown of starches in the mouth and difficulty in swallowing food.
- Dysphagia: Difficulty in swallowing. It may or may not present with painful swallowing. Dysphagia can put patients at risk for pulmonary aspiration and aspiration pneumonia, as foods that are not swallowed correctly may enter the lungs instead of the stomach.
- Gastroesophageal reflux disease (GERD): Caused by stomach contents going into the esophagus due to an incompetent lower esophageal sphincter, which causes a burning sensation in the throat (commonly referred to as "heartburn," although heartburn can occur independent of GERD). Consistent episodes can lead to severe damage to the esophagus.

- **Gallstones**: Occur when cholesterol secreted by the liver precipitate in the gallbladder. When a gallstone gets caught in a bile duct, it blocks the release of bile and interferes with normal digestion, resulting in abdominal pain and food intolerance. Generally, the gallbladder must be surgically removed to address the buildup of gallstones.

- **Pancreatitis**: Inflammation of the pancreas caused by damage to the organ due to alcohol abuse, infectious disease, or drugs that cause abdominal pain, nausea and vomiting, and fever. Jaundice may occasionally develop and in serious cases an abscess forms in the pancreas. Treatment includes diet modification, vitamins, and analgesics for pain.

- **Constipation**: Refers to infrequent bowel movements that are hard to pass where the stool is frequently hard and dry. Complications from constipation include hemorrhoids, fissures, or fecal impaction.

- **Diarrhea**: Watery feces that occurs when the mucosa of the colon is unable to maintain appropriate levels of water absorption. Food poisoning, bacteria, viruses, and protozoan infections can all cause diarrhea. If not controlled, diarrhea can lead to severe dehydration.

- **Irritable bowel syndrome**: Chronic condition that consists of a group of symptoms that affect the large intestine, such as cramping, bloating, abdominal pain, and diarrhea and/or constipation. Symptoms can be triggered by food, stress, or hormones. It can be managed with dietary and lifestyle changes, as well as medication.

- **Hemorrhoids**: Caused by the inflammation and enlargement of rectal veins. Strain during defecation causes the inflammation of these veins. A diet high in fiber produces softer stools, which lessens the amount of straining needed during defecation. Surgery is required when they become so enlarged that they remain prolapsed throughout the anal opening.

LEARNING OBJECTIVE 13.7.2 **Describe the signs, symptoms, and diagnosis of common gastrointestinal cancers.**

CANCERS OF THE GASTROINTESTINAL TRACT

Gastrointestinal cancer can affect various organs of the GI system including the mouth, esophagus, stomach, gallbladder, liver, pancreases, large intestine, and anus. Causes can vary based on the type of cancer. Some modifiable and nonmodifiable risk factors include, age, diet high in fat and processed food, smoking, alcohol use, and obesity. See Table 13-6.

Signs and Symptoms

Manifestations of GI cancers can vary based on the organ affected. Common symptoms can include mouth ulcers, changes in bowels, the presence of blood in the stool, decreased appetite, bloating, nausea and vomiting, abdominal pain or tenderness, fatigue, and weight loss.

Table 13-6 Cancers of the Gastrointestinal Tract

TYPE OF CANCER	COMMON SIGNS AND SYMPTOMS	CONTRIBUTING FACTORS	SCREENING AND DIAGNOSIS
Oral cancer (commonly the mouth, lips, or tongue)	Painless, nonhealing ulcer on the affected area	Smoking, the use of chewing tobacco, alcoholism, poor oral hygiene. Occurs more frequently in men than in women.	Review of social, familial, and medical history; document risk behaviors such as tobacco and alcohol use. A physical examination of the head, neck, oral, and pharyngeal regions is performed, including the posterior lateral tongue and tongue base. A definitive diagnosis requires a biopsy of the suspected tissue.
Esophageal cancer	Difficulty swallowing, pain with swallowing, and sometimes weight loss. Generally, symptoms do not occur until the cancer is advanced.	Smoking, alcoholism, and chronic acid reflux. Most common in people over 60 years of age.	Regular screenings for esophageal cancer are not common in the United States. Screenings for esophageal cancer usually consist of endoscopic examination that uses a small, flexible light to look for tissue that is suspected of being cancerous. This tissue will be removed for biopsy.
Stomach cancer (also known as gastric cancer)	Discomfort, loss of appetite, weight loss, and anemia	While the exact cause is unknown, dietary factors such as nitrates in meat, salted meats or fish, and consuming moldy foods are thought to be causes.	An upper endoscopy is used for people who have risk factors or signs and symptoms of stomach cancer. A small, lighted tube with a video camera attached is passed down the throat into the stomach, looking for abnormalities in the lining of the stomach. The doctor will remove any tissue that looks abnormal for biopsy.
Gallbladder cancer	Pain, indigestion, gas, weakness, loss of appetite, weight loss, and jaundice	Relatively uncommon; obesity, chronic cholecystitis, and chronic typhoid infection all increase risk factors. More common in women than in men.	An examination of the abdomen area to check for lumps, tenderness, or fluid buildup is performed. The skin and the white part of the eyes will be checked for jaundice, and lymph nodes may be checked. Lab tests will be performed to check for abnormal bilirubin levels, albumin, and liver enzymes in the blood. Imaging tests such as x-ray, ultrasound, MRI, or CT scan may be used to check for a tumor. Laparoscopic surgery may be indicated to further examine the gallbladder and remove any suspected cancerous tumors. Tissue removed during the laparoscopic surgery will be biopsied.

(continued)

TYPE OF CANCER	COMMON SIGNS AND SYMPTOMS	CONTRIBUTING FACTORS	SCREENING AND DIAGNOSIS
Hepatic cancer (liver cancer) refers to cancer that starts in the liver, not cancer begins in another part of the body but metastasizes to the liver (which is more common)	Lump or pain on the right side of the abdomen below the rib cage, abdominal swelling, yellowish skin, easy bruising, and weight loss.	The most common cause is cirrhosis due to hepatitis B, hepatitis C, or alcohol. Another cause is nonalcoholic fatty liver disease.	Screenings are not currently recommended for people who are not considered high risk for liver cancer. For people at higher risk, due to cirrhosis, hereditary hemochromatosis, or chronic Hepatitis B, screenings include alpha-fetoprotein (AFP) blood tests and ultrasounds every 6 months. Abnormal levels of AFP can indicate liver cancer. Imaging using ultrasound, MRI, and CT Scans are also used to diagnose and stage tumors. A biopsy is used to confirm diagnosis.
Pancreatic cancer	Weakness, weight loss, jaundice, gas, epigastric pain, and the onset of diabetes.	Very rare, but deadly when it does occur. It is more common in industrial areas, among smokers, people with diabetes, and people who have chronically been exposed to PBC.	Screenings are not currently recommended for people without signs and symptoms of pancreatic cancer. Screenings include imaging tests such as a CT scan, MRI, or ultrasound. A cholangiopancreatography test looks at pancreatic ducts to see if they are blocked. An endoscope can also be used to look for tumors. A PET scan injects a slightly radioactive form of sugar that collects in cancerous cells and a special camera is then used to create pictures of the radioactive areas of the body. A biopsy is performed to confirm the cancer diagnosis.
Colorectal cancer	Blood in feces, abdominal pain, and change in consistency and frequency of bowel movements.	Second most common cancer in the United States. Risk factors include high intake of fats, sugars, and red meat; obesity; smoking; and a lack of physical exercise. It is more common in men and older people.	Screenings for colorectal cancer are divided into two groups: stool-based and visual (or structural) exams. Stool-based exams check feces for signs of cancer. If any signs are detected, more invasive testing is needed. Visual exams, most commonly a colonoscopy, insert a scope with a video camera into the rectum to look for abnormal tissue. If abnormal tissue is found, it is removed and biopsied.
Anal cancer	Pain or pressure in the anus or rectum; change in bowel habits; a lump near the anus; and rectal bleeding, itching, or discharge.	HPV, smoking, immunosuppression associated with HIV, benign anal lesions, and receptive anal intercourse.	A digital rectal exam, where a doctor inserts a gloved, lubricated finger into the anus to check for lumps and other changes, is one common initial screening for anal cancer. Additionally, an endoscopy or anoscopy may be used so the doctor can view the lining of the lower rectum and anus. Any change or growth found will be removed and biopsied to determine if cancer is present.

Diagnosis

Diagnosis is specific to the organ affected. Generalized diagnostic testing can include blood sample testing, imaging, endoscopy exams, and biopsy of affected tissue. Cancer staging can be determined following diagnosis. This is used to guide the treatment plan.

UNIT OBJECTIVE 13.8

Describe common pathologies affecting structure and function of the alimentary canal.

UNIT INTRODUCTION

Different disorders can affect the structure and function of the alimentary canal. Depending on the type and severity of the disorder, digestive function may be affected.

LEARNING OBJECTIVE 13.8.1 Identify common disorders affecting the mouth and teeth.

KEY TERMS

canker sores Small, shallow ulcers that appear inside the mouth.

cold sores Painful, fluid-filled blisters that occur outside the mouth (under the nose, around the lips, or under the chin) and are caused by a virus and are highly contagious.

gingivitis Gum inflammation caused by excess plaque on the teeth.

halitosis Chronic bad breath, frequently caused by dental issues (such as cavities or gum disease); mouth, nose, or throat infections; dry mouth; or smoking or other tobacco usage.

periodontal disease An inflammatory disease of the gums that causes damage to the soft tissues and bones supporting the teeth.

COMMON DISORDERS OF THE MOUTH AND TEETH

Multiple disorders can impact the mouth and teeth. These can include:

- Dry mouth: a condition in which the salivary glands in the mouth do not make enough saliva to keep the mouth wet. Symptoms include a sticky feeling in the mouth; bad breath; difficulty chewing, speaking, or swallowing; dry or sore throat; hoarseness; or a dry, grooved tongue. It can be caused by certain medications or a condition that affects the salivary glands.
- Halitosis: chronic bad breath. It is frequently caused by dental issues (such as cavities or gum disease); mouth, nose, or throat infections; dry mouth; or smoking or other tobacco usage. Less frequently, it may be caused by gastric reflux, liver or kidney disease, or diabetes.

- **Cold sores** and **canker sores**: While similar, cold sores and canker sores are not the same thing. Cold sores are painful, fluid-filled blisters that occur outside the mouth (under the nose, around the lips, or under the chin) and are caused by a virus and are highly contagious. Canker sores are small, shallow ulcers that appear inside the mouth. Their exact cause is unknown, although stress or tissue injury is thought to be the cause of many simple canker sores.

- Yeast infection, or oral thrush: Occurs when an overgrowth of the fungus *Candida albicans* occurs in the mouth. White or yellow patches develop on the inner cheeks, tongue, tonsils, gums, or lips. This infection is typically mild and goes away when treated with the appropriate medication.

- **Gingivitis** and **periodontitis**: Gingivitis is gum inflammation caused by excess plaque on the teeth. Gingivitis is reversible; symptoms include swollen gums or gums that bleed easily when brushed or flossed. Periodontitis is another form of periodontal disease; however, it is not reversible. With periodontitis, gums inflame and recede and begin to pull away from teeth. This creates pockets where bacteria can build up and can result in increased pain, sensitivity while chewing, and tooth loss.

- Dental cavities: Damage to the tooth from tooth decay, affecting both the outer coating of the tooth (enamel) and the inner layer (dentin). Dental cavities are discussed further in the next section.

LEARNING OBJECTIVE 13.8.2 Describe the cause, signs, symptoms, and diagnosis of a dental cavity.

KEY TERM

dental cavity Area of decay or hole in a tooth.

DENTAL CAVITY

Tooth decay damages tooth enamel and causes a dental cavity or hole in the tooth. Bacteria and a diet high in sugar and starch can contribute to tooth decay. Saliva and bacteria combine with high sugar and starch food particles to form a plaque film that adheres to the tooth. Foods high in starch further promote adherence of plaque to the tooth. Failure to remove plaque promptly results in the development of tartar. This can cause gum irritation and over time leads to gingivitis or periodontitis. Cavities develop when the sugar is converted to acid by bacteria, slowly eating a hole in the enamel of the tooth (Figure 13-20).

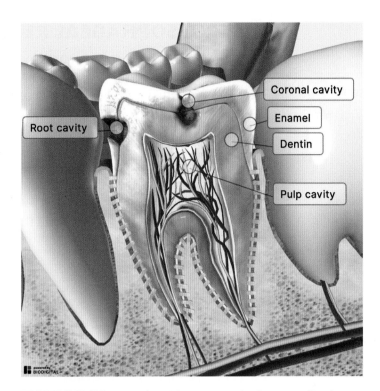

FIGURE 13-20 Dental cavities are seen in the enamel and dentin of a tooth.

Signs and Symptoms

Tooth decay may be asymptomatic. Signs and symptoms can include spots of brown discoloration, along with sensitivity to hot, cold, and sweet foods. Pain is a late symptom indicating nerve damage or fracture of the tooth. Tooth pulp can be damaged if left untreated. Tooth pain may indicate the need for a root canal.

Diagnosis

Regular dental appointments are vital to identify a cavity. Diagnosis can be made by identifying areas of softening in the tooth structure when pushing on the tooth with a sharp dental instrument. X-ray, ultrasound, fluorescence, and fiberoptic transillumination are diagnostic tests used to diagnose dental decay.

LEARNING OBJECTIVE 13.8.3 Describe the causes, signs, symptoms, and diagnosis of common stomach maladies.

KEY TERMS

gastroesophageal reflux disease Backflow of stomach acid or gastric juice, or fluids and food into the esophagus from the stomach.

manometry A test used to evaluate the motility and muscle contractions of the esophagus.

GASTROESOPHAGEAL REFLUX DISEASE

Gastroesophageal reflux disease (GERD) is a common stomach ailment. This results from failure of the lower esophageal sphincter to close completely resulting in backflow of stomach contents into the esophagus, causing irritation. Treatment is vital as over time irritation can lead to more serious diseases, including cancer.

Signs and Symptoms

Heartburn occurring more than two times in a week can indicate GERD. Interestingly, heartburn isn't always present with GERD. Difficulty swallowing, dry cough, and shortness of breath or asthma-type symptoms can indicate GERD.

Diagnosis

Symptom history and physical exam may be sufficient for diagnosis of GERD and initiation of treatment. Diagnostic testing to confirm diagnosis can include x-ray imaging with a barium swallow, endoscopy and biopsy, acid (pH) probe test, and **manometry** of the esophagus.

LEARNING OBJECTIVE 13.8.4 Describe the cause, signs, symptoms, and diagnosis of a Crohn's disease and ulcerative colitis.

INTRODUCTION TO CROHN'S DISEASE AND ULCERATIVE COLITIS

Both Crohn's disease and ulcerative colitis are inflammatory bowel diseases. While Chron's disease can affect any portion of the alimentary canal and may come and go, ulcerative colitis only occurs in the innermost portion of the colon and rectum and is consistent.

CROHN'S DISEASE

The cause of Chron's disease is unknown. An overactive immune system, genetics, and environmental factors such as bacterial or a virus are potential culprits that can cause Crohn's disease.

Signs and Symptoms

Manifestations of Chron's disease can occur anywhere along the alimentary canal from the mouth to the anus and are specific to the inflamed portion of the GI system. Symptoms can include diarrhea, rectal bleeding, weight loss, fatigue, abdominal pain, fever, persistent vomiting, and a decrease in appetite. Manifestations can also occur outside of the alimentary canal such as the eyes, skin, or joints. Symptoms can come and go or change in severity over time.

Diagnosis

No single test can be used to diagnose Crohn's disease. Diagnostic testing can include blood sampling including antibody blood tests and fecal blood tests. X-ray, CT scan, endoscopy, ultrasound, and magnetic resonance imaging can all be used to diagnose Crohn's.

ULCERATIVE COLITIS

The cause of ulcerative colitis is unknown, although factors such as genetics and stress may play a role in causing it. Environmental factors, such as a diet high in unsaturated fats and vitamin B6, not being breast-fed as a baby, and taking isotretinoin, may also cause ulcerative colitis (Figure 13-21).

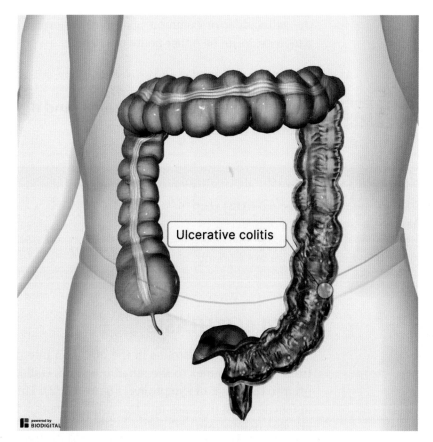

FIGURE 13-21 Example of ulcerative colitis in the colon.

Signs and Symptoms

Manifestations of ulcerative colitis are specific to the colon and rectum. Symptoms can include diarrhea, rectal bleeding, weight loss, and fatigue. Symptoms are consistent and may change in severity over time.

Diagnosis

No single test can be used to diagnose ulcerative colitis. Diagnostic testing can include blood sampling, including antibody blood tests, liver function tests, and fecal blood tests, and x-ray. An endoscopy is the best way to diagnose ulcerative colitis. An endoscopy is used to check for erythema, superficial ulceration, pseudopolyps, or change in vascular appearance of the colon.

UNIT OBJECTIVE 13.9

Describe common pathologies affecting the organs and glands of digestion.

UNIT INTRODUCTION

Cholelithiasis and pancreatitis are common pathologies that can affect the digestive system. Cholelithiasis is commonly known as gallstones, which occur in the gallbladder or common bile duct. Pancreatitis is the inflammation of the pancreas; it can be either acute or chronic.

LEARNING OBJECTIVE 13.9.1 Describe the signs, symptoms, and diagnosis of cholelithiasis.

KEY TERM

hepatobiliary iminodiacetic acid (HIDA) scan A test that uses a small amount of injected radioactive material to determine how well the gallbladder, bile ducts, and liver are working.

CHOLELITHIASIS

Cholelithiasis or gallstones in the common bile duct occlude the flow of bile from the gallbladder to the small intestine. Gallstones are commonly present prior to the onset of symptoms (Figure 13-22). This condition is more common in females than in males and the risk increases with age. Diabetes and obesity are also risk factors.

Manifestations

Cholelithiasis can be asymptomatic. Manifestations of cholelithiasis occur as a gallstone attack when flow through the bile duct is occluded or backflows to the liver. This can present as pain accompanied by nausea and vomiting. Pain is most often in the abdomen and may radiate to below the right arm and the back. Reported pain is often more intense after eating, especially when a meal is high in fat.

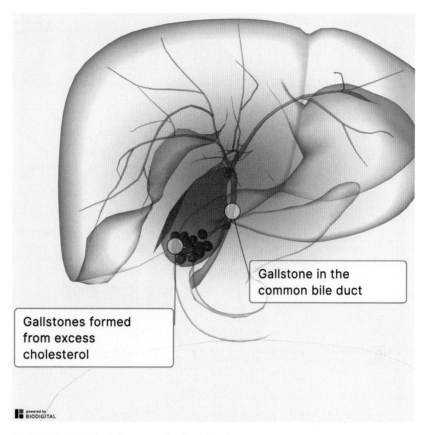

Gallstone in the common bile duct

Gallstones formed from excess cholesterol

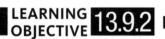

FIGURE 13-22 Gallstones in the bile duct.

Diagnosis

Diagnosis is often made incidentally during diagnostic testing for other health concerns. Ultrasound and a hepatobiliary iminodiacetic acid (HIDA) scan may be used for diagnostic testing. Liver function is assessed via blood testing.

LEARNING OBJECTIVE 13.9.2 Describe the signs, symptoms, and diagnosis of pancreatitis.

PANCREATITIS

Destruction of the pancreatic tissue by digestive enzymes results in inflammation of the pancreas or pancreatitis. It is a serious condition that can be chronic or acute (Figure 13-23).

Symptoms

Manifestations of pancreatitis can vary based on acute or chronic condition. Acute is of sudden onset and can include nausea, vomiting, and severe upper abdominal pain. Weight loss, nausea, vomiting, and oily stools are manifestations of chronic pancreatitis.

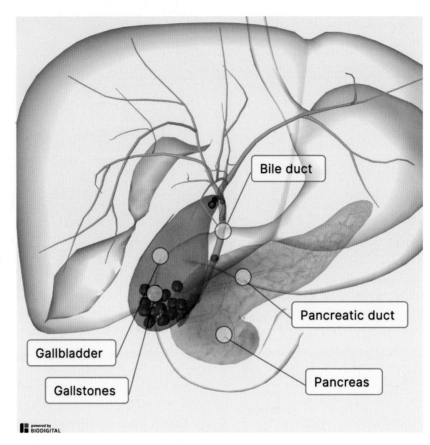

FIGURE 13-23 Pancreas with pancreatitis.

Diagnosis

Multiple diagnostic tests can be employed to diagnose pancreatitis (Table 13-7).

Table 13-7 Diagnostic Tests Used to Diagnose Pancreatitis

TEST	PANCREATITIS INDICATORS
Stool testing	Elevated fat levels
Blood testing	Elevated pancreatic enzymes
Ultrasound	Pancreas inflammation Gallstones
CT scan	Extent of pancreas inflammation Gallstones
Endoscopic ultrasound	Inflammation Bile or pancreatic duct blockage
MRI	Abnormalities in the pancreas, gallbladder, and ducts

Chapter 14

Human Nutrition

Chapter Introduction

The food that we eat contains nutrients that are converted into energy for use throughout the body. This energy helps build cellular molecules and structures and powers body processes, such as digestion, absorption, transportation, and cell metabolism. Energy, combined with certain enzymes, can also be used for growth, maintenance, and repair throughout the body.

It is imperative that we consume enough of the right nutrients to maintain homeostasis and stay healthy. Everything you eat and drink is composed of macromolecules (carbohydrates, proteins, and lipids) and micronutrients (vitamins and minerals) that are necessary to power the body. Water is also considered to be a major nutrient and critical for life.

UNIT OBJECTIVE 14.1

Describe the major sources of carbohydrates, proteins, and lipids; the energy produced by these macromolecules; and how the human body utilizes them to maintain good health.

UNIT INTRODUCTION

Essential nutrients are molecules that must be obtained from our diet because the body cannot make them. The essential nutrients include water, minerals, vitamins, certain amino acids and fatty acids, and a few carbohydrates. Essential nutrients are not the only nutrients that the body needs. Variety is important because no food contains all of the essential nutrients necessary for good health. If the proper amounts of nutrients do not exist in the body, one may suffer from diseases such as rickets.

As you work through this chapter, consider the influence of proper, balanced nutrition in caring for patients in your future role as a member of the health care team. In addition to a basic knowledge of nutrition, consider the role that guides like MyPlate have in ensuring patients receive proper nutrition.

LEARNING OBJECTIVE 14.1.1 Identify the major dietary sources of carbohydrates.

KEY TERMS

carbohydrates Organic compounds made of carbon, hydrogen, and oxygen; examples are starch, cellulose, and sugars.

starch Complex carbohydrate in plant material.

MAJOR DIETARY SOURCES OF CARBOHYDRATES

Carbohydrates are chains of sugars. They are mostly derived from plants, such as fruits and vegetables, but small amounts of carbohydrates can be found in dairy products (milk, yogurt, and cheese) and meats. After being digested, carbohydrates travel through the bloodstream as glucose and are the body's main source of energy. There are two types of carbohydrates:

- Simple carbohydrates (monosaccharides and disaccharides). These can be metabolized quickly. They include various forms of sugars, such as fructose (fruit sugar), lactose (dairy sugar), and sucrose (table sugar).
- Complex carbohydrates (polysaccharides). **Starch**, cellulose, and glycogen are complex carbohydrates.
  - ° Starch is found in grains, legumes, and root vegetables, such as potatoes and carrots.
  - ° Glycogen is a long chain of glucose molecules stored primarily in the liver and skeletal muscle (animal meat).
  - ° Nondigestible cellulose is fiber and plays an important role in health. Even though cellulose is sugar, our bodies are unable to break cellulose down into the simple sugars needed for our bodies to absorb it.

Approximately half of your MyPlate should be composed of carbohydrates (see Figure 14-1).

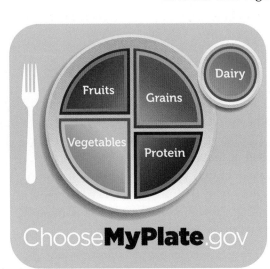

FIGURE 14-1 USDA's MyPlate shows food categories in healthy proportions on a dinner plate. You can personalize your MyPlate by going to the website *www.choosemyplate .gov*. Links for each category provide details about healthy choices for each food group.

LEARNING OBJECTIVE `14.1.2` Identify the major dietary sources of proteins.

KEY TERMS

amino acids Organic compound containing nitrogen, carbon, hydrogen, and oxygen; the building blocks of protein.

complete proteins Animal protein containing all 20 amino acids.

incomplete proteins Proteins that do not contain all 20 amino acids.

protein Organic compound made of chains of amino acids found in both animal and plant foods.

MAJOR DIETARY SOURCES OF PROTEINS

Protein is the main component of all of our cells, body tissues, and body fluids. Proteins are chains of **amino acids**. They can be found in both animal foods and plant foods. Proteins in the body are composed of 20 amino acids, which are divided into two categories: essential and nonessential.

Essential amino acids must be obtained from our food because the body cannot synthesize them. Nonessential amino acids can be synthesized from essential amino acids, so we do not need to ingest nonessential amino acids in our food. Both types of amino acids are required for our bodies to grow, maintain, and repair themselves.

Animal proteins are considered to be **complete proteins** because they contain all of the amino acids essential for the body. Eggs, milk, cheese, poultry, fish, and other meats are complete proteins. Plants, such as legumes (beans and peas), grains, and nuts, are protein rich, but they do not contain one or more of the essential amino acids that our body cannot synthesize. These are considered **incomplete proteins**. When two incomplete proteins are eaten together, such as cereal grains and legumes, they provide all of the essential amino acids our bodies need. Those people who adhere to a strictly plant-based diet (vegan, vegetarian) must make sure that they plan their meals to include all of the essential amino acids. Less than a quarter of your plate should be composed of protein (Figure 14-1).

LEARNING OBJECTIVE 14.1.3 Identify the major dietary sources of lipids.

KEY TERMS

cholesterol Steroid made by the liver; found in animal fats and body tissues.

lipids Class of molecules containing fats.

phospholipids Modified lipid made with phosphorous.

saturated fats and oils Category of triglycerides found in meats, dairy products, eggs, coconut oil, and palm oil.

triglycerides Most common type of lipid found in foods.

unsaturated fats and oils Category of triglycerides found in plant-based foods.

MAJOR DIETARY SOURCES OF LIPIDS

Lipids are fats. They are very important in maintaining a healthy body. Lipids are used for building cells and body tissues, along with aiding in the absorption of many nutrients. Just like there are essential amino acids, there are essential fatty acids (also lipids) that must come from food. We eat several different types of fats (**cholesterol** and **phospholipids**) but the main type found in most foods is **triglycerides**. They are called fats when solid at room temperature and oils when liquid at room temperature. Triglycerides can be categorized as **unsaturated fats and oils** or **saturated fats and oils**, based on their molecular structure.

- Unsaturated fats and oils are healthier lipids. They are found in fish and in plant-derived foods, such as olive oil, canola oil, nuts, and seeds.

  Saturated fats and oils are found in meat, dairy products, eggs, coconut oil, and palm oil.

Cholesterol, another type of lipid, is found in meats, dairy products, and egg yolks. It is not found in plants. Fats do not have a category on MyPlate (Figure 14-1) because they should make up a very small part of each meal.

LEARNING OBJECTIVE 14.1.4 Explain how the cells use carbohydrates.

HOW CELLS USE CARBOHYDRATES

Carbohydrates are the body's preferred fuel source. They are used to produce cellular energy molecules (called **adenosine triphosphate**, or ATP). During digestion, polysaccharides and disaccharides are split into monosaccharides (the building blocks of carbohydrates). The liver then uses monosaccharides, such as fructose and galactose, to synthesize **glucose** (see Figure 14-2A-C).

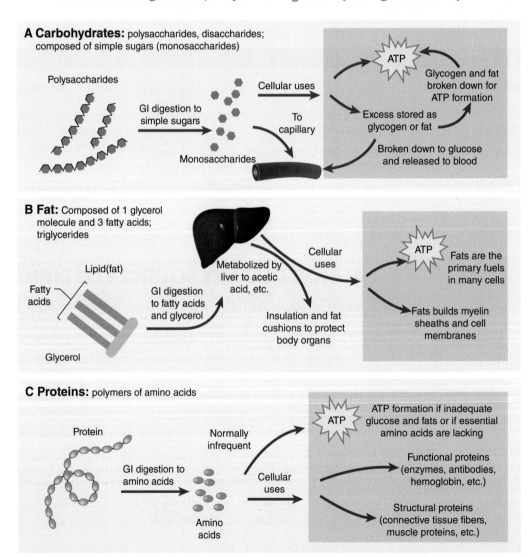

A Carbohydrates: polysaccharides, disaccharides; composed of simple sugars (monosaccharides)

Polysaccharides

GI digestion to simple sugars

Monosaccharides

Cellular uses

To capillary

ATP

Glycogen and fat broken down for ATP formation

Excess stored as glycogen or fat

Broken down to glucose and released to blood

B Fat: Composed of 1 glycerol molecule and 3 fatty acids; triglycerides

Lipid(fat)

Fatty acids

Glycerol

GI digestion to fatty acids and glycerol

Metabolized by liver to acetic acid, etc.

Cellular uses

Insulation and fat cushions to protect body organs

ATP

Fats are the primary fuels in many cells

Fats builds myelin sheaths and cell membranes

C Proteins: polymers of amino acids

Protein

GI digestion to amino acids

Amino acids

Normally infrequent

Cellular uses

ATP

ATP formation if inadequate glucose and fats or if essential amino acids are lacking

Functional proteins (enzymes, antibodies, hemoglobin, etc.)

Structural proteins (connective tissue fibers, muscle proteins, etc.)

FIGURE 14-2ABC Metabolism of carbohydrates, fats (lipids), and proteins by body cells.

Glucose may be absorbed in the small intestine if the food you are eating contains it or may be synthesized in the liver. Glucose, which is what many people refer to as blood sugar, is the major product of carbohydrate digestion. The body carefully regulates glucose levels because it is the major fuel used to make ATP and because the brain relies entirely on glucose for its energy. The liver and muscles convert excess glucose into glycogen for storage; however, a limited amount of glycogen can be stored in the cells. Any extra glucose that is not stored in cells is converted into lipids. Glycogen can quickly be converted back to glucose when the cells need energy.

Sugar molecules also play an important role in forming part of deoxyribonucleic acid (DNA), ribonucleic acid (RNA), and ATP molecules. Monosaccharides, disaccharides, and carbohydrates can also combine with proteins to form glycoproteins, which act as receptor molecules on the surface of cell membranes.

LEARNING OBJECTIVE 14.1.5 Explain how the cells use proteins.

HOW CELLS USE PROTEINS

As previously mentioned, proteins are broken down into their building blocks, amino acids. Once the liver has used all of the amino acids it needs, the remaining amino acids are released to circulate out to the rest of the cells of the body so that those cells can use them. These amino acids are the building blocks for proteins that the body needs.

Proteins make up the majority of cellular structures as well as contribute to cellular functions. They are used to synthesize protein molecules, such as enzymes, hormones, antibodies, and hemoglobin (Figure 14-2). In fact, proteins are so important that all cells actively transport them into their cytoplasm, whether they immediately need them or not. Every cell must contain the 20 amino acids in order for protein to be created within the cell. Recall that essential amino acids cannot be made and must come from food. This explains why cells hang on to amino acids in hopes of obtaining the essential ones. Proteins can be used for ATP production when carbohydrates and fats are not available; however, toxic ammonia and urea are released as a by-product and the liver must promptly remove them.

LEARNING OBJECTIVE 14.1.6 Explain how the cells use lipids.

KEY TERMS

acidosis Blood pH less than the normal lower limit of 7.35.

ketoacidosis Condition in which the blood has a decreased pH; also called acidosis.

HOW CELLS USE LIPIDS

The liver largely handles lipid metabolism. The liver cells use lipids to make ATP for their own use and to synthesize cholesterol, lipoproteins, and thromboplastin (a clotting factor). The unused lipids are released into the bloodstream where body cells remove them to build cell membranes or hormones. However, too much cholesterol or circulating fats can lead to health problems like atherosclerosis, which is a disease where the excess cholesterol sticks to the walls of arteries, causing them to become hard. Fats are also used to build myelin sheaths, fat pads for organs, and insulation under the skin (Figure 14-2). Stored fats are the body's most concentrated source of energy. When there is not enough glucose to meet the energy needs of the cells, fats are used to produce ATP. The breakdown of fats is fast, but incomplete and by-products, such as acetoacetic acid and acetone, accumulate in the blood. These by-products cause the blood to become acidic and result in a condition known as **acidosis** or **ketoacidosis**. Ketoacidosis may result from uncontrolled diabetes mellitus, starvation, or following a fad diet that eliminates carbohydrates.

LEARNING OBJECTIVE 14.1.7 Describe the process utilized to determine the energy values of foods.

KEY TERMS

calorie Unit of heat (energy); amount of energy required to raise 2 grams of water 1 degree Celsius.

kilocalorie One thousand dietary calories.

DAILY VALUES OF FOOD

The process of digestion releases the energy stored within the chemical bonds of foods. A **calorie** is the amount of energy (heat) needed to raise the temperature of 1 mL of water by 1 degree Celsius. A **kilocalorie** is 1000 calories. It is used to show the larger amounts of energy released through the metabolic process. Fats contain more energy per unit of weight than carbohydrates or proteins. Fat contains about 9 calories per gram while proteins and carbohydrates both contain about 4 calories per gram.

The daily values seen on a typical food label (Figure 14-3) help the consumer plan a healthy diet. They are based on a 2000-kcal diet and the energy-producing nutrients are determined as a percentage of daily kilocalorie intake: 60% carbohydrates, 10% proteins, 30% total fats. When using the percent daily values to determine your diet or the diet of a patient, do not forget to consider the number of servings in a package and the serving size.

Nutrition Facts

Serving Size 1 cup (228g)
Servings Per Container 2

Amount Per Serving

Calories 250	Calories from Fat 110

	% Daily Value*
Total Fat 12g	18%
Saturated Fat 3g	15%
Trans Fat 1.5g	
Cholesterol 30mg	10%
Sodium 470mg	20%
Total Carbohydrate 31g	10%
Dietary Fiber 0g	0%
Sugars 5g	
Protein 5g	

Vitamin A	4%
Vitamin C	2%
Calcium	20%
Iron	4%

* Percent Daily Values are based on a 2,000 calorie diet. Your Daily Values may be higher or lower depending on your calorie needs:

	Calories:	2,000	2,500
Total Fat	Less than	65g	80g
Sat Fat	Less than	20g	25g
Cholesterol	Less than	300mg	300mg
Sodium	Less than	2,400mg	2,400mg
Total Carbohydrate		300g	375g
Dietary Fiber		25g	30g

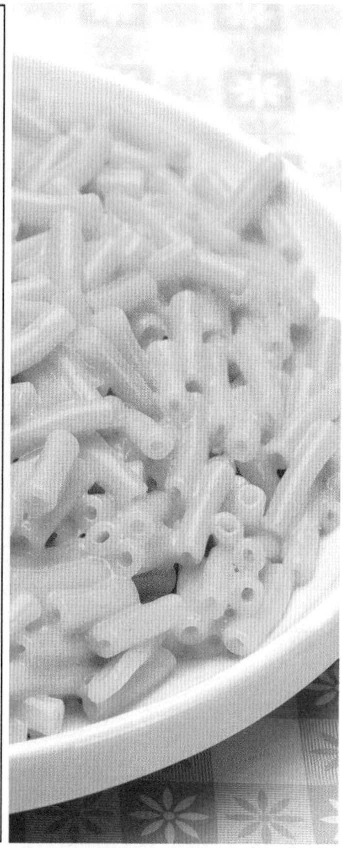

FIGURE 14-3 Food label showing energy values for macaroni and cheese. Note that 1 kcal is equal to 1 Calorie.

LEARNING OBJECTIVE 14.1.8 Explain why energy requirements differ from person to person.

VARYING ENERGY REQUIREMENTS

Energy requirements vary from person to person. There are many factors that influence the energy requirements of an individual (see Table 14-1).

These include the following:

- Age: People who are younger are still growing and developing. This means they will have higher energy needs than those who are older.
- Sex: Males tend to have higher muscle mass and, thus, require a higher level of energy.
- Lifestyle: Those with more active lifestyles require more energy than those who live more sedentary lifestyles.
- Occupation: Occupations that require higher levels of activity and body movement will require more energy. Those with jobs with long periods of sitting or inactivity will require less energy.
- Body composition: Those with higher muscle mass require more energy than those with lower muscle mass.

- Overall health: Certain health conditions and periods of illness may cause energy needs to fluctuate.
- Pregnancy: Extra nutrients are needed during pregnancy and lactation.

Taking these factors into account is an important part of determining appropriate energy requirements for each individual.

Table 14-1   Table Showing the Estimated Calories Needed for Different People Based on their Age, Sex, and Lifestyle

Estimated amounts of calories needed to maintain calorie balance for various gender and age groups at three different levels of physical activity. The estimates are rounded to the nearest 200 calories. An individual's calorie needs may be higher or lower than these average estimates

GENDER	AGE (YEARS)	PHYSICAL ACTLVITY LEVEL		
		SEDENTARY	MODERATELY ACTIVE	ACTIVE
Child (female and male)	2–3	1,000–1,200	1,000–1,400	1,000–1,400
Female	4–8	1,200–1,400	1,400–1,600	1,400–1,800
	9–13	1,400–1,600	1,600–2,000	1,800–2,200
	14–18	1,800	2,000	2,400
	19–30	1,800–2,000	2,000–2,200	2,400
	31–50	1,800	2,000	2,200
	51+	1,600	1,800	2.000–2,200
Male	4–8	1,200–1,400	1,400–1,600	1,600–2.000
	9–13	1,600–2,000	1,800–2,200	2.000–2,600
	14–18	2,000–2,400	2,400–2,800	2800–3,200
	19–30	2,400–2,600	2,600–2,800	3,000
	31–50	2,200–2,400	2,400–2,600	2,800–3,000
	51+	2,000–2,200	2,200–2,400	2,400–2,800

EER equations are from the Institue of Medicine. Dietary Reference Intakes for Energy, Carbohydrate, Fiber, Fat, Fatty Acids, Cholesterol, Protein, and Amino Acids. Washington (DC): The National Academies Press; 2002.
Source: From U.S. Department of Agriculture and U.S. Department of Health and Human Services. *Dietrary Guidelines for Americans*, 2010, 7th Edition, Washington, DC: U.S. Government Printing Office, December 2010.

LEARNING OBJECTIVE 14.1.9 Define positive energy balance and negative energy balance.

LEARNING OBJECTIVE 14.1.10 Explain the physiological consequences of negative energy balances and positive energy balances.

KEY TERMS

negative energy balance More energy is being expended than is being consumed; usually results in weight loss.

positive energy balance More nutrients (calories) are coming in than the body can use; usually result in weight gain.

ENERGY BALANCE

Energy balance is the relationship between the amount of energy consumed from food and the amount of energy used to maintain homeostasis. If energy is balanced in the body, energy intake equals energy expenditure.

- **Positive energy balance** means that more nutrients (calories) are coming in than the body can use.
- **Negative energy balance** means that more energy is being expended than is being consumed.

The relationship between the number of calories we eat and the amount of energy we use determines our body weight and overall health. An individual's entire lifestyle, including amount of exercise and the types of food consumed, must be considered in conjunction with the amount of calories they eat.

When the body is in energy balance, body weight is maintained. A positive energy balance results in weight gain and can result from overeating and/or under exercising. A negative energy balance may result in weight loss.

- Positive energy balance consequences: Many health issues are related to being overweight and not exercising. Obesity may cause sleep apnea, heart disease, high blood pressure, insulin resistance, and type 2 diabetes or increase your risk for certain cancers.
- Negative energy balance consequences: A negative energy balance results in weight loss. If the negative energy balance is too severe, it can cause such things as a decline in metabolism, an inability to concentrate, reduction in hormones, and a decrease in bone mass. All of these may contribute to more serious health issues, which are discussed in detail later in this chapter.

LEARNING OBJECTIVE 14.1.11 Describe the body mass index chart.

LEARNING OBJECTIVE 14.1.12 Identify the relationship between BMI and obesity.

KEY TERM

body mass index Value calculated by dividing a person's weight (Wt) in kilograms by the square of his or her height (Ht) in meters; indicates if a person is at a normal weight.

BODY MASS INDEX CHART

Body mass index (BMI) is a value calculated by dividing a person's weight (Wt) in kilograms by the square of his or her height (Ht) in meters:

$$BMI = Wt\ (kg)/Ht\ (m^2)$$

BMI can also be determined using a BMI chart (Figure 14-4). The higher the number, the more overweight a person may be considered. A person whose BMI is between 18 and 25 is considered to be at a normal weight. If the BMI is between 25 and 30, the person is considered to be overweight. A person with a BMI greater than 30 would be considered obese.

	Under-weight (<18.5)		Healthy Weight (18.5–24.9)						Overweight (25–29.9)									Obese (≥30)							
	18	19	20	21	22	23	24	25	26	27	28	29	30	31	32	33	34	35	36	37	38	39	40
Height											Body weight (in pounds)												
4'10"	86	91	96	100	105	110	115	119	124	129	134	138	143	148	153	158	162	167	172	177	181	186	191
4'11"	89	94	99	104	109	114	119	124	128	133	138	143	148	153	158	163	168	173	178	183	188	193	198
5'0"	92	97	102	107	112	118	123	128	133	138	143	148	153	158	163	168	174	179	184	189	194	199	204
5'1"	95	100	106	111	116	122	127	132	137	143	148	153	158	164	169	174	180	185	190	195	201	206	211
5'2"	98	104	109	115	120	126	131	136	142	147	153	158	164	169	175	180	186	191	196	202	207	213	218
5'3"	102	107	113	118	124	130	135	141	146	152	158	163	169	175	180	186	191	197	203	208	214	220	225
5'4"	105	110	116	122	128	134	140	145	151	157	163	169	174	180	186	192	197	204	209	215	221	227	232
5'5"	108	114	120	126	132	138	144	150	156	162	168	174	180	186	192	198	204	210	216	222	228	234	240
5'6"	112	118	124	130	136	142	148	155	161	167	173	179	186	192	198	204	210	216	223	229	235	241	247
5'7"	115	121	127	134	140	146	153	159	166	172	178	185	191	198	204	211	217	223	230	236	242	249	255
5'8"	118	125	131	138	144	151	158	164	171	177	184	190	197	203	210	216	223	230	236	243	249	256	262
5'9"	122	128	135	142	149	155	162	169	176	182	189	196	203	209	216	223	230	236	243	250	257	263	270
5'10"	126	132	139	146	153	160	167	174	181	188	195	202	209	216	222	229	236	243	250	257	264	271	278
5'11"	129	136	143	150	157	165	172	179	186	193	200	208	215	222	229	236	243	250	257	265	272	279	286
6'0"	132	140	147	154	162	169	177	184	191	199	206	213	221	228	235	242	250	258	265	272	279	287	294
6'1"	136	144	151	159	166	174	182	189	197	204	212	219	227	235	242	250	257	265	272	280	288	295	302
6'2"	141	148	155	163	171	179	186	194	202	210	218	225	233	241	249	256	264	272	280	287	295	303	311
6'3"	144	152	160	168	176	184	192	200	208	216	224	232	240	248	256	264	272	279	287	295	303	311	319
6'4"	148	156	164	172	180	189	197	205	213	221	230	238	246	254	263	271	279	287	295	304	312	320	328
6'5"	151	160	168	176	185	193	202	210	218	227	235	244	252	261	269	277	286	294	303	311	319	328	336
6'6"	155	164	172	181	190	198	207	216	224	233	241	250	259	267	276	284	293	302	310	319	328	336	345

FIGURE 14-4 Body mass index chart.

It is important to note that BMI calculations are strictly a comparison of height and weight and that they do not take into account muscle mass. An individual with a high muscle mass and low body fat could have an overestimated BMI. Another way to determine if these individuals are at a healthy weight is to use the waist-to-hip ratio (see Figure 14-5).

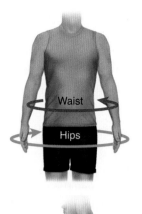
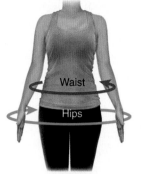
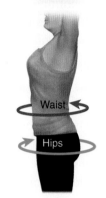

Male waist-to-hip ratio

- **Less than 0.9**
  Low risk of health problems due to weight

- **0.9 to 0.99**
  Moderate risk of health problems due to weight

- **1 or over**
  High risk of health problems due to over weight

Female waist to hip ratio

- **Less than 0.8**
  Low risk of health problems due to weight

- **0.8 to 0.89**
  Moderate risk of health problems due to weight

- **0.9 or Over**
  High risk of health problems due to over weight

FIGURE 14-5 Waist-to-hip ratio (WHR) calculation instructions.

LEARNING OBJECTIVE 14.1.13 Identify the hormones that affect appetite.

LEARNING OBJECTIVE 14.1.14 Explain how appetite is controlled by hormones.

KEY TERMS

ghrelin Hormone released mainly by the stomach believed to signal hunger or prime the body for fat absorption.

insulin Hormone that promotes the uptake of glucose (blood sugar) by cells in the body.

leptin Hormone made by fat cells that plays a role in decreasing appetite as well as maintaining body weight.

neuropeptide y Hormone produced by the hypothalamus that plays a role in increasing food intake and storing energy as fat in the body; also called NPY.

APPETITE

When thinking about the effects of eating too much or too little, it is important to consider the role that hormones play in prompting the body to eat. The hormones leptin and ghrelin affect both your hunger and your weight by sending signals to the brain.

- **Leptin** is made by fat cells and plays a role in decreasing your appetite and maintaining body weight. The more stored fat a person has, the more leptin they produce. Leptin then sends signals to the brain that enough fat has been stored. Increased levels of leptin signal to the brain that you are full. Thus, when there are low levels of leptin, your body does not think your are full, which may cause a hungry feeling. A thin person does not make as much leptin as an overweight individual.

- **Ghrelin** is released mainly in the stomach. It is believed to signal hunger or prime the body for fat absorption. Ghrelin increases if a person is undereating.

Although researchers continue to determine the exact way these hormones contribute to energy balance, it is clear that they work together to maintain energy balance. The hormones insulin and neuropeptide y (NPY) may also affect appetite and weight.

- **Insulin** promotes the uptake of glucose (blood sugar) by the cells of the body. If insulin is not present in sufficient amounts (as in type 2 diabetes) after food is ingested, then the extra glucose will be stored as fat.
- **Neuropeptide y** is produced by the hypothalamus in the brain and has many functions, including increasing food intake and storing energy as fat.

UNIT OBJECTIVE 14.2

List the vitamins and minerals needed by the human body and how they are obtained through healthy eating.

UNIT INTRODUCTION

In addition to macronutrients, the body is also fueled by a variety of vitamins and minerals. Vitamins and minerals are classified into several different types and are obtained through a variety of sources. Understanding the sources and functions of each vitamin and mineral will help you better assist in maintaining balanced nutrition for patients.

LEARNING OBJECTIVE 14.2.1 Identify the fat-soluble and water-soluble vitamins.

KEY TERMS

coenzymes Nonprotein molecule that is needed for an enzyme to function.

essential vitamins Vitamins that the body needs and cannot make.

fat-soluble vitamins Vitamins that dissolve in lipids.

organic molecules Molecules containing carbon in a ring or chain with other atoms such as hydrogen, nitrogen, and oxygen attached; commonly found in living organisms.

provitamins Substance that is converted into a vitamin in the human body.

vitamins Organic molecules that can be broken down by heat, acid, light, and oxygen; if their chemical structure is changed, they lose their function; may be changed during food preparation, which alters their function in the body.

water-soluble vitamins Vitamins that dissolve in water.

VITAMINS

Vitamins are **organic molecules** found in very small amounts in food that are necessary for normal functioning and metabolism. The best and most reliable way to ensure that you receive all the nutrients and vitamins your body needs for normal metabolism is to eat a healthy, balanced diet containing a variety of foods. Most vitamins are considered **essential vitamins**. This means that the body cannot make them in sufficient quantities to support normal body function. These vitamins must be obtained from our food in order to meet our metabolic needs. Some vitamins, referred to as **provitamins**, can be used to create vitamins by the body as long as there is an adequate level of essential vitamins available. An example of a provitamin is beta carotene. Beta carotene is found in many fruits and vegetables (most commonly carrots), and it is used by the body to make vitamin A, which is an essential vitamin.

The body uses essential vitamins in their original form or a slightly modified form for various purposes throughout the body, and they do not require digestion. Many essential vitamins function as **coenzymes**. Coenzymes are crucial because they are necessary to make enzymes functional. This is important because enzymes are the substances that trigger important reactions throughout the body. For example, vitamin K plays an important role in starting chemical reactions that are necessary for blood clotting. Vitamin B_{12} helps to trigger chemical reactions that are necessary for growth, and vitamin B_2 is necessary for producing ATP, which helps power the body and its cells.

Vitamins are either fat soluble or water soluble (Table 14-2):

- **Fat-soluble vitamins.** Fat-soluble vitamins dissolve in lipids (fats). These vitamins are absorbed in the intestines. When excess amounts of these vitamins are consumed, they are stored in the body's fat cells for long periods of time. Because the body can store these vitamins, people are at higher risk of experiencing toxicity of these vitamins than other vitamin types. This also means that the signs and symptoms of fat-soluble vitamin deficiencies may be slower to appear. Vitamins A, D, E, and K are fat-soluble vitamins. Fat-soluble vitamins can maintain their structure even after being exposed to heat (such as when they are cooked).

- **Water-soluble vitamins.** If vitamins are water soluble, they dissolve easily in water and are absorbed into the body through the intestines. Unlike fat-soluble vitamins, water-soluble vitamins cannot be stored in the body for long periods of time. Excessive amounts of these vitamins are excreted in urine. This means there is a low risk of suffering from toxicity of these vitamins. However, deficiency of these vitamins may be more likely. The signs and symptoms of water-soluble vitamin deficiencies appear quickly. Water-soluble vitamins are vitamins B and C. Unlike fat-soluble vitamins, water-soluble vitamins do not maintain their structure when they are cooked.

Table 14-2 Table Summarizing Major Vitamins, Food Sources Where those Vitamins can be Found, and their Function in the Body. It also Notes What Diseases May Occur if the Body is Deficient in that Particular Vitamin

VITAMIN	FOOD SOURCES	FUNCTION(S)	DEFICIENCY DISEASE(S)
A (fat soluble)	Butter, fortified margarine, green and yellow vegetables, milk, eggs, liver	Night vision Healthy skin Proper growth and repair of body tissues	Night blindness Dry skin Slow growth Poor gums and teeth
B1 (thiamine) (water soluble)	Chicken, fish, meat, eggs, enriched bread, whole-grain cereals	Promotes normal appetite and digestion Needed by nervous system	Loss of appetite Nervous disorders Fatigue Severe deficiency causes beriberi
B2 (riboflavin) (water soluble)	Cheese, eggs, fish, meat, liver, milk, cereals, enriched bread	Needed in cellular respiration	Eye problems Sores on skin and lips General fatigue
B3 (niacin) (water soluble)	Eggs, fish, liver, meat, milk, potatoes, enriched bread	Needed for normal metabolism Growth Proper skin health	Indigestion Diarrhea Headaches Mental disturbances Skin disorders
B12 (cyanocobalamin) (water soluble)	Milk, liver, brain, beef, egg yolk, clams, oysters, sardines, salmon	Red blood cell synthesis Nucleic acid synthesis Nerve cell maintenance	Pernicious anemia Nerve cell malfunction
Folic acid (water soluble)	Liver, yeast, green vegelables, peanuts, mushrooms, beef, veal, egg yolk	Nucleic acid synthesis Needed for normal metabolism and growth	Anemia Growth retardation
C (ascorbic acid) (water soluble)	Citrus fruits, cabbage, green vegetables, tomatoes, potatoes	Needed for maintenance of normal bones, gums, teeth, and blood vessels	Weak bones Sore and bleeding gums Poor teeth Bleeding in skin Painful joints Severe deficiency results in scurvy
D (fat soluble)*	Beef, butter, eggs, mik	Needed for normal bone and teeth development Controls calcium and phosphorus metabolism	Poor bone and teeth structure Soft bones Rickets
E (tocopherol) (fat soluble)	Margarine, nuts, leafy vegetables, vegetable oils, whole wheat	Used in cellular respiration Protects red blood cells from destruction Acts as an antioxidant	Anemia in premature infants No known deficiency in adults
K (fat soluble)	Synthesized by colon bacteria Green leafy vegetables, cereal	Essential for normal blood clotting	Slow blood clotting

*The role of vitamin D in insulin resistance, hypertension, and immune function is under investigation by researchers.

LEARNING OBJECTIVE 14.2.2 Explain the functions of the fat-soluble vitamins.

Functions of Fat-Soluble Vitamins

Fat-soluble vitamins (see Table 14-2) serve a variety of purposes throughout the body.

- Vitamin A. Vitamin A is found in butter, green and yellow vegetables, milk, eggs, and liver. They play an important part in developing and maintaining out night vision, healthy skin, and play a role in appropriate growth and repair of body tissue.
- Vitamin D. Similar to vitamin A, vitamin D can be found in beef, butter, eggs, and milk. However, the body can also produce it when absorbing ultraviolet rays from the sun. It plays an important role in how the body absorbs and uses calcium. As such, it is needed for appropriate bone and teeth development.
- Vitamin E. This is found in margarine, nuts, vegetable oils, and whole wheat. Vitamin E helps prevent red blood cells from being destroyed and is used to help form ATP (a form of energy) during cellular respiration.
- Vitamin K. As previously mentioned, vitamin K is essential to how our body clots blood. It is found in green leafy vegetables and is processed by bacteria in the colon.

Consuming fat in our food is required for absorption of these vitamins. Recall that fat-soluble vitamins can be stored in the body. This means that deficiencies of these vitamins appear slowly. Toxicity typically only occurs when someone takes high doses of supplements. Routine blood labwork can help determine and monitor the levels of these vitamins.

LEARNING OBJECTIVE 14.2.3 Explain the functions of the water-soluble vitamins.

Functions of Water-Soluble Vitamins

Water-soluble vitamins (see Table 14-2) also serve many important purposes in the body:

- Vitamin C. Also called ascorbic acid, vitamin C is needed to help support bones, gums, teeth, and blood vessels.
- Vitamin B_1. Also called thiamine, B_1 has an important role in controlling appetite and digestion. The nervous system also needs this vitamin to function properly.
- Vitamin B_2. This vitamin may also be referred to as riboflavin. It is needed in cellular respiration and has a role in maintaining skin and the eyes.

- Vitamin B_3. Also called niacin, this vitamin supports your metabolism as well as encourages growth and your skin. It also helps support appropriate digestion.
- Vitamin B_6. This vitamin, which is also called pyridoxine, plays a role in metabolism of meat protein. It also supports serotonin, which helps with mood regulation.
- Vitamin B_{12}. This vitamin, also called cobalamin, plays an important role in the production of red blood cells. It also contributes to the production of nucleic acid (which stores information used to make proteins) and helps support normal nerve cell function.
- Biotin. This vitamin is also in the vitamin B family. It plays a role in metabolizing glucose in the body.
- Folic acid. This is actually the synthetic (or man-made) version of B_9 (also called folate). Its presence in the body supports red blood cell production and production of genetic material.
- Pantothenic acid. Also referred to as vitamin B_5, pantothenic acid supports metabolism of food, adrenal function, and nerve function.

Recall that water-soluble vitamins cannot be stored in the body. This means that if you consume excessive amounts of these vitamins, the body excretes them through urine rather than storing them in your body. Because of this, deficiencies of these vitamins are more common than fat-soluble vitamins, and symptoms of deficiency appear more quickly. Routine blood labwork can determine the levels of these vitamins.

LEARNING OBJECTIVE 14.2.4 Contrast the physical properties of a mineral and a vitamin.

KEY TERMS

inorganic molecules Molecules containing no carbon that are not commonly found in living organisms.

micronutrients Vitamins and minerals needed in very small amounts by the body.

minerals Inorganic molecules whose chemical structure does not change when they are exposed to heat, acid, light, or oxygen; remain stable during food preparation.

PHYSICAL PROPERTIES OF MINERALS AND VITAMINS

Although vitamins and minerals are both micronutrients (i.e., nutrients that the body only needs in small amounts) that are necessary for normal overall metabolism, they differ in many ways. Vitamins are organic molecules that can be broken down by heat, acid, light, and oxygen. If their chemical structure is changed, they lose their function. They may be changed during food preparation, which alters their function in the body.

Minerals, on the other hand, are inorganic molecules. Their chemical structure does not change when they are exposed to heat, acid, light, or oxygen. This means that how they function in the body remains stable, regardless of how they are prepared.

LEARNING OBJECTIVE 14.2.5 List the major minerals and trace elements the human body requires for the maintenance of good health.

KEY TERMS

major minerals Minerals the body needs 100 mg or more of daily.

trace elements Minerals the body needs less than 100 mg of daily.

MINERAL AND TRACE ELEMENT REQUIREMENTS OF THE BODY

Minerals are broken down into two categories: major minerals and trace elements.

Major Minerals

The daily requirement for major minerals is 100 mg or more daily. Minerals are consumed in the food we eat. They are required for normal metabolism and they may be coenzymes or make up part of a vitamin, hemoglobin, and other organic molecules. Common major minerals are as follows (Table 14-3):

- Sodium
- Potassium
- Calcium
- Iron
- Phosphorus
- Zinc

Trace Elements

Humans only need small amounts of trace elements (less than 100 mg daily). Common trace elements are as follows (Table 14-3):

- Zinc
- Copper
- Iodine
- Cobalt
- Manganese
- Selenium
- Chromium
- Fluorine

Even though only small amounts are needed for these elements, they do help support many different functions and help maintain homeostasis in the

Table 14-3 **Dietary Sources, Functions in the Body, and Symptoms of Deficiency for the Minerals Needed by the Body to Maintain Homeostasis**

MINERAL	FOOO SOURCES	FUNCTION(S)	DEFICIENCY DISEASE(S)
Calcium	Milk, Cheese, dart green vegetables, dried legumes, sardines, shellfish	Bone and tooth formation Blood clotting Nerve transmission	Stunted growth Rickets Osteoporosis Convulsions
Chlorine	Common table salt, seafood, milk, meat, eggs	Formation of gastric juices Acid–base balance	Muscle cramps Mental apathy Poor appetite
Chromium	Fats, vegetable oils, meats, clams, wholegrain cereals	Involved in energy and glucose metabolism	Impaired ability to metabolize glucose
Copper	Drinking water, liver, shellfish, whole grains, cherries, legumes, kidney, poultry, oysters, nuts, chocolate	Constituent of enzymes involved with iron transport	Anemia incidence of disease rare
Fluorine	Drinking water, tea, coffee, seafood, rice, spinach, onions, lettuce	Maintenance of bone end tooth structure	Higher frequency of tooth decay
Iodine	Marine fish and shellfish, dairy products, many vegetables, iodized salt	Constituent of thyroid hormones	Goiter (enlarged thyroid)
Iron	Liver, lean meats, legumes, whole grains, dart green vegetables, eggs, dark molasses, shrimp, oysters	Constituent of hemoglobin involved in energy metabolism	Iron-deficiency anemia
Magnesium	Whole grains, green leafy vegetables, nuts, meats, milk, legumes	Involved in muscle and nerve function Helps with heart rhythm Maintenance of bone strength	Behavioral disturbances Weakness Spasms Growth failure Cardiac arrhythmias
Phosphorus	Milk, cheese, meat, fish, poultry, whole grains, legumes, nuts	Bone and tooth formation Acid–base balance Involved in energy metabolism	Weakness Demineralization of bone
Potassium	Meats, milk, fruits, legumes, vegetables, sweet potatoes	Acid–base and water balance Nerve transmission Helps control blood pressure	Muscular weakness Paralysis
Selenium	Fish, poultry, meats, grains, milk, vegetables (depending on amount in soil)	Necessary for vitamin E function Regulates thyroid hormone	Anemia Deficiency is rare
Sodium	Common table salt, seafood, most other foods except fruit	Acid–base balance Body water balance Nerve transmission	Muscle cramps Mental apathy
Sulfur	Meat, fish, poultry, eggs, milk, cheese, legumes, nuts	Constituent of certain tissue proteins	Related to deficiencies of sulfur-containing amino acids
Zinc	Milk, liver, shellfish, herring, wheat bran	Supports nerve and immunity functions Necessary for vitamin A metabolism	Growth failure Lack of sexual maturity Impaired wound healing

body. For example, iodine, which is only absorbed and used by the thyroid, is a key component in the creation of thyroid hormones. Thyroid hormones play key roles in how calories are burned, body temperature regulation, and digestion. Chromium, another trace element, plays an important role in regulating glucose metabolism, which provides energy to the body.

LEARNING OBJECTIVE 14.2.6 Describe the components of a healthy and adequate diet.

KEY TERM

Daily Values Recommended dietary amounts of vitamins, minerals, fat, cholesterol, carbohydrates, fiber, and protein for a healthy diet; appear on food labels and are based on a 2000-kcal diet.

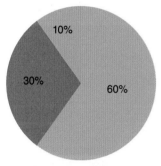

■ Carbohydrates ■ Fats ■ Proteins

FIGURE 14-6 Pie chart showing the percentage of carbohydrates, fats, and proteins that should comprise the average adult diet each day.

COMPONENTS OF A HEALTHY DIET

When health care providers refer to or encourage patients to consume a "healthy diet," they are telling patients to eat a diet that contains an appropriate balance of all needed vitamins, minerals, fat, cholesterol, carbohydrates, fiber, and protein. The specific amount of each nutrient that is required varies from person to person; however, there are some general rules that can be applied to determine the appropriate **Daily Values** of each nutrient. Daily Values appear on food labels (see Figure 14-3) and are based on a 2000-kcal diet. The Daily Values for these nutrients are determined as a percentage of your daily caloric intake. Each day, your total diet should be comprised of the following percentage of nutrients (Figure 14-6):

- 60% carbohydrates
- 30% fats
  - ° Note: No more than 10% of this amount should be saturated fats. The dietary total amount of saturated fats you eat each day should not exceed 65 grams.
- 10% proteins

In addition, you should consume the following amount of nutrients daily:

- 14 grams of fiber for each 1000 kcal ingested
- Less than 300 mg of cholesterol
- Less than 2400 mg of sodium

The percent daily value will vary among individuals and, as mentioned previously in this chapter, will depend on a person's age, weight, and lifestyle. It is also important to remember that when using the percent daily values of a food to determine how its nutrients fit into your diet, do not forget to take the serving size on the package into account. That is, many packages that seem to be a single serving (such as a bag of chips) may actually contain multiple servings, even though their nutrition label that only reflects a single serving (Figure 14-7).

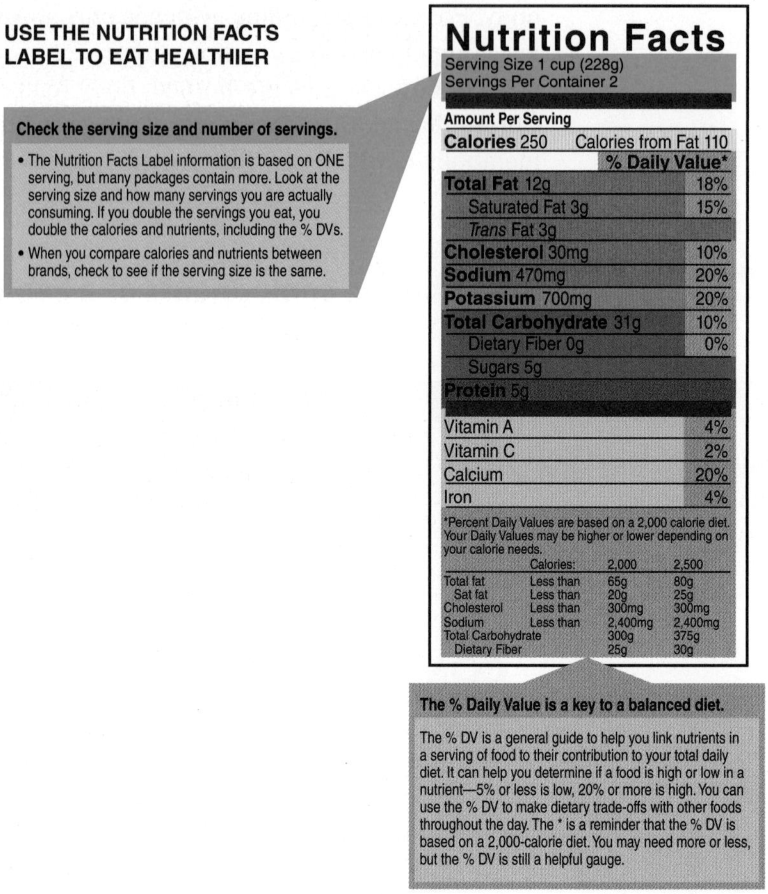

**USE THE NUTRITION FACTS
LABEL TO EAT HEALTHIER**

Check the serving size and number of servings.

- The Nutrition Facts Label information is based on ONE serving, but many packages contain more. Look at the serving size and how many servings you are actually consuming. If you double the servings you eat, you double the calories and nutrients, including the % DVs.
- When you compare calories and nutrients between brands, check to see if the serving size is the same.

Nutrition Facts

Serving Size 1 cup (228g)
Servings Per Container 2

Amount Per Serving

Calories 250   Calories from Fat 110

	% Daily Value*
Total Fat 12g	18%
Saturated Fat 3g	15%
Trans Fat 3g	
Cholesterol 30mg	10%
Sodium 470mg	20%
Potassium 700mg	20%
Total Carbohydrate 31g	10%
Dietary Fiber 0g	0%
Sugars 5g	
Protein 5g	
Vitamin A	4%
Vitamin C	2%
Calcium	20%
Iron	4%

*Percent Daily Values are based on a 2,000 calorie diet. Your Daily Values may be higher or lower depending on your calorie needs.

	Calories:	2,000	2,500
Total fat	Less than	65g	80g
Sat fat	Less than	20g	25g
Cholesterol	Less than	300mg	300mg
Sodium	Less than	2,400mg	2,400mg
Total Carbohydrate		300g	375g
Dietary Fiber		25g	30g

The % Daily Value is a key to a balanced diet.

The % DV is a general guide to help you link nutrients in a serving of food to their contribution to your total daily diet. It can help you determine if a food is high or low in a nutrient—5% or less is low, 20% or more is high. You can use the % DV to make dietary trade-offs with other foods throughout the day. The * is a reminder that the % DV is based on a 2,000-calorie diet. You may need more or less, but the % DV is still a helpful gauge.

FIGURE 14-7 This nutrition label outlines the details of a single serving; however, the package contains two servings per container.

LEARNING OBJECTIVE 14.2.7 Define primary malnutrition and secondary malnutrition.

LEARNING OBJECTIVE 14.2.8 Contrast primary and secondary malnutrition.

KEY TERMS

primary malnutrition Prolonged, inadequate dietary intake of food; due to not eating enough food, whether or not any specific nutrient deficiency is present, or eating an excess of specific nutrients.

secondary malnutrition Inadequate diet due to a secondary disease that affects growth directly or indirectly by changing the appetite or absorption of nutrients; patients are getting enough food, but a secondary disease is preventing their bodies from being able to get enough nutrients from their food.

PRIMARY AND SECONDARY MALNUTRITION

When a person is deficient in one or several nutrients and vitamins, they are said to be malnourished. There are two types of malnutrition:

- **Primary malnutrition** is prolonged, inadequate dietary intake of food. This occurs when a person does not eat enough food for a prolonged period of time. With this form of malnutrition, the person may or may not be deficient in one or several specific nutrients. This results in the body not getting enough of all of the required nutrients. When the body does not get all required nutrients, it may not be able to maintain homeostasis or function normally. For example, the person's energy levels will be decreased, as will mental functioning. The body may also become more prone to infection.
- **Secondary malnutrition** occurs due to secondary disease. This means that a person with certain diseases may have changes in appetite or have altered ability to absorb nutrients. In these cases, patients are often getting enough food and perhaps a balanced diet, but a disease is preventing their bodies from being able to absorb and use nutrients appropriately from their food.

Primary malnutrition is more likely to occur in developing countries where food supplies may be limited. Secondary malnutrition is more likely to occur in certain disease populations, such as patients with certain gastrointestinal diseases that inhibit nutrient absorption, such as Crohn's disease, and in patients with certain kidney diseases. Further discussion of pathologies that result from malnutrition and vitamin deficiencies are discussed later in this chapter.

UNIT OBJECTIVE 14.3

Describe common pathologies that relate to nutrition.

UNIT INTRODUCTION

Occasionally, a person's body may not be able to obtain, absorb, or use nutrients as expected. This may be due to not consuming enough nutrients or to underlying pathologies that decrease the body's ability to normally absorb and use nutrients that are consumed. When this occurs, a person may experience certain pathologies related to nutrient deficiencies.

LEARNING OBJECTIVE 14.3.1 Identify common pathologies affecting human nutrition.

COMMON PATHOLOGIES AFFECTING HUMAN NUTRITION

As mentioned previously, there are certain diseases that may influence the body's ability to maintain balanced nutrition. Alternatively, nutrient excesses or deficiencies in a person's diet may cause or worsen some common pathologies. Diseases and conditions that influence nutrition include the following:

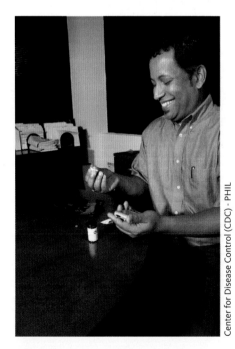

FIGURE 14-8 Adult man with diabetes checks his blood glucose levels.

Center for Disease Control (CDC) - PHIL

- **Cardiovascular disease.** In some cases, patients with decreased dietary intake of certain nutrients may show a loss of muscle, fat, and bone mass. Specifically, low intake of protein and energy may cause a loss of cardiac muscle. This can lead to heart malfunction and cause heart failure.

- **Cancer.** Patients with certain forms of cancer may struggle to consume and absorb adequate calories and nutrition. For example, gastrointestinal cancers may inhibit a person's ability to absorb and use any nutrients consumed, which would be considered a form of secondary malnutrition. This may make recovering from cancer more difficult.

- **Hypertension.** As you may recall, nutrients like potassium and vitamin D have a role in supporting certain cardiovascular functions. Therefore, patients who don't consume appropriate amounts of potassium and vitamin D may have increased blood pressure, resulting in hypertension. Alternatively, excessive consumption of certain nutrients, such as sodium, may worsen hypertension.

- **Diabetes mellitus.** Type 2 diabetes (Figure 14-8) is a condition in which a patient's pancreas may no longer produce adequate amounts of insulin or when a patient's body is no longer receptive to insulin. These malfunctions result in an excessive amount of glucose being available in the body. In addition to certain medications, managing this disease may involve reducing the level of certain foods, such as carbohydrates, in the diet. Over-restricting your diet when trying to manage this disease, however, may result in malnutrition.

- Eating disorders. Patients with eating disorders adopt unhealthy eating patterns. Two common eating disorders are **anorexia nervosa** (Figure 14-9) and **bulimia**. Those with anorexia may over restrict how much food they eat and/or over exercise. Those with bulimia binge-eat large amounts of unhealthy foods (called binging) and purge what they've eaten through self-induced vomiting and diarrhea (induced by taking laxatives). Behaviors in both of these conditions have a large impact on the patient's ability to maintain appropriate nutrition. They may be unable to absorb appropriate nutrients, consume an imbalanced diet, and suffer other conditions due to inappropriate nutrition, such as softening of the teeth and loss of muscle mass.

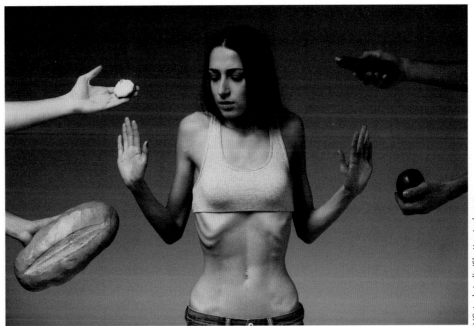

FIGURE 14-9 Patient with anorexia nervosa.

- Chronic undernutrition. This condition results when an individual is not getting enough food to meet the energy needs of the body. This may occur when a person does not eat enough, does not eat enough nutritious foods, or chronically expends more energy than they take in.
- **Hereditary metabolic disorders**. These disorders are genetic, meaning a person is born with them. They interrupt normal metabolism of food. They may lead to malnutrition when a

person does not modify their average daily intake of nutrients to accommodate their altered metabolic state.

- Food allergies and intolerances. There are many different types of food allergies and intolerances. When a person cannot consume certain foods, they may experience malnutrition or deficiency. For example, someone who is lactose intolerant (i.e., cannot digest or tolerate dairy products) may not be able to consume enough calcium and become calcium deficient. Patients with certain food allergies and intolerances may need to take vitamin/mineral supplements to manage their condition.

- Food interactions with medications. Some medications prevent the proper metabolism of food, block the absorption of nutrients from food, or affect appetite. For example, Ranitidine is commonly taken to block the production of too much stomach acid. With prolonged use, it may result in a deficiency of nutrients that require stomach acid to be broken down. If these nutrients, such as vitamin B_{12}, do not get broken down, they are not available for absorption.

- Iron deficiency. This disorder may be caused by a lack of dietary iron, which usually occurs because a patient does not eat a balanced diet.

- Obesity. Despite being the result of consuming excessive calories, obese individuals are often malnourished. This may be due to consuming an unbalanced or unhealthy diet that is deficient in all appropriate vitamins and minerals.

LEARNING OBJECTIVE 14.3.2 Identify common disorders that are associated with malnutrition.

KEY TERMS

anemia Condition caused by not having sufficient numbers of red blood cells or enough hemoglobin to carry oxygen to all of the cells.

beriberi Disease caused by vitamin B_1 (thiamine) deficiency; causes inflammation of nerves (potentially damaging neurons permanently), heart disease, and swelling.

goiter Disease that causes a swelling of the thyroid gland (seen on the anterior of the neck), chronic fatigue, low metabolic rate, and weakness; caused by a deficient amount of iodine in the diet.

hyponatremia Condition characterized by abnormally low sodium levels in the blood (lower than 136 meq/L).

rickets Bone condition due to vitamin D deficiency during childhood that causes softening and malformation of bones.

scurvy Disease that causes soft gum tissue, loose teeth, bad breath, joint pain, weakness, and blood spots under the skin; caused by a vitamin C deficiency.

COMMON MALNUTRITION DISORDERS AND DISEASES

In some instances, malnutrition results in a patient not getting enough of a few certain types of nutrients. Deficiency in certain types of nutrients may lead to several different disorders.

- **Anemia.** This common disorder is caused by deficient levels of iron and vitamin B_{12}. Some symptoms of anemia may be chronic fatigue, shortness of breath, and a change in the color of someone's skin and tongue (Figure 14-10).

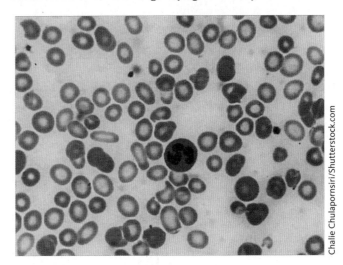

FIGURE 14-10 Blood smear of a patient with iron deficiency anemia. Notice that the RBCs have a white center due to a deficiency of iron containing hemoglobin.

- **Rickets.** This disease is caused when a person does not consume enough vitamin D during childhood. It prevents normal bone growth. The lack of vitamin D prevents the body from absorbing and depositing calcium. This means the body is unable to "grow" or lengthen bones normally (Figure 14-11). For more on this condition, review Chapter 4.

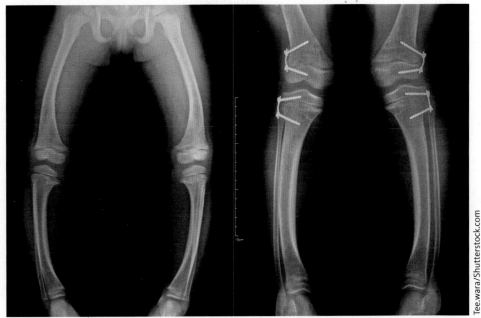

FIGURE 14-11 Child with rickets. Notice the characteristic bowing of the lower leg bones.

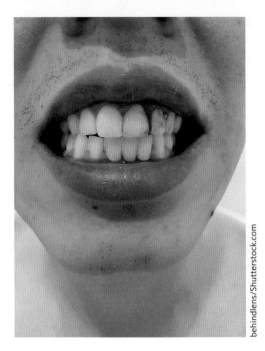

behindlens/Shutterstock.com

FIGURE 14-12 Gums of a patient with scurvy.

- **Scurvy.** This disease is caused by a deficiency of vitamin C. It is not very common in the United States, since vitamin C is widely available in our diet. After months of suboptimal vitamin C intake, a patient may experience soft gum tissue (Figure 14-12), loose teeth, bad breath, joint pain, weakness, and blood spots under the skin.

- **Beriberi.** This disease is caused by a vitamin B₁ deficiency. It causes inflammation of nerves (potentially damaging neurons permanently), heart disease, and swelling. This is common in countries where the diet primarily consists of boiled rice.

- **Hyponatremia.** A patient may be at risk for hyponatremia when they consume or do not absorb adequate amounts of sodium. This disease causes nausea, vomiting, confusion, and headache. It may also lead to convulsions and coma.

- **Goiter.** This is also sometimes referred to as an enlarged thyroid (Figure 14-13). The thyroid is the only place in the body that absorbs the trace element iodine. Thus, an iodine deficiency leads to swelling of the thyroid and altered thyroid function. This condition is common in countries that do not iodize their salt. Goiter may cause difficulty breathing, difficulty swallowing, and coughing.

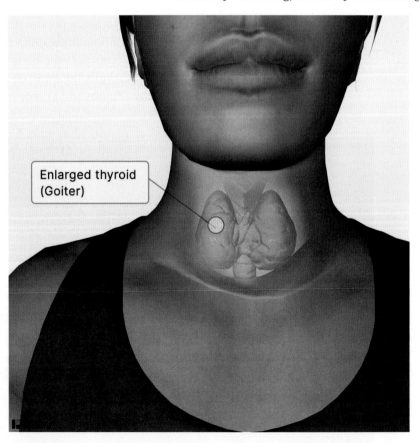

Enlarged thyroid (Goiter)

FIGURE 14-13 Enlarged thyroid, also known as a goiter.

LEARNING OBJECTIVE 14.3.3 Describe the relationship between obesity and common medical conditions.

KEY TERMS

gallbladder disease Several types of conditions that affect the flow of bile in your gallbladder including inflammation and excess fat.

gallstones An abnormal, small, hard mass that is formed in the gallbladder from bile components.

osteoarthritis Common form of arthritis that results in degeneration of joint cartilage and underlying bone.

sleep apnea Sleep disorder in which breathing repeatedly stops and starts.

stroke Occurs when blood flow (and therefore oxygen) to parts of the brain is blocked.

OBESITY'S EFFECT ON THE BODY

Obesity is the excessive accumulation of body fat. A person is generally considered obese if he or she has a body mass index (BMI) of 30 or higher (see Figure 14-4). It is usually the result of an individual consuming more calories than the body can use and the excess calories get stored as fat (adipose tissue). However, certain metabolic conditions may also contribute to obesity.

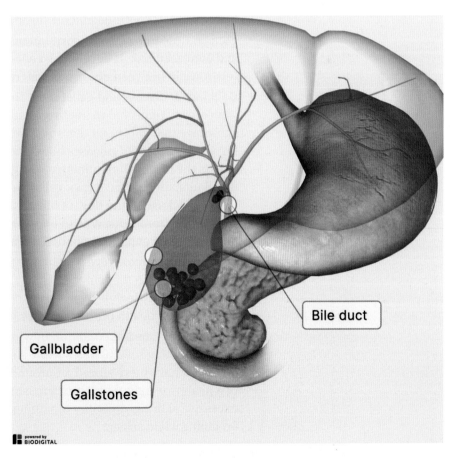

Bile duct

Gallbladder

Gallstones

powered by
BIODIGITAL

FIGURE 14-14 Inflamed gallbladder with gallstones.

Obesity increases one's risk for many diseases and may complicate recovery from certain diseases and medical procedures:

- Cardiovascular disease and **stroke**. In obese patients who consume unhealthy diets (diets high in cholesterol and fats), there is an increased risk of cardiovascular disease and stroke. These disorders are commonly due to narrowing and hardening of artery walls. This is caused by an accumulation of cholesterol in the arteries. Accumulation of cholesterol occurs when excessive amounts of cholesterol-rich foods are consumed. This decreases a person's ability to pump blood throughout their body, often preventing the heart and brain from getting the oxygen they need. Obese individuals tend to suffer from high blood pressure, high cholesterol, and high blood sugar. All of these problems increase the risk of heart disease and stroke.

- Hypertension. In obese individuals, the heart has to pump harder to supply blood to all of the cells in the body. Excess fat accumulated in the body may also cause kidney damage and decreased kidney function. Since the kidneys help regulate blood pressure, this may cause a person's blood pressure to be chronically high.

- Diabetes mellitus. Type 2 diabetes (Figure 14-18) may be genetically inherited, but it is also related to a person's weight. Patients with excess weight, low exercise levels, and a poor diet may be prone to developing this condition, which is characterized by high and uncontrolled blood sugar levels.

- Cancer. Research shows a correlation between increased weight and increased risk of developing cancer. It is unknown the exact relationship between obesity and increased cancer risk.

- **Gallbladder disease** and **gallstones**. The gallbladder (Figure 14-14) is an organ connected to the liver that stores bile, which is a substance that aids in fat digestion. When you eat meals containing fat, your gallbladder releases bile to help you digest it. Obesity affects the normal functioning of the gallbladder and may result in inflammation of the organ, gallstones, and gallbladder cancer due to blockage of the flow of bile. Excess fat may prevent the gallbladder from being able to empty properly, which results in the buildup of bile and the formation of gallstones.

- **Osteoarthritis**. Excessive weight due to obesity places extra pressure on the joints. This may lead to osteoarthritis (Figure 14-15), which is the wearing down of cartilage in the joints. This common health problem causes joint pain and stiffness.

- **Sleep apnea**. This is a condition in which a person temporarily stops breathing several times while sleeping at night. Those who are obese have more stored fat around their neck than a person of a healthy weight. This results in a smaller airway that causes excessive snoring, difficulty breathing, and temporary cessation of breathing while asleep.

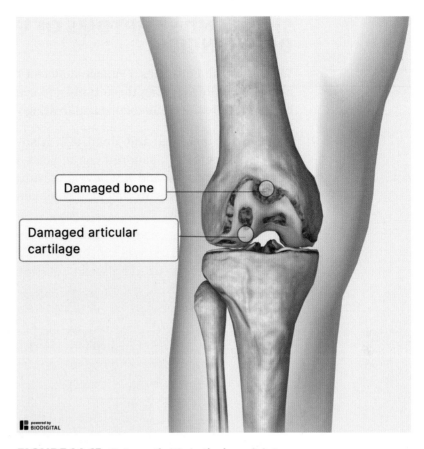

FIGURE 14-15 Osteoarthritis in the knee joint.

If there is a family history of any of these problems, it increases the risk that an obese individual will develop these conditions. Where the excess fat is stored on the body also influences which diseases an individual may develop. For example, individuals who are "apple-shaped" (carry most of his or her weight around the waist region) may be at higher risk than "pear-shaped" individuals (people who carry excess fat around the hip region) to develop these conditions. Recall the importance of the waist-to-hip-ratio discussed earlier (see Figure 14-6).

LEARNING OBJECTIVE **14.3.4** **Describe the causes, signs, and symptoms of vitamin deficiencies.**

KEY TERMS

Bitot's spots White growths on eye that result from the superficial buildup of keratin in the conjunctiva of the eye.

keratosis pilaris Red or white bumps on the skin that look like small goose bumps on the arms, thighs, buttocks, or cheeks; common in childhood (disappearing in adulthood) and tends to run in families.

seborrheic dermatitis Common skin condition that forms round, red, scaly patches and dandruff in areas where there are many sebaceous glands like the face, scalp, nose, and back.

SIGNS AND SYMPTOMS OF VITAMIN DEFICIENCIES

When a patient consumes a vitamin-deficient diet, several common symptoms may appear. Recognizing these signs and symptoms can help you assist the health care provider in detecting and treating vitamin deficiencies:

1. Scaly patches and dandruff. Also called **seborrheic dermatitis** (Figure 14-16), dandruff can indicate many common conditions. Low levels of zinc and low levels of vitamins B_2, B_3, and B_6 may cause this. Patients with this may complain of itching, but it may also be asymptomatic.

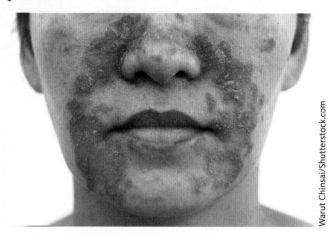

Warut Chinsai/Shutterstock.com

FIGURE 14-16 Seborrheic dermatitis of the face.

2. Bleeding gums. When due to nutritional factors, bleeding gums are usually the result of vitamin C deficiency (see Figure 14-12). Other common signs are easy bruising, dry scaly skin, frequent nosebleeds, and slow wound healing.

3. Cracks in the corners of the mouth or mouth ulcers (canker sores) (Figure 14-17). These may be caused by excessive salivation, dehydration, or insufficient amounts of B vitamins and iron. Mouth ulcers may also be the result of insufficient amounts of B vitamins and iron.

4. Poor night vision and white growths on the eyes (called **Bitot's spots**, which result from the superficial buildup of keratin in the conjunctiva of the eye). This is usually the result of a vitamin A deficiency and if left untreated can result in cornea damage and blindness.

5. Hair loss. This is also a common condition that is seen in people who are deficient in certain nutrients. It may be slowed or prevented by having sufficient dietary amounts of iron, zinc, essential fatty acids, vitamin B_3, and vitamin B_7.

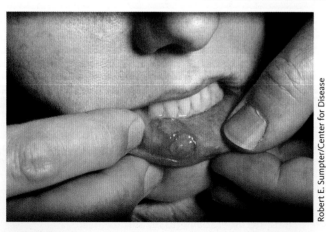

Robert E. Sumpter/Center for Disease Control (CDC) - PHIL

FIGURE 14-17 Mouth ulcers, also called canker sores.

6. Red or white bumps on the skin. These are called keratosis pilaris (Figure 14-18) and look like small goose bumps on the arms, thighs, buttocks, or cheeks. It is common in childhood (disappearing in adulthood) and tends to run in families. The causes are not fully understood but they have been observed in individuals suffering from vitamin A and C deficiencies.

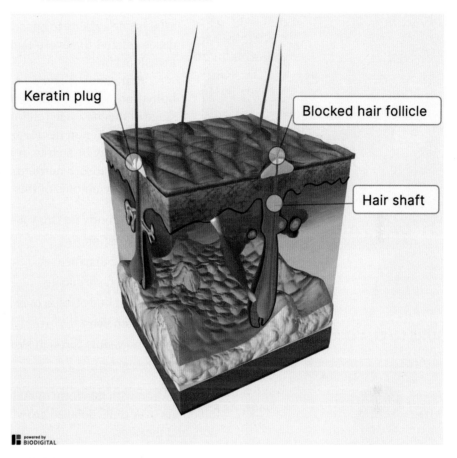

FIGURE 14-18 Keratosis pilaris.

7. Brittle hair and nails. This may be due to a biotin (vitamin B_7) deficiency. Biotin helps convert food into energy and may also cause muscle pain, cramps, tingling in hands and feet, and chronic fatigue.

See Figure Table 14-2 for more vitamin deficiencies, the associated disorder, and the signs and symptoms of each.

LEARNING OBJECTIVE 14.3.5 Describe the causes, signs, and symptoms of marasmus and kwashiorkor.

KEY TERMS

kwashiorkor Malnutrition disease, most commonly seen in young children, caused by a severe protein deficiency.

marasmus Disease of malnutrition, most commonly seen in infants and young children, caused by starvation.

MARASMUS AND KWASHIORKOR

Severe undernourishment and malnourishment in childhood or in times of famine may have short-term and long-lasting health effects. In addition to a lack of food, conditions related to malnourishment may also result from an eating disorder, taking medication that blocks the absorption of nutrients, or having a secondary medical condition that affects one's ability to absorb nutrients. Two common diseases related to severe malnutrition are marasmus and kwashiorkor.

Marasmus (Figure 14-19) is caused by severe carbohydrate and protein deficiency. It may occur at any stage of the life cycle (childhood to adulthood), but often affects children in developing countries where nutrient-rich food may be scarce. It may also occur in individuals who do not absorb nutrients normally. The most common signs and symptoms of this condition are as follows:

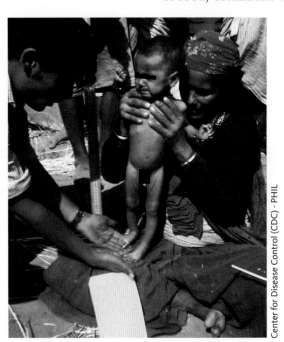

Center for Disease Control (CDC) - PHIL

FIGURE 14-19 A child with marasmus.

- Loss of body fat (may also be referred to as wasting)
- Dehydration
- Chronic diarrhea
- Stomach shrinkage
- Loss of body tissue over time
- Sunken eyes
- Bone visible through skin
- Dizziness

Children with this form of malnutrition may suffer repeated infections over time, delayed growth and development, hypotension, and measles.

Kwashiorkor (Figure 14-20) is a form of malnutrition that is caused by a severe protein deficiency. It is common in areas with food shortages and in places where the main source of food is carbohydrates. In some instances, it is possible that a person consumes adequate calories, but those calories contain little to no protein. It is usually seen in older children (unlike marasmus, which typically develops in younger children). The signs and symptoms, due to a lack of plasma proteins from an overall protein-deficient diet are:

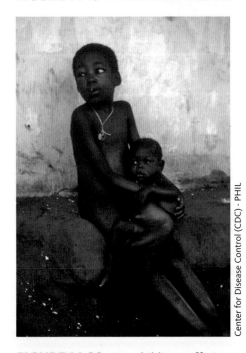

Center for Disease Control (CDC) - PHIL

FIGURE 14-20 Two children suffering from kwashiorkor.

- Fluid retention, especially in the ankles and feet
- Swollen appearance
- Bulging of the abdomen
- Inability to grow or gain weight
- Loss of hair and teeth

Chapter 15

The Renal System

Chapter Introduction

In this chapter we explore the anatomical structures and physiological mechanisms of the renal system. The renal system is involved in many different processes within the body, including the regulation of blood pressure and pH levels and the filtration of toxins and metabolic wastes. So, while the kidneys may not seem all that important, they actually serve a very vital and necessary role within the body.

UNIT OBJECTIVE 15.1

List the organs of the urinary system and their general function.

KEY TERMS

renal system Urinary system that consists of the kidneys, ureters, bladder, and urethra. The purpose of the renal system is to eliminate waste from the body, regulate blood volume and blood pressure, control levels of electrolytes and metabolites, and regulate blood pH.

urethra Canal that allows for the excretion of the urine from the urinary bladder. In males the urethra is also utilized by the reproductive system.

ureters Paired ducts that carry the urine that has been created by the kidneys to the inferior portion of the urinary bladder.

urinary bladder Membranous storage area that holds urine until it is released from the body through the urethra.

nephron One of the functional units of the kidney that filters the blood, selectively reabsorbs substances (such as glucose, ions, and amino acids), and excretes waste products, excess water, and salts in the form of urine.

UNIT INTRODUCTION

The **renal system** is comprised of a pair of kidneys where urine is created, a pair of **ureters** that transport the urine to the **urinary bladder**, the urinary bladder where urine is stored, and the **urethra** that transports urine from the urinary bladder to where it exits the body (Figure 15-1).

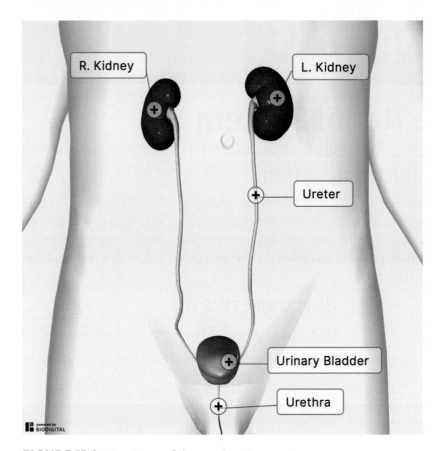

FIGURE 15-1 Structures of the renal system.

The overall function of the renal system is to filter the blood to remove toxins and waste products, as well as to maintain electrolyte, pH, and water volume homeostasis. The effect of the kidneys being unable to remove wastes or balance electrolyte and pH balance would have catastrophic consequences for the body. These consequences are evident in patients whose kidneys have failed and are now dependent on a machine to try and mimic the functions of a normal kidney. The functional unit of the kidney is known as a **nephron**. The nephrons located within the kidneys carry out all of the vital processes just mentioned, and without them the kidneys would be of no use to us.

LEARNING OBJECTIVE 15.1.1 **Identify the location of the kidneys.**

KEY TERM

retroperitoneal Situated behind the peritoneum.

ANATOMICAL LOCATION OF THE KIDNEYS

The kidneys are located in the **retroperitoneal** space along the spinal column and are partially covered by the rib cage (Figure 15-2). The left kidney is positioned about 1.5–2 cm higher than the right kidney due to the position of the renal arteries. This means that the left kidney is actually better protected by the rib cage than the kidney on the right. While the location of the kidneys may not seem important, the fact that they are in the retroperitoneal space means that any infection of the kidneys will not spread to other abdominal organs. Being covered by the rib cage and surrounded by a substantial amount of fat protects them from blunt trauma.

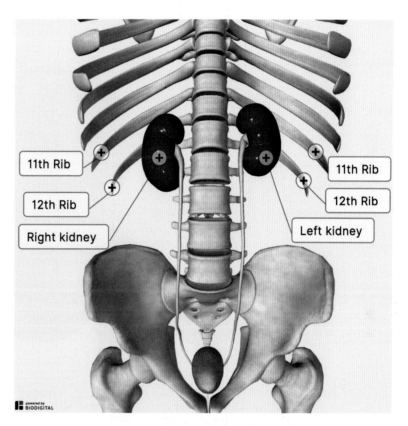

FIGURE 15-2 Anatomical location of the kidneys.

LEARNING OBJECTIVE **15.1.2** Identify the structure of the kidneys.

LEARNING OBJECTIVE **15.1.3** Describe the structure of the kidneys.

KEY TERMS

minor calyx Pathways within the kidney through which urine passes and is a portion of the urinary collecting system that drains one of the papillae. When several minor calyces merge they form a major calyx.

major calyx Portion of the urinary collecting system within the kidney that drains several minor calyces; all of the major calyces unite to form the renal pelvis.

renal capsule Tough, fibrous layer surrounding the kidney that is covered in a layer of perirenal fat.

renal cortex Outer region of the kidney found between the renal capsule and renal medulla. The renal columns that are found between the renal pyramids are extensions of the cortical tissue.

renal medulla Inner region of the kidney that contains 8–12 renal pyramids that empty into the calyx.

renal pelvis Funnel-shaped structure in each kidney that is formed by the convergence of the major calyxes and empties into the ureter.

renal pyramids Any of the somewhat triangular- or wedge-shaped masses of tissue found within the renal medulla that have a striated appearance due to the presence of collecting tubules and collecting ducts.

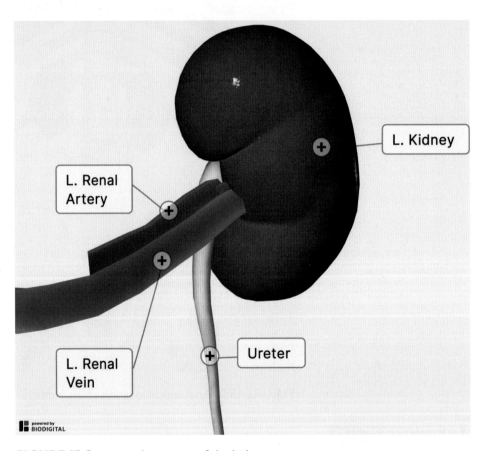

FIGURE 15-3 External anatomy of the kidney.

EXTERNAL STRUCTURE OF THE KIDNEY

The kidney is reddish-brown in color, bean shaped, and about 12 cm in length. While most diagrams show the kidney as having one renal vein, one renal artery, and one ureter, many times a kidney will actually have more than one of these structures (Figure 15-3). The outermost layer of the kidney is the **renal capsule** and is a fibrous structure that encloses and protects the kidney. It not only protects the kidney from damage or infection from the outside but also ensures that any infection of the kidney does not spread to other structures in the region.

INTERNAL STRUCTURE OF THE KIDNEY

Internally the kidney has many important structural characteristics. These structures are shown in Figure 15-4 and consist of:

- **Renal cortex**: Found immediately below the renal capsule and where most nephrons are located.
- **Renal medulla**: Layer below the renal cortex and where the renal pyramids are found; primarily composed of the nephron loops from the nephrons found in the renal cortex.
- **Renal pyramids**: Found within the renal medulla and formed by the vertical collecting ducts and nephron loops.

- Renal columns: Extensions of the renal cortex that extend downward between the renal pyramids.
- Nephron: Functional unit of the kidney that produces urine from the liquid filtered by the glomerulus; this liquid is funneled into the collecting duct, which it shares with neighboring nephrons.
- **Minor calyx**: Formed when a large number of collecting ducts come together.
- **Major calyx**: Formed when several minor calyxes join; empty the urine that is transported into the renal pelvis.
- **Renal pelvis**: Where the major calyxes drain, which then funnels the urine into the ureter.

Each of these structures has a very important role and damage to any of them will greatly alter how well the kidney functions.

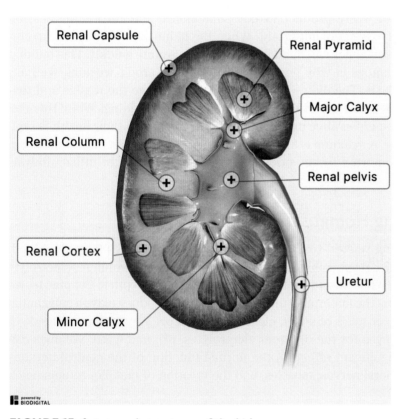

FIGURE 15-4 Internal structures of the kidney.

Labels: Renal Capsule, Renal Pyramid, Major Calyx, Renal Column, Renal pelvis, Renal Cortex, Uretur, Minor Calyx

powered by BIODIGITAL

LEARNING OBJECTIVE **15.1.4** **List the general functions of the kidney.**

KEY TERM

dialysis Medical procedure to remove wastes or toxins from the blood and adjust fluid and electrolyte levels using a semipermeable membrane.

GENERAL FUNCTIONS OF THE KIDNEY

The kidneys have two extremely important functions, which when they aren't performed or performed inadequately, leads to the improper functioning of the entire body. The first of these vital functions is the filtration of the blood and the removal of toxins, wastes, and medication metabolites. While the liver plays an important role in the detoxification of substances that enter the body through the gastrointestinal system, which includes some medications, many of the medications we take on a normal basis must be excreted through the kidneys. The other major function of the kidney is to maintain the homeostasis of body water composition, volume, and pH.

Removal of Wastes and Toxins

The removal of waste products, toxic substances, and certain medication metabolites is extremely important. When the kidney is not functioning correctly, these substances can build up to toxic levels quite quickly. This buildup of toxic substances is why people whose kidneys aren't working well are placed on **dialysis**. The dialysis machine tries to remove the wastes and toxins from the person's blood like the kidney should be doing. While this can often keep the person alive until a donor kidney is found, their health is typically very poor. A machine is a poor replacement for such an important organ and this is supported by the poor health of those forced to utilize dialysis machines.

Maintaining Homeostasis

Besides filtering wastes, toxins, and medication metabolites from the blood, the kidney is also responsible for the homeostasis of water volumes, electrolyte levels, and pH. While this information is covered in more depth in Chapter 16, we begin discussing the material in this chapter since the kidney plays a substantial role in the homeostasis of water, electrolytes, and pH. Any variance outside of the normal ranges for the different electrolytes, pH, and water volumes can have a very significant effect on the normal function of the central nervous system, peripheral nerves, muscles, and the creation of metalloproteins (such as hemoglobin).

LEARNING OBJECTIVE 15.1.5 Identify the general structure and function of the ureters.

KEY TERMS

renal calculi Calculus (kidney stone) located in the kidney, ureter, bladder, or urethra.

ureterorenal reflex Increasing peristaltic force within the ureter that attempts to force any blockage out of the ureter and into the urinary bladder; typically occurs in the presence of kidney stones.

STRUCTURE AND FUNCTION OF THE URETERS

The ureters are muscular tubes that transport urine from the renal pelvis to the inferior portion of the urinary bladder. The wall of the ureter contains three distinct layers, including from innermost to outermost the mucosa (transitional epithelium), the middle muscular layer, and the outer layer of fibrous connective tissue. While urine will often drain through the ureters due to gravity, they are also capable of creating rhythmic peristaltic waves to enhance the drainage of urine. In cases of blockage the ureters experience what is known as the **ureterorenal reflex**, which is a series of very strong peristaltic waves that try to force the blockage through the remainder of the ureter and into the urinary bladder. When this blockage is due to **renal calculi**, also known as kidney stones, strong peristaltic waves often cause intense pain and result in hematuria (blood in the urine).

LEARNING OBJECTIVE 15.1.6 Identify the general structure and function of the bladder and urethra.

KEY TERMS

detrusor muscle Outer, largely longitudinally arranged musculature of the bladder wall.

external urethral sphincter Muscle fibers that form a narrow ring of muscle around the urethra just distal to the prostate gland in males and in the female a ring of muscle more generally distributed around the urethra that controls the release of urine from the body.

internal urethral sphincter Involuntary muscle that controls the flow of urine by contracting around the internal urethral orifice; the sympathetic nervous system controls the opening and closing of the internal urethral sphincter.

micturition Act of urinating.

STRUCTURE AND FUNCTION OF THE URINARY BLADDER

The bladder functions as a urine storage container until the urine is released during **micturition** and exits the body through the urethra. The wall of the bladder has four distinct layers, which from innermost to outermost consist of a mucosal layer (transitional epithelium), submucosal layer, muscular layer, and fibrous layer. The longitudinal smooth muscle found in the muscular layer is known as the **detrusor muscle**, which contracts to both let us know that we need to urinate and to create pressure to assist in the excretion of urine.

STRUCTURE AND FUNCTION OF THE URETHRA

The purpose of the urethra is to convey urine from the urinary bladder to the external environment. In men, the urethra also plays a role in the reproductive system, as it also provides a passageway for sperm to exit the body during ejaculation.

The urethra is a muscular tube consisting of three layers, which from innermost to outermost consists of a mucosal layer, muscular layer, and outer connective tissue layer. The mucosal layer has many urethral glands that secrete mucous to help protect the urethra from the acidic nature of urine. The urethra has an **internal urethral sphincter** where the bladder and urethra join, along with an **external urethral sphincter** at the most distal portion of the urethra (Figure 15-5). The internal urethral sphincter is controlled autonomically, whereas the external urethral sphincter is controlled consciously. In women, the external urethral orifice is just anterior to the vaginal opening, while in men it is at the distal end on the penis. Females have a much shorter urethra than men do, which is one of the causes for higher rates of urinary tract infections in women than in men. The shorter the urinary tract, the easier it is for pathogens to travel up its length and cause infection.

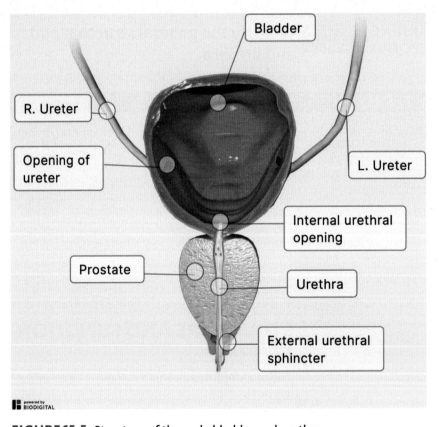

FIGURE 15-5 Structure of the male bladder and urethra.

LEARNING OBJECTIVE 15.1.7 Identify the blood vessels related to the kidney.

LEARNING OBJECTIVE 15.1.8 Trace the pathway of blood flow through the kidney.

KEY TERMS

afferent arteriole Small blood vessel in the kidney that supplies blood to glomeruli.

arcuate arteries Branches of the interlobar artery of the kidney that supply blood to the base of the pyramids.

arcuate vein Veins of the kidney that run along the arcuate arteries and receive blood from the interlobular veins, which is then emptied into the interlobar veins.

cortical radiate arteries Arteries connecting the arcuate arteries to the afferent arterioles.

cortical radiate vein Veins connecting the vasa recta and peritubular capillaries to the arcuate vein.

efferent arteriole Blood vessel that carries blood out of the glomerulus and toward the peritubular capillaries and vasa recta.

interlobar arteries Arteries leading from the renal artery to the smaller arcuate arteries within the kidney.

interlobar vein Veins leading from the arcuate veins within the kidney to the renal vein that exits the kidney.

glomerular capillaries Capillaries contained within Bowman's (glomerular) capsule that are the site of glomerular filtration.

peritubular capillaries A network of capillaries surrounding the renal tubules.

renal artery Arteries located in the abdominal cavity that supply the kidneys.

renal vein Veins carrying blood from the kidneys located in the abdominal cavity.

vasa recta Small blood vessels that arise from the efferent arteriole and play a role in the concentration of urine.

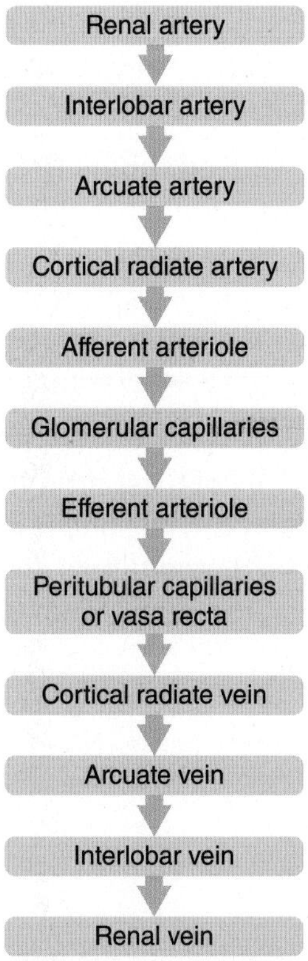

PATH OF BLOOD FLOW THROUGH THE KIDNEY

Renal artery
↓
Interlobar artery
↓
Arcuate artery
↓
Cortical radiate artery
↓
Afferent arteriole
↓
Glomerular capillaries
↓
Efferent arteriole
↓
Peritubular capillaries or vasa recta
↓
Cortical radiate vein
↓
Arcuate vein
↓
Interlobar vein
↓
Renal vein

FIGURE 15-6 Blood flow through the kidney.

If you take a look at Figure 15-6, you can trace the path of blood through the kidney as we discuss it here. The kidney receives arterial blood from the abdominal aorta through the renal artery. This blood then flows through the interlobar arteries, arcuate arteries, cortical radiate arteries, and into the afferent arteriole. From the afferent arteriole the blood flows into the glomerular capillaries (glomerulus) where it is filtered. The remaining blood moves from the glomerulus into the efferent arteriole, where it can either enter the peritubular capillaries or the capillaries of the vasa recta.

The kidney is one of the only areas in the body where blood will leave an arteriole to pass through a capillary bed, enter another arteriole, and then pass through a second capillary bed before it enters venous circulation. After the blood leaves the vasa recta or peritubular capillaries it enters the cortical radiate vein, followed by the arcuate vein, the interlobar vein, the renal vein, and finally the inferior vena cava.

LEARNING OBJECTIVE 15.1.9 Identify the structure of the nephron.

LEARNING OBJECTIVE 15.1.10 Identify the parts of the nephron.

LEARNING OBJECTIVE 15.1.11 Describe the parts of the nephron.

LEARNING OBJECTIVE 15.1.12 Identify the function of each part of the nephron.

LEARNING OBJECTIVE 15.1.13 Describe the function of each part of the nephron.

KEY TERMS

antidiuretic hormone (ADH) Also known as a vasopressin; hormone secreted by the posterior lobe of the pituitary gland or that increases blood pressure and decreases urine production.

Bowman's capsule Thin, membranous capsule that surrounds the glomerulus of a nephron through which glomerular filtrate passes to the proximal convoluted tubule. Also known as the glomerular capsule.

collecting duct Duct that receives and concentrates urine from the distal convoluted tubule of nephrons and empties into the minor calyxes.

distal convoluted tubule (DCT) Convoluted portion of the nephron between the loop of Henle and the collecting duct. Its function is to concentrate urine prior to its excretion.

renal corpuscle Part of a nephron that consists of Bowman's capsule with its included glomerulus.

glomerular capsule Thin, membranous capsule that surrounds the glomerulus of a nephron through which glomerular filtrate passes to the proximal convoluted tubule. Also known as Bowman's capsule.

glomerulus Ball of capillaries found within Bowman's capsule that is the site of glomerular filtration.

loop of Henle U-shaped part of a nephron that lies between the proximal and distal convoluted tubules that plays a role in water resorption; Also known as the nephron loop.

nephron loop U-shaped part of a nephron that lies between the proximal and distal convoluted tubules that plays a role in water resorption; Also known as the loop of Henle.

proximal convoluted tubule (PCT) Convoluted portion of the nephron that lies between Bowman's capsule and the loop of Henle; functions include resorption of glucose, electrolytes, and water from the glomerular filtrate. 70% of all tubular reabsorption occurs in the PCT.

renal tubule Part of a nephron that extends from the glomerular capsule and is composed of a proximal convoluted tubule, loop of Henle, and distal convoluted tubule and that empties into a collecting duct.

THE NEPHRON

The nephron is the functional structure of the kidney, meaning that all functions of the kidney are actually performed by the nephron. As we will see shortly, each portion of the nephron has a specific role that is vital to the normal functioning of the kidney.

The nephron is divided into two major parts, which are the renal corpuscle and renal tubule. The renal corpuscle consists of the ball of capillaries known as the glomerulus and the glomerular capsule, also known as **Bowman's capsule**, surrounding it (Figure 15-7). The second portion of the nephron is known as the **renal tubule** and consists of the proximal convoluted tubule, the nephron loop (loop of Henle), and the distal convoluted tubule. Even though the collecting duct often looks like it would be part of the nephron, it is shared by several nephrons and as such is not considered to be part of the nephron.

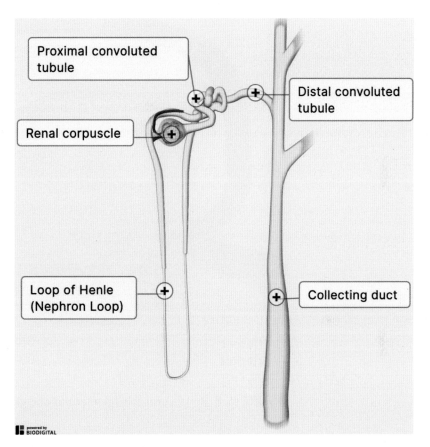

FIGURE 15-7 Structure of the nephron.

Glomerulus

The **glomerulus** is a ball of capillaries within the glomerular capsule where the filtration of blood takes place. The capillaries are surrounded by structures called podocytes, which squeeze the capillaries to increase hydrostatic pressure and forces liquid from the blood and into the glomerular capsule. This movement of fluid from the glomerular capillaries into the glomerular capsule is the act of filtration. The amount of fluid filter is directly proportional to the hydrostatic pressure. This means that when the hydrostatic pressure within the glomerular capillaries increases, the amount of fluid filtered from the capillaries will increase. This liquid that has been squeezed from the glomerular capillaries is now called filtrate. This filtrate has roughly the same composition as the interstitial fluid found around cells in our body's tissues.

Glomerular Capsule

The **glomerular capsule** surrounds the glomerulus, receives the liquid forced from the glomerular capillaries, and funnels the liquid into the renal tubule. Together, the glomerulus and glomerular capsule are known as the **renal corpuscle** (Figure 15-8).

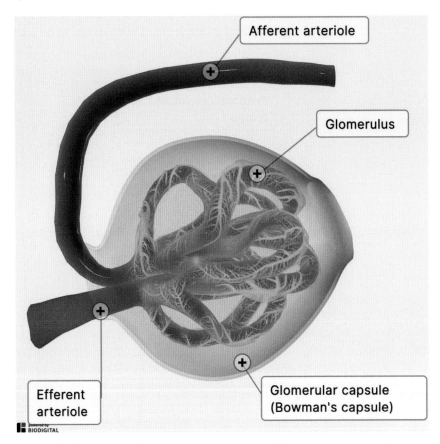

FIGURE 15-8 Renal corpuscle (glomerulus and glomerular capsule).

Proximal Convoluted Tubule

The first part of the renal tubule is known as the **proximal convoluted tubule (PCT)**. This segment of the tubule is named in this way because it is the closest and first portion of the tubule and because the tubule in convoluted, which means that it is not straight but loops around in all kinds of different ways. Of all of the substances to be reabsorbed through different portions of the renal tubule, 70% is reabsorbed in the PCT. This includes, for example, glucose, electrolytes, water, urea, amino acids, and vitamins.

Nephron Loop

The next structure in the pathway of filtrate through the renal tubule is the nephron loop. The **nephron loop**, which is also known as the **loop of Henle**, connects the proximal convoluted tubule to the distal convoluted tubule and its function is to concentrate the filtrate as it passes through. The area around the nephron loop has a salt gradient that pulls water out of the tubule, resulting in a very hypertonic filtrate by the time the fluid enters the distal convoluted tubule (Figure 15-9). The nephron loop is also the target of many diuretic medications, such as furosemide (Lasix) and bumetanide (Bumex). Loop diuretics, like the two just mentioned, work really well in patients with a reduced kidney function.

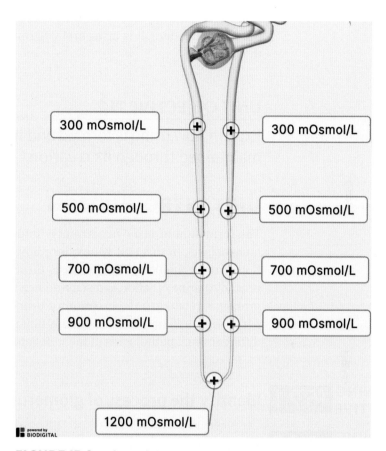

300 mOsmol/L ⊕ ⊕ 300 mOsmol/L

500 mOsmol/L ⊕ ⊕ 500 mOsmol/L

700 mOsmol/L ⊕ ⊕ 700 mOsmol/L

900 mOsmol/L ⊕ ⊕ 900 mOsmol/L

⊕

1200 mOsmol/L

powered by BIODIGITAL

FIGURE 15-9 Salt gradient surrounding the nephron loop.

Distal Convoluted Tubule

Following the nephron loop in the renal tubule is the **distal convoluted tubule (DCT)**, named because it is the last portion of the renal tubule and because it is so twisted. The DCT is the site of action for many diuretic medications, with one example being hydrochlorothiazide. The DCT, along with the collecting duct, are also the site of action for antidiuretic hormone. In the presence of **antidiuretic hormone (ADH)**, aquaporins form in the wall of the DCT and collecting duct, allowing a substantial amount of water to be reabsorbed. Unlike other areas of the renal tubule where water is reabsorbed as a result of sodium reabsorption, there is no sodium reabsorbed through the aquaporins, only pure water. This allows our body to significantly concentrate the urine to be excreted and save as much water as possible. This is especially important during times of decreased water intake when all of our body water needs to be conserved.

Collecting Duct

As we discussed earlier in this unit, the **collecting duct** is not part of the nephron, as it is shared between many different nephrons. The primary functions of the collecting duct are to help concentrate urine in the presence of antidiuretic hormone and to convey the newly created urine to the minor calyxes. Once the fluid has left the collecting duct it is no longer referred to as filtrate, as it cannot be altered in any way. No more fluid can be reabsorbed, no matter how bad your body needs the water and wants it back. Once the fluid leaves the collecting duct, it is urine and will remain in that form until excreted from the body.

UNIT OBJECTIVE 15.2

Explain how urine is formed and how homeostasis is maintained through its creation.

UNIT INTRODUCTION

The formation of urine is extremely important to the overall maintenance of homeostasis. In this unit we explore how urine is formed and how the formation of urine maintains homeostasis throughout the system. While pathologies related to urine creation is discussed in a later unit, it is important to know that problems related to the creation of urine can often have drastic effects on a person's overall health. As such, this unit provides the basis for exploring many different renal pathologies in the units ahead.

LEARNING OBJECTIVE 15.2.1 Identify the process of glomerular filtration.

LEARNING OBJECTIVE 15.2.2 Describe the process of glomerular filtration.

KEY TERMS

fenestrae Small openings in the glomerular capillaries between the pedicles of podocytes that allow for the movement of water and molecules.

glomerular filtration Process that the kidneys use to filter excess fluid and waste products out of the blood and into the nephron, so they may be eliminated from the body.

podocytes Cells with branching tentacle-shaped extensions that form the barrier through which blood is filtered in the glomerulus of the kidney.

tubular reabsorption Process by which the nephron removes water and solutes that are still needed from the tubular fluid and returns them to the blood.

tubular secretion Transfer of additional waste materials from peritubular capillaries to the glomerular filtrate found within the renal tubules.

THE CREATION OF URINE

As we discussed in the previous unit, the main function of nephrons is the filtering of blood and the creation of urine. The creation of urine is three-step process, consisting of glomerular filtration, tubular reabsorption, and tubular secretion. The liquid leaving the nephron after undergoing these three steps is what we refer to as urine. This urine we have created will contain excess water, waste, and electrolytes.

- **Glomerular filtration**: The process of forcing plasma (minus its proteins) from the glomerular capillaries and into the glomerular capsule. Once the liquid moves from the glomerular capillaries into the glomerular capsule, it is known as glomerular filtrate, or filtrate.

- **Tubular reabsorption**: The process of reabsorbing molecules that we need to remain in our bloodstream, such as nutrients, amino acids, certain electrolytes, and even certain waste products. This process also involves reabsorbing as much water as possible from the filtrate.

- **Tubular secretion**: This process involves removing certain molecules that the body needs to get rid of from the blood and secreting it directly into the nephron's filtrate in order to remove more than was originally filtered.

Here is an equation to sum these processes up.

Urine = Glomerular Filtrate + Tubular Secretion − Tubular Reabsorption

GLOMERULAR FILTRATION

Glomerular filtration is the first of three steps involved in the creation of urine and is the movement of water, electrolytes, nutrients, and wastes from the glomerular capillaries into the glomerular capsule. The movement of these substances into the glomerular capsule is due to the special structure of the glomerular capillaries and filtration pressure, both of which we discuss in more detail here.

Structure of Glomerular Capillaries

While all capillaries in the cardiovascular system allow some degree of filtration, the glomerular capillaries are created in a way to allow a much greater volume to be filtered than is possible in other capillaries. This difference between glomerular capillaries and other blood capillaries is due to the presence of **podocytes** and **fenestrae** on the glomerular capillaries (Figure 15-10). The addition of the podocyte and fenestrae increase the volume and rate at which the glomerular filtrate is produced, while still preventing the release of large proteins, such as plasma proteins, from leaving the capillaries and entering the capsular space.

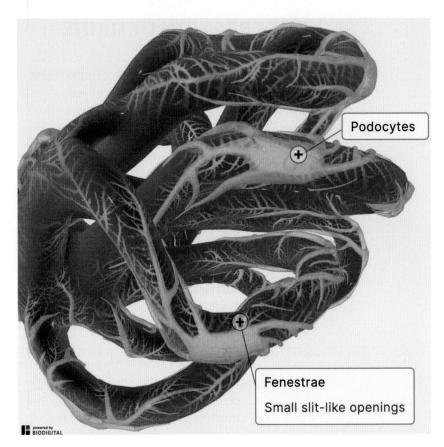

Podocytes

Fenestrae

Small slit-like openings

powered by
BIODIGITAL

FIGURE 15-10 Structure of the glomerular capillaries, showing the podocytes and fenestrae.

Fenestrae Fenestrae are small openings in the capillaries that allow plasma (minus the proteins) to leave the capillaries and enter the glomerular capsule (Figure 15-10). These openings are between the endothelial cells of the capillary, allowing fluids and molecules to pass through the wall of the capillary more easily. This structure allows for a much higher volume of plasma to leave the glomerular capillary through filtration than is normally able to move between the cells in capillaries normally. It is for this reason that glomerular capillaries are much more permeable than other capillaries.

Podocytes Podocytes are specialized structures that help control both the volume of liquid leaving the glomerular capillaries as well as making sure that plasma proteins remain in the bloodstream where they belong. The podocytes we are discussing have "feet" or pedicles that interdigitate with the pedicles of other podocytes. The very narrow spaces between the pedicles are controlled by a type of valve, very similar to your eyelids. When you want to see, you open both your top and bottom eyelids. When the podocytes want to increase the amount of liquid they are allowing through from the capillaries, the pedicles will move apart very slightly. When they want to reduce the amount of liquid leaving, they will move closer together. No matter how narrow or wide the space between the pedicles, plasma proteins will never be able to get through and into the glomerular capsule.

LEARNING OBJECTIVE 15.2.3 **Identify the composition of filtrate.**

LEARNING OBJECTIVE 15.2.4 **Describe the composition of filtrate.**

KEY TERM

pedicles Small projections originating from the podocytes that cover the glomerular capillaries. Their function is to limit the size of molecules passing from within the capillaries into the glomerular capsule.

Composition of Filtrate

The filtrate that accumulates in the glomerular capsule has the same constituents as blood plasma, with the exception of large proteins. While very small proteins are able to pass through the wall of the capillary and into the glomerular capsule to become part of the filtrate, large proteins such as albumin are too large to fit between the interwoven **pedicles** of the podocytes and remain in the blood. A list of the common constituents of filtrate is shown below.

- Water
- Electrolytes
  - Sodium (Na^+)
  - Potassium (K^+)
  - Calcium (Ca^{2+})
- Gases
  - Oxygen (O_2)
  - Carbon Dioxide (CO_2)
  - Nitrogen (N_2)
- Waste molecules
  - Urea
  - Creatinine
  - Uric Acid
- Nutrients
  - Vitamins
  - Glucose
- Amino acids
- Hydrogen ions (H^+)

While this is a general list of what is forced from the capillaries to become filtrate, many of the listed substances are either fully or partially reabsorbed into the bloodstream. This reabsorption includes not only nutrients and what we think of as useful products but also a certain amount of waste products.

LEARNING OBJECTIVE 15.2.5 Identify the factors affecting the rate of glomerular filtration.

LEARNING OBJECTIVE 15.2.6 Describe the factors affecting the rate of glomerular filtration.

KEY TERMS

capillary hydrostatic pressure Force of capillary fluids pushing against the wall of the capillary. Fluid movement is from within the capillary into the surrounding tissues; one of the forces favoring filtration.

capillary osmotic pressure Force of osmotic particles (proteins and electrolytes) within capillaries attempting to pull water into the capillary; one of the forces opposing filtration and capillary hydrostatic pressure.

capsular hydrostatic pressure Force of water within the glomerular capsule trying to push itself out of the glomerular capsule and into the glomerular capillaries; one of the forces opposing filtration and capsular osmotic pressure.

capsular osmotic pressure Force of osmotic particles (proteins and electrolytes) within the glomerular capsule trying to pull water into the capsule from the glomerular capillaries; one of the forces favoring filtration.

forces favoring filtration Forces favoring filtration that try to move water and molecules from within the glomerulus into the glomerular capsule; consist of capillary hydrostatic pressure and capsular osmotic pressure.

forces opposing filtration Forces opposing filtration that try to move water and molecules from within the glomerular capsule back into the glomerular capillaries; consist of capillary osmotic pressure and capsular hydrostatic pressure.

glomerular filtration pressure Net filtration force when the forces opposing filtration are subtracted from the forces favoring filtration; this number is almost always positive.

glomerular filtration rate Test used to check how well the kidneys are working; specifically, it estimates how much blood passes through the glomeruli each minute.

Glomerular Filtration Pressure

Glomerular filtration pressure is the way in which the liquid in the capillaries is forced through the fenestrae and between the pedicles of the podocytes. The stronger the filtration pressure, the greater the volume of filtrate created. The way in which we determine filtration pressure is shown below. This process can be seen in Figure 15-11.

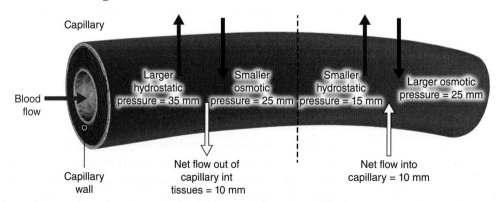

FIGURE 15-11 This process shows filtration and the creation of filtration pressure across the glomerular capillary.

Filtration Pressure = Forces Favoring Filtration − Forces Opposing Filtration

As such, forces trying to move liquid from the glomerular capillaries into the glomerular capsule would be **forces favoring filtration**, while forces trying to stop this movement would be **forces opposing filtration**. If you remember back to our discussion of the cardiovascular system in Chapter 9, typical blood capillaries will experience filtration on their arterial end due to high hydrostatic pressure and reabsorption on their venous end due to higher osmotic pressure. Glomerular capillaries are not the same due to the fenestrae and podocytes we discussed earlier, as they ensure that the forces favoring filtration are always higher than the forces opposing filtration. This prevents any movement of filtrate into the glomerular capillaries from the glomerular capsule. Below you can see the actual equation used for the calculation of filtration pressure.

Filtration Pressure = (Capillary Hydrostatic Pressure) − (Capillary Osmotic Pressure + Capsular Hydrostatic Pressure)

If you notice, the **capillary hydrostatic pressure** is really the only force favoring filtration, while the **capillary osmotic pressure** and **capsular hydrostatic pressure** are opposing filtration by trying to retain the blood plasma within the walls of the capillary. Normally, we would also add **capsular osmotic pressure** to the capillary hydrostatic pressure before subtracting the forces opposing filtration, but due to the lack of proteins in the glomerular capsule, the value is almost always negligible and we are going to ignore it.

Glomerular Filtration Rate

Glomerular filtration rate (GFR) is the rate at which the filtrate fluid is produced each minute, which is a direct result of the glomerular filtration pressure. The greater the glomerular filtration pressure, the greater the glomerular filtration rate. As we discussed, the net filtration pressure is the force favoring filtration minus the force opposing filtration. Often this results in a glomerular net filtration pressure equal to approximately 10 mmHg. This 10 mmHg of pressure is the driving force between the movement of plasma (minus the proteins) into the glomerular capsule.

The commonly accepted GFR is 125 mL/minute. This means that of the roughly 1,250 mL of blood that passes through the renal arteries every minute, 10% is forced through the walls of the glomerular capillaries and into the glomerular capsule to become filtrate. Over the course of the day the glomeruli produce roughly 180 liters of filtrate, meaning the entire volume of blood in our body is filtered 70 times a day.

Determining the Glomerular Filtration Rate The way in which we are able to estimate the glomerular filtration rate is through a renal clearance test. This test is commonly done in one of two ways. The first method is by using the creatinine clearance formula. Through a blood test we can measure a patient's creatinine level and then we measure the level of creatinine in the urine. We then divide the volume of creatinine secreted per hour by the blood concentration to determine the renal clearance. The creatinine clearance is typically around 100 mL/min and matches changes in the GFR very closely. While this test is convenient and accurate, it isn't perfect due to the fact that small amounts of creatinine are reabsorbed in the renal tubule. For this reason, physicians will at times order an inulin clearance test. Inulin is a carbohydrate from a plant root that is neither secreted or reabsorbed by the renal tubule, thus giving us an exact renal clearance amount. These patients are given intravenous inulin, their urine levels of inulin are tracked, and their blood insulin levels measured. As we did with creatinine clearance, we will divide the amount of inulin secreted in an hour by the blood inulin concentration to determine renal clearance.

Factors Affecting Glomerular Filtration Rate   There are many different factors that affect glomerular filtration rate. The rate of filtration can be impacted by a change in the size of the filtration area, hydrostatic pressure, renal plasma flow, afferent arteriolar resistance, or efferent arteriolar resistance. A decrease in glomerular filtration rate caused by the constriction in the afferent arterioles and a dilation of the efferent arterioles can imply a progression of underlying kidney disease or difficulties caused by dehydration or volume loss. In addition to this, a decreased blood volume can reduce glomerular filtration rate. An increase in glomerular filtration would then be caused by an increase in blood volume and/ or blood pressure.

LEARNING OBJECTIVE 15.2.7 Identify the methods by which glomerular filtration is controlled.

LEARNING OBJECTIVE 15.2.8 Describe the methods by which glomerular filtration is controlled.

KEY TERMS

aldosterone A steroid hormone produced by the adrenal cortex that helps regulate the salt and water balance in the body.

angiotensin I Physiologically inactive form of angiotensin that is created from angiotensinogen and can be converted by angiotensin-converting enzyme to the active form, angiotensin II.

angiotensin II Protein that can increase blood pressure by causing vasoconstriction, stimulates the release of aldosterone, and is the physiologically active form of angiotensin.

angiotensin-converting enzyme (ACE) Enzyme that converts angiotensin I to angiotensin II.

autoregulation Maintenance of a constant supply of blood to the kidney in spite of varying blood pressure.

juxtaglomerular apparatus A structure composed of juxtaglomerular cells and a macula densa that found near the glomerulus and controls the release of renin.

macula densa Group of modified epithelial cells in the distal convoluted tubule of the kidney that lie adjacent to the afferent arteriole just before it enters the glomerulus and control renin release by relaying information about the sodium concentration in the fluid passing through the convoluted tubule to the renin-producing juxtaglomerular cells of the afferent arteriole.

osmolarity Concentration of an osmotic solution, especially when measured in osmols or milliosmols per liter of solution.

renin Enzyme produced by the kidney that plays a major role in the release of angiotensin.

renin-angiotensin-aldosterone system Hormone system that regulates blood pressure and fluid and electrolyte balance, as well as systemic vascular resistance; acts as a signaling pathway and is responsible for regulating the body's blood pressure; stimulated by low blood pressure, the autonomic nervous system, or the release of renin by the kidneys.

Control of Glomerular Filtration Rate

Under normal circumstances, GFR is controlled by a combination of autoregulation, the renin-angiotensin-aldosterone system, and autonomic regulation. The purpose of these control mechanisms is to keep the filtration rate constant under normal circumstances. Without these control mechanisms in place, the body would lose its ability to closely control blood pressure, blood pH levels, compensation for blood loss, and other regulatory systems in place throughout our different organ systems. As you can see, controlling the glomerular filtration rate is of vital importance to many, if not all, of the organ systems functioning within our bodies.

Autoregulation Autoregulation involves the regulation or control of local blood flow through and around the glomerulus and the nephrons. This regulation of blood flow ensures that even in cases where there is a drop in blood pressure or changes in blood flow, there remains an adequate glomerular filtration rate. The pressure within the arterioles and capillaries, along with the degree of stretch experienced by the muscular layer of the arterioles, is monitored to detect changes in blood flow and blood pressure that will cause the filtration rate to increase or decrease. By monitoring these aspects, the smooth muscles in these arterioles are able to respond by contracting or dilating as necessary to retain an optimal filtration rate. Autoregulation is also important in responding to increases in systemic blood pressure as well as local changes. When the systemic blood pressure increases, the arterioles will be stretched and respond by constricting to prevent a large rise in glomerular filtration.

Renin-Angiotensin-Aldosterone System The renin-angiotensin-aldosterone system is a method of hormonal control over glomerular filtration rate. This system can at times be difficult for students to understand, so as we discuss it please review Figure 15-12, which is a diagram of this process. This system is initiated by the presence of hyperosmolar blood within the afferent arteriole. This is detected by the juxtaglomerular apparatus and macula densa, which together monitor the osmolarity of the blood and secrete renin in response to increases in osmolarity. Renin in return causes the creation of angiotensin I, which is converted to angiotensin II. This conversion is accomplished by angiotensin-converting enzyme (ACE), which is found within the tissues of the lungs. Once

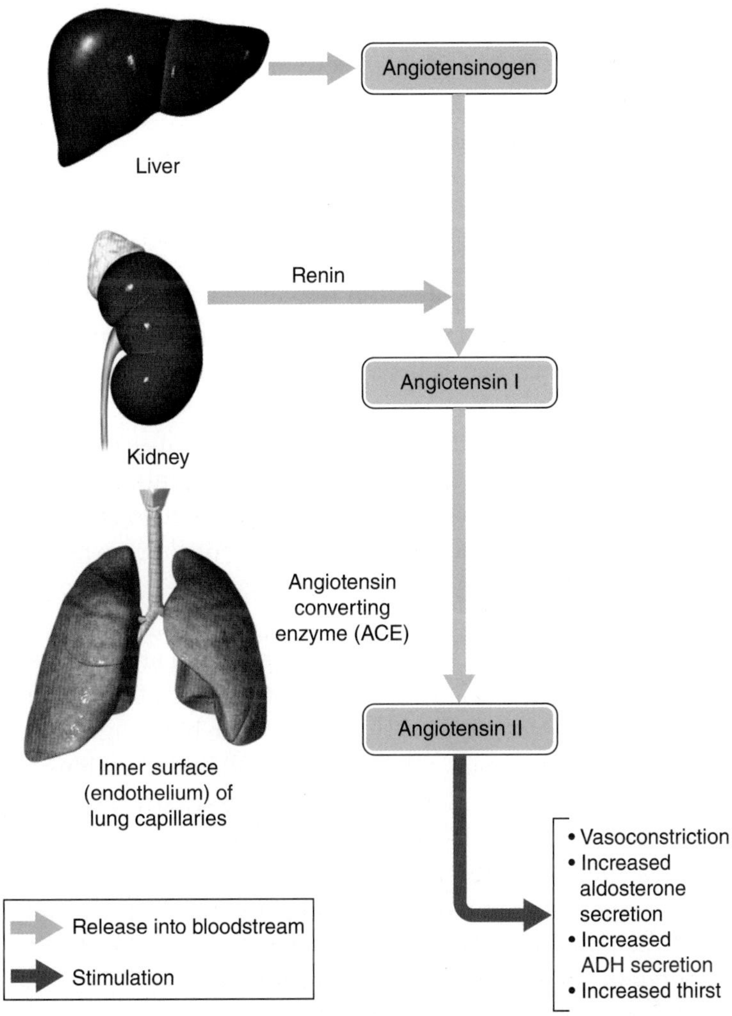

FIGURE 15-12 Progression of the renin-angiotensin-aldosterone system.

created, angiotensin II will stimulate the sympathetic nervous system to decrease glomerular filtration, while also causing the release of the hormone **aldosterone**. The presence of aldosterone causes the reabsorption of sodium, which as a result causes the reabsorption of significant amounts of water. This water is returned to the bloodstream where its presence helps to lower blood osmolarity. To assist in understanding this process, below is a numerical timeline for the progression of the renin-angiotensin-aldosterone system.

1. The juxtaglomerular apparatus and macula densa detect an increased osmolarity of blood within the afferent arteriole.
2. As a result, the juxtaglomerular apparatus creates and secretes the hormone renin into the bloodstream.
3. The presence of renin in the blood signals the need for angiotensin I to be secreted into the blood.
4. As the blood passes through the tissue of the lungs, it is converted to angiotensin II by angiotensin-converting enzyme.
5. Angiotensin II stimulates the sympathetic nervous system to decrease the glomerular filtration rate to retain water within the blood, while also stimulating the release of the hormone aldosterone.
6. Aldosterone increases the reabsorption of sodium by the renal tubule.
7. This increased reabsorption of sodium increases the reabsorption of water from the renal tubule by osmosis.
8. This reabsorbed water enters the bloodstream and assists in reducing the osmolarity of the blood.

Autonomic Regulation The glomerular filtration rate can also be controlled by the autonomic nervous system. Most of the autonomic innervation to the kidneys consists mainly of postganglionic sympathetic fibers. These sympathetic nerve fibers have extensive control over the afferent arteriole entering the glomerulus. When needed, the sympathetic nervous system can cause powerful vasoconstriction of these arterioles. This vasoconstriction will greatly decrease the blood flow to the glomerulus, which results in a drastic decrease in the glomerular filtration rate. While this may sound unhealthy or detrimental to the body, in times of significant physiological stress, this response can save our lives.

Take, for instance, a person in a car accident who is bleeding profusely. As the person begins to lose blood, the heart rate will elevate to keep blood pressure up and maintain perfusion to vital organs. However, as the bleeding continues, the body has to choose which organs are most vital and must continue to receive the limited supply of blood. The skin, muscles, gastrointestinal system, and kidneys fall toward the bottom of the list of important organs. As such, this sympathetic innervation signals the afferent arterioles to vasoconstrict significantly, greatly reducing the amount of blood that is being filtered. This not only allows the body to keep the plasma fluids in the bloodstream, but also shunt the blood away from the kidneys and toward the heart and brain.

Sympathetic innervation of the afferent arterioles also has a significant impact during times of prolonged and strenuous exercise. This response to exercise can be so drastic that it can cause mild and temporary kidney damage.

LEARNING OBJECTIVE 15.2.9 Define tubular reabsorption.

LEARNING OBJECTIVE 15.2.10 Describe tubular reabsorption and its impact on urine formation.

KEY TERMS

active transport Movement of a molecule across a membrane that requires energy because the movement is going against its concentration gradient.

co-transport Coupled transport of chemical substances across a cell membrane in which the energy required to move a substance (such as glucose) against a concentration gradient or against electrical potential is provided by the movement of another substance (such as a sodium ion) along its gradient in concentration or electric potential.

diffusion Passive movement of substances from an area of high concentration to lower concentration until reaching equilibrium.

Osmosis Movement of water through a semipermeable membrane from an area of low osmolarity to an area of high osmolarity.

TUBULAR REABSORPTION

As we briefly discussed earlier in this unit, tubular reabsorption is the process by which needed molecules and water are absorbed from the filtrate back into the peritubular capillaries and vasa recta that surround the nephron. The purpose of this reabsorption is so that we don't lose the water, nutrients, and other molecules that we need to maintain the proper functioning of our bodies. So, to prevent disease and illness, the nephron is able to transport the necessary molecules back into the bloodstream where they are so critical.

Means of Tubular Reabsorption

Reabsorption in the nephron will either be a passive or active process, and the specific permeability of each part of the nephron varies considerably in terms of the amount and type of substance reabsorbed. With that being said, over 70% of all tubular reabsorption occurs in the proximal convoluted tubule. The way in which reabsorption occurs includes osmosis, diffusion, active transport, and co-transport.

- **Osmosis** is the movement of water from areas of lower osmolarity to areas of higher osmolarity. In the nephron, this is almost always the movement of water from within the renal tubule to the peritubular capillaries and vasa recta surrounding the nephron. The osmosis of water is often caused by the active transport of sodium ions in the proximal convoluted tubule, as sodium is an osmotic particle and water will follow sodium to areas of higher osmolarity.

- **Diffusion** is the movement of solutes from an area of high concentration to an area of low concentration, which can also be stated as they are moving down a concentration gradient.

Diffusion affects many substances moving through the renal tubule, but the most prevalent will be the movement of electrolytes.

- **Active transport** requires the use of energy in the form of ATP in order to move a molecule from within the renal tubule and place it back in the bloodstream. This process is required for such molecules as amino acids, glucose, creatine, lactic acid, uric acid, and some ions.
- **Co-transport** is the last method of tubular reabsorption and involves the movement of two or more electrolytes at the same time. Co-transport can either be in the form of symport, where the ions are both traveling in the same direction, or antiport, where the ions are traveling in opposite directions. Antiport is much more common in the renal tubule than symport and can be seen extensively with sodium and potassium traveling in opposite directions. Typically, whenever sodium is being reabsorbed, potassium is being excreted, and vice versa.

Impact of Tubular Reabsorption on Urine Formation

Tubular reabsorption is going to have a significant impact on the formation of urine and the concentration of the different substances typically found in urine. A good example of these changes involves glucose and hydrogen ions. Glucose is an essential molecule in our bodies for the production of energy but is small enough that it is filtered when blood goes through the glomerular capillaries. As such, the nephron is responsible for the movement of glucose from the renal tubule back to the blood supply. This normally isn't an issue and we shouldn't see glucose present in the urine. However, in cases where the nephron is damaged and can't reabsorb the glucose properly or when the level of glucose entering the nephron is too high for it all to be reabsorbed, we will find glucose in the urine.

Similarly, the pH of urine will change based on the body's need to excrete or reabsorb hydrogen ions. If the pH of body fluids begins to rise, there will be an increased reabsorption of hydrogen ions and the result will be a more alkaline urine. Conversely, during times where the pH of our body fluids is too low, more hydrogen will be secreted into the renal tubule and not reabsorbed, leading to a more acidic urine.

LEARNING OBJECTIVE 15.2.11 **Identify the changes in the concentration of osmotic particles as they flow through the renal tubule.**

LEARNING OBJECTIVE 15.2.12 **Explain the changes in the concentration of osmotic particles as they flow through the renal tubule.**

FILTRATE CONCENTRATION

As filtrate goes through the nephron, its ion concentration or osmolarity changes as the water and ions are reabsorbed (Figure 15-13). As filtrate enters the proximal convoluted tubule, the osmolarity is 300 mOsm/L. The osmolarity of the filtrate remains constant as it leaves the tubule. The osmolarity drops to 1200 mOsm/L as water is absorbed through the descending part of the loop of Henle. When the filtrate is ascending the loop of Henle, osmolarity goes to approximately100–200 mOsm/L. After it travels through the loop of Henle, the filtrate arrives in the distal convoluted tubule and collecting duct, where varying amounts of water and ions are reabsorbed based on hormonal stimuli. The ending osmolarity of urine is dependent on these final collecting ducts—all of which is regulated by homeostasis.

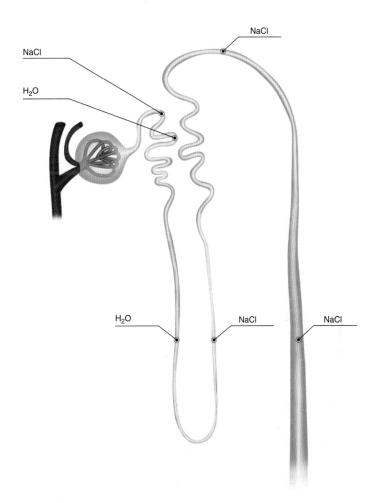

FIGURE 15-13 Movement of solutes along the renal tubule and the resulting changes in osmolarity.

LEARNING OBJECTIVE 15.2.13 Define tubular secretion.

LEARNING OBJECTIVE 15.2.14 Describe tubular secretion and its impact on urine formation.

TUBULAR SECRETION

As we stated previously, tubular secretion involves removing certain molecules that our body needs to get rid of from the blood and secreting it directly into the nephron's filtrate in order to remove more than was originally filtered. During secretion, substances will be removed from the blood through the peritubular capillaries to the renal tubular lumen and occurs by active transport and passive diffusion. Secreted substances can include hydrogen, creatinine, ions, and other substances that need to be removed from the body, such as medications and toxins.

Impact of Tubular Secretion on Urine Formation

Tubular secretion will have a direct impact on urine formation and the presence of certain substances within the urine. When a substance is secreted from the peritubular capillaries, its concentration within the blood is too high. As such, once secreted, this substance will not be reabsorbed and will be found in the urine. An example of how tubular secretion affects urine formation would be urine drug tests.

In a urine drug test, we are looking for the **metabolites** of commonly abused drugs in the person's urine. If they have used these drugs in recent days, the drug will still be breaking down into its metabolites and these metabolites will be filtered out of the blood by the kidneys through tubular secretion. Thus, the presence of the metabolite in the urine is an example of how tubular secretion can affect urine formation and would result in the drug test being positive. This is also the reason why those abusing drugs will drink copious amounts of water or take medications causing diuresis in an attempt to flush the metabolites out quicker so they don't test positive for the drug.

LEARNING OBJECTIVE **15.2.15** Identify how urine's final composition is a result of homeostatic mechanisms.

LEARNING OBJECTIVE **15.2.16** Discuss how urine's final composition is a result of homeostatic mechanisms.

COMPOSITION OF URINE

When urine exits the body, it mainly consists of water, with diluted amounts of substances. The substances that are secreted into the tubular fluid for removal from the body include potassium ions (K+), hydrogen ions (H+), ammonium ions (NH_4+), creatinine, urea, some hormones and drugs. When the presence of red blood cells, glucose, or protein is found, it is an indicator of an underlying medical condition.

Homeostatic Mechanisms Affecting Urine Composition

There are many different mechanisms that play a role, whether large or small, in the final composition of urine. As such, we discuss them in relation to their effects on glomerular filtration, tubular reabsorption, and tubular secretion. Any mechanism that plays a role in modulating filtration, reabsorption, or secretion is going to have a direct impact on the final composition of urine. This may result in a lower or higher osmolarity due to more or less water present, the presence of glucose due to changes in tubular reabsorption, or more uric acid present due to increased tubular secretion.

Mechanisms Affecting Glomerular Filtration One of the largest factors affecting glomerular filtration is the homeostatic mechanisms that regulate blood pressure. In cases where blood pressure is low due to injury or another pathology, there will be a decrease in the volume of blood filtered by the glomerulus. Moving water into the renal tubule would help to exacerbate the low blood pressure and as a result the volume of water filtered during these times is greatly decreased. In addition to less water being filtered, tubular reabsorption of water due to sodium reabsorption and the presence of antidiuretic hormone will be greatly increased. This will lead to a very concentrated urine that has a very high osmolarity.

Factors Affecting Tubular Reabsorption and Secretion Just like there are mechanisms that affect glomerular filtration, there are also homeostatic mechanisms that affect tubular reabsorption and secretion. These mechanisms are used often as one day the mechanism may require tubular reabsorption and the next day tubular secretion. We have used the regulation of pH as an example previously, so we use it again here. The mechanism that regulates pH and the amounts of hydrogen ion found in the bodily fluids may need hydrogen ions to be reabsorbed from the renal tubule today, but tomorrow there may be too much hydrogen in the bodily fluids and will cause it to undergo tubular secretion. So, the current level or concentration of a substance may cause the homeostatic mechanisms managing the substance to alternate between tubular reabsorption and tubular secretion.

UNIT OBJECTIVE 15.3

Describe the structures and functions of the urinary system organs responsible for the storage and elimination of urine.

UNIT INTRODUCTION

In addition to the kidneys and the nephrons within them creating the urine, the renal system is also composed of the structures required for the transportation, storage, and elimination of urine. The transportation of urine is the primary role of the ureters, the bladder is responsible for the storage of urine, and the urethra is responsible for the elimination of urine.

LEARNING OBJECTIVE **15.3.1** Identify the structure of the ureters.

LEARNING OBJECTIVE **15.3.2** Describe the structure of the ureters.

LEARNING OBJECTIVE **15.3.3** Identify the function of the ureters.

LEARNING OBJECTIVE **15.3.4** Describe the function of the ureters.

KEY TERMS

lithotripsy Breaking of a kidney stone (calculus) that is unable to pass using shock waves or crushing it with a surgical instrument into pieces small enough to pass through the ureters, bladder, and urethra to exit the body.

ureterorenal reflex Increasing peristaltic force within the ureter that attempts to force any blockage out of the ureter and into the urinary bladder; typically occurs in the presence of kidney stones.

STRUCTURE AND FUNCTION OF THE URETER

The ureters are a pair of long narrow ducts that carry urine from the kidneys to the urinary bladder (Figure 15-14). There is one ureter attached to each kidney and each ureter enters the inferior portion of the bladder on its posterior side. Together with the exit for the urethra, the entry of the ureters into the bladder form an area on the floor of the bladder known as the trigone.

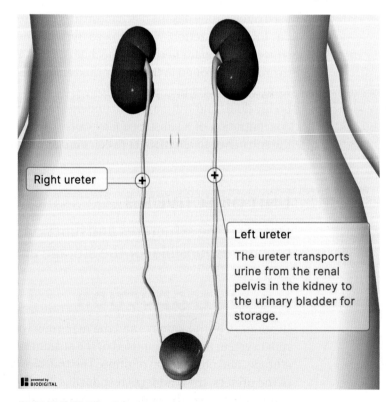

Right ureter ⊕

⊕ Left ureter

The ureter transports urine from the renal pelvis in the kidney to the urinary bladder for storage.

powered by
BIODIGITAL

FIGURE 15-14 The ureter.

The ureter is a long muscular tube around 25 cm in length that connects the renal pelvis of the kidney to the urinary bladder. Each kidney has its own ureter that conveys urine to the bladder, where it will be stored until release. The wall of the ureter is composed of three layers, consisting of an inner mucous coat in the form of transitional epithelium, a middle muscular coat, and an outer fibrous coat.

The function of the ureter is to transport the urine produced by the kidneys to where it is stored in the urinary bladder. Since the urinary bladder is inferior to the kidneys, the urine will be affected by gravity and flow downward passively. While the urine can flow passively, the ureter also exhibits peristalsis, which propels the urine downward more quickly and efficiently into the bladder. In cases of a renal calculus, also known as a "kidney stone," where the ureter is blocked and urine is unable to pass, the ureter will experience what is known as the **ureterorenal reflex**. This reflex causes increasingly powerful waves of peristalsis in an attempt to clear the blockage and allow urine to move freely again. These strong peristaltic waves often cause the prototypical pain associated with a kidney stone that radiates from the patient's flank toward the groin and comes in waves. These strong peristaltic waves also commonly cause the blood found in the urine, as the renal calculi are sharp and often lacerate the renal pelvis and ureter as they move through the structures. If the stones cannot be passed by the body's natural mechanisms, often the patient will require procedures such as **lithotripsy**, where the stones are broken up with intense sound waves projected through the affected area. This is very similar to an ultrasound, but at a much greater intensity, which often leaves bruises on the patient following the procedure.

LEARNING OBJECTIVE 15.3.5 Identify the structure of the urinary bladder.

LEARNING OBJECTIVE 15.3.6 Describe the structure of the urinary bladder.

LEARNING OBJECTIVE 15.3.7 Identify the function of the urinary bladder.

LEARNING OBJECTIVE 15.3.8 Describe the function of the urinary bladder.

KEY TERM

trigone Smooth triangular area on the inner surface of the bladder formed by the ureters entering the bladder and the urethra leaving the bladder.

STRUCTURE AND FUNCTION OF THE URINARY BLADDER

The urinary bladder is a hollow, distensible muscular organ that stores the urine created by the kidneys (Figure 15-15). The bladder is located within the pelvic cavity, posterior to the pubic symphysis and inferior to the parietal peritoneum.

Urine is transported from the kidneys to the urinary bladder by the ureters, which enter the bladder through the inferior portion of its posterior wall. The bladder then holds the urine until it is released to the external environment during the process of micturition, which is discussed in more depth shortly.

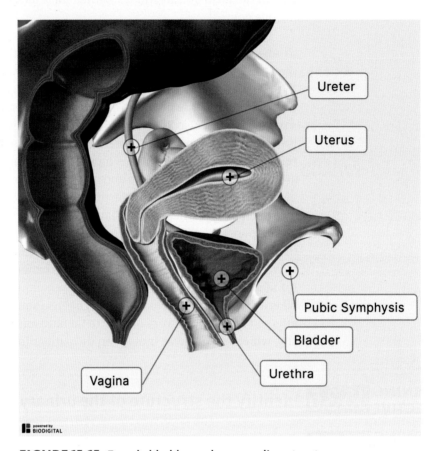

FIGURE 15-15 Female bladder and surrounding structures.

As stated previously, the urinary bladder is a hollow muscular organ and is shaped like a balloon or grapefruit. It sits in the center of the pelvis and is held in place by a combination of ligaments and the pelvic bones. In the female, the bladder contacts the anterior walls of the uterus and vagina, while in a male it rests posteriorly against the rectum. At the floor of the bladder is the **trigone**, a triangular-appearing area of tissue with a slightly different appearance than the rest of the wall of the bladder. The corners of the trigone are formed by the entrance of the two ureters and the exit of the urethra. The wall of the bladder has four layers, consisting of an innermost mucous coat that is transitional epithelium, the submucosal coat, the muscular coat that forms the detrusor muscle, and an outermost serous coat. The presence of transitional epithelium and elastic fibers within the wall of the bladder allow it to stretch as it fills with urine.

The urinary bladder stores urine that is transported by the ureters from the kidneys where it was produced. The urinary bladder stores the urine until enough urine accumulates within the bladder to alert the conscious mind of the need to release it from the body through the process of micturition (urination). When the volume of urine within the bladder reaches approximately

150 mL, stretch receptors begin to signal the need to micturate. This process is discussed in more detail later in this unit. A normal urinary bladder usually holds 300–350 mL of urine but can hold much larger volumes when required. The bladder should empty completely upon discharge and when this does not occur, the elasticity of the bladder has been compromised.

LEARNING OBJECTIVE 15.3.9 Identify the structure of the urethra.

LEARNING OBJECTIVE 15.3.10 Describe the structure of the urethra.

LEARNING OBJECTIVE 15.3.11 Identify the function of the urethra.

LEARNING OBJECTIVE 15.3.12 Describe the function of the urethra.

KEY TERMS

membranous urethra Part of the male urethra that is situated between the prostatic urethra and the penile urethra.

penile urethra Portion of the male urethra contained within the corpus spongiosum of the penis.

prostatic urethra Part of the male urethra that passes through the prostate gland.

STRUCTURE AND FUNCTION OF THE URETHRA

The urethra is a muscular tube between the urinary bladder and outside of the body that is responsible for facilitating the movement of urine from the urinary bladder to the external environment. The urethra has no action in the creation of urine, but it does assist in the storage and facilitates the elimination of urine. The storage function of the urethra is quite simple and entirely related to the action of the internal and external urethral sphincters, which prevents the urinary bladder from releasing its contents until the body is ready. The primary role of the urethra is related to the elimination of urine and is discussed in more detail shortly.

As stated previously, the urethra is a muscular tube that connects the urinary bladder to the outside environment and controls the flow of urine. The wall of the urethra consists of four layers: the inner mucous layer that consists of transitional epithelium, a submucosa that supports the mucosal layer, a muscular layer composed of thick longitudinal smooth muscle, and an outer connective tissue layer. The urethra has many mucous glands that are known as urethral glands.

While the anatomy of the wall of the urethra is the same for men and women, the remaining urethral anatomy is very different due to the male body's use of the urethra for both the urinary and reproductive systems.

The function of the urethra is very simply to transport urine from the bladder to the external environment. As part of this task, it also controls the release of urine from the bladder and body by means of the internal and external urethral sphincters. The internal urethral sphincter surrounds the neck of the bladder where the bladder and urethra join and is composed of smooth muscle. As this sphincter is composed of smooth muscle, it means it is controlled autonomically and will open when the nervous system decides that it is time to urinate. The sphincter that prevents us from urinating whenever our bladder is full like we did as a child is the external urethral sphincter. The external urethral sphincter is composed of skeletal muscle and thus is controlled consciously. When a child is being toilet-trained, the objective is for the brain to exert more of an influence over this sphincter and to be able to control its opening until the desired time. This process takes time, which is why children often wet the bed even after they are toilet-trained when awake. The brain needs to further enhance its control over the external urethral sphincter until it can keep the sphincter closed even while asleep and the conscious mind is at rest.

Female Urethra

The female urethra begins at the bottom of the bladder, which is also known as its neck, and extends downward through the muscular pelvic floor. Before urine passes out of the urethral opening, it must pass through the urethral sphincters. The urethral sphincters are muscular structures within the urethra that help to hold urine inside the body until a person is ready to urinate. The female urethra opens into the vestibule (discussed in more depth in chapter 17) and sits just anterior to the vaginal opening. The female urethra is significantly shorter than the male's, with the female urethra measuring approximately 4 cm in length, compared to the 19.5 cm of the male urethra. The short length of the female urethra leads to an increased risk for urinary tract infections for females, as pathogens have a much shorter distance to traverse in females than they do in males.

Male Urethra

The male urethra connects the urinary bladder to the penis where urine exits the penis through the urethral meatus (Figure 15-16). The male urethra acts as both a urinary duct to eliminate urine and as a conduit for semen and sperm to exit the body from the reproductive system during intercourse. The role of the urethra in the male reproductive system is discussed further in Chapter 17. The male urethra is comprised of three main segments, which consist of the prostatic urethra, membranous urethra, and penile urethra.

- The **prostatic urethra** is where the urethra and urinary bladder connect and is where the internal urethral sphincter resides. This section of the urethra runs through the male prostate gland, hence termed the *prostatic urethra*. This is also where the urethra and ejaculatory duct connect, allowing the male sex cells and semen a means of exiting the body.
- The **membranous urethra** begins where the prostatic urethra ends and passes through the urogenital diaphragm of the pelvic floor.

The urogenital diaphragm also forms the male external urethral sphincter, which is composed of skeletal muscle and can be consciously controlled. The bulbourethral gland, which provides lubrication for the head of the penis during sexual intercourse, connects to the membranous urethra.

- The **penile urethra** is the final portion of the male urethra. This section of the urethra begins where the corpus spongiosum of the penis begins to form the outer wall of the urethra and continues the length of the penis to where the urethra terminates at the external urethral orifice, located at the distal tip of the penis.

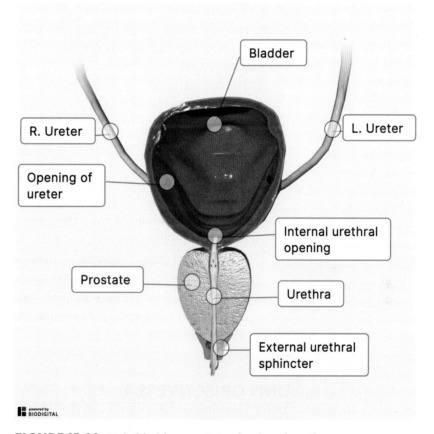

FIGURE 15-16 Male bladder, prostate gland, and urethra.

LEARNING OBJECTIVE 15.3.13 Identify the process of micturition.

LEARNING OBJECTIVE 15.3.14 Explain the process of micturition and how it is controlled.

KEY TERM

micturition Act of urinating.

MICTURITION

Micturition is the process of releasing urine stored within the bladder to the outside environment, often also referred to as urination. This process is one of the more complex processes that you will learn about, as it involves not only the autonomic nervous system but also the need for the conscious mind to realize that there is the need to release the stored urine. Thus, the action will require the autonomic nervous system, spinal reflexes, and the somatic nervous system. Below we walk through the process step by step and try to make it as easy to understand as possible.

Below are the steps involved in the process of micturition.

1. Urinary bladder distends as it fills with urine.
2. Stretch receptors in the bladder wall are stimulated at a volume of around 150 mL, and they signal the micturition center in the sacral spinal cord.
3. Parasympathetic nerve impulses travel to the detrusor muscle, which responds by contracting rhythmically.
4. The need to urinate is perceived by the conscious mind.
5. Voluntary contraction of the external urethral sphincter and inhibition of the micturition reflex by impulses from the brainstem and the cerebral cortex prevent urination.
6. Following the decision to urinate, the external urethral sphincter is relaxed, and impulses from the pons and the hypothalamus facilitate the micturition reflex.
7. The detrusor muscle contracts, the internal urethral sphincter relaxes, and urine is expelled through the urethra.
8. The micturition reflex subsides, the detrusor muscle relaxes, the internal urethral sphincter contracts, and the bladder begins to fill with urine again.

UNIT OBJECTIVE 15.4

Describe common pathologies affecting the organs of the urinary system.

UNIT INTRODUCTION

There are many different pathologies that affect the urinary system and do so in a variety of ways. They may affect the blood flow to the kidneys; alter the processes of filtration, reabsorption, and secretion; or interfere with the excretion of urine once created. In this unit we discuss a variety of different pathologies related to structural abnormalities of the urinary system, including their signs, symptoms, and diagnosis.

Identify common disorders affecting the organs of the urinary system.

Describe the following conditions: polycystic kidney disease, horseshoe kidney, and renal agenesis.

KEY TERMS

horseshoe kidney Congenital partial fusion of the kidneys resulting in a horseshoe shape.

polycystic kidney disease Hereditary disease characterized by gradually enlarging cysts within the kidney that lead to renal failure.

renal agenesis Failure of the body to develop part of the renal system while developing in the uterus. This most likely takes the form of a person only having one kidney instead of two.

COMMON DISORDERS AFFECTING RENAL SYSTEM ORGANS

There are many different conditions that affect the organs of the renal system. These include infections, cancers, congenital abnormalities, and structural changes to the organs due to injury or disease. When we think of infections, the most common are urinary tract infections (UTIs), infections of the bladder, and infections of the kidney. Cancer is also a common pathology affecting the renal system and will often necessitate the removal of the affected kidney. Lastly are congenital abnormalities and inherited disorders, with some of the more common ones being discussed in more detail below.

Polycystic Kidney Disease

Polycystic kidney disease (PKD) is a congenital disease that results in the spontaneous development of cysts throughout the structure of the kidneys (Figure 15-17). Polycystic kidney disease is one of the most common life-threatening inherited diseases worldwide and affects all races and ethnicities equally. There are two primary forms of PKD: autosomal dominant and autosomal recessive. The autosomal dominant form is primarily seen in adults who develop the condition, whereas autosomal recessive is primarily a childhood disease. Diagnosis and screening for the condition will consist of both genetic testing, as it is an inherited disease, along with the use of diagnostic imaging to look for the presence of cysts within the kidneys. This disease often leads to kidney failure and the need for the patient to be placed on dialysis. The only cure for this condition is a kidney transplant.

Horseshoe Kidney

Horseshoe kidney is the most common fusion anomaly affecting the kidneys and is a birth defect in which the kidneys are joined at the midline of the abdomen (Figure 15-18). They will either be fused at the superior or inferior poles of the kidneys, with fusion at the inferior pole being the most common and causing the resulting horseshoe shape. This condition does not typically affect the normal functioning of the kidneys and thus they are often left as is and not separated.

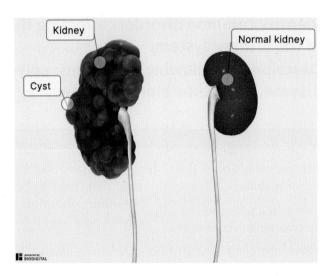

FIGURE 15-17 Pair of kidneys affected by polycystic kidney disease.

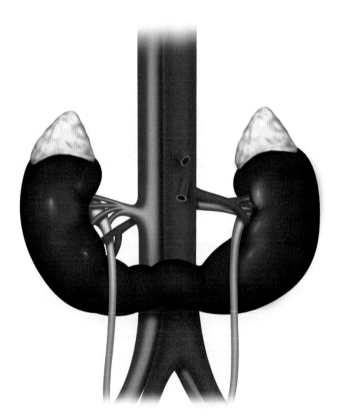

FIGURE 15-18 Fusion of the right and left kidney at their inferior pole.

Renal Agenesis

Renal agenesis is a condition in which one of the kidneys fails to form, leaving the affected person with only one kidney. Due to the body's ability to function just fine with only one kidney, many people who have this condition do not find out about it until an imaging study is done of the abdomen and only one kidney can be visualized. While the body is able to function normally with only one kidney, if the only kidney is damaged or begins to fail, there is no second kidney to assist the first. This will lead to the need for dialysis or a kidney transplant.

UNIT OBJECTIVE 15.5

Describe common pathologies related to the creation of urine.

UNIT INTRODUCTION

In this unit we explore some of the different pathologies that affect the creation of urine, including their signs, symptoms, and diagnosis. As we discussed in Unit 15.2, the creation of urine is extremely important to the overall homeostasis of the body. As such, these pathologies can cause issues not only within the kidney, but for the rest of the body as well.

LEARNING OBJECTIVE 15.5.1 Identify common pathologies related to the creation of urine.

PATHOLOGIES RELATING TO URINE CREATION

There are many different conditions that affect the creation of urine, with pathologies affecting all aspects of the process in a variety of ways. While the discussion of these pathologies could go on indefinitely, we focus on chronic kidney disease, acute renal failure, and diabetes insipidus.

Chronic kidney disease and acute renal failure share some similarities and also have some key differences. While both conditions result in the kidneys not functioning properly to filter the blood, acute renal failure has a rapid onset and is due to some form of damage to the kidney, while chronic kidney disease is the slow, progressive decline in kidney function that results in dialysis or a kidney transplant.

LEARNING OBJECTIVE 15.5.2 Describe the signs, symptoms, and diagnosis of chronic kidney disease.

LEARNING OBJECTIVE 15.5.3 Describe the signs, symptoms, and diagnosis of acute renal failure.

KEY TERMS

acute renal failure Occurs when the kidneys suddenly become unable to properly filter the blood and remove waste products.

azotemia Excess urea and other nitrogenous wastes in the blood as a result of kidney disease.

blood urea nitrogen (BUN) Concentration in the blood of nitrogen in the form of urea.

end-stage renal disease (ESRD) Final stage of kidney failure is characterized by the complete or nearly complete irreversible loss of renal function.

glomerulopathies Diseases that affect the structure and function of the renal glomeruli.

hypertensive nephrosclerosis Hardening of the walls of the small arteries and arterioles of the kidney that is caused by hypertension.

metabolic syndrome Syndrome consisting of the presence of three or more of a group of factors (such as high blood pressure, abdominal obesity, high triglyceride levels, low HDL levels, and high fasting levels of blood sugar) that are linked to increased risk of cardiovascular disease and type 2 diabetes.

nocturia The need to frequently urinate at night.

renal insufficiency Inability of kidney to function normally.

Chronic Kidney Disease

Chronic kidney disease is a long-standing, progressive deterioration in renal function (Figure 15-19). The most common cause of chronic kidney disease in the United States is diabetic neuropathy, which is closely followed by **hypertensive nephrosclerosis**, **glomerulopathies**, and **metabolic syndrome**. Chronic kidney disease starts as **renal insufficiency**, which then will often progress to renal failure and **end-stage renal disease (ESRD)**.

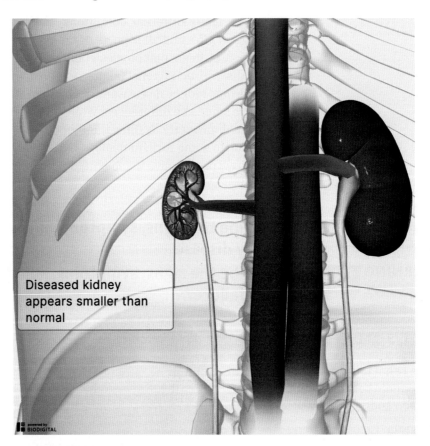

Diseased kidney appears smaller than normal

FIGURE 15-19 Small kidney typical of chronic kidney disease.

The five stages of renal disease are:

- Stage 1: Normal or high GFR (GFR > 90 mL/min)
- Stage 2: Mild CKD (GFR = 60–89 mL/min)
- Stage 3A: Moderate CKD (GFR = 45–59 mL/min)

- Stage 3B: Moderate CKD (GFR = 30–44 mL/min)
- Stage 4: Severe CKD (GFR = 15–29 mL/min)
- Stage 5: End Stage CKD (GFR < 15 mL/min)

Signs and Symptoms Signs and symptoms of chronic kidney disease include anorexia, nausea and vomiting, **nocturia**, fatigue, reduced mental acuity, muscle spasms, water retention, undernutrition, neuropathies, and seizures. These signs and symptoms are related to electrolyte imbalances, water imbalances, and the buildup of waste products in the blood. Many times, these signs and symptoms due not initially present, despite the patient having increased **blood urea nitrogen (BUN)** and fitting the criteria for renal insufficiency and the initial stages of renal failure.

Diagnosis To diagnose CKD, the following tests are typically performed.

- Blood tests: electrolytes, BUN, creatinine, phosphate, calcium, CBC
- Urinalysis (including urinary sediment examination)
- Quantitative urine protein (24-hour urine protein collection or spot urine protein to creatinine ratio)
- Ultrasonography of kidneys (often shows small kidneys)
- Renal biopsy (if required)

The most reliable evidence of CKD is decreased kidney function (estimated GFR of less than 60 mL/min) for greater than 3 months.

Acute Renal Failure

Acute renal failure is a rapid decrease in renal function over a couple days to a couple of weeks that leads to the accumulation of nitrogen products in the blood, which is called **azotemia**. If not treated quickly, fluid and electrolyte imbalances will develop and cause a myriad of other problems. The most serious fluid and electrolyte imbalances that may occur are hyperkalemia and fluid overload. Hyperkalemia can lead to cardiac dysrhythmias and disorders of the nervous system, while fluid overload can lead to pulmonary edema. The causes of acute renal failure are classified as either prerenal, renal, or postrenal. See Table 15-1 for more information on these classifications.

Table 15-1 Classifications of Acute Renal Failure

CAUSE	EXAMPLE
Prerenal	
ECF volume depletion	• Hemorrhage • Dehydration • Diabetes insipidus
Low cardiac output	• Heart failure • Cardiac tamponade • Myocardial infarction • Pulmonary embolism

CAUSE	EXAMPLE
Low systemic vascular resistance	• Anaphylactic shock • Septic shock • Antihypertensive medications
Vasoconstriction of afferent and glomerular arterioles	• Cyclosporine • Hypercalcemia • Nonsteroidal anti-inflammatory drugs (NSAIDs)
Renal	

Acute tubular injury	Ischemia
	• Vascular obstruction
	• Hemorrhage
	• Surgery
	• Medications
	   ◦ Amphotericin B
	   ◦ Cyclosporine
	   ◦ NSAIDs
	Toxins
	• Ethylene glycol
	• Heavy metals
	• Radiology contrast agents
	• Hemoglobin (as in hemoglobinuria)
	• Methotrexate

Acute glomerulonephritis	• Microscopic polyangiitis • Lupus

Acute tubulointerstitial nephritis	• Drug reactions
	   ◦ Beta-lactams (amoxicillin, penicillin, ampicillin)
	   ◦ NSAIDs
	   ◦ Sulfonamides
	   ◦ Ciprofloxacin
	   ◦ Thiazide diuretics
	   ◦ Furosemide
	   ◦ Cimetidine
	• Papillary necrosis
	• Pyelonephritis

Acute vascular nephropathy	• Atheroembolism • Malignant hypertension • Vasculitis
Infiltrative disease	• Leukemia • Lymphoma • Sarcoidosis
Postrenal	
Ureteral obstruction	Intrinsic • Calculi • Cancer • Clots • Congenital defects Extrinsic • Cancer • Retroperitoneal fibrosis • Ureteral trauma during surgery or high impact injury

CAUSE	EXAMPLE
Bladder obstruction	Mechanical • Benign prostatic hyperplasia (BPH) • Bladder cancer • Prostate cancer • Urethral valves Neurogenic • Anticholinergic drugs • Upper or lower motor neuron lesion

Signs and Symptoms The signs and symptoms of acute renal failure include:

• Anorexia
• Nausea
• Vomiting
• Weakness
• Muscle twitching
• Seizures
• Confusion
• Coma

Diagnosis The diagnosis of acute renal failure will include the following exams:

• Clinical evaluation, including review of prescription and over-the-counter drugs and exposure to iodinated IV contrast
• Serum creatinine
• Urinary sediment
• Urinalysis and assessment of urine protein
• Postvoid residual bladder volume if a postrenal cause is suspected

Acute renal failure is suspected when urine output falls or serum BUN and creatinine rise and is diagnosed when any one of the following are present:

• Increase in the serum creatine value of > 0.3 mg/dL in 48 hours
• Increase in serum creatine of > 1.5 times baseline within the prior seven days
• Urine volume of < 0.5 mL/kg/hour for six hours

LEARNING OBJECTIVE 15.5.4 Describe the causes, signs, symptoms, and diagnosis of diabetes insipidus.

KEY TERMS

diabetes insipidus Disorder of the pituitary gland that results in extremely low levels of ADH being produced causing intense thirst and the excretion of large amounts of dilute urine.

nephrogenic Originating in the kidney.

neurogenic Originating in the brain or spinal cord.

Diabetes Insipidus

Diabetes insipidus (DI) is a condition in which the kidneys produce very large amounts of dilute urine due to the lack of influence by antidiuretic hormone on the production of urine. This can either be in the form of **neurogenic** or **nephrogenic**. The difference between the two forms of the condition relates to whether antidiuretic hormone (ADH) is not produced by the pituitary gland (neurogenic) or whether it is produced but the kidneys are lacking receptors for it (nephrogenic).

Cause While the signs and symptoms of the two forms of DI are almost identical, the cause of the symptoms is very different. As stated above, neurogenic or central DI is caused by the pituitary gland not producing sufficient quantities of antidiuretic hormone. This could be a complete absence of ADH production or an insufficient quantity produced. Central DI can be caused by a genetic defect where the ADH gene on chromosome 20 is damaged or missing, causing the person to be unable to produce ADH. It can also be caused by damage to the hypothalamus or pituitary stalk from severe head trauma, tumors, granulomas, and other conditions affecting these structures. The development of central DI is often a sign of brain death in those who have experienced severe head trauma or a severe intracranial hemorrhage.

In patients with nephrogenic DI, while they produce sufficient quantities of ADH, their renal tubules and collecting ducts lack the necessary receptors to be signaled by the ADH. This leads to similar results as central DI, as not producing ADH will have essentially the same clinical presentation as having ADH and not knowing it is present. Nephrogenic DI can either be inherited (congenital) or acquired during a patient's lifetime. The congenital form is an X-linked trait that will severely affect men, but often has little effect on women due to the presence of a second X chromosome. Acquired nephrogenic DI is often the result of a previous disease the patient experienced, such as cancer, polycystic kidney disease, Sjögren syndrome, amyloidosis, or pyelonephritis.

Signs and Symptoms The hallmark sign of DI is the production of vast quantities of dilute urine, usually within the range of 3–20 liters a day. The kidneys normally produce about 2 liters of urine a day, so this is an increase of 50–1000% of normal. This will can lead to severe dehydration, hypernatremia, and death in those who are unable to consume or communicate their need (infants, older adults, those with a disability) to consume large amounts of water to replace the massive volume of water they are losing. Those that develop hypernatremia are also at risk of developing an altered mental status, coma, seizures, and death due to the significantly higher levels of sodium within the blood.

Diagnosis Diabetes insipidus is diagnosed through a combination of tests, including a 24-hour urine volume and osmolality test, serum electrolytes, and a water deprivation test. If the physician is thinking that the DI is nephrogenic in origin, they will often administer ADH to the patient via injection or intranasally and monitor urine output to determine if the urine volume decreases and the osmolarity increases. If the urine volume is relatively unchanged and the osmolarity only changes minimally, the patient is most likely experiencing nephrogenic DI. However, if urine volume decreases and osmolarity markedly changes, it is most likely central/neurogenic DI and ADH or a similar medication must be given regularly.

UNIT OBJECTIVE 15.6

Describe common disorders related to the storage and elimination of urine.

UNIT INTRODUCTION

There are many pathological conditions that affect the normal storage and elimination of urine from the body. These can be due to structural abnormalities, whether congenital or acquired, as well as physiological abnormalities. In this unit we discuss the pathologies that affect both the structures and physiological mechanisms related to the normal storage and elimination of urine.

LEARNING OBJECTIVE 15.6.1 Identify common disorders associated with the storage and elimination of urine.

KEY TERMS

urinary incontinence Inability of the body to control the release of urine from the bladder.

urinary retention Abnormal retaining of urine within the bladder despite attempting to urinate and empty the bladder.

DISORDERS ASSOCIATED WITH THE STORAGE AND ELIMINATION OF URINE

There are several different disorders related to urine storage and elimination, primarily affecting the urinary bladder and urethra. The most frequent conditions that affect storage and elimination of urine are urinary incontinence and urinary retention. While older adults suffer from these conditions on a much more frequent basis, there are many pathologies that can cause them in younger people as well.

LEARNING OBJECTIVE 15.6.2 Describe the causes, signs, symptoms, and diagnosis of urinary retention.

Urinary Retention

Urinary retention is the inability to fully release all of the urine stored in the bladder and is often a symptom of another condition, rather than the primary issue. This ranges in severity from a small amount of urine retained in the bladder following the patient urinating, to the complete inability to pass any urine. Thus, the condition can be more an annoyance to the patient or may actually be a medical emergency that needs prompt attention.

Causes There are many causes of urinary retention, including weakness of the detrusor muscle, damage to the nerves that signal the internal and external urethral sphincter to open, certain medications, and as a result of surgery on the bladder, urethra, or muscles of the pelvis floor. Urinary retention is very common after general anesthesia, due to the combination of opiate pain medications and anticholinergic medications used for nausea that are given during the procedure. The urinary retention usually disappears as the medications wear off in the hours following the procedure.

Diagnosis The diagnosis of urinary retention involves three steps: verifying urinary retention exists, determining the severity of the retention, and determining the underlying cause. Verifying that urinary retention exists is done through obtaining a patient history or the patient being unable to void while under medical care. To determine the severity of the retention, an ultrasound of the pelvis is often performed to visualize the bladder and get a rough measurement of the volume of urine within it. A urine volume over 400 mL is typical in cases of urinary retention and volumes over 900 mL can be seen as well. Determining the cause of urinary retention is often not very difficult, as the patient will have either just come out of anesthesia or will have a significant clue to the cause in the medical history. If the underlying cause for the retention cannot be resolved to alleviate the situation, the patient will often be catheterized using a Foley catheter or straight catheter to relieve the situation temporarily.

Chapter 16

Water, Electrolyte, and pH Homeostasis

Chapter Introduction

As we have learned throughout the previous chapters, maintaining homeostasis within the body is of extreme importance. In this chapter we will be specifically looking at the homeostasis of the body's water levels, electrolyte levels, and pH of the body fluids and tissues. If these elements fall out of balance, it can have drastic effects on the proper functioning of the entire body.

UNIT OBJECTIVE 16.1

Explain the importance of water and electrolyte balance.

UNIT INTRODUCTION

As we have seen throughout the study of the human body so far, it is a finely tuned but delicate machine. It is important to understand that even though this chapter is not discussing an organ system in particular, the physiology and processes we discuss are just as important as any organ system covered so far or yet to be discussed. The proper balance of water and electrolytes enables the proper functioning of every system in our bodies and even a small deviation from normal levels can cause catastrophic events. If there is too little water in the body, it will result in organ failure and death. If there is a level of potassium in the blood that is too high, it can be just as fatal. So, as we move through this chapter covering water, electrolyte, and water balance, don't forget their importance to the human body as a whole.

LEARNING OBJECTIVE	16.1.1	**Identify the water compartments present in the human body.**
LEARNING OBJECTIVE	16.1.2	**Describe the water compartments present in the human body.**

KEY TERMS

extracellular fluid (ECF) Fluid located outside of cells.

intracellular fluid (ICF) Fluid within the body that is contained within a cell.

transcellular fluid (TCF) Portion of extracellular fluid that is separated from other extracellular fluids by an epithelial membrane; examples are synovial fluid, the aqueous and vitreous humor of the eye, cerebrospinal fluid, and synovial fluid.

WATER CONTENT OF THE HUMAN BODY

As we know from Chapter 15, the body of an infant is approximately 75–78% water. While the amount of water present in our body decreases as we age, adults are still almost two-thirds water, with a total body water volume of 42 liters. It is important to understand though that this water is not homogenously spread throughout the body. Some organ systems in the body have a higher water content than others. For example, the muscles and kidneys are 79% water, while the bones are only 31% water. Because adult men have a larger proportion of muscle to adipose tissue than adult women do, men are typically 60% water and women are 55% water, Figure 16-1 illustrates the differences between the male body water content and the female body water content. The same concept holds true when comparing someone with a larger proportion of adipose tissue to someone with a normal amount of adipose tissue. The adipose tissue does not hold as much water as other structures, so the person with a normal amount of adipose tissue will have a higher proportion of water.

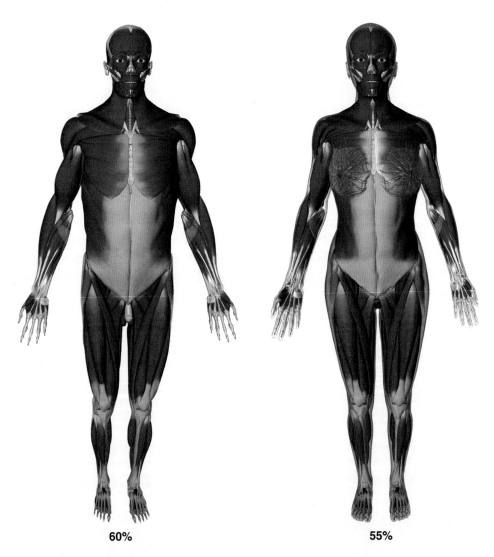

60%   55%

FIGURE 16-1 Proportion of water in both the male and female body.

WATER COMPARTMENTS OF THE BODY

Now that we have discussed the amount of water present in the body and factors that increase and decrease that amount, it is time to find out where that water is actually located. Within our bodies we have two large water compartments. The first water compartment contains the water located inside of our cells and is known as the **intracellular fluid (ICF)** compartment. The ICF contains the water stored within every cell in our bodies and accounts for about 65%, or two-thirds of the total water content.

The second water compartment in our bodies is known as the **extracellular fluid (ECF)** compartment. The ECF contains all of the rest of the water in the body that is not located within our cells and totals one-third of the total body water. Unlike the ICF, the extracellular fluid volume can be further broken down into more precise compartments. These compartments within the ECF consist of interstitial fluid, blood plasma, lymph fluid, and transcellular fluid. Each of the body water compartments can be seen in Table 16-1. As we learned in Chapter 8, blood plasma is the liquid portion of the blood and is composed of water, proteins, electrolytes, nutrients, and wastes. When the blood plasma is forced out of our capillaries by hydrostatic pressure, the fluid moves in the interstitial space and becomes interstitial fluid. Interstitial fluid is the fluid that bathes and surrounds the cells found in the tissues throughout the body. When interstitial fluid enters lymphatic capillaries for transport back to the circulatory system, the fluid becomes known as lymph fluid. Once the lymph fluid is emptied into the bloodstream, it resumes being called blood plasma. The last type of extracellular fluid is known as **transcellular fluid (TCF)**. Transcellular fluid is fluid that is separated from other extracellular fluids by a layer of epithelium and consists of the aqueous humor in the eye, synovial fluid, and cerebrospinal fluid.

Table 16-1 **Extracellular and Intracellular Water Compartments; The Extracellular Compartment is then Further Split between Blood Plasma, Interstitial Fluid, Lymph Fluid, and Transcellular Fluid**

TOTAL BODY WATER				
Intracellular fluid (28 L or 65%)	Extracellular fluid (14 L or 35%)			
	Interstitial fluid (25%)	Blood plasma (7%)	Lymph fluid (2%)	Transcellular fluid (1%)

LEARNING OBJECTIVE 16.1.3 **Explain how the composition of fluids varies between compartments.**

KEY TERMS

albumin Plasma protein found in the blood that creates and maintains blood's colloid osmotic pressure.

ions Chemical compound possessing an overall charge that is less than or greater than zero.

DIFFERENCES IN THE COMPOSITION OF FLUIDS BETWEEN WATER COMPARTMENTS

It may be easy to assume that the composition of fluids in the body is the same whether it is in the intracellular compartment or the extracellular compartment, but that assumption would be incorrect. While the fluid in both compartments is almost entirely made up of water, there are important differences between the molecules and electrolytes present in the fluid of each compartment. It is these differences that make such physiological actions like resting membrane potential, cardiac conduction, and nerve impulse transmission possible.

Composition of Water in the Extracellular Compartment

The fluid making up the extracellular compartment can vary greatly depending on which part of the extracellular compartment we are talking about. For example, blood plasma is going to have high concentrations of the protein **albumin** to assist in maintaining the osmotic pressure required to keep the liquid inside the blood vessels where it belongs. If you compare blood plasma to another extracellular fluid known as interstitial fluid, you won't find the great quantities of albumin that was so prominent in the blood plasma. Interstitial fluid is also different from lymph fluid, in that lymph fluid will have high levels of lipids that are being transported away from the gastrointestinal tract. So even though blood plasma is forced out of our capillaries to become interstitial fluid and interstitial fluid is absorbed into lymphatic capillaries to become lymph fluid, there are some components of extracellular fluid that are different depending on their specific location.

Even though there are differences between the compositions of different extracellular fluids, there are some aspects that are almost identical no matter which area of the extracellular compartment you are looking at. Probably the most important aspect of the fluid in the extracellular compartment to remember is which electrolytes are found in relative abundance. The reason these are so important is that they and the electrolytes of the intracellular compartment are what control the resulting membrane potential, cellular depolarization, and cellular repolarization. In the extracellular compartment the most abundant electrolytes are sodium (Na^+), chloride (Cl^-), calcium (Ca^{2+}), and bicarbonate (HCO_3^-) **ions**. High concentrations of positive sodium and calcium ions give the outside of the cell membrane a slight positive charge.

Composition of Water in the Intracellular Compartment

The composition of the fluid within our cells contains the electrolytes, proteins, and sugar molecules that are necessary for the proper functioning of a cell. While the intracellular fluid composition may change slightly from one cell type to the next, most aspects of the fluid composition are the same no matter which cell type you are studying. Just like with the extracellular fluid we just discussed, one of the most important components of the intracellular fluid is the electrolyte concentrations. Within the cell the most abundant electrolytes are potassium (K^+), magnesium (Mg^{2+}), phosphate (PO_4^{3-}), and sulfate (SO_4^{2-}) ions. The relative differences between intracellular electrolyte concentrations and extracellular concentrations can be seen in Figure 16-2. Even though there are positive ions within the cell, the number of positively charged ions inside the cell is much less than the number of positively charged ions outside of the cell. This disparity between the number of positively charged ions outside the cell versus the number inside of the cell results in a slight negative charge to the inside of the cell membrane. The difference in charges between the outside and inside of the cell membrane makes depolarization and repolarization of the cell membrane possible.

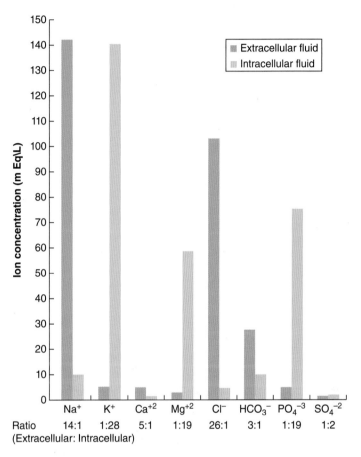

FIGURE 16-2 Comparing intracellular and extracellular electrolyte concentrations.

LEARNING OBJECTIVE **16.1.4** **Identify how fluids move between compartments based on physiological factors.**

LEARNING OBJECTIVE **16.1.5** **Describe how fluids move between compartments based on physiological factors.**

KEY TERMS

hydrostatic pressure Pressure of liquid pushing outward against the walls of its container. In the blood this would be the pressure of the liquid plasma pushing outward against the walls of the blood vessel.

osmotic pressure Pressure created by electrolytes and other osmotic molecules pulling water inward toward themselves; in the blood, the osmotic pressure is trying to pull liquid from the tissues into the blood vessels.

MOVEMENT OF WATER BETWEEN COMPARTMENTS

When we discuss the water compartments of the body it is easy to assume that they are static and there is no water movement between the intracellular and extracellular spaces. While it may seem this way, there is actually a constant movement of water between these spaces. Even though there is a constant movement of water between the intracellular and extracellular spaces, there is no net movement from one space to the other. This means that as the water moves between the spaces there is no change in the overall volume of either compartment. In instances where the body needs to cause a net movement of water, it has to rely on either hydrostatic pressure or osmotic pressure.

Hydrostatic Pressure

Hydrostatic pressure is the force created by the liquid pushing outward against the walls of the container or tube that it is in. For instance, let's imagine a garden hose with a small leak; the pressure that is forcing the water out of the small hole in the hose and up into the air is hydrostatic pressure. Just like the garden hose, hydrostatic force is due to the liquid portion of the blood that is contained within the arteries, veins, and capillaries exerting pressure against the walls of the blood vessels. The hydrostatic force found within the large arteries is also known as the blood pressure.

There are two ways in which the body can alter the naturally occurring hydrostatic forces within us. The body can either change the size of the container or the volume within the container. If the nervous system signals the arteries to contract and make the lumen of the vessel smaller, this is an example of changing the size of the container. If you were to measure the blood pressure, or hydrostatic pressure, following this change in blood vessel diameter you would find that the pressure has increased. The second way that the body is able to control hydrostatic pressure is by changing the volume. When the volume inside a container is really high, the pressure against the walls of the container is high as well. If we measured the pressure within the container as we slowly decrease the volume, we will see that as the volume decreases, the hydrostatic pressure within the container will decrease as well. For example, if you are getting a cup of water from a water dispenser with the jug on the top you will notice that when the jug is full the water coming out is more forceful and fills your cup quickly. If you were to come back later when the jug is almost empty you will notice that the flow of water isn't as strong and it takes longer to fill your cup.

Osmotic Pressure

The second type of pressure within the human body is osmotic pressure. **Osmotic pressure** is what we would consider to be a pulling pressure. This pressure is created by solid particles pulling water toward themselves. Examples of molecules that pull water toward themselves and thus increase osmotic pressure are electrolytes (e.g., sodium, potassium, and calcium), proteins such as albumin, and the sugar molecule glucose. While osmotic pressure is much weaker than the force of hydrostatic pressure, it is still important and drives many physiological processes. One example where we can really observe the effects of osmotic pressure is within our blood capillaries. At the arterial or beginning of the capillary, hydrostatic pressure forces a large volume of fluid out of the capillary. By the venous end of the capillary, the loss of fluid has greatly decreased the hydrostatic pressure, allowing the osmotic pressure that is pulling the fluid back into the capillary to become the dominant force. Despite the ability of osmotic pressure to pull some of the liquid back into the capillaries, it is not as strong as hydrostatic pressure and reabsorbs all of the water forced out. As a result, there is a net water loss of approximately 20–25% of the original volume of fluid over the length of the capillary. The fluid that is not reabsorbed by the capillary contributes to the volume of interstitial fluid until it absorbs into the lymphatic capillaries to be transported back to the bloodstream. We can see these four forces and their effects on the movement of water into and out of a blood capillary in Figure 16-3.

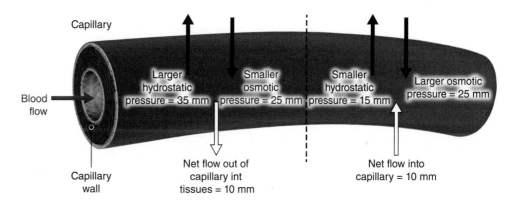

FIGURE 16-3 Four forces that affect water movement between the blood plasma and the interstitial fluid along the length of a capillary. These forces consist of capillary hydrostatic pressure, capillary osmotic pressure, interstitial hydrostatic pressure, and interstitial osmotic pressure.

LEARNING OBJECTIVE 16.1.6 List the routes that water uses to enter and exit the body.

MAINTAINING THE BALANCE OF WATER

As you have probably gathered from the information so far, the maintenance of the water balance in our bodies is very important. It only takes a small change in the intake or output of water to cause a disturbance in the normal functioning of the body. For that reason, it is important to know how water can enter the body and how it typically leaves the body.

Water Intake

The intake of water on a daily basis is extremely important and the lack of this water can quickly cause problems with several different systems within our bodies. This is the reason that the current health recommendations state a person should drink eight 8-oz. glasses of water each day in order to ensure our bodies get enough water to function properly. While 64 oz. of water each day can seem like a lot, this volume can also include, for example, soda, juice, coffee, and sports drinks. In addition to drinking fluids, we are also able to absorb the water contained in moist foods. Foods that are soft and moist will supply a small amount of water to our system when they are consumed, and while the volume of water supplied is small when compared to the volume obtained from drinking liquids, it is still an important contributor to our body's water content. The last route of water intake is the water created by biochemical reactions constantly occurring within the body. There are many reactions that occur in the body that create water as a by-product. An example of a water-producing reaction is the bicarbonate buffering system that we learned about in Chapter 15.

$$H_2O + CO_2 \longleftrightarrow H_2CO_3 \longleftrightarrow H^+ + HCO_3^-$$

As you can see, when this equation shifts to the left, it creates both a carbon dioxide molecule and a water molecule. Like the volume of water contributed to the system by moist foods, it's a small amount, but it is a factor that we need to remember. We can see the different means of water intake in Figure 16-4AB.

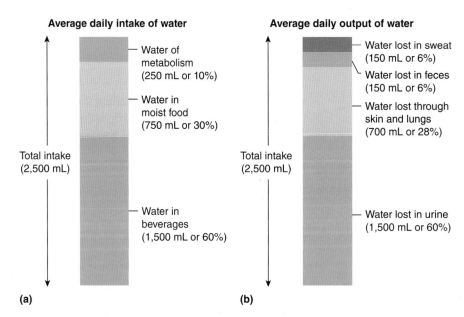

FIGURE 16-4AB Approximate volume and percentage of each form of daily water intake and each form of daily water output.

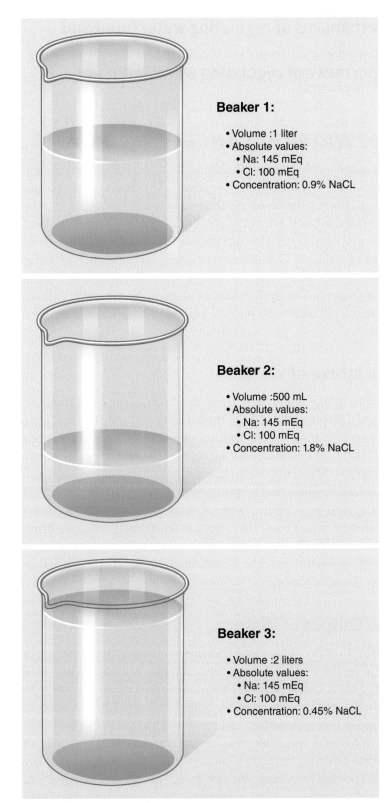

Beaker 1:

- Volume :1 liter
- Absolute values:
  - Na: 145 mEq
  - Cl: 100 mEq
- Concentration: 0.9% NaCL

Beaker 2:

- Volume :500 mL
- Absolute values:
  - Na: 145 mEq
  - Cl: 100 mEq
- Concentration: 1.8% NaCL

Beaker 3:

- Volume :2 liters
- Absolute values:
  - Na: 145 mEq
  - Cl: 100 mEq
- Concentration: 0.45% NaCL

FIGURE 16-5 Beaker 1 is normal electrolyte concentrations. The effects of dehydration (Beaker 2) and overhydration (Beaker 3) on the concentration of electrolytes in extracellular fluids.

Water Output

Just like there were a few different ways for water to enter the body, there are also a few different ways that water can leave the body. Some of these routes you may not have even considered when we start discussing them. The first route that the body uses to remove excess water is through the process of urination. The average adult should create around 30–40 mL of urine every hour, which is approximately 850 mL per day. While the average amount of urine created each day is 850 mL, normal urinary output differs from person to person. Some people may only create 500 mL per day, while others may produce up to 2 liters of urine each day. When examining a patient, it is important to remember that every person is different and just because they put out more or less urine than the adult average does not indicate that something is wrong with them. Always remember when examining patients, we always need to ask what their normal urinary output per day is.

The next way that water can leave the body is through the creation and defecation of feces. Despite the fact that feces are typically compacted and formed into a solid by the colon, they are still 85% water. So, in a healthy adult the amount of water that exits the body in the form of feces is significant. We can see the normal routes of water output illustrated in Figure 16-5. In someone with a type of infectious diarrhea, the amount of water lost can be extreme and life-threatening at times. Prior to the 1940s and 1950s, people with dysentery (infectious diarrhea) were in danger of dying due to a lack of antibiotics and intravenous fluids to treat the infection and keep the person hydrated. Because of the creation of antibiotics and intravenous fluids, most people in first-world countries will never need to worry about dying from infectious diarrhea.

Identify the mechanisms of regulating water input and output.

Explain the importance of regulating water input and output.

CONTROL OF WATER BALANCE HOMEOSTASIS

When we think of how the level of water is balanced between compartments and in the organism as a whole, it is important to recognize that the way in which it is controlled is through the regulation of the amount of water coming in and the amount of water leaving the body. When the amount of water entering our bodies is equal to the amount of water leaving our bodies, the water level throughout the body is in a state of balance. Conditions that cause an imbalance of water between compartments and in the body as a whole will also cause other organ systems to not work properly. The dysfunction of multiple systems will cause a much larger problem overall than most people would attribute to an imbalance of body water levels.

Regulating the Intake of Water

The regulation of water intake is almost entirely the result of the body monitoring the concentration of electrolytes and the modulation of thirst. The body has an amazing ability to monitor the concentration of electrolytes in body fluids and when the concentration or osmolality increases, the thirst center in the hypothalamus is triggered. When the thirst center is triggered, humans and animals alike experience a sensation that is interpreted as the need to drink. This thirst sensation is triggered by a 1% drop in total body water and the increased osmolality associated with water loss. This signal is terminated when we drink and water stretches our stomach, triggering stretch receptors that tell our hypothalamus that we have ingested water. The cessation of this signal is what makes us feel like we aren't thirsty anymore.

Regulating the Output of Water

The regulation of water output is just as important as the regulation of water intake. In order to keep the levels of water, electrolytes, and electrolyte concentration stable, the body controls how water leaves and when it leaves. As we discussed earlier, the main routes of water output consist of the creation of urine, the water found in feces, sweating, and the moisture lost through breathing. Our bodies have become quite adept at controlling the water content of feces and the creation of urine, primarily because it is unable to control the amount of water lost through breathing and sweating. The amount of water lost through breathing and sweating is often in response to the environment's heat and humidity. If the environment is humid and saturated with water, our bodies tend to lose less water through the process of respiration. On the other hand, if the air is very hot and dry, we will lose a larger volume of water through respiration. The same environmental concept typically holds true for the amount of water lost through sweating.

The amount of water lost through feces is controlled by the gastrointestinal system. When we ingest food and water it is transported through the alimentary canal. On its way through the alimentary canal there are many secretions added to the digested material and any nutrients present are primarily absorbed by the small intestine. Even after the small intestine has absorbed most of the nutrients, the digested material still has a large amount of water present. As the digested material enters the large intestine and travels through the colon, almost all of the water is absorbed through the walls of the colon. By the time it reaches the end of the colon almost all of the water has been absorbed. In cases where the colon has been irritated or the presence of increased parasympathetic stimulation causes the contents to pass through the colon too quickly, the result is often a watery diarrhea. Naturally, if the colon had less time to absorb the water and the feces were a watery diarrhea, the volume of water lost would be higher. There are also cases where the digested contents are slowed on their way through the colon and spend more time having the water absorbed. This situation will result in constipation due to the feces being overly dry and unable to move through the colon normally.

The last, and most significant form of water loss is through urination. Our kidneys are very adept at precisely controlling the amount of water lost through the process of creating and excreting urine. The amount of urine produced is going to vary based on a couple of different components. As we discussed earlier in the chapter and in Chapter 15, adults typically create 30–40 mL of urine each hour, or approximately 1 liter each day. While this is the average amount created, there are many situations that will result in a greater or lesser amount of urine created. If a person has ingested a much larger amount of water than normal that day, they will typically create more urine to help balance the amount of water present in the body. The opposite would occur in someone who has not ingested much water in the last couple of days, as they will create a smaller amount of urine than normal to preserve body water. Many outdoor adventurers and members of the military have learned that if they have not felt the need to urinate recently, they most likely are not drinking enough liquids. The other factor affecting the volume of urine created is the concentration of electrolytes and presence of osmotic molecules. The creation of osmotic pressure is typically related to the level of albumin present in the blood and electrolyte levels throughout the body water compartments. There are other osmotic molecules present in body fluids, but they are typically found in small amounts that do not appreciably change osmotic pressure. One instance where we see these molecules cause a change in osmotic pressure is in diabetics with chronic hyperglycemia. Glucose is an osmotic substance that can affect overall fluid balances when present in high amounts. This is one of the major reasons that people with diabetes that have poorly controlled blood glucose levels feel like they are always thirsty and always urinating.

Importance of Regulating Water Input and Output

Regulating the amount of water that enters and leaves the body is very important, as it has an effect on each and every organ system. The imbalance of water between compartments and in the body as a whole will not just affect the volume of water in our blood or how much urine our body makes to try and compensate for the imbalance. An increase or decrease in total body water or the water volume in a specific compartment can change the viscosity of the blood, the concentration of electrolytes in body fluids, and can also cause pathological conditions that result from these changes.

In years past, when a student wanted to join a fraternity or sorority, there were times when they would be made to drink copious amounts of alcohol as a form of hazing. In recent years the hazing changed as people became increasingly aware of the dangers of binge drinking and many universities banned the possession or drinking of alcohol on their campuses. When this occurred, some of the fraternities and sororities stopped using alcohol as a hazing method and switched to drinking water, as they thought this was a safer option. This belief was quickly shattered when several students died from water toxicity on campuses across the United States. The massive ingestion of water dilutes the concentrations of many important electrolytes, neurotransmitters, hormones, and plasma proteins. This dilution can cause nerves to misfire, fluid to accumulate in the lungs and around the brain, and the inability of the cardiac pacemaker cells to create and conduct the normal electrical signal that causes the heart to beat. It is for these reasons that our bodies try to carefully control the input and output of water.

LEARNING OBJECTIVE 16.1.9 List the ways that electrolytes enter and leave the body.

LEARNING OBJECTIVE 16.1.10 Explain the importance and mechanisms of regulating electrolyte input and output.

KEY TERM

pica Eating disorder that involves ingesting items that are not typically thought of as food, such as paint or clay.

ELECTROLYTE HOMEOSTASIS

Maintaining a constant concentration and level of electrolytes throughout the body is extremely important for several reasons. First, we need to remember that electrolytes are responsible for the creation and maintenance of the resting membrane potential of muscle cells, signal conduction in neurons, and maintaining cell membrane permeability. If there is even a small change in the concentration of electrolytes such as sodium, potassium, and calcium, it can really affect the ability of muscle cells to create the resting membrane potential or depolarize normally when signaled to do so. Just like an imbalance can affect the normal function of muscle cells, it can also interfere with signal transductions in neurons throughout the central and peripheral nervous systems. This interference may cause the inability for a neuron to transmit its signal or it may cause the creation of an aberrant signal, both of which may cause significant problems for the affected person. Lastly, electrolytes are responsible for maintaining the permeability of the cell membrane. Figure 16-5 depicts the change in extracellular compartment fluid osmolarity during times of dehydration and overhydration.

Mechanisms of Maintaining Electrolyte Homeostasis

Now that we have discussed the importance of electrolyte homeostasis, we are now going to discuss how this state of homeostasis is maintained. As with water, the body keeps electrolyte levels in balance through the regulation of electrolyte input and output. The regulation of electrolyte input centers around the control of hunger and thirst sensations. Once electrolytes have entered the body, the output of these ions is controlled even more tightly than their input. While it can be difficult to precisely control the exact amount of the different electrolytes entering the body through food and water, the kidneys are quite adept at getting rid of any excess and hanging on to those in short supply.

Electrolyte Input As we discuss electrolyte input, keep in mind that there is really only two ways in which they enter the body. The only way that electrolytes enter the body is by their presence in the food we eat and the fluids we drink. These two routes typically provide the body with more than sufficient amounts of the needed ions. As the body cannot control the amount of electrolytes in the food and liquids ingested, it instead modulates the creation and resolution of our hunger and thirst sensations. If you remember our discussion of hunger in Chapter 13, the sensation our mind interprets as hunger is caused by the neurotransmitter neuropeptide Y that is secreted by the hypothalamus in response to the presence or absence of the hormones leptin and ghrelin. Leptin is the hormone secreted by adipocytes while eating and inhibits the release of neuropeptide Y, which causes us to no longer feel hungry. Ghrelin, on the other hand, stimulates the release of neuropeptide Y and causes us to feel hungry.

Earlier in this chapter we discussed the control of water input by the sensation of thirst. Just like how the body regulates water input through the feeling of thirst, the entry of electrolytes is a result of the body feeling thirsty and the liquid we choose to ingest to suppress this action. While the hypothalamus does not cause the thirst sensation in response to an insufficient concentration of electrolytes in the water compartments of the body, an increase in the concentration of electrolytes through the body's water will cause the sensation of thirst. As we discussed previously, when learning about the regulation of water input, the sensation of thirst is caused by the increased concentration of electrolytes in the extracellular fluids. In cases where a person is not ingesting enough of the needed electrolytes, they may experience salt craving, leading to the condition known as pica. While **pica** is typically thought of as a psychological disorder that causes the affected people to eat nonfood items, in rare instances it may occur due to severe insufficiency of electrolytes in the body.

Electrolyte Output While the regulation of electrolyte input is a consequence of hunger and thirst sensations and the amount of electrolytes present in the food we eat and the liquids we drink cannot be strictly controlled, the kidneys monitor and control electrolyte output very precisely. In Chapter 15 we discussed the functions of the nephron and how it filters, reabsorbs, and secretes a variety of substances and electrolytes. The amount of each electrolyte that is reabsorbed or secreted is almost always a direct result of the concentration of that specific electrolyte in the extracellular fluid. So, if the concentration of sodium in the extracellular fluids is higher than normal, the nephron will allow more of the filtered sodium to be excreted in the form of urine. However, if the concentration of sodium in the plasma or the liquid filtered by the nephron is too low, the nephron will reabsorb all of the filtered sodium to prevent the concentration from getting any lower. While the nephrons found in the kidneys cannot increase the amount of an electrolyte in the body, it is able to effectively prevent any further loss. Figure 16-6 shows the regions of the nephron where different electrolytes are reabsorbed and secreted.

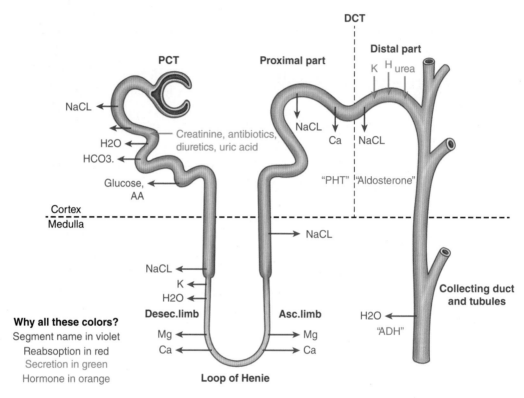

FIGURE 16-6 Cross-section of a nephron depicting the regions where different electrolytes are reabsorbed and secreted.

UNIT OBJECTIVE 16.2

Explain the importance of acid-base balance and the physiological mechanisms used to maintain this balance.

UNIT INTRODUCTION

In this unit we discuss acids and bases, how they relate to the pH scale, and how they relate to the normal homeostasis of the body. Acid-base imbalances within the human body are very severe and can quickly lead to a patient's death. To ensure that the pH of our bodily fluids stays within the normal range, the body has developed several different methods of regulating pH. These mechanisms involve the kidneys, the respiratory system, and a variety of buffering agents.

LEARNING OBJECTIVE 16.2.1 Identify the pH scale and its relationship to acids and bases.

LEARNING OBJECTIVE 16.2.2 Explain how the pH number relates to the substance's acidity or alkalinity.

KEY TERMS

acid Chemical compound that ionizes when placed in a liquid and releases hydrogen ions (H^+).

acidity Measurement of how strong or weak an acid solution is.

acidosis Blood pH less than the normal lower limit of 7.35.

alkaline Chemical compound that ionizes when placed in a liquid and has the ability to bind to free hydrogen ions. The solution could also be called a base and has a pH greater than 7 (7.45 when used in reference to the human body).

alkalinity Measurement of how strong or weak an alkaline solution is.

alkalosis Blood pH greater than 7.45.

base Chemical compound that ionizes when placed in a liquid and has the ability to bind to free hydrogen ions. The solution could also be called alkaline and has a pH greater than 7 (7.45 when used in reference to the human body).

logarithmic scale Scale in which each whole number above or below zero (seven in the case of the pH scale) is 10 times greater than the preceding whole number; the pH scale for the measurement of acids/bases and the Richter scale used to measure the force of earthquakes are common logarithmic scales. For example, a pH of 5 is ten times more acidic than a pH of 6.

pH scale Logarithmic scale numbered from 1 to 14 that is used to measure the concentration of hydrogen ions within a solution; tells us how acidic or basic a solution is. When using the pH scale, a pH of 7 is neutral, a pH less than 7 is acidic and a pH greater than 7 is basic (alkalotic). When used in reference to the human body, a pH of 7.35 to 7.45 is normal. Thus, a pH less than 7.35 is considered acidic and a pH greater than 7.45 is considered alkalotic.

THE pH SCALE

Understanding how the pH scale works is extremely important, but before we get into how it works, we are going to review some of the terminology utilized when discussing acids and bases.

- **Acid**: Acid is any substance that releases an ionized hydrogen molecule (H^+) when placed in solution.
- **Acidity**: Measure of how acidic a chemical or substance is.
- **Acidosis**: Condition in which a person's bodily fluids have a pH less than 7.35.
- **Base**: Chemical or substance having a pH of greater than 7 that is able to accept and bind to one or more free hydrogen ions.
- **Alkaline**: Another term for base that is commonly used in medicine and the study of anatomy and physiology.
- **Alkalinity**: Measure of how alkaline a substance or chemical is.
- **Alkalosis**: Condition in which the person's bodily fluids have a pH greater than 7.45.

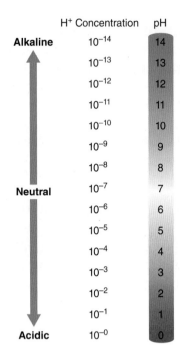

FIGURE 16-7 The pH scale with hydrogen ion concentration.

Now returning to the discussion of acids and bases, it is so important to know how acidic or basic a substance is that scientists developed a scale to measure it, known as the **pH scale**. The pH of a substance is based on the concentration of hydrogen ions present within that substance. In more technical terms, the pH of a substance is the negative log of the hydrogen ion concentration, which can be calculated through the following equation:

$$pH = -Log[H^+]$$

If you look at Figure 16-7, you will notice that the pH scale is numbered from 0 to 14. At the middle of the scale is pH 7.0, which is considered to be neutral. The only truly neutral substance is distilled water, which we discuss in more detail shortly. Any other substance will be higher or lower than pH 7.0. Any substance with a pH lower than 7.0, or having a pH between 0 and 6.99, is considered to be an acid. On the other hand, any pH greater than 7.0, or having a pH between 7.01 and 14, is considered to be a base.

Since the pH scale is a **logarithmic scale**, it means that a pH of 5 is 10 times stronger, or the concentration of hydrogen ions is 10 times greater than a pH of 6. If you were to compare a substance with a pH of 5 to a substance with a pH of 7, there is a 100 times difference in the hydrogen ion concentration between the two. So, whenever the pH moves more than one number, we multiply the difference in strength or acidity by 10. As such, a difference of 3 on the pH scale represents a 1,000 times difference in the acidity of the substances.

Acids

When looking at the pH scale seen in Figure 16-8, you will notice that any substance that lies below the neutral pH of 7.0 is considered to be an acid. The lower the pH number, the greater the hydrogen ion concentration, and the stronger the acid is. So, if we use a pH of 5.0 as an example, any acid with a number lower than 5.0 will be more acidic and any number greater than 5.0 will be less acidic.

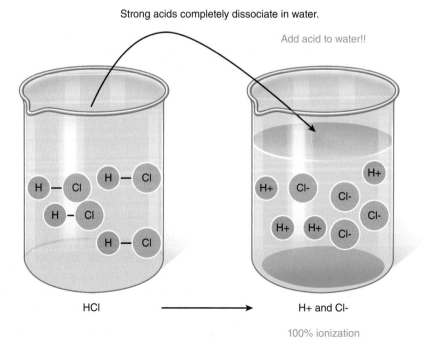

FIGURE 16-8 Ionization of hydrochloric acid (HCl) when placed in water.

Bases

Just like we used the pH scale to determine a substance's acidity level, we can also use the scale to determine how alkaline or basic a substance is. Bases fall between 7.01 and 14 on the pH scale and, similar to acids, the further the number is from pH 7 the more basic or alkaline the substance is. While acids donate a hydrogen ion when they ionize in solution, bases ionize to become a hydrogen ion recipient when placed in solution. An example of a strong base is sodium hydroxide, with the chemical formula of NaOH. When sodium hydroxide is put in water, it ionizes to form sodium ions (Na^+) and hydroxide ions (OH^-). The hydroxide ions are looking for a positively charged ion like hydrogen to bond with and return to a neutral charge. The combination of a hydrogen ion (H^+) and hydroxide ion (OH^-) results in water (H_2O), which is neutral. If we were to mix hydrochloric acid (strong acid) with sodium hydroxide (strong base), the result would be water (H_2O) and sodium-chloride salt (NaCl). So, whenever we mix an acid with a base, we will get some water and some salt.

LEARNING OBJECTIVE 16.2.3 Explain acid-base balance.

ACID-BASE BALANCE

The idea of acid-base balance refers to the need to keep the acids and bases found within our bodies in check. If the acidity or alkalinity of the fluids within our bodies strays very far above or below the normal range for humans, the results can be fatal. Our normal pH range is between a pH of 7.35 and 7.45, but during times of illness or when experiencing a disease, the body's pH may stray outside of this range. However, there is a limit to how acidic or alkalotic our bodily fluids can become and still remain alive. The minimum and maximum pH for human life to occur are generally thought to be between a pH of 6.5 and 6.6 and a pH of 7.7 and 7.8. In order to minimize large changes in the pH of our bodily fluid and to remain within the normal range of 7.35–7.45, the body utilizes several different physiological mechanisms, which are discussed in the coming sections.

LEARNING OBJECTIVE 16.2.4 Describe the relationship between the pH and hydrogen ion concentration.

LEARNING OBJECTIVE 16.2.5 List the major sources of hydrogen ions in the body.

SOURCES OF HYDROGEN IONS

There are two primary sources for the hydrogen ions found within our bodies. These two sources consist of the hydrogen ions found in the foods we consume and the hydrogen ions created as the product of metabolic processes that are continually occurring within our bodies. While the vast majority of the hydrogen ions found in our bodies come from metabolic reactions, the gastrointestinal (GI) tract's absorption of hydrogen ions and compounds containing hydrogen is also an important source.

Hydrogen Ions from the Gastrointestinal Tract

As we just mentioned, while the amount of hydrogen absorbed from the gastro-intestinal tract is limited, it is still an important source. Hydrogen can be found in a variety of food sources, along with the absorption of hydrogen ions secreted higher in the GI tract. As explained in Chapter 13, the stomach secretes gastric juice, which not only contains pepsinogen and intrinsic factor, but contains hydrochloric acid as well. As we discuss in the next section, hydrochloric acid is a strong acid and releases almost all of the hydrogen molecules that it contains.

Hydrogen Ions from Metabolic Processes

As you can see in Table 16-2, there are several different metabolic processes that create different acids and the hydrogen molecules found within them. The processes include respiration, the oxidation of fats and amino acids, and the breakdown of phosphoproteins and nucleic acids.

Table 16-2 Acids are Important Hydrogen Ion Contributors and When Found in Normal Quantities they Allow us to Maintain Our Normal pH of 7.35–7.45

METABOLIC PROCESSES THAT PRODUCE HYDROGEN IONS IN THE FORM OF ACID	
Metabolic Reaction	**Resulting Acid**
Aerobic respiration	Carbonic acid
Anaerobic respiration	Lactic acid
Oxidation of amino acids containing sulfur	Sulfuric acid
Incomplete oxidation of fatty acids	Acidic ketone bodies
Metabolism of phosphoproteins	Phosphoric acid
Metabolism of nucleic acids	Uric acid

LEARNING OBJECTIVE 16.2.6 Identify strong acids and weak acids.

LEARNING OBJECTIVE 16.2.7 Explain the difference between strong acids and weak acids.

KEY TERMS

acetic acid Weak acid that is also known as vinegar.

ionize Process by which chemical compounds dissociate when placed in water.

COMPARING STRONG ACIDS AND WEAK ACIDS

The relative strength of an acid is determined by the degree to which the substance **ionizes** when placed in water (Figure 16-8). Those substances that ionize fully or very close to fully release a large number of hydrogen ions and are considered strong acids. Substances that do not ionize or ionize very little when placed in water release a small number of hydrogen ions and are considered to be weak acids.

Strong acids are those substances that ionize fully, or close to fully, when added to water. When put in solution the hydrogen molecule will dissociate from the rest of the compound, creating an H^+ ion and some other negatively charged ion. For example, hydrochloric acid is a strong acid that ionizes well when put in solution. As such, the solution will contain large amounts of H^+ and Cl^- ions, while containing very small amounts of the nonionized HCl compound. The large number of free hydrogen ions leads to a pH that is much closer to 0 than it is to 7.

While strong acids will completely ionize or almost completely ionize, weak acids ionize to a much smaller extent when placed in water. An example of a weak acid is acetic acid, also known as vinegar, which has the chemical structure of CH_3COOH. When placed in water there will be a small amount of ionization that occurs and creates H^+ and CH_3COO^- ions, but most of the compound will remain in its nonionized form. This results in fewer free hydrogen ions and results in a pH closer to 7.

LEARNING OBJECTIVE 16.2.8 Identify chemical buffer systems in the body.

LEARNING OBJECTIVE 16.2.9 Describe the bicarbonate buffering system.

KEY TERMS

amino groups Portion of a chemical substance that contains an amine group ($-NH3$).

carboxylic groups Portion of a chemical compound that contains a carboxyl group (-COOH).

PHYSIOLOGICAL BUFFERS

Physiological buffers are very important within the human body and are composed mainly of protein buffers. Protein buffers consist of proteins like albumin, hemoglobin, and intracellular proteins that can use their amino groups ($-NH_2$) and carboxylic groups (–COOH) to accept or release hydrogen ions. This ability to gain or lose a hydrogen ion is how they are able to buffer or prevent large changes in our pH.

CHEMICAL BUFFERS

Chemical buffers are fast and allow our body to quickly compensate for changes in the pH of our bodily fluids. There are two major chemical buffering systems within our body, consisting of a phosphate buffering system and a bicarbonate a buffering system. The phosphate buffering system is less complex and involves the reversible release of a hydrogen ion to form HPO_4^{2-} or reversible binding of a hydrogen ion to form $H_2PO_4^-$.

The bicarbonate buffering reaction is one of the most widely used and important biochemical reactions that occur within the body. The reaction that occurs, shown below, can reversibly combine water (H_2O) and carbon dioxide

(CO_2) to carbonic acid (H_2CO_3), which can then be reversibly broken down into hydrogen ions (H^+) and bicarbonate ions (HCO_3^-).

$$H_2O + CO_2 \longleftrightarrow H_2CO_3 \longleftrightarrow H^+ + HCO_3^-$$

This reaction is always in motion and moving in one direction or the other to maintain equilibrium. If there is a high level of CO_2 in our bodily fluids, the reaction will begin combining it with water to form carbonic acid, which can then be broken down into hydrogen ions and bicarbonate ions. If the amount of hydrogen ions is too large, the reaction will move in the opposite direction to create water and carbon dioxide. In short, the reaction will always move in the direction that is away from where a buildup of reactants is occurring.

The ability of this reaction to reversibly convert hydrogen ions to carbonic acid and then to carbon dioxide allows the body to use two different mechanisms to keep acids and bases in check. These two vital mechanisms consist of the respiratory system and renal system, which is discussed further in the next section.

LEARNING OBJECTIVE 16.2.10 **Explain how chemical buffers, the respiratory system, and the urinary system help control the pH of the body.**

KEY TERMS

diabetic ketoacidosis Complication of diabetes that occurs when the body produces high levels of acidic ketones due to the increased breakdown of fats for energy use.

Kussmaul's respirations Breathing pattern typically seen in patients experiencing diabetic ketoacidosis; characterized by very deep, rapid breathing.

pH HOMEOSTASIS

The ability of our bodies to maintain a state of pH homeostasis is both incredible and absolutely necessary. As we just learned, our bodies utilize physiological buffers and chemical buffers to maintain pH, but that isn't the end of the story. Once we have converted excess hydrogen ions to carbon dioxide and water, or excess carbon dioxide to hydrogen ions and bicarbonate, we need to be able to get rid of the newly created molecules. If we were to just leave these molecules in the body, they would keep increasing in number and become a large issue, rather than the solution to our pH problems. As such, the body uses two different organ systems to eliminate these products, the respiratory system and renal system.

There are two primary buffering systems found within the body. The first is the bicarbonate buffering system, which we have discussed and will continue throughout this chapter. The second buffering system is the phosphate buffering system, which we will not be covering as deeply. Chemical buffers are absolutely vital to the body's ability to maintain a normal pH range, as they are able to respond to changes in the pH of the blood and bodily fluids. Physiological buffers, like the respiratory system and the renal mechanism for regulating pH, take much longer to respond to these changes. As a result, there is a time gap between the time with the pH is changing and the time when our physiologic buffers are actually able to respond to this change. This is why chemical buffers are so vital to pH homeostasis.

By manipulating the bicarbonate buffering system, our body is able to quickly adapt and convert excess hydrogen ions into carbonic acid and then to carbon dioxide. Chemical buffers are also able to run in reverse and can convert excess carbon dioxide into carbonic acid, and then convert the carbonic acid into free hydrogen ions and bicarbonate ions. Not only can we buffer any changes that are increasing the acidity in the body, we can also use these buffers to resist changes that would make the blood more alkalotic or basic. When a person is vomiting, there is a loss of hydrogen ions in the form of stomach acid that would normally be absorbed and used to maintain blood pH. In response, the body is able to force the bicarbonate buffering equation to the right, creating more hydrogen ions to replace what was lost and reduce the effects of having too much unopposed bicarbonate ions. As you can see, chemical buffers are incredibly important to the maintenance of a normal pH range in our bodily fluids and the overall health of our bodies.

Respiratory Compensation

One of the two primary ways the body is able to compensate for pH changes is by changing the rate and/or depth of breathing. The faster we breathe, the more carbon dioxide that is expelled from the lungs, which typically equates to a lower partial pressure of carbon dioxide and blood pH. This decrease in carbon dioxide is going to force the bicarbonate buffering system equation to the left, causing more hydrogen ions to combine with bicarbonate ions and form carbonic acid, which is then converted to carbon dioxide. By doing so, the body has reduced the number of free hydrogen ions present in the blood, which results in a decreasing acidity of the blood and an increased pH.

So, when examining a patient that has been found to be experiencing acidosis, it's common for the respiratory rate and depth of breathing to be higher than normal. A prime example of this respiratory pattern change is a diabetic patient who cannot transport glucose into the cells for energy, and as a result begins burning fat for energy instead. This use of fat as a primary energy source results in high levels of acidic ketones building up in the body. These ketones increase the number of free hydrogen ions, forcing the equation to the left and creating excess carbon dioxide. This excess carbon dioxide leads to an increased respiratory rate and increased depth of breathing. This increased rate and depth of breathing is known as **Kussmaul's respirations** and is highly indicative of a patient experiencing **diabetic ketoacidosis**. In comparison to the renal system's mechanism for compensating for a change in pH, the speed in which the respiratory system takes action is relatively fast.

Renal Compensation

The second physiological mechanism that assists the body in the maintenance of pH homeostasis is renal compensation. Just like the respiratory system can increase or decrease the carbon dioxide levels found on the left side of the bicarbonate buffering system equation, the renal system is able to directly affect the levels of free hydrogen ions found on the right side of the equation. At times when there are too many free hydrogen ions present in the blood and the filtered fluid of the renal tubule, the body is able to channel the excess hydrogen ions into the urine. This functions to decrease the number of free hydrogen ions found in the blood and lower its pH. In addition to the ability to increase and decrease hydrogen ion levels within the blood and filtered fluids, the kidneys are also able to absorb or excrete excess bicarbonate ions as needed. So, through an increased reabsorption of hydrogen ions and a decreased reabsorption of bicarbonate ions, the kidneys are able to increase the acidity and decrease blood pH. Not only can the kidneys increase blood acidity and decrease pH, but they can also decrease the acidity of the blood by excreting more hydrogen ions and reabsorbing more bicarbonate ions from the filtered fluid. Due to the kidneys' ability to manipulate both the hydrogen ion concentration and the bicarbonate ion concentration within the blood and filtrate, the kidneys are able to exert a significant amount of control over pH homeostasis.

LEARNING OBJECTIVE 16.2.11 Identify the causes of acid-base increases and decreases.

LEARNING OBJECTIVE 16.2.12 Explain the causes and resulting consequences of acid-base increases and decreases.

ACID-BASE IMBALANCES

Acid-base imbalances are typically very severe and can affect the health of the entire body. There are four primary categories of acid-base imbalances. These imbalances consist of respiratory acidosis, respiratory alkalosis, metabolic acidosis, and metabolic alkalosis. Of these different imbalances, metabolic acidosis and metabolic alkalosis are typically more severe and much more difficult to treat than respiratory-induced imbalances.

Respiratory Acidosis

Respiratory acidosis is defined as a pH less than 7.35 with a respiratory pathology. When examining an arterial blood gas for a patient with respiratory acidosis, not only will you see a pH of less than 7.35, but you will also typically see an arterial pCO_2 of greater than 45 mmHg. As we discussed earlier in this chapter, excess CO_2 can be converted to carbonic acid and then to free hydrogen ions and bicarbonate ions. This process is how the increased CO_2 in a patient with certain respiratory conditions results in a state of respiratory acidosis. Typically, this condition is brought on by respiratory diseases that result in a decreased respiratory rate or decreased tidal volume. This results in a decreased alveolar minute volume (as explained in Chapter 10), which leads to increased levels of CO_2 in the blood. Common causes of respiratory acidosis include opiate overdoses (heroin), chronic obstructive pulmonary disease, and pathologies that may cause respiratory arrest.

Respiratory Alkalosis

Respiratory alkalosis is defined as a pH greater than 7.45 and is caused by a respiratory pathology. When examining an arterial blood gas from these patients, you'll see a pH that is greater than 7.45 and an arterial pCO_2 of less than 35 mmHg. Due to a decrease in the amount of CO_2 present in the blood, the bicarbonate buffering system shifts the equation to the left, which uses free hydrogen ions and bicarbonate ions to form carbonic acid, which will then be split to create carbon dioxide and water. The reason the blood becomes alkalotic is because when the equation shifts to the left, there is a resulting decrease in the number of free hydrogen ions. This loss of hydrogen ions is the cause for the alkalosis and the pH to rise above the normal pH of 7.45. Common conditions that cause respiratory alkalosis include hyperventilation syndromes and traumatic head injuries that damage the respiratory center and result in an increased respiratory rate and depth of breathing.

Metabolic Acidosis

Metabolic acidosis is defined as a pH less than 7.35 due to a metabolic pathology. When examining an arterial blood gas from a patient with metabolic acidosis, you will find that the pH is often much less than 7.35, the CO_2 levels will be on the high side of normal or slightly increased, and the bicarbonate ion level will be severely decreased. This decrease in bicarbonate ions is caused by the body trying to buffer the excess hydrogen ions that are in the blood by combining the free hydrogen ions and bicarbonate ions to form carbonic acid, which can then be converted to CO_2 and water. On average, metabolic acidosis is much more severe than respiratory acidosis and can be significantly harder to treat. Pathologies that result in metabolic acidosis include diabetic ketoacidosis and renal failure. We discuss these pathologies in more detail in the next unit.

Metabolic Alkalosis

Metabolic alkalosis is defined as a pH of greater than 7.45 due to a metabolic, or nonrespiratory, pathology. When examining an arterial blood gas from a patient with metabolic alkalosis, the pH will typically be much greater than 7.45 and the bicarbonate level will also typically be much higher than normal. This increase in bicarbonate can be caused by either an excess intake of bicarbonate ions or a loss of free hydrogen ions. Conditions causing metabolic alkalosis include severe vomiting and medication overdoses. Older adults who present to the emergency department with metabolic alkalosis is frequently due to ingestion of numerous calcium-bicarbonate tablets. They use the tablets to increase their calcium levels and think that bicarbonate is just a harmless filler. In actuality, the bicarbonate is the medication used to treat excess stomach acid and by taking too much of it they have severely decreased the amount of free hydrogen ions present in the blood, causing metabolic alkalosis. Table 16-3 sums this information up in the form of a table.

Table 16-3 Arterial Blood Gas Changes During Acid-Base Imbalances

ARTERIAL BLOOD GAS INTERPRETATION		
	Acidosis	**Alkalosis**
Respiratory	pH: < 7.35 P_aCO_2 : > 45 mmHg HCO_3^- : Normal (22–28 mEq/L)	pH: > 7.45 P_aCO_2 : < 35 mmHg HCO_3^- : Normal (22–28 mEq/L)
Metabolic	pH: < 7.35 P_aCO_2 : Normal (35–45 mmHg) HCO_3^- : < 22 mEq/L	pH: >7.45 P_aCO_2 : Normal (35–45 mmHg) HCO_3^- : > 28 mEq/L

UNIT OBJECTIVE 16.3

Describe the common pathologies affecting water and electrolyte balances.

UNIT INTRODUCTION

In this unit we explore the common pathologies that can cause water and electrolyte imbalances. The information covered includes the types of imbalances, their cause, and the signs and symptoms of these conditions. By the end of the unit you will know more about a few of the common disorders affecting water and electrolyte homeostasis.

LEARNING OBJECTIVE 16.3.1 **Identify common disorders associated with water and electrolyte imbalances.**

KEY TERMS

dehydration State in which the extracellular fluids are significantly reduced and their osmolarity has increased to the point that it is outside the body's normal range. Typically dehydration is due to a lack of water entering the body or too much water leaving the body.

overhydration Excessive intake of liquids that results in the dilution of the body's fluids and results in a large decrease in osmolarity.

DISORDERS ASSOCIATED WITH WATER AND ELECTROLYTE IMBALANCES

There are many different disorders associated with water and electrolyte imbalances. As we discuss some electrolyte imbalances in detail in the next section, we concentrate on water imbalances here. When thinking about water homeostasis, there are two major problems we become concerned about: underhydration or dehydration and overhydration. In overhydration there is a markedly increased water intake, while in dehydration there is not enough water intake.

Dehydration

In **dehydration**, there is either a lack of water coming into the body, there is too much water leaving the body, or a combination of the two. Maintaining a normal body water balance is extremely important, which is illustrated well in the fact that we can only live for a few days without water. On the other hand, we can live for a few weeks without food.

In dehydration the extracellular fluid is depleted to a point where the osmolarity is increased and has become much greater than the intracellular fluid osmolarity. This causes the intracellular water to begin moving into the extracellular space to try and equalize the two different osmolarities. This water movement is not sufficient to fix the loss of extracellular fluid and further compounds the problem by depriving the cells of the fluid they need to work normally. The loss in extracellular fluid will cause a decrease in blood pressure, an increased heart rate, poor peripheral perfusion, and can even lead to a loss of consciousness and death. As such, it is vitally important that we regulate the amount of water entering our bodies to maintain body water homeostasis.

Overhydration

Overhydration did not gain widespread attention until a few years ago when several deaths were reported in conjunction with fraternity/sorority initiation. Public awareness of the dangers of binge drinking had increased and clubs that were notorious for alcohol abuse wisely decided to move away from activities including alcohol. Instead, they decided to have initiates ingest a large amount of spring water in a very short amount of time (think gallons of water in 15–30 minutes). Thinking that ingesting large volumes of water was okay, in actuality they diluted the osmolarity of the extracellular fluids so greatly that the excess extracellular water began rushing into intracellular spaces and interstitial spaces. This caused edema, or the buildup of water, within vital areas like the brain and lungs. The students who had ingested this massive quantity of water suffered the effects of pulmonary edema, cerebral edema, and the rupturing of cells that were overfilled with water. This resulted in the death of some students and a new public awareness campaign regarding the danger of consuming massive quantities of water in a very short period of time.

LEARNING OBJECTIVE 16.3.2 Discuss the cause, signs, symptoms, and diagnosis of hyperkalemia, hypokalemia, hypercalcemia, hypocalcemia, hypernatremia, and hyponatremia.

KEY TERMS

hypercalcemia Blood calcium levels in excess of the body's normal range (> 10.3 mg/dL).

hyperkalemia Blood potassium levels in excess of the body's normal range (> 4.5 mg/dL).

hypernatremia Blood sodium levels in excess of the body's normal range (> 145 mg/dL).

hypocalcemia Blood calcium levels lower than the body's normal range (< 8.5 mg/dL).

hypokalemia Blood potassium levels lower than the body's normal range (< 3.5 mg/dL).

hyponatremia Condition characterized by abnormally low sodium levels in the blood (lower than 136 meq/L).

polydipsia Excessive thirst typically seen in diabetic patients with an elevated blood glucose level.

SODIUM, POTASSIUM, AND CALCIUM IMBALANCES

Electrolyte imbalances within the body can be extremely serious and even lethal. This is especially true when the imbalances are related to the blood plasma levels of calcium, sodium, and potassium. These electrolytes are vital to the proper functions of our heart, nerves, muscles, and any cell that maintains an electrical potential across its membrane. We discuss the cause, signs and symptoms, and diagnosis of imbalances related to sodium, potassium, and calcium ions.

Hypernatremia

Hypernatremia is a condition in which the blood level of sodium is higher than the normal range for sodium of 135–145. This increased sodium level can have many effects on the body, including causing seizures, cardiac arrhythmias, coma, and even death. Hypernatremia is not typically due to excess input of sodium ions in our bodies, but rather a decrease in the overall level of water within the body and blood. This can be seen in conditions where a person has exercised strenuously over the course of several hours without replacing any of the lost fluids.

Hyponatremia

Hyponatremia is a condition in which the blood level of sodium is less than the normal range of 135–145. Causes of hyponatremia include the excess intake of water, a diet deficient in sodium, and strenuous athletic activities where there is a significant loss of sodium through sweat without being properly replaced. It is for this reason that many athletes will drink liquids high in electrolytes or will use salt tablets to maintain normal electrolyte levels. Hyponatremia can cause a variety of problems, including seizures, cardiac arrhythmias, and the loss of water from the blood vessels into the surrounding tissues (edema).

Hyperkalemia

Hyperkalemia is a condition where the blood plasma level of potassium is greater than the normal range of 3.5–5.0 mEq/L. Causes of hyperkalemia are typically related to renal dialysis and medical conditions causing insufficient secretion of the hormone aldosterone. If you remember from our discussion in Chapter 15, aldosterone leads to the reabsorption of sodium from the renal tubule and the secretion of potassium into the renal tubule. Low or insufficient secretion of aldosterone prevents sodium from being reabsorbed and results in potassium retention. This retention of potassium on a chronic basis will lead to a significantly increased blood potassium level, or hyperkalemia. The other frequent cause of hyperkalemia is renal dialysis. As dialysis is not as good as the kidney when it comes to regulating electrolyte levels in our bodies, patients on dialysis experience a variety of electrolyte imbalances. It is for this reason that their blood is tested very frequently and any imbalances treated immediately. Consequences of moderate hyperkalemia (6.01–7.0 mEq/L) and severe hyperkalemia (> 7.0 mEq/L) can include muscle spasms, nerve impulse conduction delays and/or interruption, and cardiac arrhythmias. Cardiac arrhythmias resulting from hyperkalemia are severe and can lead to death quite quickly.

CLINICAL TIP	When performing an electrocardiogram (ECG) on a patient with hyperkalemia, the T-wave will be very tall and pointed. If the T-wave looks like a tack that you would be afraid to sit on, hyperkalemia should be at the top of your list of suspects. Severe hyperkalemia can also lead to the presence of a sine-wave, which can be seen in Figure 16-9. The treatment in this case is the administration of IV calcium chloride, bicarbonate, glucose, and insulin.

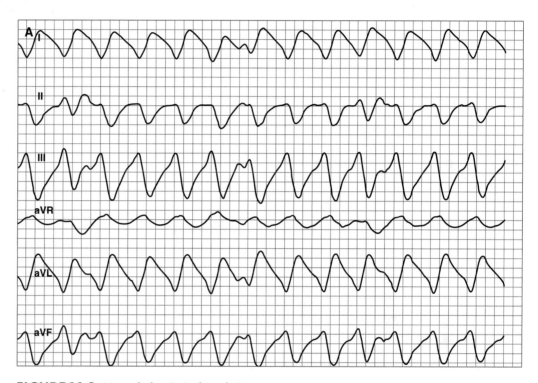

FIGURE 16-9 Hyperkalemia-induced sine-wave ECG.

Hypokalemia

When the blood plasma level of potassium is lower than the normal 3.5–5.0 mEq/L, the patient is said to be experiencing **hypokalemia**. Hypokalemia can be caused in a variety of ways, including dialysis, potassium-wasting diuretics like the "thiazides," and the over secretion of aldosterone. Just like the under secretion of aldosterone can result in hyperkalemia, over secretion can lead to hypokalemia. While discussing hyperkalemia, we mentioned that dialysis can cause a variety of electrolyte imbalances, one of which could be hypokalemia. Hypokalemia can also be caused by certain medications, the most prominent and well known being the potassium-wasting diuretic thiazide. These diuretics work on the distal convoluted tubule and result in the over secretion of potassium into the renal tubule, resulting in their excretion from the body in the form of urine. The group of people most commonly affected with hypokalemia are older adults, as they are more commonly on diuretics and/or dialysis than other age groups. Hypokalemia is often non-symptomatic, but it can cause muscle weakness, **polydipsia**, confusion, and cardiac arrhythmias.

Hypercalcemia

When blood tests reveal a total blood calcium level greater than the normal 8.5–10.3 mg/dL, the patient is said to be experiencing **hypercalcemia**. This condition may be due to the over ingestion of calcium supplements, hyperparathyroidism, and vitamin D toxicity. Hyperparathyroidism is a condition in which parathyroid hormone is oversecreted into the bloodstream and is the leading cause of hypercalcemia. This increase in parathyroid hormone causes excess calcium absorption from the intestinal lumen, increased reabsorption of calcium from the renal tubule, and the excessive release of calcium from bone tissue. Vitamin D toxicity results from the excessive ingestion of vitamin D supplements and causes a marked increase in the amount of dietary calcium absorbed from the intestinal lumen. The results of hypercalcemia include constipation, anorexia, and nausea and vomiting when total blood calcium levels are mildly increased. As the levels of calcium continue to rise, the patient will begin experiencing muscle weakness, confusion, stupor, cardiac arrhythmias, coma, and death.

Hypocalcemia

The last electrolyte imbalance we discuss here is **hypocalcemia**. Hypocalcemia is a condition in which the blood plasma total calcium level is less than 8.5 mg/dL. Hypocalcemia can be caused by vitamin D deficiency, dialysis, and the under secretion or absence of parathyroid hormone seen in hypoparathyroidism. Without vitamin D, the levels of dietary calcium absorbed from the gastrointestinal tract will be significantly reduced. A lack of parathyroid hormone will also lead to a decreased absorption of dietary calcium from the GI tract, decreased reabsorption of calcium from the renal tubule, and the inability to access calcium reserves in bone tissue. These low levels of blood plasma total calcium will cause paresthesia and tetany when mildly decreased, followed by seizures, encephalopathy, and heart failure when significantly decreased. Treatment includes IV replacement of calcium and supplemental vitamin D.

UNIT OBJECTIVE 16.4

Describe common pathologies affecting the pH of the body.

UNIT INTRODUCTION

In this unit we explore a few of the common pathologies affecting the body's pH homeostasis. An imbalance in our normal pH can be linked to many different diseases, whether the cause, or a result, of the pathologies. While there are many pathologies that could be considered minor or insignificant, those affecting pH homeostasis are severe and can result in death without proper treatment.

LEARNING
OBJECTIVE **16.4.1** **Identify common disorders associated with acid-base imbalances.**

opiates Naturally occurring substances that are able to stimulate opioid receptors in the human body and produce pain relief and/or a feeling of euphoria. Examples of common opiates are opium, and such medications as morphine, hydrocodone, oxycodone, hydromorphone, and heroin.

COMMON DISORDERS ASSOCIATED WITH ACID-BASE IMBALANCES

There are many disorders that can cause an acid-base imbalance in the body, but we only discuss four of them. These four pathologies consist of opiate overdoses and chronic obstructive pulmonary disease, both types of respiratory acidosis, and hyperventilation which is a type of respiratory alkalosis. In the next section we also talk about diabetic ketoacidosis in depth, which is a type of metabolic acidosis. Metabolic alkalosis is a bit rarer and we won't be covering a specific pathology related to it. These conditions will hopefully give you a better understanding of what types of pathologies cause each of the pH imbalances.

Opiate Overdose

Opiates are a common medication that you may have heard quite a bit about recently. For roughly the last 150 years they have been used throughout the world as a potent painkiller. Even today they are one of the most effective medications for relieving acute pain or the pain of chronic debilitating conditions and cancers. Prior to their use as a remedy for pain, they were used for their euphoric effects throughout Asia, the Middle East, and Europe. This class of medications includes morphine, codeine, heroin, hydrocodone, opium, hydromorphone, and many others.

While these medications are effective for pain relief and can produce euphoria for those who abuse them, they cause significant respiratory depression. Often those who abuse opiates will have a markedly reduced respiratory rate and depth of breathing once the opiate has reached its maximum effect. While the body develops a tolerance to opiates, which requires a progressively higher dose to achieve the same feeling of euphoria, the respiratory system does not exhibit this same development of tolerance. As such, when these patients take a higher dose to get high, the respiratory system is even more depressed than it previously was with a lower dose. Eventually the person will get to the point where they will only be breathing two to three times a minute and may actually stop breathing altogether. This is why opiate overdoses are so serious, as the patient is euphoric and unable to realize that they aren't breathing and will soon experience cardiac arrest. During this period of a markedly reduced respiratory rate, carbon dioxide is building up in the bloodstream and is being converted to hydrogen ions. This leads to decreased blood pH and respiratory acidosis condition. Thankfully, prompt reversal of the opiates with naloxone or artificial ventilation will often correct this imbalance and return the patient's PCO_2 levels and pH to within normal ranges.

Hyperventilation

Hyperventilation is a condition in which the patient is breathing rapidly and deeply, without a physiological need to do so. While hyperventilation is often tied to anxiety, there are other causes. When there is no physiological need to be breathing deeply and rapidly, the increased rate and depth of the breathing will result in an unnecessary and possibly harmful reduction in the blood's PCO_2 level. This will result in a PCO_2 level below the normal range of 35 to 45 mmHg and will pull the bicarbonate buffering system equation to the left. When it does so, there will be a decrease in the concentration of H^+ ions in the blood and the pH will begin to rise. Often hyperventilation will cause the individual to become dizzy and lose consciousness, allowing the body to "reset" and resume a normal breathing pattern. Soon after, the effects of a decreased blood PCO_2 will wear off and the person will regain consciousness without any lasting impacts.

Chronic Obstructive Pulmonary Disease

Chronic obstructive pulmonary disease (COPD) is a family of respiratory pathologies that includes chronic bronchitis and emphysema. Chronic bronchitis is considered to be an "air trapping" disease, as patients with this condition can inhale without a problem, but they have difficulty forcing the air out of their lungs and are often left with a larger volume of air than normal trapped inside their lungs. Emphysema is the exact opposite in that due to the loss in the lung's elasticity, the patient often has a hard time inhaling and bringing air into the lungs, but has no problem exhaling. Despite the difference between the two diseases, the end result of not being able to remove enough carbon dioxide from the blood is the same. As a result, these patients experience a chronic respiratory acidosis due to the constantly higher than normal PCO_2 and the resulting decrease in blood pH.

LEARNING OBJECTIVE 16.4.2 Describe the cause, signs, symptoms, and diagnosis of diabetic ketoacidosis.

DIABETIC KETOACIDOSIS

Diabetic ketoacidosis is a pathology that affects primarily people with insulin-dependent diabetes, formerly known as type 1 diabetes. The pathology results from their cells being unable to access the glucose in their blood, which causes them to begin burning fat molecules for energy. While this provides the cell with energy, our bodies are unable to fully burn the molecules and as a result we produce acidic ketones. While burning fat during exercise or dieting causes the creation of ketones, the sheer quantity produced during diabetic ketoacidosis becomes the problem.

Cause

As stated above, diabetic ketoacidosis is the result of the body being unable to access the glucose found in the bloodstream like it normally would. This inability to access the glucose is due to the hormone insulin being in very low supply or completely absent. Most tissues in our bodies require insulin to be present in order to move glucose into its cells, where it can metabolize it to create energy in the form of ATP. When insulin isn't present, or in this case can't be utilized, most cells begin to use a backup energy source in the form of fat molecules. As discussed above, these fat molecules cannot be completely metabolized by the cells and the resulting by-products are ketones. As we said, the creation of ketones during dieting or exercise is a quantity that our bodies can handle without any negative side effects. However, when the entire body is using fat as an energy source, the amount of ketones produced is more than we can handle. This leads to an accumulation of the acidic ketones in the bloodstream and body fluids, resulting in a drop in pH.

Signs and Symptoms

The signs and symptoms of DKA are primarily linked to the presence of unusually high levels of ketones in the body. If you recall from our discussion of the bicarbonate buffering system, the presence of excess hydrogen ions (acid) leads to the creation of carbonic acid, which is then broken down to water and carbon dioxide (CO_2). In patients experiencing DKA, the amount of carbon dioxide is excessive and their body tried to get rid of it quickly by increasing the rate and depth of breathing. When evaluating these patients, you will notice that both their rate and depth of breathing are increased dramatically, until it seems like they are taking a deep breath 40–60 times a minute. This respiratory pattern is known as Kussmaul's respirations, which we briefly mentioned earlier in Unit 16.2. In addition to the rapid and deep breathing, the presence of excessive ketones in their bodily fluids will also give their breath a noticeable "fruity" odor.

Diagnosis

Diagnosis of these patients is primarily based on blood glucose levels, arterial blood gas levels, patient medical history, and signs/symptoms present during patient evaluation. As this is a form of metabolic acidosis, the pH will be much less than 7.35 and there will be a very low bicarbonate level. However, as this is not an acute condition and normally takes a week or more to develop, the body will have had time to begin compensating, resulting in a markedly increased carbon dioxide level. Blood glucose levels in patients with diabetic ketoacidosis are often greater than 700 mg/dL, while the blood glucose of a nondiabetic is less than 120 mg/dL. The patient's medical history will often show a diagnosed history of insulin-dependent diabetes mellitus, but this condition can at times be seen in those with a new onset of diabetes.

Treatment

Treatment for diabetic ketoacidosis will focus around correcting the acid-base imbalance and on decreasing the blood glucose level. These patients will typically be given medication to reverse the acidosis, such as bicarbonate, which will help to buffer the effects of the ketones present in their bodies. Patients will also receive intravenous insulin, glucose, and potassium to assist in correcting the pH and to also correct the hyperglycemia. The insulin is given intravenously, as it allows for greater control of the amount being given, while the glucose is given to prevent an overcorrection to a hypoglycemia state. The patient is treated with potassium, as the blood levels of potassium will often decrease when insulin is given in large amounts.

Chapter 17

The Reproductive System

Chapter Introduction

The reproductive system is one of the most fascinating systems within the human body. Without this system, the human race would not exist.

Studying this content provides a better understanding of how the body is able to replicate cells and create another living being (Figure 17-1).

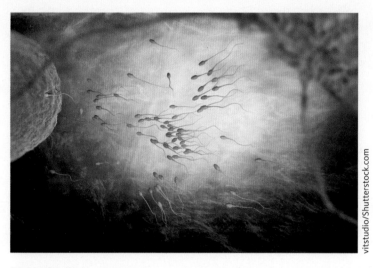

vitstudio/Shutterstock.com

FIGURE 17-1 Human sperm penetrates an egg.

UNIT OBJECTIVE 17.1

Explain the process of meiosis and how it provides genetic variability.

UNIT INTRODUCTION

This unit explains the process of meiosis, or division of reproductive cells (Figure 17-2). There are numerous stages of meiosis that occur in two phases. During meiosis, chromosomes from the two parents divide twice and reconnect in different ways to make each person a unique individual.

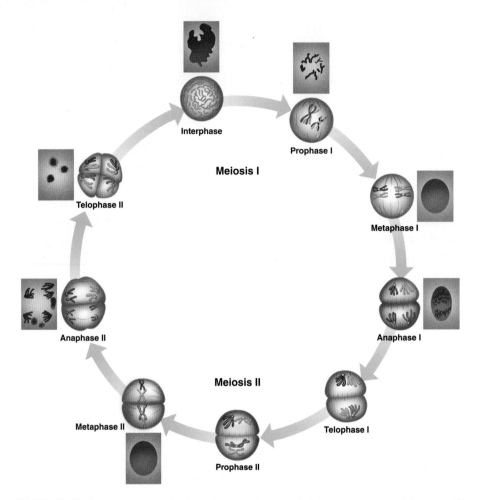

FIGURE 17-2 Stages of meiosis and the behavior of chromosomes, as illustrated here.

LEARNING OBJECTIVE **17.1.1** Identify the process of meiosis.

LEARNING OBJECTIVE **17.1.2** Explain the process of meiosis.

KEY TERMS

anaphase I Stage during meiosis I when the spindle fibers are pulling the homologues apart to opposite ends of the cell.

anaphase II Stage during meiosis II when the spindle fibers are pulling the sister chromatics apart to opposite ends of the cell.

centromere Region of a chromosome where sister haploids connect; also the site where spindle fibers attach.

chromosome String of DNA that contains genetic material.

crossing over (recombination) Trading of bits of DNA that occurs between homologous chromosomes during prophase I.

cytokinesis Proteins that play a regulatory function in the immune system.

DNA Content of a cell that contains proteins that make up genetic material.

fertilization Outcome when a sperm cell penetrates an ovum.

first polar body Small haploid cell formed during meiosis of the female sex cell that does not have the ability to be fertilized.

gametes Sperm and oocytes, or the sex cells.

germ cells Embryonic cell that can develop into a gamete through meiosis.

homologue pairs Also called homologous pairs; chromosome pairs that contain one chromosome from each parent and align at each gene location and centromere.

interphase Resting phase in mitosis between successive divisions, or the phase between meiosis I and II when the cell copies its DNA.

meiosis Division of the sex cell that results in half (23) of the total pairs of chromosomes.

metaphase I Phase when the homologous chromosomes arrange themselves on the metaphase plate while the spindle fibers attach to them at the centromeres.

metaphase II Occurs during the second stage of meiosis when the daughter cells align at the metaphase plate while the spindle fibers attach from opposite poles and prepare to separate the sister chromatids.

mitosis Process of cell duplication so that each cell has the same number of chromosomes.

oocytes Immature gamete within the ovary.

ova Haploid female gametes of animals develop into new individuals after fertilization with sperm during reproduction.

ovaries Female reproductive organ located in the pelvic cavity responsible for the secretion of hormones involved in secondary-sex characteristic development and menstruation.

ovum Mature female reproductive cell.

prophase I Phase during meiosis I when the homologous chromosomes line up with each other and bits of DNA cross over between them.

prophase II Phase during meiosis II when the two already divided daughter cells (with nonhomologous chromosomes) condense and the nuclear membrane disintegrates.

sister chromatids Two sides of a chromosome; each is joined to the other by the centromere.

sperm Gamete within the male anatomy that fertilizes the female egg in reproduction.

spermatogenesis Production and development of mature sperm.

telophase I Phase of meiosis I in which a nuclear membrane forms around each set of 23 chromosomes that were formed when the homologous chromosomes split in anaphase I.

telophase II Phase of meiosis II in which a nuclear membrane forms around each set of chromosomes.

testes Structure within the male anatomy that creates and stores sperm.

zygote Cell that results from fertilization of the ovum by the sperm; it contains 46 chromosomes, 23 from the ovum and 23 from the sperm.

MEIOSIS

Knowing the ways cells divide is essential to understanding the physiology of the reproductive system. One way that cells divide is through the process of **meiosis**. This process occurs in **germ cells**. Unlike other cells in the body, germ cells are the only type that can develop into sex cells. Meiosis has just one purpose—to produce **gametes** (sex cells) called **sperm** and **oocytes** that are stored in the **testes** and **ovaries**, respectively.

Chromosomes

First, let's look at the parts of a **chromosome**, which is the genetic material within a body cell. Every cell has 23 pairs of chromosomes. The two sides of each chromosome are called **sister chromatids**. Joining them together is a **centromere** (Figure 17-3).

We look at the process of meiosis and see that the sperm or oocyte that are end products of meiosis contain only one half of each pair of 23 chromosomes. Later, when these two cells meet during **fertilization**, the result, called a **zygote** (Figure 17-4), is a complete cell containing half of the chromosome pairs from the oocyte and half from the sperm. The fertilized egg now has 23 pairs of chromosomes.

Process of Meiosis

During meiosis, a cell with 23 pairs of chromosomes splits twice to form four daughter cells that contain one of each pair of chromosomes. Meiosis occurs in two stages with phases (Figure 17-5).

Meiosis stage I has five phases:

1. Interphase I: the 23 chromosomes in a cell are copied, making two identical sets of 23 chromosomes, or a total of 46 chromosomes.
2. Prophase I: identical sets of chromosomes line up as pairs, called homologues, and exchange some pieces.
3. Metaphase I: the chromosome pairs line up along the metaphase plate and spindle fibers attach to the centromeres of each pair.
4. Anaphase I: the spindle fibers pull apart the homologue pairs, which then move to opposite sides of the cell.
5. Telophase I: a nuclear membrane begins to form around each half of the cell.

Meiosis stage II has four phases:

1. Prophase II: the cell splits into two daughter cells with 23 chromosomes each, one from each pair, and a nuclear membrane forms around each daughter cell.
2. Metaphase II: single chromosomes line up along the metaphase plate.

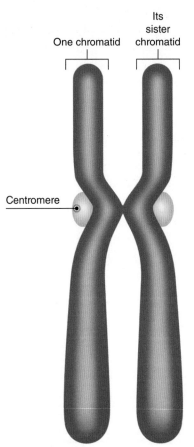

One chromatid   Its sister chromatid

Centromere

One chromosome in the duplicated state

FIGURE 17-3 This chromosome has copied itself during interphase, forming duplicate chromosomes, each with two chromatids that are attached to each other with a centromere.

3. Anaphase II: this time, the sister chromatids separate and are pulled to the opposite sides of the cells.
4. Telophase II: a nuclear membrane forms around each side of both daughter cells, forming four new cells.

Let's now look more closely at the process of meiosis.

Meiosis I: Interphase During meiosis I, a cell with 23 pairs of chromosomes (46 in total) first goes through **interphase**, when the **DNA** (the molecules that are the blueprints for how a living being is built) in the 23 chromosomes of a cell are copied (replicated) to make two identical full sets of chromosomes (23 chromosome pairs), called **homologue pairs** (Figure 17-6).

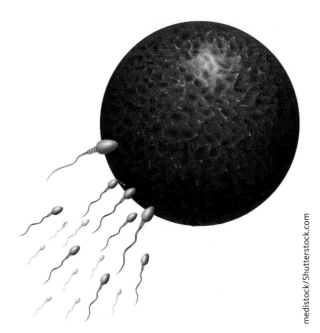

medistock/Shutterstock.com

FIGURE 17-4 Process of fertilization shows the oocyte surrounded by sperm. If fertilization occurs, the result is a zygote.

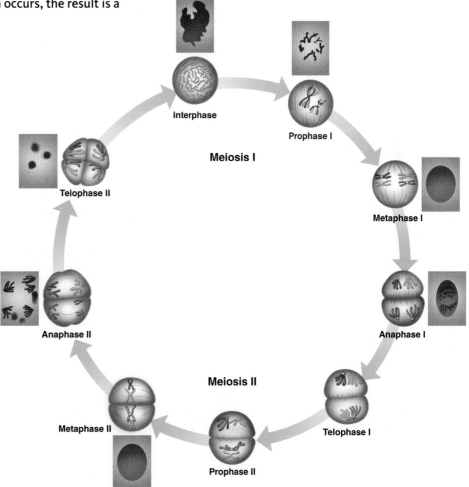

FIGURE 17-5 Stages and phases of meiosis as a circular process, in which one cell results in four cells.

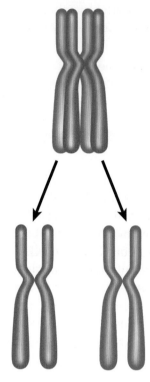

FIGURE 17-6 Two homologue pairs are created during interphase. They will line up in prophase I.

Meiosis I: Prophase I During the next phase, prophase I, the chromosomes pair up, aligning with their homologue partner along their full length. The homologue pairs then trade some bits of DNA during a process called **crossing over** (also called **recombination**) (Figure 17-7). Why are the bits of DNA switched on the chromosome pairs? So that each of us receives some of the same and some different genes from our parents. We become unique. This process accounts for siblings looking similar in some ways but different in others.

Meiosis I: Metaphase During metaphase I of meiosis I, the homologous pairs line up at the metaphase plate. Spindle fibers from the centrosomes attach to one of each chromosome (Figure 17-8).

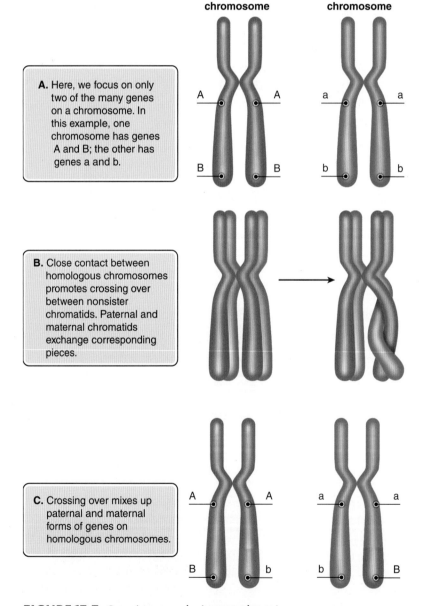

A. Here, we focus on only two of the many genes on a chromosome. In this example, one chromosome has genes A and B; the other has genes a and b.

B. Close contact between homologous chromosomes promotes crossing over between nonsister chromatids. Paternal and maternal chromatids exchange corresponding pieces.

C. Crossing over mixes up paternal and maternal forms of genes on homologous chromosomes.

One duplicated chromosome

One duplicated chromosome

FIGURE 17-7 Crossing over during prophase I.

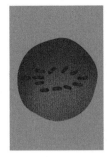

Metaphase I. The homologous chromosome pairs are aligned midway between spindle poles.

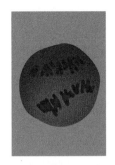

Anaphase I. The homologous chromosomes separate and begin heading toward the spindle poles.

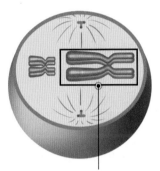

One pair of homologous chromosomes

FIGURE 17-8 Homologous pairs line up at the metaphase plate. Spindle fibers attach to one of each chromosome.

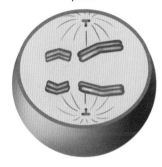

FIGURE 17-9 During anaphase I the homologues separate to opposite ends of the cells. The spindle fibers then pull apart the homologues at the centromeres.

Meiosis: Anaphase I Next is **anaphase I**, still a phase of meiosis I. The homologues now separate to opposite ends of the cells as the spindle fibers pull apart the homologues at the centromeres. Meanwhile, the sister chromatids of each chromosome stay together. The nuclear membrane around the single cell begins to disintegrate (Figure 17-9).

Meiosis: Telophase I and Cytokinesis Finally, in **telophase I**, a nuclear membrane forms around each chromosome at the opposite ends of the original parent cell with 23 pairs of chromosomes, creating two cells that each have 23 chromosomes, one from each homologue pair. This is **cytokinesis**, and the two resulting daughter cells have half the chromosomes (23) of the parent cell.

Figure 17-10 shows the process of the parental chromosomes being reduced by half.

Meiosis II The two daughter cells created in meiosis I undergo another division in which the sister chromatids separate to make cells that have nonhomologous chromosomes (Figure 17-11). During **prophase II**, the chromosomes condense, and the nuclear membrane begins to disintegrate. In **metaphase II**, the chromosomes line up as individuals along the metaphase plate. During **anaphase II**, the sister chromatids separate and are pulled to opposite ends of the cell by the spindle fibers of the centrosomes. Finally, in **telophase II**, new nuclear membranes surround each set of chromosomes. Cytokinesis splits the chromosome sets into four new cells in which each chromosome has just one chromatid. These cells are zygotes, or sperm and oocytes.

Differences Between Meiosis in Male and Female Germ Cells

Although male and female gametes are created through meiosis, there are some differences in certain stages. In women, the process of producing an oocyte is called **oogenesis**. In men, the production of sperm is called **spermatogenesis** (Figures 17-12 and 17-13).

Both processes begin the same way in meiosis, although not at the same time. Spermatogenesis begins at puberty in men. Oogenesis begins before birth. Spermatogenesis produces four haploid gametes per each male germ cell that undergoes meiosis. The process is continuous. In oogenesis, only one ovum is produced from one oocyte. Why does this occur?

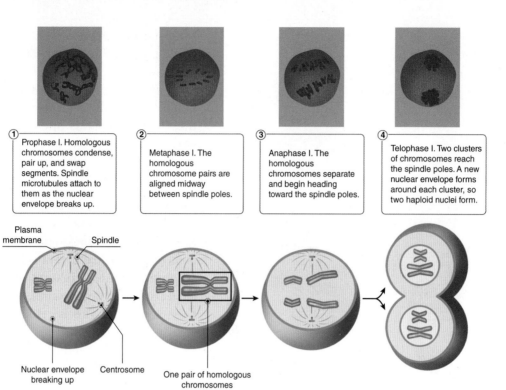

① Prophase I. Homologous chromosomes condense, pair up, and swap segments. Spindle microtubules attach to them as the nuclear envelope breaks up.

② Metaphase I. The homologous chromosome pairs are aligned midway between spindle poles.

③ Anaphase I. The homologous chromosomes separate and begin heading toward the spindle poles.

④ Telophase I. Two clusters of chromosomes reach the spindle poles. A new nuclear envelope forms around each cluster, so two haploid nuclei form.

Plasma membrane

Spindle

Nuclear envelope breaking up

Centrosome

One pair of homologous chromosomes

FIGURE 17-10 Meiosis I.

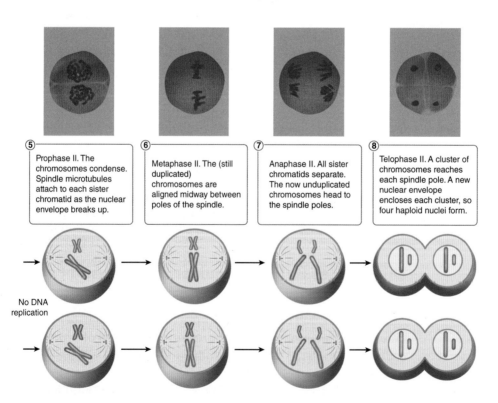

⑤ Prophase II. The chromosomes condense. Spindle microtubules attach to each sister chromatid as the nuclear envelope breaks up.

⑥ Metaphase II. The (still duplicated) chromosomes are aligned midway between poles of the spindle.

⑦ Anaphase II. All sister chromatids separate. The now unduplicated chromosomes head to the spindle poles.

⑧ Telophase II. A cluster of chromosomes reaches each spindle pole. A new nuclear envelope encloses each cluster, so four haploid nuclei form.

No DNA replication

FIGURE 17-11 Meiosis II.

Stages of
spermatogenesis

Chromosomes
in each cell

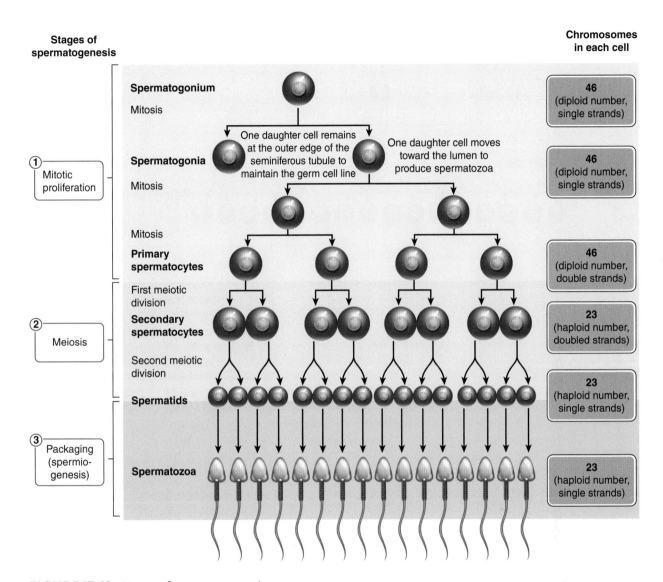

FIGURE 17-12 Stages of spermatogenesis.

In oogenesis, the metaphase plate is not in the middle of the oocyte but instead is in the margin of the dividing oocyte. As a result, the first division of meiosis in the oocyte results in two unevenly sized cells. One is large and contains most of the cytoplasm and organelles of the cell, as well as half the chromosomes of the parent cell. The small cell contains half the genetic material and very little cytoplasm; it is called the **first polar body**. During meiosis II, an **ovum** and an additional polar body form. Unlike the sperm, whose purpose is to fertilize the ovum, the ova's purpose is to provide the other structures, that is, the organelles and other cellular parts, to support the cell after fertilization. Therefore, the large ova contain the necessary structures, and the two polar bodies disintegrate.

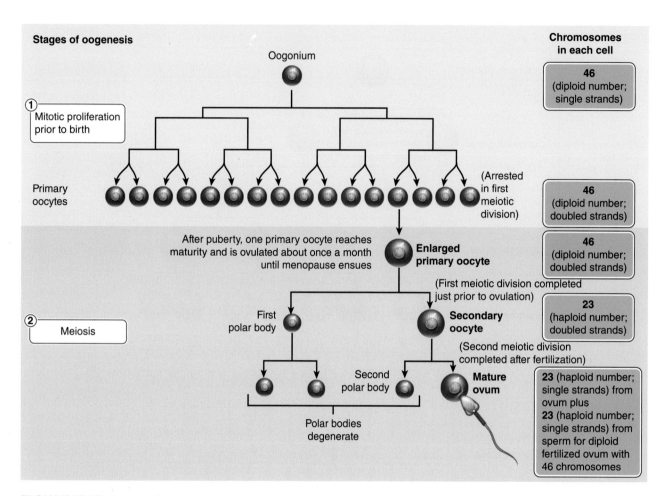

Stages of oogenesis

Oogonium

Chromosomes in each cell

① Mitotic proliferation prior to birth

| 46 (diploid number; single strands) |

Primary oocytes

(Arrested in first meiotic division)

| 46 (diploid number; doubled strands) |

After puberty, one primary oocyte reaches maturity and is ovulated about once a month until menopause ensues

Enlarged primary oocyte

| 46 (diploid number; doubled strands) |

(First meiotic division completed just prior to ovulation)

② Meiosis

First polar body

Secondary oocyte

| 23 (haploid number; doubled strands) |

(Second meiotic division completed after fertilization)

Second polar body

Mature ovum

Polar bodies degenerate

| 23 (haploid number; single strands) from ovum plus 23 (haploid number; single strands) from sperm for diploid fertilized ovum with 46 chromosomes |

FIGURE 17-13 Stages of oogenesis.

LEARNING OBJECTIVE 17.1.3 Contrast mitosis and meiosis.

KEY TERMS

mitosis Process of cell duplication so that each cell has the same number of chromosomes.

somatic cells Any cell that is not a reproductive cell.

DIFFERENCES BETWEEN MITOSIS AND MEIOSIS

The other way that a cell replicates is through the process of **mitosis**, an asexual process that produces two daughter cells with identical genetic information (Figure 17-14). In mitosis, which occurs in all body cells except gametes, the two daughter cells each have a full 23 pairs of chromosomes (46 total).

The purpose of mitosis is to create more cells that are duplicates of each other. These are used to repair damaged cells or to grow tissue. As previously explained, the purpose of meiosis is to create sex cells for reproduction (Table 17-1).

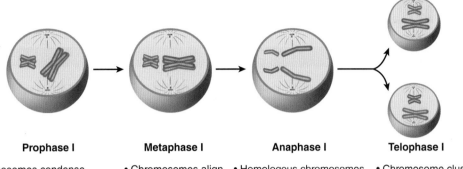

| Prophase I | Metaphase I | Anaphase I | Telophase I |

- Chromosomes condense.
- Homologous chromosomes pair.
- Crossovers occur (not shown).
- Spindle forms and attaches chromosomes to spindle poles.
- Nuclear envelope breaks up.

- Chromosomes align midway between spindle poles.

- Homologous chromosomes separate and move toward opposite spindle poles.

- Chromosome clusters arrive at spindle poles.
- New nuclear envelopes form.
- Chromosomes decondense.

FIGURE 17-14 Similarities between mitosis and meiosis.

Table 17-1 Differences between Mitosis and Meiosis

DIFFERENCES	MITOSIS	MEIOSIS
Purpose	To create duplicate **somatic cells**	To create sex cells from germ cells
Reproduction type	Asexual	Sexual
Number of divisions	One	Two
Phases	Prophase, metaphase, anaphase, telophase	Meiosis I: prophase I, metaphase I, anaphase I, telophase I Meiosis II: prophase II, metaphase II, anaphase II, telophase II
Number of daughter cells	Two	Four
Change in chromosome number	Stays the same	Reduces by half
Genetic outcome of daughter cells	Similar; crossing over does not occur so that all cells are duplicates	Different; crossing over occurs to provide genetic variation

Mitosis is an asexual process, whereas meiosis is a sexual process. One division of cells occurs in mitosis through four phases; two divisions occur in meiosis through either phase. Each daughter cell produced by mitosis contains the same genetic material. Each daughter cell produced by meiosis contains different genetic material.

Crossing over (recombination) does not occur during prophase in mitosis. In the metaphase of mitosis, individual chromosomes (pairs of *chromatids*) line up along the metaphase plate, whereas in meiosis pairs of *chromosomes* line up along the metaphase plate. During the anaphase of mitosis, sister chromatids separate toward opposite poles, whereas in meiosis, sister chromatids move together to the same pole and are then separated during anaphase II.

In sex cells, meiosis causes two divisions that produce four cells each with only 23 chromosomes. Each of these cells is genetically different from the parent cell and from each other.

LEARNING OBJECTIVE 17.1.4 Define haploid, diploid, and euploid.

KEY TERMS

diploid Cell that contains 23 pairs of chromosomes for a total of 46 chromosomes.

haploid Cell that contains half of the pairs of chromosomes.

euploid Cell that contains 23 full pairs or 46 total chromosomes.

HAPLOID, DIPLOID, AND EUPLOID

Oocytes and sperm cells are called haploid: they contain half of the 23 pairs of chromosomes. The daughter cells that are made during mitosis are referred to as diploid because they contain the full 23 pairs of chromosomes, for a total of 46 chromosomes. A cell that contains a full set of chromosomes, such as a parent cell, is also termed euploid, meaning that the cell has an exact multiple of the haploid number of chromosomes.

LEARNING OBJECTIVE 17.1.5 Explain how the process of meiosis leads to the creation of haploid sex cells.

Creation of Haploid Cells Through Meiosis

Through the steps and phases of meiosis, as explained in Section 17.1.1, four haploid cells each with half of the full set of chromosomes are created. It's worthwhile to review the process in a shortened form.

During meiosis, a germ cell first duplicates all of its chromosomes to form 23 homologue pairs. Each set of homologue pairs has identical sister chromatids.

During metaphase I, pairs of chromosomes are tightly coiled so that the genes line up with the same genes on each pair. While they are tightly coiled, bits of chromosomes cross over, or exchange places with each other, at the same location on their sister chromatid.

Next, they line up along the metaphase plate. The sorting of chromosomes to one side of the cell or the other is done randomly. In anaphase I, when the homologues are pulled apart, the sister chromatids remain attached. Cytokinesis occurs at the end of meiosis I, forming two daughter cells that now contain only one chromatid from each pair of chromosomes. These are haploid cells.

The haploid cells enter the second phase of meiosis having just one chromosome from each homologue pair. During metaphase II, the chromosomes line up individually along the metaphase plate. This time, the sister chromatids separate and are pulled to opposite sides of the cell during anaphase II. This separation is also done randomly.

Then during telophase II and cytokinesis, the two haploid daughter cells created during meiosis I become four haploid cells with 23 chromosomes, or half the set of 46.

Figure 17-15 illustrates and reviews the sequences of meiosis that results in four haploid cells in both male and female germ cells.

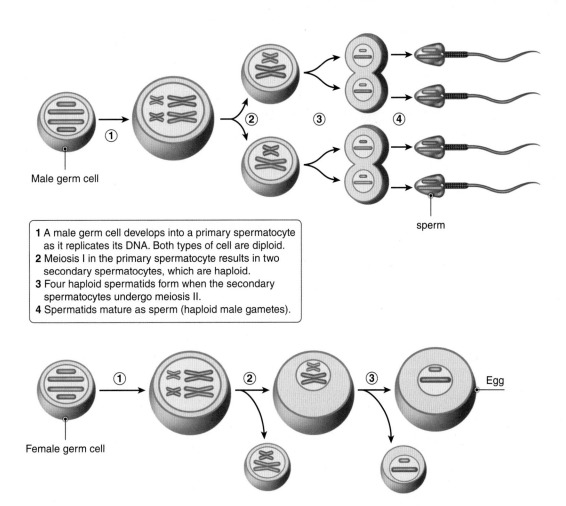

1 A male germ cell develops into a primary spermatocyte as it replicates its DNA. Both types of cell are diploid.
2 Meiosis I in the primary spermatocyte results in two secondary spermatocytes, which are haploid.
3 Four haploid spermatids form when the secondary spermatocytes undergo meiosis II.
4 Spermatids mature as sperm (haploid male gametes).

FIGURE 17-15 Creation of four haploid cells in male and female germ cells during meiosis.

LEARNING OBJECTIVE 17.1.6 Explain the relationship between haploid sex cells and the resulting genetic variability.

KEY TERMS

genes Series of DNA and proteins located on a chromosome that provides material to create body's traits and characteristics.

independent assortment Process during meiosis in which the homologous pairs of chromosomes randomly separate to form haploid cells, enabling genetic variation.

Genetic Variability in Haploid Cells

Let's look at how pieces of genes get traded and scrambled during meiosis.

Each human body cell contains DNA that holds the code for building other specific proteins in the body. Segments of DNA make up specific **genes**. Hundreds to thousands of these genes are contained in chromosomes, long strands of DNA. The 23 pairs of chromosomes in the human body consist of two sister haploids (i.e., sister chromatids that each contain 23 chromosomes) connected at the center by a centromere.

During sexual reproduction, half of the male's and half of the female's DNA contributes to the new zygote.

Meiosis I As previously explained, the creation of the haploid cells, or gametes, occurs during meiosis. Just before prophase I of meiosis (which occurs after the chromosomes have been copied into two identical, or homologous, pairs of 23 chromosomes), these homologous chromosomes tightly coil. In doing so, bits of chromosomes that contain genes cross over between the two chromosomes, recombining to form chromatids that have pieces of the other chromatid. The way the pieces cross over is random. This is where genetic variability begins.

During late prophase I, the chromosomes move to the metaphase plate and the spindle fibers attach to the centromeres. Then during anaphase I, the sister chromatids stay together while the homologous pairs of chromosomes are pulled to opposite sides of the cell—this is the opposite of what occurs during anaphase I in mitosis. This random sorting during telophase I produces two haploid cells with genetic variation that occurred during crossover.

Meiosis II During meiosis II (anaphase II), the sister chromatids separate and independently move to the opposite sides of the cell in what is called **independent assortment.** Thus, the four haploid cells that result during telophase II and cytokinesis each have nonhomologous chromosomes. They are gametes with different sets of DNA that formed during crossing over (recombination) and independent assortment. The gametes have different combinations of chromosomes, meaning some traits are similar and some are not (Figure 17-16).

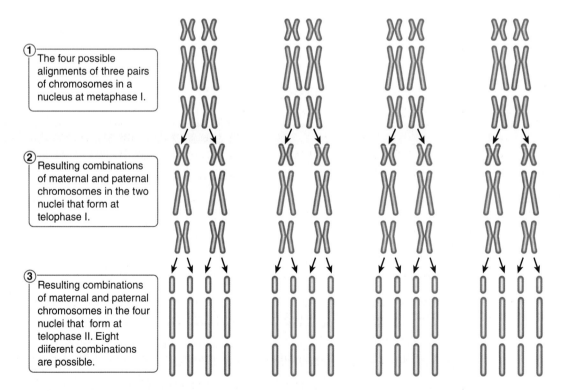

① The four possible alignments of three pairs of chromosomes in a nucleus at metaphase I.

② Resulting combinations of maternal and paternal chromosomes in the two nuclei that form at telophase I.

③ Resulting combinations of maternal and paternal chromosomes in the four nuclei that form at telophase II. Eight diiferent combinations are possible.

FIGURE 17-16 Telophase I and II.

UNIT OBJECTIVE 17.2

Describe the organs of the male reproductive system and their functions.

UNIT INTRODUCTION

The anatomy of the male reproductive system can be divided into structures that are either inside or outside of the body. These structures serve to create, store, and transport semen.

LEARNING OBJECTIVE 17.2.1 Identify the structure of each part of the male reproductive system.

LEARNING OBJECTIVE 17.2.2 Describe the structure of each part of the male reproductive system.

LEARNING OBJECTIVE 17.2.3 Identify the function of each part of the male reproductive system.

LEARNING OBJECTIVE 17.2.4 Describe the function of each part of the male reproductive system.

KEY TERMS

bulbourethral gland Glands in the male reproductive system located beneath the prostate that adds fluids to semen.

circumcision Procedure conducted to remove the foreskin of the penis.

corpus cavernosa Spongy tissue within the penis that becomes engorged with blood to cause an erection.

corpus spongiosum Mass of erectile tissue that runs along the penis.

ducts Long coiled tubes where sperm are created, matured, and stored.

ejaculation Expulsion of sperm through the penis.

epididymis Long tube that attaches to each testis where sperm mature and are stored.

erection Results when the corpora cavernosa within the penis becomes engorged with blood and causes the penis to become stiff.

flagellum Appendage that allows the sperm to swim.

foreskin Fold of skin that covers the glans of the penis.

glans External region of the clitoris (the female reproductive organ); also the head of the penis (the male reproductive organ).

Leydig cells Cells responsible in the male for the production of testosterone.

lobules Small lobes.

male sex hormones Substances that are secreted by specialized organs and glands that impact the maturation of specific body tissues.

penis Main organ of the male reproductive system.

prostate gland Gland that sits at the base of the male urinary bladder and wraps around the urethra in order to secrete a fluid that contributes to the development of semen.

scrotum Pouch of skin containing the testicles.

semen Fluid from the glands and epididymis that contains sperm.

seminal vesicles Gland within the male reproductive system.

seminiferous tubules Structures within the testes that make sperm.

Sertoli cells Cells responsible in the male for spermatogenesis.

sperm Gamete within the male anatomy that fertilizes the female egg in reproduction.

spermatogenesis Production and development of mature sperm.

testes Structure within the male anatomy that creates and stores sperm.

testosterone Steroid hormone that stimulates the development of male sexual characteristics.

urethra Canal that allows for the excretion of the urine from the urinary bladder. In males the urethra is also utilized by the reproductive system.

vas deferens Structure that transports semen.

THE MALE REPRODUCTIVE SYSTEM

The male reproductive system has both internal and external structures that are responsible for reproduction. The main external organs are the **scrotum** and **penis**. Internal structures are the **prostate gland**, **urethra**, **seminal vesicles**, **bulbourethral gland**, **vas deferens**, and **epididymis**.

Let's first take a look at the external structures (Figure 17-17).

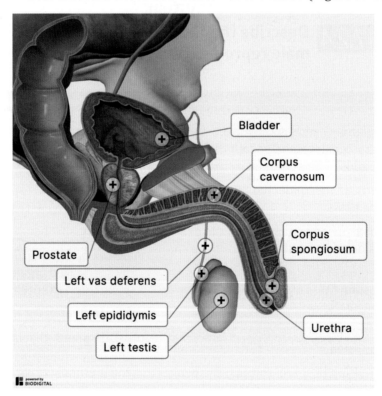

FIGURE 17-17 Cross-section of the penis shows the corpus cavernosa and corpus spongiosum around the urethra.

External Male Reproductive Structures

The penis is the major male external organ; it contains the urethra, which carries both urine and semen out of the body. The ejection of semen is called **ejaculation**. The scrotum is the other main external organ; it holds and protects the testes and hangs on either side of the penis. One testis may appear lower in the scrotum than the other, and this is normal.

The main portion of the penis is the shaft. The tip of the penis is the **glans**. At birth, the penis is covered with loose tissue called the **foreskin.** It is this tissue that is removed during a **circumcision**. The urethra, corpus cavernosa, and the corpus spongiosum are located within the penis (Figure 17-17). The **corpus cavernosa** are columns within the penis that contain blood vessels; these blood vessels fill up during sexual stimulation and cause the penis to become erect. **Corpus spongiosum** is a column of sponge-like tissue running along the front of the penis. It also fills with blood during arousal and keeps the urethra open for ejaculation.

Internal Male Reproductive Structures

The **testes** are the primary sex organs in the male reproductive system. They produce **sperm** (which are the male sex gametes produced during meiosis) and the **male sex hormones**. In the next section, you learn more about the testes and the other structures in the internal male reproductive system.

Testes The testes are oval-shaped glands housed within an external structure called the scrotum. Before birth, the testes are formed within the abdominal cavity and then descend through the inguinal canal. The scrotum is a part of the abdominal wall that pouches outward during development of the male fetus. Its location on the outside of the body keeps the sperm and male sex hormones in an environment that is about three degrees cooler than normal body temperature. This lower temperature is essential for healthy sperm.

Each testis has about 30 lobes that contain structures called **seminiferous tubules** (Figure 17-18)**.** These tubules, which are about 400 meters in length, begin to produce sperm once a male reaches puberty. Sperm are produced continuously thereafter.

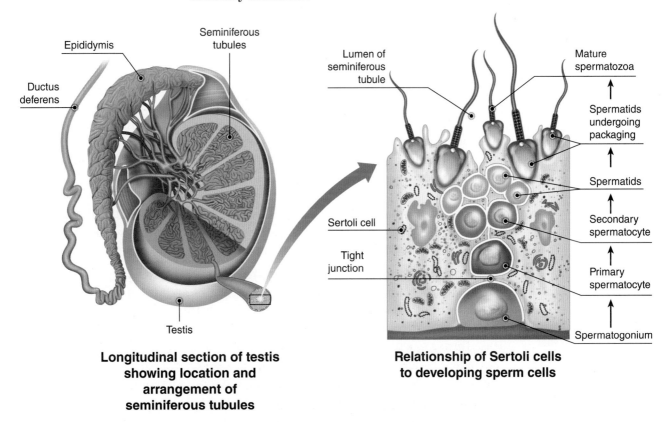

Longitudinal section of testis showing location and arrangement of seminiferous tubules

Relationship of Sertoli cells to developing sperm cells

FIGURE 17-18 Testis and its seminiferous tubules where sperm develop in varying stages.

The process of spermatogenesis was discussed in the first part of this chapter, but let's briefly review. Spermatogonia are diploid cells contained in the seminiferous tubules. They develop into spermatocytes and then spermatids during meiosis (Figure 17-19).

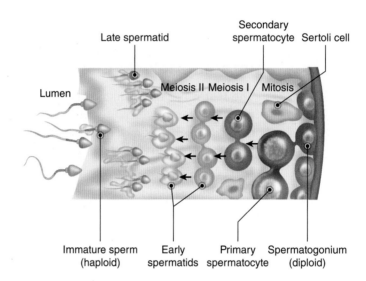

FIGURE 17-19 Spermatogenesis.

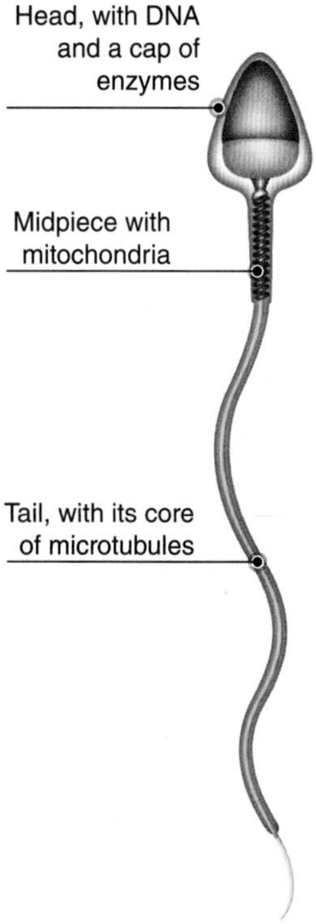

Head, with DNA and a cap of enzymes

Midpiece with mitochondria

Tail, with its core of microtubules

Spermatids become sperm, which develop tails, or **flagellum**, toward the end of development, which takes about 9–10 weeks (Figure 17-20). While sperm are maturing, they receive nutrients and chemicals from **Sertoli cells** in the seminiferous tubules.

The **Leydig cells** in the tissue surrounding the seminiferous tubules produce **testosterone**, the hormone that matures and governs the male reproductive system, including the development of secondary sexual characteristics (e.g., hair, a deeper voice).

The epididymis is a long and coiled tube on the back of each testis. The sperm that develop within the seminiferous tubules move to the epididymis where they mature and are stored. During ejaculation, the mature sperm move from the epididymis through the vas deferens and eventually out of the penis. Accessory glands produce **semen**, a secretion that helps carry the sperm. We'll learn more about them further in the chapter.

The Prostate Gland, Ducts, and Other Structures The **prostate gland**, found only in men, is a muscular gland about the size of an apricot that produces ingredients of semen. These ingredients protect the sperm and the genetic material they carry.

During ejaculation, sperm from the testes travel through two tubes called vas deferens (also called ductus deferens) to the seminal vesicles. These vesicles are attached to the prostate gland and add more ingredients to semen. As

FIGURE 17-20 Parts of the mature sperm that carry mitochondria and DNA.

the semen exits the prostate gland, the bulbourethral glands (also called Cowper's glands) add lubricant to the semen, which continues through the urethra (Figure 17-21).

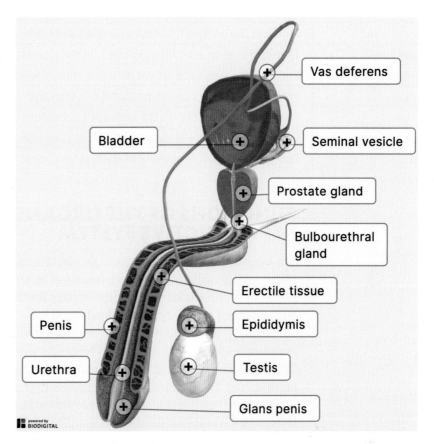

FIGURE 17-21 Vas deferens, prostate gland, bulbourethral gland, and seminal vesicle.

PURPOSE OF THE ORGANS OF THE MALE REPRODUCTIVE SYSTEM

Sexual reproduction is the way in which humans (and other animals) create another being like themselves. This method of reproduction requires both the male and the female and their reproductive systems.

The male reproductive system has three main purposes:

1. To produce, maintain, and transport sperm and protective fluid (semen).
2. To expel sperm within the female reproductive tract during intercourse.
3. To produce and secrete male sex hormones that maintain the male reproductive system.

To this end, each organ within the male reproductive system has a specific function in reproduction. The penis and urethra have an additional purpose, and that is to expel urine from the bladder. Let's take a look at the functions in Table 17-2.

Table 17-2 Structures of the Male Reproductive System

STRUCTURE	FUNCTION
Seminal vesicles	Produces and stores fluid that will become semen
Prostate gland	Produces the seminal fluid that nourishes and transports sperm
Vas deferens	Transports sperm from the epididymis to the ejaculatory ducts
Epididymis	Connects the testicle to the vas deferens; stores sperm until it undergoes maturation
Testes	Produces and stores sperm; produces testosterone
Scrotum	Contains the testes; keeps the testes at a consistent temperature
Urethra	Connects the urinary bladder to the penis; structure semen is ejaculated out of
Penis	Contains the external opening of the urethra to expel urine and semen

FUNCTIONS OF THE ORGANS OF THE MALE REPRODUCTIVE SYSTEM

The overall function of the male reproductive system is to produce sperm to fertilize ova that will develop into a fetus—in other words, to reproduce. The male hormones it produces regulate the system itself and elicit male characteristics, such as facial and body hair and a deep voice.

Briefly, the function of the penis is to eliminate urine and expel semen. The scrotum houses and protects the testes to ensure optimal sperm production. The testes are equivalent to the female ovaries in that they produce, mature, and store sperm. The **ducts** join the epididymis to transport the sperm to the prostate gland where fluids and ingredients are added from the prostate, the seminal vesicles, and the bulbourethral gland to make semen, the fluid that helps move and protects the sperm through the urethra and out of the penis during **ejaculation**.

When a man is sexually aroused, blood enters the penis, which fills the corpus spongiosum and cavernosa, an **erection** in which the penis stands upward. The connective tissue of the scrotum ensures that the temperature of the testes remain two to three degrees below body temperature. This temperature is required for optimal sperm production and health. If the temperature of the testes drops too low, the scrotal tissue will contract to bring the testes closer to the body. If the temperature of the testes is too high, the scrotal tissue will relax to place the testes further away from the body.

Whether aroused or not, the testes are busy making a continuous supply of sperm once a male has reached puberty. Each testis has hundreds of **lobules** that contain seminiferous tubules. Within each tubule Sertoli cells provide nutrients to the developing sperm, and the Leydig cells produce the hormone testosterone. During sexual stimulation, the epididymis, which lies on each testis, contracts to propel the sperm forward through the vas deferens to the seminal vesicles, prostate gland, and bulbourethral glands that add ingredients and fluids that nourish sperm, reduce acidity in the urethra, and provide a mucus-like substance to transport sperm during ejaculation.

The semen must be alkaline to transport the sperm and to fertilize the ovum. In preparation for ejaculation, the semen enters the urethra at the prostate gland. The amount of ejaculate varies between 2 and 6 mL and contains between 20 and 150 million sperm per milliliter.

Prior to ejaculation, the prostate gland secretes fluid that enters the urethra through several ducts. The prostate fluid activates the sperm to propel it through the urethra upon ejaculation.

Let's review (Figure 17-22):

- Penis: eliminates urine and expels semen
  - Corpus cavernosa: two columns of tissue on either side of the urethra containing blood vessels that fill up during sexual stimulation, causing the penis to become erect
  - Corpus spongiosum: sponge-like tissue along the front of the penis that fills with blood and keeps the urethra open when the penis is erect
  - Urethra: ejects urine or semen
  - Glans penis: head of the penis that is particularly sensitive to stimulation
- Scrotum: houses and protects the testes, keeping the testes from getting too warm
- Testes: produce, mature, and store sperm
  - Seminiferous tubules: produce sperm in the process of spermatogenesis
    - Sertoli cells: provide nutrients and chemicals to the developing sperm in the seminiferous tubules

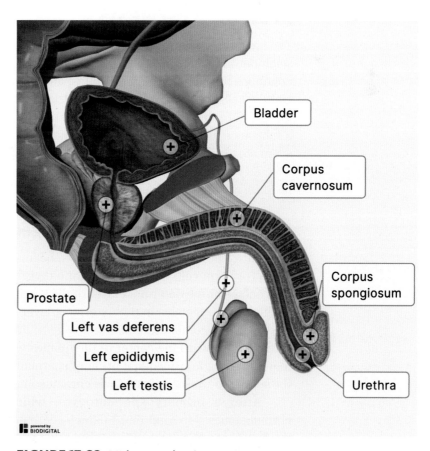

FIGURE 17-22 Male reproductive system.

- Leydig cells: produce testosterone that helps sperm and the male reproductive system to mature
  - ° Epididymis: matures and stores sperm until ejaculation
- Vas deferens (ductus deferens): transports sperm from the epididymis to the prostate gland
- Seminal vesicles: secrete components of semen
- Prostate gland: produces ingredients for semen that protects and nourishes sperm and activates its travel through the urethra
- Bulbourethral glands (or Cowper's glands): produce a mucus-like fluid to lubricate the urethra and neutralize acidity

LEARNING OBJECTIVE 17.2.5 Identify the process of spermatogenesis.

LEARNING OBJECTIVE 17.2.6 Describe the process of spermatogenesis.

KEY TERM

spermatogonia Male germ cells.

SPERMATOGENESIS

The creation of male germ cells is spermatogenesis. This process occurs in the seminiferous tubules within the testes, begins before the onset of puberty, and continues throughout the male's lifespan. Spermatogenesis begins within specialized cells called Sertoli and spermatogenic cells in the seminiferous tubules. The Sertoli and spermatogenic cells are tightly packed. The Sertoli cells secrete a substance that attracts the male hormone testosterone to feed the developing spermatozoa. The spermatogenic cells are interspersed between the Sertoli cells.

As you've previously learned in this chapter, sperm are produced through meiosis, as shown in Figure 17-23AB.

What Occurs During Spermatogenesis

Spermatogenesis, which takes 64 days, begins when the immature spermatogonia (or germ cells) engage in mitotic division to create two daughter cells. This occurs at the outermost layer of the seminiferous tubules. One of the two daughter cells remains in the outermost layer of the tubule as an undifferentiated spermatogonium to maintain the germ line. The other primary spermatocyte moves toward the center of the tubules where it divides mitotically twice more, forming four identical primary spermatocytes. Before entering meiosis, the spermatocytes duplicate their chromosomes so that each has 23 pairs.

After a primary spermatocyte, which has a diploid number of chromosomes—46 total or 23 pairs—is created during mitosis, it undergoes the first phase of meiosis. During the first meiotic division, the diploid primary spermatocyte forms two secondary spermatocytes that are haploid, meaning

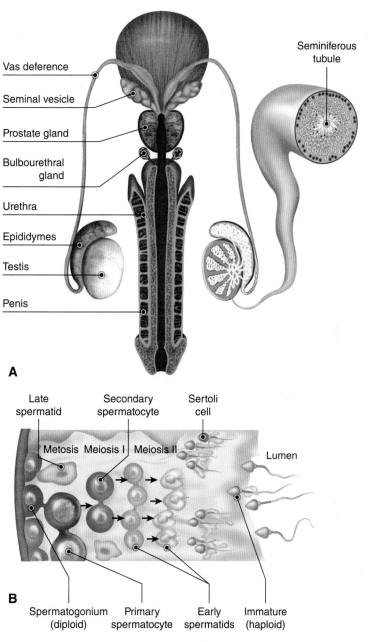

A

B

FIGURE 17-23AB Spermatogenesis begins in the seminiferous tubules where Leydig cells produce testosterone, needed for the developing sperm to move beyond meiosis. Receptors in the Sertoli cells receive testosterone signals that support spermatogenesis.

they each have 23 chromosomes or one of each pair of 46 chromosomes. During the second meiotic division, four spermatids with 23 chromosomes each form. You'll recall that meiosis produces cells with a randomly distributed haploid set of chromosomes. At this point, remodeling of the spermatids occurs to form sperm cells (Figure 17-24).

Once sperm cells are created, they are transported to the epididymis for storage and maturation. Sperm can be stored in the epididymis for several months before they are destroyed by other body cells.

Stages of
spermatogenesis

Chromosomes
in each cell

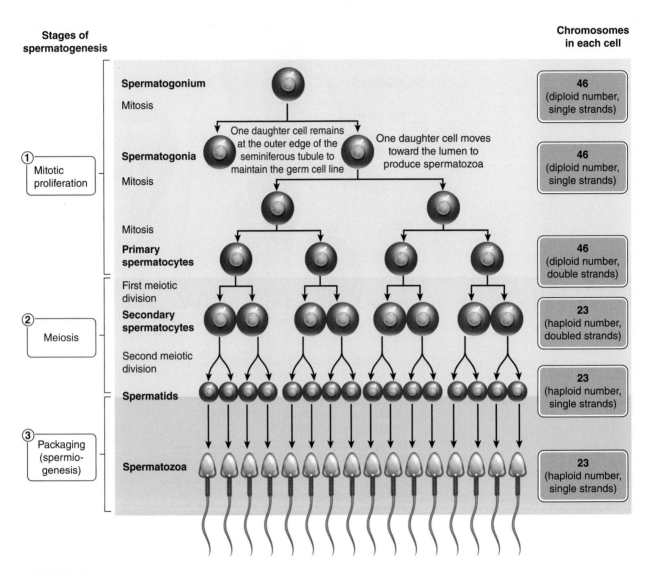

FIGURE 17-24 Process of spermatogenesis.

LEARNING
OBJECTIVE **17.2.7** Describe semen production.

KEY TERMS

ejaculatory duct Duct formed by the seminal vesicle as it enters the prostate gland.

fructose Sugar substance used for sperm motility.

prostaglandins Hormone-like substance that propels the sperm toward the ovary.

PRODUCTION OF SEMEN

Semen is produced by the testes, epididymis, prostate gland, seminal vesicles, and the bulbourethral glands. Included in semen are sperm cells created in the testes and liquid secretions from these other organs. The testes also produce testosterone and inhibin. Inhibin is a hormone that inhibits production of follicle-stimulating hormone in the pituitary gland.

The seminal vesicles, located on the posterior portion of the urinary bladder, are lined with cells that secrete fructose, prostaglandins, and proteins. The fructose provides the energy for sperm motility. The prostaglandins move the sperm toward the female ovary. The proteins provide nourishment to the sperm. Fluid from the seminal vesicles supplies about 70% of semen volume.

Each seminal vesicle has a duct that meets to form the ejaculatory duct. This duct enters the posterior portion of the prostate gland and ends at the urethra. The prostate gland secretes a thin milky fluid that includes acid phosphatase, enzymes, and immunoglobulin. The fluid is about 20% of the volume of semen. The bulbourethral glands, located on either side of the urethra, secrete a clear mucus-like fluid, which accounts for about 5% of semen.

LEARNING OBJECTIVE 17.2.8 Identify the pathway semen follows when exiting the body.

PATHWAY FOR SEMEN TO EXIT THE BODY

In order for the ejaculation process to occur, semen follows the following pathway to leave the body:

- During sexual stimulation, the sperm leave the epididymis, where they have been stored, and enter the vas deferens.
  - From the vas deferens, they travel to the prostate gland.
  - Before sperm enter the prostate gland, they are first mixed with the fructose, prostaglandins, and proteins from the seminal vesicles; once mixed, they flow into the prostate gland through the ejaculatory duct.
  - Once in the prostate gland, the sperm mixes with the milky fluid secreted by the prostate gland and other chemicals.
  - From the prostate, the sperm and forming semen enter the bulbourethral glands, which secretes mucus-like liquid. The sperm and this liquid combine to form semen.
  - The semen enters the urethra and travels to the end of the penis, from which it is expelled during ejaculation (Figure 17-25).

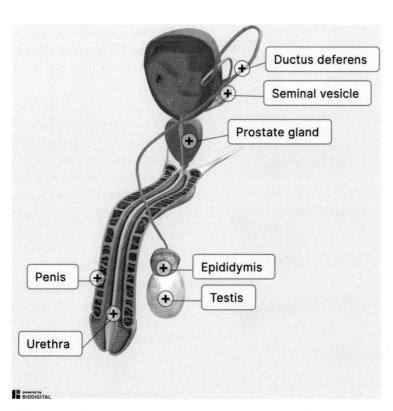

FIGURE 17-25 Pathway of semen.

LEARNING OBJECTIVE 17.2.9 Explain the physiological mechanisms that lead to erection.

KEY TERMS

detumescence Penis's return to a flaccid state.

neurotransmitters Molecule secreted by neurons that produces changes in other neurons or organs.

parasympathetic nervous system Portion of the autonomic nervous system (ANS) that promotes digestive and excretory processes.

sympathetic nervous system Region of the autonomic nervous system that activates the fight-or-flight response.

PROCESS OF AN ERECTION

An erection is a complex neurophysiological process that is controlled by hormones, neurotransmitters, and the vascular system. Coordination of the sympathetic, parasympathetic, and somatic pathways is required. Sensory or mental sexual stimulation signals the parasympathetic nervous system in the sacral spine to send stimulatory input to the neurotransmitters in the corpus cavernosa, causing the smooth muscles of this area to relax and arteries to dilate. The impulses from the parasympathetic nervous system also cause release of nitric oxide, which further relaxes the corpus cavernosa. At the same time, veins constrict to block the outflow of blood from the penis.

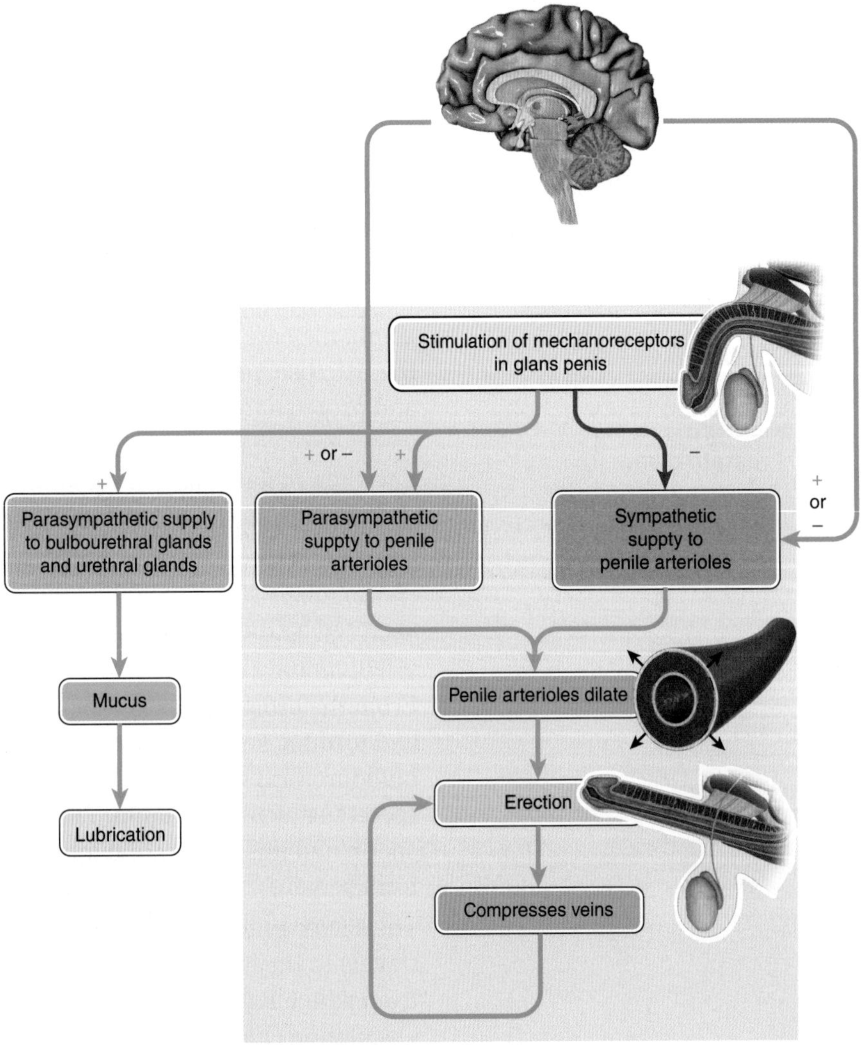

Blood flow to the corpus cavernosa increases, filling the empty spaces. The engorged penis elongates and begins to point outward or upward. The pressure in the corpus cavernosa increases above diastolic blood pressure, and the penis becomes rigid (Figure 17-26).

Detumescence, or a return to the flaccid state of the penis, requires the sympathetic nervous system to contract the smooth muscle of the penis. Contraction of the arteries pushes the blood back out of the corpus cavernosa, and the penis returns to its flaccid state.

FIGURE 17-26 Erection reflex.

LEARNING OBJECTIVE 17.2.10 Identify the hormones that control the activity and development of male secondary sex characteristics.

KEY TERMS

androgens Hormones that regulate the growth and development of the male reproductive system.

follicle-stimulating hormone (FSH) Stimulates spermatogenesis in males and ovarian follicle maturation in females while also producing estrogen.

gonadotropin-releasing hormone (GnRH) Controls the release of gonadotropins, follicle-stimulating hormone, and luteinizing hormone.

hypothalamus Region of the cerebrum that controls body states such as hunger, thirst, and body temperature and regulates hormone release from the pituitary gland.

inhibin A hormone that is produced from the testis and ovary prevents the production of follicle-stimulating hormone (FSH) from the pituitary gland.

luteinizing hormone (LH) Promotes testosterone production in males and ovulation in females while also producing estrogen and progesterone.

pituitary gland A pea sized gland that is housed in the sella turcica and is the master regulator of the endocrine system, controlling the activity of numerous hormone secreting glands.

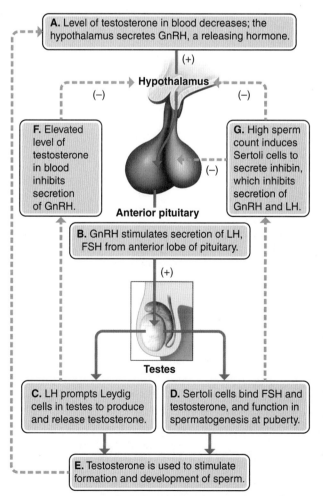

A. Level of testosterone in blood decreases; the hypothalamus secretes GnRH, a releasing hormone.

(+)

Hypothalamus

(−)   (−)

F. Elevated level of testosterone in blood inhibits secretion of GnRH.

G. High sperm count induces Sertoli cells to secrete inhibin, which inhibits secretion of GnRH and LH.

(−)

Anterior pituitary

B. GnRH stimulates secretion of LH, FSH from anterior lobe of pituitary.

(+)

Testes

C. LH prompts Leydig cells in testes to produce and release testosterone.

D. Sertoli cells bind FSH and testosterone, and function in spermatogenesis at puberty.

E. Testosterone is used to stimulate formation and development of sperm.

FIGURE 17-27 Role of hormones in the male reproductive system.

HORMONES OF THE MALE REPRODUCTIVE SYSTEM

Hormones from the **hypothalamus** and anterior **pituitary gland**, as well as the testosterone produced by the testes, control the male reproductive system. At puberty, the hypothalamus sends **gonadotropin-releasing hormone (GnRH)** to the pituitary. The pituitary then releases **follicle-stimulating hormone (FSH)** and **luteinizing hormone (LH)** into the blood. FSH enters the testes to stimulate Sertoli cells to start spermatogenesis. LH enters the testes and stimulates Leydig cells to make and release the **androgen** testosterone. Testosterone stimulates spermatogenesis and begins the development of secondary sex characteristics.

A negative feedback loop prevents the overproduction of sperm. As testosterone levels increase, they act on the hypothalamus and pituitary to decrease the release of GnRH, FSH, and LH. The Sertoli cells also produce the hormone **inhibin** when the sperm count gets too high. Inhibin inhibits the release of GnRH and LH by the hypothalamus and LH and FSH by the pituitary. This negative feedback loop slows spermatogenesis (Figure 17-27).

LEARNING OBJECTIVE 17.2.11 Explain how hormones control the activity and development of male sex characteristics.

Action of Hormones on Male Sex Characteristics

At the onset of **puberty**, the hypothalamus and pituitary gland in the brain increase the production of androgens, or male hormones.

From the hypothalamus comes GnRH, which stimulates the pituitary to secrete LH and FSH. LH causes the testes to produce testosterone. FSH and testosterone together kick-start spermatogenesis. Testosterone also spurs the development of secondary sex characteristics such as axillary, chest, facial, and pubic hair. The male vocal cords lengthen and thicken, deepening the voice. Testosterone also enhances bone growth and increases the number and thickness of muscle fibers in the male body.

Through the action of these hormones, sexual development then occurs in the following sequence and usually within the timeframes listed:

- The scrotum and testes enlarge (ages 10½–17 years)
- The penis lengthens (ages 11–13)
- The seminal vesicles and prostate gland enlarge (ages 11–13)
- Pubic hair grows (ages 11–15)
- Growth spurt occurs (ages 13–17)
- Axillary and facial hair grows (ages 13–18)
- Ejaculation becomes possible (ages 12½–14)

UNIT OBJECTIVE 17.3

Describe the organs of the female reproductive system and their functions.

UNIT INTRODUCTION

The anatomy of the female reproductive system can be divided into structures that are either inside or outside of the body. These structures serve two functions. The first is to create, store, and release ovum. The second function is to nurture and grow the fetus after fertilization occurs and continue to provide nutrients for the baby after birth.

LEARNING OBJECTIVE 17.3.1 Identify the structure of each part of the female reproductive system.

LEARNING OBJECTIVE 17.3.2 Describe the structure of each part of the female reproductive system.

LEARNING OBJECTIVE **17.3.3** Identify the function of each part of the female reproductive system.

LEARNING OBJECTIVE **17.3.4** Describe the function of each part of the female reproductive system.

KEY TERMS

mammary alveoli Glands within the ducts of breast tissue that secrete milk.

ampullae (also called lactiferous sinuses) Expanded areas at the ends of the mammary ducts that are close to the nipple.

antrum Term used to describe the cavity that is formed when an oocyte is maturing.

areola Area of pigmented tissue that surrounds the breast nipple and contains sebaceous and sweat glands.

Bartholin's glands Gland that provides lubrication to the vagina during sexual stimulation.

body of the uterus Large central area of the uterus that tapers to the cervix.

cervical canal Interior portion of the cervix.

cervix Projects into the vagina and forms a pathway between the uterus and the vagina.

cilia Hair-like projections that move in a wavelike manner that support movement.

clitoris Erectile organ like the male penis that is highly sensitive and distends during sexual arousal.

coitus Sexual intercourse.

embryo After fertilization, the zygote or fertilized egg forms into an embryo, an unborn offspring; early stages of fetal growth approximately from the second week to the eighth week.

endometrium Inner layer of the uterus.

estrogen

external os Cervix's opening into the vagina.

fallopian tubes Thin structures that are attached to the uterus on one end and are open to the ovaries on the other end.

fertilization Outcome when a sperm cell penetrates an ovum.

fetus Infant before birth that develops from the embryo and remains in the uterus for approximately 40 weeks.

fimbriae Finger-like projections attached to one end of the fallopian tubes that hover over the ovary.

fornix The recessed area of the vagina that is close to the cervix.

uterine fundus Top portion of the uterus.

germinal epithelium Outermost covering of the ovaries.

glans Exposed portion of the clitoris; also the head of the penis.

Graafian follicle Mature ova.

hymen Thin layer of tissue that partially covers the vestibule.

infundibulum End of the fallopian tubes nearest the ovary.

internal os Cervix's external upper connection to the uterus.

isthmus Area between the body of the uterus and the cervix.

labia majora Outermost folds of skin and fat tissue covered with hair that begins at the mons pubis and ends at the anus.

labia minora Folds of skin tissue that are pink, hairless, and are located between the clitoris and the base of the vagina.

lactation Production of breast milk.

lactiferous ducts Duct that leads to the nipple and opens to the outside

mammary glands Enlarged, modified sweat glands found in the breasts of females.

menstruation First phase of the female reproductive cycle where contents of the uterus are discharged as menstrual fluid.

mons pubis Pad of fat tissue located on top of the symphysis pubis bone and is covered with skin and hair.

myometrium Middle layer of the uterine wall comprised of muscle tissue.

nipple Tissue of the breast where milk is excreted.

oocytes Immature gamete within the ovary.

oogenesis Development of an ovum.

ovarian follicles Follicles found in the ovaries that secrete hormones that influence the stages of the menstrual cycle.

ovaries Female reproductive organ located in the pelvic cavity responsible for the secretion of hormones involved in secondary-sex characteristic development and menstruation.

ovulation Release of an ovum from the ovaries.

perimetrium Outer layer of uterine tissue.

perineum Area between the buttocks and thighs.

prepuce Layer of skin that covers the clitoris.

progesterone Steroid hormone that stimulates the uterus to prepare for pregnancy.

pudendum External female reproductive organs including the mons pubis, clitoris, labia major,

labia minora, hymen, Bartholin's glands, Skene's glands, and vaginal and urethral orifices.

Skene's glands Gland that provides lubrication to the vagina during sexual stimulation.

tunica albuginea Collagenous connective tissue that makes up the germinal epithelium.

urethral orifice Opening of the urethra within the vestibule.

uterine cavity Interior of the uterus.

uterus Hollow pear-shaped organ located between the bladder and rectum.

vagina Fibromuscular tube located behind the bladder and urethra and in front of the rectum.

vaginal orifice Opening of the vagina within the vestibule.

vestibule Area of the female anatomy that contains the openings to the vagina and urethra and glands.

vulva Also called pudendum; refers to the external female genitalia.

zygote Cell that results from fertilization of the ovum by the sperm; it contains 46 chromosomes, 23 from the ovum and 23 from the sperm.

STRUCTURES AND FUNCTIONS OF THE PARTS OF THE FEMALE REPRODUCTIVE SYSTEM

Like the male reproductive system, the female system has both internal and external parts. External parts contain stimulatory organs and lubricating glands to prepare the female for sexual intercourse. The internal female reproductive system does the work of creating an ovum, preparing the uterus for implanting of a fertilized egg, and growing the fetus until it is born.

Internal Female Reproductive Structures

The internal organs of the female reproductive system are primarily located inside the pelvic cavity (Figure 17-28). The primary sex organs of the female reproductive system are the ovaries. This pair of glands are the size of walnuts. They are located in the upper pelvic cavity on each side of the uterus. Holding them in place are ligaments. The function of the ovaries is to produce the female gametes, or ova.

Ovaries The ovaries are the primary female sex glands where ova develop. They're rather complicated glands. First is the external covering, called the germinal epithelium. This is made of collagenous connective tissue, or tunica albuginea. The tunica albuginea has two areas, including the outer cortex where ovarian follicles develop. The inner area is the stroma of the medulla.

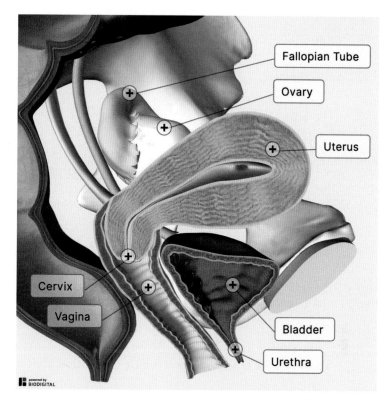

FIGURE 17-28 Organs of the female reproductive system.

The ovarian follicles contain immature ova, called **oocytes**, and surrounding tissues. The ova develop within the ovarian follicles that increase in size. The follicle develops a fluid-filled center called the **antrum** and is now called a secondary follicle. Once this follicle matures, it is called a **Graafian follicle**, and it begins to secrete the female hormone **estrogen**. The Graafian follicle expels the ova during **ovulation** (Figure 17-29). The ovaries also secrete the female hormone **progesterone**.

Fallopian Tubes The **fallopian tubes** are attached to the uterus on one end and opened on the other end to align with the ovaries. They are made of smooth muscle and lined with mucus and cilia. Each end of the fallopian tube hovers over an ovary like a funnel, to capture ova released from the ovaries and transport them to the uterus. The end of the fallopian tube nearest the ovary is called the **infundibulum**, which is shaped like a funnel. It is not attached to the ovary, but it has finger-like projections called **fimbriae** that create a wavelike motion that sweeps the ova into the fallopian tube when it is released during ovulation. The **cilia** within the fallopian tube create a wavelike motion that continues as the smooth muscle of the tube contracts and moves the ova into the uterus.

Uterus The **uterus** is an organ shaped like a pear with the wider end at the top. It lies between the rectum and bladder. Within the uterus the fertilized ovum is planted, the fetus develops, and labor begins.

The uterus is held in place by four ligaments: the broad ligaments attach the uterus to the left and right pelvic bones; the round ligaments support the

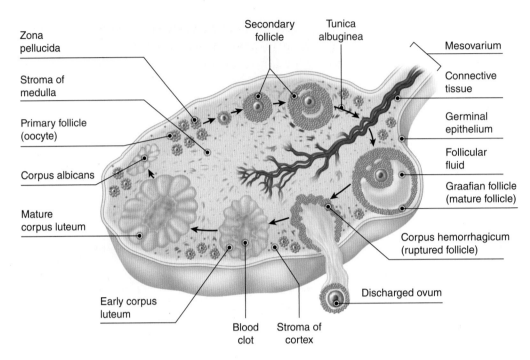

FIGURE 17-29 Stages of follicle maturation, starting with the primary follicle.

fundus; the uterosacral ligaments support the uterus at the sacrum; and the cardinal ligaments support the sides of the uterus. The uppermost, bigger end of the uterus is the **uterine fundus**. The central area that tapers is the **body of the uterus**. The connecting ring at the bottom of the uterus that leads into the vagina is the cervix. Between the body and cervix is an area called the **isthmus**. The interior of the uterus is the **uterine cavity**, and the interior of the cervix is the **cervical canal**. The cervix's external upper connection to the uterus is the **internal os**, and the opening into the vagina is called the **external os**.

The wall of the uterus has an innermost layer called the **endometrium**, a middle layer called the **myometrium**, and the outermost layer called the **perimetrium**. The three layers of tissue in the uterus have specific functions. The perimetrium is similar to the other tissue within the abdominal cavity. The myometrium consists of muscle tissue and makes up the major part of the uterine wall. The contraction of this muscle layer is what expels menstrual blood or a baby during childbirth. The endometrium is the innermost layer that changes in amount and consistency during the menstrual cycle and pregnancy. During menstruation, the endometrial lining is shed. If fertilization occurs, the fertilized ovum is implanted in this layer during pregnancy.

Vagina A passageway, called the **vagina**, connects the uterus to the external female genitalia. Menstrual flow departs the uterus and flows through the vagina. The vagina is where the penis is inserted during sexual intercourse. During birth, the vagina is part of the birth canal where the fetus passes to the outside world.

Between the uterus and the vagina is the **cervix**, a neck-like circle of fibro-muscular tissue. The cervix is located at the end of the vagina and is considered the lower portion of the uterus. The cervix produces mucus that changes consistency during the menstrual cycle to promote or prevent fertilization. The area of the vagina that is close to the cervix is a recess called the **fornix**. The cervix has a small opening through which semen enters the uterus during sexual intercourse. Menstrual blood flows through the cervix during menstruation. During pregnancy, a mucus plug forms at the cervix to protect the uterus.

External Female Reproductive Structures

External female reproductive organs include the mons pubis, clitoris, labia majora, labia minora, hymen, Bartholin's glands, Skene's glands, and vaginal and urethral orifices (Figure 17-30). This portion of the female reproductive system is sometimes collectively referred to as the **vulva**, or the **pudendum**.

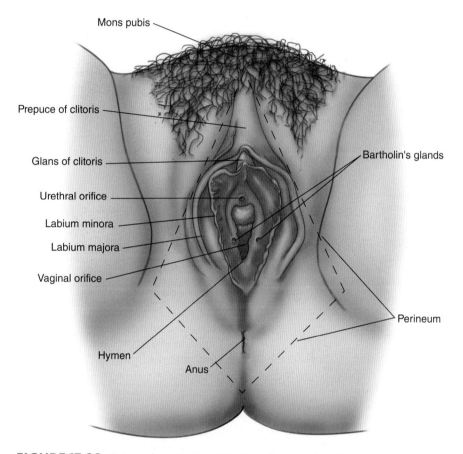

FIGURE 17-30 External genitalia of the female reproductive system.

Covering the pubic symphysis is the **mons pubis**, a mound of fat tissue that at puberty becomes covered with pubic hair. Two folds of hair-covered skin containing fat and sweat glands are called the **labia majora**. The folds extend from the mons pubis longitudinally toward the anus. Within the labia majora are the **labia minora**, folds of skin without hair but containing a few sweat glands and numerous sebaceous glands. The function of the mons pubis, including the labia majora and labia minora, are to protect the internal structures.

At the top of the labia minora is the **clitoris**, a small mass of erectile tissue that can enlarge when blood flows into it during sexual stimulation. The clitoris provides sexual stimulation to the female during intercourse, or **coitus**. A layer of skin, the **prepuce**, covers part of the clitoris; the exposed part of the clitoris is the **glans**. The area between the labia minora is the **vestibule**, partially covered by a thin layer of tissue called the **hymen.** The **vaginal orifice** and **urethral orifice** open within the vestibule. The **Skene's glands** are located on either side of the urethral orifice and secrete mucus, as do the **Bartholin's glands,** which are located on either side of the vaginal orifice. Secretions from these two pairs of glands lubricate the vagina to facilitate the entry of the penis during sexual intercourse. The **perineum** is the area between the buttocks and thighs of both men and women.

Mammary Glands Although both men and women have **mammary glands,** they normally function only in women. Estrogen causes the mammary glands to grow larger during puberty. Each mammary gland contains 15–20 lobes surrounded by fat tissue. This fat is what determines the size of the breast.

Within the lobes are small compartments, or lobules. The lobules contain **mammary alveoli,** cells that secrete milk. The alveoli look like grape clusters and they connect to the **nipple** of the breast with ducts. At the ends of these ducts closest to the nipple there are expanded areas called **ampullae** or **lactiferous sinuses.** These ampullae contain stored milk and connect to the nipple via **lactiferous ducts** (Figure 17-31).

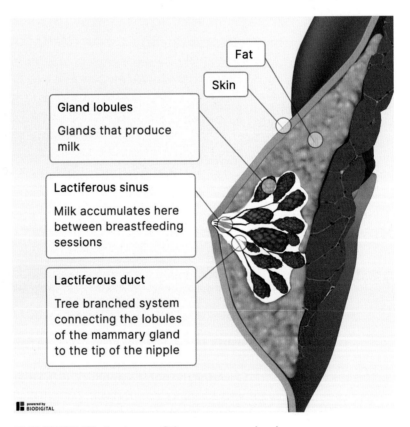

FIGURE 17-31 Anatomy of the mammary glands.

The pigmented area that encircles the nipple of the breast is the **areola.** It contains sebaceous glands.

The process of secreting milk from the mammary glands is called **lactation.** Lactation occurs so that the mother can provide nutrients for survival to her newborn baby after birth and during the beginning of the child's life.

Table 17-3 summarizes the functions of the internal and external organs of the female reproductive system.

Table 17-3 Internal and External Structures of the Female Reproductive System

STRUCTURE	FUNCTION
Mons pubis	Protects the internal structures of the female reproductive system
Clitoris	Provides sexual stimulation to the female
Vagina	Receives penis and ejaculate during sexual intercourse; expands during labor to provide a path for the newborn from the uterus; route for expulsion of menstrual blood
Cervix	Opening through which semen enters the uterus and menstrual blood is expelled from the uterus
Uterus	Provides a place for a fertilized ovum to implant and for the fetus to develop during gestation
Fallopian tubes	Pathway for a mature ova to travel from the ovaries to the uterus
Ovaries	Produce ovum and female reproductive hormones
Mammary Glands	Secrete milk during lactation to provide nutrients to a newborn

PURPOSE OF THE STRUCTURES OF THE FEMALE REPRODUCTIVE SYSTEM

The female reproductive system, much like the male system, exists for the purpose of procreation. It is the way in which humans reproduce. An ovum erupts from the ovary every month and travels down the fallopian tube where it may or may not be fertilized by a male sperm. If not fertilized, the uterus sheds its innermost layer of tissue and blood, a process called **menstruation**.

If a sperm penetrates the ovum, **fertilization** occurs—usually in the upper two-thirds of the tube. An **embryo** and then a **fetus** develop within the uterus and is born approximately 40 weeks after fertilization.

LEARNING OBJECTIVE 17.3.5 Identify the process of oogenesis.

KEY TERMS

oogenesis Development of an ovum.

oogonia Female germ cells.

primary oocytes Oocyte that has divided mitotically and contains 46 chromosomes.

OOGENESIS

Oogenesis is the generation of female eggs or ova. In Unit 1 of this chapter, we discussed the process of oogenesis, but here we follow the ova through the steps of becoming a mature ovum.

Oogenesis involves both mitosis and meiosis, much like what happens during spermatogenesis. But there are some big differences. The germ cells of females are called **oogonia**. Oogenesis occurs before birth in the female fetus. First, mitotic division produces about 7 million oogonia by the time the fetus is about five months old. Then toward the end of gestation, the oocytes begin, but do not complete, meiosis.

The oocytes that have divided mitotically contain the diploid number of chromosomes, 46, or 23 pairs. They are now called **primary oocytes**. Meiosis stops in these primary oocytes until ovulation occurs many years later (Figure 17-32).

In the next section, we'll see how the primary oocytes continue their journey to becoming ova.

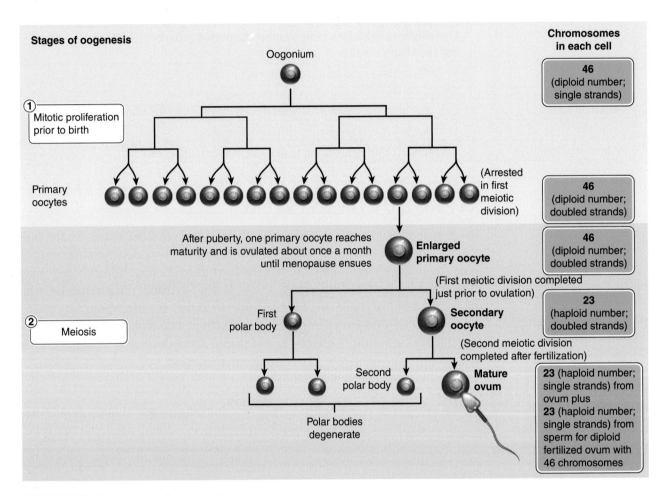

FIGURE 17-32 Process of oogenesis.

LEARNING OBJECTIVE **17.3.6** Describe the process of oogenesis.

KEY TERMS

atresia Degeneration of a follicle.

first polar body Small haploid cell formed during meiosis of the female sex cell that does not have the ability to be fertilized.

gestation Pregnancy; conception to birth.

granulosa cells Single layer of connective tissue that covers the primary oocyte.

mature ovum (also called ootid) Secondary oocyte.

menopause End of the reproductive capability of the female.

primordial follicles Immature ova.

second polar body One of the female daughter cells that are created during the second phase of meiosis that disintegrates.

secondary oocytes Female daughter cell formed during the second phase of meiosis and becomes an ovum.

zygote Cell that results from fertilization of the ovum by the sperm; it contains 46 chromosomes, 23 from the ovum and 23 from the sperm.

Process of Oogenesis

The primary oocyte is enclosed in a single layer of connective tissue, called granulosa cells. Together the primary oocyte and granulosa cells are called the primordial follicles. Some primary oocytes don't reach this stage, however, and instead self-destruct. By the time of birth, only about 2 million primordial follicles are still alive. After birth, no new oocytes are created. The primordial follicles hold the primary oocytes until ovulation occurs. Over the lifespan, these primordial follicles begin to disintegrate.

The developing follicles will either reach maturity and ovulate or they will degenerate, forming scar tissue. This latter process is called atresia. By the time of puberty, only about 300,000 follicles remain, and only about 400 will release ova. The rest have undergone atresia. By menopause, few remain, and a woman's ability to reproduce ends.

Starting at puberty, some of the primary oocytes will mature into secondary oocytes. Why some do not mature is unknown.

The primary oocytes that mature will enlarge and the cell layers will differentiate. Just before ovulation occurs, a primary oocyte completes the first phase of meiosis that had been halted at the end of gestation. Its division during meiosis produces two daughter cells with a haploid number of chromosomes 23.

Nearly all of the cytoplasm surrounding the primary oocyte stays with just one daughter cell. This cell is called the secondary oocyte, which will become an ovum. The 23 chromosomes of the other daughter cell and the remaining amount of cytoplasm form what is called the first polar body. This first polar body disintegrates.

If the secondary oocyte is fertilized by a sperm, it will become an ovum and begin the second phase of meiosis. If unfertilized, the remaining secondary oocyte does not divide.

Meanwhile, the fertilized secondary oocyte divides again during the second phase of meiosis. Again, a half set of the chromosomes and a small amount of cytoplasm form a second polar body. The other half set of chromosomes and larger amount of cytoplasm become the mature ovum. The second polar body disintegrates.

Fertilization is complete when the 23 chromosomes of the ovum and the 23 chromosomes of the sperm unite to form a zygote with the full set of 46 chromosomes.

LEARNING OBJECTIVE 17.3.7 List the steps that occur in the process of oogenesis.

Steps in Oogenesis

The steps in the process of oogenesis are as follows (Figure 17-33AB):

1. In the sixth week of intrauterine life, the ovaries and oocytes are developed.
2. Upon birth the oocytes remain as primary/primordial follicles.
3. At puberty, FSH and LH are released from the pituitary gland.
4. FSH and LH cause primary/primordial follicles to mature by increasing the size and granulosa tissue develops a wall around the oocytes.
5. A membrane called the zona pellucida develops and surrounds the ovum for fluid to accumulate.
6. FSH causes the cells in the oocyte to develop a sheath of connective tissue or the theca folliculi.
7. Theca folliculi divide into an internal layer called the theca interna and an outer layer called the theca externa.
8. The theca interna produces androgens and the theca externa serves as connective tissue.
9. As the oocyte enlarges, a cavity or antrum is formed that causes the oocyte to be moved to one side of the follicle. The oocyte is surrounded by granulosa cells called the corona radiata.
10. The granulosa cells begin to produce estrogen. At this time, the selection of a dominant oocyte occurs.
11. Oocytes that are not dominant degenerate. The dominant oocyte accumulates more granulosa cells as the theca become more vascular.
12. The release of estrogen stops the secretion of FSH and increases the secretion of LH.
13. The increase in LH causes the oocyte to burst and be ejected from the follicle at which time it is picked up by the fallopian tube for transport to the uterus.

14. The empty follicle collapses and is filled with blood and fluid called the **corpus luteum**.

15. The corpus luteum secretes progesterone to maintain the integrity of the ovum if fertilization occurs.

16. If fertilization does not occur, the corpus luteum atrophies and is replaced by scar tissue called the **corpus albicans**.

17. Progesterone stops being excreted and menstruation occurs.

18. If fertilization occurs, the embryo produces the **human chorionic gonadotropin hormone** to maintain LH levels.

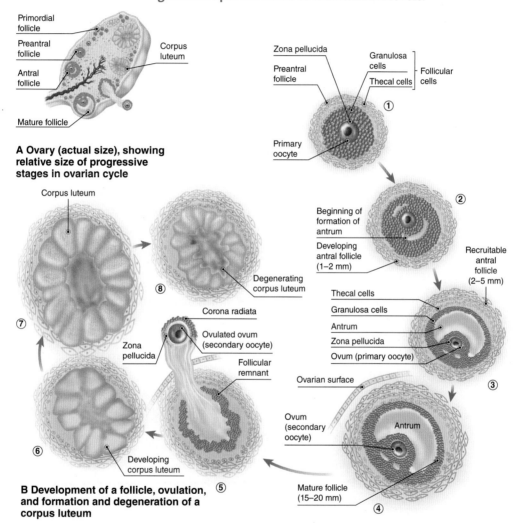

A Ovary (actual size), showing relative size of progressive stages in ovarian cycle

B Development of a follicle, ovulation, and formation and degeneration of a corpus luteum

1 During development of a preantral follicle, under the influence of local paracrines, granulosa cells proliferate, the zona pellucida forms around the oocyte, and surrounding ovarian connective tissue cells differentiate into thecal cells.

2 During early development of an antral follicle, an estrogen-rich antrum starts to form and the follicle continues to enlarge.

3 Antral follicles that have reached a given size at the beginning of the follicular phase of the ovarian cycle are recruited for further rapid development and antrum expansion under the influence of FSH.

4 After about 2 weeks of rapid growth under the influence of FSH, the follicle has developed into a mature follicle, which has a greatly expanded antrum; the oocyte, which by now has developed into a secondary oocyte, is displaced to one side.

5 At midcycle, in response to a burst in LH secretion, the mature follicle, bulging on the ovarian surface, ruptures and releases the oocyte, resulting in ovulation and ending the follicular phase.

6 Ushering in the luteal phase, the ruptured follicle develops into a corpus luteum under the influence of LH.

7 The corpus luteum continues to grow and secrete progesterone and estrogen that prepare the uterus for implantation of a fertilized ovum.

8 After 14 days, if a fertilized ovum does not implant in the uterus, the corpus luteum degenerates, the luteal phase ends, and a new follicular phase begins under the influence of a changing hormonal milieu.

FIGURE 17-33AB Follicular phases.

LEARNING OBJECTIVE **17.3.8** Identify the hormones that control the activity and development of female sexual characteristics.

LEARNING OBJECTIVE **17.3.9** Explain how hormones control the activity and development of female sexual characteristics.

KEY TERMS

estradiol One of three estrogen hormones; the most abundant.

estriol One of three estrogen hormones.

estrone One of three estrogen hormones.

menarche First menstrual period.

menstrual cycle Cycle of physiological changes that occur from the beginning of one menstrual period to the beginning of the next.

prolactin Hormone within the female reproductive system that stimulates breast tissue to produce breast milk.

HORMONES OF THE FEMALE REPRODUCTIVE SYSTEM

Although quite a few hormones have already been explained during the previous section, additional information is reviewed here. Estrogens are a group of sex hormones that are necessary for normal female development and maintenance of female characteristics in the human body. Levels of these hormones vary through a woman's lifespan.

There are three estrogen hormones: estrone, estradiol, and estriol. Estradiol is the most abundant. These hormones are produced mainly by the ovaries, with additional amounts produced in fat tissue. Progesterone is also produced by the ovaries, in the corpus luteum. It prepares the endometrium for potential implantation with a fertilized ovum. Low progesterone levels can make pregnancy difficult to attain or maintain.

Estrone is a weak form of estrogen and is present in most body tissues, but mostly in fat and muscle. The female body can convert estrone into estradiol and estradiol to estrone.

Estradiol is the strongest type of estrogen. It may contribute to disorders such as endometriosis, fibroid tumors, and cancers in women.

Estriol is the weakest estrogen and is actually a waste product of estradiol. During pregnancy, estriol plays a larger role.

Action of Hormones on Female Sex Characteristics

The three estrogens cause prolactin release from the pituitary gland to promote breast development and milk production. Estrogen influences the structural differences between men and women, including a wider pelvis and more permanent hair on the head in females, growth of hair on the genitals and underarms, increased body fat, and maturity of the genitals and uterus.

Estrogens are released from the ovaries at puberty, coinciding with the onset of the menstrual cycle. This first instance of the menstrual cycle is called menarche. Rising levels of estrogen trigger the release of an ovum and growth of the uterine lining. The level quickly decreases after ovulation. If the ovum is fertilized, estrogen and progesterone work together to stop ovulation.

Estrogens also travel through the bloodstream and have a role in blood clotting, maintaining the vaginal wall and urethral lining, and producing vaginal lubrication. Estrogen works with vitamin D and calcium to break down and rebuild bones. However, lessening estrogen levels are part of aging, and women become susceptible to osteoporosis (Figure 17-34).

At menopause, when women stop menstruating, estrogen levels fall, causing symptoms of hot flashes, vaginal dryness, and loss of sex drive.

Low levels of estrogen are related to depressed mood, irregular menstrual periods, infertility, weak bones, and increased urinary tract infections.

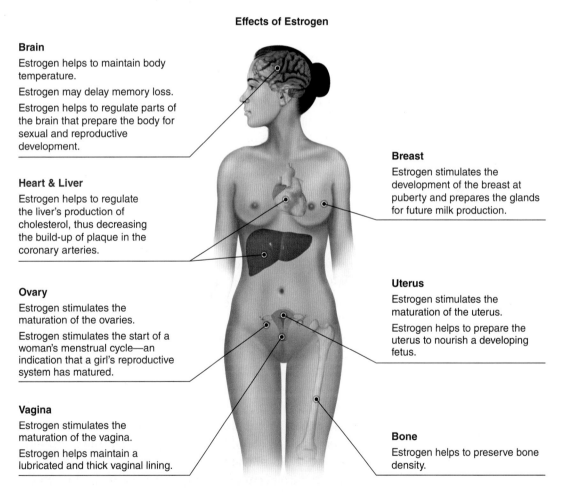

Effects of Estrogen

Brain
Estrogen helps to maintain body temperature.
Estrogen may delay memory loss.
Estrogen helps to regulate parts of the brain that prepare the body for sexual and reproductive development.

Heart & Liver
Estrogen helps to regulate the liver's production of cholesterol, thus decreasing the build-up of plaque in the coronary arteries.

Ovary
Estrogen stimulates the maturation of the ovaries.
Estrogen stimulates the start of a woman's menstrual cycle—an indication that a girl's reproductive system has matured.

Vagina
Estrogen stimulates the maturation of the vagina.
Estrogen helps maintain a lubricated and thick vaginal lining.

Breast
Estrogen stimulates the development of the breast at puberty and prepares the glands for future milk production.

Uterus
Estrogen stimulates the maturation of the uterus.
Estrogen helps to prepare the uterus to nourish a developing fetus.

Bone
Estrogen helps to preserve bone density.

FIGURE 17-34 Female secondary sexual characteristics caused by estrogen.

LEARNING OBJECTIVE 17.3.10 Identify the major events that occur during the female reproductive cycle.

LEARNING OBJECTIVE 17.3.11 Describe the major events that occur during the female reproductive cycle.

KEY TERMS

corpus luteum stage Stage in which the cells of the follicle divide quickly and the corpus luteum secretes progesterone to build up the endometrium.

follicle stage Stage of the female reproductive cycle during which follicle-stimulating hormone is secreted from the pituitary gland and circulates to the ovary, stimulating the growth of a follicle.

lactation Production of breast milk.

luteal stage Stage in which the cells of the follicle divide quickly and the corpus luteum secretes progesterone to build up the endometrium.

menstruation stage First phase of the female reproductive cycle where contents of the uterus are discharged as menstrual fluid.

ovulation stage When the ova are released by a follicle in the ovary and begins to travel along the fallopian tube to the uterus.

THE FEMALE REPRODUCTIVE CYCLE

The female reproductive cycle occurs in stages or phases. These include the luteal stage, follicle stage, menstruation stage, and ovulation stage (Figure 17-35). These stages encompass the stimulation of the ovary and preparation of the uterus in the follicle stage. Next is the corpus luteum stage when the cells of the follicle divide rapidly, and progesterone is released to prepare the uterus. The ovulation stage is when the ova is released by a follicle in the ovary and begins to travel along the fallopian tube to the uterus. The menstruation phase occurs when an ovum is not fertilized and the uterus sheds its blood and tissue.

The first stage is the **follicle stage**, lasting about 10 days, when FSH is secreted from the pituitary gland on about day 5 of the menstrual cycle. FSH circulates to the ovary through the bloodstream. At the ovary, it stimulates follicles. One of them will mature. The follicle will grow, as will the egg cell. At the same time, estrogen causes the endometrium to thicken and prepare for implantation of an embryo.

Cervical mucus changes to a thin substance to facilitate the movement of sperm into the uterus to fertilize the maturing ovum. While all of this is going on, another hormone, prolactin, is secreted by the anterior pituitary gland. This hormone stimulates lactation, or the production of breast milk in anticipation of a developing embryo.

High levels of circulating estrogen cause a halt of FSH secretion. The pituitary secretes LH. At about 14 days, the follicle ruptures and a mature egg is released in what is termed the **ovulation stage**.

After ovulation comes the **corpus luteum stage**. LH causes the cells of the follicle (corpus luteum) to divide quickly. The corpus luteum secretes progesterone, which helps maintain the growth of the endometrium and prevents formation of a new follicle by blocking the release of FSH. This stage lasts about 14 days. The mucus within the cervix also thickens in anticipation of creating a cervical mucus plug.

MENSTRUAL CYCLE

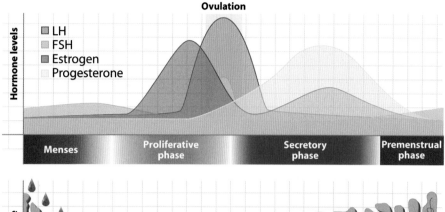

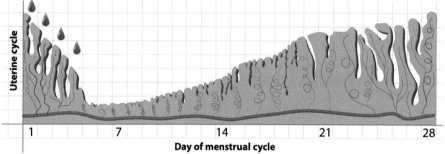

FIGURE 17-35 Four phases of the female reproductive cycle.

If the egg is not fertilized, the menstruation stage occurs and lasts one to five days. The increased progesterone levels in the blood blocks LH secretion, causing the corpus luteum to break down and progesterone levels to decrease. The endometrium thins and peels away from the uterus. It and the unfertilized egg are expelled through the vagina. During menstruation, the production of estrogen decreases, which stimulates the pituitary gland to secrete FSH, restarting the cycle.

LEARNING OBJECTIVE 17.3.12 Identify the structure of the mammary glands.

KEY TERMS

Cooper ligaments Structures that support the breast from the outer region to the nipple like the spokes of a wheel.

mammary glands Enlarged, modified sweat glands found in the breasts of females.

pectoris muscles Muscles on the anterior chest that support the mammary glands.

THE MAMMARY GLANDS

The mammary glands are housed within the breasts, which are fat and connective tissue. Estrogen is responsible for the development of the fat tissue. The mammary glands are located on the anterior chest wall, between the third and seventh ribs. They are held in place by the **pectoris muscles** and the **Cooper ligaments** that support the entire breast from the outer region to the nipple (Figure 17-36). Although both men and women have mammary glands, only the female's normally function.

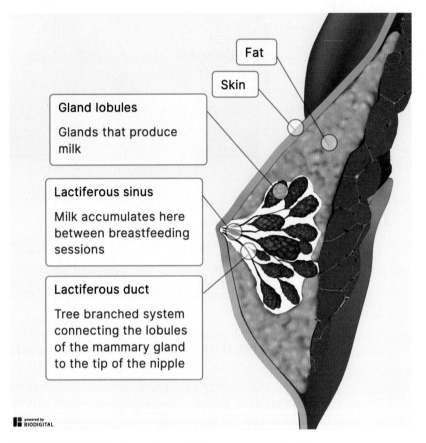

Fat

Skin

Gland lobules

Glands that produce milk

Lactiferous sinus

Milk accumulates here between breastfeeding sessions

Lactiferous duct

Tree branched system connecting the lobules of the mammary gland to the tip of the nipple

powered by
BIODIGITAL

FIGURE 17-36 Basic anatomy of the mammary gland.

LEARNING OBJECTIVE 17.3.13 Describe the structure of the mammary glands.

KEY TERMS

alveolar glands Glands within the ducts of breast tissue that secrete milk.

lactiferous duct Duct that leads to the nipple and opens to the outside.

sebaceous glands Exocrine gland located in the skin that produces sebum, or oil; usually associated with hair follicles.

Structure of the Mammary Glands

The mammary glands evolved from sweat glands hundreds of million years ago. They are unique to mammals. These specialized structures consist of fat and fibrous and glandular tissue. The fibrous tissue is attached to the skin. Each breast contains a nipple at the tip, which is surrounded by pigmented skin or the areola. The areola contains both **sebaceous glands** and sweat glands.

The Cooper ligaments divide the breast tissue into 15–20 lobes each. Each lobe consists of grapelike clusters of glands called alveolar glands and a duct called a lactiferous duct that leads to the nipple and opens to the outside.

The breast structure changes during the menstrual cycle and pregnancy. In response to estrogen, the ductal system grows. Progesterone stimulates the development of the glands. This creates the feeling of fullness and discomfort during the menstrual cycle.

During pregnancy, prolactin is released; however, milk production does not occur until after the birth.

LEARNING OBJECTIVE 17.3.14 **Identify the function of the mammary glands.**

LEARNING OBJECTIVE 17.3.15 **Describe the function of the mammary glands.**

KEY TERMS

colostrum Thins watery liquid that is ejected from the mammary glands at the start of lactation.

luminal epithelial Type of cell within the female breast that is capable of producing breast milk.

myoepithelial Cell within the lobes of the female breast.

oxytocin Hormone that stimulates uterine contractions and causes the ejection of milk.

placenta Structure within the pregnant uterus that is attached to the lining of the uterus and serves to nourish the developing fetus.

Purpose of the Mammary Glands

The mammary glands are considered organs of sexual stimulation; however, their primary function is to provide breast milk for the newborn. In addition to providing breast milk, they also provide important immune protection to the infant and defense against infection for the breast itself (Figure 17-37AB).

Function of the Mammary Glands

During pregnancy, the mammary glands develop their internal structure and milk-producing function. Estrogen promotes the development of the duct system; progesterone promotes development of the lobes and alveoli. Prolactin and a placental hormone (human chorionic somatomammotropin, or hCS) induce the development of milk-producing enzymes. While a woman is pregnant, estrogens and progesterone block prolactin so that lactation will not start.

The lobes within each breast are lined with myoepithelial and luminal epithelial cells that produce milk. Prolactin is what causes the luminal epithelial cells to produce milk. After birth, prolactin stimulation reaches the breast tissue cells and milk production (lactation) begins.

Two hormones maintain lactation: oxytocin, which causes ejection of milk, and prolactin, which promotes secretion of milk.

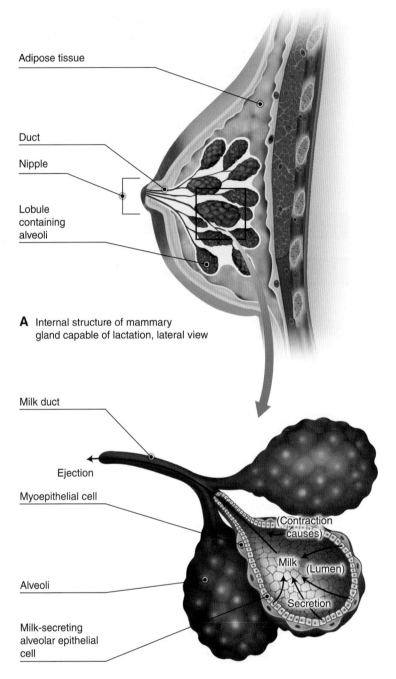

A Internal structure of mammary gland capable of lactation, lateral view

B Alveoli within mammary gland

FIGURE 17-37AB Structure (A) and function (B) of mammary glands.

As a baby suckles, nerve signals from the nipple travel to the hypothalamus, which, in turn, releases oxytocin. Oxytocin causes the myoepithelial cells that surround each alveolus to contract, which causes milk ejection. Suckling also increases prolactin secretion by the pituitary gland, which maintains milk production (Figure 17-38).

The breast also secretes a substance called **colostrum** at the start of breast-feeding. It has high concentrations of B and T lymphocytes and neutrophils that produce antibodies to harmful microorganisms. Breast milk itself contains immunoglobulin A, lactoferrin, bifidus factor, and other components to further protect the infant from microorganisms.

It is believed that breastfeeding helps prevent the infant from getting asthma, autoimmune diseases like type 1 diabetes, and certain cancers.

The release of oxytocin from the hypothalamus also helps to decrease the size of the mother's uterus, while prolactin helps to prevent menstruation so that pregnancy does not occur.

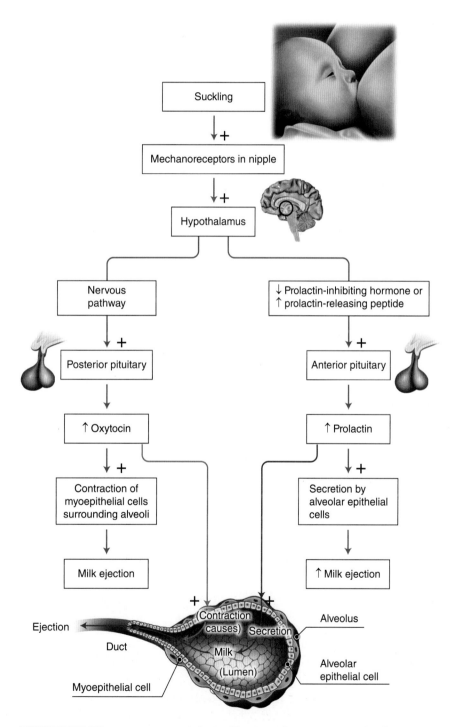

FIGURE 17-38 Hormones and their effects on the mammary glands.

When a woman stops breastfeeding, the suckling mechanism stops prolactin secretion, which halts milk production. Oxytocin release is halted to prevent milk ejection. Milk remaining in the alveoli builds up pressure in the cells, which further lowers milk production.

UNIT OBJECTIVE 17.4

Describe the common methods of birth control and common sexually transmitted diseases.

UNIT INTRODUCTION

This lesson begins with a review of the different types of birth control and the effectiveness of each to prevent pregnancy and sexually transmitted infections (STIs). The lesson concludes with a review of the signs, symptoms, and treatment of the most common STIs.

LEARNING OBJECTIVE 17.4.1 Identify the different types of birth control.

LEARNING OBJECTIVE 17.4.2 Describe the different types of birth control.

KEY TERMS

abstinence Avoidance of sexual intercourse as a method of birth control.

basal body temperature (BBT) method Type of fertility awareness-based method of birth control that uses the female body temperature to determine ovulation.

cervical cap Method of birth control where a soft cup-shaped device is placed over the base of the cervix.

cervical mucus ovulation method Type of fertility awareness-based method of contraception where the cervical mucus is examined to determine periods of fertility.

condom Method of birth control where a sheath is placed over the male penis or a sheath is inserted into the female vagina.

coitus interruptus Method of birth control where the penis is withdrawn before ejaculation.

cervical diaphragm cap Method of birth control where a cup is placed over the cervix.

emergency contraceptive Method of birth control where a pill containing hormones is ingested within 72 hours after unprotected intercourse.

fertility awareness-based methods Method of birth control where sexual intercourse is avoided during periods of fertility.

implanted contraceptive Method of birth control where a pellet containing hormones to suppress ovulation is placed under the skin.

intrauterine contraceptive Method of birth control where a T-shaped device is inserted into the uterus and releases hormones to suppress ovulation.

lactational amenorrhea method (LAM) Method of birth control where lactation is used to prevent pregnancy.

oral contraceptive Method of birth control that suppresses ovulation by ingesting a pill that contains estrogen and progestin.

spermicide Chemical used to destroy sperm as a method of birth control.

sponge Method of birth control where a disk-shaped device containing spermicide is inserted into the vagina and becomes activated by wetting with water.

sterilization Surgical procedure to prevent pregnancy accomplished through a vasectomy or tubal ligation.

transdermal patch Method of birth control where a patch is placed on the skin that contains estrogen and progestin to suppress ovulation.

tubal ligation Method of birth control where the fallopian tubes are blocked to prevent conception.

vaginal ring Method of contraception where a ring containing estrogen and progestin is inserted into the vagina to suppress ovulation.

vasectomy Method of contraception where the male vas deferens is sealed, tied, or cut.

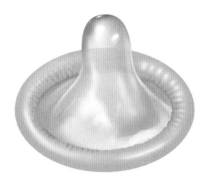

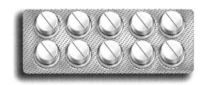

FIGURE 17-39 A condom is an example of the barrier method of contraception and birth control pills are an example of a hormonal method of contraception.

BIRTH CONTROL METHODS

The types of birth control can be categorized according to method. Reversible methods include behavioral interventions, the use of barriers, or the application or ingestion of hormones (See Figure 17-39). Irreversible birth control includes vasectomy for men or tubal ligation for women.

The reasons for birth control are several. There may be health risks for the woman that would make the pregnancy dangerous to both mother and infant. Some couples prefer to space out the birth of their children. Couples may also be at risk for passing along genes that cause birth defects. Often a couple wants to delay pregnancy early in a relationship, perhaps while each begins a career. A couple may also want to limit the number of children in their own family as well as in the world. Finally, those couples who are unmarried may want to avoid causing single parenthood.

Behavioral Methods

Behavioral interventions include abstinence, fertility awareness-based methods, withdrawal or coitus interruptus, and the lactational amenorrhea method (LAM).

Barrier Methods

Barrier methods for birth control include the male or female condom, the cervical diaphragm cap, the cervical cap, the sponge, or the intrauterine device (IUD).

Hormonal Methods

Hormonal contraceptives can be used orally, through injection, by a transdermal patch, vaginal ring, implanted, placed in the uterus, or taken orally for an emergency.

Permanent Methods

Permanent methods of birth control include **tubal ligation** for females or a **vasectomy** for males (Figure 17-40AB).

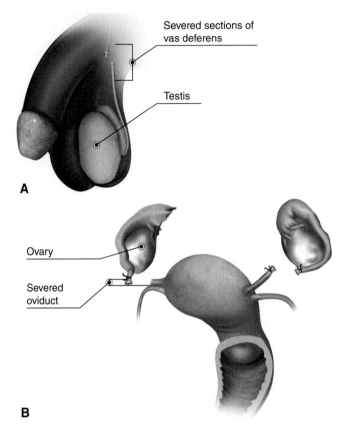

FIGURE 17-40AB Permanent methods of birth control are (A) vasectomy and (B) tubal ligation.

DESCRIPTION OF THE TYPES OF BIRTH CONTROL

The following describes the different types of birth control. Couples choose birth control methods based on cost, ease of use, effectiveness, and possible side effects. Religious beliefs may also influence choice.

Behavioral Methods

Abstinence is the complete avoidance of sexual intercourse. This method has no associated cost; however, both parties must cooperate and it can be a difficult method to maintain. Fertility awareness-based methods advocate the avoidance of sexual intercourse during periods of fertility, often days 10–17 of the woman's menstrual cycle. This method has a high failure rate and requires cooperation from both parties. Examples of fertility awareness-based methods include the **cervical mucus ovulation method,** in which the cervical mucus is examined to determine fertility. Another fertility-awareness method, the **basal body temperature (BBT) method,** uses the female body temperature to determine ovulation. The morning body temperature will be low before ovulation and will peak and stay elevated after ovulation (Figure 17-41).

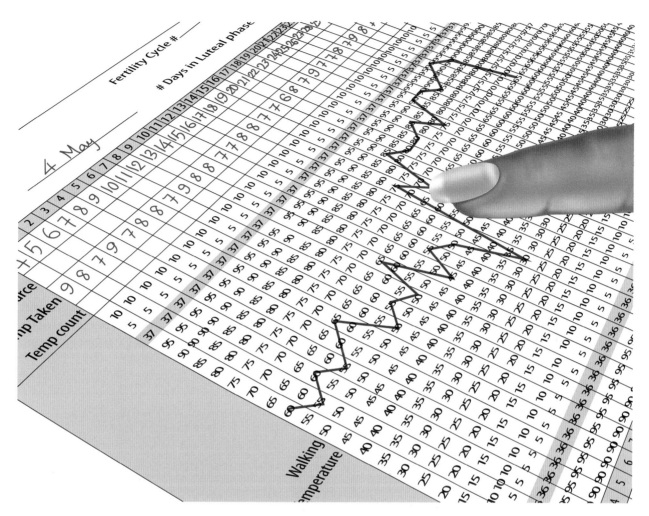

FIGURE 17-41 Basal body temperature method charts female body temperature.

Coitus interruptus is a method whereby the penis is withdrawn before ejaculation during sexual intercourse. This is one of the oldest methods of birth control and also the least effective, particularly if a few drops of pre-ejaculate fluid escapes from the penis. This fluid will contain sperm and pregnancy can result. With the lactational amenorrhea method (LAM), the breastfeeding female is able to prevent pregnancy because the hormone prolactin prevents ovulation.

Barrier Methods

The condom is a method of birth control in which a sheath is placed over the male penis or a sheath is inserted into the female vagina. The diaphragm is the placement of a cup placed over the cervix to prevent the introduction of semen into the uterus. This device can be inserted up to four hours before sexual intercourse. Another barrier method uses a cervical cap or soft-shaped device that is coated with **spermicide** and placed over the base of the cervix. This device is smaller than a diaphragm and can be inserted up to 36 hours before sexual intercourse. The sponge is a soft device that covers the cervix and releases a spermicide. The sponge is saturated with water before insertion, which can be done up to 24 hours before sexual intercourse. It can also be used for more than one sexual encounter without having to add additional spermicide. The device does need to be removed within 30 hours to prevent the development of an infection. Spermicides are about 70–75% effective. That percentage is increased when the spermicide is used with a diaphragm.

The IUD is a T-shaped device that can use copper or hormones. The device is inserted into the uterus by a healthcare provider. The copper type emits a small amount of copper that causes inflammation that prevents the sperm from reaching the egg and also prevents implantation of a fertilized egg. A hormonal IUD releases progesterone, which thickens the cervical plug to prevent sperm from entering the uterus.

Hormonal Methods

Oral contraceptives are the most commonly used method of birth control (Figure 17-42). A daily pill contains hormones that prevent ovulation. There are over 30 different formulations of oral contraceptives available. Injected contraceptives provide effective birth control for up to three months. In contrast, the transdermal patch contains hormones that are absorbed through the skin. The patch needs to be applied once a week for three weeks followed by one week without the patch.

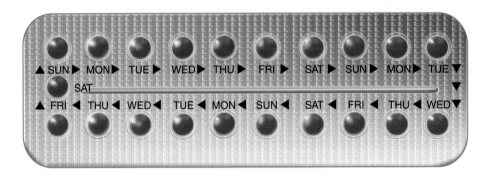

FIGURE 17-42 Oral contraceptives.

The vaginal ring is a device inserted into the vagina that releases estrogen and progestin to prevent ovulation. Similar to the transdermal patch, the vaginal ring is inserted once for three weeks followed by one week without the ring. An implanted contraceptive is a subdermal time-release method that provides hormones to suppress ovulation. The implanted device lasts for three years.

An intrauterine contraceptive (IUC) or IUD is a T-shaped object that is inserted into the uterus (Figure 17-43). The device prevents pregnancy by making the endometrial lining of the uterus difficult for a fertilized ovum to implant. It also interrupts the potential union between an ovum and potential sperm. Depending on the type of device, it can stay in the uterus up to seven years before needing to be replaced.

The last type of hormonal contraception is used in an emergency as the "morning-after" pill. This oral contraceptive is ingested within 72 hours after unprotected intercourse and serves to prevent a pregnancy.

Intrauterine Device (IUD)

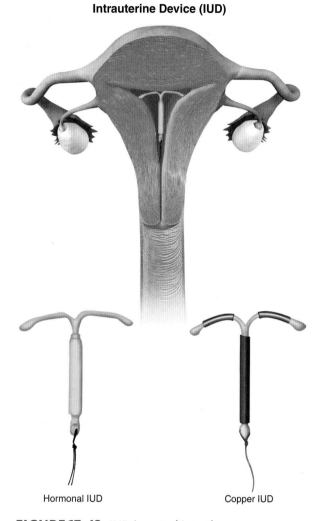

Hormonal IUD   Copper IUD

FIGURE 17-43 IUD inserted into the uterus.

Permanent Methods

Sterilization is a permanent method of contraception indicated for people who do not want to have any more children. Tubal ligation is the method for females where the fallopian tubes are blocked, tied, or cut to prevent conception. A vasectomy is the only procedure available for males. In this procedure the vas deferens is accessed through the scrotum and cut, preventing sperm from entering semen.

LEARNING OBJECTIVE 17.4.3 Identify the effectiveness of each type of birth control.

EFFECTIVENESS OF BIRTH CONTROL

The effectiveness of a birth control method may depend on the willingness of the partners to comply with the method or adhere to taking prescribed oral or transdermal hormone therapy. See Table 17-4 for failure rates by method.

Table 17-4 Failure Rates by Method of Conception

CONTRACEPTIVE METHOD	AVERAGE FAILURE RATE (ANNUAL PREGNANCIES/100 WOMEN)
None	90%
Natural (rhythm) methods	20–30%
Coitus interruptus	23%
Chemical contraceptives	20%
Barrier methods	10–25%
Intrauterine device	4%
Oral contraceptives	2–2.5%
Implanted contraceptives	1%
Sterilization	>1%

Behavioral Methods

The only reversible contraceptive method with 100% effectiveness against pregnancy is abstinence. However, this approach is difficult to maintain and takes consistent cooperation by both parties. Fertility awareness-based methods also take a high level of commitment. Because of this, they have an estimated 20–30% failure rate. Coitus interruptus places the female in a trusting and dependent role and has a failure rate of 23%. The lactational amenorrhea method has an estimated 20–30% failure rate; the female must engage in uninterrupted breast-feeding for six months for the method to be effective.

Barrier Methods

The condom method is effective only if the device is properly placed over the penis or inserted into the vagina. The failure rate for the male or female condom is 10–20%. The diaphragm requires the female to learn how to properly insert the device before sexual intercourse and has a failure rate of 16%. The cervical cap also has a high failure rate of 24%, primarily because of inadequate insertion. The sponge is a popular contraceptive device even though it has a failure rate of 25%. Spermicides have a failure rate of about 20%.

Hormonal Methods

The failure rates for hormonal methods of contraception are much lower. Oral and transdermal contraception has a failure rate of 2–2.5%. The contraceptive injection has a failure rate of 3%, while the implant has a failure rate of 0.05%. An IUD has a failure rate of 4%.

Even though emergency contraception is promoted as preventing a pregnancy after unprotected intercourse, this method has an 80% failure rate. This could be because the female waited too long to take the pill or the complete dose was not taken. Emergency contraception also includes insertion of an IUD within five days of intercourse, but this must be done by a healthcare provider.

Permanent Methods

Permanent methods of birth control have some of the lowest failure rates. In the United States, surgical birth control methods are the second most common form of preventing pregnancy. One of the reasons for its popularity is because surgical birth control methods do not require periodic taking of hormones or require sex be interrupted to insert a diaphragm or put on a condom. Because of this, permanent methods of birth control such as a vasectomy or tubal litigation typically have a failure rate of less than 1%.

LEARNING OBJECTIVE 17.4.4 List the types of birth control that also prevent the transmission of sexually transmitted diseases.

BIRTH CONTROL METHODS THAT PREVENT SEXUALLY TRANSMITTED INFECTIONS

A common misconception is that an effective birth control method will also prevent the contraction or transmission of an STI. This is not the case for all methods. The birth control methods that provide protection against STIs include abstinence, the male condom (latex only), and the female condom. Every other form of birth control, including sterilization, carries a risk of contracting an STI.

LEARNING OBJECTIVE 17.4.5 Describe the signs, symptoms, and treatment of common sexually transmitted diseases.

KEY TERMS

acquired immunodeficiency syndrome (AIDS) Exacerbation of the human immunodeficiency virus (HIV) that causes the development of opportunistic infections.

acyclovir Oral medication used to treat the genital herpes virus.

azithromycin Antibiotic used to treat a chlamydia infection.

chlamydia Type of STI caused by the bacterium *Chlamydia trachomatis*.

doxycycline Antibiotic used to treat chlamydia infection.

genital herpes Viral sexually transmitted infection that causes lesions on the genitalia; there is no cure.

gonorrhea Sexually transmitted infection caused by *Neisseria gonorrhoeae*; infection occurs in the genitals and rectum.

gummas Soft tumors that develop in tertiary syphilis.

human immunodeficiency virus (HIV) Virus transmitted by intimate sexual contact, use of drug paraphernalia, inoculation with infected blood or blood products, or to the newborn during birth; affects CD4 cells that support immunity and leads to acquired human immunodeficiency syndrome (AIDS).

human papillomavirus (HPV) Hundred different types of viruses, the majority of which affect the genital area and cause genital warts.

imiquimod Topical medication used to treat genital warts caused by human papillomavirus.

opportunistic infections Infection that occurs in immunocompromised individuals due to opportunistic pathogens.

pelvic inflammatory disease (PID) Infection that affects pelvic organs.

syphilis Sexually transmitted infection that is transmitted through a spirochete and has three distinct phases.

trichomoniasis vaginalis Protozoan parasite responsible for the common STI Trichomoniasis.

SEXUALLY TRANSMITTED INFECTIONS

STIs are caused by viruses and bacteria and are transmitted through exchange of body fluids such as semen, vaginal fluid, and blood. The symptoms primarily affect the organs of reproduction; however, they may also have systemic effects. Some STIs can cause long-term complications that include sterility, chronic infection, fallopian tube scarring, ectopic pregnancy, cancer, and death. Many STIs have no symptoms and are therefore easy to spread unknowingly.

Many people feel embarrassed about being checked for an STI and may avoid diagnosis by a healthcare professional. Diagnosis can include physical examination, blood tests, or other laboratory tests.

The major STIs are discussed below.

Genital Herpes

Genital herpes is caused by herpes simplex viruses HSV-1 and HSV-2. The HSV-1 virus typically causes oral cold sores, whereas the HSV-2 virus causes lesions located on the genitalia. It is transmitted through sexual contact (oral, vaginal, or anal) with an infected person or through childbirth. There is no cure for genital herpes.

Signs and Symptoms After exposure to the virus, painful red papules appear within 2–10 days on the genital area (Figure 17-44). Lesions will appear on the male penis and on the labia, vagina, and cervix of the female. These papules turn into blisters that break and shed additional virus. The areas of the broken blisters turn into ulcers that can last up to six weeks before healing. Touching these areas can cause the virus to spread to other body parts or other people.

The first episode of an infection can last up to 12 days. Repeated episodes have less severe symptoms that last between four and five days. During the latency period between outbreaks, the virus settles in the nerve fibers and remains dormant until the next outbreak.

In addition to the ulcerations, herpes simplex causes lymph node swelling, headache, fever, painful urination, urinary retention, vaginal discharge in females, and penile discharge in males. Symptoms that occur before a repeated outbreak include burning, itching, tingling, or throbbing at the site of a potential lesion.

Treatment There is no cure for genital herpes. However, there are medications that can help reduce the symptoms and shorten the length of time it takes the lesions to heal. The drug of choice is the antiviral **acyclovir** (Zovirax). This medication is taken orally for 7–10 days or until the lesions heal. It is used for both the initial infection and

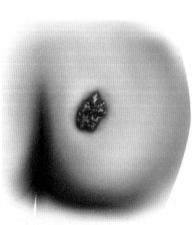

FIGURE 17-44 Herpes lesions on the buttocks.

repeated episodes. During outbreaks, those affected should keep the sores clean and dry, not touch the sores, wash hands after contact with the sores, and avoid all sexual contact until the sores have healed.

Human Papillomavirus

Human papillomavirus (HPV) is actually more than 100 different types of viruses, the majority of which affect the genital area and may cause genital warts. The types numbered 16 and 18 are the ones that cause cervical, penile, vulvar, vaginal, and some types of oropharyngeal cancers. The virus is most often transmitted through genital and oral sexual intercourse.

Signs and Symptoms Most people with HPV have no symptoms, and the infection resolves without treatment. The period of time between the initial exposure and the development of symptoms is between six weeks and eight months. For those who have no symptoms, the infection resolves within one to two years. In others, HPV causes single or multiple painless soft, moist, pink swellings in the genital area, penis, urethra, anus, groin, or thigh. HPV is also responsible for the development of genital warts that can appear as cauliflower-shaped lesions, hard lesions, or flat smooth lesions on the skin of the genitalia.

Treatment Treatment of HPV includes topical application of imiquimod or through removal of the warts through cryotherapy, electrocautery, laser vaporization, or surgical removal. Currently there is a vaccine to prevent the transmission of HPV. This vaccine guards against the most common types of HPV that cause genital cancer; however, it is limited in use to those whose age is between preadolescence and young adult. Children ages 11–12 should be vaccinated to prevent this disease. The vaccine has no effect on a current infection.

Human Immunodeficiency Virus

The STI that has the most devastating effects is **human immunodeficiency virus (HIV)**. This infection is transmitted by intimate sexual contact, use of paraphernalia to inject drugs, newborn exposure to the virus during birth, or inoculation with infected blood or blood products. This virus affects the CD4 cell that supports body immunity. If this level drops extremely low, the person with HIV can develop **acquired human immunodeficiency syndrome** or **AIDS**.

Signs and Symptoms The development of HIV has three different phases. The first phase is termed acute seroconversion. This begins about two to six weeks after exposure to the virus. Symptoms at this time include fever, sore throat, rash, and body aches that can be confused with the flu. After the initial symptoms dissipate, the virus continues to replicate in the body. CD4 cell level changes occur from 3 to 12 months after seroconversion. The infected person has no symptoms during this time. The progression to AIDS is the final phase and is characterized by an extremely low CD4 cell count and the onset of **opportunistic infections** or cancers. Symptoms of AIDS include fatigue, fever, night sweats, weight loss, skin dryness and rash, diarrhea, and oral lesions. Some individuals with AIDS may develop pneumonia, tuberculosis, and have outbreaks similar to those caused by genital herpes. Other individuals may develop cancers of the lymph system, skin, and cervix.

Treatment Currently there is no cure for HIV, although research is ongoing for a vaccination to prevent and treat the disorder. Medication therapy is started early in the disease process in efforts to preserve the number of CD4 cells and prevent the deterioration of the person's immune functioning. The medications used to treat HIV are antiviral drugs and are taken at specific times when the virus is replicating. Many people with HIV are treated with multiple different drugs that need to be taken at specific times during the day. The medications are costly and have many side effects. Those who adhere to the prescribed medication regimen are able to delay the development of AIDS and further deterioration of the immune function.

Vaginal Infections

A vaginal infection is one of the most common STIs. This infection can be caused by the bacteria *Gardnerella vaginalis*, the Trichomonas vaginalis protozoa (Figure 17-45), or the yeast *Candida albicans*.

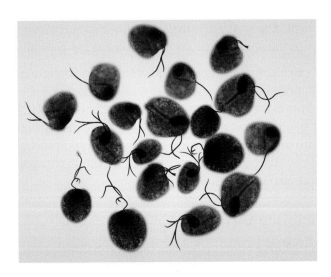

FIGURE 17-45 *Trichomonas vaginalis.*

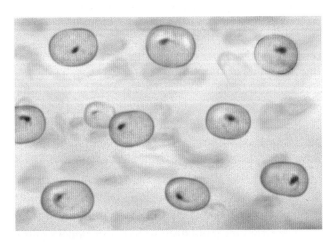

FIGURE 17-46 *Chlamydia trachomatis.*

Signs and Symptoms The symptoms of a vaginal infection will depend on the offending organism. For a bacterial infection, a thin, grayish-colored, and foul-smelling vaginal discharge will develop. Discharge often smells fishy. Symptoms of a *Trichomonas* infection include a frothy green-yellow vaginal discharge with a foul fishy odor. Men with a *Trichomonas* infection may have painful urination and pain in the urethra. Symptoms of a *Candida* infection include an odorless, thick cheese-like vaginal discharge accompanied with vaginal itching and painful urination.

Treatment The treatment of a vaginal infection will also depend on the causative organism. A bacterial infection will be treated with an antibiotic. Antifungal agents are used to treat a *Candida* infection. Specific medication is required to treat a *Trichomonas* infection. All sexual partners will also need to be treated to prevent reinfection of the same organism.

Chlamydia

A chlamydia infection is really a group of STIs caused by the *Chlamydia trachomatis* bacterium (Figure 17-46). This infection is transmitted through oral, vaginal, or anal intercourse or during childbirth through the vagina of an infected female. This infection is the most commonly reported STI.

Signs and Symptoms This bacterium has an incubation period of one to three weeks. However, it may be dormant for months or years before producing symptoms in a female. For some people, symptoms never occur. For others, symptoms include painful urination, urinary frequency, vaginal discharge in females, and penile discharge in males. A person with chlamydia can transmit the disease to others even when symptoms are not present.

Treatment Treatment of a chlamydia infection is through the antibiotic **azithromycin** (Zithromax) in a single oral dose or **doxycycline** (Adoxa), which is to be taken by mouth for seven days. All sexual partners must be treated at the same time or before having sexual intercourse.

Gonorrhea

Gonorrhea is caused by the bacteria *Neisseria gonorrhoeae* and is the second most commonly reported communicable disease. The infection is transmitted through direct sexual intercourse or during birth through the vagina of a female who is infected.

Signs and Symptoms The incubation period for gonorrhea is two to seven days after exposure. After this, the female experiences painful urination, urinary frequency, and a vaginal discharge. Males with the infection experience painful urination and a milky or purulent drainage from the penis.

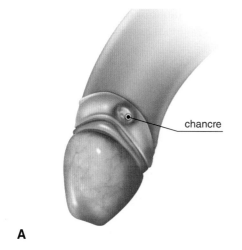

chancre

Treatment Gonorrhea is treated with two antibiotics: ceftriaxone and azithromycin. Individuals need to take the full course of the medication, and all sexual partners should also be treated before resuming sexual intercourse.

Syphilis

Syphilis is an STI caused by the spirochete *Treponema pallidum*. This organism can enter the body through any route including sexual contact or open lesions. The incubation period is 10–90 days with an average of three weeks. This STI rarely exists alone and is most often diagnosed in those with HIV/AIDS or a chlamydia infection.

Signs and Symptoms Syphilis has three stages: primary, secondary, and tertiary. During the primary stage, a chancre sore develops along with swollen lymph nodes (Figure 17-47AB). The sore appears at the site where the infection was introduced into the body and develops three to four weeks after exposure. The sore will spontaneously heal within four to six weeks and the person will have no further symptoms.

Symptoms of secondary syphilis begin two weeks to six months after the chancre sore heals. Symptoms at this time include rash on

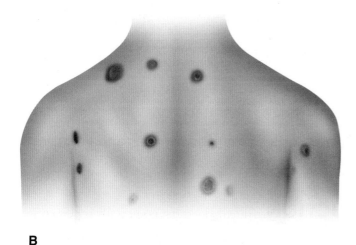

A

B

FIGURE 17-47AB Chancre of syphilis.

the palms of the hands and soles of the feet, patches on the oral tissue, a sore throat, swollen glands, development of flat wartlike growths on the genitalia, flulike symptoms, and hair loss. These symptoms also will disappear after two to six weeks at which time a period of latency begins. This period can last from 2 to 50 years until the final stage of syphilis appears. During the latency period the infection cannot be transmitted through sexual contact but is transmissible through exposure to blood.

Tertiary syphilis is the final stage and can take two forms. The first form is characterized by small tumors called **gummas** that develop in the skin, bones, and liver. The second form affects the cardiovascular and neurological systems.

Treatment The medication used to treat all stages of syphilis is an intramuscular injection of penicillin G. This is given as one single dose. For those allergic to penicillin, the oral medication doxycycline or tetracycline is taken for 28 days. Depending on the length of time the infection has been present in the body, additional medication doses may be required. Those who are being treated for syphilis are prone to developing a severe reaction after receiving the antibiotic treatment. This is because of the sudden destruction of the microorganism flooding the bloodstream. The adverse effects of this reaction may begin within 24 hours of starting treatment and end after another 24 hours. Individuals with the second form of tertiary syphilis may have residual cardiac and neurological effects even after being treated.

Pelvic Inflammatory Disease

Pelvic inflammatory disease (PID) is considered an STI because the infection affects the pelvic organs, including the fallopian tubes, ovaries, cervix, and endometrium. This disease can be caused by the same organisms that cause gonorrhea and chlamydia.

Signs and Symptoms Symptoms of PID include a fever, purulent vaginal discharge, and abnormal vaginal bleeding. Some people with the infection have mild symptoms that go undetected and untreated. If left undiagnosed and untreated, PID can cause abscesses, infertility, and chronic pelvic pain.

Treatment PID is treated with at least two broad-spectrum antibiotics that are given by mouth or intravenously. If the infection and symptoms are severe, the patient may need to be hospitalized and given intravenous fluids and pain medication. Surgery may be required to drain an abscess if one develops.

UNIT OBJECTIVE 17.5

Describe common pathologies affecting meiosis and genetic variability.

UNIT INTRODUCTION

The process of meiosis is complex and can lead to alterations that affect the resulting cell structure. The following section describes some of the alterations that can occur.

LEARNING OBJECTIVE **17.5.1** **Identify common errors during meiosis that cause disorders and genetic variability.**

KEY TERMS

deletion Alteration that occurs when a part of a chromosome is missing.

deoxyribonucleic acid (DNA) Content of a cell that contains proteins that make up genetic material.

Down syndrome Another name for trisomy 21.

duplication Alteration that occurs when a part of a chromosome is replicated.

inversion (chromosomal) Chromosome alteration that occurs when a part of a DNA strand breaks and reattaches upside down in the same chromosome.

Klinefelter's syndrome Another name for monosomy that occurs in males.

monosomy Absence of a chromosome after the cell divides through meiosis.

mutation Change in hereditary material: either a change in the sequence of a gene's codon or a change in chromosome number or structure.

nondisjunction Failure of a cell to split completely during meiosis that results in an inaccurate number of chromosomes.

translocation Alteration that occurs when a part of a chromosome moves and attaches to another chromosome.

trisomy 21 Additional chromosome that occurs after the cell divides through meiosis and causes Down syndrome.

Turner syndrome Another name for monosomy that occurs in females.

GENETIC ALTERATIONS

Information that determines genetic traits is coded within the deoxyribonucleic acid (DNA) strands. These multiple strands make up the genes and chromosomes. As we learned earlier in this chapter, through meiosis, the strands split so that half of the contents of the chromosome are in each cell. At times, there is a change in the structure of the strands, or the strands do not completely split, causing a change in the number of chromosomes. These are errors in meiosis, and they can cause mutations. As errors occur during meiosis, a mutated gene is then inherited by the fetus. Sometimes these mutations can be harmful or sometimes beneficial or harmless. Beneficial mutations cause biological changes that can help a species evolve and better adapt to the environment. Let's take a look at the types of mutations.

Change in Structure

A chromosome can be altered in four different ways. Through inversion (chromosomal), a portion of a chromosome is broken and reversed. This can happen if the DNA strand breaks and then becomes reattached upside down in the same chromosome.

A deletion occurs when a piece or segment of a chromosome is missing. A repeated piece of a chromosome causes a duplication. In both deletion and duplication, the lack of or too much genetic material will adversely affect the entire organism. These errors are not compatible with life or may cause severe physical or mental developmental problems.

The last type of change in chromosome structure is **translocation**. This occurs when a segment or part of a chromosome reattaches to another chromosome (Figure 17-48).

Types of DNA mutations

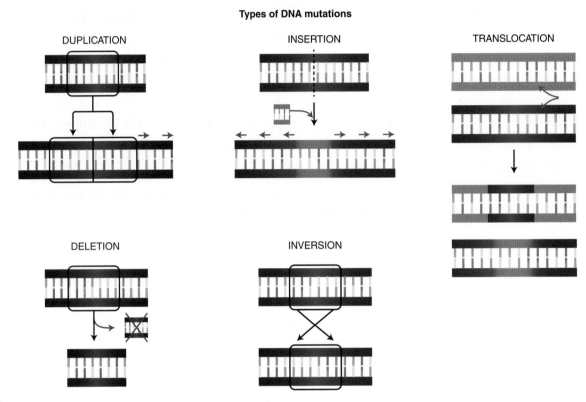

FIGURE 17-48 There are five common types of DNA mutations: duplication, insertion, deletion, translocation, and inversion.

Failure to Split

If a cell fails to split completely during meiosis, the result is a cell with an inaccurate number of chromosomes. This is called **nondisjunction**. If the cell then becomes fertilized, the resulting number of chromosomes will not equal 23 pairs. If one chromosome is missing, it can cause **monosomy** of the sex chromosome. In a female, this is known as **Turner syndrome**; in a male it is known as **Klinefelter's syndrome**. Another outcome could be an additional chromosome resulting in **trisomy 21**, or **Down syndrome**.

LEARNING OBJECTIVE 17.5.2 Describe the cause, signs, symptoms, and diagnosis of trisomy 21.

KEY TERMS

amniocentesis Use of amniotic fluid to test for trisomy 21.

chorionic villi sampling (CVS) Testing of the tissue that makes up the placenta to determine the presence of a genetic anomaly.

fecal nuchal translucency (FNT) test Ultrasound test completed between weeks 11 and 13 of gestation to determine the amount of fluid behind the neck of the developing fetus.

TRISOMY 21

Trisomy 21 is the most common genetic anomaly. It is caused by the addition of a single chromosome, resulting in a total of three copies of chromosome 21. Trisomy 21, or Down syndrome, is the most common chromosomal cause of intellectual disability that occurs in the fetus of a mother whose age is greater than 35.

Signs and Symptoms

The most characteristic feature of a newborn with trisomy 21 is that of a depressed nasal bridge and slanted eyes (Figure 17-49). Other signs are a short neck, a tongue that may stick out, small hands and feet, small pinky fingers, and poor muscle tone or loose joints. Cognitive development is delayed, resulting in some degree of intellectual disability. Other health problems that can occur from trisomy 21 include heart defects, impaired vision and hearing, malformation of the intestines, and an alteration in immune function. The degree of disability that the child experiences will vary.

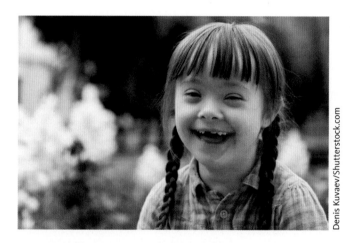

FIGURE 17-49 Child with trisomy 21.

Diagnosis

Trisomy 21 can be diagnosed while the fetus is in utero or after birth. Early diagnostic tests to identify the disorder include **chorionic villi sampling (CVS)** and **amniocentesis**. In CVS, a small sample of the tissue that makes up the fetal portion and maternal portion of the placenta is analyzed for chromosome number. An extra chromosome validates the presence of trisomy 21. Completed between weeks 7–11 of gestation, CVS is the earliest genetic test that can be performed, and the results can be available within 24 hours.

An amniocentesis is the removal of amniotic fluid to test for genetic anomalies. This test is performed after week 15 of gestation and is also used to diagnosis trisomy 21. Even though an amniocentesis is the most common test performed to detect genetic anomalies, the results may take 7–10 days to obtain.

One additional test used to determine trisomy 21 is the **fetal nuchal translucency (FNT) test**. This test uses ultrasound to determine the amount of fluid behind the neck of the developing fetus. Performed between weeks 11 and 13 of gestation, a large amount of fluid indicates a genetic anomaly. Other indications that the developing fetus has trisomy 21 include a change in the nasal bones, changes in the length of the femur or humerus, and bright spots on the heart. When examined with the results of blood hormone tests, the FNT predicts the risk of having a baby born with trisomy 21.

UNIT OBJECTIVE 17.6

Describe common pathologies affecting the male reproductive system.

UNIT INTRODUCTION

As we recall the organs and tissues that make up the male reproductive system, it is easy to see how these body areas can be adversely affected by infections, obstructions, and injuries. This section focuses on the most prevalent disorders that can affect the male reproductive system.

LEARNING OBJECTIVE 17.6.1 Identify common disorders affecting the male reproductive system.

KEY TERMS

benign prostatic hyperplasia (BPH) Nonmalignant enlargement of the prostate gland.

epididymitis Infection of the epididymis, usually caused by an STI.

erectile dysfunction Inability to attain and maintain an erection to perform sexual intercourse.

hydrocele Swelling in the scrotum that occurs when fluid collects in the tissue surrounding the testicle.

orchitis Acute infection of the testes usually caused by a urinary tract infection or the mumps.

phimosis Constriction of the foreskin in an uncircumcised male.

premature ejaculation Release of sperm before the achievement of the male orgasm.

priapism Involuntary sustained erection not associated with sexual arousal.

prostate cancer Cancer that affects the prostate gland.

prostatitis Inflammation or infection of the prostate gland.

retrograde ejaculation Release of semen into the bladder.

spermatocele Swelling in a duct of the epididymis.

testicular cancer Cancer of the testicles.

testicular torsion Twisting of the spermatic cord that inhibits blood supply to a testicle, which is a medical emergency.

varicocele Swelling or an increase in size of the veins that supply the scrotum and testicles.

COMMON DISORDERS OF THE MALE REPRODUCTIVE SYSTEM

Disorders of this body system can be divided into those that affect the penis, scrotum and testes, and the prostate.

Disorders of the Penis

One of the most common disorders is that of **erectile dysfunction**. This disorder affects the neurovascular integrity of the organ in that an erection cannot be achieved or maintained. It has many causes: a side effect of a medication, a chronic disease affecting the cardiovascular or neurological status, and lifestyle factors such as smoking and alcohol intake.

There are other disorders that affect the ability to ejaculate. These include retrograde ejaculation where the sperm are released into the urinary bladder and premature ejaculation.

Additional disorders of the penis include priapism, a prolonged erection, and phimosis, a condition in which a tight foreskin cannot be pulled over the head of the penis. Priapism can be caused by another health problem or as a side effect of medications used to treat erectile dysfunction. Although rare, phimosis can occur especially if an illness or infection causes the foreskin of an uncircumcised male to constrict.

As we read at the beginning of this chapter, the penis can also be the site of a STI. These infections can cause open sores, swelling, pain, and drainage of the organ.

Although rare, cancer of the penis can occur. It most often occurs in older men who are uncircumcised.

Disorders of the Scrotum and Testes

A mass in the scrotum can either be benign or malignant. Benign disorders include hydrocele, spermatocele, and varicocele. A hydrocele is the most common cause of scrotal swelling and is caused by fluid accumulating in the scrotal tissue. A spermatocele is a mass in one of the ducts of the epididymis. A varicocele is an enlarged vein within the spermatic cord.

Epididymitis, an infection within the epididymis, is usually caused by an STI such as *Chlamydia trachomatis* or *Neisseria gonorrhea*.

Orchitis, an acute infection of the testes, is caused by a urinary infection or mumps. And testicular torsion is the twisting of the spermatic cord. This health problem causes a sudden severe onset of scrotal swelling and pain. It is considered a medical emergency.

A cancer that affects young men is testicular cancer. It is the most common cancer in males between the ages of 13 and 35 and, when treated, it has a 95% cure rate.

Disorders of the Prostate

Disorders of the prostate gland include prostatitis, an infection or inflammation of the prostate gland, benign prostatic hyperplasia (BPH), and prostate cancer. More information about BPH and prostate cancer appears later in this lesson.

LEARNING OBJECTIVE 17.6.2 Describe the cause, signs, symptoms, and diagnosis of cryptorchidism.

KEY TERM

cryptorchidism Undescended testicle.

CRYPTORCHIDISM

An undescended testicle, or cryptorchidism, occurs when one or both testicles do not enter the scrotal sac during fetal development. While in utero, the testes develop in the abdomen and usually descend during the last trimester of pregnancy. In cryptorchidism, the testis may remain in the abdomen or somewhere along the canal leading to the scrotum.

Causes

Causes of cryptorchidism include premature birth or a fetus who is small for gestational age. The health problem may also occur in a fetus that is full term; however, the reasons for the disorder are usually genetic or hormonal factors.

Signs and Symptoms

The primary sign of the disorder is the absence of a testis in the scrotum. Depending on the location of the testis, it may be felt low in the abdomen (Figure 17-50). At times, the testis will descend spontaneously by three months of age; however, if it is not descended by age four months, intervention will be required.

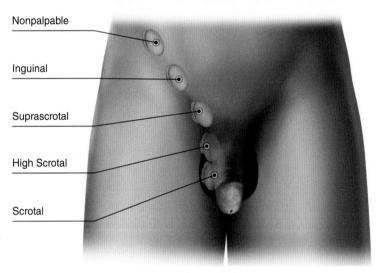

Nonpalpable

Inguinal

Suprascrotal

High Scrotal

Scrotal

FIGURE 17-50 In cryptorchidism, the undescended testis may be present in various areas of the abdomen or scrotum.

At birth the undescended testis is considered normal. However, if the testis is left undescended, changes in the cells and spermatic tubules occur. If the disorder only affects one testis, the descended one will also begin to change.

The long-term effects of cryptorchidism can include infertility, testicular torsion, risk for testicular cancer, and psychosocial issues because of a misshaped scrotum. Those with this disorder will have decreased sperm counts and poor quality of sperm, both of which can cause infertility.

Diagnosis

The diagnosis of cryptorchidism is made through examination of the male infant's genitalia at birth. If the testis cannot be located through palpating the abdomen and inguinal ring, surgery may be required to locate the organ and move it to the scrotum. There is no specific test that is used to diagnose cryptorchidism. Treatment should occur before one year of age to prevent infertility and any further deterioration of testicular tissue. A male with a history of cryptorchidism should be carefully followed through the lifespan because of the increased risk of testicular cancer.

LEARNING OBJECTIVE 17.6.3 Describe the signs, symptoms, and diagnosis of benign prostatic hyperplasia.

KEY TERMS

bladder distention Enlarged bladder caused by retention of urine.

digital rectal examination Examination of the prostate gland performed through direct palpation of the gland through the rectum.

nocturia The need to frequently urinate at night.

overflow incontinence Uncontrolled release of urine that occurs if the bladder is distended.

prostate-specific antigen (PSA) Blood test that measures the presence or absence of cancer in the prostate gland.

BENIGN PROSTATIC HYPERPLASIA

Benign prostatic hyperplasia (BPH) is the benign enlargement of the prostate gland (Figure 17-51). It is a disorder that affects more than 50% of all men over the age of 60. Although there are many theories as to why the disorder occurs, the most prominent explanation is an imbalance between prostate cell growth and cell death. Other theories for the development of BPH include a hormone imbalance that also affects cell growth and death.

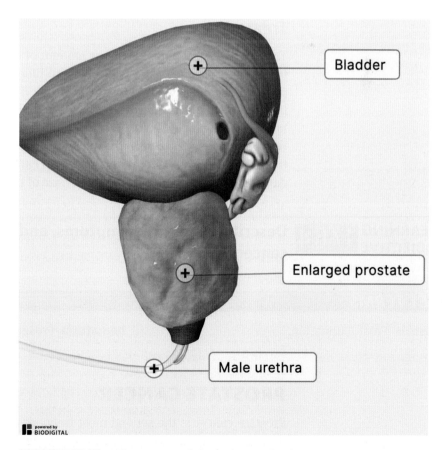

powered by
BIODIGITAL

FIGURE 17-51 Enlargement of the prostate gland.

Signs and Symptoms

As a review, the prostate gland wraps around the urethra at the base of the urinary bladder. Once the tissue begins to overgrow, pressure increases on the urethra. This is the reason for the primary symptoms of weak urine stream, dribbling, increased frequency to urinate, and nocturia. As the prostate tissue continues to grow, urinating becomes progressively more difficult, which can lead to bladder distention and an increased risk for bladder infections. The over-filled bladder can also cause overflow incontinence if any pressure is placed on the abdomen. If left untreated, BPH can cause changes to the tissue within the bladder wall. With the inability to empty the bladder, urine can back up into the ureters and kidneys, leading to structural changes and infections.

Diagnosis

The decision to assess a male for BPH depends on the responses to questions about bladder emptying, frequency, urgency, strength of the stream, and nocturia. BPH is diagnosed through a physical examination, digital rectal examination, urinalysis, and blood tests for kidney function and prostate-specific antigen (PSA). The digital rectal examination is done to determine the size of the enlarged gland. A urinalysis determines if there is any infection or inflammation of the bladder. Kidney function tests are done to determine if there are any changes to kidney function because of incomplete bladder emptying of urine. The PSA is used to rule out cancer as a cause for the urinary tract symptoms.

Treatment

Treatment of BPH depends on the amount of obstruction and associated symptoms. There are medications available to block the effects of hormones on the prostate gland tissue and effectively shrink the size of the gland. The result of these medications is improved urine output. For those whose symptoms do not improve with medication, surgery to remove a part of the enlarged prostate can be done. Techniques have improved and now include laser, microwave, vaporization, and needle ablation. Individuals who cannot have surgery may be a candidate for a urethral stent to increase the size of the urethra and facilitate urination.

LEARNING OBJECTIVE 17.6.4 Describe the signs, symptoms, and diagnosis of prostate cancer.

KEY TERMS

dysuria Painful urination.

hematuria Presence of blood in the urine.

PROSTATE CANCER

Prostate cancer is the second most frequent type of cancer in men; frequency development increases after age 50. The risk for the development of prostate cancer is higher for those who have a family history of the disorder and consume a high-fat diet. Factors that protect against the development of prostate cancer include a low-fat diet, soy, green tea, and vitamin D and E supplements. Because prostate tissue responds to androgens, controlling the amount of this type of hormone also helps prevent the development of the disease.

Signs and Symptoms

The early stage of prostate cancer causes no symptoms. The presence of symptoms may indicate the disease has spread to the urinary bladder, lungs, and bone. Because of this, bone pain may be the first sign of the disease. Depending on the size and location of the cancer in the prostate, the first symptom might be a change in urination such as urgency, frequency, nocturia, dysuria, hematuria, or blood in the ejaculate. Bone metastasis may cause back pain. Additional symptoms of metastasis include weight loss, anemia, and shortness of breath. A digital rectal examination may find a fixed, nodular, and firm prostate (Figure 17-52).

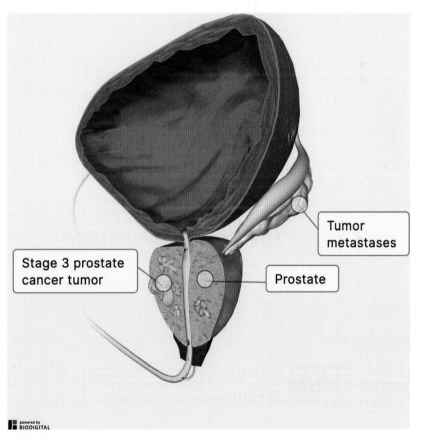

Stage 3 prostate cancer tumor

Tumor metastases

Prostate

powered by BIODIGITAL

FIGURE 17-52 Stage III prostate cancer.

Diagnosis

Although it is used as a screening tool, a positive PSA test does not definitively indicate that prostate cancer is present. The actual diagnosis of the disease is determined through a physical examination and results of a prostate biopsy. If present, the biopsy tissue will help determine the stage of the disease so that treatment, such as surgery, radiation, and hormone therapy, can be prescribed. Cancer of the prostate that produces no symptoms may not be treated at all but rather undergo a course of "watchful waiting."

LEARNING OBJECTIVE 17.6.5 Contrast the signs and symptoms associated with benign prostatic hyperplasia and prostate cancer.

COMPARING BENIGN PROSTATIC HYPERPLASIA AND PROSTATE CANCER

Unfortunately, the signs and symptoms of BPH and prostate cancer are very similar. Depending on the size and location of a prostate mass, urinary symptoms such as urgency, frequency, and nocturia can occur as in BPH. In prostate cancer, however, there is painful urination, hematuria, and blood in the ejaculate. These symptoms do not occur in BHP.

In prostate cancer, pain from the disease or metastasis is a major sign. In BPH, pain does not occur, but there is discomfort caused by bladder distention and possible backing up of urine into the ureters and kidneys. There may be no symptoms in the early stage of prostate cancer. However, similar to BPH, the first symptoms may be a weak urinary stream, frequency, dribbling, and nocturia.

Because the beginning symptoms of these disorders are so similar, it is essential for a complete diagnostic evaluation, including digital rectal examination and PSA level, to be completed when any of these symptoms occur.

UNIT OBJECTIVE 17.7

Describe common pathologies affecting the female reproductive system.

UNIT INTRODUCTION

As we recall the organs and tissues that make up the female reproductive system, it is easy to see how these body areas can be adversely affected by infections or cancer. This section focuses on the most common disorders that can affect the female reproductive system.

LEARNING OBJECTIVE 17.7.1 Identify common disorders of the female reproductive system.

KEY TERMS

abscess Infection of a gland and surrounding tissue that causes pain, swelling, and inflammation.

amenorrhea Absence of menstruation.

breast cancer Cancer of the breast; the most common type of cancer that affects the female reproductive system.

endometrial cancer Cancer that occurs from the lining of the uterus or the endometrium of the female reproductive system causes bleeding in postmenopausal females.

endometriosis Health problem where endometrial tissue grows outside of the uterus.

endometritis Inflammation of the endometrium.

fibrocystic breast changes Changes in the cell structure of breast tissue.

hypomenorrhea Scant menstruation.

leiomyomas Benign growth in the uterus.

mastitis Inflammation of breast tissue.

menometrorrhagia Heavy bleeding during and between menstrual periods.

menorrhagia Excessive menstruation.

oligomenorrhea Infrequent menstruation or periods that occur more than 35 days apart.

polycystic ovary syndrome (PCOS) Condition in women where higher than normal levels of male hormones are produced leading to hirsutism, diabetes, and possible infertility.

polymenorrhea Frequent menstruation or periods that occur less than 21 days apart.

postmenopause Stage in which a female stops maturing ova and menstruation ceases.

purulent Drainage that is white and thick; often referred to as pus.

COMMON DISORDERS OF THE FEMALE REPRODUCTIVE SYSTEM

The disorders of the female reproductive system can be divided into those that affect the external genitalia, the internal genitalia, the menstrual cycle, and the breasts.

External Genitalia

Disorders of the external genitalia include infections or **abscesses** of the Bartholin's or Skene's glands. Infection may block the glands, which become enlarged. The abscess may need to be drained to remove the infection and reduce the pain and swelling. The skin of the mons pubis may become inflamed and cause itching and skin breakdown. Cancer of the mons pubis is rare and can be caused by HPV. Any lesion that appears like a wart or fails to heal should be evaluated for cancer.

Internal Genitalia

Disorders of the vagina include vaginitis, or an infection of the vaginal tissue, and vaginal cancer. Vaginitis can be caused by local irritation or an infection from a microorganism that lives on the body. Although rare, vaginal cancer can occur. It has also been linked to HPV.

The cervix can also become inflamed or develop cancer. With inflammation, or cervicitis, the tissue is exposed to a pathogen that causes **purulent** drainage. If the cervix is repeatedly exposed to HPV, cancer can develop.

The uterus is prone to developing inflammation, infection, and cancer. **Endometritis** is an acute inflammation of the endometrium and is often caused by instrumentation or an intrauterine device used for birth control. In contrast, **endometriosis** is a health problem in which functional endometrial tissue is found in areas outside the uterus. Additional information about endometriosis will occur later in this chapter.

Endometrial cancer is the most common cancer of the female reproductive tract and causes **postmenopausal** bleeding. Benign growths or **leiomyomas** can also occur within the uterus.

Within the ovaries, cysts can develop at the site of a ruptured ovum. These cysts may be singular or develop into polycystic ovary syndrome (PCOS). Additional information about PCOS appears later in this chapter.

The ovaries are also prone to developing cancer. Ovarian cancer is the second most common type of cancer that affects the female reproductive system. Unfortunately, this type of cancer is often detected late in the disease process when metastasis has most likely occurred.

Menstrual Cycle

Disorders of the menstrual cycle can take many forms. The first of these is amenorrhea or the absence of menstruation, which is reviewed later in this chapter. Other disorders include hypomenorrhea, oligomenorrhea, polymenorrhea, menorrhagia, and menometrorrhagia.

Breasts

Benign disorders of the breast include mastitis or inflammation of the breast tissue. This most often occurs during breastfeeding. Another benign disorder of the breast is fibrocystic breast changes. These changes make up the most common breast disorders. Breast cancer remains the most common cancer of the female reproductive system.

LEARNING OBJECTIVE 17.7.2 Describe the signs, symptoms, and diagnosis of endometriosis.

KEY TERMS

adhesions Areas of body tissue that are stuck together.

chocolate cysts Endometriotic lesions that contain old blood and appear like chocolate syrup.

retrograde menstruation Menstrual blood that flows upward in the uterus and through the fallopian tubes.

ENDOMETRIOSIS

Endometriosis is a chronic inflammatory disease in which functional endometrial tissue is found outside the uterus. These areas include the ovaries, behind the broad ligaments, around the other uterine ligaments, the pelvic cavity, the vagina, or the intestines. The cause of the disorder is unknown; however, one reason might be from retrograde menstruation or menstrual blood that flows upward toward the fallopian tubes. Other theories for the development of this disorder include endometrial tissue entering the lymph system and reaching other organs.

Signs and Symptoms

The displaced endometrial tissue responds to the same hormone influence as the tissue in the uterus. This means that at the beginning of the menstrual cycle, the tissue begins to slough. It will proliferate and thicken during the proliferative and secretory phases of the cycle. These changes are the reason for the symptoms of endometriosis that include pelvic pain, pelvic adhesions, back pain, and pain with defecation and urination. Endometriosis can cause infertility because the adhesions distort the normal anatomy and physiology of the ovaries. Some of the endometriotic lesions may form cysts and contain old blood that resembles chocolate syrup. These types of cysts are termed chocolate cysts.

Diagnosis

Endometriosis is challenging to diagnose because the symptoms are similar to other disorders of the female reproductive system. A definite diagnosis can only be made through laparoscopic examination of the tissue and pelvic organs. Depending on the extent of the disease, ultrasound or magnetic resonance imaging may be used. Treatment may include pain management, hormone therapy to reduce the growth of endometrial tissue, and surgery to remove the areas or organs affected by the endometrial tissue.

LEARNING OBJECTIVE 17.7.3 **Describe the signs, symptoms, and diagnosis of polycystic ovaries.**

KEY TERMS

hirsutism Condition of male-pattern hair growth in the female population. Usually occurring on the face.

type 2 diabetes mellitus Most common type of diabetes where an individual's body no longer responds to insulin due to an overall increase in glucose levels.

POLYCYSTIC OVARIAN SYNDROME

Polycystic ovarian syndrome (PCOS) is considered an endocrine disorder that affects a large number of females of childbearing age. The health problem causes irregular menstruation and is believed to be caused by an abnormally elevated testosterone level. The elevated testosterone level prohibits the full maturation of oocytes, which leads to infertility in the female. The immature oocytes do not rupture but develop cysts over the surface of the ovaries.

Signs and Symptoms

The most common signs and symptoms of PCOS are the results of elevated testosterone levels and include hirsutism, acne, and obesity. Over the long-term, PCOS can lead to type 2 diabetes mellitus.

Diagnosis

PCOS is diagnosed through physical examination, irregular menstruation, physical manifestations, and select laboratory tests to measure hormone levels and blood glucose level. Ultrasound and laparoscopic visualization of the ovaries may be done; however, it is not required to make a definitive diagnosis. Treatment is through weight reduction and medication to improve ovulatory functioning and prevent the long-term effects of the disorder.

17.7.4 **Describe the causes, signs, symptoms, and diagnosis of amenorrhea.**

primary amenorrhea Absence of menstruation by age 15 or the failure to menstruate and the absence of secondary sex characteristics by age 13.

secondary amenorrhea Absence of menstruation for six months after routine menstruation has been established.

AMENORRHEA

Amenorrhea is the absence or failure to menstruate and can be of two types. The first type is considered **primary amenorrhea**, in which a female does not menstruate by age 15, or fails to menstruate and has no secondary sex characteristics by age 13. The other type, **secondary amenorrhea**, is the stopping of menstruation for six months or longer after routine menstruation has been established.

Causes

Primary amenorrhea is usually caused by a genetic malformation of the reproductive tissue or a hormone imbalance. Secondary amenorrhea can be caused by hormone imbalances, ovarian or pituitary dysfunction, adhesions in the uterus, infections, and tumors of the pituitary gland. Anorexia nervosa or strenuous physical exercise can also cause the disorder because the amount of body fat needed to support menstruation is altered.

Signs and Symptoms

The only symptom of the disorder is the failure of menstruation to begin or the stopping of menstruation when it has been established.

Diagnosis

The diagnosis of amenorrhea is made from a complete physical examination and a test to rule out pregnancy. Other tests that are used to diagnose the disorder include hormone blood levels and possibly computed tomographic scans or magnetic resonance imaging to exclude the presence of a pituitary tumor. Treatment will depend on the findings but may include surgery to remove a tumor and hormone therapy.

Chapter 18

Pregnancy and Childbirth

Chapter Introduction

In this chapter, we discuss the many changes that occur throughout fetal development from conception to birth and in the surrounding period afterward. Included in the discussion are the many anticipated maternal physiological changes that also occur throughout pregnancy, birth, and the postpartum period. We also explore the many maternal and fetal pathological conditions and their implications that can occur throughout this time period.

UNIT OBJECTIVE 18.1

Describe the process of fertilization.

UNIT INTRODUCTION

Fertilization is when a sperm fuses with an ovum, forming a zygote. In order for fertilization to occur, a sperm must unite with a mature ovum within 12–24 hours after ovulation occurs. This unit describes the human fertilization process, beginning with the movement of sperm through the female reproductive tract. We then discuss how fertilization occurs once sperm reach the ovum. The causes of monozygotic and dizygotic twins and the process for in vitro fertilization are also discussed.

LEARNING OBJECTIVE 18.1.1 **Trace the movement of the sperm along the female reproductive tract toward an egg.**

KEY TERMS

ampulla Third portion of the fallopian tube, which curves over the ovary; most common site for human fertilization.

bactericidal Capable of killing bacteria.

pathogenic Capable of causing illness or disease.

spermatozoa Motile male gamete with a rounded or elongated head and a long posterior flagellum.

MOVEMENT OF SPERM

During sexual intercourse, the seminal fluid that contains sperm is expelled through ejaculation into the female reproductive tract and is deposited in the posterior vaginal fornix. Under normal conditions, semen is slightly alkaline. This acts as a buffer to protect the spermatozoa from the acidic vaginal fluid, which generally serves as bactericidal function in safeguarding the cervical canal from pathogenic organisms. The passage through the cervical canal is a crucial phase for the selection of sperm cells. The cervical mucus barrier functions as a filter, which protects the entrance to the uterus. Only sperm that are normal with the greatest motility can travel through the layers of cervical mucus. During ovulation, the cervical barrier becomes thinner, and the changes in acidity create a friendlier environment for the sperm. During ejaculation, an average of 200 million sperm enter the vagina. As the sperm travel from the vagina to the cervix, and from the cervix to the uterus, only about 1 million sperm will make it to the top of the uterus. The rest are either killed by the acidic nature of the vagina, attacked by white blood cells, or swim into dead-end channels in the walls of the cervix. Once the sperm has entered the uterus, prostaglandins in the semen may increase uterine smooth muscle contractions, which enhances the passage of the sperm through the uterine cavity. These contractions and the flagellar movement of their tails propel the sperm through the uterine tube junctions to reach the fallopian tubes. Approximately 1,000 sperm will reach the fallopian tubes. For fertilization to take place, the ovary must release a mature ovum while this is occurring. That ovum is also making its way through the fallopian tubes, traveling from the ovary to the uterus. Fertilization usually takes place in the **ampullary** portion of the fallopian tube (Figure 18-1). Approximately 200 sperm will reach the ovum; only one will penetrate it (Figure 18-2).

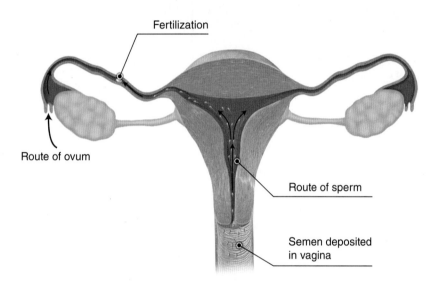

FIGURE 18-1 Fertilization takes place in the ampullary portion of the fallopian tube.

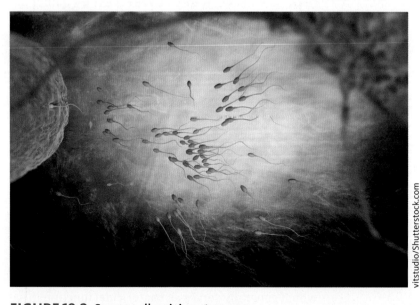

vitstudio/Shutterstock.com

FIGURE 18-2 Sperm cell arriving at an egg.

LEARNING OBJECTIVE 18.1.2 Describe fertilization in detail.

FERTILIZATION PROCESS

The corona radiata, which is the outer layer of follicular cells surrounding the ovum, release chemicals that attract the sperm that has undergone capacitation. The acrosome of the sperm must penetrate the corona radiata, which surrounds the oocyte, and the underlying protective layer known as the zona pellucida, which is a thick glycoprotein membrane surrounding the cell's plasma membrane (Figure 18-3). The sperm initially burrows through the cells on the corona radiata and upon contact with the zona pellucida bind to the receptor sites. Once the sperm successfully penetrates the corona radiata, the sperm and ovum become enclosed with a membrane that becomes impenetrable to other sperm. An acrosomal reaction then occurs in which enzymes allow the sperm to dissolve and penetrate the zona pellucida. At this point, the tail of the sperm is lost and only the nucleus of the sperm reaches the plasma membrane of the oocyte. The entrance of the sperm stimulates the oocyte to undergo a second meiotic division that produces the ovum and forms a second polar body. The nuclei fuse and the chromosomes combine, restoring the diploid number of 46 chromosomes, which now allow for meiotic division (Figure 18-4). At this point in conception, the formation of the zygote has been achieved. Mitotic cellular replication, called cleavage, begins as the zygote travels the length of the uterine tube into the uterus. Figure 18-5A-C shows the steps in fertilization and meiosis in detail.

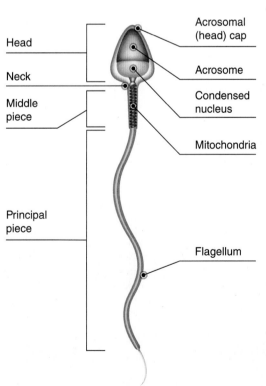

Head

Neck

Middle piece

Principal piece

Acrosomal (head) cap

Acrosome

Condensed nucleus

Mitochondria

Flagellum

FIGURE 18-3 Acrosome of a sperm.

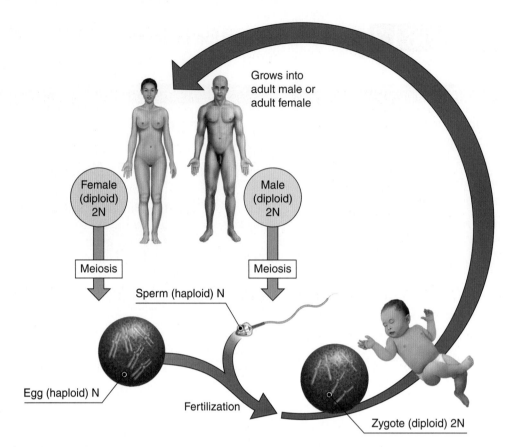

FIGURE 18-4 The egg and sperm each have a single set of unpaired chromosomes, or haploid. During fertilization, they combine, resulting in two complete sets of chromosomes, or diploid.

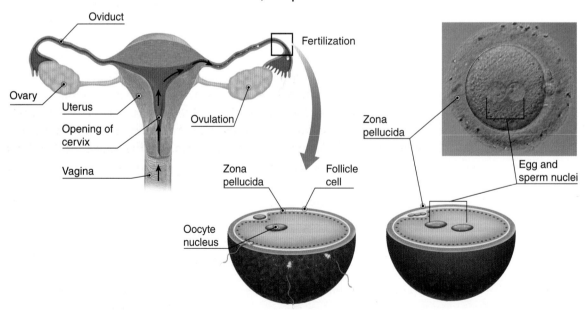

A Fertilization most often occurs in the oviduct. Many sperm swim through the vagina into oviducts (blue arrows).
Inside an oviduct, the sperm surround a secondary oocyte that was released by ovulation.

B Enzymes released from the cap of each sperm clear a path through the zona pellucida. Penetration of the secondary oocyte by a sperm causes the oocyte to release substances that prevent other sperm from binding.

C The oocyte completes meiosis II. The sperm's tail and other organelles degenerate.
Later, the egg and sperm nuclei will fuse and the zygote will form.

FIGURE 18-5A-C Fertilization and meiosis.

LEARNING OBJECTIVE 18.1.3 **Explain the mechanisms that cause monozygotic and dizygotic twins.**

KEY TERMS

amnion Innermost fetal membrane.

assisted reproductive technology (ART) Any fertility treatment in which eggs or embryos are handled outside of the body.

chorion Outermost fetal membrane.

dichorionic-diamniotic Twins who do not share a chorion, amnion, or placenta while in utero.

dizygotic Twins derived from two separate ova; also known as fraternal or nonidentical twins.

embryo After fertilization, the zygote or fertilized egg forms into an embryo, an unborn offspring;

early stages of fetal growth approximately from the second week to the eighth week.

monozygotic Twins derived from a single ovum; also known as identical twins.

monochorionic-diamniotic Twins who share a placenta but do not share a chorion or amnion while in utero.

monochorionic-monoamniotic Twins who share a chorion, amnion, and placenta while in utero.

placenta Structure within the pregnant uterus that is attached to the lining of the uterus and serves to nourish the developing fetus.

MONOZYGOTIC AND DIZYGOTIC TWINS

Monozygotic twins develop from one fertilized ovum, which then divides. This division takes place after the zygote consists of thousands of cells. The twins will be the same gender and have identical genotypes. Most often, division occurs between four and eight days after fertilization, and there are two embryos, two amnions, one chorion, and one placenta. These are known as monochorionic-diamniotic twins. Less common are dichorionic-diamniotic twins (where there are two amnions, two chorions, and two placentas) or monochorionic-monoamniotic twins (where there is one amnion, one chorion, and one placenta; this occurs rarely). There is no conclusive research on why the fertilized ovum divides. Monozygotic twins generally do not run in families, so it is not thought to have a genetic cause. It is hypothesized that the fertilized ovum divides as a result of an environmental trigger or it may be a random, spontaneous event.

Dizygotic twins develop when two mature ova are produced in one ovarian cycle. When two ova are fertilized by two separate sperm, the result is two zygotes or dizygotic twins. There are two amnions, two chorions, and two placentas. Because dizygotic twins originated from two separate ova and sperm, they do not have identical genotypes. Dizygotic twins are essentially siblings that are born at the same time. Dizygotic twins are most likely to occur in women over age 35, women undergoing assisted reproductive technology (ART), and women who have a mother or sister who gave birth to dizygotic twins. Figure 18-6 shows how fertilization differs for monozygotic and dizygotic twins.

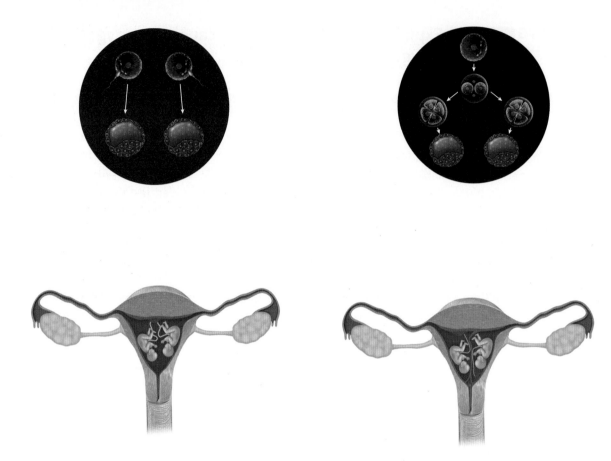

FIGURE 18-6 In dizygotic twins, two different eggs are fertilized by two different sperm. In monozygotic twins, one sperm fertilizes one egg, which then divides. Monozygotic twins frequently share a placenta and may share a chorion and amnion. Dizygotic twins always have their own placenta, chorion, and amnion.

LEARNING OBJECTIVE 18.1.4 Describe the process of in vitro fertilization.

KEY TERMS

blastocyst Early form in the development of an embryo that consists of a circular layer of cells filled with fluid.

hCG (human chorionic gonadotropin) Hormone produced by the placenta after implantation; can be detected in the urine of a pregnant woman;

most pregnancy tests check for the presence of hCG in urine; in the presence of one or more mature ovaries, can be used clinically to induce ovulation in the ovaries.

intracytoplasmic sperm injection When a single sperm is injected into an egg.

IN VITRO FERTILIZATION

In vitro fertilization (IVF) is an assisted reproductive technology used to treat infertility. During IVF, an ova is fertilized by a sperm outside of a woman's body and then placed back inside her uterus after normal embryo development has begun.

The first step in IVF is ovarian hyperstimulation. Injectable follicle-stimulating hormones are used to overstimulate the ovaries, with the goal of producing multiple viable ova. During this process, follicular growth is closely monitored through ultrasounds. After the doctor determines that the ovum is mature enough, the patient is given an **hCG (human chorionic gonadotropin)** injection to trigger ovulation (colloquially, this is known as the "trigger shot"). The next step of IVF is egg retrieval. Between 34 and 36 hours after the hCG injection is given and before ovulation occurs, mature ovum are surgically removed from the woman's body. This procedure is usually done transvaginally, using ultrasound guidance. A needle aspirates the vaginal walls to reach the ovaries. Many follicles can be aspirated with one puncture; depending on the success of ovarian hyperstimulation from the first step, as many as 20–30 eggs can be removed. At some point during this process, prior to fertilization, the semen is prepared in a process called sperm washing, which is the separating of individual sperm from the seminal fluid.

After both the ovum and sperm have been prepared, insemination takes place. Generally, sperm and ovum are incubated together in a culture media. Sometimes, often in instances of low sperm count or motility, a single sperm is injected into an egg in a process known as **intracytoplasmic sperm injection**, or ICSI (pronounced ICK-SEE; Figure 18-7). Fertilization is assessed 16–18 hours after insemination and again on the second and third day. These embryos are then incubated until they reach the stage of a **blastocyst**. At this point, a grading system is used to assess the quality of the embryos, and the ones that are considered the highest quality will be transferred to the woman's uterus. The embryos are inserted through the woman's cervix into her uterus. Most clinics have a maximum number of embryos they will transfer at a time; any unused, high-quality embryos can be frozen for use in another cycle. Figure 18-8 illustrates the steps in the IVF process.

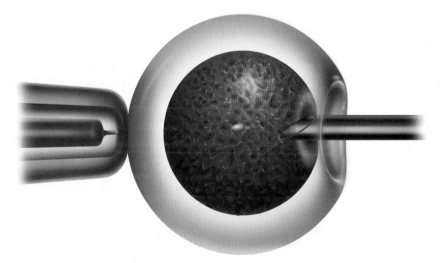

FIGURE 18-7 During intracytoplasmic sperm injection, a single sperm is injected into an egg.

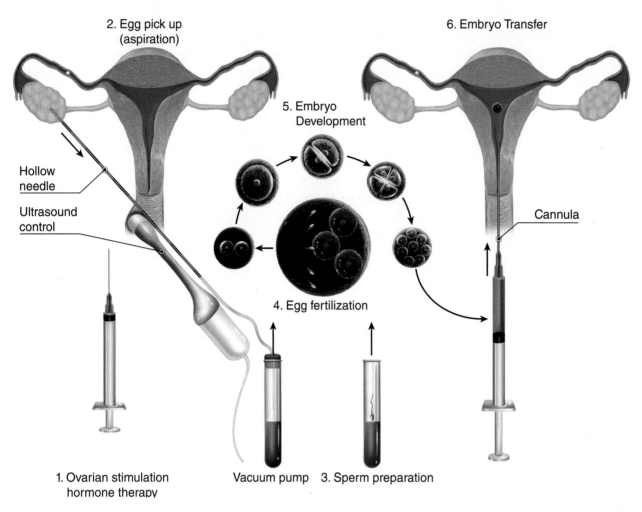

FIGURE 18-8 Steps in the in vitro fertilization process.

UNIT OBJECTIVE 18.2

Describe the fetal stages and prenatal period.

UNIT INTRODUCTION

The prenatal period is the time between when an ovum is fertilized and a baby is born. It is a time of great change! During the prenatal period, the fertilized ovum will go from a single diploid cell to a fully formed baby. Changes occur that change a zygote to an embryo, an embryo to a fetus, and a fetus to a living baby. This chapter describes the different fetal stages and the changes that occur during each stage.

LEARNING OBJECTIVE 18.2.1 Describe the major events of cleavage.

KEY TERMS

blastomeres Type of cell produced after cleavage of the zygote; it is essential in the formation of the blastula.

blastocoel Fluid-filled cavity that forms during the cleavage stage of embryonic development.

blastocyst Early form in the development of an embryo that consists of a circular layer of cells filled with fluid.

stem cells Type of cell that is undifferentiated and can produce other cells that are able to develop into any kind of cell in the body.

trophoblast Outer layer of the blastocyst that supplies nutrition to the embryo and facilitates implantation.

EMBRYONIC DEVELOPMENT: CLEAVAGE

The mitotic cellular replication that occurs within the zygote as it travels the length of the uterine tube toward the uterus is referred to as cleavage. Throughout the process of cleavage, the fertilized egg develops rapidly with no increase in size to form **blastomeres** with each cellular division. Within three days of fertilization, a morula forms (Figure 18-9). A morula is a solid ball of 12–32 cells surrounded by the protective zona pellucida; these cells continue to divide. Around the fifth day after fertilization, the morula enters the uterus and these cells organize themselves into a fluid-filled cavity known as the **blastocoel**. At this point, the zygote is known as a **blastocyst**. **Stem cells**, from which the embryo will form, make up the inner cell mass of the blastocyst. The cells that form the outer portion of the blastocyst are called a **trophoblast**, which will develop into a chorionic sac and the fetal portion of the placenta.

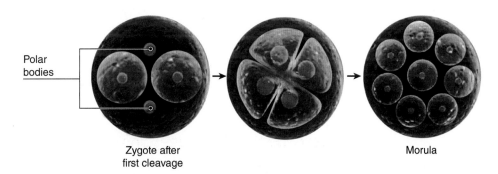

Polar bodies

Zygote after first cleavage

Morula

FIGURE 18-9 Zygote after the first cleavage.

LEARNING OBJECTIVE 18.2.2 Describe the process of embryo implantation.

KEY TERMS

endometrium Inner layer of the uterus.

fundal Larger upper part of the uterus.

EMBRYO IMPLANTATION

As the blastocyst forms, the trophoblast secretes enzymes that begin to degrade the zona pellucida, and the trophoblast cells displace the cells of the **endometrium**, beginning the process of implantation (Figure 18-10). Protrusions from trophoblast cells penetrate the endometrium, allowing adhesion to occur. The blastocyst secretes immunosuppressive agents so that the mother's immune system does not mistake it for a parasite and reject it. Progesterone causes the endometrium to thicken below the blastocyst. The process of implantation is complete when the blastocyst is burrowed into the endometrium and entirely covered (Figure 18-11). Implantation usually occurs in the anterior or posterior **fundal** region of the uterus between 6 and 10 days after conception.

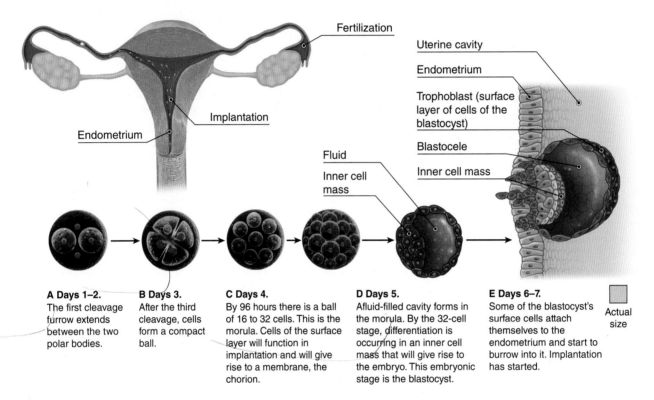

Fertilization

Uterine cavity

Endometrium

Trophoblast (surface layer of cells of the blastocyst)

Blastocele

Inner cell mass

Fluid

Inner cell mass

Implantation

Endometrium

A Days 1–2.
The first cleavage furrow extends between the two polar bodies.

B Days 3.
After the third cleavage, cells form a compact ball.

C Days 4.
By 96 hours there is a ball of 16 to 32 cells. This is the morula. Cells of the surface layer will function in implantation and will give rise to a membrane, the chorion.

D Days 5.
A fluid-filled cavity forms in the morula. By the 32-cell stage, differentiation is occurring in an inner cell mass that will give rise to the embryo. This embryonic stage is the blastocyst.

E Days 6–7.
Some of the blastocyst's surface cells attach themselves to the endometrium and start to burrow into it. Implantation has started.

Actual size

FIGURE 18-10 Embryo implantation.

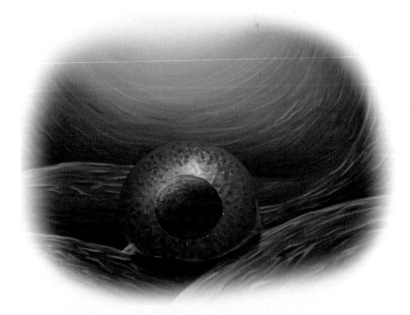

FIGURE 18-11 Blastocyst implants in the endometrium of the uterus.

LEARNING
OBJECTIVE **18.2.3** Describe the formation of the placenta.

KEY TERM

chorionic villi Found on the surface of the
chorion of the embryo, they implant within the
endometrium to provide a maximal contact area
with maternal blood.

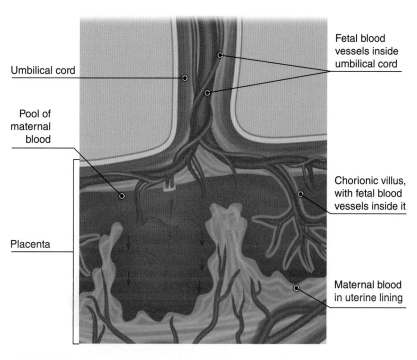

Umbilical cord

Pool of
maternal
blood

Placenta

Fetal blood
vessels inside
umbilical cord

Chorionic villus,
with fetal blood
vessels inside it

Maternal blood
in uterine lining

FIGURE 18-12 Maternal and fetal blood vessels of the placenta.

FORMATION OF THE PLACENTA

The trophoblast cells are the precursor for the placenta. Chorionic villi, which are finger-like projections, develop out of the trophoblast and extend into the blood-filled spaces of the endometrium. These villi are vascular processes that will form the fetal portion of the placenta, obtaining oxygen and nutrients from the maternal bloodstream and disposing of carbon dioxide and waste products into the maternal blood. Fetal blood remains in the vessels of the chorionic villi and the maternal blood in the intervillous spaces, so there is no mixing of maternal and fetal blood (Figure 18-12).

LEARNING
OBJECTIVE **18.2.4** List the functions of the placenta.

PLACENTAL FUNCTION

The functions of the placenta include:

- Fetal nutrition—the placenta transfers nutrients from the mother to the fetus.
- Fetal respiration—the placenta allows for exchange of oxygen from the mother to the fetus.
- Fetal excretion—the fetus is able to transfer waste products and carbon dioxide back to the mother through the placenta.
- Hormone production—the placenta secretes hCG, progesterone (both of which aid in implementation), and estrogen (to enlarge the breasts and uterus of the mother).

LEARNING OBJECTIVE 18.2.5 Explain the process of blood flow and gas exchange through the placenta.

PLACENTAL BLOOD FLOW

Oxygen and carbon dioxide diffuse across the placenta in response to differences in partial pressure. The **mean partial pressure** of oxygen (pO_2) in the maternal blood is higher than the fetal blood, allowing for the oxygen to readily **diffuse** across the placenta from maternal to fetal blood. The partial pressure of carbon dioxide ($PaCO_2$) is higher in the fetal blood, allowing it to diffuse from the fetal blood through the placenta into the maternal circulation. Transfer of oxygen occurs as maternal blood enters the spiral arteries and perfuses the intervillous spaces. The intervillous spaces are where the exchange of oxygen and nutrients take place. The maternal blood passes through the intervillous spaces and drains back through the venous orifices, which return the blood to the maternal systemic circulation via the uterine veins. The umbilical cord carries deoxygenated blood and fetal waste through two umbilical arteries. Nutrients and oxygen are transported from the mother to the fetus through the single umbilical vein (Figure 18-13). Fetal hemoglobin has a higher affinity for oxygen then adult hemoglobin. Because of this, the developing fetus has better access to oxygen in the mother's blood than the mother does.

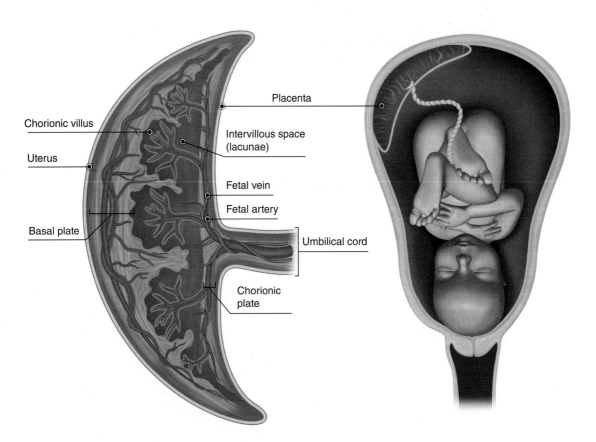

FIGURE 18-13 Placental structure and circulation.

LEARNING
OBJECTIVE **18.2.6** Contrast the circulatory system of the fetus with that of an adult.

FETAL CIRCULATORY SYSTEM

The circulatory pathways of the fetus differ from that of an adult. It uses two shunts that allow for bypass of fetal body parts (particularly the lungs and the liver) that are not fully developed while the fetus is in the womb. Oxygenated and nutrient-rich blood flows from the mother, across the placenta, and through the umbilical cord to the fetal liver. When this blood reaches the fetal liver, it is divided into two branches. One branch circulates some of the oxygenated blood through the liver, but the majority of the blood is shunted through the **ductus venosus** into the inferior vena cava where it mixes with deoxygenated blood from the fetal legs and abdomen on its way to the right atrium. The majority of the blood entering the right atrium is shunted through the **foramen ovale** to the left atrium. There it mixes with a small amount of deoxygenated blood returning from the fetal lungs through the pulmonary veins. The blood then flows into the left ventricle in which the majority of the oxygen-rich blood is pumped out of the aorta, to the heart, head, neck, and arms. Deoxygenated blood returning from the head and arms enters the right atrium through the superior vena cava. The blood is then directed downward into the right ventricle, where it is squeezed into the pulmonary artery. A small amount of blood circulates through the resistant lung tissue, but the majority flows through the **ductus arteriosus** into the aorta, distal to the point of exit of the arteries supplying the head and arms with oxygenated blood. The oxygen-poor blood that flows through the abdominal aorta into the internal iliac arteries is where the umbilical arteries direct most of it back through the umbilical cord to the placenta. It is at this point the waste in the blood and carbon dioxide are exchanged for nutrients and oxygen. The blood remaining in the iliac arteries flows through the fetal abdomen and legs, ultimately returning through the inferior vena cava to the heart (Figure 18-14).

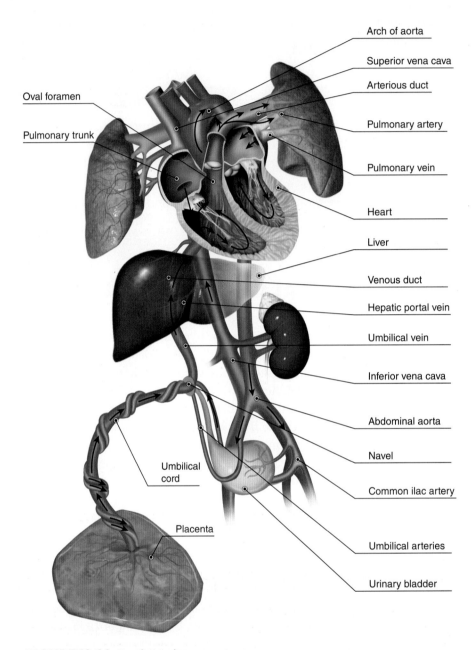

Arch of aorta

Superior vena cava

Arterious duct

Oval foramen

Pulmonary artery

Pulmonary trunk

Pulmonary vein

Heart

Liver

Venous duct

Hepatic portal vein

Umbilical vein

Inferior vena cava

Abdominal aorta

Navel

Umbilical cord

Common iliac artery

Placenta

Umbilical arteries

Urinary bladder

FIGURE 18-14 Fetal circulatory system.

ADULT CIRCULATORY SYSTEM

The circulatory system of the adult does not have right to left shunts in the circulatory system; the shunts close soon after birth so that the adult circulatory system can function correctly. The foramen ovale that bypasses blood flow to the lungs by **shunting** the blood from the right to the left atrium and the ductus arteriosus that moves the blood from the pulmonary artery to the aorta is not present in the adult circulatory system. The circulatory system of an adult also does not have the ductus venosus shunt in which highly oxygenated blood flows through the liver to the inferior vena cava and then to the right atrium of the heart. In an adult, oxygenation and removal of carbon dioxide take place in the lungs and waste is removed by the kidneys (Figure 18-15).

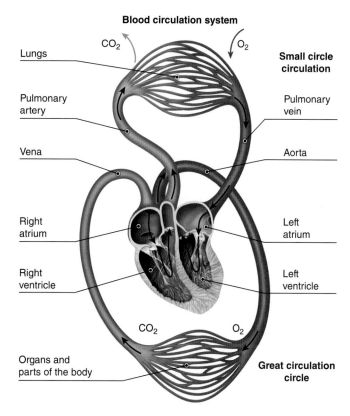

Blood circulation system

FIGURE 18-15 Adult circulatory system.

LEARNING OBJECTIVE	**18.2.7**	**Identify the stages of development between fertilization and delivery.**
LEARNING OBJECTIVE	**18.2.8**	**Describe the stages of development between fertilization and delivery.**

KEY TERMS

canalicular period Period of lung development that occurs between 16 and 26 weeks of gestation; during this period, basic structures of the gas-exchanging parts of the lungs form, and the terminal saccules begin to form.

herniating Protruding through an abnormal body opening; in the case of fetal development, the intestine temporarily herniates into the umbilical cord until there is enough room for it in the abdomen.

lanugo Fine, downy hair is present in almost all parts of the body of the fetus after 20 weeks of gestation.

ossification Calcification of soft tissue into bone-like material or bone formation.

pharyngeal arches Series of externally observable anterior tissue bands located below the early brain and that will eventually form the structural features of the head and neck.

preembryonic stage First two weeks of development after fertilization; during this time, cleavage, implantation, and embryogenesis occur.

pseudoglandular Embryonic stage of growth of lung tissue before the ciliated cells are differentiated.

somite Divisions of the body of an embryo.

terminal saccular stage Last generation of air spaces in the respiratory system are formed.

transvaginal Assessment through the vagina.

STAGES OF DEVELOPMENT

After conception, there are three stages of development:

- Preembryonic stage—occurring during weeks 1–4 of gestation
- Embryonic stage—occurring during weeks 5–8 of gestation
- Fetal stage—occurring during weeks 9–40 of gestation

Preembryonic Stage

The first stage of development is the preembryonic stage (one to four weeks' gestation). During the first two weeks after the last menstrual period, the egg follicles mature in the ovaries and are released at the end of the second week. This time is considered the first two weeks of the pregnancy, even though the woman is not yet pregnant at this time. During the third week, if fertilization occurs, the zygote will begin producing the pregnancy hormone hCG. This hormone becomes detectable in the mother's blood and urine 6–14 days after fertilization. During the third week of gestation, the sex of the fetus is determined by the father's sperm, and during this time twins may be formed. The embryo is the size of a pinhead and most pregnancy tests will be positive at this time. During the fourth week of gestation, **somites** form on either side of the embryo's midline. A tailbud as well as the **pharyngeal arches** are present (Figure 18-16).

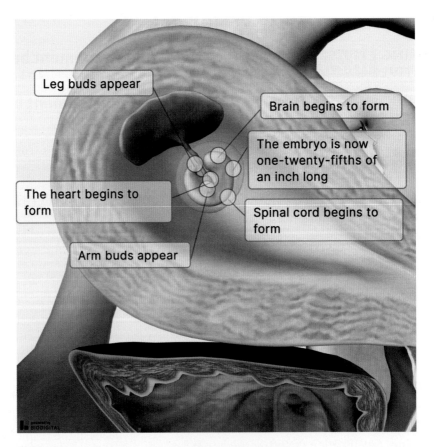

Leg buds appear

Brain begins to form

The embryo is now one-twenty-fifths of an inch long

The heart begins to form

Spinal cord begins to form

Arm buds appear

FIGURE 18-16 Embryonic Development—Week 4
Embryo inside of the uterus at week 4 of gestation.

Embryonic Stage

The second stage of development is the embryonic stage (five to eight weeks' gestation). During this stage, tissues differentiate into organs and external features develop. The major milestones that occur during this stage are:

- Five weeks: The brain, spine, and heart have begun to form. By the end of the fifth week, the heart will start beating. During this critical period, the embryo is at risk for many birth defects; most of them will have no known cause or will be due to multiple factors.
- Six weeks: the embryo is about the size of a pea, and the eyes, nostrils, arms, and legs are taking shape. Both the arms and legs have digits, although they may be webbed. The heartbeat is about 110 beats per minute and can be seen during a **transvaginal** ultrasound. The liver begins to produce blood cells.
- Seven weeks: the embryo is about 0.4 inches, and the hands, feet, mouth, and face are forming. The trachea and bronchi have formed, and the heart is beating about 120 beats per minute. The beginnings of all important external and internal structures are now present.
- Eight weeks: the embryo is 0.6 inches and weighs less than ½ ounce. The embryo is about the size of a bean and the fingers and toes are developing. The intestine elongates and becomes too large to fit inside the baby's abdomen; it temporarily moves outside the abdomen, **herniating**, or bulging, the outside of the umbilical cord and rotating counter-clockwise. (The intestines will return into the abdomen at about 12 weeks' gestation.) Large bones are forming and muscles can contract (Figure 18-17).

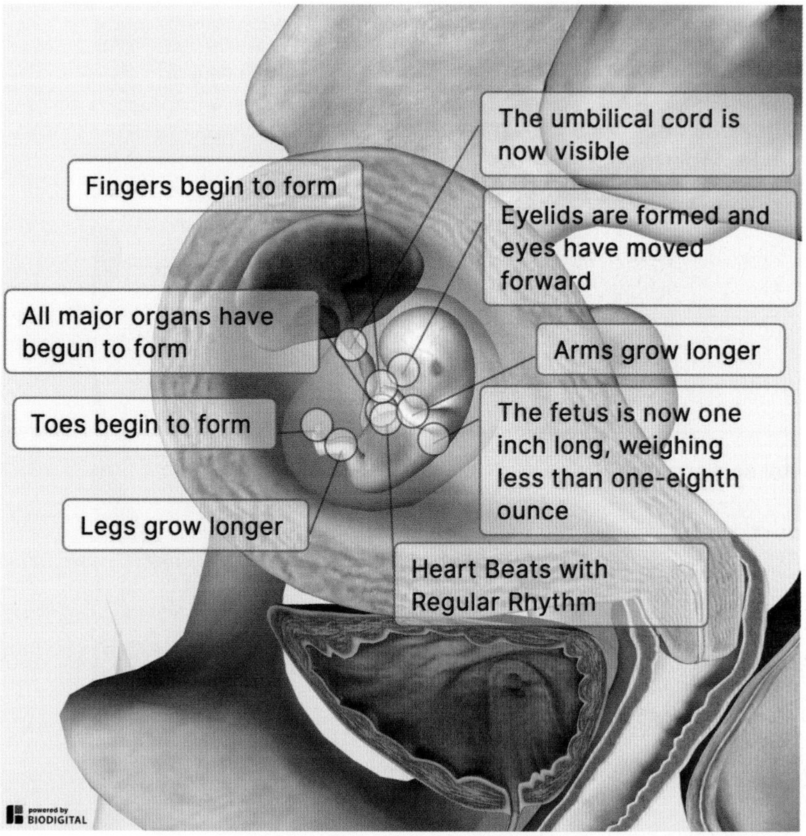

FIGURE 18-17 The embryo inside of the uterus at week 8 of gestation.

Fetal Stage

The third and final stage is the fetal stage (9–40 weeks' gestation). At the beginning of the fetal stage, every organ system and external structure is present. During this stage, rapid growth and tissue and organ differentiation occur. Because all of the major organs have already begun to develop during the embryonic phase, the fetus is less susceptible to environmental abnormalities during this period. While toxins or nutritional defects can cause physiological abnormalities, they are unlikely to cause miscarriage. The major milestones that occur during this stage are:

- Nine weeks' gestational age: the heart is beating at about 170 beats per minute, the average embryo is 0.9 inches long and weighs about ½ ounce. The head is large, almost half the entire size of the fetus.
- Ten weeks' gestational age: the tail of the embryo has disappeared by the end of the tenth week. Fingerprints are forming, and bone cells are replacing cartilage. The eyelids have formed and closed. The average fetus at 10 weeks is 1.2 inches long and 1.2 ounces.
- Eleven weeks' gestation age: the fetus is starting to produce breathing movements and can open its mouth and swallow. The average fetus at 11 weeks is 1.6 inches long and weighs 1.6 ounces.
- Twelve weeks' gestational age: the fetus is starting to make random movements and producing thyroid hormone. Its pancreas is making insulin, the liver is making red blood cells, and the kidneys are producing urine. The heartbeat can usually be heard by now, and tooth buds have formed for all 20 baby teeth. The fetus is able to curl its fingers toward the palm to make a fist. The fetus is 12.1 inches and weighs 2 ounces. This marks the end of the first trimester (Figure 18-18).

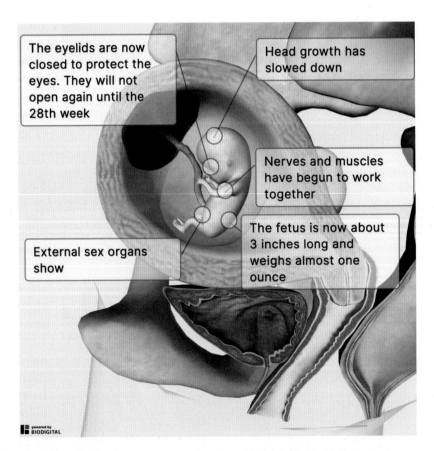

FIGURE 18-18 Fetus inside the uterus at week 12 of gestation.

- Thirteen weeks' gestational age: all of the major organs are formed, but are too immature for the fetus to survive outside the womb. **Lanugo** begins to develop on the head and bones are beginning to harden. The fetus is 2.5 inches and weighs 2.6 ounces.

- Fourteen weeks' gestational age: the fetus's toenails are appearing, and the gender may be apparent. Skin is still transparent, making the blood vessels visible. The fetal length is 3.1 inches with a weight of 3.3 ounces.

- Fifteen weeks' gestational age: the mother may sense fetal movements, referred to as quickening. The fetus can make sucking movements, swallowing amniotic fluid. The average fetus is 6.4 inches and weighs 4.1 ounces.

- Sixteen to seventeen weeks' gestational age: the **canalicular period** of lung development has started, with bronchial tubes branching out into the lungs; it will continue through 25 weeks' gestation. By the end of 17 weeks, the **pseudoglandular** stage of lung development ends; however, there are no alveoli developed. Hearing has also begun to occur. The fetus is now 7.9 inches long and weighs 6.4 ounces. The fetus grows rapidly between weeks 17 and 20 (Figure 18-19).

- Eighteen weeks' gestational age: the ears stand out, and the fetus begins to respond to sound. A layer of fat begins to accumulate underneath the skin. The average length is 8.6 inches and a weight of 7.9 ounces.

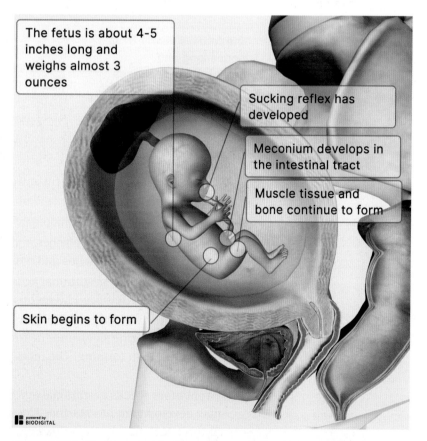

The fetus is about 4–5 inches long and weighs almost 3 ounces

Sucking reflex has developed

Meconium develops in the intestinal tract

Muscle tissue and bone continue to form

Skin begins to form

powered by
BIODIGITAL

FIGURE 18-19 Fetus inside the uterus at week 16 of gestation.

- Nineteen weeks' gestational age: the nose, ears, and lips are recognizable. The fetus begins to experience somewhat regular periods of sleeping and wakefulness. The average length is 9.3 inches and average weight is 9.6 ounces.
- Twenty weeks' gestational age: the body of the fetus is now covered in lanugo and has some scalp hair. The fetus is now capable of producing IgG and IgM antibodies. The average fetus is 9.9 inches and weighs 11.7 ounces (Figure 18-20).

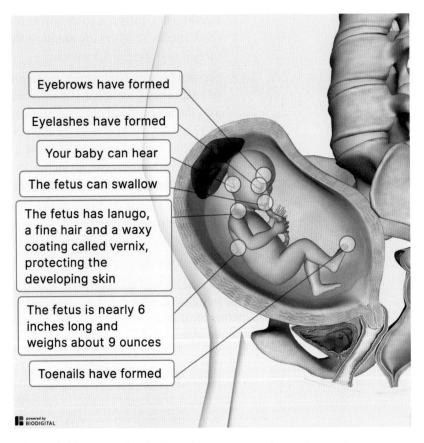

Eyebrows have formed

Eyelashes have formed

Your baby can hear

The fetus can swallow

The fetus has lanugo, a fine hair and a waxy coating called vernix, protecting the developing skin

The fetus is nearly 6 inches long and weighs about 9 ounces

Toenails have formed

FIGURE 18-20 Fetus inside the uterus at week 20 of gestation.

- Twenty-one weeks' gestational age: the fetus can suck and grasp and may get hiccups. Eyelashes and fingernails are forming. The average fetus is 10.6 inches and weighs 14.1 ounces.
- Twenty-two weeks' gestational age: in boys, the testes have begun to descend. The fetus is 11.2 inches and weighs 1.1 pounds.
- Twenty-three weeks' gestational age: the fetus has rapid eye movements during sleep and the foundation for fingerprints and footprints begin forming. The fetus is 11.9 inches long weighing 1.2 pounds.
- Twenty-four weeks gestational age: the **terminal saccular stage** of lung development has started. The skin is coated in vernix caseosa. At this point, the startle reflex is present. The average fetus is about 12.5 inches long and weighs 1.5 pounds (Figure 18-21).

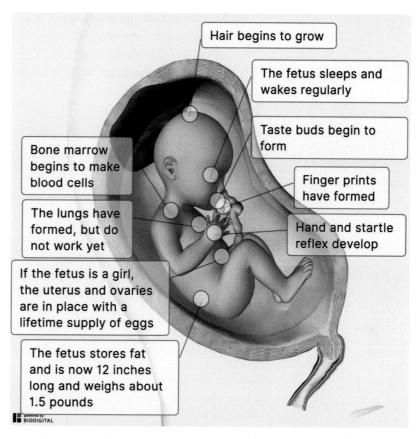

Hair begins to grow

The fetus sleeps and wakes regularly

Taste buds begin to form

Finger prints have formed

Hand and startle reflex develop

Bone marrow begins to make blood cells

The lungs have formed, but do not work yet

If the fetus is a girl, the uterus and ovaries are in place with a lifetime supply of eggs

The fetus stores fat and is now 12 inches long and weighs about 1.5 pounds

FIGURE 18-21 Fetus inside the uterus at week 24 of gestation.

- Twenty-five weeks' gestational age: by the 25th week, respirations are possible and the survival rate outside the womb is good. By the end of this week, the fetus heartbeat can be heard through a stethoscope. The brain is developing rapidly and the nervous system is able to regulate some body functions. The average fetus is 13.1 inches long and weighs about 1.7 pounds.

- Twenty-six weeks' gestational age: the fetus can respond to sound that occurs in the mother's surroundings and the eyelids open and close. The average fetus is 13.7 inches and 2 pounds. Survival outside of the womb is expected.

- Twenty-seven weeks' gestational age: the fetus is developing additional fat, which makes skin look smoother. The average fetus is 14.2 inches long and weighs 2.3 pounds. This marks the end of the second trimester.

- Twenty-eight weeks' gestational age: the fetus has eyelashes. The central nervous system can control rhythmic breathing movements and body temperature. The average fetus is now 14.8 inches long and weighs 2.7 pounds.

- Twenty-nine through thirty-one weeks' gestational age: the fetus continues to grow and gain weight. Bones are fully developed, although still soft and flexible. At the end of this period, the average fetus is 16.4 inches long and weighs 3.9 pounds.

- Thirty-two through thirty-three weeks' gestational age: the fetus begins to form muscle and store body fat. **Ossification** can be seen on the distal femoral epiphysis. The fetus at the end of this period is 17.3 inches long and weighs 4.8 pounds (Figure 18-22).

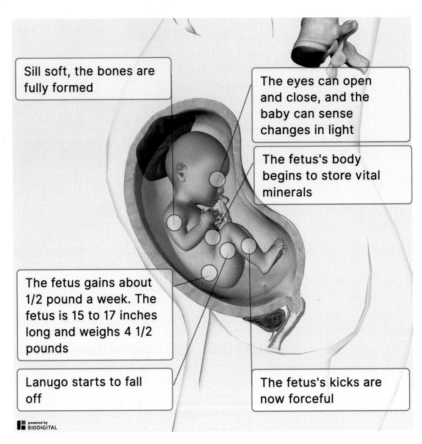

Sill soft, the bones are fully formed

The eyes can open and close, and the baby can sense changes in light

The fetus's body begins to store vital minerals

The fetus gains about 1/2 pound a week. The fetus is 15 to 17 inches long and weighs 4 1/2 pounds

Lanugo starts to fall off

The fetus's kicks are now forceful

powered by BIODIGITAL

FIGURE 18-22 Fetus inside the uterus at week 32 of gestation.

- Thirty-four through thirty-six weeks' gestational age: the tibial epiphysis ossification center may be seen. Lanugo begins to disappear, replaced by vellus hair. At this point, the fetus takes up most of the amniotic sac. At the end of this period the fetus is 18.6 inches long weighing 5.2 pounds. A baby born at 36 weeks has a very good chance for survival, although some medical intervention may be necessary (Figure 18-23).
- Thirty-seven through thirty-eight weeks' gestational age: the proximal humerus epiphysis ossification center can be seen. At around 37 weeks, the baby may turn so that its head points toward the pelvis. The fetus is 19.5 inches long weighing 7.1 pounds.
- Thirty-nine through forty-one weeks' gestational age: the fetus is considered full term. The fetus is gaining up to a half a pound a week at this point. At the end of this period, the average fetus is 20.5 inches and weighs 8.3 pounds (Figure 18-24).

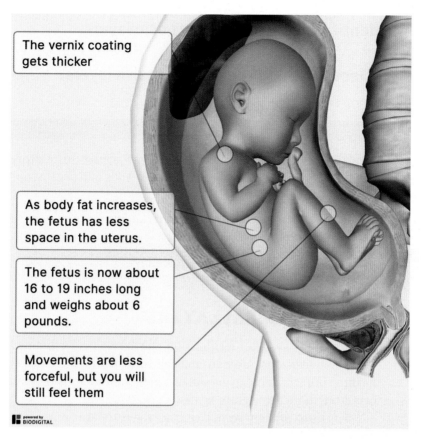

The vernix coating gets thicker

As body fat increases, the fetus has less space in the uterus.

The fetus is now about 16 to 19 inches long and weighs about 6 pounds.

Movements are less forceful, but you will still feel them

FIGURE 18-23 The fetus inside the uterus at week 36 of gestation.

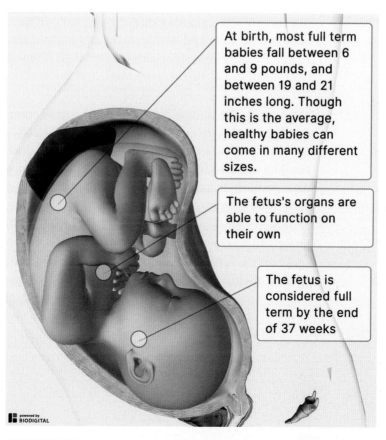

At birth, most full term babies fall between 6 and 9 pounds, and between 19 and 21 inches long. Though this is the average, healthy babies can come in many different sizes.

The fetus's organs are able to function on their own

The fetus is considered full term by the end of 37 weeks

FIGURE 18-24 Fetus inside the uterus at week 40 of gestation.

LEARNING OBJECTIVE 18.2.9 Identify the three primary germ layers.

LEARNING OBJECTIVE 18.2.10 Describe the three primary germ layers.

KEY TERMS

ectoderm Outermost germ layer in the early embryo; it will go on to form the nervous system; tooth enamel; epidermis; and lining of the mouth, nose, anus, and sweat glands.

endoderm Innermost germ layer in the early embryo; it will go on to form much of the gastrointestinal tract, respiratory tract, endocrine glands and organs, and urinary system.

mesoderm Middle germ layer in the early embryo; it will go on to form muscle and connective tissue.

PRIMARY GERM LAYERS

Prior to 10–14 days after fertilization, the mass of cells that make up the blastocyst is homogeneous. After around day 14, however, these cells differentiate into the three primary germ layers. All of a person's tissues and organs will eventually form from these three germ layers.

The three primary germ layers are the ectoderm, mesoderm, and endoderm (Figure 18-25):

- **Ectoderm:** This outer germ layer gives rise to the epidermis, pigmented cells, glands (anterior pituitary, cutaneous, and mammary), nails and hair, central and peripheral nervous systems, endocrine structures, adrenal gland medullary cells, the lens of the eyes, tooth enamel, and floor of the amniotic cavity.

- **Mesoderm:** The middle germ layer that forms connective tissues and muscle throughout the body, except the head. The connective tissues include cartilage, bone, blood vessel endothelium, dermis, etc. The muscles formed include cardiac, skeletal, and smooth. Also developed are the cardiovascular system, spleen, and urogenital system.

- **Endoderm:** The inner germ layer that contributes the epithelial lining and glands of the gastrointestinal tract, respiratory tract, oropharynx, urethra, bladder, vagina, and the liver and pancreas (Figure 18-26).

Germ layers

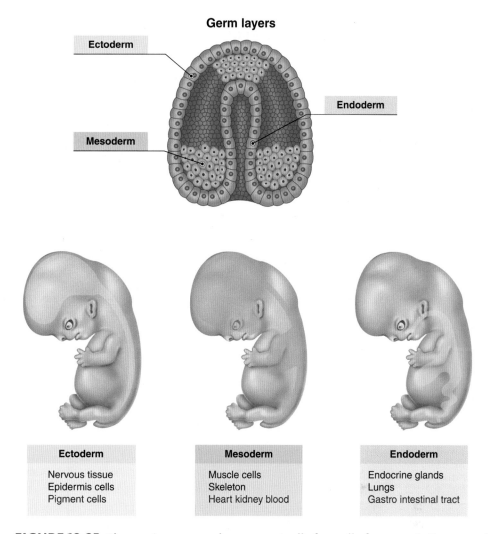

Ectoderm	Mesoderm	Endoderm
Nervous tissue	Muscle cells	Endocrine glands
Epidermis cells	Skeleton	Lungs
Pigment cells	Heart kidney blood	Gastro intestinal tract

FIGURE 18-25 Three primary germ layers eventually form all of a person's tissues and organs.

Stem cell

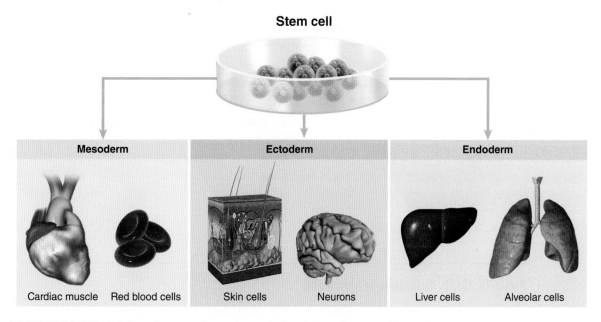

Mesoderm		Ectoderm		Endoderm	
Cardiac muscle	Red blood cells	Skin cells	Neurons	Liver cells	Alveolar cells

FIGURE 18-26 Origins of organs from the endoderm, ectoderm, and mesoderm.

LEARNING OBJECTIVE 18.2.11 Identify the major events of the fetal period.

LEARNING OBJECTIVE 18.2.12 Describe the major events of the fetal period.

KEY TERM

organogenesis Formation and development of organs.

MAJOR EVENTS OF THE FETAL PERIOD

Pregnancy is divided into three trimesters:

First trimester: 1–12 weeks' gestation

Second trimester: 13–27 weeks' gestation

Third trimester: 28–41 weeks' gestation (Figure 18-27)

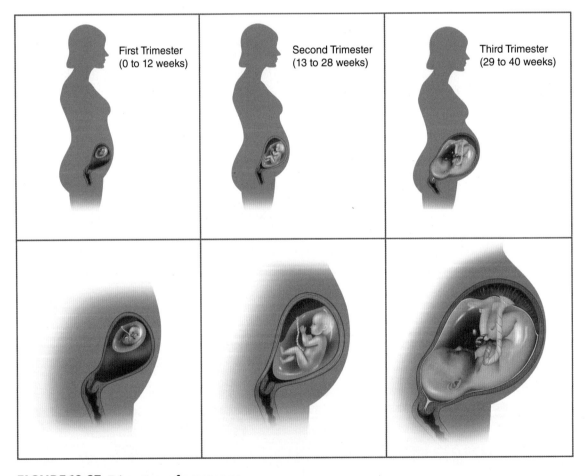

FIGURE 18-27 Trimesters of pregnancy.

The major events that occur during each trimester are:

- First trimester: **Organogenesis** is completed. A doppler can detect the heartbeat by the end of the 12th week of gestation (Figure 18-28).
- Second trimester: Fetal movement can be felt. At 24 weeks' gestation, the fetus has reached an age of viability wherein there is a possibility of survival (Figure 18-29).
- Third trimester: Lung maturity continues to develop, the fetus stores adipose tissue, and the basic reflex responses are developed; at the end of the trimester the fetus is considered full term (Figure 18-30).

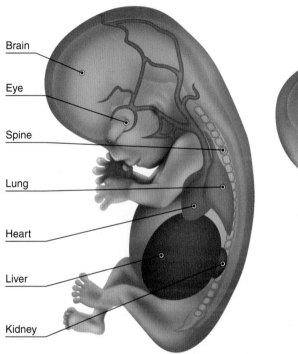

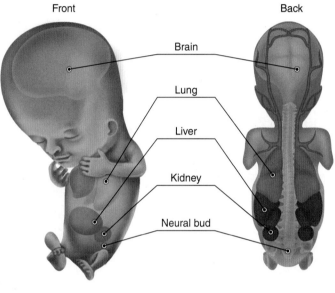

FIGURE 18-28 Embryo anatomy—week 10.

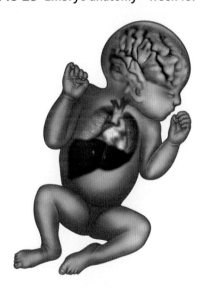

Fetus at week 24

FIGURE 18-29 Fetus—week 24.

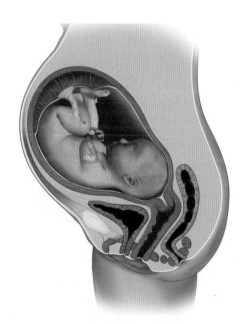

FIGURE 18-30 Fetus—week 40.

UNIT OBJECTIVE 18.3

Describe female hormonal, physiological, and anatomical changes during pregnancy.

UNIT INTRODUCTION

There are many physiological and anatomical changes that occur during pregnancy. Hormones play a large role in sustaining the pregnancy and facilitates physiological and anatomical changes that are necessary to support the pregnancy. Other changes result from the fetus growing inside the uterus and the reaction of the mother's body to that growth. In the following section, you will find a description of the changes that occur prior to conception up until delivery, as well as the changes that support lactation.

LEARNING OBJECTIVE 18.3.1 List female hormonal changes during pregnancy.

LEARNING OBJECTIVE 18.3.2 Describe female hormonal changes during pregnancy.

KEY TERMS

linea nigra Linear hyperpigmentation that occurs during pregnancy midline on the abdomen from the symphysis pubis to the top of the uterus (fundus).

melasma Dark spots that form on the face during pregnancy due to hormonal fluctuations.

LIST OF HORMONAL CHANGES DURING PREGNANCY

Female hormonal changes during pregnancy include:

Increased insulin

Increased relaxin

Increased estrogen

Increased cortisol

Increased oxytocin

Parathyroid hormone

Increased aldosterone

Increased progesterone

Increased melanotropin

Increased serum prolactin

Increased human chorionic gonadotropin (hCG)

Increased human chorionic somatomammotropin

Increased thyroxine-binding globulin, thyroxine, triiodothyronine

DESCRIPTION OF HORMONAL CHANGES DURING PREGNANCY

- Increased insulin: Production increases to compensate for insulin antagonism caused by placental hormones; effect of insulin antagonists is to decrease tissue sensitivity to insulin or ability to use insulin.
- Increased relaxin: Promotes loosening of the ligaments of the pubic symphysis and sacroiliac joints to facilitate labor and birth.
- Increased estrogen: Suppresses secretion of follicle-stimulating hormone (FSH) and luteinizing hormone (LH) by the anterior pituitary gland; causes fat to deposit in subcutaneous tissues over the maternal abdomen, back, and upper thighs; promotes enlargement of genitals, uterus, and breasts; increases vascularity; relaxes pelvic ligaments and joints; interferes with folic acid metabolism; increases the level of total body proteins; promotes retention of sodium and water; decreases secretion of hydrochloric acid and pepsin; decreases mother's ability to use insulin.
- Increased cortisol: Stimulates production of insulin and increases the peripheral resistance to insulin.
- Increased oxytocin: Stimulates uterine contractions and milk ejection from the breasts.
- Parathyroid hormone: Responsible for balancing calcium and magnesium; any abnormal maternal levels will also be found in the fetus.
- Increased aldosterone: Stimulates reabsorption of excess sodium from the renal tubules.
- Increased progesterone: Suppresses secretion of FSH and LH by the anterior pituitary gland; maintains pregnancy by relaxing smooth muscles, decreasing uterine contractility; causes fat to deposit in subcutaneous tissues over the maternal abdomen, back, and upper thighs; decreases mother's ability to use insulin.
- Increased melanotropin: Responsible for the darkening of the nipples, areola, axilla, and vulva that occurs in the second trimester; melasma and linea nigra occur as a result of the increased release of the hormone.
- Increased serum prolactin: Prepares breasts for lactation.
- Increased human chorionic gonadotropin (hCG): Produced only during pregnancy and almost exclusively by the placenta. The hormone maintains the corpus luteum production of estrogen and progesterone until the placenta takes over.
- Increased human chorionic somatomammotropin: Acts as a growth hormone; contributes to breast development; decreases maternal metabolism of insulin; and increases the amount of fatty acids for metabolic needs.
- Increased thyroxine-binding globulin, thyroxine, triiodothyronine: With adequate iodine intake, levels are increased slightly to maintain metabolic function.

LEARNING OBJECTIVE **18.3.3** List female anatomical changes during pregnancy.

LEARNING OBJECTIVE **18.3.4** Describe female anatomical changes during pregnancy.

KEY TERMS

diastasis recti abdominis Gap between the two sides of the rectus abdominis muscle, caused by the stretching of the expanding uterus in pregnancy.

Montgomery tubercles Sebaceous oil glands embedded in the areola that secrete anti-infective and lubricating properties to protect the nipples and areola during breastfeeding.

LIST OF ANATOMICAL CHANGES DURING PREGNANCY

The female body goes through many anatomical changes during pregnancy. The maternal anatomical changes that occur during pregnancy take place in the:

Breasts
Vagina
Reproductive system
Cardiovascular system
Renal system
Integumentary system
Respiratory system
Musculoskeletal system

DESCRIPTION OF ANATOMICAL CHANGES DURING PREGNANCY

As pregnancy progresses, the female body will begin experiencing anatomical changes that will continue to change her body throughout pregnancy.

Breast changes. Sensitivity and heaviness occur due to the increased levels of estrogen and progesterone. The Montgomery tubercles hypertrophy around the areola. Breast size increases due to glandular growth and an increase in adipose.

Vaginal changes. Changes occur as a result of hormonal changes; the vaginal mucosa thickens, connective tissue loosens, smooth muscle hypertrophies, and the vaginal vault lengthens.

Reproductive system. Occurrence of Hegar's sign, which is a softening of the lower uterine segment. Goodell's sign, which is the softening of the cervical tip, also occurs as a result of the increased vascularity and tissue hyperplasia.

Cardiovascular system. Slight cardiac hypertrophy occurs as a result of the changes in the cardiovascular volume and cardiac workload. Slight cardiac elevation and rotation to the left occurs as the diaphragm is displaced upward by the growing uterus.

Renal system. Changes occur in the renal system in relation to the blood volume, estrogen and progesterone, and pressure from the enlarging uterus. These changes include dilation of the pelvis and ureters, hyperplasia, hypertrophy, and decreased muscle in the ureters, which also become elongated. These changes place the client at risk for urinary stasis and stagnation, which can result in unwanted growth of bacteria.

Integumentary system. Hair and nail growth may be accelerated.

Respiratory system. Structural changes occur to meet the need for oxygen consumption, changes in maternal organs, and the needs of the fetus and placenta. The diaphragm rises, the costal angle of the ribs increases, the lower ribs flare out, and ligaments of the rib cage relax.

Musculoskeletal system. Due to the physical changes, including increasing weight, an increase in the lumbosacral curve develops, which is known as lordosis (Figure 18-31). A compensatory change in the cervicodorsal region also develops to help the client maintain balance. This change appears as an exaggerated anterior flexion of the head. A **diastasis recti abdominis** may occur due to the loss of abdominal muscle tone and stretching of the abdominal wall.

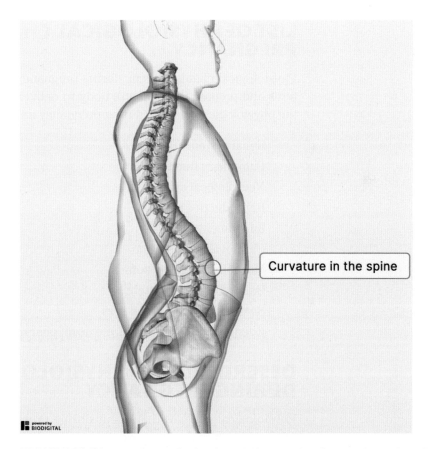

Curvature in the spine

FIGURE 18-31 Increase in the lumbosacral curve develops and can alter the gait and posture of a pregnant woman.

LEARNING
OBJECTIVE **18.3.5** List female physiological changes during pregnancy.

LEARNING
OBJECTIVE **18.3.6** Describe female physiological changes during pregnancy.

KEY TERMS

acroesthesia Extremely abnormal sensitivity to pain, heat, cold, or touch.

hypoglycemia Low blood sugar.

microbiome Microorganisms in a particular environment.

mucus plug Plug formed by a small amount of cervical mucus that fills and seals the cervical canal during pregnancy.

nocturia The need to frequently urinate at night.

striae gravidarum Stretch marks on the skin.

thromboembolic Formation of a blood clot in a vessel.

vasomotor Controlling the diameter of a blood vessel.

LIST OF PHYSIOLOGICAL CHANGES DURING PREGNANCY

Physiological changes occur during pregnancy to accommodate the growing fetus and prepare the woman's body to deliver the child. Systems affected by the physiological changes during pregnancy are:

Renal system
Pulmonary function
Neurological system
Reproductive system
Integumentary system
Cardiovascular system
Musculoskeletal system
Gastrointestinal system
Sense of fullness in the ears
Edema and hyperemia of the nose, pharynx, larynx, trachea, and bronchi

DESCRIPTION OF PHYSIOLOGICAL CHANGES DURING PREGNANCY

Physiological changes that occur during pregnancy include changes to most organ systems in the body. We discuss these changes one system at a time.

Renal system. During the first and third trimesters, nocturia, urinary frequency, and urgency occur as a result of the influence of pressure of the uterus. During the second trimester, the bladder is out of the pelvis of the abdomen so the symptoms are not as prevalent. The plasma renal flow and glomerular filtration rate increases due to the maternal metabolic and circulatory demands and the excretion of fetal waste. The tubular absorption of the kidneys is also increased to manage the increased fluids and electrolytes. Decreased motility of the ureters, caused by increased progesterone, can lead to urine stasis and increase the risk of a urinary tract infection.

Pulmonary function change. Tidal volume of air increases and the volume of gas expelled from the lungs increases. This results in a state of chronic mild hyperventilation or a state of respiratory alkalosis occurring. Oxygen consumption increases to meet the needs of the mother, as well as the fetus and placenta.

Neurological system. Some physiological alterations may result in sensory changes in the legs from compression of the pelvic nerves. Pain may occur as a result of the exaggerated lordosis and carpal tunnel syndrome can occur during the last trimester from edema. Additionally, a pregnant woman may experience **acroesthesia** caused by a stooped shoulder stance; tension headache, lightheadedness, or syncope as a result of postural hypotension; **vasomotor** instability; **hypoglycemia**; and a corneal thickening and decreased intraocular pressure.

Reproductive system. During pregnancy, the pH of the vagina decreases from a decline in vaginal **microbiome** and anaerobic bacteria. Goodell's sign, which occurs at around four weeks' gestation, is the softening of the cervical tip that occurs as a result of the increased vascularity and tissue hyperplasia. Chadwick sign, which occurs as early as six to eight weeks after conception, is an increase in vascularity that results in bluish discoloration of the vaginal mucosa and cervix. Leukorrhea is an increase in mucoid vaginal discharge in response to estrogen and progesterone. Estrogen also causes an increase in activity of the endocervical glands in the cervix. These secrete a thick mucus, which will thicken and accumulate, forming the **mucus plug**.

Integumentary system. Changes occurring due to the hormone melanotropin include a darkening of the nipples, areola, axilla, and vulva that occurs in the second trimester. Melasma may occur; this is characterized by a blotchy brown hyperpigmentation over the forehead, nose, and cheeks. Linea nigra is a pigmented line that extends form the symphysis pubis midline to the top of the fundus (Figure 18-32). These changes occur frequently in clients with darker skin. **Striae gravidarum** may appear as a result of the separation of the underlying connective tissue on the abdomen and breasts. Angiomatas are spider-like dilated vessels that are a result of the increased vascularity of the skin and occur on the neck, arms, and chest. Pink or red mottled blotches may appear on the palms of the hands and acne may worsen.

Cardiovascular system. The heart rate increases from the fifth week of gestation by 10–15 beats a minute over the pre-pregnancy baseline by 32 weeks' gestation and will remain elevated throughout the pregnancy. Cardiac output increases 30–50% by the end of the second and the beginning of the third trimester. Blood volume increases by 1200–1500 mL. There may be a slight decrease in systolic blood pressure and

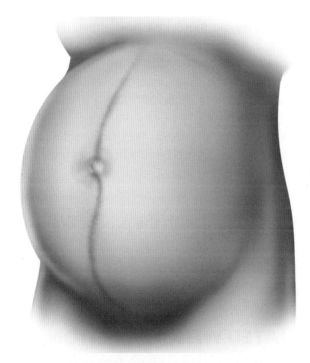

FIGURE 18-32 Linea nigra is the pigmented line extending from the symphysis pubis midline to the top of the fundus.

a slight decrease in diastolic blood pressure in mid-pregnancy with a gradual return to the pre-pregnancy baseline by term. Vasodilation occurs as a result of progesterone to allow the maternal circulatory system to compensate for the increased blood volume. A decrease in hematocrit and hemoglobin occurs due to the disproportionate increase of red blood cells in relation to plasma volume. This effect results in a hemodilution known as physiological anemia of pregnancy. Increased clotting factors and decreased clotting time is a protective mechanism that decreases the client's chance of bleeding but also places the client at risk for thromboembolic disease.

Musculoskeletal system. A woman's body posture will change during pregnancy to accommodate the fetus growing inside of her. Generally, the pelvis will tilt while the lower back arches. As pregnancy progresses, the mother will arch the lumbar region of the vertebral column to maintain balance. The change in the mother's center of gravity causes an accentuation in the lumbodorsal spinal curve. During the later parts of pregnancy, the sacroiliac, sacrococcygeal, and the pubic joints of the pelvis relax.

Gastrointestinal system. Increased levels of human chorionic gonadotropin (hCG) are associated with nausea and vomiting in the first trimester (known as "morning sickness," although it can occur at any time). Gum tissue becomes hyperemic and swollen, resulting in tissue that easily bleeds. Decreased tone and motility of the gastrointestinal tract causes constipation and esophageal regurgitation, acid reflux, and heartburn. A hiatal hernia may occur as a result of the upward displaced stomach. The gall bladder becomes distended due to decreased muscle tone increasing the emptying time, which may cause increased incidence of gallstones in some women. Intra-abdominal alterations are responsible for general discomfort such as pelvic heaviness or pressure, round ligament tension, increased flatulence, bowel distension and cramping, and uterine contractions.

Sense of fullness in the ears. This occurs due to the increased vascularity of the upper respiratory airway. The Eustachian tubes and tympanic membranes can swell, resulting in earaches, a sense of fullness in the ear, or symptoms associated with impaired hearing.

Edema and hyperemia of the nose, pharynx, larynx, trachea, and bronchi. The congestion of the respiratory tissues results in nasal congestion and stuffiness, epistaxis, and voice change.

LEARNING OBJECTIVE **18.3.7** Identify the hormones associated with the production and expression of milk.

LEARNING OBJECTIVE **18.3.8** Describe the anatomical, physiological, and hormonal changes necessary for milk production.

HORMONES ASSOCIATED WITH LACTATION

A woman's body starts producing hormones that will help with lactation during the 18th week of pregnancy. These hormones will stimulate the growth of milk ducts in the breasts. Hormones that are associated with lactation are insulin, cortisol, prolactin, and oxytocin.

CHANGES NECESSARY TO FACILITATE MILK PRODUCTION

Because of the effects of estrogen, progesterone, human placental lactogen, and other hormones of pregnancy, changes occur in the breasts in preparation for lactation. These hormones stimulate the growth of the ductules, alveoli, and lobules during pregnancy (Figure 18-33). During the latter part of the pregnancy, the alveoli begin producing colostrum. Colostrum will be the first milk the baby receives. Colostrum is easily digested and contains high amounts of nutrients and protective maternal antibodies. After birth, there is a decrease in progesterone that triggers the release of prolactin from the anterior pituitary gland. Additionally, prolactin is produced in response to infant suckling and emptying of the breasts. As the nipple is stimulated by the suckling infant, the posterior pituitary gland is prompted by the hypothalamus to produce oxytocin. This hormone is responsible for the milk ejection reflex. The myoepithelial cells surrounding the alveoli respond to oxytocin by contracting and sending the milk forward through the ducts to the nipple. The nipple-erection reflex is an important part of lactation. When the infant cries, suckles, or rubs against the breast, the nipple becomes erect, which aids in the propulsion of milk through the ducts to the nipple pores. Other hormones associated with milk production include insulin and cortisol, although their roles in milk production are not fully understood.

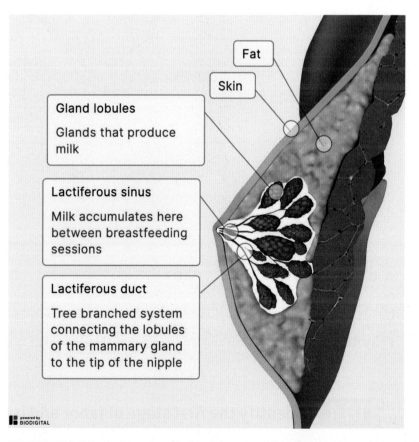

FIGURE 18-33 During pregnancy, hormones stimulate the breast to prepare for lactation.

UNIT OBJECTIVE 18.4

Describe the stages of labor and fetal postnatal changes.

UNIT INTRODUCTION

The onset of labor is considered to have occurred once a woman begins to experience regular contractions as well as the occurrence of cervical dilation, effacement, and the station of the fetus. These last three are evaluated and the woman is assigned a Bishop Score, which is used by healthcare providers to determine if further intervention (such as induction) will be needed to assist with labor. Once labor has begun, it is divided into three stages (Figure 18-34ABCD). The first stage of labor, which is usually the longest, is subdivided into three phases. Once the baby is born, it quickly experiences two major anatomical and physiological changes so that it can survive outside of the uterus.

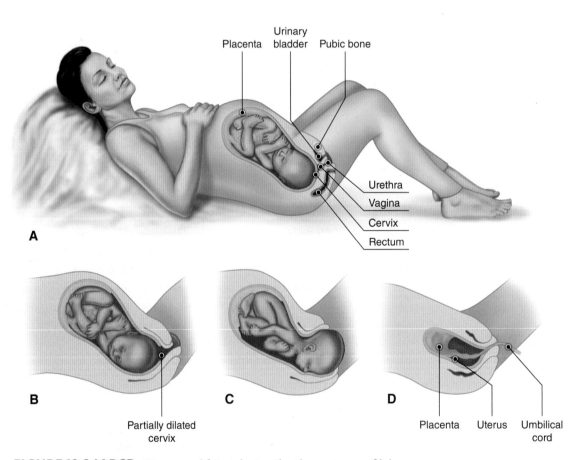

FIGURE 18-34ABCD Uterus and fetus during the three stages of labor.

LEARNING OBJECTIVE 18.4.1 Identify the first stage of labor and its three phases.

LEARNING OBJECTIVE 18.4.2 Describe the first stage of labor and its three phases.

FIRST STAGE OF LABOR

The first stage of labor begins with the onset of regular uterine contractions and ends with complete cervical dilation at 10 centimeters. The first stage of labor is divided into three phases: latent, active, and transition.

Latent Phase

During this phase of labor, the cervical dilation is 0–4 cm and effacement begins (Figure 18-34). The uterine contractions during this phase may be irregular or regular and are mild to moderate in palpation, occurring 5–20 minutes apart and lasting 30–40 seconds in duration. Vaginal discharge may consist of a mucus discharge that is brown in color or slightly mixed with blood. The mother may not notice this phase or experience mild discomfort such as backache or menstrual cramps. For first-time mothers, this phase lasts an average of eight hours; it should not be allowed to continue for longer than 20 hours. Prolonged labor can be dangerous for the baby, potentially causing low oxygen levels, abnormal heart rhythm, or abnormal substances in the amniotic fluid. Prolonged labor also increases the chance that the mother will need a C-section.

Active Phase

During this phase of labor, the cervical dilation is 4–8 cm and the cervix continues to efface or may be completely effaced (Figure 18-34). The intensity of uterine contractions continues to get stronger, closer together, and longer in duration. On average, they will occur every 2 to 5 minutes and last for between 40 and 60 seconds. The fetus continues to descend into the pelvis. During this phase the mother may become restless and anxious. For first-time mothers, this phase lasts an average of five hours; it generally does not last longer than 10 hours.

Transition Phase

During this phase of labor, cervical dilation is 8–10 cm, which is a complete cervical dilatation, and the cervix achieves 100% effacement (Figure 18-35). This is also the phase in which there is a more rapid descent of the fetus lower in the pelvis and into the birth canal. The uterine contractions are very strong, occurring every minute to a minute and a half and lasting 60–90 seconds in duration. The client will have an increased amount of vaginal bloody show. If the amniotic membranes have not ruptured prior to this phase, they will rupture spontaneously or be ruptured by the healthcare provider. The client usually feels anxious, exhausted, and irritable and has the urge to bear down and push during this phase. For first-time mothers, the transition phase should last no longer than three hours.

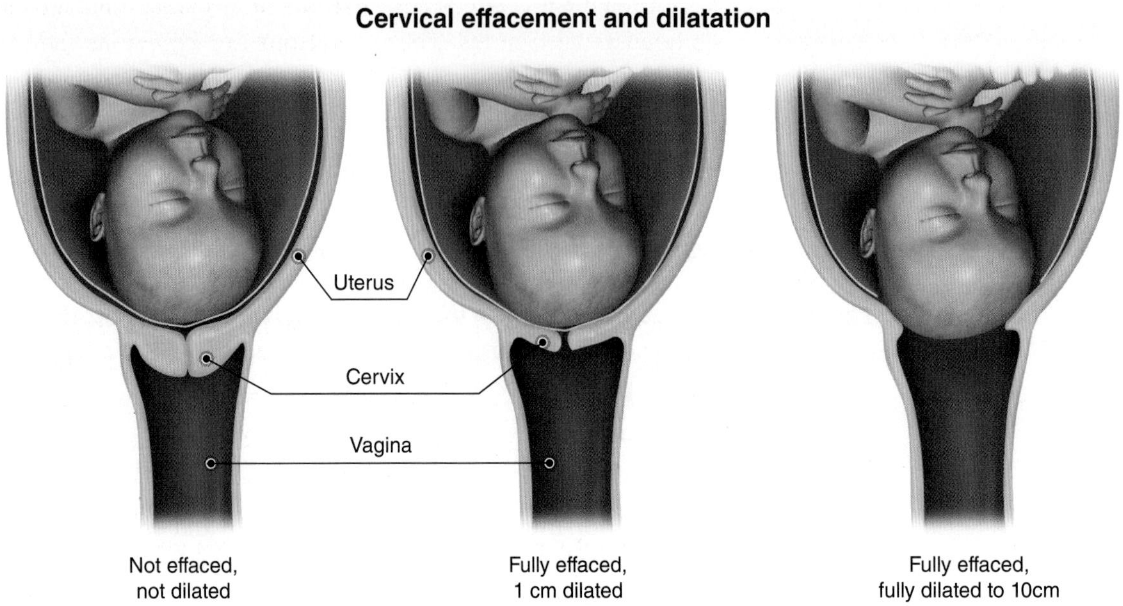

Cervical effacement and dilatation

| Not effaced, not dilated | Fully effaced, 1 cm dilated | Fully effaced, fully dilated to 10cm |

FIGURE 18-35 Cervix goes from not being effaced or dilated to being 100% effaced and 10 cm dilated.

LEARNING OBJECTIVE 18.4.3 Identify the second stage of labor and related physiological changes.

LEARNING OBJECTIVE 18.4.4 Describe the second stage of labor and related physiological changes.

KEY TERMS

cardinal movements Positional changes of the fetus inside the womb of the mother when it moves during the process of labor and birth through the birth canal.

crowning Appearance of the head of the fetus at the vagina during labor.

SECOND STAGE OF LABOR

The second stage of labor begins with complete cervical dilation of 10 cm and 100% effacement and ends with the delivery of the infant. During the second stage of labor the force of the uterine contractions, maternal pushing, and gravity help facilitate fetal decent.

At this stage, strong, intense contractions occur every 1.5–2 minutes for a duration of 60–90 seconds. The pressure of the fetal head on the sacral and obturator nerves causes a sensation of pelvic pressure and the urge to begin pushing. As the contractions and maternal pushing continue, the fetal head continues to descend. **Crowning** occurs when the fetal head is surrounded by the external opening of the vagina.

In order for the fetus to successfully exit the birth canal, it must rotate the position of its head several times. These rotations are known as the **cardinal movements** of labor. They are:

- Engagement occurs when lowermost part of the fetus passes below the ischial spine of the pelvis of the mother. For first time mothers, this generally occurs two to three weeks before labor begins. For mothers who have previously given birth, it may not occur until labor actually begins.

- Descent and flexion—During descent, the fetal head moves down into the pelvic cavity in the transverse position. During flexion, the fetal head meets resistance from the soft tissues of the pelvis, causing the chin to flex downward onto the chest.

- Internal rotation—As the head reaches the pelvic floor, it must rotate from left to right so that the sagittal suture is in the anteroposterior pelvic diameter. Without this rotation, the head's position would make it wider than the pelvic cavity and make it difficult for the shoulders to pass through the widest part of the pelvic inlet.

- Extension—At this point, the birth canal curves upward and the head, face, and chin curve under and past the pubic symphysis. The fetal head extends as it passes under the pubic symphysis. At this point, the occiput is born, followed by the head, face, and chin.

- External rotation—At this point, in order for the shoulders to fit underneath the pubic arch, the baby needs to rotate from a face-down position to one where he or she is facing either of the mother's inner thighs. This positions the baby's shoulders anterior-posterior, which positions them in the widest diameter of the pelvis.

- Expulsion—Almost immediately after external rotation, the mother pushes and the anterior shoulder is born, followed by the posterior shoulder. Once both shoulders have been born, the body quickly follows.

After the birth of the baby, the umbilical cord will be clamped and cut. The second stage of labor is usually completed in under three hours; this time can be significantly less for mothers giving birth to subsequent children.

LEARNING OBJECTIVE 18.4.5 Identify the third stage of labor.

LEARNING OBJECTIVE 18.4.6 Describe the third stage of labor.

KEY TERM

retained placenta Condition in which all or part of the placenta or membranes are retained in the uterus of a female during the final stage or third stage of labor after the baby has been delivered.

THIRD STAGE OF LABOR

The third stage of labor begins with the delivery of the infant and ends with the expulsion of the placenta.

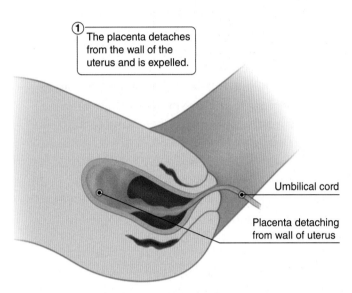

① The placenta detaches from the wall of the uterus and is expelled.

Umbilical cord

Placenta detaching from wall of uterus

FIGURE 18-36 Placenta detaching from wall of the uterus. After the baby is born, the placenta will detach from the wall of the uterus and be expelled from the woman's body.

After the birth of the baby, the uterus contracts, decreasing its size and volume. This reduces the surface area for placental attachment, which helps facilitate the separation of the placenta from the uterine wall (Figure 18-36). Small contractions will begin again as the placenta is separating from the uterine wall, signaling that it is ready to be delivered. Signs of placental separation usually occur 5 minutes after the baby's delivery but may occur as much as 30 minutes later. Separation that takes longer than 30 minutes causes concern that **retained placenta** may be occurring.

Once the placenta separates it is expelled from the vagina. A woman can aid in this expulsion by pushing. If this fails to expel the placenta, a doctor may gently pull on the umbilical cord while pressing down on the fundus. However, it is important to ensure that the placenta has separated from the uterine wall before doing this, or else hemorrhage may occur.

LEARNING OBJECTIVE 18.4.7 Identify major anatomical and physiological changes to the newborn immediately after birth.

LEARNING OBJECTIVE 18.4.8 Describe major anatomical and physiological changes to the newborn immediately after birth.

KEY TERMS

chemoreceptors Sensory proteins that detect chemicals in bodily fluids; also related to the perception of smell and taste.

lymphatic circulation Network of vessels through which lymph drains from the tissues into the blood.

ANATOMICAL AND PHYSIOLOGICAL CHANGES TO THE NEWBORN AFTER BIRTH

Major anatomical and physiological changes in the newborn after birth occur in the respiratory and circulatory systems. These two systems must undergo major physiological and anatomical changes in order for the fetus to survive extrauterine life.

Changes to the Respiratory System

Respirations in the newborn are stimulated by the following factors:

- Thermal: The changes in the newborn temperature occur after birth due to the fact that the environmental temperature is significantly lower. This change stimulates the receptors in the skin, which stimulates the respiratory center in the brain (medulla).
- Sensory: Sensory stimulation such as suctioning and drying the newborn stimulate the respiratory center in the brain (medulla).
- Chemical: Decreased levels of oxygen, increased levels of carbon dioxide, and a decrease in the blood pH stimulate the fetal aortic and carotid chemoreceptors, which activate the respiratory center (medulla) in the brain to initiate respirations.
- Mechanical: Mechanical compression of the chest that occurs during a vaginal birth forces fluid from the fetal lungs, allowing the chest to re-expand after delivery. This re-expansion generates negative pressure, which draws air into the lungs. When the infant cries, a positive intrathoracic pressure is established that keeps the alveoli open and forces the remaining fluid in the lungs into the lymphatic circulation.

Changes to the Circulatory System

During the infant's first breath and increased oxygen level, there is an increased blood flow to the lungs, which results in the closure of the foramen ovale. The ductus arteriosus constricts in response to increased oxygenation. When the infant's umbilical cord is clamped and cut, the umbilical arteries, vein, and ductus venosus are functionally closed.

UNIT OBJECTIVE 18.5

Describe pathologies of the fetus occurring during development, the prenatal period, childbirth, and the postnatal period.

UNIT INTRODUCTION

While the fetus is growing in utero, there are a number of conditions that can happen when development doesn't occur normally. If the abnormal development is not compatible with life, the woman may experience a spontaneous abortion when fetal development ceases. Other developmental abnormalities may not be so severe as to cease any further development of the fetus, but may result in conditions outside the womb after birth.

LEARNING OBJECTIVE 18.5.1 Identify common pathologies of the fetus occurring during development, prenatal period, childbirth, and postnatal period.

LEARNING OBJECTIVE 18.5.2 Describe common pathologies of the fetus occurring during development, prenatal period, childbirth, and postnatal period.

KEY TERMS

cleft lip and palate Cleft lip is the opening in the upper lip of a baby and that can extend up to the nose; the cleft palate is the opening in the roof of a baby's mouth.

congenital cardiac defects Defect in the structure of the heart or great vessels that is present at birth.

congenital diaphragmatic hernia Birth defect of the diaphragm that allows the abdominal organs to push into the chest cavity; hinders proper lung formation.

gastroschisis Birth defect in which the baby's intestines extend outside of the abdomen through a hole near the belly button.

hip dysplasia Abnormality of the hip joint where the socket does not fully cover the ball portion.

neural tube defects Group of birth defects in which the opening in the spine or cranium remains; spina bifida and anencephaly are examples.

omphalocele Abdominal wall defect in which the liver, intestines, and other abdominal organs remain outside of the abdomen in a sac because of failure of return of the intestines and other organs back into the abdominal cavity.

retractions Drawn backward movement of the body.

talipes equinovarus Condition where the foot appears rotated inward at the ankle. Also known as clubfoot.

LIST OF COMMON FETAL PATHOLOGIES

Common fetal pathologies that occur during development and the prenatal period include:

- Hip dysplasia
- Omphalocele
- Gastroschisis
- Cleft lip and palate
- Neural tube defects
- Talipes equinovarus
- Congenital cardiac defects
- Congenital diaphragmatic hernia and choanal atresia

Common pathologies that occur during the postnatal period include:

- Hypothermia
- Hypoglycemia
- Respiratory distress syndrome
- Transient tachypnea of the newborn

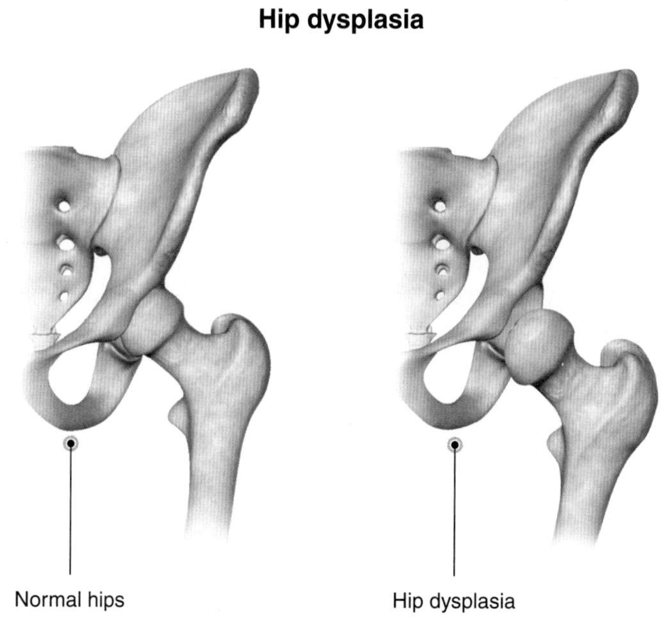

Hip dysplasia

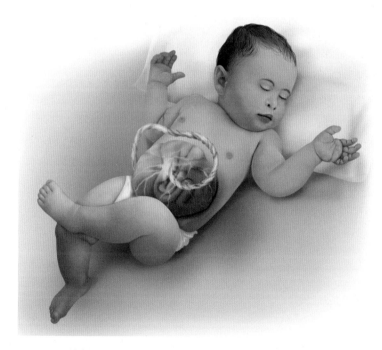

Normal hips   Hip dysplasia

FIGURE 18-37 In hip dysplasia, the ball-and-socket fails to fit together snugly.

COMMON FETAL PATHOLOGIES DURING THE PRENATAL PERIOD

Hip Dysplasia

In **hip dysplasia**, the fetus's ball-and-socket hip joint doesn't fully develop and fails to fit together snugly (Figure 18-37). While the cause of hip dysplasia is not clear, it is more likely to occur in babies born in the breech position, births of multiples, and when amniotic fluid in the womb is deficient. It is more common in females than in males. Additionally, a baby is more likely to have hip dysplasia if a parent or sibling had it as well. Hip dysplasia is treatable, and most babies diagnosed with it go on to have normal lives.

Omphalocele

An **omphalocele** is a birth defect of the abdominal wall in which the infant's intestines, liver, and other abdominal organs are outside of the body because of a hole in the naval area (Figure 18-38). The intestines are covered by a thin layer of membranes and can easily be seen. This occurs as a result of the failure of the normal return of these organs back into the abdominal cavity that occurs around the ninth week of fetal development. An omphalocele can often be detected through an ultrasound. Unless the sac containing the organ bursts, there is no need for any prebirth intervention. After birth, surgery is needed to place the organs back in the abdominal cavity. For small omphaloceles, surgery can be done all at once. For larger omphaloceles, staged closure is needed so intra-abdominal pressure is not raised. Prognosis depends on if there are any

FIGURE 18-38 Infants with an omphalocele have their abdominal organs, intestines, and liver outside of their body due to a hole in the naval area.

other fetal abnormalities; the mortality rate for large omphaloceles is higher than that of small omphaloceles. Most surviving infants grow up to have no long-term problems.

Gastroschisis

Gastroschisis is an abdominal wall defect, similar to an omphalocele, in which the anterior abdomen does not close properly, allowing the intestines to protrude outside the fetus (Figure 18-39). In gastroschisis, the hole from which the intestines (and sometimes the stomach and liver, although this is rare) protrude is usually to the right of the belly button. Unlike an omphalocele, these organs are not covered by a thin membrane and are directly exposed to air after the baby is born. Gastroschisis is usually diagnosed during a prenatal ultrasound screening. Surgery is required after birth to return the exposed intestines to the abdominal cavity. Surgery may or may not be done immediately after birth; if it is not done immediately, the exposed intestines will be covered with sterile bandages. For larger gastroschises, more than one surgery is generally required. Gastroschisis is fatal if left untreated, but surgery is usually very successful. Recovery is usually a few weeks, while the bowel heals and adjusts to normal functioning. Long-term prognosis is very good for infants whose surgery is successful; most do not experience any complications.

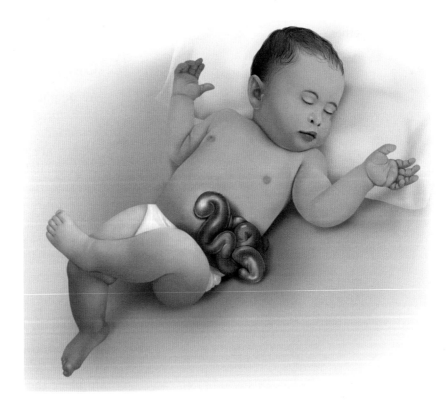

FIGURE 18-39 Intestines protrude from the abdominal wall in an infant suffering from gastroschisis.

Cleft Lip and Palate

Cleft lip and **cleft palate** are birth defects that occur when a fetus's lip or mouth do not form properly during pregnancy (Figure 18-40). A cleft lip happens if the tissue that makes up the lip does not join completely before birth. This results in an opening in the upper lip that can be a small slit or a large opening that goes through the lip into the nose. A cleft lip can be on one or both sides of the lip or in the middle of the lip, which occurs very rarely. A cleft palate happens if the tissue that makes up the roof of the mouth does not join together completely during pregnancy. Both the front and back parts of the palate may be open or only part of the palate is open. Cleft lip and cleft palate are usually diagnosed during an ultrasound screening. Surgery is required to treat both cleft lip and cleft palate. The first surgery to repair a cleft lip usually occurs within the first two to three months after birth. The first surgery to repair a cleft palate usually occurs when the infant is between 6 and 12 months old. Multiple surgeries are normally needed to fix a cleft palate. Children born with cleft palates are frequently treated for the condition throughout their childhood. Even after corrective surgery, children with a cleft palate often have speech impairments.

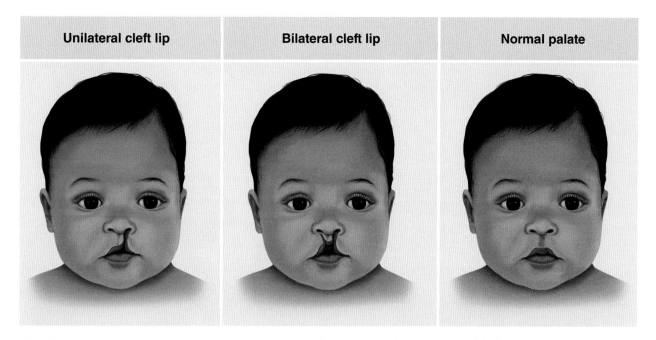

FIGURE 18-40 A unilateral cleft lip affects one side of the mouth while a bilateral cleft lip affects both sides of the mouth.

Neural Tube Defects

Neural tube defects (NTD) are one of the most common birth defects, affecting the brain, spine, or spinal cord during fetal development (Figure 18-41AB). In neural tube defects, an opening remains in the spinal cord or brain. There are several types of neural tube defects which include spina bifida and anencephaly. Inadequate levels of folic acid and B12 during pregnancy lead to an increased risk of NTD. There is no treatment for anencephaly; infants born with this condition usually only survive a few hours. Aggressive surgery increases the survival and function of infants born with spina bifida. Both spina bifida and anencephaly are discussed further later in this chapter.

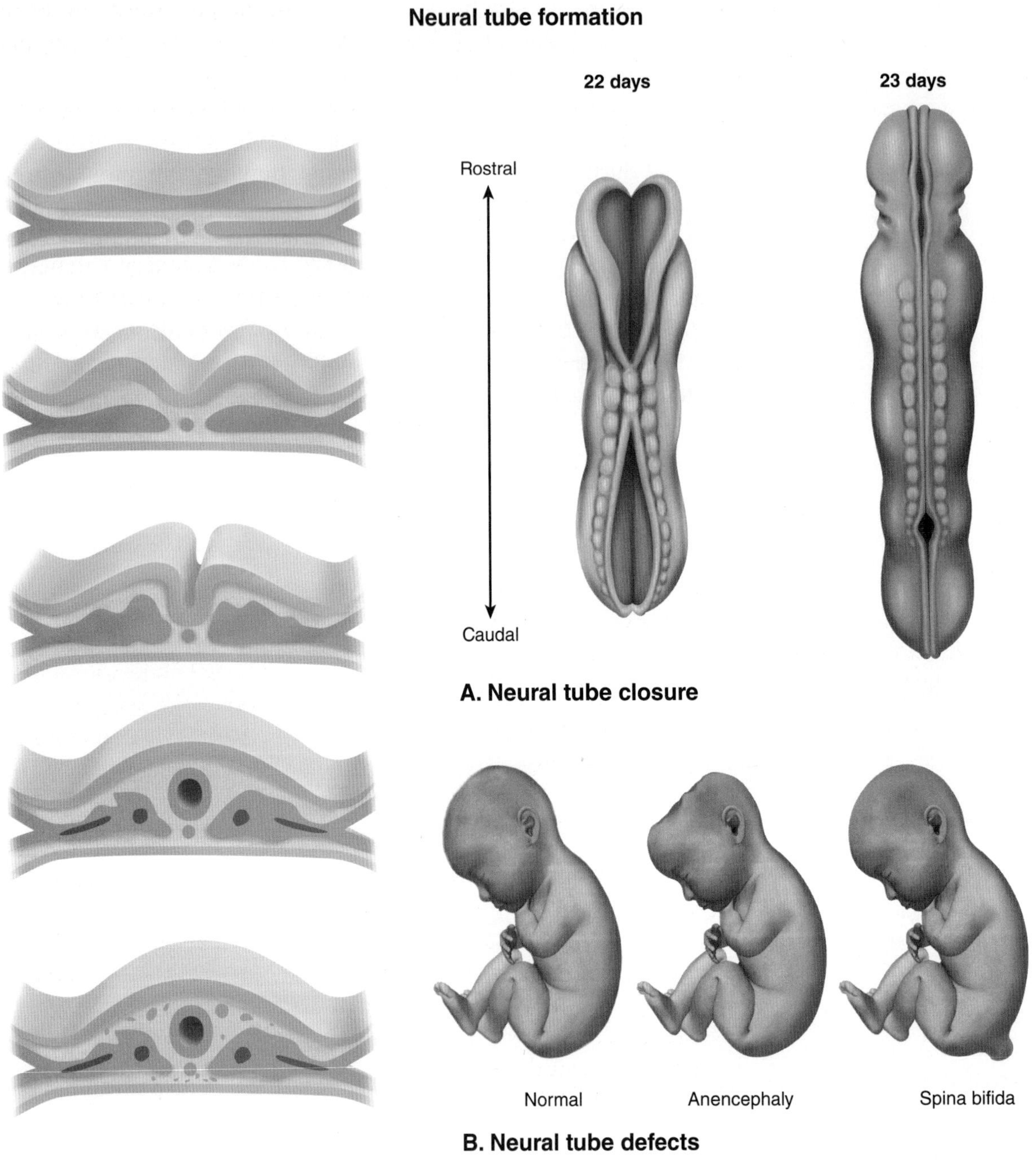

Neural tube formation

22 days   23 days

Rostral

Caudal

A. Neural tube closure

Normal   Anencephaly   Spina bifida

B. Neural tube defects

FIGURE 18-41AB In a neural tube defect, an opening remains in either the spinal cord or brain.

Talipes Equinovarus

Talipes equinovarus is a fixation of the foot in a hand-like orientation—in adduction, supination, and oblique displacement toward the midline—with concomitant soft tissue abnormalities. It is also known as clubfoot (Figure 18-42). Talipes can affect one or both feet. It is diagnosed either by ultrasound or physical examination after the baby is born. The four components of deformity that exist with talipes are a higher arch on the inside of the foot, the

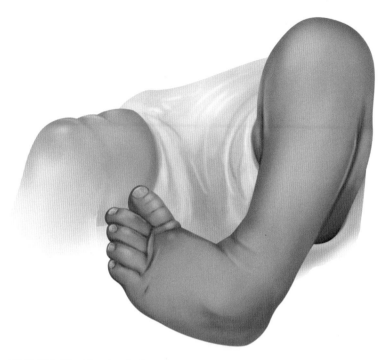

FIGURE 18-42 This baby's foot is clearly turned inward, a symptom of talipes equinovarus.

forefoot curved inward toward the big toe, the heel turned inward, and the ankle pointed downward. Treatment can take one of two forms. The Ponseti method involves positioning the foot correctly and casting it to hold it in place. This is repeated about once a week for several months. At the end of the process, a surgery to lengthen the Achilles tendon is performed. Braces are worn afterward for up to three years to maintain the proper alignment. If the Ponseti method doesn't work, surgery is required to reposition the foot.

Congenital Cardiac Defects

A **congenital cardiac defect** is a defect on the structure of the heart that is present at birth; they are the most common type of birth defect. They can affect the shape of the baby's heart, how it functions, or both. Some congenital cardiac defects will not need treatment or can be treated easily. Other, more critical congenital cardiac defects will require surgery and treatment during the first year of life.

Hypoplastic Left Heart Syndrome In hypoplastic left heart syndrome, the left side of the heart is not fully formed; therefore, the heart cannot properly pump blood. The aorta and left ventricle are underdeveloped and the aortic and mitral valves are too small to allow proper blood flow or may be completely closed (Figure 18-43). This results in the left ventricle being unable to pump blood to the rest of the body after it returns from the lungs. Without a series of surgical interventions, the baby will die within a few weeks of birth. When surgery is successful (or a heart transplant is performed), prognosis is good, although patients will need lifelong cardiac monitoring.

Pulmonary Atresia In pulmonary atresia, the pulmonary valve does not form properly; therefore, enough blood cannot flow from the heart to the lungs (Figure 18-44). There are two classifications of pulmonary atresia: pulmonary atresia with intact ventricular septum, which involves complete blockage of the pulmonary valve, and pulmonary atresia with ventricular septal defect, which is the underdevelopment of the right ventricle. Because oxygenated blood is unable to be circulated, babies with this condition will be bluish once born since they are no longer receiving oxygenated blood from their mother. Surgical treatment is required, although the type and number of surgeries depends on the size of the right ventricle and pulmonary artery. If left untreated, pulmonary atresia is fatal; prognosis after surgery is generally good, although complications may arise.

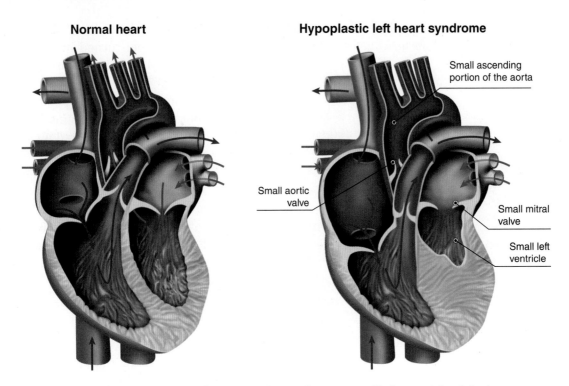

Normal heart

Hypoplastic left heart syndrome

Small ascending
portion of the aorta

Small aortic
valve

Small mitral
valve

Small left
ventricle

FIGURE 18-43 In hypoplastic left heart syndrome the aorta and left ventricle of the heart are severely underdeveloped.

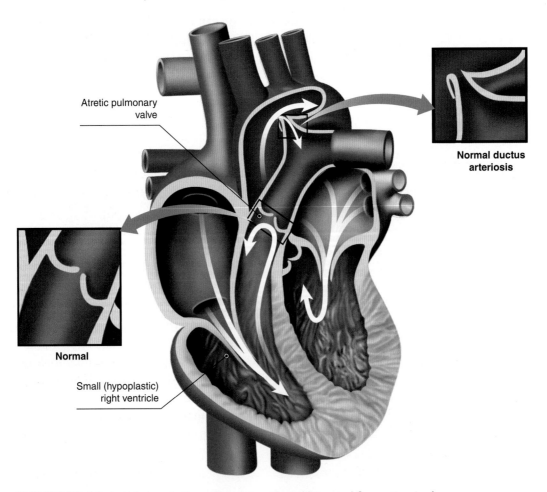

Atretic pulmonary
valve

Normal ductus
arteriosis

Normal

Small (hypoplastic)
right ventricle

FIGURE 18-44 In this heart, the pulmonary valve's abnormal formation is shown.

Tetralogy of Fallot Tetralogy of Fallot (TOF) is a condition in which there are four heart defects that include:

- Ventricle septal defect—a hole between the two bottom chambers of the heart; this allows deoxygenated blood to mix with oxygenated blood, reducing the supply of oxygenated blood to the body.
- Pulmonary stenosis—a narrowing of the ventricular outflow tract that can occur at or below the pulmonary valve; signs and symptoms vary based on the rate of obstruction and include heart murmur, fatigue, shortness of breath, chest pain, or loss of consciousness.
- Right ventricular hypertrophy—a more muscular, enlarged right ventricle that gives the heart a bootlike shape; left untreated it can cause the heart to weaken and stiffen and may lead to heart failure.
- Aortic displacement—the aorta is placed directly over the ventricle septal defect instead of the left ventricle, which causes the aorta to receive some blood from the right ventricle and results in a mixing of oxygenated and deoxygenated blood (Figure 18-45).

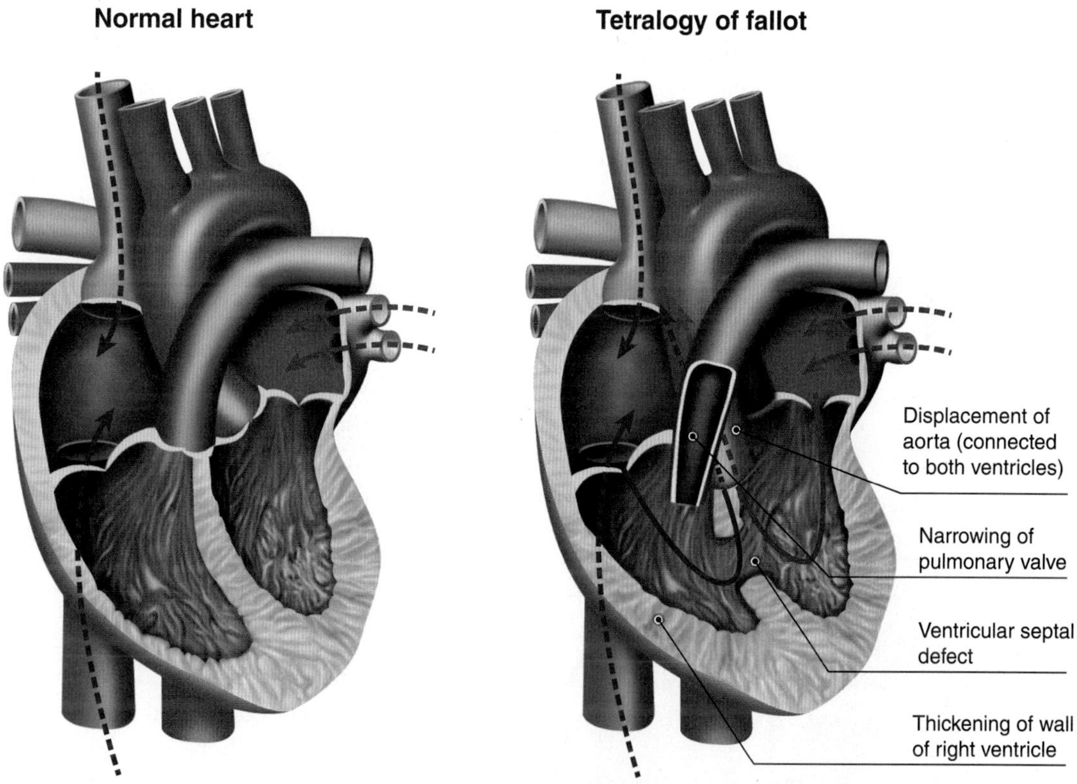

Normal heart   **Tetralogy of fallot**

Displacement of aorta (connected to both ventricles)

Narrowing of pulmonary valve

Ventricular septal defect

Thickening of wall of right ventricle

FIGURE 18-45 Tetralogy of Fallot is a condition that includes four heart defects: ventricle septal defect, pulmonary stenosis, right-ventricular hypertrophy, and aortic displacement.

TOF is usually treated with open heart surgery to increase the size of the pulmonary valve and arteries and repair the ventricular septum defect. Surgery usually occurs within the first year of life; most people who undergo successful surgeries can expect to live to adulthood with no or minor complications.

Normal heart

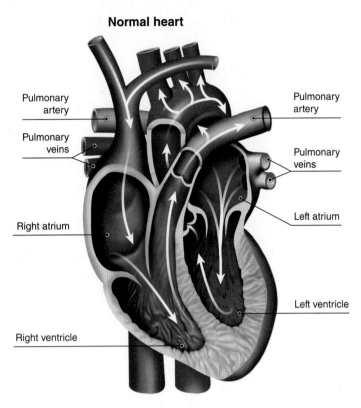

Total anomalous pulmonary venous return

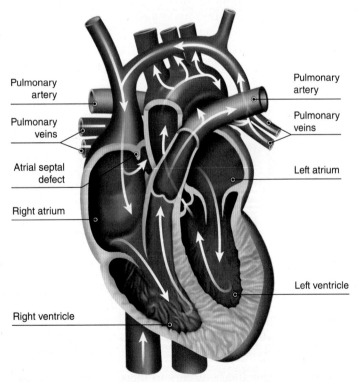

FIGURE 18-46 In total anomalous pulmonary venous return, the pulmonary veins are not attached to the upper left chamber of the heart.

"Tet spells" can occur in people who have not undergone surgery to repair TOF. These can be triggered by anxiety, pain, dehydration, or fever and are characterized by shortness of breath, cyanosis, agitation, and loss of consciousness. Untreated, TOF can progress to heart failure. People with untreated TOF rarely progress to adulthood.

Total Anomalous Pulmonary Venous Return Total anomalous pulmonary venous return is a condition in which the pulmonary veins do not attach to the upper left chamber of the heart and instead attach at an incorrect location (Figure 18-46). This causes blood to circulate back and forth between the lungs and heart but does not flow out to the body. There may be an atrial septal defect that allows some blood to move to the left atrium, to the left ventricle, and then out to the rest of the body; however, there is less oxygen in this blood than is needed. This lack of oxygen may result in babies having a bluish color. This condition is generally treated by surgery that connects the pulmonary veins to the left atrium and closes up the holes between the atrium. Surgery usually occurs during the first month of life.

Transposition of the Great Arteries In transposition of the great arteries, the two main arteries leaving the heart are transposed, which changes the way blood flows through the body and results in a shortage of oxygen in the rest of the body (Figure 18-47). It can be diagnosed prenatally; if it goes undetected until birth, it is usually diagnosed within a few hours after birth. Symptoms include cyanosis, shortness of breath, lack of appetite, and poor weight gain. In most cases, surgery is required to move the arteries so they are connected to the correct heart valve. Although there is a good prognosis after a successful surgery, heart problems may arise later in life.

Tricuspid Atresia In tricuspid atresia, the heart's tricuspid valve (which connects the right atrium to the right ventricle) is missing or does not develop properly (Figure 18-48). This prevents blood from flowing properly into the lungs to become oxygenated.

Transposition of the great arteries

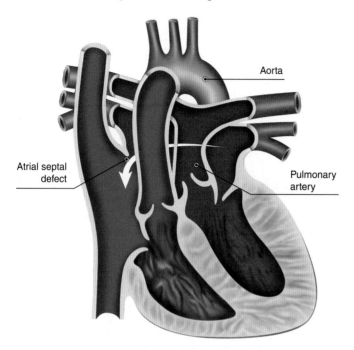

FIGURE 18-47 Two main arteries of the heart are transposed.

Tricuspid Atresia

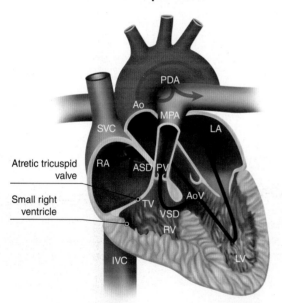

RA - Right Atrium   MPA - Main Pulmonary Artery
RV - Right Ventricle   Ao - Aorta
LA - Left Atrium   SVC - Superior Vena Cava
LV - Left Ventricle   IVC - Inferior Vena Cava

TV - Tricuspid Valve   ASD - Atrial Septal Defect
MV - Mitral Valve   VSD - Ventricular Septal Defect
AoV - Aortic Valve   PDA - Patent Ductus Arteriosus
PV - Pulmonary Valve

FIGURE 18-48 In tricuspid atresia, the heart's tricuspid valve is missing or does not connect properly.

Instead, blood moves from the right atrium to the left atrium through a hole between them. Symptoms include blue-tinged skin; difficulty breathing; tiring easily, especially during feedings; and slow growth and poor weight gain. Diagnosis usually occurs during a prenatal ultrasound or shortly after birth. Because the missing tricuspid valve cannot be replaced, treatment usually involves multiple surgeries to ensure adequate blood flow from the heart into the lungs. Types of surgeries include shunting and creating or enlarging the hole between the right and left atrium. When surgeries are successful, the outlook is generally promising, although lifelong follow-up care will be required.

Truncus Arteriosus Truncus arteriosus causes the infant to have only one artery that leaves the heart instead of two (Figure 18-49). It results in blood with oxygen mixing with blood that does not contain oxygen. An echocardiogram is used to diagnose this condition after birth. Surgery is needed to separate the pulmonary arteries from the truncus arteriosus (the shared artery) and connect them to the right ventricle using a conduit, allowing the shared artery to act as the aorta. This surgery generally takes place during the first month of life. Follow-up surgery may be required as the child gets older and regular follow-up care is required.

Atrial Septal Defects In atrial septal defects (ASD), there is a hole in the septum between the right and left atria (Figure 18-50). This allows oxygenated blood from the left atrium to flow into the right atrium, mixing with deoxygenated blood and flowing back into the lungs. Small defects may never cause a problem and may only be found incidentally. Larger defects can result in extra blood overfilling the lungs and overworking the right side of the heart, eventually enlarging and weakening it. Small atrial septal defects may not require any treatment beyond monitoring; larger ones can be corrected with surgery that closes the hole between the atria. Follow-up care is generally recommended for all patients to monitor the condition; for those who have surgery, the follow-up care is recommended

Healthy heart

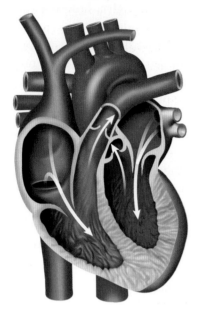

Truncus arteriosus

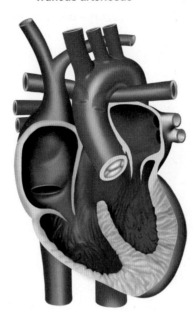

FIGURE 18-49 In truncus arteriosus, only one artery leaves the heart instead of two.

**Congenital heart disease
atrial septal defect**

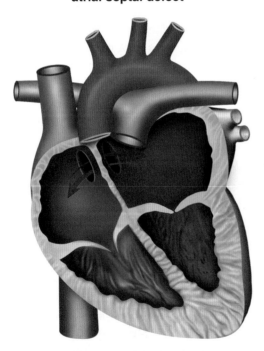

FIGURE 18-50 In atrial septal defect, there is a hole in the septum between the right and left atria that allows oxygenated blood to mix with deoxygenated blood.

on a yearly basis to check for complications.

Ventricular Septal Defects

In a ventricular septal defect (VSD), there is a hole in the septum between the right and left ventricles, causing oxygen-rich blood to get pumped back through the lungs, making the heart work harder (Figure 18-51). A small VSD may cause no problems and may close on its own. VSDs often cause a heart murmur that can be heard through a stethoscope; it is then confirmed by either an echocardiogram or an electrocardiogram. Most small VSDs are not treated; larger ones may require surgery to close the hole between the ventricles. Most people with VSDs go on to lead normal lives, although regular lifelong follow-up care is usually required.

**Congenital heart disease
*Ventricular septal defect***

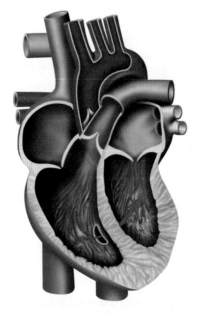

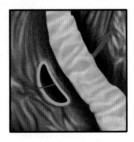

FIGURE 18-51 In a ventricular septal defect, there is a hole in the septum between the right and left ventricles.

Coarctation of the Aorta Coarctation of the aorta is the narrowing of the aorta, which causes the heart to work harder to get the blood out of the aorta (Figure 18-52). If the aorta is not significantly narrowed, this condition may not be diagnosed until adulthood. Less severe cases of coarctation of the aorta may not have any symptoms; in more severe cases symptoms include pale skin, heavy sweating, difficulty breathing, and difficulty feeding. Treatment for coarctation of the aorta includes surgery to remove or expand the narrow aorta or balloon angioplasty with stenting to stretch the aorta. The prognosis for mild cases, or for those who successfully undergo surgery, is quite positive, although high blood pressure is a common, long-term side effect.

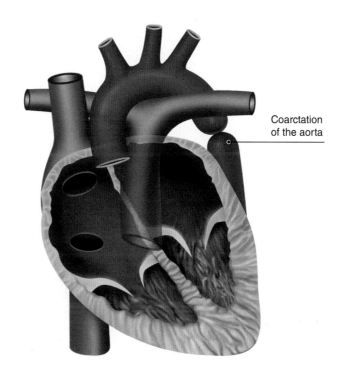

Coarctation
of the aorta

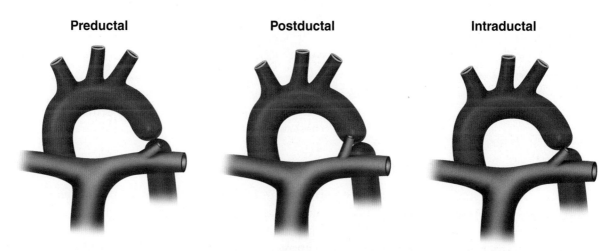

Preductal   **Postductal**   **Intraductal**

FIGURE 18-52 In coarctation of the aorta, the aorta is narrower, causing the heart to work harder to get the blood out of the aorta. Coarctation of the aorta can be preductal, intraductal, or postductal depending on where the narrowing occurs in relation to the ductus arteriosus.

Heart Valve Anomalies Finally, there are various conditions where the heart valves do not close properly, or are narrow or blocked so blood cannot flow smoothly within and out of the heart.

Congenital Diaphragmatic Hernia

In a congenital diaphragmatic hernia (CDH), there is a hole in the diaphragm that allows the intestines to enter the chest cavity; this affects proper lung formation (Figure 18-53). Newborns with CDH often have severe, potentially life-threatening respiratory distress. Pulmonary hypoplasia and pulmonary hypertension are two common complications that occur as a result of CDH. This condition can be diagnosed via ultrasound while the fetus is in utero. Infants born with CDH must be intubated and placed on a ventilator. At that point, abdominal surgery can occur to correct any organ displacement and close the hernia. The heart and lungs will generally move back into their correct positions once the other organs are out of the way. However, while decreasing, the mortality rate for CDH is still high. Survival rates depend on the size of the hernia and the number of abdominal organs that are in the incorrect position.

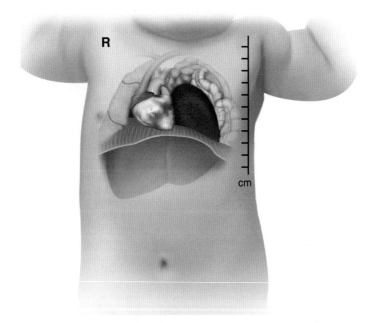

FIGURE 18-53 Illustration of congenital diaphragmatic hernia showing the abdominal visceral in the chest cavity.

Choanal Atresia

Choanal atresia is a narrowing or blockage of the nasal airway (Figure 18-54). Choanal atresia can be unilateral or bilateral. A unilateral choanal atresia may not be diagnosed until later in life if the person is able to breathe through one nostril. Bilateral choanal atresia is serious and life-threatening after birth, since babies primarily breathe through their noses. Resuscitation after birth may be required. The only treatment for this condition is to surgically create holes in the atresia. This surgery will need to be redone later in life.

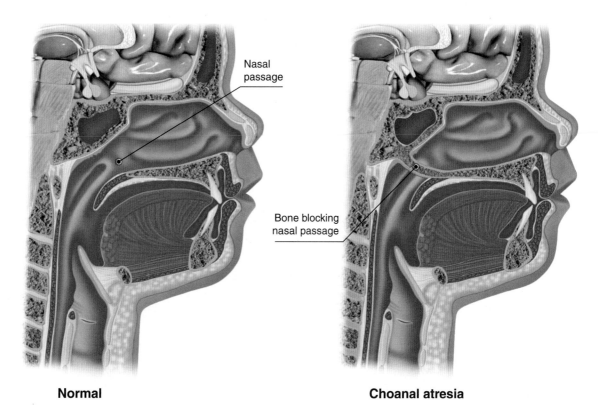

Normal   **Choanal atresia**

FIGURE 18-54 In choanal atresia, the nasal airway is either narrowed or blocked.

COMMON FETAL PATHOLOGIES DURING THE POSTNATAL PERIOD

Common pathologies that occur during the postnatal period are hypothermia, hypoglycemia, respiratory distress syndrome, and transient tachypnea of the newborn. While these pathologies can be serious if not treated—possibly even life-threatening—once diagnosed they are able to be treated and should not cause lifelong problems for the child.

Hypothermia

Hypothermia occurs due to the inability of the newborn to maintain body temperature due to a large surface body mass, little subcutaneous fat, thin skin, and blood vessels close to the surface of the skin. The treatment for hypothermia is warming the infant in an incubator or radiant warmer.

Hypoglycemia

Hypoglycemia occurs when the glucose levels in the infant are less than the body requires. This can be caused by limited glycogen stores, increased use of glucose, and depleted glycogen stores. Elevated maternal glucose levels prior to birth that stimulate the fetal production of insulin can also cause hypoglycemia, since after the umbilical cord is cut the infant no longer receives high levels of glucose to compensate for the insulin produced. In the United States, all hospitals screen for hypoglycemia after birth, testing the neonate every two to four hours for the first 24 hours after birth. Hypoglycemia is treated with intravenous infusions of glucose or (in less severe cases) early introduction of breast milk.

Respiratory Distress Syndrome

Respiratory distress syndrome (RDS) occurs in premature infants and is the inadequate production of surfactant necessary to keep the alveoli open. Symptoms are fast breathing, fast heart rate, chest wall **retractions**, nasal flaring, and blue discoloration of skin. If time permits before a baby is delivered prematurely, steroids are given to the mother to improve lung maturity. Treatment after birth includes surfactant replacement therapy, oxygen therapy, and breathing support using a ventilator or CPAP machine. The condition usually gets worse after two to four days but improves after that. Recent therapies have improved the prognosis for RDS, and most babies survive.

Transient Tachypnea of the Newborn

Transient tachypnea of the newborn (TTN) is caused by retained fetal lung fluid due to the impaired clearance of fluid from the lungs at birth. Symptoms include rapid, labored breathing; nostril flaring; cyanosis; and chest retractions during breathing. Treatment includes supplemental oxygen. Oral feeding may need to be delayed until breathing is easier for the newborn. TTN is most common in babies born before 38 weeks, babies delivered by C-section, and babies of mothers with diabetes. Symptoms of TTN usually resolve within one to three days of birth.

LEARNING OBJECTIVE 18.5.3 **Identify the possible causes of a spontaneous abortion.**

SPONTANEOUS ABORTION

Spontaneous abortion, also known as a miscarriage, is the natural death of a fetus or embryo before it can survive independently outside of the uterus. The most common symptom is vaginal bleeding, which may or may not be accompanied by abdominal pain and cramping. Spontaneous abortion most frequently occurs during the first trimester. Good prenatal care, including avoiding drugs and alcohol, can reduce the risk for spontaneous abortion. Possible causes associated with spontaneous abortion include:

- Maternal age greater than 35 years
- History of spontaneous abortion
- Cigarette smoking
- Substance abuse, such as using cocaine, alcohol, amphetamines, and other narcotics while pregnant
- Chronic disorders, such as diabetes, hypertension, and thyroid disease

- Uterine anomalies, such as an abnormally shaped uterus
- Genetic malformation of the fetus, resulting in a physical defect that is caused by abnormal genetic sequencing
- Incompetent cervix; weak cervical tissue causes the cervix to open too soon
- Deficiencies in hormones, such as progesterone and estrogen
- Maternal infection, such as sexually transmitted infections, parasitic infections, and maternal systemic infections

LEARNING OBJECTIVE 18.5.4 Identify the pathologies anencephaly and spina bifida.

KEY TERMS

alpha-fetoprotein Protein secreted by the fetus; it is present in the mother's bloodstream and amniotic fluid.

laminae Plates of bone that form the walls of each vertebra, enclosing the spinal cord.

neocortex Part of the mammalian brain where sensory perception, conception, motor

commands, spatial reasoning, and language occur.

neural tube Embryonic precursor to the central nervous system (CNS) and is composed of the brain and spinal cord; generally, during the fourth week of pregnancy, the neural tube closure occurs.

ANENCEPHALY

Anencephaly is the complete absence of major portions of the brain, skull, and scalp resulting from the upper part of the neural tube not closing during fetal development.

Signs, Symptoms, and Diagnosis

An infant with anencephaly is born without parts of the brain and the skull. Fetuses with anencephaly usually lack the largest part of the brain that contains the **neocortex**, which is responsible for cognition. The parts of the brain that do remain are covered by a thin membrane. The diagnosis of this condition occurs during pregnancy or after the baby is born. There is no known cure or standard treatment for anencephaly. Infants with this disorder are frequently stillborn; if they are not stillborn, they will not survive longer than a few hours to a few days after birth.

SPINA BIFIDA

Spina bifida is part of a group of **neural tube** defects that occurs early during embryonical development. Spina bifida is caused by a defect in the neural arch, generally in the lumbosacral region. There are three types of spina bifida: spina bifida occulta, meningocele, and myelomeningocele.

Signs, Symptoms, and Diagnosis

Spina bifida is a failure of the posterior laminae of the vertebrae to close; this leaves an opening through which the spinal meninges and spinal cord may protrude. Screening for this condition is performed during the prenatal period by obtaining a maternal blood sample to evaluate the level of alpha-fetoprotein. An ultrasound can also be done in the prenatal period to detect signs of spina bifida. Diagnosis can be made after obtaining a sample of the amniotic fluid and evaluating the level of alpha-fetoprotein. Treatment for spina bifida is based on the type and condition of the client. The classifications of spina bifida include spina bifida occulta, meningocele, and myelomeningocele (Figure 18-55).

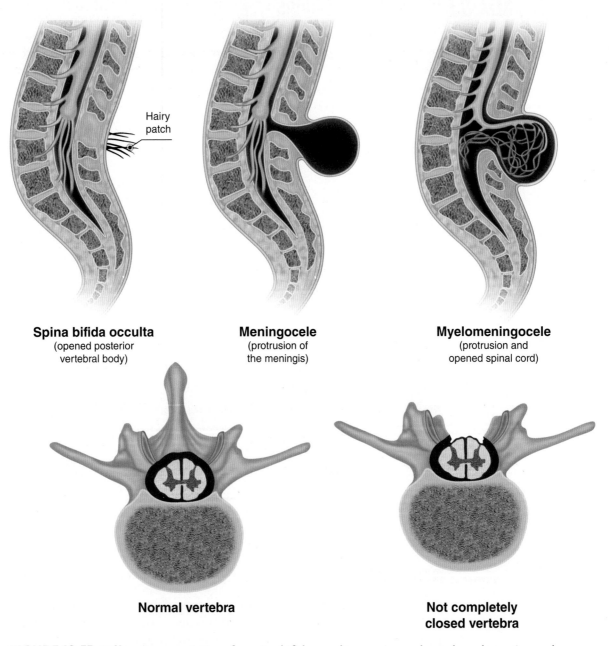

Spina bifida occulta
(opened posterior
vertebral body)

Meningocele
(protrusion of
the meningis)

Myelomeningocele
(protrusion and
opened spinal cord)

Normal vertebra

**Not completely
closed vertebra**

FIGURE 18-55 Different presentations for spina bifida occulta, meningocele, and myelomeningocele.

Spina Bifida Occulta Spina bifida occulta is the mildest form of spina bifida, where the outer part of some of the vertebrae are not completely closed. It presents with a hairy patch, dimple, dark spot, or swelling on the back at the site of the gap in the spine. Frequently, no other symptoms occur with this form of spina bifida.

Meningocele This is the least common form of spina bifida and occurs when part of the spinal meninges protrude through the bony defect and forms a cystic sac. Because the nervous system remains undamaged, there are unlikely to be long-term health problems associated with meningocele.

Myelomeningocele The most severe symptoms and complications affecting the meninges and nerves occur with this type of spina bifida. In spina bifida with myelomeningocele, the unfused portion of the spinal column allows a sac of fluid to come through an opening in the baby's back. Part of the spinal cord and nerves are in this sac and are damaged, resulting in paralysis and loss of sensation below the spinal defect. Treatment for myelomeningocele is usually surgery to put the spinal cord and nerves back inside the spine and close the hole in the back. There is no cure for the nerve and spinal damage that has taken place; the goal of surgery is to prevent further damage of the nervous tissue and prevent infections.

LEARNING OBJECTIVE 18.5.5 Contrast the signs, symptoms, and diagnosis of anencephaly and spina bifida.

ANENCEPHALY VERSUS SPINA BIFIDA

Put simply, anencephaly is the absence of a closed cranial cavity, and spina bifida is the incomplete closure of the neural tube. Because anencephaly is essentially being born without a functional brain and with much of the skull missing or malformed, anencephaly is not compatible with life. Most fetuses with anencephaly will either be born stillborn or die shortly after birth. Brain function or development is not impaired due to spina bifida, although the incomplete closure of the neural tube generally causes nerve damage and some paralysis.

LEARNING OBJECTIVE 18.5.6 Identify common pathologies related to newborn anatomical and physiological adjustments.

KEY TERMS

ductus arteriosus Fetal circulatory pathway between the aorta and pulmonary trunk.

foramen ovale Opening in the septum that pushes blood between the left and right atrium that is present in the fetal heart; normally closes on its own shortly after birth.

COMMON PATHOLOGIES RELATED TO NEWBORN ANATOMICAL AND PHYSIOLOGICAL ADJUSTMENTS

After birth, the neonate undergoes physical transitions that allow it to live outside of the uterus. The liver stops acting as storage for sugar and iron and begins to break down wastes and produce a protein that breaks down bilirubin. Once the first breath is taken, fluid drains from the lungs and they inflate and begin to work on their own. Meconium is passed from the GI system as the baby's first stools and the urinary system begins to work. However, sometimes these physiological and anatomical adjustments do not occur. Two of the most common are:

- Patent foramen ovale (an opening in the heart between the left and right atrium)
- Patent ductus arteriosus (the ductus arteriosus, which allows the fetus' heart to bypass its nonfunctioning lungs in utero, does not close after birth)

LEARNING OBJECTIVE 18.5.7 Describe the signs, symptoms, and diagnosis of patent foramen ovale and patent ductus arteriosus.

Patent Foramen Ovale and Ductus Arteriosus

The foramen ovale is an opening between the right and left atrium that closes after the initiation of respirations. Most infants do not have any symptoms associated with a patent foramen ovale. In some cases, an infant may experience cyanosis when crying. Generally, a patent foramen ovale will not cause complications.

The ductus arteriosus is a blood vessel that connects the main pulmonary artery to the proximal descending aorta during fetal life. After birth a functional closing of this duct occurs. The ductus arteriosus that does not close is called a patent ductus arteriosus (PDA). A PDA produces a left-to-right shunting of the blood mixing both oxygenated and deoxygenated blood. This is described as blood flowing from the aorta (the main artery in the body) into the pulmonary artery. This extra blood flow into the lungs can overload the lungs and put a greater burden on the heart to pump the extra blood. A small patent ductus arteriosus will often not cause problems or require treatment. However, larger ones can result in complications, such as congestive heart failure. Symptoms of this include:

- Poor eating, which leads to poor growth
- Sweating with crying or eating
- Persistent fast breathing or breathlessness
- Easy tiring
- Rapid heart rate

UNIT OBJECTIVE 18.6

Describe pathologies associated with pregnancy and childbirth that affect the mother.

UNIT INTRODUCTION

Pregnancy can introduce different complications in the mother's body even if she was healthy before becoming pregnant. These complications may be minor or life-threatening (to the mother and the fetus) and may develop gradually or suddenly without warning. One of the goals of prenatal care is to evaluate the mother during pregnancy to determine if she is developing any condition that could affect her or her fetus and to prevent or treat such conditions before they become life-threatening.

LEARNING OBJECTIVE 18.6.1 Identify common pathologies associated with pregnancy and childbirth that affect the mother.

LEARNING OBJECTIVE 18.6.2 Describe common pathologies associated with pregnancy and childbirth that affect the mother.

KEY TERMS

choriocarcinoma Malignant tumor of the uterus that originates in the cells of the chorion of the fetus.

ketonuria Excretion of an abnormally large number of ketones in the urine.

proteinuria Excretion of a large number of protein molecules in the urine.

suction dilation and curettage (D&C) Medical procedure where the uterine cervix of a female is dilated and the curette is inserted into the uterus for the scraping and the removal of the endometrium.

PATHOLOGIES OF PREGNANCY AND CHILDBIRTH THAT AFFECT THE MOTHER

There are a wide variety of health issues that can arise for a woman while she is pregnant. These issues include:

- Anemia
- Ectopic pregnancy
- Hydatidiform mole
- Gestational diabetes mellitus
- Cervical insufficiency
- Hyperemesis gravidarum

- Gestational hypertension
- HELLP syndrome
- Preeclampsia
- Eclampsia
- Placental abruption
- Placenta previa
- Preterm labor
- Miscarriage

Anemia

A physiological anemia occurs during pregnancy due to the increased plasma volume. This is not pathological, but many women lack the iron stores in the second and third trimester of pregnancy to make hemoglobin, which results in a pathological anemia. Symptoms include weakness, fatigue, trouble concentrating, rapid or irregular heartbeat, chest pain, and cold hands and feet. Treatment usually consists of taking vitamin or iron supplements. Severe cases may require a blood transfusion.

Ectopic Pregnancy

An ectopic pregnancy occurs when the fertilized ovum is implanted outside of the uterine cavity, with the majority implanting in the fallopian tube (Figure 18-56). This places the client at a high risk for hemorrhage. At first, there may not be any symptoms; later symptoms include pelvic pain and may include light vaginal bleeding. A transvaginal ultrasound is generally used to diagnose an ectopic pregnancy. An ectopic pregnancy cannot be allowed to continue. Early ectopic pregnancies can be removed through an injection of methotrexate. Laparoscopic or abdominal surgery is required to remove ectopic pregnancies that cannot be treated with medication.

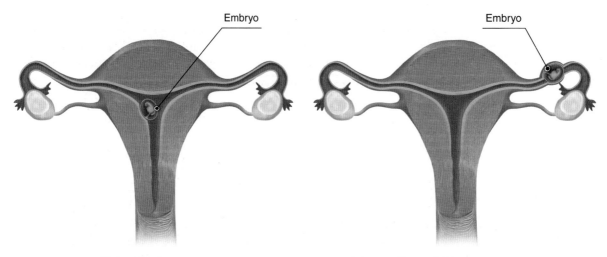

Embryo   Embryo

Normal pregnancy   **Ectopic pregnancy**

FIGURE 18-56 In an ectopic pregnancy, the fertilized ovum implants outside of the uterine cavity, most frequently in the fallopian tube.

Gestational Diabetes Mellitus

Gestational diabetes mellitus (GDM) occurs when elevated blood sugars develop during pregnancy. GDM can be treated with diet modifications, increased exercise, and insulin. Complications that can result from GDM are babies that are large for their gestational age, resulting in increased incidence of forceps, vacuum extraction, or caesarean section during delivery and neonates with hypoglycemia, jaundice, high red blood cell mass, and low blood calcium. GDM generally resolves after the baby is born, although women who have had GDM are at a higher risk for developing diabetes mellitus.

Cervical Insufficiency

Cervical insufficiency is the painless cervical dilation that occurs and results in a miscarriage in the second trimester of pregnancy. There are usually no symptoms of cervical insufficiency in early pregnancy; later symptoms include mild abdominal pressure, mild cramping, and slight vaginal bleeding. Diagnosis can be difficult; a transvaginal ultrasound and pelvic examination can be used to determine the length of the cervix and check for prolapsed fetal membranes. Treatment may include a cervical cerclage, which uses strong sutures to close the cervix.

Hyperemesis Gravidarum

Hyperemesis gravidarum is excessive vomiting during pregnancy that causes weight loss, electrolyte imbalance, nutritional deficiencies, and **ketonuria**. The exact cause of hyperemesis gravidarum is not known, although it is hypothesized to be an adverse reaction to the hormones that occur during pregnancy. Hyperemesis gravidarum is treated with fluids and a balanced, bland diet. An IV or medication is sometimes required.

Gestational Hypertension

Gestational hypertension is the onset of elevated blood pressure without **proteinuria** during the second half of the pregnancy in a client who has never had high blood pressure. There is no specific treatment for gestational hypertension, although it will be closely monitored to make sure other life-threatening conditions (such as preeclampsia) do not occur. Labor may be induced if blood pressure is consistently high and the fetus has reached viability.

HELLP Syndrome

HELLP is an acronym for hemolysis, elevated liver enzymes, and low platelets. This life-threatening condition occurs during the last trimester or shortly after birth and can be a variant of preeclampsia. Symptoms include abdominal pain accompanied by nausea, vomiting, backache, hypertension, headache, and vision impairment. The only effective treatment is delivery of the baby; signs and symptoms will usually disappear after the baby and placenta have been delivered. Maternal mortality is low with treatment, although there is increased risk for placental abruption, acute renal failure, and liver damage.

Preeclampsia

Preeclampsia is hypertension with proteinuria that develops after 20 weeks' gestation in a client that does not have hypertension. In the absence of proteinuria, preeclampsia may be defined as hypertension along with either thrombocytopenia, impaired liver function, new-onset renal insufficiency, pulmonary edema, or new-onset cerebral or visual disturbances. Preeclampsia can cause damage to other organs, specifically the liver and kidneys, may result in seizures, and is associated with abruptio placenta and HELLP syndrome. Eclampsia is defined as the presence of new-onset grand mal seizures in a woman with preeclampsia.

Placental Abruption

Placental abruption is the detachment of part or all of the placenta from the uterine wall after 20 weeks' gestation. This places the mother and fetus at risk for hemorrhage.

Placenta Previa

Placenta previa occurs when the placenta is implanted into the lower uterine segment, which may completely or partially cover the cervical opening.

Preterm Labor

Preterm labor is generally diagnosed clinically as regular contractions that occur between 20 weeks and 36 weeks, 6 days of gestation, along with a change in cervical effacement or dilation (or both), or presentation with regular uterine contractions and cervical dilation of at least 2 cm. Symptoms include contractions; pelvic pressure; vaginal bleeding; preterm rupture of membranes; or a watery, mucous-like, or bloody vaginal discharge. A pelvic exam, ultrasound, or uterine monitor may be used to diagnose preterm labor. While there is no treatment or procedure to stop preterm labor, medicine can be given that will stop it for up to two days. During this time, corticosteroids can be administered to aid in fetal lung development.

Miscarriage

A pregnancy that ends before 20 weeks' gestation is referred to as a miscarriage or spontaneous abortion. It places the client at risk for bleeding and infection. Most miscarriages occur before the 12th week of pregnancy and are usually a result of abnormal fetal development. Symptoms of miscarriage include vaginal spotting or bleeding, pain or cramping in the lower back, and tissue passing from the vagina. Risk for miscarriage is increased for women older than age 35; those who have had previous miscarriages; chronic illnesses, such as diabetes; those who smoke, drink, or use drugs while pregnant; and those who are overweight. The client can let the miscarriage occur naturally, take medication to speed the process of the miscarriage, or undergo a surgical procedure, typically a **suction dilation and curettage (D&C)**.

Hydatidiform Mole

Also known as a molar pregnancy, a hydatidiform mole is a partial or full abnormal growth of trophoblast cells that normally develop into the placenta. There is an absence of a formation of fetal tissue. A full hydatidiform molar pregnancy places the client at risk for **choriocarcinoma**. In a complete molar pregnancy, the placental tissue is swollen and appears to form fluid-filled cysts and there is no fetal formation. In an incomplete molar pregnancy, there is both normal and abnormal placental tissue. There may be a fetus, but it is not able to survive. An incomplete molar pregnancy is caused by an empty egg (with no chromosomes from the mother) being fertilized by one or two sperm. In an incomplete molar pregnancy, there are chromosomes from the mother, but two sets of chromosomes from the father. This results in 69, instead of 46, chromosomes in the embryo. While a molar pregnancy may initially appear normal, the client will eventually experience symptoms, such as dark brown or bright red vaginal bleeding, severe nausea and vomiting, pelvic pressure or pain, and vaginal passage of grape-like cysts. A molar pregnancy is generally treated with a D&C. HCG monitoring may continue for six months to one year to ensure that there is no remaining molar tissue.

LEARNING OBJECTIVE 18.6.3 Identify common causes of female infertility.

FEMALE INFERTILITY

Infertility is defined as trying to get pregnant for a year without conception occurring. Infertility can result from male or female factors. There are many causes for female infertility; the most common are:

- Age: Women over 35 are more likely to experience infertility than younger women. Female infertility accelerates after age 35 until a woman reaches **menopause**.
- Sexually transmitted infections: Untreated conditions, such as gonorrhea and chlamydia, can lead to pelvic inflammatory disease, which results in scarring of the fallopian tubes and uterus.
- Obesity: Too much body fat can cause the production of too much estrogen, causing the body to act as if it were on hormonal birth control.
- Anorexia: Eating disorder in which individuals starve themselves. This interferes with estrogen production and disrupts the menstrual cycle.
- Developmental anomalies: Structural anomalies of the uterus, fallopian tubes, or vagina can make it difficult for the sperm to fertilize the egg.
- Tubal factors: The descent of a fertilized or unfertilized ovum can be impeded by inflammation, adhesions, disruption, or scarring caused by an ectopic pregnancy or congenital factors.

- Nutritional deficiencies
- Thyroid dysfunction: In **hypothyroidism**, low levels of thyroid hormones can impair the release of a mature ovum. **Hyperthyroidism** can cause **anovulation**, resulting in irregular menstrual cycles and difficulties conceiving.
- Endometriosis: Tissue that normally makes up the uterine lining is present on other organs in the body, most frequently the ovaries, fallopian tubes, and tissue around the uterus (Figure 18-57). In early-stage endometriosis, it is believed that an inflammatory response affects conception. In advanced endometriosis, infertility is a result of the adhesions and scarring caused by the tissue growth. Infertility occurs in up to half of the women who suffer from endometriosis.
- Polycystic ovarian syndrome (PCOS): A hormonal abnormality that results in the ova's inability to mature fully; this results in an incomplete ovulation process that prohibits conception from occurring (Figure 18-58). This cause of the disorder is unknown.
- Pituitary or hypothalamic hormone disorders: Hypothalamic dysfunction is the decreased secretion of hormones normally produced by the pituitary gland. Commonly, there is an insufficiency in FSH and LH, which results in light or nonexistent menstrual periods.

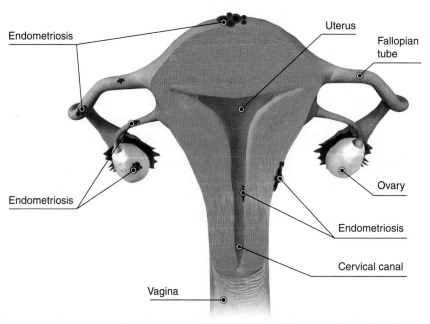

Endometriosis

Endometriosis

Uterus

Fallopian tube

Endometriosis

Ovary

Endometriosis

Cervical canal

Vagina

FIGURE 18-57 In endometriosis, tissue that normally makes up the uterine lining is present on other organs of the body.

- Medications: Certain medicines, such as antidepressants, oral contraceptives, corticosteroids, and chemotherapy, can cause infertility.
- Uterus: An abnormally shaped uterus may cause problems becoming or remaining pregnant. Submucosal fibroid tumors may disrupt implantation and embryo growth.
- Cervical: Cervical stenosis may prevent the sperm from traveling through the cervix to fertilize the egg. Sometimes, the mucous produced by the cervix also prevents sperm from traveling through the cervix to the uterus.

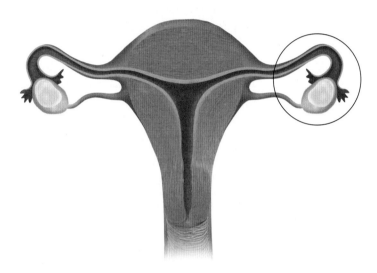

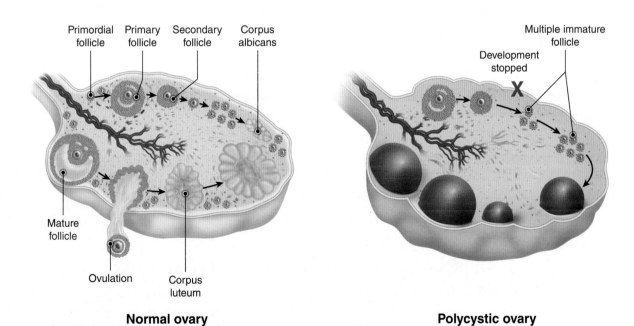

Normal ovary

Polycystic ovary

FIGURE 18-58 In PCOS, ova do not fully mature, resulting in cystic ovaries.

LEARNING OBJECTIVE 18.6.4 Identify common pathologies associated with vaginal bleeding during pregnancy.

VAGINAL BLEEDING DURING PREGNANCY AND CHILDBIRTH

Vaginal bleeding during pregnancy can have many different causes, some serious and others not. The causes of vaginal bleeding include:

- Implantation bleeding: A small amount of light spotting or bleeding that occurs 10–14 days after conception. This is considered normal and not cause for alarm.
- Molar pregnancy: An abnormal mass of cells develops instead of the fetus (and sometimes the placenta) can cause vaginal bleeding.
- Ectopic pregnancy: When the embryo implants outside of the uterus, usually in the fallopian tubes. Light vaginal bleeding is often a sign of an ectopic pregnancy.
- Placenta previa: The placenta is implanted into the lower uterine segment which may completely or partially cover the cervical os (opening), resulting in bleeding.
- Placentae abruption: Detachment of part or all of the placenta from the uterine wall after 20 weeks' gestation. This places the mother and fetus at risk for hemorrhage.
- Incompetent cervix: Light vaginal bleeding may accompany the opening of the cervix.
- Miscarriage: A pregnancy that ends before 20 weeks' gestation is referred to as a miscarriage or spontaneous abortion. All types of miscarriages place the client at risk for bleeding and infection.

LEARNING OBJECTIVE 18.6.5 Describe the signs, symptoms, and diagnosis of placenta previa and abruptio placenta.

KEY TERM

hysterectomy Surgical removal of the uterus.

PLACENTA PREVIA AND ABRUPTIO PLACENTA

Both placenta previa and abruptio placenta are complications that can result in vaginal bleeding and fetal distress. Both require monitoring of the mother and fetus by a physician, and they may require an emergency c-section to deliver the fetus.

Placenta previa occurs when the placenta is implanted into the lower uterine segment, which may completely or partially cover the cervical opening (Figure 18-59). The most common symptom is painless, bright red vaginal bleeding, which commonly occurs around 32 weeks. There are three classifications of placenta previa: complete (when the placenta completely covers the cervix), partial (when the placenta only partially covers the cervix), and marginal (when the placenta occurs near the edge of the cervix). Placenta previa is confirmed with an ultrasound. If the fetus and mother are not in distress, the condition can be managed at home. If the gestational age of the fetus is more than 30 weeks, or if the mother or fetus is in distress, immediate delivery may be warranted.

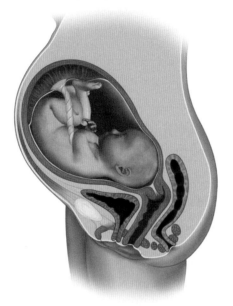
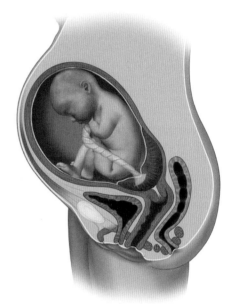

Normal   **Total placenta previa**

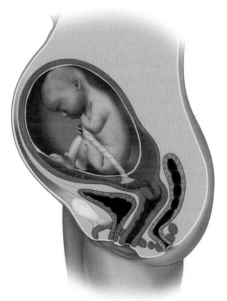
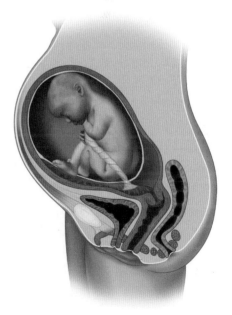

Partial placenta previa   **Marginal placenta previa**

FIGURE 18-59 Placenta previa is a condition in which the placenta completely or partially covers the cervical opening.

Abruptio placenta is the detachment of part or all of the placenta from the uterine wall after 20 weeks' gestation. This places the mother and fetus at risk for hemorrhage. Symptoms include vaginal bleeding, lower back pain, and very low blood pressure. These symptoms are sometimes accompanied by contractions. If neither the fetus nor mother is in distress and the fetus is less than 36 weeks, treatment will most likely be hospital monitoring to detect a change in condition. If the fetus or mother is in distress, immediate delivery of the fetus is warranted, even if the fetus is not yet at 36 weeks. If treatment occurs, the long-term prognosis for the mother is positive, although excessive bleeding may require blood transfusions or, when blood loss cannot be controlled, a **hysterectomy** may be required. Fetal complications include low birth weight, asphyxia, or stillbirth. Fetal prognosis depends on its gestational age at birth; babies closer to full term will have fewer complications.

LEARNING OBJECTIVE 18.6.6 Describe the signs, symptoms, and diagnosis of preeclampsia and eclampsia.

PREECLAMPSIA AND ECLAMPSIA

Preeclampsia and eclampsia are pregnancy-related high blood pressure disorders. Untreated preeclampsia can develop into eclampsia, which puts both the mother and baby at risk and can be fatal.

Preeclampsia is hypertension with proteinuria that develops after 20 weeks' gestation in a client that does not have hypertension. In the absence of proteinuria, preeclampsia may be defined as hypertension along with either thrombocytopenia, impaired liver function, new-onset renal insufficiency, pulmonary edema, or new-onset cerebral or visual disturbances. A diagnosis of preeclampsia requires blood pressure greater than or equal to 140 mm Hg systolic or greater than or equal to 90 mm Hg diastolic on two occasions at least four hours apart. Preeclampsia is also indicated by proteinuria levels greater or equal to 300 mg per 24-hour urine collection. Preeclampsia can cause damage to other organs, specifically the liver and kidneys, may result in seizures, and is associated with abruptio placenta and HELLP syndrome. The treatment for preeclampsia is the delivery of the baby and placenta, timed to aim for optimal outcomes for the baby while reducing risks for the mother.

Eclampsia is defined as the presence of new-onset grand mal seizures in a woman with preeclampsia. Eclampsia can reduce blood flow to the placenta, which may result in a low-birth-weight baby. The delivery of the baby and placenta is the only treatment that will resolve eclampsia. Most grand mal seizures that occur will happen within the first 48 hours after delivery. Treatment after delivery is designed to control convulsions and elevated blood pressure and monitor the client for indication of multiorgan failure. Medications may be needed to prevent seizures and to manage hypertension.

LEARNING OBJECTIVE 18.6.7 **Describe the signs, symptoms, and diagnosis of postpartum depression.**

POSTPARTUM DEPRESSION

Postpartum depression (PPD) is an intense and pervasive sadness with severe and labile mood swings. It is more serious and persistent than postpartum blues (colloquially known as the "baby blues"), lasting more than two weeks. Intense fears, anger, anxiety, and despondency that persist past the baby's first few weeks are not a normal part of postpartum blues. Eventually, symptoms may interfere with caring for the baby or completing other daily tasks. These symptoms rarely disappear without outside help. Most mothers suffering from PPD seek help only after reaching a crisis point.

The symptoms of postpartum depression are very similar to those of adult depression except that the mother's self-reflection of guilt and inadequacy feed her worries about being an incompetent and inadequate parent. In PPD, there can be loss of appetite or odd food cravings (often sweet desserts) and binges with abnormal appetite and weight gain. Sleep disturbance is common. Sleep deprivation is a factor in the development of PPD, and it can worsen the symptoms, which include:

- Anger
- Sadness
- Excessive crying
- Isolation
- Irritability
- Mood swings
- Poor appetite
- Hopelessness
- Sleep impairment
- Fatigue or energy loss
- Feeling overwhelmed
- Feeling worthless or inadequate
- Physical pain and muscle aches
- Trouble bonding with the baby
- Disinterest in caring for the baby
- Severe anxiety
- Difficulty maintaining relationships
- Inability to concentrate and make decisions
- Thoughts of harming the baby
- Thoughts of suicide

Diagnosis occurs based on an evaluation by your healthcare provider about your feelings, thoughts, and mental health. The doctor may have the patient fill out a questionnaire to screen for depression and to help distinguish PPD from the baby blues. Recently, proactive measures have been taken to diagnose PPD in new mothers; screenings usually occur at the initial follow-up appointment at the OBGYN, and may occur during regular visits to the baby's pediatrician. Treatment usually includes psychotherapy and antidepressants.

Glossary

A

A-bands Dark regions in sarcomeres where the contractile proteins, actin and myosin, overlap.

abdominal aorta Portion of the aorta just after it passes below the diaphragm and before it divides into the common iliac arteries.

abdominal aponeurosis Flat, sheetlike tendinous structure located at the anterior abdominal wall and formed by the tendons of three abdominal muscles: internal obliques, external obliques, and transversus abdominis.

abdominal ultrasound Imaging test of the abdominal region using high-frequency sound waves.

abdominals Referring to the abdominal musculature.

abducens nerve Cranial nerve VI; controls eye movement.

abduction Movement away from the midline of the body.

abductor digiti minimi Muscle located in the first layer of the foot.

abductor hallucis Muscle located in the first layer of the foot that is connected to the big toe.

abrasions Scrapes caused by rubbing the skin against another surface that are on the surface of the skin and do not bleed.

abscess Infection of a gland and surrounding tissue that causes pain, swelling, and inflammation.

absorption Passage of digested food materials from the digestive tract of an individual into the cardiovascular and lymphatic systems for distribution to the body's cells.

abstinence Avoidance of sexual intercourse as a method of birth control.

accessory hemiazygos vein Vein located on the left side of the vertebral column.

accessory nerve Cranial nerve XI; controls muscles of head and neck.

acetabulofemoral joint Ball-and-socket joint of the hip, located between the femur and acetabulum.

acetic acid Weak acid that is also known as vinegar.

acetylcholine receptors Cellular receptors located on the motor end plate of skeletal muscles that respond to acetylcholine.

acetylcholine Neurotransmitter secreted by motor neurons that promotes contraction of skeletal muscle.

Achilles Large tendon in the back of the lower leg, also known as the calcaneal tendon.

achondroplasia Most common form of dwarfism.

acid Chemical compound that ionizes when placed in a liquid and releases hydrogen ions (H^+).

acidic Pertaining to an acid; a value lower than 7 on the pH scale.

acidity Measurement of how strong or weak an acid solution is.

acidosis Blood pH less than the normal lower limit of 7.35.

acquired immunodeficiency syndrome (AIDS) Exacerbation of the human immunodeficiency virus (HIV) that causes the development of opportunistic infections.

acquired Something a person develops.

acroesthesia Extremely abnormal sensitivity to pain, heat, cold, or touch.

acromegaly Condition causing excessive growth in adulthood.

acromioclavicular joint Gliding joint located at the upper portion of the shoulder, between the clavicle and acromion of the scapula.

acromion process Large process extending off the superior portion of the scapula.

acromion Outward end of the shoulder blade or scapular spine that forms the upper section of the shoulder socket and articulates with the collarbone or clavicle.

acrosome Organelle that covers the anterior portion of the head of the sperm and contains enzymes that penetrate the ovum.

actin Double-helix contractile protein found in muscle tissue.

action potential Rapid change in voltage generated by muscle and nervous tissue.

active immunity Immune condition where a person produces antibodies.

active transport Movement of a molecule across a membrane that requires energy because the movement is going against its concentration gradient.

acupuncture Healing modality characterized by the insertion of needles or manipulation of points along lines known as meridians running throughout the body.

acute renal failure Occurs when the kidneys suddenly become unable to properly filter the blood and remove waste products.

acyclovir Oral medication used to treat the genital herpes virus.

Addison's disease A disorder that occurs when your body produces too little of cortisol.

adduction Movement toward the midline of the body.

adductor brevis Muscle located in the medial thigh region that perform adduction of the hip; part of the adductor group of muscles.

adductor hallucis Muscle in the third layer of the foot that maintains the transverse arch of the foot; part of the adductor group of muscles.

adductor longus Muscle located in the medial thigh region that performs adduction of the hip; part of the adductor group of muscles.

adductor magnus Muscle located in the medial thigh region that performs adduction of the hip; part of the adductor group of muscles.

adenocarcinoma Type of lung cancer that forms in glands.

adenosine triphosphate Compound that provides cellular energy; also called ATP.

adhesions Areas of body tissue that are stuck together.

adipocytes Specialized cells found in adipose connective tissue that store fat.

adipose cells Specialized cells that store fat and make up adipose connective tissue.

adipose Loose connective tissue commonly known as fat.

ADP Adenosine diphosphate; molecule consisting of the amino acid adenosine and two phosphates; an additional phosphate can be added to form adenosine triphosphate.

adrenal glands Triangular-shaped glands located superior to the kidneys. These glands are responsible for the production and secretion of hormones involved in cellular metabolism and the regulation of water.

adrenergic receptors Receptor on the surface of cells that cause a sympathetic response.

adrenocorticotropic hormone (ACTH) Promotes release of glucocorticoids and androgens.

afferent arteriole Small blood vessel in the kidney that supplies blood to glomeruli.

afferent vessels Lymphatic vessels leading to a lymph node.

Agammaglobulinemia No detectable antibodies in the blood.

Agglutination Clumping of blood particles that are of differing types. Usually a result of a mismatched transfusion.

agonist muscles Muscles performing a specific movement.

agranulocytes White blood cells that do not contain packets of chemicals that can activate the immune system. Examples include leukocytes and monocytes.

albinism Group of genetic disorders where there is partial or complete loss of melanin in the hair, eyes, and skin.

albumin Plasma protein found in the blood that creates and maintains blood's colloid osmotic pressure.

aldosterone A steroid hormone produced by the adrenal cortex that helps regulate the salt and water balance in the body.

alimentary canal The long muscular tube of the digestive system that transports ingested materials from the mouth to anus; site of mechanical and chemical digestion.

alkaline Chemical compound that ionizes when placed in a liquid and has the ability to bind to free hydrogen ions. The solution could also be called a base and has a pH greater than 7 (7.45 when used in reference to the human body).

alkalinity Measurement of how strong or weak an alkaline solution is.

alkalosis Blood pH greater than 7.45.

allergens Antigens that stimulates allergic reactions.

alloantigens Antigens on the cell surface of other humans; antigens from the same species.

all-or-none rule Contraction of a muscle fiber once the threshold for voltage is reached.

alopecia Partial or complete loss of hair from parts of the body that would normally have hair; male and female pattern baldness is an example.

alpha motor neurons Large motor neurons of the brainstem and spinal cord that extend to skeletal muscle.

alpha-fetoprotein Protein secreted by the fetus; it is present in the mother's bloodstream and amniotic fluid.

alveolar epithelium Tissue lining the inside of the alveolus (simple squamous epithelium).

alveolar minute volume Amount of air reaching the alveoli during a one-minute duration.

alveoli Smallest functional units of the lung; structures in which the exchanges of gases occur.

alveolus Bony socket for the root of a tooth.

Alzheimer's disease A chronic, progressive neurological disorder resulting in dementia, language and mood problems, and other behavioral changes.

amenorrhea Absence of menstruation.

amines Small modified amino acids.

amino acids Organic compound containing nitrogen, carbon, hydrogen, and oxygen; the building blocks of protein.

amino groups Portion of a chemical substance that contains an amine group ($-NH_3$).

amniocentesis Use of amniotic fluid to test for trisomy 21.

amnion Innermost fetal membrane.

amniotic membranes Fluid-filled membrane or sac that protects the fetus.

ampulla of Vater Cavity where the common bile duct and the pancreatic duct open into the major duodenal papilla.

ampullae Expanded areas at the ends of the mammary ducts that are close to the nipple.

ampullary Third portion of the fallopian tube, which curves over the ovary; most common site for human fertilization.

amygdala Region of the limbic system involved in processing emotion.

amylin Peptides that are secreted from beta cells that inhibit glucagon synthesis.

amyotrophic lateral sclerosis (ALS) A chronic, progressive neurological disease that affects the motor neurons of the brain and spinal cord. Also known as Lou Gehrig's disease.

anaconeus Small muscle of the elbow that attaches to the humerus and ulna.

anaphase I Stage during meiosis I when the spindle fibers are pulling the homologues apart to opposite ends of the cell.

anaphase II Stage during meiosis II when the spindle fibers are pulling the sister chromatics apart to opposite ends of the cell.

anaphylaxis Systemic, rapid reaction to an allergen that causes life-threatening respiratory and circulatory dysfunction.

anatomical dead space Air in the lungs that does not contribute to gas exchange.

anatomical neck Bony landmark found between the head and shaft of the bone.

anchoring filaments Structure in skin containing elastic fibers that have a role in fluid movement throughout the body.

androgen Hormones that regulate the growth and development of the male reproductive system.

anemia Condition caused by not having sufficient numbers of red blood cells or enough hemoglobin to carry oxygen to all of the cells.

aneurysms Defect in a blood vessel usually caused by a weakened wall and characterized by bulging of the vessel.

angina Chest pain occurring from ischemia of heart muscle.

angiography Imaging of blood vessels using contrast media and x-rays.

angiotensin I Physiologically inactive form of angiotensin that is created from angiotensinogen and can be converted by angiotensin-converting enzyme to the active form, angiotensin II.

angiotensin II Protein that can increase blood pressure by causing vasoconstriction, stimulates the release of aldosterone, and is the physiologically active form of angiotensin.

angiotensin-converting enzyme (ACE) Enzyme that converts angiotensin I to angiotensin II.

anhidrosis Disorder of the sweat gland that inhibits normal sweating.

anorexia nervosa Eating disorder in which a patient may severely limit food intake and/or compulsively overexercise to avoid weight gain; leads to abnormally low body weight and malnutrition.

antagonist muscles Muscles opposing a specific joint movement.

anterior and posterior tibial arteries Arteries extending below and continuing from the popliteal artery.

anterior chamber Fluid-filled cavity in the front of the eye.

anterior cruciate ligament (ACL) One of the major ligaments in the human knee; provides rotational stability for the knee; it is also the most frequently injured ligament of the knee.

anterior horn Anterior portions of the gray matter of the spinal cord.

anterior superior iliac spine Bony landmark located on the anterior portion of the ilium of the pelvis.

antibodies Immune system proteins produced in response to a specific antigen that non-self cells for destruction.

anticoagulants Molecules that decrease clotting.

anticonvulsants Drug used to prevent brain seizures from epilepsy or other brain disorders.

antidepressants duloxetine Drug used to prevent depression and other brain disorders including anxiety, pain, and addictions.

antidiuretic hormone (ADH) Also known as a vasopressin; hormone secreted by the posterior lobe of the pituitary gland or that increases blood pressure and decreases urine production.

antigen presentation Process in which MHC molecules along with antigen attach to the cell surface of the phagocyte to allow immune cells to distinguish between self-cells and other cells.

antigen Surface protein that creates a certain label on the cell. Usually used to distinguish differing blood types.

antigen-presenting cells Phagocytic cells that have engulfed foreign invaders and placed the foreign invaders' antigens on their own cell surface to present it to other cells in the immune system.

antigens Chemical groups, such as proteins and polysaccharides, on the surface of a cell that can stimulate an immune response.

antithrombin III Molecule that inhibits the coagulation pathway by decreasing the number of co-factors that are needed to stimulate clotting.

antrum Term used to describe the cavity that is formed when an oocyte is maturing.

anucleate Cells that are without a nucleus.

aorta Large blood vessel exiting the left ventricle, known as a great vessel of the heart.

aortic bodies Series of chemoreceptors located in the aortic arch.

aortic sinus Widening of the aorta just above the aortic valve that serves as a location for baroreceptors.

aortic valve Semilunar valve located near the junction of the aorta and left ventricle.

apex Apex of the heart is the inferior point of the heart.

apical surface Side of epithelial tissue that is exposed to the cavity of an internal organ or exterior of the body.

apnea Stopped breathing.

apneustic center Respiratory center in the pons portion of the brainstem.

apocrine Type of sweat gland found only in the axillary and genital areas that does not function until puberty; also secretes proteins and fatty acids.

aponeurosis of the sacrospinalis Flat, broad, tendinous structure that attaches to the sacrospinalis muscles.

appendicular skeleton Division of bones in the human skeleton where muscles can attach and move the body.

arachnodactyly Condition in which the fingers and toes are abnormally long and slender and the thumb is pulled in toward the palm.

arachnoid matter Middle, spongy layer of the meninges permeated by cerebrospinal fluid.

arcuate arteries Branches of the interlobar artery of the kidney that supply blood to the base of the pyramids.

arcuate popliteal ligament Y-shaped extracapsular ligament that attaches to the posterior portion of the head of the fibula.

arcuate vein Veins of the kidney that run along the arcuate arteries and receive blood from the interlobular veins, which is then emptied into the interlobar veins.

areola Area of pigmented tissue that surrounds the breast nipple and contains sebaceous and sweat glands.

areolar Loose connective tissue with predominantly fibroblast cells, collagen, and elastic fibers; has a large amount of ground substance around the cells.

arrector pili muscles Small smooth muscles located in the integument that can move hair follicles.

arrhythmias Abnormal heart rhythms.

arrhythmogenic right-ventricular dysplasia Type of cardiomyopathy that occurs in the right ventricle and causes arrhythmias.

arteries Thick tubular structures that carry blood away from the heart.

arterioles Smaller vessels branching from arteries.

articular capsule Double-layered capsule that surrounds the synovial joint.

articular cartilage Hyaline cartilage covering bone ends at movable joints.

articular cavity Joint cavity bounded by the synovial membrane and articular cartilage of all synovial joints; normally only contains synovial fluid.

articular process Helps bones connect to one another and is associated with movable joints.

articulating bones Bones that move around a connecting joint.

artificially acquired active immunity Immune condition where a person is introduced to a microorganism through medical means and develop their own antibodies to the microorganism.

artificially acquired passive immunity Immune condition where a person is given someone else's antibodies through a medical procedure.

arytenoid Small paired cartilage on the posterior portion of the larynx.

asbestos Silicate substance that acts as a carcinogen in lung tissue.

ascending aorta Portion of the aorta between the left ventricle and aortic arch.

ascending lumbar veins Veins located in the thoracic cavity that contribute to the azygos vein.

ascending pathways Region of the spinal cord consisting of the axons transmitting sensory information up to the brain.

aspiration Inhalation of nonair substances into the trachea.

Aspirin Pain reliever and blood thinner used for minor aches and its anticoagulation properties via the inhibition of COX 1 and 2 receptors.

assisted reproductive technology (ART) Any fertility treatment in which eggs or embryos are handled outside of the body.

association cortex Highly developed regions of the cerebral cortex that processes sensory information to a greater extent than the primary areas.

Asthma Disease characterized by constriction of the bronchial air passages resulting in a decrease in airflow into and out of the lungs.

astrocytes Glial cell of the CNS involved in making the blood-brain barrier and altering synaptic function.

asymptomatic Showing no signs or symptoms.

asystole ECG reading indicating no contraction of the heart.

athlete's foot Fungal infection affecting the skin around the toes and toenails.

atlantoaxial joint Pivotal joint formed between the first (atlas) and second (axis) cervical vertebrae in the upper part of the neck.

atlanto-occipital joint Joint formed between the occipital bone of the skull and the first cervical vertebra.

ATP Adenosine triphosphate; energy-storing molecule consisting of the amino acid adenosine and three phosphate molecules.

atresia Degeneration of a follicle.

atria Hollow chamber of the heart that acts as a receiving chamber for blood entering the heart.

atrial fibrillation Abnormal heart rhythm characterized by chaotic contractions of the atria.

atrial septal defect Perforation of the atrial septum allowing blood to flow between atria.

atrioventricular (AV) node Section of nodal tissue located at the inferior portion of the right atrium at the junction of the right atrium and ventricles capable of generating action potentials at 40–60 bpm.

atrioventricular bundle Section of nodal tissue located inferior to the atrioventricular node and at the superior junction of the ventricles capable of generating action potentials at 20–40 beats per minute.

atrioventricular valves Heart valves located between the atria and ventricles.

auricle Irregularly shaped structure overlying the atria.

auscultation Examination of the sounds of the heart.

autoantibodies Antibodies directed against self-antigens.

autoantigens "Self" antigens; antigens on our own body cells.

autoimmune disease Disease caused by your immune system mistakenly attacking your own body.

autoimmune disorders Disorders in which the immune system mistakenly attacks the body.

autoimmune syndrome Syndrome in which the body's antibodies destroy tissue.

autoimmune Immune condition that results from making antibodies that attack self-antigens.

autonomic nervous system neurons Nervous system cells (neurons) belonging to the autonomic nervous system.

autonomic nervous system Division of the peripheral nervous system that regulates organ function; composed of the sympathetic and parasympathetic nervous systems.

autoregulation Maintenance of a constant supply of blood to the kidney in spite of varying blood pressure.

autosomal recessive Trait that requires two genes in order to be expressed.

avulsions Occurs when the skin is torn away and the tissues below are exposed, causing extensive bleeding.

axes Imaginary lines about which parts of the body rotate; in anatomy, an axis is termed as the three anatomical planes, namely frontal, transverse, and sagittal.

axial skeleton Division of bones in the human skeletal system that functions as an anchor or base for the body and provides protection to vital organs.

axillary artery Lateral continuation of the subclavian artery.

axillary vein Lateral continuation of the subclavian vein.

axon bulbs End of the axon where neurotransmitters are released.

axon terminal buds Specialized region of the neuron that releases neurotransmitters and serves as the output zone.

axon terminal Portion of a neuron located at the end of an axon that releases neurotransmitter into the synaptic cleft.

axon Single, long extension of the cell membrane of a neuron; carries outgoing signals to other cells.

axons Long processes extending from the cell bodies of neurons; can be myelinated or unmyelinated.

azithromycin Antibiotic used to treat a chlamydia infection.

azotemia Excess urea and other nitrogenous wastes in the blood as a result of kidney disease.

azygos vein Vein that runs along the right side of the thoracic vertebrae. It empties into the superior vena cava.

B

Babinski reflex Reflex in infants that involves the big toe flexing and the toes spreading in response to a stroke of the bottom of the foot.

bactericidal Capable of killing bacteria.

balance Sense processed by vestibular organs and proprioception that allows us to remain upright.

ball-and-socket joint Spheroidal joint that allows for extension, flexion, abduction, and internal and external rotation.

barium contrast Thick solution of barium sulfate used to enhance x-ray images, particularly of the digestive tract.

baroreceptor Sensory receptor that senses pressure.

barrel chest Thoracic deformity produced in chronic obstructive pulmonary disease from the hypertrophy of respiratory muscles.

Bartholin's glands Gland that provides lubrication to the vagina during sexual stimulation.

basal body temperature (BBT) method Type of fertility awareness-based method of birth control that uses the female body temperature to determine ovulation.

basal cell carcinoma Most common type of skin cancer; appears as flattened, round spots that are shiny and pale; rarely spreads.

basal metabolic rate The smallest amount of energy over a period of time that a person needs to maintain body function.

base Chemical compound that ionizes when placed in a liquid and has the ability to bind to free hydrogen ions. The solution could also be called alkaline and has a pH greater than 7 (7.45 when used in reference to the human body).

basement membrane Material secreted by both the epithelial cells above it and the connective tissue cells below it; forms the basal surface and anchors epithelium in place.

basilar artery Artery formed by the union of the vertebral arteries.

basilic vein Medial superficial vein of the upper extremity.

basophils Granulocytic white blood cells which function in allergic responses and inflammation.

Beau's lines Horizontal grooves across the nails caused by a temporary disruption in nail growth from things such as illness, malnutrition, or chemotherapy.

Becker MD Type of muscular dystrophy characterized by low levels of dystrophin protein in muscle cells.

benign prostatic hyperplasia (BPH) Nonmalignant enlargement of the prostate gland.

beriberi Disease caused by vitamin B_1 (thiamine) deficiency; causes inflammation of nerves (potentially damaging neurons permanently), heart disease, and swelling.

biaxial Allows movement within two principal axes; the wrist and ankles are examples.

bicarbonate ion Ionic form of bicarbonate (HC_3^-).

biceps brachii Muscle in the upper arm attaching to the scapula and humerus.

biceps femoris Muscle in the posterior portion of the leg and part of the hamstring group.

bicipital tuberosity Broad eminence on the anterior portion of the radius bone.

bicuspid Also known as the mitral valve, located between the left atrium and ventricle and containing two cusps.

bifid Spinous process that splits into two smaller processes so that it resembles a Y-shaped projection from the vertebral arch.

bile Yellow or greenish alkaline fluid secreted by the liver and passed into the duodenum where it aids in the absorption of fat.

biliary tree Bile ducts and gallbladder.

bilirubin Pigment formed by the breakdown of hemoglobin and excreted in the bile.

biliverdin Byproduct of heme synthesis.

bipennate Feather-like arrangement of fascicles in muscle tissue attaching to a central structure.

bisphosphonates Group of drugs used to limit the loss of bone density.

Bitot's spots White growths on eye that result from the superficial buildup of keratin in the conjunctiva of the eye.

bladder distention Enlarged bladder caused by retention of urine.

blastocoel Fluid-filled cavity that forms during the cleavage stage of embryonic development.

blastocyst Early form in the development of an embryo that consists of a circular layer of cells filled with fluid.

blastomeres Type of cell produced after cleavage of the zygote; it is essential in the formation of the blastula.

blood plasma Watery ground substance containing dissolved proteins, of the fluid connective tissue called blood.

blood pressure Fluid (hydrostatic) pressure in the vascular system.

blood typing Testing of a sample of blood to determine an individual's blood group.

blood urea nitrogen (BUN) Concentration in the blood of nitrogen in the form of urea.

blood urea nitrogen Blood test that measures urea nitrogen, a waste product, in the blood and can help to indicate organ disease.

BNP B-type natriuretic peptide; produced by the heart and tends to rise with heart damage.

Body mass index Value calculated by dividing a person's weight (Wt) in kilograms by the square of his or her height (Ht) in meters; indicates if a person is at a normal weight.

body of the uterus Large central area of the uterus that tapers to the cervix.

body Central and the largest portion of the stomach.

bohr effect Changes in hemoglobin's affinity for oxygen binding from changes in pH.

bone marrow Substance found in medullary cavity that primarily produces new blood cells.

bony landmarks Individual parts of bones.

Botulinum toxin Substance produced from the bacterium *Clostridium botulinum* that paralyzes muscles.

Bowman's capsule Thin, membranous capsule that surrounds the glomerulus of a nephron through which glomerular filtrate passes to the proximal convoluted tubule. Also known as the glomerular capsule.

Boyle's Law Law stating that the pressure of a gas is inversely proportional to its volume.

brachial plexus Network of interconnected nerves formed by four cervical nerves and one thoracic spinal nerve.

brachial vein Continuation of the axillary vein.

brachialis Muscle in the upper arm that attaches to the humerus and extends to the radius.

brachiocephalic artery Artery branching off the aorta.

brachiocephalic trunk Artery branching off the aorta on the right side and dividing into the right subclavian and right common carotid arteries.

brachioradialis Muscle in the forearm that attaches to the humerus and extends to the radius.

breast cancer Cancer of the breast; the most common type of cancer that affects the female reproductive system.

Broca's area Region of the (typically) left frontal lobe associated with the production of speech.

Brodmann areas Fifty-two distinct areas of the brain organized based on the shapes and sizes of neurons.

bromhidrosis Condition of offensive body odor, usually associated with the breakdown of sweat from apocrine sweat gland secretion.

bronchi Air passages extending from the trachea and entering the lungs.

bronchial Referring to the lungs. For example, the bronchial arteries supply the lungs with oxygenated blood.

bronchioles Smaller branches from tertiary bronchi that attach to alveoli.

buccinator Muscle located in the cheek that compresses the cheek against the teeth.

bulbourethral gland Glands in the male reproductive system located beneath the prostate that adds fluids to semen.

bulimia Eating disorder in which a patient may cycle through periods of compulsive and excessive food intake (binge) and then purge through vomiting or use of laxatives.

bursae Small sacs filled with lubricating fluid to reduce friction in the moving body joints.

C

calcifies To harden by depositing calcium.

calcitriol Synthetic version of vitamin D_3.

calmodulin Calcium-binding protein found in smooth muscle.

calorie Unit of heat (energy); amount of energy required to raise 2 grams of water 1 degree Celsius.

canalicular period Period of lung development that occurs between 16 and 26 weeks of gestation; during this period, basic structures of the gas-exchanging parts of the lungs form, and the terminal saccules begin to form.

canaliculi Small ducts found in between lacunae that help route nutrients to cells in lacunae and lamellae.

cancellous bone Also called spongy or trabecular bone, found at the ends of long bones, in parts of the pelvis, ribs, skull, and spinal column.

cancer Disease caused by uncontrolled division of abnormal cells in the body.

canker sores Small, shallow ulcers that appear inside the mouth.

capacitation Process by which the sperm becomes capable of fertilizing an egg.

capillaries Smallest blood vessels consisting of one layer of simple squamous epithelium.

capillary epithelium Thin tissue lining capillaries consisting of simple squamous epithelium.

capillary hydrostatic pressure Force of capillary fluids pushing against the wall of the capillary. Fluid movement is from within the capillary into the surrounding tissues; one of the forces favoring filtration.

capillary osmotic pressure Force of osmotic particles (proteins and electrolytes) within capillaries attempting to pull water into the capillary; one of the forces opposing filtration and capillary hydrostatic pressure.

capsular hydrostatic pressure Force of water within the glomerular capsule trying to push itself out of the glomerular capsule and into the glomerular capillaries; one of the forces opposing filtration and capsular osmotic pressure.

capsular osmotic pressure Force of osmotic particles (proteins and electrolytes) within the glomerular capsule trying to pull water into the capsule from the glomerular capillaries; one of the forces favoring filtration.

carbaminohemoglobin Hemoglobin molecule formed by the attachment of carbon dioxide.

carbohydrates Organic compounds made of carbon, hydrogen, and oxygen; examples are starch, cellulose, and sugars.

carbon monoxide poisoning Condition that occurs when carbon monoxide builds up in the blood from inhalation of carbon monoxide.

carbonic anhydrase Enzyme in red blood cells that promotes the formation of carbonic acid from carbon dioxide and water.

carboxylic groups Portion of a chemical compound that contains a carboxyl group (–COOH).

cardia Part of the stomach that encloses the gastroesophageal sphincter.

cardiac accelerator nerves Group of sympathetic nervous system nerves arising from thoracic spinal nerve roots that travel to the sinoatrial node.

cardiac cycle Sequence of mechanical and electrical events allowing the heart to contract and move blood.

cardiac muscle cells Tissue cells of cardiac muscle.

cardiac muscle tissue Involuntary, striated, branched type of muscle tissue found in the heart; the cells have a single nucleus and are tightly adhered to each other by intercalated discs.

cardiac muscle Type of striated muscle tissue found in the heart.

cardiac notch Indentation in the area where the heart contacts the left lung; also known as a cardiac impression.

cardiac plexus Group of nerves that connect the autonomic nervous system to the heart.

cardinal movements Positional changes of the fetus inside the womb of the mother when it moves during the process of labor and birth through the birth canal.

cardio selective Receptors or hormones that are only located on the myocardium of the heart.

cardiomyopathy Disease characterized by damage to heart muscle tissue.

Cardiovascular disease Conditions of narrow, blocked, or hardened arteries.

carotid artery stenosis Narrowing of the carotid artery.

carotid bodies Chemoreceptors located in the carotid arteries near the bifurcation where the common carotid becomes the internal and external carotid arteries.

carpometacarpal joint Saddle joint that allows movement of the thumb; connects the trapezium to the first metacarpal bone.

Cartilage cells Cells involved in endochondral ossification.

cartilaginous joints Joints connected by fibrocartilage or hyaline cartilage that allow for movement.

cataract Clouding of the lens of the eye leading to a reduction in the sharpness of vision.

catecholamines Monoamine hormones composed of a catechol and a side-chain amines. These hormones are usually involved in the up or downregulation of the sympathetic and central nervous system.

cavernous sinuses Cavities that serve the venous system by draining the ophthalmic veins.

celiac trunk Branch of the abdominal aorta.

cell membrane junctions Hold cells tightly together to prevent loss of chemicals and water and cells from being pulled apart and allow chemicals and water to pass between cells; three common types are tight junctions, desmosomes, and gap junctions.

cell-mediated immunity Action of the adaptive immune system mediated by T cells.

cellular respiration Series of reactions occurring in the cell that converts glucose to ATP.

cementum Substance that encloses the dentin of the root of a tooth.

central (haversian) canal Central canal of bone that contains nerve fibers and blood vessels.

centromere Region of a chromosome where sister haploids connect; also the site where spindle fibers attach.

cephalic vein Lateral superficial vein of the upper extremity.

cerebellum Portion of the brain located in the posterior region and inferior to the cerebrum. Processes fine motor movements, balance, coordination, and proprioception.

cerebral aqueduct One of four fluid-filled cavities in the brain.

cerebral cortex Uppermost layers of the cerebrum involved in sensory, motor, and higher-order processing.

cerebrospinal fluid (CSF) Fluid produced in the lateral ventricles of the brain that surrounds the brain and spinal cord to protect and remove waste products.

cerebrovascular accident (CVA) The sudden death of neurons and neuroglia in the brain due to a lack of blood supply to the region. Also known as a stroke.

cerebrum Largest portion of the brain; located above the brainstem.

cerumen Also called ear wax, secreted by ceruminous glands in the external ear canal and helps protect the skin there.

ceruminous glands Found in the skin that lines the external ear canal; modified apocrine sweat glands that produce a substance called cerumen, also known as earwax.

cervical canal Interior portion of the cervix.

cervical cap Method of birth control where a soft cup-shaped device is placed over the base of the cervix.

cervical diaphragm cap Method of birth control where a cup is placed over the cervix.

cervical mucus ovulation method Type of fertility awareness-based method of contraception where the cervical mucus is examined to determine periods of fertility.

cervical plexus Network of interconnected nerves formed by the first 4 cervical nerves.

cervical spinal nerves Eight pairs of peripheral nerves that exit from the uppermost region of the spinal cord.

cervix Projects into the vagina and forms a pathway between the uterus and the vagina.

chemical digestion Molecular breakdown of food by bile and enzymes secreted throughout the digestive system.

chemical senses Senses that allow us to detect chemicals in the world around us; smell and taste.

chemical stress Any molecule or substance that can create a stress response in the body. These stressors lead to a disruption in homeostasis.

chemoreceptors Sensory proteins that detect chemicals in bodily fluids; also related to the perception of smell and taste.

Cheyne-Stokes breathing Abnormal breathing pattern characterized by cycles of deep and shallow breathing.

chiasmatic groove The upper surface of the sphenoid bone that contains the pituitary gland.

chiropractic Healing modality characterized by manipulation of joints and soft tissues of the body.

chlamydia Type of STI caused by the bacterium *Chlamydia trachomatis*.

chloride shift Movement of chloride ions into red blood cells as bicarbonate ions exit.

chocolate cysts Endometriotic lesions that contain old blood and appear like chocolate syrup.

cholecalciferol Substance produced by the kidneys that helps the body absorb calcium. This compound can be used as a dietary supplement to enhance calcium levels.

cholesterol Steroid made by the liver; found in animal fats and body tissues.

chondrocytes Mature cells found in cartilage.

chordae tendineae Tendinous structures that connect the atrioventricular valves to papillary muscles on the inner walls of the ventricles.

choriocarcinoma Malignant tumor of the uterus that originates in the cells of the chorion of the fetus.

chorion Outermost fetal membrane.

chorionic villi sampling (CVS) Testing of the tissue that makes up the placenta to determine the presence of a genetic anomaly.

chorionic villi Found on the surface of the chorion of the embryo, they implant within the endometrium to provide a maximal contact area with maternal blood.

chromaffin cells Cells located in the adrenal cortex that are responsible for the production and secretion of catecholamines.

chromosome String of DNA that contains genetic material.

chronic bronchitis Chronic inflammation of the bronchial air passages characterized by a productive cough lasting greater than three months.

chronic obstructive pulmonary disease (COPD) Chronic lung disease that includes chronic bronchitis and emphysema.

chylomicrons Protein and fat globules found in lymph and blood.

chyme Digested, viscous, semifluid contents of the intestine.

cilia Hair-like projections that move in a wavelike manner that support movement.

ciliated pseudostratified columnar epithelium Type of epithelium characterized by one row of columnar cells that contain cilia.

circadian rhythm Internal body clock that regulates the sleep–wake pattern.

Circle of Willis (cerebral arterial circle) System of arteries that provides blood to the brain.

circulatory circuits Blood vessel pathways.

circumcision Procedure conducted to remove the foreskin of the penis.

circumduction Movement of the distal end of a limb in a circular motion.

circumflex artery Branch of the left coronary artery that wraps around the left side of the heart.

cisterna chyli Enlarged sac in the abdomen that eventually leads to the thoracic duct.

cisternae Tiny membranous channels located around muscle cells that combine to form the sarcoplasmic reticulum.

citric acid cycle System of reactions located in the mitochondrion that convert acetyl-coenzyme A into ATP, FADH2, and NADH for providing energy to the body.

clavicle Bone of the shoulder connecting the scapula and the sternum; also called the collarbone.

cleft lip and palate Cleft lip is the opening in the upper lip of a baby and that can extend up to the nose; the cleft palate is the opening in the roof of a baby's mouth.

cleft palate Genetic condition that results in incomplete closure of the hard or soft palate.

clitoris Erectile organ like the male penis that is highly sensitive and distends during sexual arousal.

Clostridium botulinum Bacterium that produces the botulinum toxin.

Clostridium tetani Bacterium that produces the tetanus toxin.

clotting factor III Surface glycoprotein that can initiate the clotting cascade when activated.

clotting factors Substances in blood plasma that are involved in the clotting process.

coagulation The process by which the blood thickens to form blood clots.

coarctation of the aorta Narrowing of the aorta.

coccygeal spinal nerves One pair of peripheral nerves that exit from the lowermost region of the spinal cord.

coccyx Small bone attached to the inferior portion of the sacrum.

cochlea Sensory structure of the inner ear that detects sound.

coenzymes Nonprotein molecule that is needed for an enzyme to function.

cognitive-behavioral therapy Type of psychotherapy that works to change negative behaviors.

coitus interruptus Method of birth control where the penis is withdrawn before ejaculation.

coitus Sexual intercourse.

cold sores Painful, fluid-filled blisters that occur outside the mouth (under the nose, around the lips, or under the chin) and are caused by a virus and are highly contagious.

collagen An abundant structural protein found throughout the body.

collecting duct Duct that receives and concentrates urine from the distal convoluted tubule of nephrons and empties into the minor calyxes.

colloid Substance that is dispersed evenly throughout another substance.

colony-stimulating factors Chemicals that can increase the growth of certain white blood cells in the bone marrow.

colostrum Thins watery liquid that is ejected from the mammary glands at the start of lactation.

columnar cells Epithelial cells that are taller than they are wide with elongated, oval-shaped nuclei.

comedo A follicle on the skin that becomes clogged with sebum, dead skin cells, and bacteria. Usually occurring in the setting of acne and over-production of androgens that may increase bodily secretions.

common carotid artery Arteries branching from the brachiocephalic artery on the right and aorta on the left carrying blood to the internal and external carotid arteries.

common hepatic arteries Arteries in the abdominal cavity that supply the stomach and liver.

common iliac arteries Paired inferior branches off the abdominal aorta.

common iliac vein Inferior branch of the inferior vena cava.

compact bone Also called cortical bone, most rigid bone type in the body.

complement cascade Set of reactions that occur after the complement system is activated in which protein triggers the activation of the next protein.

complete proteins Animal protein containing all 20 amino acids.

compliance Pertaining to the elastic property of the lungs; ability of lung tissue to stretch and relax.

compliant Referring to the elastic component of a structure.

compound fracture Broken bones that puncture the skin and are significantly displaced.

computed tomography Imaging test in which x-rays are used to produce a three-dimensional image.

concave Curve inward.

concentration gradient Difference in concentration between two sides of a membrane.

concentric contractions Contractions in which a muscle shortens while moving a load.

conchae Protrusions located on the inner surface of the nasal cavity that help to create turbulent air flow.

concussion Injury to the brain that results in a temporary change in the function of the brain.

condom Method of birth control where a sheath is placed over the male penis or a sheath is inserted into the female vagina.

conduct Ability of nerves to transmit impulses.

conduction Process of losing heat by directly contacting another object.

conductive hearing loss Decrease or complete loss of the ability to hear due to something, such as a blockage or infection, preventing sound waves from affecting the inner ear structure.

condyle Rounded prominence at the point where two bones meet.

cones Visual sensory cells specialized to detect color.

congenital cardiac defect Defect in the structure of the heart or great vessels that is present at birth.

congenital diaphragmatic hernia Birth defect of the diaphragm that allows the abdominal organs to push into the chest cavity; hinders proper lung formation.

congenital heart disease Form of heart disease that is inherited.

congenital hypertrichosis Rare genetic disease resulting in hair growth that covers the entire body.

congenital Something a person is born with.

congestive heart disease Disease characterized by damage to heart muscle and enlargement of the ventricles of the heart.

congestive heart failure Type of heart disease characterized by damage to heart muscle resulting in the inability of the heart to pump blood.

connective tissue One of the four primary tissue types, forms and functions vary and include support, storage, and protection.

constipation Infrequent bowel movement or difficulty emptying bowels.

contractile proteins Proteins located in muscle cells that assist in muscle contraction.

contracture Type of scar common in burn patients that tightens the skin and may extend deeper, affecting muscles and nerves, which results in impaired movement.

control center Area in which the input from the receptor is analyzed in the negative feedback loop. Usually the control center is the central nervous system.

convection Transfer of heat to the air surrounding the body.

convex Curve outward.

Cooper ligaments Structures that support the breast from the outer region to the nipple like the spokes of a wheel.

cor pulmonale Enlargement of the right side of the heart occurring from lung disease.

coracobrachialis Muscle in the upper arm extending from the coracoid process of the scapula to the humerus.

coracohumeral ligament Broad ligament that strengthens the upper part of the capsule of the shoulder joint.

coracoid process Bony extension on the anterior portion of the scapula just inferior to the acromion process.

cornea Thin, transparent membrane covering the eye.

corniculate Small paired cartilage on the posterior portion of the larynx.

corona radiata Granulosa cells that surround the oocyte during the maturation process.

coronal suture Immovable, fibrous joint between the frontal bone and the right and left parietal bones.

coronary arteries Branches off the aorta that carry blood to heart muscle.

coronary artery disease (CAD) Narrowing of the inner lumen of coronary arteries usually from atherosclerotic plaquing.

coronary circulatory pathways Blood vessel pathway that brings blood to the heart.

coronary sinus Cardiac vein that empties into the right atrium.

coronoid process Bony triangular process located on the ulna.

corpus albicans White scar tissue on an ovary after the corpus luteum atrophies.

corpus callosum Axon pathways that travel between and functionally connect the two cerebral hemispheres.

corpus cavernosa Spongy tissue within the penis that becomes engorged with blood to cause an erection.

corpus luteum stage Stage in which the cells of the follicle divide quickly and the corpus luteum secretes progesterone to build up the endometrium.

corpus luteum Mass that develops in the area of a ruptured oocyte follicle on an ovary.

Corpus spongiosum Mass of erectile tissue that runs along the penis.

cortex Outer layer of an organ.

cortical radiate arteries Arteries connecting the arcuate arteries to the afferent arterioles.

cortical radiate vein Veins connecting the vasa recta and peritubular capillaries to the arcuate vein.

corticospinal tract Spinal cord pathway containing the axons of neurons controlling skeletal muscle.

corticotropin-releasing hormone (CRH) Stimulates both the synthesis and the secretion of ACTH.

costal cartilages Areas of hyaline cartilage extending from the anterior portion of the ribs to the sternum.

co-transport Coupled transport of chemical substances across a cell membrane in which the energy required to move a substance (such as glucose) against a concentration gradient or against electrical potential is provided by the movement of another substance (such as a sodium ion) along its gradient in concentration or electric potential.

cranial nerves Sensory and motor neurons that primarily control and detect stimuli of the head and neck but do not arise from the spinal cord.

cranial plates Bones of the skull.

cranium Flat bones that surround the brain and make up the head.

C-reactive protein Protein blood marker that is used to indicate inflammation.

creatine kinase Enzyme found in muscle tissue that is released into the blood when muscles become damaged.

creatine phosphate Energy-storing molecule located around muscle tissue that can lend its phosphate for phosphorylation of ADP to make ATP.

crescendo murmurs Abnormal heart sounds characterized by an increase in loudness.

crescendo–decrescendo murmurs Abnormal heart sounds characterized by an increase followed by a decrease in loudness.

Crest Raised edge of a bone.

cricoid cartilage Cartilage located on the anterior portion of the larynx just below the thyroid cartilage.

cross-bridge cycling Cycle in which myosin attaches to actin, moves actin, then releases from actin while powered by ATP.

cross-bridge Connections in muscle tissue formed by the binding of myosin to actin.

crossed extensor reflex Reflex that involves the extension of one leg and the simultaneous retraction of the other.

crossing over Trading of bits of DNA that occurs between homologous chromosomes during prophase I.

crown Portion of the tooth that found over the gum line.

crowning Appearance of the head of the fetus at the vagina during labor.

cryoprecipitate Type of prepared plasma that contains fibrinogen, von Willebrand factor, Factor 8, Factor 9, and fibronectin. Usually used to substitute significant blood loss or a decrease in clotting factors.

cryptorchidism Undescended testicle.

CT Computed tomography. Imaging study in which x-rays are used to produce a three-dimensional image.

cuboidal cells Epithelial cells that are cube-shaped with nuclei that are round and central in the cell.

cuneiform Small paired cartilage on the posterior portion of the larynx.

curvatures Curves in the spinal column.

cusps Leaflet structures that comprise the heart valves.

cuticle Edge of the skinfold covering the proximal nail.

cystic fibrosis transmembrane conductance regulator Defective gene in cystic fibrosis that results in a decrease in water content in mucous.

cystic fibrosis Genetic disease characterized by the production of thick and salty mucous.

cystic veins Veins in the abdominal cavity that drain the gallbladder.

cytokines Proteins that play a regulatory function in the immune system.

cytotoxic T cells T cells that kill virally infected cells and cancer cells.

D

Daily Values Recommended dietary amounts of vitamins, minerals, fat, cholesterol, carbohydrates, fiber, and protein for a healthy diet; appear on food labels and are based on a 2000-kcal diet.

dandruff Small pieces or flakes of dead skin on the scalp or in the hair.

D-dimer test Test used to measure the by-products of clot destruction. Usually carried out when there is a suspicion for a hypercoagulable; estate in the blood.

deep palmar arch Arteries located in the palms of the hands.

deep vein thrombosis (DVT) Blood clot that forms in a vein deep in the body.

defensins Peptides that kill foreign cells by poking holes in cell membranes and cell walls.

degenerative Progressive, often irreversible deterioration.

deglutition Process of swallowing.

degranulation Cellular process that causes release of histamine, which enables immune response.

dehydration State in which the extracellular fluids are significantly reduced and their osmolarity has increased to the point that it is outside the body's normal range. Typically dehydration is due to a lack of water entering the body or too much water leaving the body.

deletion Alteration that occurs when a part of a chromosome is missing.

deltoid Superficial muscle of the shoulder.

dendrites Specialized regions of the neuron that have neurotransmitter receptors and serve as the input zone.

dense connective tissue Type of fibrous connective tissue found in ligaments and tendons.

dental cavity Area of decay or hole in a tooth.

dentin Bonelike substances found in teeth.

deoxygenated blood Blood containing low oxygen levels after passing through tissue capillaries.

deoxyhemoglobin Hemoglobin molecule that forms when oxygen is released by hemoglobin.

depolarization Change in voltage from a negative resting membrane potential toward a positive state from the movement of sodium ions inside of a cell.

depolarizes Process of depolarization such as in a cell membrane becoming less polarized.

depression Downward movement of body structures.

depth Ability to see an object three-dimensionally.

dermal papillae Projections of the dermis that push upward into the epidermis; increase surface area and allow for more diffusion of nutrients and oxygen into the epidermal cells.

dermatome Area of the skin of which a particular spinal nerve is influencing.

dermis Deepest layer of skin that is composed of irregular connective tissue.

dermoid cystic teratomas Tumor made up of several different types of tissues.

descending genicular artery Branch of the femoral artery supplying the area around the knee.

descending pathways Region of the spinal cord consisting of the axons transmitting motor information from the brain.

desmopressin Synthetic version of ADH. Usually used to replace ADH or to clinically determine ADH levels.

desmosomes Junctions that are scattered throughout the cell membrane and act as anchors to prevent cells from being pulled apart due to mechanical stress.

detrusor muscle Outer, largely longitudinally arranged musculature of the bladder wall.

detumescence Penis's return to a flaccid state.

diabetes insipidus Disorder of the pituitary gland that results in extremely low levels of ADH being produced causing intense thirst and the excretion of large amounts of dilute urine.

diabetes mellitus Disease caused by the body's inability to process glucose normally; body's inability to produce or respond to the hormone insulin results in the abnormal metabolism of sugar.

diabetic autonomic neuropathy Nerve damage of neurons in the autonomic nervous system due to complications of diabetes resulting in autonomic dysregulation.

diabetic ketoacidosis (DKA) Complication of diabetes that occurs when the body produces high levels of acidic ketones due to the increased breakdown of fats for energy use.

dialysis Medical procedure to remove wastes or toxins from the blood and adjust fluid and electrolyte levels using a semipermeable membrane.

diapedesis Process of white blood cells squeezing through blood vessel walls to enter the tissues.

diaphragm Large skeletal muscle located at the base of the thoracic cavity that contracts to increase the volume of the thoracic cavity.

diaphysis Shaft in the middle of a long bone.

diarrhea Increased frequency of defecation, usually with liquid stools.

diastasis recti abdominis Gap between the two sides of the rectus abdominis muscle, caused by the stretching of the expanding uterus in pregnancy.

diastolic heart failure Type of heart failure that affects ventricular filling.

diastolic murmurs Abnormal heart sounds occurring during diastole.

dichorionic-diamniotic Twins who do not share a chorion, amnion, or placenta while in utero.

differentiate Specialization of cells.

diffusion Passive movement of substances from an area of high concentration to lower concentration until reaching equilibrium.

digastric Muscle in the region of the neck.

digestion Breakdown of the large food materials into smaller particles by mechanical and chemical digestion.

digital rectal examination Examination of the prostate gland performed through direct palpation of the gland through the rectum.

dilated cardiomyopathy Type of heart disease in which the ventricles become enlarged and are unable to adequately move blood.

diploid Cell that contains 23 pairs of chromosomes for a total of 46 chromosomes.

direct antagonist Ligand or drug that decreases a biological process by binding to and blocking a receptor.

dissecting abdominal aortic aneurysm Weakening of the wall of the abdominal aorta causing bulging and eventual tearing of the artery.

disseminated intravascular coagulopathy (DIC) Widespread hemorrhaging after clots are destroyed or used up. Usually a condition that is preceded by massive trauma where the body needs to quickly use clotting factors in attempts to stop blood loss.

distal convoluted tubule (DCT) Convoluted portion of the nephron between the loop of Henle and the collecting duct. Its function is to concentrate urine prior to its excretion.

distance Ability to determine how far away an object is.

dizygotic Twins derived from two separate ova; also known as fraternal or nonidentical twins.

DNA Content of a cell that contains proteins that make up genetic material.

dopamine Hormone that inhibits prolactin release from the anterior pituitary. This hormone can also affect heart rate, pleasure reception in the brain, and learning.

dorsal and plantar arches Arteries supplying the inferior portion (plantar) and superior portion (dorsal) of the foot.

dorsal column Region of the spinal cord containing ascending neurons encoding information about touch.

dorsal interossei Small muscles located on the back or dorsal region of the hand.

dorsal respiratory group Paired group of neurons located in the posterior portion of the medulla oblongata that work to regulate breathing rate and rhythm.

dorsal root ganglion Enlargement of the dorsal root in which the sensory neuron cell bodies reside.

dorsal root Region of the spinal cord that sensory neurons enter.

dorsalis pedis artery Branch of the tibial artery located in the ankle.

dorsalis pedis vein Vein in the ankle that becomes the anterior tibial vein.

dorsiflex Movement of the ankle in which the toes are extended upward as if walking on the heels.

dorsiflexion Bending at the ankle such that the toes are lifted toward the shin.

dorsum Pertaining to the back or posterior region of the body.

Down syndrome Another name for trisomy 21.

doxycycline Antibiotic used to treat chlamydia infection.

d-transposition of the great arteries Condition characterized by reversal of the aorta and pulmonary trunk.

Duchenne MD Most common type of muscular dystrophy affecting young boys between the ages of 3 and 5 years old characterized by the absence of the muscle dystrophin protein.

ducts Long coiled tubes where sperm are created, matured, and stored.

ductus arteriosus Fetal circulatory pathway between the aorta and pulmonary trunk.

ductus venosus Carries oxygenated blood from the umbilical vein in the fetus to the inferior vena cava, bypassing the fetal liver.

duloxetine Antidepressant medication used to treat nerve pain, depression, and anxiety.

duodenorenal flexure Border between the duodenum and the jejunum.

duplication Alteration that occurs when a part of a chromosome is replicated.

dura matter Thick, leathery outermost layer of the meninges.

dural sac Membranous sheath that surrounds the spinal cord and the cauda equina.

dural sinuses Hollow areas in the meninges that carry venous blood.

dyskinesia Involuntary, uncontrollable movement of the body typically associated with prolonged treatment for neurological disorders.

dysphagia Inability to swallow normally.

dystrophin Type of structural protein in muscle tissue that helps to provide strength to muscle fibers.

dysuria Painful urination.

E

eardrum Also known as the tympanic membrane. Boundary membrane between the middle and outer inner that vibrates in response to sound waves.

eccentric contractions Muscle contraction in which a muscle lengthens while supporting a load.

eccrine Type of sweat gland that is more common than apocrine sweat glands and found everywhere on the body; the sweat that they secrete plays an important role in preventing bacterial growth and thermoregulation.

ECG Electrocardiogram; test that measures electrical impulses generated by the heart.

echocardiogram Imaging test using high-frequency sound waves (ultrasound).

ectoderm Outermost germ layer in the early embryo; it will go on to form the nervous system; tooth enamel; epidermis; and lining of the mouth, nose, anus, and sweat glands.

edema Localized area of excess fluid.

edrophonium test Medical test incorporating the use of edrophonium, an acetylcholinesterase inhibitor, performed to help diagnose myasthenia gravis.

effacement Cervical softening, shortening, and thinning.

effector Area or cells that are responsible for carrying out the response from the control center in the negative feedback pathway.

efferent arteriole Blood vessel that carries blood out of the glomerulus and toward the peritubular capillaries and vasa recta.

efferent vessels Lymph vessels that leave the lymph nodes.

ejaculation Expulsion of sperm through the penis.

ejaculatory duct Duct formed by the seminal vesicle as it enters the prostate gland.

ejection Referring to ejection fraction which is a measure of the blood exiting the left ventricle with each contraction.

elastic Type of cartilage found in the epiglottis and external ear that contains many elastic fibers in its extracellular matrix.

electrolyte imbalance Abnormalities of concentration of electrolytes such as sodium, potassium, and calcium.

electrolytes Minerals, typically salts, that carry a charge and are responsible for many essential processes in the body.

electromyography Medical test measuring the electrical activity in muscle and nerve tissues.

elevation Upward movement of body structures.

ellipsoidal joint Joint shaped like a ball and socket that can rotate on two axes but does not allow for rotation.

embolism Condition resulting from material (e.g., clot, lipid, gas) lodged in a blood vessel.

embryo After fertilization, the zygote or fertilized egg forms into an embryo, an unborn offspring; early stages of fetal growth approximately from the second week to the eighth week.

emergency contraceptive Method of birth control where a pill containing hormones is ingested within 72 hours after unprotected intercourse.

eminences Bumps in bones.

emotional stress Mental state that can increase a stress response and disruption in homeostatic balance.

emphysema Lung disease characterized by damage to the alveoli resulting in large air pockets.

enamel Hard, a calcareous substance that is used for the formation of a thin layer capping the teeth to protect the teeth from wear and acids.

encapsulated Input zones of sensory nerves of the skin which consist of specialized membrane structures used to detect mechanical stimuli.

endocardium Inner layer of the heart.

endochondral ossification Process through which bone is created from a cartilage model.

endocrine gland Ductless gland that secretes a hormone into the bloodstream.

Endoderm Innermost germ layer in the early embryo; it will go on to form much of the gastrointestinal tract, respiratory tract, endocrine glands and organs, and urinary system.

endometrial cancer Cancer that occurs from the lining of the uterus or the endometrium of the female reproductive system causes bleeding in postmenopausal females.

endometriosis Health problem where endometrial tissue grows outside of the uterus.

endometritis Inflammation of the endometrium.

endometrium Inner layer of the uterus.

endomysium Thin, loose connective tissue membrane surrounding muscle cells.

endoplasmic reticula Network of tubes within the cytoplasm of the cell with a role in synthesizing proteins and lipids.

endoscopy Medical procedure incorporating the use of a device called an endoscope for visualizing internal anatomical structures.

endothelium Simple squamous epithelium found lining blood vessels, lymphatic vessels, and the heart.

end-stage renal disease (ESRD) Final stage of kidney failure is characterized by the complete or nearly complete irreversible loss of renal function.

enteric nervous system One of the main part of the autonomic nervous system, consisting of a meshlike system of neurons that govern the functions of the gastrointestinal tract.

eosinophils Granulocytic white blood cells which function in the destruction of helminths and participate in allergic responses.

ependymal cells Glial cell of the CNS that lines the ventricles and produces cerebral spinal fluid.

epicardium Outer fibrous layer of the heart.

epicondyle Area of the bone between the condyle and the shaft of the bone.

epicranial aponeurosis Flat, broad area of fibrous connective tissue located on the superior portion of the skull.

epidermis Superficial layer of skin that covers the dermis; composed of stratified squamous epithelium.

epidermolysis bullosa Rare genetic disorder that causes the skin to become loose and very thin, forming large red areas that blister and peel away.

epididymis Long tube that attaches to each testis where sperm mature and are stored.

epididymitis Infection of the epididymis, usually caused by an STI.

epiglottis Cartilaginous structure in the larynx that closes it off when swallowing to prevent the movement of substances into the trachea.

epilepsy A group of chronic neurological disorders in which brain activity becomes abnormal, resulting in seizures.

epimysium Thin connective tissue membrane surrounding a muscle.

epiphyseal line Junction line of long bone end part (epiphysis) and central part of the long bone (diaphysis), where growth in length occurs.

epiphyseal plate During bone development, hyaline cartilage is replaced by bone at the epiphyseal plate.

epiphysis Flared ends of a long bone.

epithelial tissue The center of the artery, called the tunica interna endothelium.

epithelium One of four primary tissue types, lines and covers all free body surfaces, both inside and out; functions are protection, absorption, filtration, and secretion.

Erb's point Auscultation point heard at the third left intercostal space at the left border of the sternum.

erectile dysfunction Inability to attain and maintain an erection to perform sexual intercourse.

erection Results when the corpora cavernosa within the penis becomes engorged with blood and causes the penis to become stiff.

erector spinae group Group of back muscles that function in extension of the trunk that consist of the spinalis, longissimus, iliocostalis, and semispinalis muscles.

erythroblastosis fetalis Abnormal presence of erythroblasts in the blood usually found in newborns or mothers with nonmatching Rh surface proteins.

erythrocytes Red blood cells found in blood that contain hemoglobin and carry oxygen throughout the body.

erythropoiesis Process of creating red blood cells.

erythropoietin (EPO) Hormone that increases red blood cell production.

esophageal artery Arteries supplying the esophagus.

esophageal dysphagia Type of swallowing abnormality that affects the esophagus.

esophageal hiatus An opening in the diaphragm, the esophagus passes through the esophageal hiatus and joins the stomach.

esophageal sphincter Sphincters that close the esophagus when food is not being swallowed; the upper esophageal sphincter surrounds the upper part of the esophagus, and the lower esophageal sphincter surrounds the lower part of the esophagus at the junction between the esophagus and stomach.

esophageal Pertaining to the esophagus.

esophagus Smooth muscle structure located between the pharynx and stomach that is part of the alimentary canal that carries substances from the mouth to the stomach.

essential vitamins Vitamins that the body needs and cannot make.

estradiol One of three estrogen hormones; the most abundant.

estriol One of three estrogen hormones.

estrogen Steroid hormone that promotes the development and maintenance of female characteristics of the body.

estrone One of three estrogen hormones.

ethmoid Deep bone in the skull that contributes to the nasal septum and orbit.

euploid Cell that contains 23 full pairs or 46 total chromosomes.

Eustachian tubes Small passageways between the middle ear and nasal cavity.

evaporation Transfer of heat through the vaporization of water.

eversion Act of turning the feet outwards or inside out.

evert To move the ankle so the sole of the foot is pointing away from the midline of the body.

excitatory neuron Presynaptic neuron that makes its post-synaptic partner more likely to fire an action potential.

excitatory neurotransmitter Neurotransmitter that promotes the opening of sodium channels on adjacent tissue.

excitatory post-synaptic potentials Secretion of neurotransmitters that promote depolarization of the post-synaptic membranes of tissues.

excretion Discharge of waste from the body.

excursion Range of motion regularly repeated.

exocrine glands Gland that secretes a substance onto the surface of the body using a duct.

exocytosis Process where products are moved from the cytoplasm of the cell to the plasma membrane where they are packaged and ultimately released from the cell.

exogenous External source or administration of a substance.

exophthalmos Abnormal protrusion of the eyeballs.

expiratory reserve volume Lung volume representing the amount of air leaving the lungs during a maximal exhalation in addition to tidal volume.

extension Straightening movement that increases the angle between the bones of the joint.

extensor carpi radialis brevis Muscle in the posterior forearm that attaches to the humerus and extends to the radius.

extensor carpi radialis longus Muscle in the posterior forearm that attaches to the humerus and extends to the radius.

extensor carpi ulnaris Muscle on the posterior forearm that attaches to the humerus and extends to the ulna.

extensor digiti minimi Muscle located in the posterior hand region that moves the fingers or digits into extension.

extensor digitorum longus Muscle in the lower leg located deep to the tibialis anterior and works to dorsiflex the ankle.

extensor digitorum Muscle in the posterior forearm that moves the fingers or digits into extension.

extensor hallucis longus Deep muscle of the lower leg that works to extend the big toe.

external acoustic meatus Opening in temporal bone that allows for the ear canal.

external epithelial root sheath External layer of the epithelial root sheath.

external iliac vein Vein in the pelvis that connects the femoral and common iliac veins.

external intercostals Superficial muscles located between the ribs that work to spread apart the ribs.

external obliques Superficial muscles located on the lateral abdominal region that work to rotate and flex the trunk.

external os Cervix's opening into the vagina.

external respiration Process by which gas exchange occurs between the alveoli and the blood.

external rotation Outward or lateral rotation.

external urethral sphincter Muscle fibers that form a narrow ring of muscle around the urethra just distal to the prostate gland in males and in the female a ring of muscle more generally distributed around the urethra that controls the release of urine from the body.

extracellular fluid (ECF) Fluid located outside of cells.

extracellular matrix Ground substance and protein fibers found in connective tissue that make up the extracellular matrix.

extracellular space Fluid surrounding tissue or cells within the body.

extrinsic anemias Acquired forms of anemia not related to genetic components.

eye muscles Muscles that attach to the eyelid to cause it to close.

eyebrows Short strip of hair above each eye.

eyelashes Row of hairs that grow on the end of the eyelids.

eyelids Layer of skin that covers the eye to control light, particle, and sweat access to the eyes.

F

facial nerve Cranial nerve VII; motor control and sensory detection of the face.

facioscapulohumeral MD Form of muscular dystrophy in teenage boys that affects the muscles of the shoulder, chest, face, arms, and legs.

factor X Clotting factor involved in the common pathway that is responsible for initiating the common pathway.

factor XIII (fibrin-stabilizing factor) Molecule that increases the stability of the fibrin clot.

fallopian tubes Thin structures that are attached to the uterus on one end and are open to the ovaries on the other end.

false ribs Three pairs of ribs inferior to true ribs that attach to sternum indirectly.

falx cerebri Section of dura mater located in the longitudinal fissure that separates the right and left hemispheres of the brain.

farsightedness Inability to focus on relatively close objects.

fascia Band of connective tissue that separates or surrounds anatomical structures.

fascicles Small bundles of muscle fibers.

fast-twitch fibers Small groups of muscle fibers that can generate a high degree of force for a short duration.

fat-soluble vitamins Vitamins that dissolve in lipids.

fatty acid molecules Fat molecules that are digested in the small intestines.

fecal nuchal translucency (FNT) test Ultrasound test completed between weeks 11 and 13 of gestation to determine the amount of fluid behind the neck of the developing fetus.

feces Semisolid mass of indigestible food materials in the large intestine.

feed-forward regulation The release of insulin before the rise of blood glucose. This event usually occurs before ingestion of food or continued digestion of food.

femoral arteries Continuation of the external iliac arteries located in the thighs.

femoral circumflex artery Branch of the femoral artery located in the upper thigh.

femoral vein Continuation of the external iliac vein located in the thigh.

femur Long bone of the upper leg; longest bone in the body.

fenestrae Small openings in the glomerular capillaries between the pedicles of podocytes that allow for the movement of water and molecules.

ferritin Blood cell protein that contains iron.

fertility awareness-based methods Method of birth control where sexual intercourse is avoided during periods of fertility.

fertilization Outcome when a sperm cell penetrates an ovum.

fetus Infant before birth that develops from the embryo and remains in the uterus for approximately 40 weeks.

fibers Muscle cells containing strands of contractile proteins.

fibrin A protein that is activated the clotting cascade that binds to platelets, forming a plug around the area of blood vessel damage.

fibrinolysis Breakdown of fibrin in blood clots leading to thinning of the blood.

fibrocartilage Type of durable cartilage with many fibers and very little extracellular matrix found in the intervertebral discs, the menisci of the knee, and the pubic symphysis; acts as a shock absorber and resists compression.

fibrocystic breast changes Changes in the cell structure of breast tissue.

fibromyalgia Diffuse pain syndrome extending throughout the body and producing sleep disturbances and cognitive problems along with muscle pain.

fibrous connective tissue Tough connective tissue containing collagen fibers.

fibrous joints Fixed or immobile joints that are connected by dense, tough connective tissue.

fibrous pericardium Outer portion of the heart containing fibrous connective tissue.

fibula Bone in the lateral portion of the lower leg.

fibular artery (peroneal artery) Inferior and lateral branch of the popliteal artery.

fibularis tertius One of the fibularis group of muscles located in the lateral portion of the lower leg.

fifth metatarsal Most lateral metatarsal bone in the foot.

fimbriae Finger-like projections attached to one end of the fallopian tubes that hover over the ovary.

first metatarsal Most medial metatarsal bone in the foot.

first polar body Small haploid cell formed during meiosis of the female sex cell that does not have the ability to be fertilized.

first-degree burns Superficial burns that only affect the epidermis. Skin may look red, swollen and be sensitive.

fissure Openings for nerves, blood vessels, and tendons to pass through. Usually elongated and larger than foramina.

fixator Muscle that assists in holding a joint immobile, such as in maintaining posture.

flagellum Appendage that allows the sperm to swim.

flat bones Relatively thin bones that are responsible for protecting inner organs.

flatus Gas generated in the stomach or bowels.

flexion Bending of the joint decreasing the angle of the bones at the joint.

flexor carpi radialis longus Muscle located in the anterior forearm extending from the humerus to the radius.

flexor carpi radialis Muscle on the anterior portion of the forearm extending from the radius to the carpals.

flexor carpi ulnaris Muscle located in the anterior forearm extending from the humerus to the ulna.

flexor digiti minimi brevis Muscle located in the third layer of foot muscles producing flexion of the toes.

flexor digitorum brevis Muscle located in the first layer of foot muscles producing flexion of the toes.

flexor digitorum longus Muscle in the posterior leg that produces flexion of the toes.

flexor digitorum profundus Muscle in the anterior forearm that produces flexion of the toes.

flexor digitorum superficialis Muscle in the anterior forearm that produces flexion of the toes.

flexor hallucis brevis Muscle in the lower leg that flexes the big toe.

flexor retinaculum Band of connective tissue in the wrist that forms the carpal tunnel.

floating ribs Two pairs of ribs that do not connect with the sternum.

follicle stage Stage of the female reproductive cycle during which follicle-stimulating hormone is secreted from the pituitary gland and circulates to the ovary, stimulating the growth of a follicle.

follicles Small secretory cavity, sac, or gland usually found on the surface of the skin.

follicle-stimulating hormone (FSH) Stimulates spermatogenesis in males and ovarian follicle maturation in females while also producing estrogen.

follicular keratosis Skin condition caused by excessive production of keratin that results in blocked hair follicle openings and tiny, rough bumps on the skin.

folliculitis Inflammation of the hair follicles from something like a bacterial infection.

fontanelles Spaces between bones of the skull seen in infants.

fontanels Soft, membranous gaps between the cranial bones of an infant.

foramen magnum Bony landmark that is a large hole that transmits the spinal cord.

foramen ovale Opening in the septum that pushes blood between the left and right atrium that is present in the fetal heart; normally closes on its own shortly after birth.

foramen Openings for nerves, blood vessels, and tendons to pass through. Usually round or ovoid in shape and smaller than fissures.

foramina of brain case Opening inside the skull that allows arteries, veins, and cranial nerves to pass through.

forced expiratory volume Test performed with a spirometer in which a subject performs a maximal exhalation directly after a maximal inhalation as quickly as possible.

forced vital capacity Amount of air measured by a forced expiratory volume test.

forces favoring filtration Forces favoring filtration that try to move water and molecules from within the glomerulus into the glomerular capsule; consist of capillary hydrostatic pressure and capsular osmotic pressure.

forces opposing filtration Forces opposing filtration that try to move water and molecules from within the glomerular capsule back into the glomerular capillaries; consist of capillary osmotic pressure and capsular hydrostatic pressure.

foreskin Fold of skin that covers the glans of the penis.

formed elements Living cellular components of the blood.

fornix The recessed area of the vagina that is close to the cervix

fossa ovalis Indentation located in the interatrial septum that is a remnant of fetal circulation.

fossa Depression in a bone.

fourth ventricle One of four fluid-filled cavities within the brain.

fracture Any type of break in a bone.

fragment antigen binding (Fab) Part of the immunoglobulin molecule that binds to antigens.

fragment constant (Fc) Bottom portion of the immunoglobulin that attaches to the B cells to form receptors.

free edge Distal end of the nail that appears white.

free nerve endings Input zones of sensory neurons which rely on specialized proteins, rather than membrane specializations, to detect stimuli.

fresh frozen plasma Blood product made from the plasma portion of the blood that can be unfrozen in the hospital during an emergency situation and provided to a patient that may be deficient of clotting factors.

frontal lobes Anterior portion of the cerebrum that processes motor information and higher-level brain functions such as concentration, planning, problem solving, and personality.

frontalis Muscle located in the anterior portion of the skull that attaches to the epicranial aponeurosis.

fructose Sugar substance used for sperm motility.

fulcrum In a lever, the fulcrum is the pivot point in which a load is attached to a structure on each side.

functional residual capacity Volume of air residing in the lungs after a passive exhalation.

fundal Larger upper part of the uterus.

fusiform Shape of a muscle that is wider in the middle and narrower on each end.

G

gag reflex Reflex in which the throat contracts in response to an object coming in contact with the back of the mouth.

gait How a person walks.

gala aponeurotica Alternative name for the epicranial aponeurosis.

gallbladder disease Several types of conditions that affect the flow of bile in your gallbladder including inflammation and excess fat.

gallstones An abnormal, small, hard mass that is formed in the gallbladder from bile components.

gallstones A small, hard, mass formed in the gallbladder from bile components such as cholesterol, bile salts, and bilirubin.

gametes Sperm and oocytes, or the sex cells.

gap junctions Hollow, water-filled cylinders that allow things like nutrients and ions to pass between neighboring cells; most commonly found in cardiac cells and embryonic cells.

gastric emptying The time it takes for food to empty from the stomach and into the small intestines.

gastric fundus Round portion of the stomach located above and to the left of the cardia.

gastric pit Indentations in the stomach that denote entrances to the gastric glands.

gastrocnemius Muscle on the posterior portion of the lower leg that crosses both the knee and ankle joint.

gastroesophageal reflux disease (GERD) Backflow of stomach acid or gastric juice, or fluids and food into the esophagus from the stomach.

gastroschisis Birth defect in which the baby's intestines extend outside of the abdomen through a hole near the belly button.

general senses Senses that can be detected throughout the body without specialized organs or other structures.

genes Series of DNA and proteins located on a chromosome that provides material to create body straits and characteristics.

genital herpes Viral sexually transmitted infection that causes lesions on the genitalia; there is no cure.

germ cells Embryonic cell that can develop into a gamete through meiosis.

germinal centers Central areas of lymph nodes where a small number of B lymphocytes are produced.

germinal epithelium Outermost covering of the ovaries.

gestation Pregnancy; conception to birth.

gestational diabetes Condition where there is an elevated level of glucose in the blood during pregnancy.

ghrelin Hormone released mainly by the stomach believed to signal hunger or prime the body for fat absorption.

gigantism Growth disorder causing excessive growth in children prior to growth plate closure.

gingiva tissue Area around the root of the tooth that helps keep the tooth in place.

gingivitis Gum inflammation caused by excess plaque on the teeth.

ginglymus joint Hinge joint; another name for the elbow joint.

glandular epithelium Tissue type that makes up endocrine and exocrine glands.

glans Exposed portion of the clitoris; also the head of the penis

glans External region of the clitoris (the female reproductive organ); also the head of the penis (the male reproductive organ).

glaucoma Group of disease characterized by increase pressure in the eye that can result in vision loss due to damage to the optic nerve.

glenohumeral joint Ball-and-socket joint between the scapula and humerus.

glenohumeral ligament Three ligaments on the anterior position of the shoulder joint.

glia Support cells of the nervous system that directly and indirectly help all neurons to function properly.

gliding joint Also known as a plane or planar joint, allows the bones to glide past one another in any direction along the plane of a joint; directions include left and right, up and down, and diagonally.

globular proteins Protein structures containing small protein chains and large globular proteins.

glomerular capillaries Capillaries contained within Bowman's (glomerular) capsule that are the site of glomerular filtration.

glomerular capsule Thin, membranous capsule that surrounds the glomerulus of a nephron through which glomerular filtrate passes to the proximal convoluted tubule. Also known as Bowman's capsule.

glomerular filtration pressure Net filtration force when the forces opposing filtration are subtracted from the forces favoring filtration; this number is almost always positive.

glomerular filtration rate (GFR) Test used to check how well the kidneys are working; specifically, it estimates how much blood passes through the glomeruli each minute.

glomerular filtration Process that the kidneys use to filter excess fluid and waste products out of the blood and into the nephron, so they may be eliminated from the body.

glomerulopathies Diseases that affect the structure and function of the renal glomeruli.

glomerulus Ball of capillaries found within Bowman's capsule that is the site of glomerular filtration.

glossopharyngeal nerve Cranial nerve IX; sensory and motor information of the throat and neck.

glottis Triangular space formed in the larynx when the vocal cords are relaxed.

glucose Monosaccharide that is the primary sugar in the blood.

gluteus maximus Large muscle in the posterior pelvis region that attaches to the femur and produces flexion of the leg.

gluteus medius Muscle located in the posterior pelvis deep to the gluteus maximus that works to stabilize the sacroiliac joint.

gluteus minimus Muscle located in the posterior pelvis deep to the gluteus medius.

glycogen Molecule that is the storage form of glucose.

glycolysis Metabolic process in which one molecule of glucose is converted to two molecules of pyruvic acid while producing a net gain of two molecules of ATP.

goiter Disease that causes a swelling of the thyroid gland (seen on the anterior of the neck), chronic fatigue, low metabolic rate, and weakness; caused by a deficient amount of iodine in the diet.

golfer's elbow Also known as medial epicondylitis and characterized by inflammation of the wrist flexor tendons near their insertion at the medial epicondyle of the humerus bone.

Golgi tendon organ Sensory structure in the tendon that detects stretch in the tendon.

Golgi tendon reflex Reflex which prevents the muscle from pulling so hard it separates from the bone.

gomphosis Fibrous joint that holds the teeth in their sockets and is found on the maxilla and mandible.

gonadal arteries Arteries located in the abdominal and pelvic cavities.

gonadal veins Veins located in the pelvis that drain the testes and ovaries.

gonadotropin-releasing hormone (GnRH) Controls the release of gonadotropins, follicle-stimulating hormone, and luteinizing hormone.

gonorrhea Sexually transmitted infection caused by *Neisseria gonorrhoeae*; infection occurs in the genitals and rectum.

Graafian follicle Mature ova.

gracilis Muscle located in the medial thigh that works to produce hip adduction.

granulocytes White blood cells that contain immunologic chemicals packaged in small granules. Examples include neutrophils, eosinophils, and basophils.

granulomas Small mass of inflamed tissue that is granular in appearance.

granulosa cells Single layer of connective tissue that covers the primary oocyte.

gray matter Region of the CNS that consists primarily of connections between neurons.

great cardiac vein Large vein located on the heart that connects with the coronary sinus.

great saphenous vein Superficial medial vein in the upper portion of the lower extremity.

great vessels Large vessels entering and exiting the heart.

greater curvature Boundary of the stomach that forms a long, convex curve on the left from the opening for the esophagus to the opening of the duodenum.

greater trochanter of the femur Large bony prominence located on the lateral femur.

greater tubercle of humerus Bony prominence located on the lateral humerus.

Groove Deep depression in the bone.

ground substance Nonliving material secreted by connective tissue cells; along with the protein fibers in connective tissue, it makes up the extracellular matrix.

growth hormone (GH) Stimulates somatic growth multiple organs while also increasing the levels of insulin growth factors.

growth hormone-inhibiting hormone (somatostatin) Inhibits the secretion of growth hormone.

growth hormone-releasing hormone (GHRH) Stimulates the secretion of growth hormone.

Guillain-Barre syndrome Autoimmune disorder in which the body attacks the peripheral nerve, resulting in pain or muscle weakness.

gummas Soft tumors that develop in tertiary syphilis.

gynecomastia Enlargement of breast tissue usually related to hormone imbalance or hormone therapy.

H

hair bulb Swelling at the base where the hair originates in the dermis.

hair follicle Tube that surrounds the root hair.

Haldane effect Changes in hemoglobin's affinity for carbon dioxide binding from changes in pH.

halitosis Chronic bad breath, frequently caused by dental issues (such as cavities or gum disease); mouth, nose, or throat infections; dry mouth; or smoking or other tobacco usage.

hallucinations Sensory sensation that appear real but are created without the appropriate sensory input.

hamstring One muscle of a group of muscles located in the posterior thigh.

haploid Cell that contains half of the pairs of chromosomes.

Hartmann's pouch Mucosal fold at the junction of the neck of the gallbladder and the cystic duct.

Hashimoto's thyroiditis Autoimmune disorder that leads to the destruction of the thyroid gland causing a hypothyroid state.

Haustra Pouches in the colon.

hCG (human chorionic gonadotropin) Hormone produced by the placenta after implantation; can be detected in the urine of a pregnant woman; most pregnancy tests check for the presence of hCG in urine; in the presence of one or more mature ovaries, can be used clinically to induce ovulation in the ovaries.

hearing Ability to detect sound in the world.

heart valve disease Disease affecting one or more of the four valves of the heart.

heat illness Category of hyperthermia; signs and symptoms include normal to elevated core temperature; fatigue; nausea; vomiting; increased heart rate; signs of dehydration; mental status intact; and responsiveness to a cool environment, electrolytes, and fluids.

heat stroke Category of hyperthermia; patient usually has an elevated core temperature greater than 40.5°C; hot, dry skin; increased heart rate; weakness; vomiting, nausea, headache; the blood's ability to coagulate may be impaired; and skeletal muscle may be injured, leading to renal failure.

helix protein Protein structure in the shape of a helix.

helper T cells T cells that help activate B cells by secreting cytokines.

hematocrit (Hct) Blood test that measures the volume percentage of red blood cells in blood.

hematoma Swelling in one area that is filled with blood.

hematopoiesis Process of creating new blood cells.

hematopoietic factors Chemical messengers that can increase or decrease the clotting ability of the blood.

hematopoietic stem cells (HSCs) Immature cell that can develop into the formed elements of blood.

hematuria Presence of blood in the urine.

heme Iron-containing portion of hemoglobin.

hemiazygos vein Vein located on the left side of the vertebral column that originates from the posterior intercostal and left ascending lumbar veins.

hemisphere dominance Concept that some functions are performed better by one cerebral hemisphere than the other.

hemispheres Symmetric halves of the cerebrum that preferentially process the opposite side of the body.

hemochromatosis Disorder where the body holds onto too much iron. These iron molecules are stored in the liver and skin causing liver damage, diabetes mellitus, and bronze discoloration of the skin.

hemoglobin buffer system Chemical process that hemoglobin undergoes in order to balance blood pH.

hemoglobin Protein containing a red pigment that can bind and transport oxygen.

hemolysis Breakdown of red blood cells.

hemophilia Rare disorder in which the blood doesn't clot normally.

hemorrhoids The inflammation and enlargement of rectal veins.

hemosiderin A deposits or collection of iron after it has been broken down from RBCs.

hemostasis Stoppage of bleeding and the first step in wound healing.

Henry's Law Law stating the amount of gas in a liquid is proportional to its partial pressure.

heparin Anticoagulant that is used to decrease the clotting ability of the blood.

hepatic portal system System of veins carrying digestive substances from the digestive system to the liver.

hepatic veins Vein located in the abdominal cavity that drains blood from the liver.

hepatobiliary iminodiacetic acid (HIDA) scan A test that uses a small amount of injected radioactive material to determine how well the gallbladder, bile ducts, and liver are working.

hepatopancreatic ampulla Cavity where the common bile duct and the pancreatic duct open into the major duodenal papilla; also known as the ampulla of Vater.

Hereditary metabolic disorders Genetic disorders that interrupt the normal metabolism of food.

Hering-Breuer reflex Protective reflex in the lungs preventing overinflation by inhibiting neural respiratory centers.

herniating Protruding through an abnormal body opening; in the case of fetal development, the intestine temporarily herniates into the umbilical cord until there is enough room for it in the abdomen.

heteroantigens Antigens on the cell surface of a microorganism; antigens from another species.

hinge joint Joint formed from two or more bones where the bones can only move along one axis to flex or extend.

hip dysplasia Abnormality of the hip joint where the socket does not fully cover the ball portion.

hippocampus Region of the limbic system involved in memory storage.

hirsutism Condition of male-pattern hair growth in the female population. Usually occurring on the face.

histamine Chemical released during inflammation that causes smooth muscle contraction and blood vessel dilation.

hives Also called urticaria, red, round, itchy welts on the skin usually in response to an allergic reaction.

homeostasis A dynamic equilibrium that keeps the internal state of the body balanced.

homologue pairs Also called homologous pairs; chromosome pairs that contain one chromosome from each parent and align at each gene location and centromere.

hormonal stimuli Relying on the presence of a certain hormone to be activated and create a response within surrounding or distant tissues.

hormones Chemical substances, secreted by endocrine glands, that target another tissue in the body.

horseshoe kidney Congenital partial fusion of the kidneys resulting in a horseshoe shape.

human chorionic gonadotropin hormone Hormone produced by the developing embryo.

human immunodeficiency virus (HIV) Virus transmitted by intimate sexual contact, use of drug paraphernalia, inoculation with infected blood or blood products, or to the newborn during birth; affects CD4 cells that support immunity and leads to acquired human immunodeficiency syndrome (AIDS).

human papillomavirus (HPV) Hundred different types of viruses, the majority of which affect the genital area and cause genital warts.

humeral circumflex artery Branch of the brachial artery.

humerus Long bone of the upper arm extending from the shoulder to the elbow.

humoral immunity Action of the adaptive immune system mediated by antibodies.

Huntington's disease A progressive neurological disorder characterized by uncontrollable movements of the body.

hyaline cartilage Type of connective tissue that is to some degree flexible and found in areas of the body, such as the nose, ears, and ribs.

hyaline Most common type of cartilage but also the weakest; flexible and resilient; found in the fetal skeleton, nose, trachea, larynx, costal cartilage, and articular ends of long bones.

hydroceles Swelling in the scrotum that occurs when fluid collects in the tissue surrounding the testicle.

hydrochlorothiazide Loop diuretic that can help in removing water via the kidneys.

hydrolyze Catabolic chemical reaction in which water is removed and a larger molecule is split into smaller molecules.

hydrophilic Polar molecules that attract water.

hydrophobic Nonpolar molecules that repel water.

hydrostatic pressure Pressure of liquid pushing outward against the walls of its container. In the blood this would be the pressure of the liquid plasma pushing outward against the walls of the blood vessel.

hymen Thin layer of tissue that partially covers the vestibule.

hyoid bone U-shaped bone in the anterior portion of the neck just inferior to the mandible.

hypercalcemia Blood calcium levels in excess of the body's normal range (>10.3 mg/dL).

hypercapnia Condition characterized by abnormally high carbon dioxide levels in the blood.

hypercoagulable state Increased predisposition to form clots.

hyperextension Continuation of the extension movement beyond the natural anatomical position.

hyperhidrosis Condition in which patient experiences excessive sweating.

hyperkalemia Blood potassium levels in excess of the body's normal range (>4.5 mg/dL).

hypernatremia Blood sodium levels in excess of the body's normal range (>145 mg/dL).

hyperpolarization Changing the membrane potential of a neuron to make it more negative than at rest.

hypersensitivity Increased sensitivity of the immune system leading to an elevated immune response.

hypertension High blood pressure as indicated by a systolic pressure greater than 130/80 mm Hg.

hypertensive nephrosclerosis Hardening of the walls of the small arteries and arterioles of the kidney that is caused by hypertension.

hyperthermia Having a core temperature greater than 38.5°C.

hyperthyroidism A disease state where the thyroid gland produces increased amounts of thyroid hormones.

hypertrophic cardiomyopathy Type of heart disease characterized by thickening of the muscular walls of the heart.

hypertrophic scarring Type of scar resulting from excessive collagen deposits; appear as raised, red scars that do not grow beyond the boundary of the wound.

hypertrophic Increasing in size.

hyperventilation Increase in breathing rate greater than the normal rate of 12–25 breaths per minute.

hypocalcemia Blood calcium levels lower than the body's normal range (<8.5 mg/dL).

hypocapnia Condition characterized by lower than normal carbon dioxide levels in the blood.

hypodermis Layer of loose areolar connective tissue below the layer of dermis, mainly adipose tissue, that connects skin to muscle and bone.

hypogammaglobulinemia Low levels of antibodies in the blood.

hypoglossal nerve Cranial nerve XII; controls motor movements of the tongue.

hypoglycemia Low blood sugar.

hypokalemia Blood potassium levels lower than the body's normal range (<3.5 mg/dL).

hypomenorrhea Scant menstruation.

hyponatremia Condition characterized by abnormally low sodium levels in the blood (lower than 136 meq/L).

hypoperistalsis Wavelike smooth muscle contraction that is weaker than normal.

hypophyseal fossa Depression within the sella turcica bone indicates where the pituitary gland is located.

hyposecretory Decreased secretory capacity.

hypothalamic hypophyseal portal system (HHPS) Collection of capillaries that absorbs the hormones from the neuroendocrine cells of the hypothalamus and ensures that they arrive at the anterior pituitary gland.

hypothalamic infundibulum Cavity connecting the hypothalamus and posterior pituitary gland.

hypothalamus Region of the cerebrum that controls body states such as hunger, thirst, and body temperature and regulates hormone release from the pituitary gland.

hypothermia Having a core temperature below 36°C.

hypothyroidism Disease state where the thyroid gland produces decreased amounts of thyroid hormones.

hypotonic bladder Loss of smooth muscle tone in the urinary bladder.

hypoventilation Abnormally low breathing rate less than the normal rate of 12–25 breaths per minute.

hypoxia Condition characterized by low oxygen levels in the blood.

hysterectomy Surgical removal of the uterus.

H-zone Portion of a sarcomere at the center of an A-band consisting of myosin filaments.

I

I-bands Regions of the sarcomere containing only actin filaments.

IgA Immunoglobin present on mucous membranes and body secretions, such as tears, saliva, and breast milk; prevents bacterial cells from attaching to mucous membranes.

IgD Antibody found in low numbers throughout the body. Most commonly found on surface of B cells.

IgE Antibody found on certain white blood cells; plays a role in allergic reactions and inflammation.

IgG Smallest immunoglobulin; most predominant antibody secreted into serum; secondary response antibody.

IgM Largest antibody; primary response antibody and is the first released when exposure to pathogen occurs.

ileocecal sphincter Valve that separates the small intestine from the large intestine.

iliac crest Superior portion of the ilium of the coxal bone.

iliacus Deep pelvic muscle connecting to the ilium and extending to the femur causing hip flexion.

iliocostalis Muscle in the back; part of the erector spinae group of back muscles.

iliopsoas Combination of two muscles, the iliacus and psoas major, that extend from the pelvis to the femur.

iliotibial band Broad band of fibrous connective tissue located on the lateral portion of the thigh.

ilium Most superior portion of the coxal bone.

imiquimod Topical medication used to treat genital warts caused by human papillomavirus.

immune system Diverse system of the body that protects it from foreign invaders; includes white blood cells and lymphoid organs.

immunity Body's ability to defend itself.

immunocompetent Immune system that functions normally.

immunocompromised Immune system that isn't functioning properly.

immunodeficiency Decrease in immune function leading to low levels of immune cells or chemicals.

immunoglobulin Immune system protein; another name for an antibody.

immunoreactive trypsinogen Blood test for cystic fibrosis; immunoreactive trypsinogen is usually elevated in cystic fibrosis.

impetigo Highly contagious bacterial skin infection that forms blisters and yellow, crusty sores.

implanted Method of birth control where a pellet containing hormones to suppress ovulation is placed under the skin.

impotence Inability of a male to achieve an erection.

incomplete proteins Proteins that do not contain all 20 amino acids.

independent assortment Process during meiosis in which the homologous pairs of chromosomes randomly separate to form haploid cells, enabling genetic variation.

indolamine Monoamine hormone that has a similar structure to catecholamines. Examples include serotonin.

infant rooting reflex Reflex in which an infant attempts to suckle in response to stroking the cheek.

infarctions The reduction or loss of blood supply to a specific organ.

infection Condition arising from having a microorganism living in and reproducing in the body.

infectious disease Condition arising from an infection that is damaging the body.

inferior gemellus Deep muscle of the posterior pelvis that functions as an external rotator of the hip.

inferior oblique One of six eye muscles connected to the inferior and lateral portions of the eyeball.

inferior phrenic veins Veins in the abdominal cavity that drain the diaphragm.

inferior phrenic Small artery branching from the aorta that supplies the diaphragm.

inferior rectus One of six eye muscles connected to the inferior portion of the eyeball.

inferior rotation Rotation downward.

inferior sagittal sinus Hollow area that is part of the venous system located between the hemispheres of the brain.

inferior vena cava Large vein carrying blood to the right atrium.

inflammation Generalized, localized response to cellular injury in order to prevent the spread of infection.

inflammatory Second step in wound healing resulting in a red, hot, painful, swollen area.

infrared Heat loss from radiating heat in the infrared spectrum.

infraspinatus One of the rotator cuff muscles connected to the scapula and extending to the humerus; produces external rotation of the shoulder.

infundibulum End of the fallopian tubes nearest the ovary.

inhibin A hormone that is produced from the testis and ovary prevents the production of follicle-stimulating hormone (FSH) from the pituitary gland.

inhibiting Act of stopping something.

inhibitory neuron Presynaptic neuron that makes its post-synaptic partner less likely to fire an action potential.

inhibitory neurotransmitter Neurotransmitter that inhibits the generation of an action potential in a post-synaptic neuron by promoting the opening of potassium and chloride gates.

inhibitory post-synaptic potentials Potential that inhibits the generation of an action potential in a post-synaptic neuron.

innate Natural and inborn such as innate immunity.

inner ear Region of the ear that contains the cochlea and vestibular organs.

inner epithelial root sheath Internal layer of the epithelial root sheath; surrounds the hair but does not extend the length of the hair follicle.

inorganic molecules Molecules containing no carbon that are not commonly found in living organisms.

insertions Point of a muscle attachment on the relatively more moveable end of a joint.

insomnia Inability to sleep.

inspiratory capacity Amount of air that can be inhaled after a normal exhalation.

inspiratory reserve volume Amount of air that enters the lungs during a maximal inhalation in addition to tidal volume.

insular lobe Region of the cerebrum involved in processing taste and emotions.

insulin growth factors (IGFs) Hormone that plays an important role in growth when stimulated by increased levels of growth hormone.

insulin Hormone that promotes the uptake of glucose (blood sugar) by cells in the body.

integumentary Skin and its accessory organs.

intercalated disks Specialized cell junctions found in cardiac muscle.

Intercarpal joint Gliding joint that allows for movement of the wrist.

intercostal space The space between two ribs.

interferons Innate immune system chemicals which inhibit viral replication.

interleukins Chemical messengers that attract will enhance the immune response.

interlobar arteries Arteries leading from the renal artery to the smaller arcuate arteries within the kidney.

interlobar vein Veins leading from the arcuate veins within the kidney to the renal vein that exits the kidney.

intermediate fibers Muscle fibers exhibiting characteristics of both fast- and slow-twitch fibers.

internal and external carotid arteries Branches of the common carotid arteries.

internal and external iliac arteries Inferior branches of the common iliac arteries.

internal and external jugular veins Veins located in the neck draining structures of the head and neck and connecting to the subclavian veins.

internal iliac vein Branch of the common iliac vein.

internal intercostals Deep muscles locate between the ribs that function to pull the ribs together.

internal obliques Deep muscles of the abdomen that act as synergists in trunk flexion.

internal os Cervix's external upper connection to the uterus.

internal respiration Movement of oxygen and carbon dioxide into and out of cells by way of diffusion.

internal rotation Inward or medial rotation of a joint.

internal urethral sphincter Involuntary muscle that controls the flow of urine by contracting around the internal urethral orifice; the sympathetic nervous system controls the opening and closing of the internal urethral sphincter.

international normalized ratio (INR) A measurement on how much time it takes for a patient's blood to clot. An elevated INR means that the patient's blood is too thin while a decreased level means that the blood is too prone to clotting.

internodal pathways Specialized pathways in cardiac muscle that carry electrical impulses between nodes.

interosseous membrane Broad, thick, and dense fibrous tissue between many bones in the body.

interphase Resting phase in mitosis between successive divisions, or the phase between meiosis I and II when the cell copies its DNA.

interstitial fluid Fluid found in interstitial spaces (space between cells).

interstitial space Fluid compartment surrounding cells.

intertarsal joint Joints between the tarsal bones of the foot.

intertubercular groove Groove between the greater and lesser tubercle of the humerus.

interventricular septum Heart muscle located between the ventricles.

interventricular sulcus Indentation or groove between the ventricles on the anterior portion of the heart.

intracellular fluid (ICF) Fluid within the body that is contained within a cell.

intracytoplasmic sperm injection When a single sperm is injected into an egg.

intramembranous ossification Process through which flat bones, short bones, and irregular bones are formed.

intrathoracic pressure Gas pressure inside of the thoracic cavity.

intrathoracic Area inside of the thoracic cavity.

intrauterine device (IUD) Method of birth control where a T-shaped device is inserted into the uterus and releases hormones to suppress ovulation.

intrinsic anemias Inherited disorders that can lead to anemia. The most common inherited anemias are sickle cell anemia and thalassemia.

intrinsic factor Substance secreted by the stomach that enables the body to absorb vitamin B_{12}.

inversion (chromosomal) Chromosome alteration that occurs when a part of a DNA strand breaks and reattaches upside down in the same chromosome.

inversion Movement of the soles of the feet inward toward the midline of the body.

involuntary contraction Muscle contraction produced without volition or intention.

ionize Process by which chemical compounds dissociate when placed in water.

ions Chemical compound possessing an overall charge that is less than or greater than zero.

iris Thin membrane between the anterior and posterior chambers of the eye that has the pupil at its center.

irregular bones Complex bones of varying shapes that do not fit into other bone classifications.

irritable bowel syndrome Chronic condition of a group of symptoms such as cramping, bloating, abdominal pain, constipation, and diarrhea, that affect the large intestine.

ischemic heart disease Disease of heart tissue resulting from a lack of blood flow to heart muscle.

ischemic Decrease in blood supply.

ischial tuberosity Broad eminence of bone located on the posterior portion of the ischium.

isoelectric line Reference line in the ECG representing the baseline or zero voltage.

isometric contractions Muscle contraction characterized by the length of the contracting muscle not changing while the load the muscle pulls or pushes can change.

isotonic contractions Muscle contraction characterized by the length of the contracting muscle changing while the load the muscle pulls or pushes does not change.

isthmus Area between the body of the uterus and the cervix.

J

jumper's knee Disorder characterized by inflammation of the patellar tendon usually caused by jumping.

juxtaglomerular apparatus A structure composed of juxtaglomerular cells and a macula densa that found near the glomerulus and controls the release of renin.

K

keloid Scar resulting from an overly aggressive healing process; grow larger than the wound and are usually smooth on top and pink or purple in color; more common in dark-skinned individuals.

keratin Insoluble and resilient protein found in hair, nails, and the epidermis of the skin.

keratinization Addition of keratin to epidermal cells as they move to the surface of the epidermis.

keratinocytes Cells in the epidermis that produce keratin.

keratosis pilaris Red or white bumps on the skin that look like small goose bumps on the arms, thighs, buttocks, or cheeks; common in childhood (disappearing in adulthood) and tends to run in families.

ketoacidosis Condition in which the blood has a decreased pH; also called acidosis.

ketonuria Excretion of an abnormally large number of ketones in the urine.

kilocalorie One thousand dietary calories.

Klinefelter's syndrome Another name for monosomy that occurs in males.

Kussmaul's respirations Breathing pattern typically seen in patients experiencing diabetic ketoacidosis; characterized by very deep, rapid breathing.

kwashiorkor Malnutrition disease, most commonly seen in young children, caused by a severe protein deficiency.

kyphosis Exaggeration of the primary curvature of the thoracic spine.

kyphotic curvature Primary curvature of the spine.

L

labia majora Outermost folds of skin and fat tissue covered with hair that begins at the mons pubis and ends at the anus.

labia minora Folds of skin tissue that are pink, hairless, and are located between the clitoris and the base of the vagina.

lacerations Cut that is a deep tear in the skin; bleeding is common.

lacrimal glands Gland near the eye that produces tears.

lactation Production of breast milk.

lactational amenorrhea method (LAM) Method of birth control where lactation is used to prevent pregnancy.

lacteals Vessels in the small intestine that are part of the lymphatic system.

lactic acid By-product of glycolysis resulting from the production of pyruvic acid.

lactiferous duct Duct that leads to the nipple and opens to the outside

lacunae Small spaces within the extracellular matrix of bone and cartilage where osteocytes and chondrocytes are found.

Lambert-Eaton syndrome Autoimmune disease in which antibodies attack the neuromuscular junction.

lamellae Layers of compact bone tissue that resemble the layers of a tree trunk.

lamellar bone Mature bone.

lamina propria Thin layer of loose connective tissue located beneath epithelial cells.

lamina propria Thin layer of loose connective tissue that lies beneath the epithelium.

laminae Plates of bone that form the walls of each vertebra, enclosing the spinal cord.

lanugo Fine, downy hair is present in almost all parts of the body of the fetus after 20 weeks of gestation.

large cell carcinoma A type of lung cancer that accounts for a small portion of lung cancers and originates from epithelial tissue.

laryngitis Condition characterized by inflammation of the larynx.

laryngopharynx Lowermost portion of the pharynx.

larynx Portion of respiratory system located between the pharynx and trachea that contains the vocal cords.

lateral (fibular) collateral ligament Ligament located on the lateral side of the knee, stretching from the femur to the fibula. Because it does not fuse with the capsular ligament or the lateral meniscus, it is more flexible.

lateral condyle of the tibia Large rounded process on the proximal portion of the tibia on the lateral side.

lateral epicondyle Small, bony protuberance located on the distal lateral portion of the humerus and femur.

lateral pterygoid Muscle contributing to chewing or mastication located lateral to the medial pterygoid muscle.

lateral rectus One of six eye muscles attached to the lateral portion of the eyeball.

lateral rotation Movement away from the body.

lateral ventricles C-shaped cavities located in the center of each cerebral hemisphere in which cerebrospinal fluid is produced.

latissimus dorsi Large muscle in the back that extends to the intertubercular groove of the humerus.

left anterior descending artery Branch of the left coronary artery that extends along the interventricular sulcus.

left anterior descending artery Branch of the left coronary artery located in the interventricular sulcus.

left atrium Hollow chamber of the heart that receives oxygenated blood from the lungs carried by the pulmonary veins.

left coronary artery Artery originating from the aorta to supply the left side of the heart.

left gastric artery Arteries in the abdominal cavity that supply the stomach and liver.

left ventricle Hollow chamber in the heart that contracts and pushes blood out of the heart.

leiomyomas Benign growth in the uterus.

lens Gelatinous region of the eye that can change shape to help focus light in the eye.

leptin Hormone made by fat cells that plays a role in decreasing appetite as well as maintaining body weight.

lesser curvature Part of the stomach that extends between the cardiac and pyloric orifices, forming the right border.

lesser trochanter of the femur Bony eminence on the proximal portion of the lateral femur just inferior to the greater trochanter.

lesser tubercle of the humerus Small bony eminence located on the proximal portion of the humerus anterior and medial to the greater tubercle of the humerus.

leukocytes White blood cell; circulates throughout the body and plays an important part in the body's immune response and reaction to foreign bodies and disease.

leukocytosis Increased white blood cell counts usually due to an immune response or neoplastic syndrome.

leukopoiesis Process of creating new white blood cells within the bone marrow.

levator scapula Muscle in the back connected to the superior portion of the scapula and extending to the skull that functions to elevate the scapula.

Leydig cells Cells responsible in the male for the production of testosterone.

ligament Fibrous connective tissue that supports and holds the bones and internal organs in a stable position.

ligamentous laxity Loose ligaments.

ligamentum arteriosum Remnant of fetal circulation, a ligament that forms from the ductus arteriosum.

ligand-gated transport proteins Transport proteins that are activated by other molecules that bind to them.

limbic system Deep brain region often called the emotional brain that processes emotion, memory, and reward.

Line Ridge of bone that is less prominent than a crest.

linea alba White fibrous structure that extends from superior to inferior in the abdomen.

linea aspera Protruding ridge of bone located on the posterior portion of the femur.

linea nigra Linear hyperpigmentation that occurs during pregnancy midline on the abdomen from the symphysis pubis to the top of the uterus (fundus).

lipid soluble Dissolves in lipids.

lipids Class of molecules containing fats.

lipoprotein Molecules that contain lipids and proteins.

lithotripsy Breaking of a kidney stone (calculus) that is unable to pass using shock waves or crushing it with a surgical instrument into pieces small enough to pass through the ureters, bladder, and urethra to exit the body.

lobules Small lobes.

lockjaw Result of the disease tetanus in which the muscles of the jaw contract.

logarithmic scale Scale in which each whole number above or below zero (seven in the case of the pH scale) is 10 times greater than the preceding whole number; the pH scale for the measurement of acids/bases and the Richter scale used to measure the force of earthquakes are common logarithmic scales. For example, a pH of 5 is ten times more acidic than a pH of 6.

long bones Hard, dense bones responsible for bearing most of the body's weight, providing support to the skeletal system, and enabling the body's mobility.

longissimus Muscle located in the back that is part of the erector spinae group of muscles.

long-term memories Maintaining information in the mind on the order of a lifetime.

loop of Henle U-shaped part of a nephron that lies between the proximal and distal convoluted tubules that plays a role in water resorption; also known as the nephron loop.

loose connective tissue Contains fewer cells and fibers than dense connective tissue; types are areolar, adipose, and reticular.

lordosis Exaggeration in the curvature of the lumbar spine.

lordotic curvature Secondary curvature of the spine.

lumbar artery Parietal branches of the abdominal aorta.

lumbar spinal nerves Five pairs of peripheral nerves that exit from the lower-back region of the spinal cord.

lumbricales Deep muscles of the hand that flex the hand and extend the fingers.

luminal epithelial Type of cell within the female breast that is capable of producing breast milk.

lung carcinoid Cancerous lung tumor made of cells from the neuroendocrine system.

lunula Whitish area at the proximal end of the nail.

luteal stage Stage in which the cells of the follicle divide quickly and the corpus luteum secretes progesterone to build up the endometrium.

luteinizing hormone (LH) Promotes testosterone production in males and ovulation in females while also producing estrogen and progesterone.

lymph nodes Encapsulated ovoid structures found along lymph vessels.

lymphadenitis Inflammation of lymph nodes.

lymphangitis Bacteria and debris that accumulate in the sinuses of a lymph node, resulting in inflammation of the superficial lymph nodes.

lymphatic circulation Network of vessels through which lymph drains from the tissues into the blood.

lymphatic trunks Vessels that lead to larger lymphatic structures.

lymphocytes Agranulocytic white blood cells which primarily function in the adaptive immune system; T cells and B cells.

lymphoma Also called lymphatic cancer; condition in which lymphocytes begin to mutate and duplicate rapidly and out of control.

lysis Popping or bursting of a cell.

lysozyme Enzyme in tears and saliva that can poke holes in bacterial cell walls.

M

macrophages Type of white blood cell found in areolar connective tissue; functions as part of the body's immune system and engulfs and breaks down cells and cellular debris.

macula densa Group of modified epithelial cells in the distal convoluted tubule of the kidney that lie adjacent to the afferent arteriole just before it enters the glomerulus and control renin release by relaying information about the sodium concentration in the fluid passing through the convoluted tubule to the renin-producing juxtaglomerular cells of the afferent arteriole.

macular degeneration Vision loss due to breakdown of the region of the retina that we most rely on for our most accurate vision.

major calyx Portion of the urinary collecting system within the kidney that drains several minor calyces; all of the major calyces unite to form the renal pelvis.

major duodenal papilla Rounded projection at the opening of the common bile duct and pancreatic duct that is the primary mechanism for the secretion of bile and other digestive enzymes.

major minerals Minerals the body needs 100 mg or more of daily.

malabsorption Disorder characterized by the inability of the digestive tract to absorb nutrients.

male sex hormones Substances that are secreted by specialized organs and glands that impact the maturation of specific body tissues.

mammary alveoli Glands within the ducts of breast tissue that secrete milk.

mammary glands Enlarged, modified sweat glands found in the breasts of females.

mandible Lower jaw.

manometry A test used to evaluate the motility and muscle contractions of the esophagus.

marasmus Disease of malnutrition, most commonly seen in infants and young children, caused by starvation.

marginal arteries Refers to a branch of the right coronary artery.

masseter Chewing (mastication) muscle located in the cheek area that works to close the jaw.

mast cells Type of cell found in areolar connective tissue; contains structures rich in histamine and heparin, which have important functions in immune response and blood thinning, respectively.

mastication Chewing.

mastitis Inflammation of breast tissue.

mastoid process Bony protuberance off of the temporal bone.

matrix Intracellular substance that makes bones dense and builds up bone during mineralization.

mature ovum (also called ootid) Secondary oocyte.

maxilla Upper jaw.

Mechanical digestion Physical breakdown of food.

mechanoreceptors Sensory proteins which detect physical deformations of the cellular membrane.

medial and lateral plantar arteries Arteries in the foot.

medial and lateral plantar veins Veins in the foot.

medial collateral (tibial) ligament Ligament found on the medial side of the knee; its primary function is to resist the outward turning of the knee.

medial condyle of tibia Large, rounded process on the proximal medial portion of the tibia.

medial cuneiform One of three cuneiform bones of the foot located just anterior to the navicular bone.

medial epicondyle Small, bony protuberance located in the distal medial portion of the humerus and femur.

medial rectus One of six eye muscles attaching to the medial portion of the eyeball.

medial rotation Movement toward the midline of the body.

medial One of the muscles of mastication located in the deep lateral portion of the jaw.

median cubital vein Vein located in the anterior portion of the elbow.

median sacral arteries Parietal branches of the abdominal aorta.

mediastinal arteries Branch of the thoracic aorta.

mediastinum Area in the thoracic cavity between the lungs.

medulla oblongata Region of the brainstem that controls respiratory and cardiovascular functions.

medulla Inner layer of an organ.

medullary cavity Hollow inner cavity of bones.

medullary chords Inner region of a lymph node where lymphocytes are arranged in strands.

medullary respiratory center Area in the medulla oblongata that contains the ventral and dorsal groups of neurons that contribute to respiratory control.

megakaryocytes Large bone marrow cell that acts as the precursor to platelets.

meiosis Division of the sex cell that results in half (23) of the total pairs of chromosomes.

melanin Pigments ranging from yellow to black that are found in the retina, skin, and hair.

melanocytes Cells found in the stratum basale that produces melanin.

melanoma Type of skin cancer that develops from melanocytes; appears as a freckle or mole that changes in color, size, or shape and grows quickly; may also look like a blood blister; commonly spread and if left untreated may be fatal.

melasma Dark spots that form on the face during pregnancy due to hormonal fluctuations.

melena Blood-tinged feces usually containing a dark red or brown hue.

membrane attack complex (MAC) Group of proteins that form to drill holes and small pores in the membranes of foreign cells to cause lysis of foreign cells.

membrane permeability Property of a membrane that allows substances to pass through.

membrane potential Electrical charge of a membrane.

membranous urethra Part of the male urethra that is situated between the prostatic urethra and the penile urethra.

memory T cells T cells that remember how to fight a particular antigen.

menarche First menstrual period.

meninges Layers of three membranes that surround and protect the nervous system.

meningitis Swelling of the protective layers surrounding the brain and spinal cord.

menisci Fibrous cartilage within a joint, especially the knee.

menometrorrhagia Heavy bleeding during and between menstrual periods.

menopause End of the reproductive capability of the female.

menorrhagia Excessive menstruation.

menstrual cycle Cycle of physiological changes that occur from the beginning of one menstrual period to the beginning of the next.

menstruation First phase of the female reproductive cycle where contents of the uterus are discharged as menstrual fluid.

mesenchymal cells Type of stem cell that is not yet specialized from which all connective tissue is derived.

mesenchyme Viscous tissue consisting of mesenchymal cells and watery matrix.

mesoderm Middle germ layer in the early embryo; it will go on to form muscle and connective tissue.

mesothelium Single layer of epithelial cells that forms part of serous membranes in the body.

metabolic demand Referring to the action of cell metabolism.

metabolic syndrome Syndrome consisting of the presence of three or more of a group of factors (such as high blood pressure, abdominal obesity, high triglyceride levels, low HDL levels, and high fasting levels of blood sugar) that are linked to increased risk of cardiovascular disease and type 2 diabetes.

metabolites A molecule that is the result of the breakdown of a large substance. Metabolites are typically the active form of the parent substance.

metacarpophalangeal joint Ellipsoidal joints that allow movement of the fingers.

metaphase I Phase when the homologous chromosomes arrange themselves on the metaphase plate while the spindle fibers attach to them at the centromeres.

metaphase II Occurs during the second stage of meiosis when the daughter cells align at the metaphase plate while the spindle fibers attach from opposite poles and prepare to separate the sister chromatids.

metaphysis Narrow portion of a long bone between the epiphysis and diaphysis.

metarteriole Area between arteriole and capillary containing a precapillary sphincter muscle.

metastasis When cancer cells from tumors near lymphatic vessels enter lymph and spread to and infect other locations in the body.

metatarsals Bones of the foot located just anterior to the tarsal bones and posterior to the phalanges.

MHC molecule Unique molecules that help the immune system to recognize self versus non-self.

microbiome Microorganisms in a particular environment.

microglia Glial cell of the CNS that serves immune and protective functions.

micronutrients Vitamins and minerals needed in very small amounts by the body.

micro-thrombosis Small thrombosis usually affecting small capillaries that can lead to infarctions.

microvilli Cellular membrane profusions that increase the absorptive area of the cell for diffusion.

micturition Act of urinating.

midbrain Region of the brainstem that allows for identifying the source of a sound and coordinating body movements.

mid-clavicular line Imaginary anatomical line extending inferior along the thorax from the middle of the clavicle.

middle cardiac vein Vein extending from the apex of the heart along the posterior interventricular sulcus that drains into the cardiac sinus.

middle cerebral arteries One of three major paired arteries that supply the cerebrum.

middle ear Air-filled cavity of the ear that contains the ossicles.

middle sacral arteries Small artery that branches from the posterior portion of the abdominal aorta and extends along the lower lumbar vertebrae and sacrum.

middle and posterior cardiac veins Veins of the coronary circuit that drain the area supplied by the marginal and circumflex arteries.

migraine A painful or throbbing sensation in the head which is often accompanied by nausea, vomiting, or sensitivity to light.

milnacipran Medication used to treat fibromyalgia and nerve pain and functioning as a selective serotonin and norepinephrine reuptake inhibitor.

mineralization Process of making bones more rigid.

minerals Inorganic molecules whose chemical structure does not change when they are exposed to heat, acid, light, or oxygen; remain stable during food preparation.

minor calyx Pathways within the kidney through which urine passes and is a portion of the urinary collecting system that drains one of the papillae. When several minor calyces merge they form a major calyx.

minute volume Amount of air reaching the alveoli in one minute found by multiplying the tidal volume by the number of breaths per minute.

mitochondria Organelle of the cell that produces energy by way of aerobic metabolism.

mitosis Process of cell duplication so that each cell has the same number of chromosomes.

mitral valve Also known as the bicuspid valve, a valve containing two cusps located between the left atrium and ventricle.

M-line Portion of the sarcomere where myosin filaments attach.

molecular mimicry Body is exposed to, and makes antibodies against, an antigen that is similar in structure to a self-antigen, which can result in cross-reactivity of the antibody.

monochorionic-diamniotic Twins who share a placenta but do not share a chorion or amnion while in utero.

monochorionic-monoamniotic Twins who share a chorion, amnion, and placenta while in utero.

monocytes Agranulocytic white blood cells which perform phagocytosis.

mononucleosis Contagious disease typically caused by the Epstein-Barr virus that causes swollen lymph nodes and swollen liver or spleen.

monosomy Absence of a chromosome after the cell divides through meiosis.

monozygotic Twins derived from a single ovum; also known as identical twins.

mons pubis Pad of fat tissue located on top of the symphysis pubis bone and is covered with skin and hair.

Montgomery tubercles Sebaceous oil glands embedded in the areola that secrete anti-infective and lubricating properties to protect the nipples and areola during breastfeeding.

motilin Hormones secreted in the small intestine that control interdigestive contractions.

motor end plate Specialized area in muscle tissue where neurons connect.

motor neuron Neuron that connects to and sends impulses to muscle tissue.

motor system Division of the nervous system involved in stimulating muscle contraction or regulating organ function.

mucosa Innermost layer of the alimentary canal.

mucosa-associated lymphatic tissues Groups of lymphocytes called lymphoid nodules within mucosa throughout the body.

mucus plug Plug formed by a small amount of cervical mucus that fills and seals the cervical canal during pregnancy.

multiaxial Allows movement along all the three axes; the hip joint is an example.

multidisciplinary approach Treatment approach characterized by a combination of different healing modalities.

multinucleated cells Cells containing more than one nucleus such as in skeletal muscle cells.

multipennate Arrangement of muscle fibers consisting of multiple feather-like structures connecting to a central structure.

multiple sclerosis A presumptive autoimmune disorder resulting in breakdown of the myelin-producing cells of the brain and spinal cord.

multisystemic smooth muscle dysfunction syndrome Disorder affecting smooth muscle throughout the body.

multi-unit Arrangement of smooth muscle characterized by interconnected motor units.

muscalaris Part of the alimentary canal that covers the submucosa, consisting of a double layer of smooth muscle that promotes contractions and the movement of chyme.

muscle fibers Long, cylindrical cells that make up skeletal muscle tissue.

muscle spindle Sensory structure embedded in skeletal muscle that detects changes in the stretch of the muscle.

muscle tissue One of four primary tissue types, contracts and creates a force resulting in movement.

muscle tone Degree of continuous muscle contraction in a muscle.

muscle twitch Single contraction of a muscle fiber.

muscular Dystrophy Genetic disorder that includes several variants, with Duchenne muscular dystrophy being the most common form; characterized by the lack of the muscle protein dystrophin, which results in muscle weakness.

mutation Change in hereditary material: either a change in the sequence of a gene's codon or a change in chromosome number or structure.

myalgia Muscle pain.

myasthenia gravis Autoimmune neuromuscular disorder characterized by antibodies destroying acetylcholine receptors in muscle tissue.

myelin sheath Insulating layer around parts of an axon that greatly increases the speed of an action potential.

myelin Wrapping of glial cell membrane around an axon that acts to speed up conduction of action potentials.

mylohyoid Muscle in the anterior cervical region connecting to the hyoid bone.

myocardial biopsy Test of cardiac muscle performed by inserting a device in a blood vessel that collects a small amount of heart muscle tissue.

myocardium Thick middle layer of the heart wall consisting of cardiac muscle.

myocytes Muscle cells.

myoepithelial Cell within the lobes of the female breast.

myofascial pain syndrome Muscular pain syndrome characterized by the presence of painful areas called trigger points in muscle tissue.

myofibrils Contractile proteins found in skeletal muscle tissue.

myoglobin Reddish-colored molecule found in muscle tissue that carries oxygen.

myometrium Middle layer of the uterine wall comprised of muscle tissue.

myopia Nearsightedness.

myosin binding site Area on the thin actin filament where myosin can bind to form a cross-bridge.

myosin Thick protein filament containing globular protein heads found in muscle tissue.

myositis Inflammation of muscle tissue.

myotonic MD Type of muscular dystrophy that can affect adults, causing muscle spasms, heart problems, endocrine problems, and cataracts.

N

nail bed Layer of living epidermis below the nail body.

nail body Part of the nail we see.

nailfold capillaroscopy Test performed with special optical equipment on fingernails or toenails to investigate the circulatory function of the small capillaries.

nasal cavity Air passageway located behind the maxillary bones and above the hard palate.

nasal polyps Small, noncancerous growths on the inside of the nasal cavity.

nasal septum Bony structure consisting of the perpendicular plate of the ethmoid bone and vomer bone.

nasopharynx Portion of the pharynx that extends from the posterior portion of the nasal cavity to the soft palate.

natriuretic peptide Hormone secreted by the atria that promotes reduction of sodium reabsorption in the kidneys with a net effect of water loss.

natural killer (NK) cell Specialized type of lymphocyte that functions in the second line of defense.

naturally acquired active immunity Immune condition where a person is exposed to a microorganism in the course of daily life and make antibodies to the microorganism.

naturally acquired passive immunity Immune condition where a person is given someone else's antibodies through the course of natural life.

nearsightedness Inability to focus on relatively distant objects.

negative energy balance More energy is being expended than is being consumed; usually results in weight loss.

negative feedback When a product of the stimulus leads to the decrease or inhibition of the original stimulus that caused the original increase in the product.

neocortex Part of the mammalian brain where sensory perception, conception, motor commands, spatial reasoning, and language occur.

neoplastic A collection of cells that have developed due to abnormal cell or tissue growth.

nephrogenic Originating in the kidney.

nephron loop U-shaped part of a nephron that lies between the proximal and distal convoluted tubules that plays a role in water resorption; also known as the loop of Henle.

nephron One of the functional units of the kidney that filters the blood, selectively reabsorbs substances (such as glucose, ions, and amino acids), and excretes waste products, excess water, and salts in the form of urine.

nephropathy Disease or dysfunction of the kidneys.

nerve plexus Branching network of intersecting nerves.

nervous tissue Tissue that consists of neurons and supporting neuroglial cells and makes up the central and peripheral nervous system.

neural control centers Groups of neurons located in the pons and medulla oblongata of the brainstem that work to regulate respiration.

neural tube defects Group of birth defects in which the opening in the spine or cranium remains; spina bifida and anencephaly are examples.

neural tube Embryonic precursor to the central nervous system (CNS) and is composed of the brain and spinal cord; generally, during the fourth week of pregnancy, the neural tube closure occurs.

neuralgia Nerve pain.

neurocranium Upper and back part of the skull.

neuroendocrine Pertaining to the nervous and endocrine systems.

neurogenic Originating in the brain or spinal cord.

neuroglia Supporting cells found in nervous tissue.

neuromuscular junction Areas between motor neurons and the point of attachment to muscles.

neurons Cells found in nervous tissue that detect stimuli, process information, and transmit electrical impulses from one area of the body to another.

neuropathy Weakness, numbness, or pain resulting from peripheral nerve damage.

neuropeptide y Hormone produced by the hypothalamus that plays a role in increasing food intake and storing energy as fat in the body; also called NPY.

neurotransmitter Molecule secreted by neurons that produces changes in other neurons or organs.

neutrophils Agranulocytic white blood cells with segmented nuclei which perform phagocytosis.

nipple Tissue of the breast where milk is excreted.

nociception Ability to detect painful stimuli.

nociceptors Sensory proteins that activate pain neurons.

nocturia The need to frequently urinate at night.

nodal cells Specialized cardiac muscle cells that can generate action potentials.

nodal tissue Tissue capable of producing action potentials.

nodes of Ranvier Small spaces in between areas of myelination on an axon; nerve impulse jumps from node to node.

nonaxial Allows for gliding movement between bones.

nondisjunction Failure of a cell to split completely during meiosis that results in an inaccurate number of chromosomes.

non-small cell lung cancer Most common type of lung cancer consisting of subtypes including squamous cell carcinoma, adenocarcinoma, and large cell carcinoma.

nonsteroid hormones Hormones created by molecules and chemicals that do not contain a cholesterol compound in the basic structure of the hormone.

notch Small indentation in bone.

nuclei Portions of cells that contain DNA.

nucleus accumbens Region of the limbic system involved in processing reward and reinforcement.

O

obesity Excessive accumulation of body fat; a person is considered obese if he or she has a body mass index (BMI) of 30 or higher.

oblique popliteal ligament Ligament that originates at the tibia and connects to the femur, crossing in back of the knee joint; provides a reinforcing structure, acting as a stabilizing force for the posterior of the knee.

obstructive cardiomyopathy Enlargement of a heart ventricle that obstructs blood flow out of the ventricle.

obturator externus Deep posterior pelvic muscle that produces external rotation of the hip.

obturator internus Deep posterior pelvic muscle that produces external rotation of the hip.

occipital bone One of the bones of the skull located in the posterior inferior region of the skull.

occipital lobe Region of the cerebrum that processes visual information.

occipitalis Muscle located on the posterior portion of the skull that attaches to the epicranial aponeurosis.

oculomotor nerve Cranial nerve III; controls movements of the eye.

olecranon process Bony protuberance on the proximal portion of the ulna commonly referred to as the elbow.

olfactory nerve Cranial nerve I; contains neurons that detect the sense of smell.

oligodendrocytes Specialized neuroglial cells that myelinate the axons of neurons in the brain and spinal cord.

oligomenorrhea Infrequent menstruation or periods that occur more than 35 days apart.

omohyoid Muscle located in the anterior cervical region connecting to the hyoid bone.

omphalocele Abdominal wall defect in which the liver, intestines, and other abdominal organs remain outside of the abdomen in a sac because of failure of return of the intestines and other organs back into the abdominal cavity.

one-way valves Valves in the venous system that only allow blood flow toward the heart.

onychomycosis Fungal infection of the nail resulting in nail discoloration, thickening, and crumbling.

oocytes Immature gamete within the ovary.

oogenesis Development of an ovum.

oogonia Female germ cells.

ophthalmic artery Artery supplying the eye.

ophthalmic veins Veins in the skull draining the eye.

opiates Naturally occurring substances that are able to stimulate opioid receptors in the human body and produce pain relief and/or a feeling of euphoria. Examples of common opiates are opium, and such medications as morphine, hydrocodone, oxycodone, hydromorphone, and heroin.

opisthotonos Type of severe tetanic contraction that occurs from untreated tetanus in which the back muscles spasm and bend into extension.

opportunistic infections Infection that occurs in immunocompromised individuals due to opportunistic pathogens.

opportunistic pathogens Microorganisms that do not usually cause disease but can in immunocompromised patients.

opposition Rotation of the thumb touching each of the fingers of the same hand.

opsonins Groups of proteins that coat foreign cells during opsonization.

opsonization Coating of foreign cells with proteins to help with phagocytosis.

optic chiasm Location in the brain where visual fibers cross and the optic nerve becomes the optic tract.

optic nerve Cranial nerve II; visualizes sensory information.

optic radiation Axon pathway from the thalamus to the occipital lobe.

optic tract Axon pathway from the optic chiasm to the thalamus.

oral contraceptive Method of birth control that suppresses ovulation by ingesting a pill that contains estrogen and progestin.

orbicularis oculi Circular muscle surrounding the eye and causing the action of blinking the eye.

orbicularis oris Circular muscle surrounding the mouth and causing the action of puckering the lips.

orchitis Acute infection of the testes usually caused by a urinary tract infection or the mumps.

organic molecules Molecules containing carbon in a ring or chain with other atoms such as hydrogen, nitrogen, and oxygen attached; commonly found in living organisms.

organogenesis Formation and development of organs.

organophosphate poisoning A complex response to ingestion of a class of chemicals which prevents the breakdown of acetylcholine in the neuromuscular synapse.

origins Muscle attachment on the relatively immoveable end of a joint.

oropharyngeal dysphagia Type of swallowing disorder affecting the smooth muscles of the oropharynx.

oropharynx Portion of the pharynx extending from the soft palate to the epiglottis.

osmolarity Concentration of an osmotic solution, especially when measured in osmols or milliosmols per liter of solution.

osmosis Movement of water through a semipermeable membrane from an area of low osmolarity to an area of high osmolarity.

osmotic pressure Pressure created by electrolytes and other osmotic molecules pulling water inward toward themselves; in the blood, the osmotic pressure is trying to pull liquid from the tissues into the blood vessels.

osmotic Liquid that has the tendency to absorb through a semipermeable structure or membrane.

ossicles Small bones found in the middle ear that amplify the sound collected by the outer ear.

ossification Calcification of soft tissue into bone-like material or bone formation.

osteoarthritis Common form of arthritis that results in degeneration of joint cartilage and underlying bone.

osteoblasts Immature bone cells found around the perimeter of bone tissue that help build new bone tissue and contribute to the density of bones.

osteoclasts Cells that help break down old bone tissue; phagocytic bone cells that are formed from white blood cells.

osteocytes Specialized bone cells that maintain bone tissue.

osteogenesis Process through which bones are formed.

osteoid Organic component of bone matrix comprised of protein mixture, matrix vesicles, and collagen that helps to grow new bone.

osteomalacia Condition caused by prolonged, severe vitamin D deficiency, which leads to softening and weakening of bones in adulthood.

osteon Circular areas where bone tissues come together.

osteoprogenitor cells Cells that are considered precursors to fully formed bone cells.

outer ear Region of the ear that collects the sound and funnels it toward the sensory structures.

ova Haploid female gametes of animals develop into new individuals after fertilization with sperm during reproduction.

ovarian follicles Follicles found in the ovaries that secrete hormones that influence the stages of the menstrual cycle.

ovaries Female reproductive organ located in the pelvic cavity responsible for the secretion of hormones involved in secondary-sex characteristic development and menstruation.

overflow incontinence Uncontrolled release of urine that occurs if the bladder is distended.

overhydration Excessive intake of liquids that results in the dilution of the body's fluids and results in a large decrease in osmolarity.

ovoid Oval shaped.

ovulation stage When the ova are released by a follicle in the ovary and begins to travel along the fallopian tube to the uterus.

ovulation Release of an ovum from the ovaries.

ovum Mature female reproductive cell.

oxygen debt Use of oxygen in the conversion of lactic acid to pyruvic acid and glucose.

oxygenated blood Blood containing high oxygen levels after passing though capillaries in the lungs.

oxygenation Process of increasing oxygen levels in the blood.

oxygen-hemoglobin saturation (dissociation) curve Mathematical curve representing the percent saturation of hemoglobin on the vertical axis and the partial pressure of oxygen on the horizontal axis.

oxyhemoglobin Molecule that forms when oxygen combines with hemoglobin.

oxytocin Hormone that stimulates uterine contractions and causes the ejection of milk.

P

pacemaker cells Cells in the heart that produce action potentials that govern the rhythm of the heart.

pacesetter cells Cells located in the digestive system that undergo spontaneous depolarization and promote smooth muscle contraction.

pachyonychia congenita Rare genetic disorder that causes skin and nails to become thick and abnormally shaped.

pain Perception of damaged cells or tissues.

palatine bones Bones of the skull contributing to the posterior portion of the hard palate.

palmaris longus Muscle located in the anterior forearm that connects to the flexor retinaculum and is absent in about 14% of the population.

palpation Act of examining by touching.

palpitations Heartbeats that are fast, strong, or irregular that can be felt.

pancreas Gland that regulates multiple hormones involved in glucose control and digestion.

pancreatic ducts Small ducts that traverse through the pancreas and combine with the common bile duct at the hepatopancreatic ampulla.

pancreatitis Disorder characterized by inflammation of the pancreas.

papillary muscles Small muscles located on the inner walls of the ventricles that attach to the atrioventricular valves by way of chordae tendineae.

parasympathetic nervous system Portion of the autonomic nervous system (ANS) that promotes digestive and excretory processes.

parathyroid glands Small glands located within the thyroid glands that are involved in regulating serum levels of calcium.

parenchyma Tissue of an organ that enables the organ to function.

paresthesia Abnormal sensation in part of the body. Sometimes referred to as numbness or tingling.

parietal lobe Region of the cerebrum that processes touch, pain, and temperature information.

parietal pericardium Outer layer of the fibrous structure that contains the heart known as the pericardium.

parietal pleural membrane Membrane of the lungs that attaches to the inside of the thoracic cavity.

Parkinson's disease A chronic, progressive movement disorder caused by the degradation of the dopamine producing cells in the area of the brain that initiates movement.

paroxysmal supraventricular tachycardia Rapid heart rate that originates from tissue located above the ventricles.

partial pressure gradient Difference in partial pressure on both sides of a membrane.

partial pressures Pressure exerted by a single gas in a mixture of gases.

passive immunity Immune condition where a person is given someone else's antibodies.

patella alta X-ray sign in which the patella is located in a superior position resulting from rupture of the patellar ligament.

patella Small sesamoid bone commonly called the kneecap.

patellar tendon Dense connective tissue structure that anchors the distal patella to the tibial tuberosity of the tibia.

patellofemoral joint One of the joints that form the knee, for which the hinge joint allows for movement.

patent ductus arteriosus Hollow tubular structure between the aorta and pulmonary trunk that should close after birth but remains open.

pathogen Microorganism that can cause disease.

pathogenic Capable of causing illness or disease.

pectineus Muscle located on the medial portion of the thigh that works to adduct the hip.

pectoral girdle Clavicle and scapula bones.

pectoralis major Superficial muscle in the anterior thorax connecting to the ribcage, clavicle, and humerus.

pectoralis minor Deep muscle in the anterior thorax connecting to the rib cage and scapula.

pectoris muscles Muscles on the anterior chest that support the mammary glands.

pedicles Small projections originating from the podocytes that cover the glomerular capillaries. Their function is to limit the size of molecules passing from within the capillaries into the glomerular capsule.

pelvic inflammatory disease (PID) Infection that affects pelvic organs.

penile urethra Portion of the male urethra contained within the corpus spongiosum of the penis.

penis Main organ of the male reproductive system.

pennate Feather-like arrangement of muscle fibers in which many fibers connect in an oblique fashion to a central tendon.

perforins Chemicals released by NK cells that kill foreign cells.

pericardial tamponade Condition arising from fluid buildup in the pericardium that inhibits ventricular contraction.

pericardial Referring to the pericardium.

pericarditis Inflammation of the pericardium.

pericardium Fibrous tissue structure that contains the heart.

perimetrium Outer layer of uterine tissue.

perimysium Membrane covering a muscle fascicle.

perineum Area between the buttocks and thighs.

periodontal disease An inflammatory disease of the gums that causes damage to the soft tissues and bones supporting the teeth.

periodontal ligament Group of specialized connective fibers that attach a tooth to the alveolar bone.

periosteum Fibrous outer layer of bone.

peripheral edema Swelling that occurs when lymphatic vessels are unable to drain excess interstitial fluid.

peripheral nerve Bundle of sensory and motor neurons traveling to a common location outside the vertebral column.

peripheral nervous system Division of the nervous system that extends off the brain and spinal cord.

peristalsis Process of smooth muscle contraction along the GI tract that forces material to move further along the tract.

peritubular capillaries A network of capillaries surrounding the renal tubules.

permeability Quality of a membrane that allows molecules to pass through it.

perpendicular process of the ethmoid bone Bony process of the ethmoid bone extending inferior.

petechiae Tiny, circular, nonraised patches that appear on the skin or in a mucous or serous membrane. Usually is a sign of bleeding under the skin.

Peyer's patches Aggregated lymphatic follicles found at the region of the small intestine.

pH scale Logarithmic scale numbered from 1 to 14 that is used to measure the concentration of hydrogen ions within a solution; tells us how acidic or basic a solution is. When using the pH scale, a pH of 7 is neutral, a pH less than 7 is acidic and a pH greater than 7 is basic (alkalotic). When used in reference to the human body, a pH of 7.35 to 7.45 is normal. Thus, a pH less than 7.35 is considered acidic and a pH greater than 7.45 is considered alkalotic.

pH Exponential (logarithmic) scale measuring the acidity or alkalinity of a substance.

phagocytic Cell possessing the ability to absorb or "eat" another cell.

phagocytosis Process by which white blood cells engulf, digest, and excrete foreign cells.

phagolysosome Phagosome that has joined together with a lysosome to digest a foreign cell.

phagosome Endocytic vesicle within a phagocytic cell containing an engulfed foreign cell.

phalanges Fingers or toes.

phantom limb Perceived sensation that an amputated limb is present.

pharyngeal arches Series of externally observable anterior tissue bands located below the early brain and that will eventually form the structural features of the head and neck.

pharyngeal tonsils Masses of lymphoid tissue located in the pharynx.

pharyngitis Inflammation of the pharynx.

pharynx Partially shared passageway for the respiratory and digestive systems beginning at the posterior nasal cavity and extending to the trachea.

pheochromocytoma Noncancerous tumor on the adrenal gland that results excess hormone release causing high blood pressure, headaches, sweating, and other symptoms.

phimosis Constriction of the foreskin in an uncircumcised male.

phosphocreatine Molecule that can lend a phosphate molecule to ADP to produce ATP.

phospholipid bilayer Cell membrane consisting of an arrangement of two layers of phospholipids.

phospholipids Modified lipid made with phosphorous.

phosphorylation Chemical process by which a phosphate molecule is added to adenosine diphosphate to produce one molecule of adenosine triphosphate.

photoreceptor Sensory proteins in the eye that respond to light.

phrenic nerve Paired nerves consisting of cervical nerve roots (C3, C4, C5) that innervate the diaphragm.

pia matter Innermost thin layer of the meninges that clings tightly to the brain and spinal cord surface.

pica Eating disorder that involves ingesting items that are not typically thought of as food, such as paint or clay.

pineal gland Gland located near the posterior portion of the brain that is primarily involved in regulating the sleep–wake cycle. Secretes melatonin.

pinnae External portion of the out ear.

piriformis Deep posterior pelvic muscle in close proximity to the sciatic nerve that produces external rotation of the hip.

pitcher's shoulder Type of shoulder tendinitis that occurs from throwing a ball.

pituitary dwarfism Genetically inherited condition in which the pituitary gland does not release an adequate amount of growth hormone.

pituitary gland A pea sized gland that is housed in the sella turcica and is the master regulator of the endocrine system, controlling the activity of numerous hormonesecreting glands.

pivot joint Type of joint that permits rotation around a single axis.

placenta Structure within the pregnant uterus that is attached to the lining of the uterus and serves to nourish the developing fetus.

plantar aponeurosis Band of fibrous connective tissue located at the sole of the foot.

plantar interossei Small muscles between the toes located in the fourth layer of the foot muscles.

plantarflexion Bending at the ankle when the heel is lifted, flexing the foot or toes downward.

plasma cell Activated B cell that secretes antibodies.

plasma Liquid portion of blood that contains proteins and clotting factors.

plasmin Enzyme that degrades blood plasma proteins.

plasminogen Precursor to plasmin.

platelet-derived growth factor (PDGF) Growth factors that regulate cell growth and division of platelets.

platelets Formed elements that help to form blood clots.

platysma Superficial muscle of the neck that produces frowning.

pleural cavity Space between the visceral and parietal pleural membranes surrounding the lungs.

pleural effusion Fluid buildup in the pleural cavity.

pleural fluid Fluid secreted by the parietal pleural membrane.

pluripotential Undifferentiated stem cell.

pneumoconiosis Lung disease caused by inhaling toxic substances such as coal dust resulting in lung fibrosis.

pneumonia Lung infection caused by viruses or bacteria characterized by fluid buildup in the lungs.

pneumotaxic center Neural control center located in the pons that works to inhibit inhalation.

pneumothorax Lung condition whereby air becomes trapped between the pleural membranes of the lungs.

P_{O2} Partial pressure of oxygen.

P_{CO2} Partial pressure of carbon dioxide.

podocytes Cells with branching tentacle-shaped extensions that form the barrier through which blood is filtered in the glomerulus of the kidney.

polarized Pertaining to a difference in electrical potential on either side of a membrane.

polycystic kidney disease Hereditary disease characterized by gradually enlarging cysts within the kidney that lead to renal failure.

polycystic ovarian syndrome (PCOS) Condition in women where higher than normal levels of male hormones are produced leading to hirsutism, diabetes, and possible infertility.

polydipsia Excessive thirst typically seen in diabetic patients with an elevated blood glucose level.

polymenorrhea Frequent menstruation or periods that occur less than 21 days apart.

polysomnogram Sleep study in which physiological processes such as blood oxygen levels, brain waves, pulse, and breathing are monitored during sleep.

pons Region of the brainstem regulating breathing, heart rate, blood pressure, hearing, equilibrium, and other functions.

pontine respiratory group Group of respiratory control neuron; also known as the pneumotaxic center.

popliteal artery Artery located behind the knee.

popliteal vein Vein located behind the knee.

popliteus Muscle located on the posterior portion of the knee.

positive energy balance More nutrients (calories) are coming in than the body can use; usually result in weight gain.

posterior cardiac vein Vein extending along the posterior wall of the left ventricle and draining into the cardiac sinus.

posterior chamber Fluid-filled cavity between the iris and the lens of the eye.

posterior communicating arteries Arteries that are part of the Circle of Willis that supply blood to the brain.

posterior cruciate ligament (PCL) One of the major ligaments in the human knee, connecting the posterior intercondylar area of the tibia to the medial condyle of the femur.

posterior intercostal artery Veins located in the posterior thorax.

posterior interventricular artery Coronary artery located in the posterior interventricular sulcus connecting with the left anterior descending artery.

posterior tibial vein Vein located in the lower leg.

postganglionic neuron Second of two autonomic neurons that leave the spinal cord before innervating an organ.

postmenopausal Stage in which a female stops maturing ova and menstruation ceases.

post-synaptic neuron Neuron at a synapse that has receptors on dendrites being activated by neurotransmitters.

power stroke Portion of the sliding filament model of muscle contraction in which a myosin molecule moves an actin molecule while powered by ATP.

PR interval The section on an ECG between the beginning of the P-wave and beginning of the R-wave.

PR segment The section on an ECG between the end of the P-wave and beginning of the R-wave.

precapillary sphincter Circular smooth muscle located between an arteriole and capillary.

precentral gyri Gyrus in the frontal lobe just anterior to the central sulcus that processes motor information.

preembryonic stage First two weeks of development after fertilization; during this time, cleavage, implantation, and embryogenesis occur.

pregabalin Medication used to treat fibromyalgia.

preganglionic neuron First of two autonomic neurons that leave the spinal cord before innervating an organ.

premature ejaculation Release of sperm before the achievement of the male orgasm.

prepuce Layer of skin that covers the clitoris.

pressure Deeper form of touch requiring a heavy, but nondamaging physical stimulus.

presynaptic neuron Neuron at a synapse that releases neurotransmitters from the axon terminal buds.

pretibial myxedema Localized lesions of the skin around the tibia as a result of increase in fat deposits due to Graves' disease.

priapism Involuntary sustained erection not associated with sexual arousal.

primary amenorrhea Absence of menstruation by age 15 or the failure to menstruate and the absence of secondary sex characteristics by age 13.

primary curvatures Curvature of the thoracic and sacral vertebrae that forms during fetal development.

primary immune response Immune responses that occur the first time the immune system comes in contact with a pathogen.

primary lymphatic organs Sites where new lymphatic cells are formed and matured.

primary malnutrition Prolonged, inadequate dietary intake of food; due to not eating enough food, whether or not any specific nutrient deficiency is present, or eating an excess of specific nutrients.

primary motor cortex Area of the frontal lobe that contains neurons that lead to physical movements.

primary oocytes Oocyte that has divided mitotically and contains 46 chromosomes.

primary sensory cortex First region of a cortical lobe that undergoes sensory processing of the most basic forms of that sense.

prime movers Muscle most responsible for a specific joint movement.

primordial follicles Immature ova.

process Projection from a bone.

progesterone Steroid hormone that stimulates the uterus to prepare for pregnancy.

pro-insulin Prohormone precursor to insulin.

prolactin Hormone within the female reproductive system that stimulates breast tissue to produce breast milk.

prolapse Bulging or collapsing of a heart valve.

proliferation Cloning and increase in number of cells.

proliferative Third step in wound healing when cells generate quickly to fill in and cover an injured area.

pronate To rotate the hand so that the palm is facing downward or to turn the sole of the foot outward.

pronation Rotation of the hand and forearm so that the palm faces downward.

pronator quadratus Muscle located in the distal forearm between the ulna and radius that works to pronate the forearm and wrist.

pronator teres Muscle located in the proximal forearm between the humerus, ulna, and radius that works to pronate the forearm and wrist.

prophase I Phase during meiosis I when the homologous chromosomes line up with each other and bits of DNA cross over between them.

prophase II Phase during meiosis II when the two already divided daughter cells (with nonhomologous chromosomes) condense and the nuclear membrane disintegrates.

proprioception Sense of the position of a joint.

prostacyclin Platelet aggregation inhibitor.

prostaglandins Hormone-like substance that propels the sperm toward the ovary.

prostate cancer Cancer that affects the prostate gland.

prostate gland Gland that sits at the base of the male urinary bladder and wraps around the urethra in order to secrete a fluid that contributes to the development of semen.

prostate-specific antigen (PSA) Blood test that measures the presence or absence of cancer in the prostate gland.

prostatic urethra Part of the male urethra that passes through the prostate gland.

prostatitis Inflammation or infection of the prostate gland.

protein C Blood coagulation factor involved in creating a hypercoagulable state.

protein filaments Contractile proteins in muscle tissue.

protein Organic compound made of chains of amino acids found in both animal and plant foods.

proteinuria Excretion of a large number of protein molecules in the urine.

prothrombin activator Complex of a dozen blood coagulation factors usually occurring as a result of blood loss or trauma.

protracting Extension of a part of the body.

protraction Movement of a body part in an anterior direction.

provitamins Substance that is converted into a vitamin in the human body.

proximal convoluted tubule (PCT) Convoluted portion of the nephron that lies between Bowman's capsule and the loop of Henle; functions include resorption of glucose, electrolytes, and water from the glomerular filtrate. 70% of all tubular reabsorption occurs in the PCT.

pseudoglandular Embryonic stage of growth of lung tissue before the ciliated cells are differentiated.

pseudopods Extensions of a cell's membranes to make "false feet."

pseudostratified epithelium Layer of epithelium that appears to be multilayered but is only one cell layer thick; cells vary in height but all touch the basement membrane.

psoas major Deep muscle of the abdominopelvic region that attaches to the lumbar spine and extends to the femur.

psoriasis Skin disease characterized by shiny, silver or red patches.

PTT test Measurement that calculates the time it takes for a blood clot to form.

puberty Stage in which the reproductive system matures and secondary sex characteristics develop.

pubic bone One of three fused coxal bones located on the anterior–inferior portion of the coxal bone.

pudendum External female reproductive organs including the mons pubis, clitoris, labia major, labia minora, hymen, Bartholin's glands, Skene's glands, and vaginal and urethral orifices.

pull With respect to levers, the pull is the load.

pulmonary arteries Arteries branching off the pulmonary trunk that carry deoxygenated blood to the lungs.

pulmonary circuit System of blood vessels that bring deoxygenated blood from the heart to the lungs for oxygenation and then transport oxygenated blood back to the heart.

pulmonary fibrosis Formation of scar tissue in the lungs.

pulmonary function testing Measurement of volumes of air using a spirometer.

pulmonary trunk Great vessel of the heart exiting the right ventricle.

pulmonary tuberculosis Disease caused by a bacterium (*Mycobacterium tuberculosis*) that produces an infection with a chronic cough containing bloody sputum.

pulmonary valve Semilunar valve located in the pulmonary trunk near its connection to the right ventricle.

pulmonary veins Blood vessels carrying oxygenated blood from the lungs to the left atrium.

pulmonary ventilation Movement of air into and out of the lungs.

pulmonary Referring to the lungs.

pulp Center of the tooth that contains blood and nerves.

punctures Wound caused by a small, pointed object that results in a hole in the skin; do not always bleed.

pupil Opening of the iris that controls the amount of light entering the eye.

pupillary light reflex Reflex in which the pupil rapidly constricts in response to a bright light.

Purkinje fibers Specialized muscle fibers containing cells that conduct electricity located in the walls of the ventricles.

purpura Tiny raised patches that can appear on the skin. Usually a result of bleeding under the skin.

purulent Drainage that is white and thick; often referred to as pus.

P-wave ECG waveform that represents ventricular repolarization.

pyloric sphincter Connection or link between the stomach and the starting point of the duodenum that controls the emptying of the stomach contents into the small intestine.

pylorus Narrow inferior part of the stomach; also known as the antrum.

pyrogens Chemicals that raise the temperature set point of the hypothalamus.

pyruvic acid Product of glycolysis.

Q

QRS complex ECG waveform that represents ventricular depolarization and atrial repolarization.

quadratus femoris Muscle located on the posterior portion of the hip joint that works to produce external rotation of the hip.

quadratus plantus Muscle of the second layer of foot muscles.

quadriceps Group of four muscles on the anterior thigh that includes the rectus femoris, vastus medialis, vastus lateralis, and vastus intermedius.

R

radial artery Arteries in the forearm that originate from the brachial arteries.

radial vein Veins in the forearm that transport blood to the brachial vein.

radiation Loss of internal heat by infrared (or energy) waves.

radius Tubular bone located in the lateral forearm.

Raynaud's phenomenon Circulatory disorder characterized by reduced circulation to the hands or feet.

reaction pathways Systems of chemical reactions.

receptor Type of sensor that monitors the environment and responds to changes in the equilibrium in the negative feedback loop.

recruitment Action of additional firing of motor units.

rectal ampulla Place in the rectum where feces is stored before their release via the anal canal.

rectal valves Crescent-like folds located in the rectal ampulla caused by infoldings of the circular muscle and submucosa.

rectus abdominis One of the abdominal muscles located in the center of the abdomen.

rectus femoris One of the quadriceps muscles located in the anterior thigh.

red bone marrow Bone marrow reddish in appearance that produces platelets, red blood cells, and white blood cells.

referred pain Perception of pain in one region of the body when the actual source of the pain is at a distance.

reflex arc Neurons that create the circuit that starts with a stimulus and ends with reflexive behavior.

reflex Involuntary behavior that is processed entirely in the spinal cord.

refraction Bending of light as it passes through different mediums.

refractory period Period of time shortly after the contraction of a motor unit during which it is unresponsive to further stimulation.

regurgitation Abnormality of heart valves characterized by leaking.

relaxation phase Period during a muscle twitch in which myosin releases from actin and the muscle lengthens.

relaxin Hormone; in pregnant women, the placenta secretes relaxin and relaxes the pelvic ligaments.

remodeling Process in which osteoblasts and osteoclasts work together to reshape the repair site of a broken bone so that it resembles original bone before fracture.

renal agenesis Failure of the body to develop part of the renal system while developing in the uterus. This most likely takes the form of a person only having one kidney instead of two.

renal artery Arteries located in the abdominal cavity that supply the kidneys.

renal calculi Calculus (kidney stone) located in the kidney, ureter, bladder, or urethra.

renal capsule Tough, fibrous layer surrounding the kidney that is covered in a layer of perirenal fat.

renal corpuscle Part of a nephron that consists of Bowman's capsule with its included glomerulus.

renal cortex Outer region of the kidney found between the renal capsule and renal medulla. The renal columns that are found between the renal pyramids are extensions of the cortical tissue.

renal insufficiency Inability of kidney to function normally.

renal medulla Inner region of the kidney that contains 8–12 renal pyramids that empty into the calyx.

renal pelvis Funnel-shaped structure in each kidney that is formed by the convergence of the major calyxes and empties into the ureter.

renal pyramids Any of the somewhat triangular- or wedge-shaped masses of tissue found within the renal medulla that have a striated appearance due to the presence of collecting tubules and collecting ducts.

renal system Urinary system that consists of the kidneys, ureters, bladder, and urethra. The purpose of the renal system is to eliminate waste from the body, regulate blood volume and blood pressure, control levels of electrolytes and metabolites, and regulate blood pH.

renal tubule Part of a nephron that extends from the glomerular capsule and is composed of a proximal convoluted tubule, loop of Henle, and distal convoluted tubule and that empties into a collecting duct.

renal veins Veins carrying blood from the kidneys located in the abdominal cavity.

renin Enzyme produced by the kidney that plays a major role in the release of angiotensin.

renin-angiotensin-aldosterone system Hormone system that regulates blood pressure and fluid and electrolyte balance, as well as systemic vascular resistance; acts as a signaling pathway and is responsible for regulating the body's blood pressure; stimulated by low blood pressure, the autonomic nervous system, or the release of renin by the kidneys.

repolarization Phase of the action potential in which the neuron is returning back to its negative resting membrane potential.

reposition Movement of the thumb and fingers away from each other.

residual volume Amount of air remaining in the lungs after a maximal exhalation.

respiratory acidosis Blood pH lower than 7.35 caused by a decrease in breathing rate or inability of the lungs to expel carbon dioxide.

respiratory cycle Cycle consisting of inhalation and exhalation.

respiratory membrane Membrane consisting of the alveolar and capillary membrane in which gas exchange occurs.

resting membrane potential Electrically polarized state of muscle and nerve cells during an absence of stimulation.

restrictive cardiomyopathy Type of cardiomyopathy characterized by stiffness of the heart's muscular walls.

retained placenta Condition in which all or part of the placenta or membranes are retained in the uterus of a female during the final stage or third stage of labor after the baby has been delivered.

reticular cells Cells found in a netlike structure containing fibers, fibroblasts, and white blood cells that forms an internal framework for the spleen, thymus, lymph nodes, and bone marrow.

reticular formation Collection of brainstem neurons that are involved in maintaining attention.

reticular Netlike structure containing fibers, fibroblasts, and white blood cells that forms an internal framework for the spleen, thymus, lymph nodes, and bone marrow.

reticulocyte Precursor to a red blood cell.

reticulospinal tract Region of the spinal cord containing the axons of neurons originating in the brainstem (reticular formation).

retina Rear layer of the eyeball that contains photosensitive neurons.

retinopathy Disease or dysfunction of the retinas.

retraction Drawn backward movement of the body.

retrograde ejaculation Release of semen into the bladder.

retrograde menstruation Menstrual blood that flows upward in the uterus and through the fallopian tubes.

retroperitoneal Situated behind the peritoneum.

Rh factor Protein found on the surface of red blood cells.

rheumatoid arthritis Autoimmune disorder causing destruction of the joints of the body.

RhoGAM Medication used to prevent Rh antibody development in an Rh negative mother after childbirth.

rhomboid major Deep muscle of the back that attaches to the medial border of the scapula and extends to the spine.

rhomboid minor Deep muscle of the back located just superior to the rhomboid major muscle.

rickets Bone condition due to vitamin D deficiency during childhood that causes softening and malformation of bones.

rider's bone Also known as cavalry bone, sesamoid bone that forms in individuals who ride horses often that causes repeated strain on the upper thighs.

right and left common iliac arteries Arteries branching inferior from the abdominal aorta.

right and left coronary arteries Part of the coronary circuit or circulatory pathway.

right and left pulmonary arteries Arteries carrying deoxygenated blood from the pulmonary trunk to the lungs.

right and left pulmonary veins Veins extending from the lungs to the left atrium carrying oxygenated blood.

right and left suprarenal arteries Arteries carrying blood to the adrenal glands.

right atrium Hollow chamber on the right side of the heart that receives blood from the superior and inferior vena cavae.

right lymphatic duct Short vessel that begins just inferior to the clavicle on the right side of body.

right posterior descending artery Artery branching off the right coronary artery.

right posterior descending artery Artery that is a branch of the right coronary artery.

right ventricle Hollow chamber in the right side of the heart that pushes blood to the pulmonary trunk.

rods Visual sensory neurons specialized to detect low light, but only in black and white.

root Found at the proximal end of the nail.

rotation Movement around a single longitudinal axis.

rubrospinal tract Region of the spinal cord containing the axons of neurons originating in the brainstem (red nucleus of midbrain).

rugae Large mucosal folds of the stomach.

Rule of Nines Standardized method used to quickly assess the extent of burns on the surface area of the body; applied to second- and third-degree burns and divides the body into 11 areas, each accounting for 9% of the total body surface area, with one additional area around the genitals, accounting for 1%.

S

saccharolytic fermentation Breakdown of carbohydrates by bacteria.

sacral plexus Network of interconnected nerves formed by the lower lumbar and sacral nerves.

sacral spinal nerves Five pairs of peripheral nerves that exit from the lowest region of the spinal cord.

sacrum Triangular bone located just below the spine that articulates with the lowest lumbar spinal segment and both coxal bones.

saddle joint Joint that allows for abduction, adduction, flexion, and extension.

sagittal suture Immovable, fibrous joint between the right and left parietal bones.

sarcoidosis Chronic disease of unknown cause that results in the enlargement of lymph nodes in many parts of the body and the widespread deposition of immune complexes. This abnormal tissue can cause scar tissue formation and destruction of normal tissue within the pulmonary and cardiovascular system leading to respiratory or cardiac failure.

sarcolemma Membrane covering muscle cells (myocytes).

sarcomere Arrangement of contractile protein filaments forming a contractile unit in muscle tissue.

sarcoplasm Fluid portion of a muscle cell (myocyte).

sarcoplasmic reticulum Network of membranous channels surrounding a muscle cell.

sartorius Superficial muscle of the thigh attached to the ilium and extending to the medial knee.

satellite cells Glial cell of the PNS that supports the PNS neuron.

satiety Feeling of fullness after eating.

saturated fats and oils Category of triglycerides found in meats, dairy products, eggs, coconut oil, and palm oil.

scalene group Group of muscles in the neck.

scapula Triangular-shaped bone in the back that articulates with the posterior rib cage, humerus, and clavicle.

scapulothoracic joint An articulation between anterior scapula and posterior thoracic rib.

schizophrenia A chronic mental disorder that alters the way a person thinks, feels, acts, and interrupts sensory processing.

Schwann cells Specialized neuroglial cells that myelinate neurons outside of the brain and spinal cord.

sclera Opaque, the fibrous, protective outer layer of the human eye; also known as the white of the eye.

scoliosis Lateral bending of the spinal column caused by birth defects or other conditions.

scrotum Pouch of skin containing the testicles.

scurvy Disease that causes soft gum tissue, loose teeth, bad breath, joint pain, weakness, and blood spots under the skin; caused by a vitamin C deficiency.

Sebaceous glands Exocrine gland located in the skin that produces sebum, or oil; usually associated with hair follicles.

sebaceous hyperplasia Disorder characterized by enlarged sebaceous glands that appear as bumps on the face.

seborrheic dermatitis Common skin condition that forms round, red, scaly patches and dandruff in areas where there are many sebaceous glands like the face, scalp, nose, and back.

sebum Oily substance secreted by sebaceous glands that helps keep the skin soft and moist and prevents the hair from becoming too brittle.

second messengers Molecules within the cell that respond to a change in environment due to hormonal activation. These signals are responsible for carrying out the specific job of the hormone that attached to the surface of the target cell.

second polar body One of the female daughter cells that are created during the second phase of meiosis that disintegrates.

secondary amenorrhea Absence of menstruation for six months after routine menstruation has been established.

secondary curvatures Curvature of the lumbar and cervical vertebrae that develops once a child learns to walk.

secondary immune response Immune response that occurs with secondary and subsequent exposures to pathogen; response begins almost immediately and includes a higher amount of antibodies than primary immune response.

secondary lymphatic organs Organs that monitor and filter extracellular fluids.

secondary malnutrition Inadequate diet due to a secondary disease that affects growth directly or indirectly by changing the appetite or absorption of nutrients; patients are getting enough food, but a secondary disease is preventing their bodies from being able to get enough nutrients from their food.

secondary oocyte Female daughter cell formed during the second phase of meiosis and becomes an ovum.

second-degree burns Burns that affect the epidermis and dermis. Skin is red, painful, and blistered.

secretion Discharge of enzymes to aid in the breakdown of bolus materials.

segmentation Mixing movement that combines chyme with gastric solutions.

sella turcica Depression within the sphenoid bone that allows for the housing of the pituitary gland.

semen Fluid from the glands and epididymis that contains sperm.

semilunar valves Valves located in the pulmonary trunk and aorta containing three cusps.

semimembranosus One of three hamstring muscles located on the medial portion of the posterior thigh.

seminal vesicles Gland within the male reproductive system.

seminiferous tubules Structures within the testes that make sperm.

semispinalis capitis Muscle located in the posterior cervical region connecting to the skull.

semispinalis muscles Muscles located in the back that are part of the erector spinae group.

semitendinosus One of three hamstring muscles located on the medial portion of the posterior thigh and superficial to the semimembranosus.

sensation Mental experience following stimulation of a sensory structure.

sensitization First exposure to an allergen.

sensorineural hearing loss Decrease or complete loss of the ability to hear due to damage to the cochlea or vestibulocochlear nerve.

sensory adaptation Changing perception of a continued sensory stimulus.

sensory processing disorder Condition in which one or more senses are improperly processed by the brain.

sensory receptors Specialized proteins that change a sensory stimulus and convert it into a neuronal signal.

sensory system Division of the nervous system involved in detecting stimuli from outside.

serosa Outermost layer or external covering of the wall of the alimentary canal.

serous pericardium Portion of the pericardium that contains the visceral and parietal pericardium.

serratus anterior Muscle located on the lateral rib cage and extending to the anterior portion of the scapula.

Sertoli cells Cells responsible in the male for spermatogenesis.

serum antitoxin blood test Medical test used to diagnose tetanus.

sesamoid bones Bones that form within tendons.

short bones Bones, found in the wrists and ankles, that are roughly as wide as they are long.

short-term memories Maintaining information in the mind on the order of minutes.

shunt Act of moving blood to other parts of the body.

shunting Redirection of something such as the blood flow.

Shy-Drager syndrome See multiple systems atrophy.

sickle cell anemia Inherited form of anemia in which there aren't enough healthy red blood cells to carry adequate oxygen throughout the body.

sigmoid sinuses Hollow areas in the skull that carry venous blood from the posterior venous sinus.

silica dust Dust occurring from working with materials containing silica such as quartz.

simple epithelium Epithelium that is one cell layer thick.

simple fracture Also called closed fractures, breaks in the bone that do not protrude through the skin.

simple squamous epithelium Epithelial tissue consisting of one layer of flat squamous cells.

sinoatrial (SA) node Area of specialized cardiac muscle that can generate action potentials; sets the heart's rhythm.

sinus bradycardia Heart rate lower than the normal 60–100 beats per minute.

sinus tachycardia Regular heart rhythm greater than 100 beats per minute.

sinus Space (cavity) within a bone.

sinuses Hollow chambers within the bones of the skull.

sinusitis Inflammation of the sinuses of the skull.

sister chromatids Two sides of a chromosome; each is joined to the other by the centromere.

skeletal muscle tissue Voluntary, striated, multinucleated type of muscle tissue; its contraction causes movement of the skeleton.

Skene's glands Gland that provides lubrication to the vagina during sexual stimulation.

skin grafting Surgical procedure that involves removing skin from one area of the body and attaching it to another injured area; common procedure for burned areas.

sleep apnea Sleep disorder in which breathing repeatedly stops and starts.

sliding filament theory Theory explaining the physiology of skeletal muscle contraction.

slow-twitch fibers Type of muscle fiber capable of producing low force over long durations while relying on aerobic sources of energy.

small cardiac vein Refers to a portion of the coronary circulatory circuit that drains blood into the great cardiac vein.

small cardiac vein Vein draining blood from the right side of the heart to the coronary sinus.

small cell lung cancer Type of lung cancer originating from neuroendocrine cells that can spread rapidly.

small saphenous vein Vein located in the lower leg.

smell Ability to detect chemical in the nose.

smooth muscle tissue Involuntary, nonstriated type of muscle tissue with tapered cells that contain a single nucleus; found in the hollow organs of the body.

smooth muscle One of three types of muscle tissues characterized by the lack of striations and involuntary control.

sodium-potassium pump Type of transport protein located in cell membranes that requires energy (ATP) to move three sodium ions outside and two potassium ions into a cell.

soleus Muscle located on the posterior lower leg just deep to the gastrocnemius muscle.

solubility coefficient Volume of a substance that can be dissolved by a unit volume of solvent at a specified pressure and temperature.

solubility Ability of a substance to dissolve in water.

soma Cell body of a neuron containing the nucleus and other cell organelles.

somatic cells Any cell that is not a reproductive cell.

somatic growth Growth and multiplication of cells in the body responsible for creating tissues.

somatic nervous system Portion of the nervous system innervating the skin, muscles, and viscera.

somatotropic cells Cells that create growth hormone.

somatotropinoma Mass that has developed in the pituitary gland that is oversecreting growth hormone.

somite Divisions of the body of an embryo.

somnolence Sleepy, drowsy.

special senses Senses of the head that use specialized organs or structures to detect stimuli.

sperm Gamete within the male anatomy that fertilizes the female egg in reproduction.

spermatocele Swelling in a duct of the epididymis.

spermatogenesis Production and development of mature sperm.

spermatogonia Male germ cells.

spermatozoa Motile male gamete with a rounded or elongated head and a long posterior flagellum.

spermicide Chemical used to destroy sperm as a method of birth control.

sphenoid bone Bone of the skull located near the anterior and middle portion of the cranium. This bone houses and protects the pituitary gland along with the hypothalamus.

sphincter of Oddi Muscular valve that controls the flow of digestive juices through the hepatopancreatic duct into the second part of the duodenum.

sphincters Type of muscle with a circular shape that functions to constrict and dilate an area of the body.

spinal nerve Bundle of sensory and motor neurons traveling to a common area outside the spinal cord but within the vertebral column.

spinalis Muscles of the back that are part of the erector spinae group.

spinocerebellar tract Region of the spinal cord containing the axons of sensory neurons sending information to the cerebellum.

spinothalamic tract Region of the spinal cord containing the axons of sensory neurons sending information to the thalamus.

spinous process Sharp edge or point in a bone.

spirometer Device used to measure volumes of air entering and exiting the lungs.

splenic artery Branch of the abdominal aorta that brings blood to the spleen.

splenic vein Vein that takes deoxygenated blood away from the spleen.

splenius capitis Muscle located in the upper posterior portion of the cervical area connecting to the occipital bone.

sponge Method of birth control where a disk-shaped device containing spermicide is inserted into the vagina and becomes activated by wetting with water.

spoon nails Nail disease resulting in spoon-shaped nails that look scooped out; usually caused by iron-deficiency anemia.

spray and stretch Type of therapy used to treat muscles in which a coolant is sprayed on a muscle just before manually stretching it.

squamous cell carcinoma Type of skin cancer that appears as scaly, red, painful areas that bleed and do not heal and that grow slowly and rarely spread.

squamous cells Epithelial cells that are flat and hexagonal shaped with disc-shaped nuclei.

ST segment ECG measurement that begins at the end of the QRS complex and ends at the beginning of the T-wave.

staphylococcus scalded skin syndrome is a serious bacterial skin infection that is usually caused by *Staphylococcal aureas bacteria*.

starch Complex carbohydrate in plant material.

stem cells Type of cell that is undifferentiated and can produce other cells that are able to develop into any kind of cell in the body.

stenosis Narrowing, usually refers to narrowing of a vessel or heart valve.

sterilization Surgical procedure to prevent pregnancy accomplished through a vasectomy or tubal ligation.

sternoclavicular joint Gliding-type joint between the sternum and the clavicle.

sternocleidomastoid Muscle located in the lateral cervical region extending from the mastoid process to the clavicle and sternum.

sternohyoid Muscle located in the anterior portion of the cervical region attaching to the sternum and hyoid bones.

sternothyroid Muscle located in the anterior portion of the cervical region attaching to the sternum and thyroid cartilage.

sternum Bone located in the anterior portion of the thorax that has three divisions (manubrium, body, xiphoid process) and connects to the ribs and clavicles.

steroid hormones Chemical messengers derived from a cholesterol molecule.

stimulated Ability to respond to a stimulus and change it into an impulse.

stimulus Substance or event invoking a change in a system.

straight sinus Hollow vascular area that drains the inferior sagittal sinus.

stratified epithelium Epithelium that consists of more than one layer of cells.

stratum basale Also called the stratum germanitivum; deepest layer of the epidermis.

stratum corneum The outer dead layer of the skin.

stratum granulosum Layer in the epidermis filled with keratin granules.

stratum lucidum Translucent layer of epidermis between the stratum granulosum and stratum corneum; only present in thick skin.

stratum spinosum Layer of epidermis above the stratum basale.

stress Feeling of emotion or physical tension.

stretch receptors Specialized sensory structures that detect changes in the size of structures.

stretch reflex Reflex that maintains muscle at a constant length.

striae gravidarum Stretch marks on the skin.

striated Light and dark areas in muscle tissue formed by overlapping contractile protein filaments.

striations Ridges or visible lines.

stroke Occurs when blood flow (and therefore oxygen) to parts of the brain is blocked.

stylohyoid Muscle in the anterior portion of the cervical region attaching to the styloid process of the temporal bone and hyoid bone.

styloid process Sharp, pointed process located on several bones of the body.

subclavian arteries Arteries located below the clavicle.

subclavian vein Vein located below the clavicle.

subcostal Referring to below the ribs.

subcutaneous bursa Under the skin.

subcutaneous tissue Same tissue as the hypodermis.

submucosa Layer of connective tissue located below a mucous membrane.

Submuscular bursa Under the muscles.

subscapularis One of four rotator cuff muscles located on the anterior portion of the scapula and extending to the humerus.

subtendinous bursa Found between a tendon and a bone.

suction dilation and curettage (D&C) Medical procedure where the uterine cervix of a female is dilated and the curette is inserted into the uterus for the scraping and the removal of the endometrium.

sudoriferous glands Also called sweat glands; eccrine and apocrine are the two types.

superficial arch Arteries located in the palms of the hands.

superficial dorsal venous arch System of veins in the foot that drain into the Great Saphenous vein.

superior and inferior mesenteric arteries Arteries in the abdominal cavity supplying the mesentery with blood.

superior and inferior vena cava Large veins carrying deoxygenated blood to the right atrium.

superior gemellus Deep muscle of the pelvis that functions to externally rotate the hip.

superior oblique One of six eye muscles, with a tendon that attaches to the superior portion of the eyeball then forms an angle as it passes through a structure called the trochlea and works to abduct, depress, and internally rotate the eye.

superior phrenic arteries Arteries located in the thoracic cavity that branch from the thoracic aorta.

superior rectus One of six eye muscles attaching to the superior portion of the eyeball that functions to rotate the eye upward.

superior rotation Rotation upward.

supinate To hold a hand, foot, or limb so that the palm or sole is facing upward or outward.

supination Rotation of the forearm and hand so that the palm faces upward.

supinator Muscle in the posterior portion of the forearm that functions to supinate the forearm.

supracondylar ridge of the humerus Roughed area on the distal, medial portion of the humerus.

supraglenoid tubercle Small rounded eminence located on the superior portion of the glenoid cavity that serves as an attachment point for the biceps brachii muscle.

suprascapular fossa Groove located on the scapula just superior to the spine of the scapula.

supraspinatus One of four rotator cuff muscles that attaches to the scapula and extending to the humerus that functions to externally rotate the humerus.

supraventricular tachycardia Fast but regular heartbeat caused by nodal tissue located above the ventricles.

surfactant Substance secreted by type II alveolar cells that decreases surface tension in the alveoli.

surgical neck Bony landmark in the humerus where breaks often occur.

sutures Immovable joints between skull bones.

swanlike neck Long, thin neck resulting from a form of muscular dystrophy called myotonic MD.

sweat chloride test Test measuring the amount of chloride in sweat used to diagnose cystic fibrosis.

swimmer's shoulder Syndrome of the shoulder resulting from the action of swimming causing overuse of the muscles, tendons, and bursae of the shoulder.

sympathetic chain Structure that runs parallel to the spinal cord and is the site of the preganglionic and postganglionic synapses for the sympathetic nervous system.

sympathetic nervous system Region of the autonomic nervous system that activates the fight-or-flight response.

symphyses Fibrocartilaginous joint fusion between two bones.

symphysis pubis Cartilaginous joint that joins the left and right superior rami of the pubic bone.

synapses Specialized site of communication between the axon terminal bud of one neuron and a receptor found on another neuron, gland, or muscle.

synaptic cleft Fluid-filled space located between a neuron and another neuron or organ.

synchondrosis Slightly moveable joint between bones that is composed of hyaline cartilage.

syncope Commonly known as fainting and characterized by a loss of consciousness from decreased blood flow to the brain.

syncytia Group of motor units in muscle that contract together.

syndesmoses Fibrous joint in which connective tissue joins the bones such as fibula and tibia.

synergist muscles Muscles that work together to perform a specific movement.

synesthesia Abnormal sensory processing in which stimulation of one sensory modality causes a different sensory modality (or cognitive process) to be stimulated.

synostoses Fusion of two bones.

synovial fluid Viscous fluid found in the cavities of the joints that permits smooth movement and provides nourishment to the joints.

synovial joints Diarthrosis joint, a connection between two existing bones that consists of fluid-filled cartilage-lined cavity; common joint in mammals.

synovial membrane Connective tissue that lines the inner surface of capsules of synovial joints.

syphilis Sexually transmitted infection that is transmitted through a spirochete and has three distinct phases.

systemic circuit System of blood vessels carrying blood from the heart to the body.

systemic lupus erythematosus Autoimmune disorder, commonly referred to as lupus, characterized by inflammation of body tissues.

systemic Referring to throughout the body such as in the systemic circulatory circuit.

systolic heart failure Type of heart failure that affects contraction of the ventricles.

systolic murmurs Abnormal heart sounds occurring during contraction, or systole, of the ventricles of the heart.

T

T cells Specialized immune cells created in the thymus.

tachycardia Heart rate greater than 100 beats per minute.

tachypnea Rapid breathing greater than 20 breaths per minute.

talipes equinovarus Condition where the foot appears rotated inward at the ankle. Also known as clubfoot.

target cells Cells that can be affected by hormones.

target receptors Molecules inserted into or on the surface of the plasma membrane of a target cell. These compounds allow for hormone activation of the cell.

taste Ability to detect chemical on the tongue.

tear ducts Nasal portion of the orbit that excretes a protective fluid.

tectospinal tract Region of the spinal cord containing descending neurons encoding information about head and eye movement.

telophase I Phase of meiosis I in which a nuclear membrane forms around each set of 23 chromosomes that were formed when the homologous chromosomes split in anaphase I.

telophase II Phase of meiosis II in which a nuclear membrane forms around each set of chromosomes.

temperature Ability to detect changes in the amount of heat in the body.

temporal bone One of the bones of the skull located on the lateral sides.

temporal lobe Region of the cerebrum that processes auditory information.

temporalis Muscle located on the lateral portion of the skull.

temporomandibular joint Joint formed by the temporal bone and mandible often referred to as the jaw joint.

tendon A tough fibrous connective tissue that connects muscle to bone to withstand tension.

tenesmus Painful defecation.

tenia coli Three smooth muscle strips on the outside of the ascending, transverse, descending, and sigmoid colon; contract lengthwise to produce the bulges in the colon.

tennis elbow Tendinitis of the wrist extensor tendons near their attachment at the lateral epicondyle of the humerus; also known as lateral epicondylitis.

tensor fascia latae Muscle located on the superior and lateral side of the thigh.

teres major Shoulder muscle that attaches to the lateral portion of the scapula and extends to the humerus.

teres minor One of four rotator cuff muscles that attaches to the lateral portion of the scapula and extends to the humerus; functions to externally rotate the humerus.

terminal cisternae Tubular channel located in the sarcoplasmic reticulum.

terminal ganglia Structures in or near an organ that is the site of the preganglionic and postganglionic synapses for the parasympathetic nervous system.

terminal saccular stage Last generation of air spaces in the respiratory system are formed.

testes Structure within the male anatomy that creates and stores sperm.

testicular cancer Cancer of the testicles.

testicular torsion Twisting of the spermatic cord that inhibits blood supply to a testicle, which is a medical emergency.

testis Male reproductive organ located in the groin region responsible for the secretion of hormones involved in secondary-sex characteristic development and overall growth.

testosterone Steroid hormone that stimulates the development of male sexual characteristics.

tetanic contraction Muscle contraction in which motor units completely contract without relaxing.

tetanospasmin toxin Toxin produced by the bacterium *Clostridium tetani* that produces tetanus.

tetanus Muscular disorder characterized by muscle spasms resulting from the tetanospasm toxin produced by the bacterium *Clostridium tetani*.

tetralogy of Fallot Genetic heart defect characterized by four abnormalities: ventricular septal defect (hole between the ventricles), stenosis of the pulmonary valve, enlargement of the right ventricle (right-ventricular hypertrophy), and an aorta that is positioned to receive blood from both ventricles (overriding aorta).

thalamus Region of the cerebrum that is the first stop for all sensory information entering the brain prior to going to areas involved in their processing.

thalassemia Blood disorder that decreases the proper formation of hemoglobin within the red blood cell structure.

theca externa Outer layer of the theca folliculi.

theca folliculi Connective tissue that develops during the maturation of an oocyte.

theca interna Internal layer of theca folliculi.

thermoreceptors Proteins that detect changes in temperature.

thermoregulation Regulation of body temperature.

third ventricle One of four connected fluid-filled cavities within the brain.

third-degree burns Burns that affect the epidermis, dermis and underlying tissues such as fat and muscle. Area appears blistered and black. Skin regeneration is not possible and skin grafts are needed.

thoracic aorta Portion of the aorta below the arch extending into the thoracic cavity.

thoracic cavity Hollow area of the body located in the chest or thoracic area.

thoracic duct Large lymph duct of the lymphatic system; begins as the cisterna chyli.

thoracic spinal nerves Twelve pairs of peripheral nerves that exit from the chest region of the spinal cord.

threshold Voltage in muscle or nervous tissue that results in the generation of an action potential when reached.

thrombin Principal enzyme in hemostasis that continues that activation of the coagulation pathway and formation of stable fibrin complex.

thrombocytes Commonly called platelets, found in the blood and play a role in blood clotting and wound healing.

thrombocytopenia Condition of low blood platelet count.

thrombocytosis Increase in clot formation.

thromboembolic disorders Formation of blood clots in blood vessels. Usually caused by a hypercoagulable state.

thromboembolic Formation of a blood clot in a vessel.

thrombophilia Abnormality of blood coagulation that increases the risk of thrombosis by having too many platelets produced.

thrombopoietin Hormone that controls platelet production.

thymus gland Bilobed gland located just deep to the manubrium of the sternum that produces T-lymphocytes.

thyroglobulin Protein present in the thyroid gland from which thyroid hormones are synthesized.

thyrohyoid Muscle located in the anterior cervical region connecting to the thyroid cartilage and hyoid bone.

thyroid cartilage Large cartilage wrapping around the larynx.

thyroid gland Gland located superior to the clavicles in the midline of the body responsible for the secretion of hormones involved in metabolism.

thyroid-releasing hormone (TRH) Controls the release of thyroid-stimulating hormone from the pituitary gland that will increase production of thyroid hormones (T3/T4) in the thyroid gland. Usually regulates energy balance, eating patterns, heat production, and prolactin levels.

thyroid-stimulating hormone (TSH) Stimulates the thyroid gland to release triiodothyronine (T3) and thyroxine (T4).

tibia Anterior long bone in the lower leg that articulates with the femur, fibula, and talus.

tibial tuberosity Broad eminence located on the anterior proximal portion of the tibia that serves as an attachment point of the patellar tendon.

tibialis anterior Muscle located in the anterior portion of the lower leg just lateral to the tibia that works to dorsiflex the ankle.

tibialis posterior Deep muscle located deep to the soleus muscle that works to stabilize the lower leg.

tibiofemoral joint The synovial joint between the femur, tibia, and patella bones; another name for the knee joint.

tidal volume Amount of air entering or exiting the lungs during resting breathing.

tight junctions Junctions that encircle cells, fusing them together into leakproof sheets; prevent substances from leaking into spaces between cells and, in the small intestine, prevent digestive enzymes from getting into the bloodstream.

Tinnitus Perception of ringing, or other repetitive sounds, in the ears without the sound being present.

tissue plasminogen activator (tPA) Treatment for the destruction of emboli within the body. Mostly used for the breakdown of emboli in the setting of strokes.

titer Laboratory test to check the number of a particular antibody in the blood.

Total lung capacity Amount of air residing in the lungs including residual volume.

Touch Sense of a normal, nondamaging light physical stimulus to the skin.

trabeculae Tissue that provides structural support to spongy bone.

trace elements Minerals the body needs less than 100 mg of daily.

trachea Respiratory air passage containing C-shaped hyaline cartilage rings beginning at the inferior border of the larynx and extending to the primary bronchi.

trachealis muscle Smooth muscle located in the trachea that helps to regulate air flow into the lungs by constricting or dilating the trachea.

transcellular fluid (TCF) Portion of extracellular fluid that is separated from other extracellular fluids by an epithelial membrane; examples are synovial fluid, the aqueous and vitreous humor of the eye, cerebrospinal fluid, and synovial fluid.

transdermal patch Method of birth control where a patch is placed on the skin that contains estrogen and progestin to suppress ovulation.

transfusion reaction Inappropriate blood destruction due to the mismatch of surface antigens and antibodies between the donor and the host.

translocation Alteration that occurs when a part of a chromosome moves and attaches to another chromosome.

transvaginal Assessment through the vagina.

transverse process Lateral prominence of bone.

transverse sinuses Hollow venous area on the outside of the brain.

transverse thoracic Thin muscle located on the inner surface of the anterior thoracic wall.

transversus abdominis Deepest abdominal muscle with fibers running anterior to posterior that act to stabilize the trunk.

trapezius Superficial muscle of the back that extends from the occipital bone to the 12th thoracic vertebra and laterally to the spine of the scapulae.

traumatic brain injury Injury to nervous tissues of the brain resulting from head trauma.

triceps Muscle located on the back of the upper arm with three heads that work to extend the elbow.

Trichomonas vaginalis Protozoan parasite responsible for the common STI Trichomoniasis.

tricuspid valve Atrioventricular valve containing three cusps and located between the right atrium and ventricle.

trigeminal nerve Cranial nerve V; sensory and motor information of the jaw and ear.

trigger point injection Medical procedure in which a medication such as a steroid or anesthetic is injected into a trigger point.

trigger points Localized, painful areas in muscles that refer pain to other areas of the body.

triglycerides Most common type of lipid found in foods.

trigone Smooth triangular area on the inner surface of the bladder formed by the ureters entering the bladder and the urethra leaving the bladder.

trismus Spasm of the jaw muscles, commonly referred to as lockjaw, that results from tetanus.

trisomy 21 Additional chromosome that occurs after the cell divides through meiosis and causes Down syndrome.

trochlea Fibrocartilaginous pulley through which the tendon of the superior oblique muscle of the eye passes.

trochlear nerve Cranial nerve IV; controls movements of the eye.

trophoblast Outer layer of the blastocyst that supplies nutrition to the embryo and facilitates implantation.

tropomyosin Double-stranded helical protein located in muscle cells.

troponin–tropomyosin complex Structure containing troponin and tropomyosin that is capable of undergoing a conformational change in response to the binding of calcium to troponin.

troponin Protein complex consisting of three units that function to cover the myosin binding site on actin.

true pathogens Microorganisms that can cause disease in healthy patients with fully functioning immune systems.

true rib Seven most superior pairs of ribs that connect directly with sternum.

true vocal chords Thick portions of the vocal cords (vocal folds) that vibrate and produce sound.

t-tubules Membranous tubular channels that result from the enfolding of the sarcolemma extending into the sarcoplasm of muscle cells.

tubal ligation Method of birth control where the fallopian tubes are blocked to prevent conception.

tubercle Small rounded eminences in bones.

tuberosity Small rounded eminences in bones. Significantly larger than tubercles.

tubular necrosis Breakdown and damage to the nephron tubule of the kidney.

tubular reabsorption Process by which the nephron removes water and solutes that are still needed from the tubular fluid and returns them to the blood.

tubular secretion Transfer of additional waste materials from peritubular capillaries to the glomerular filtrate found within the renal tubules.

tunica albuginea Collagenous connective tissue that makes up the germinal epithelium.

tunica externa Outer layer of an artery or vein.

tunica interna Inner layer of an artery or vein.

tunica intima Inner layer of an artery or vein.

tunica media Middle muscular layer of an artery or vein.

Turner syndrome Another name for monosomy that occurs in females.

T-wave Portion of an ECG just after the QRS complex that represents ventricular repolarization.

type 1 diabetes mellitus Autoimmune disorder that affects the beta cells in the pancreas, leading to decreased insulin production and subsequent uncontrolled hyperglycemia.

type 2 diabetes mellitus Most common type of diabetes where an individual's body no longer responds to insulin due to an overall increase in glucose levels.

type I pneumocytes Mucous-producing cells located in alveoli that form part of the respiratory membrane through which gas exchange occurs between the alveoli and capillaries.

type II pneumocytes Surfactant-secreting cells located in the alveoli.

U

ubiquitous State of being in many places in the earth.

ulnar arteries Arteries in the forearm that originate from the brachial arteries.

ulnar collateral arteries Small arteries branching off the ulnar arteries.

ulnar vein Veins in the forearm that transport blood to the brachial vein.

uniaxial Allows movement in a single plane or axis; the elbow is an example.

unipennate Arrangement of muscle fascicles in which fascicles connect to one side of a tendon.

unsaturated fats and oils Category of triglycerides found in plant-based foods.

ureterorenal reflex Increasing peristaltic force within the ureter that attempts to force any blockage out of the ureter and into the urinary bladder; typically occurs in the presence of kidney stones.

ureters Paired ducts that carry the urine that has been created by the kidneys to the inferior portion of the urinary bladder.

urethra Canal that allows for the excretion of the urine from the urinary bladder. In males the urethra is also utilized by the reproductive system.

urethral orifice Opening of the urethra within the vestibule.

uric acid A breakdown or a waste product generated from the metabolism (nitrogenous) of purine nucleotides; a normal component of urine.

urinary bladder Membranous storage area that holds urine until it is released from the body through the urethra.

urinary incontinence Inability of the body to control the release of urine from the bladder.

urinary retention Abnormal retaining of urine within the bladder despite attempting to urinate and empty the bladder.

urticaria Also called hives, red, round, itchy welts on the skin usually in response to an allergic reaction.

uterine cavity Interior of the uterus.

uterine fundus Top portion of the uterus.

uterus Hollow pear-shaped organ located between the bladder and rectum.

V

vagina Fibromuscular tube located behind the bladder and urethra and in front of the rectum.

vaginal orifice Opening of the vagina within the vestibule.

vaginal ring Method of contraception where a ring containing estrogen and progestin is inserted into the vagina to suppress ovulation.

vagus nerve Cranial nerve X; sensory and motor nerves extending to the visceral organs.

Valsalva maneuver Action that involves closure of the glottis while contracting abdominal and diaphragm muscles to induce defecation.

valves Structures in the heart and veins that only allow blood flow in one direction.

varicoceles Swelling or an increase in size of the veins that supply the scrotum and testicles.

varicosities Small eminences on axons of neurons innervating smooth muscle that release neurotransmitters.

vas deferens Structure that transports semen.

vasa recta Small blood vessels that arise from the efferent arteriole and play a role in the concentration of urine.

vascular circuits Systems of blood vessels that work together to carry blood to specific parts of the body.

vascular collapse Failure of circulation most likely due to volume issues.

vascular spasm A quick tightening of a blood vessel that happens immediately after vessel damage in attempts to prevent significant blood loss.

vasectomy Method of contraception where the male vas deferens is sealed, tied, or cut.

vasoconstricting Process of constricting or narrowing a blood vessel.

vasoconstriction Narrowing of blood vessels.

vasodilating Dilating or widening of a blood vessel from relaxation of smooth muscle.

vasodilation Process of dilating or widening a blood vessel through relaxation of smooth muscle.

vasomotor Controlling the diameter of a blood vessel.

vasovagal and syncope A loss of consciousness from decreased blood flow to the brain caused by an emotional stimulus.

vasovagal Parasympathetic stimulus carried by the vagus nerve: cranial nerve X.

vastus intermedius One of four quadriceps muscles located in the anterior thigh just deep to the rectus femoris muscle that works to extend the knee joint.

vastus lateralis One of four quadriceps muscles located in the lateral thigh that works to extend the knee joint.

vastus medialis One of four quadriceps muscles located in the medial thigh that works to extend the knee joint.

veins Tubular structures carrying blood toward the heart.

ventilation Movement of air into and out of the lungs.

ventral respiratory group Group of neurons located in the anterior portion of the medulla oblongata that work to control forceful breathing.

ventral root Region of the spinal cord in which motor neurons exit.

ventricle Hollow structure in the heart that pushes blood out.

ventricular fibrillation Chaotic abnormal heart rhythm in which the ventricles do not contract.

ventricular filling Portion of cardiac cycle characterized by filling of the ventricles with blood.

ventricular septal defect Birth defect characterized by perforations in the ventricles.

ventricular systole Contraction of the ventricles.

ventricular tachycardia Regular heart rhythm greater than 100 beats per minute.

venules Vascular structures of the venous system that are smaller than veins and connect veins with capillaries.

vertebral arteries Arteries located in the transverse foramen of vertebrae.

vertebral veins Veins located in the transverse foramen of vertebrae.

vesicles Spheres of cell membrane that contain a high concentration of neurotransmitters in preparation for their release at the synapse from the axon terminal bud.

vestibular organs Sensory structures in the inner ear that detect equilibrium and balance.

vestibular schwannoma Noncancerous tumor on the Schwann cells surrounding the vestibulocochlear nerve which can result in disruption of auditory or vestibular senses.

vestibular senses The sensation of body orientation and movement.

vestibule Area of the female anatomy that contains the openings to the vagina and urethra and glands.

vestibulocochlear nerve Cranial nerve VIII; sensory information of the inner ear structures.

vestibulospinal Region of the spinal cord containing the axons of neurons originating in the brainstem (vestibular nucleus).

vibration Ability to detect rapid physical oscillations.

villi Projections or small, finger-like structures located on the plicae circulares of the small intestine to promote the absorption of digested food; a villus is composed of numerous microvilli which are used for increasing the surface area of the wall of the intestine.

viscera Organs in cavities of the body.

visceral pericardium Portion of the pericardium located on the surface of the heart.

visceral pleural membrane Portion of the pleural membrane attached to the surface of the lungs.

Visceral smooth muscle Type of smooth muscle characterized by sheetlike layers that contract as a unit.

visceral Pertaining to the organs of the body.

viscerocranium All bones not included in the neurocranium.

viscous Watery or sticky.

vision Ability to detect light and create images.

vital capacity Amount of air entering and exiting the lungs during a maximal inhalation and exhalation; sum of tidal volume, inspiratory reserve volume, and expiratory reserve volume.

vitamins Organic molecules that can be broken down by heat, acid, light, and oxygen; if their chemical structure is changed, they lose their function; may be changed during food preparation, which alters their function in the body.

vitiligo Skin condition in which a loss of pigment occurs in areas of skin or hair that result in white patches.

vitreous chamber Largest of three fluid-filled cavities of the eye between the lens and retina.

voltage-gated calcium channels Transport proteins located in muscle tissue, particularly in the sarcoplasmic reticulum, that open in response to depolarization and release calcium into the cell.

voltage-gated ion channels Proteins in the axon that open in response to a change in membrane potential and allow ions to cross the membrane once activated.

vomer Bone located in the nasal cavity that, along with the perpendicular plate of the ethmoid bone, forms the nasal septum.

vulva Also called pudendum; refers to the external female genitalia.

W

waddling gait Type of shuffling gait exhibited by people suffering from muscular dystrophy.

warfarin (coumadin) Anticoagulant that is used to decrease the clotting ability of the blood by inhibiting the metabolism of vitamin K and its production of clotting factors.

water soluble Dissolves in water.

water-soluble vitamins Vitamins that dissolve in water.

Wernicke's area Region of the (typically) left temporal lobe that is associated with understanding language.

white matter Region of the CNS that consists of primarily myelinated axons.

withdrawal reflex Reflex in which a limb is rapidly pulled away in response to a painful stimulus.

woven bone Temporary bone that forms after a bone breaks.

X

xiphoid process Most inferior portion of the sternum just below the body of the sternum.

Y

yellow bone marrow Bone marrow yellow in color that contains a high number of fat cells and contributes to formation of bones and cartilage.

yellow nail syndrome Rare medical syndrome caused by the underdevelopment of lymphatic vessels, respiratory disease, and possibly titanium exposure; nails stop growing and appear yellowish-green.

Z

Z-disks Portion of the sarcomere where actin filaments attach, marking the ends of a sarcomere.

zona fasciculata Middle portion of the adrenal gland responsible for the production of glucocorticoids.

zona glomerulosa Most superficial layer of the adrenal gland responsible for the production of mineralocorticoids.

zona pellucida Membrane that surrounds an oocyte.

zona reticularis Deepest layer of the adrenal gland responsible for the production of androgens.

zygapophyseal joint Apophyseal joint between the superior and inferior articular process of adjacent vertebrae; hingelike joints link the vertebrae together.

zygomaticus Muscle of facial expression that moves the ends up the mouth superior as if in smiling.

zygote Cell that results from fertilization of the ovum by the sperm; it contains 46 chromosomes, 23 from the ovum and 23 from the sperm.

Index